D1605316

ISCHEMIC CEREBROVASCULAR DISEASE

HAROLD P. ADAMS, Jr., M.D.
Professor and Director
Division of Cerebrovascular Diseases
Department of Neurology
University of Iowa College of Medicine
Iowa City, Iowa

VLADIMIR HACHINSKI, M.D., D.Sc.
Professor of Neurology
Department of Clinical Neurological Sciences
University of Western Ontario London Health Science Center
University Campus
London, Ontario, Canada

JOHN W. NORRIS, M.D.
Professor of Neurology
University of Toronto Sunnybrook Health Science Center
Stroke Research Unit
Toronto, Ontario, Canada

OXFORD
UNIVERSITY PRESS
2001

OXFORD
UNIVERSITY PRESS

Oxford New York
Athens Auckland Bangkok Bogotá Buenos Aires Calcutta
Cape Town Chennai Dar es Salaam Delhi Florence Hong Kong Istanbul
Karachi Kuala Lumpur Madrid Melbourne Mexico City Mumbai
Nairobi Paris SãoPaulo Shanghai Singapore Taipei Tokyo Toronto Warsaw

and associated companies in
Berlin Ibadan

Published by Oxford University Press, Inc.
198 Madison Avenue, New York, New York 10016

Oxford is a registered trademark of Oxford University Press

Library of Congress Cataloging-in-Publication Data
Adams, Harold P., Jr., 1944-
Ischemic cerebrovascular disease/Harold P. Adams, Jr., Vladimir Hachinski, John W. Norris.
p.;cm. – (Contemporary neurology series; 62)
Includes bibliographical references and index.
ISBN 0-19-513289-0
1. Cerebrovascular disease. I. Hachinski, Vladimir. II. Norris, John W. III. Title. IV-Series-
[DNLM: 1. Cerebrovascular Accident, WL 355 A21402001]
RC388.5 A325 2001
616.8'1-dc21 00-062432

9 8 7 6 5 4 3 2 1

Printed in the United States of America
on acid-free paper

This book is dedicated to
the memory of
Harold P. Adams, M.D.—a father and
role model and
a victim of
ischemic cerebrovascular disease

PREFACE

The diagnosis and treatment of patients with ischemic cerebrovascular disease is an important component of the practice of medicine for physicians of all specialties and, in particular, neurologists. The high incidence of stroke likely will not decline greatly in the 21st century largely because of the aging of the population, especially in industrialized countries. Physicians will make an impact on the impending public health crisis of stroke only with continued advances in diagnosis and treatment. This book is the successor to *The Acute Stroke*, which was published in 1985 by Drs. Hachinski and Norris. This book is organized differently and reflects the tremendous changes in diagnosis and treatment that have occurred since 1985.

Advances in stroke management have occurred at a particularly rapid pace since 1985. Newly identified causes of stroke, such as CADASIL and antiphospholipid antibodies, have been added to the differential diagnosis. Information about the pathogenesis and course of other vascular diseases, such as atherosclerosis, continues to expand. The identification and treatment of risk factors for premature and advanced atherosclerosis or heart disease are having an important effect on the incidence of stroke. Improvements in imaging of the brain, heart, and blood vessels are affecting physicians' ability to rapidly diagnose and treat patients. Finally, therapies of proven value to prevent or treat stroke now are available. Additional advances in treatment can be anticipated. Thus, the timing of this book is opportune. We have aimed the contents of the book at the busy physician who is seeing patients with stroke and who is seeking a reference that provides up-to-date information. The authors have added to this book information and references at the last possible moment to make this book as current as possible. The book's very large number of references (almost 4000) emphasizes recent publications. These references are provided so that the reader can pursue topics of interest.

The book is organized in a chronological manner that corresponds to a physician's interaction with a patient. The first chapter deals with stroke as a public health problem, general terminology, and prognosis. It also includes a brief review of the pathophysiology of brain ischemia. The second chapter deals with the identification and treatment of risk factors for premature atherosclerosis and stroke. The subsequent chapters follow the sequence of clinical evaluation, diagnostic studies, determination of the likely cause of stroke, and treatment. The spectrum of presentations of brain ischemia is described in Chapter 3. Chapter 4 includes description of the diagnostic studies that are commonly performed in assessing a patient. Chapters 5 through 8 focus on atherosclerotic cerebrovascular disease, heart diseases leading to embolism to the brain, non-atherosclerotic vasculopathies, and disorders of coagulation that lead to stroke. Chapter 9 deals with the problem of ischemic stroke in children and young adults because these patients represent a different diagnostic and treatment challenge than older persons. A review of the genetic and inherited causes of stroke also is included in Chapter 9. The medical or surgical interventions to prevent stroke are discussed in Chapters 10 and 11. Although these chapters are presented before those related to acute stroke management, the authors want to emphasize that measures to prevent recurrent stroke are the same as those used to forestall the first stroke.

Chapter 12 is the longest in the book and reflects the marked changes that are occurring in initial care of stroke—*The Acute Stroke*. The goal of this chapter is to provide information about identification, transport, urgent evaluation, and treatment of patients with acute ischemic stroke. Although the chapter highlights the issues related to the early administration of intravenous rt-PA, the only medication currently approved for treatment of ischemic stroke itself and the other components of emergent stroke care also are included. These other aspects of treatment are important for improving outcomes, regardless of whether the patient receives rt-PA. Chapter 13 involves the next logical step in treatment. It focuses management of the patient in the acute in-patient hospital setting, including preventing or treating acute or subacute medical or neurological complications. In particular, the effects of specialized stroke unit care in lowering mortality and morbidity after stroke are stressed, and the components of a successful stroke care unit are outlined. The issues of rehabilitation and return to society are reviewed in the concluding chapter. Chapter 14 was a challenge for the authors to write because of the diverse issues and the limited amount of data about the usefulness of some of interventions. Still, the importance of the issues to patients should not be ignored. A physician is well served by addressing these aspects of his or her patient's care. In addition, this area of care probably will be a major focus of research during the new century because society will demand ways to improve the quality of life of survivors of stroke.

The authors have many people to thank. We thank our patients who have taught us much about stroke. We thank our colleagues and families for their sage advice and patience. We thank Ms. Cheryl Moores, Maribeth Klimek, Daneita Harmon, Julie Adams, Brenda Herzberg, and Nelda Dierickx for their assistance in the collection of the references and in preparation of the manuscript. Their efforts were critical for the timely completion of this book. The authors also thank Lauren Enck at Oxford University Press and Dr. Sid Gilman, the editor-in-chief of this series, for their sound advice and numerous and important suggestions.

Iowa City, Iowa H.P.A.
London, Ontario V.H.
Toronto, Ontario J.W.N.

CONTENTS

ISCHEMIC CEREBROVASCULAR DISEASE

Chapter 1

INTRODUCTION TO ISCHEMIC CEREBROVASCULAR DISEASE

ISCHEMIC STROKE AS A PUBLIC HEALTH PROBLEM

Ischemic cerebrovascular disease (ischemic stroke) is a leading public health problem. Every 53 seconds, someone in the United States has a stroke.[1] Annually, approximately 750,000 Americans have an initial or recurrent ischemic stroke.[2] Stroke incidence is even higher in most other countries.[3,4] Rates are particularly high in Asia and Eastern Europe.[5–9] Changes in the rates of stroke vary considerably among regions; for example, the incidence of stroke is declining in Western Europe and North America while it is rising in Eastern Europe.[10–14] Although definitive data from many third-world countries are not available, stroke likely is a major health care problem in these nations.[15–17] Poungvarin[18] recently reported that stroke is a rising problem in the developing world. With the advancing life expectancy of people in developing countries, the importance of ischemic stroke likely will grow as a worldwide problem.

Mortality

Stroke is second to heart disease as a worldwide cause of death.[16] In the United States, stroke is the third most common cause of death, following heart disease and cancer. Annually, 150,000 Americans die of stroke, *and* it contributes to the death of another 140,000 people.[1,19]

Disability

Since the late 1990s, there has been an increase in survival after stroke and, therefore, it has become a common cause of human suffering and the leading cause of long-term disability.[20–22] The 1996 American Heart Association Heart and Stroke Statistical Update reports that there are more than 4.4 million stroke survivors in the United States. Similarly high prevalence rates are noted in men and women of all ages in Europe.[23]

A stroke often precludes patients' abilities to return to work or to regain their role in a family. Thus, by affecting both patients and loved ones, stroke is a family illness.[24,25] Family relationships and dynamics often are changed irrevocably. Disability may require a spouse or other relative to assume a new role or become a full-time caregiver. Stroke is second only to dementia as a neurological disorder leading to long-term institutionalized care.[26] Recurrent stroke produces dementia, and its effects exacerbate cognitive impairments from degenerative dementias, such as Alzheimer's disease. Stroke is expensive in terms in human suffering.

Economic Consequences of Stroke

Due to the high incidence of stroke and the high costs expended for each individual patient, it accounts for a sizeable amount of the health care costs in the United States (see Table 1–1). The economic consequences of stroke likely are as high or higher in other countries.[15,27,28] A study from The Netherlands found that stroke accounts for approximately 3% of the Dutch national health care budget.[29] However, direct, per-patient health care costs of stroke have fallen in some countries. For example, in Canada, the direct costs declined from $27,000 (CD) in 1993 to $10,000 (CD) in 1998 largely due to changes in hospital and rehabilitation services.[30] Information is needed to determine whether increased long-term expenses negate the savings in direct costs of stroke care. Thus, stroke and its sequelae are important issues for health care planners in governments, insurance companies, and medical services everywhere. Because the costs of treatment and the economic consequences of lost productivity are so great, prevention of stroke will be a very cost-effective strategy.[31]

Annually, the economic costs of stroke in the United States amount to approximately $30 billion (U.S.).[19,32] In 1996, Taylor et al[32] estimated that the lifetime economic consequences for strokes that occurred in 1990 in the United States would be approximately $40 billion (U.S.). The costs per patient with ischemic stroke amount to approximately $100,000 (U.S.).[32] These expenses include the financial costs of acute hospital care and rehabilitation as well as losses in the patient's and the family's productivity.[32–35] A major factor in health care costs is early care in acute care hospital facilities.[30] Leibson et al[36] reported that medical costs in the first year after stroke are approximately 3.4 times those expended in the year before the ischemic event. The costs of long-term care are less for men than for women because men typically have family caregivers at home (usually a wife), whereas women more commonly leave an empty house and are placed in long-term facilities.[30]

Table 1–1. **Causes of Economic Costs of Ischemic Stroke**

Direct Costs
Medical treatment
Physicians' fees
Medical care
Surgery
Diagnostic tests
Medications
Risk factor reduction
Stroke prevention
Acute hospitalization (in-patient) care
Hospitalization
Medications
Diagnostic tests
Consultations
Rehabilitation
Professional fees
Orthotic devices
Modification of home environment
Long-term care—nursing home
Indirect Costs
Loss of productivity of patient
Disability payments—welfare
Loss of productivity of caregiver

Health Care Systems

Ongoing changes in health care systems and evolving priorities in care likely will have an effect on the future treatment of patients with stroke.[37] As advances in the understanding of prevention and treatment of stroke build and new developments occur on a regular basis, health care systems must adjust their priorities to give stroke its proper due. This process must be ongoing. It should emphasize both the availability and quality of care. Important statements on stroke care in Europe and the Asia-Pacific have prescribed broad guidelines for management that, one hopes, will influence decisions of health care planners.[38–40] (See Tables 1–2 and 1–3.) Unfortunately, some governmental health care systems do not have well-developed stroke services, and patients may be sent to medical institutions that do not even have computed tomography (CT) available.[41] In addition, reimbursement for expensive procedures and therapies is becoming an issue. For example, a physician might not receive adequate compensation for going to an emergency department to urgently administer thrombolytic therapy to a patient with acute ischemic stroke. Economic disincentives to provide such care must be overcome.

Development of health maintenance organizations (HMOs) in the United States is already having an impact on stroke care, some of which may not be best for patient care. Retchin et al[42] reported that persons with stroke who are enrolled in an HMO are likely to go to a nursing home for treatment after hospitalization, whereas patients in a fee-for-service system are likely to be referred to an inpatient rehabilitation program. Webster and Feinglass[43] noted that the care of patients with stroke might not be optimal in an HMO setting largely because of payer status. A minority of HMOs have a policy that advises their participants to call an emergency number or to go to the nearest emergency department if they are experiencing signs of a stroke.[44] Stroke prevention and acute treatment strategies must be incorporated in health care plans. Both health care providers and the public must demand inclusion of aggressive stroke care programs in insurance plans and HMOs.

Governmental and regulatory issues, such as the inaccuracy of the *International Classification of Diseases* (ICD-9) coding system in identifying the diagnosis of ischemic stroke, also affect health care planning.[45] Hospital discharge diagnoses often are incorrect, and these records do not give an accurate accounting of stroke.[46] For example, the diagnosis of stroke remains elusive; coding of stroke at discharge may denote only 78%–98% of cases with cerebrovascular events.[47] The size and expertise of the hospital likely will be reflected in the number of coding errors.

Table 1–2. **Summary of Recommendations of European and Asia-Pacific Conferences on Stroke Care**

The high economic costs of stroke should receive more attention.
Primary prevention is critical for lowering the incidence of stroke.
Organization of stroke services locally, regionally, and nationally—
Acute care
Stroke units
Rehabilitation services
Community support
Special plans for rural and developing regions
Goal of seamless flow from one setting to another
Management of acute stroke
Awareness
Diagnosis
Basic care
Medical treatment
Surgical treatment
Prevention of thromboembolism
Mortality at 1 month
Use of evidence-based therapies
Rehabilitation after stroke
Rehabilitation services
Patient education
Unbroken chain of care
Advocacy groups
Mortality at 2 years
Activities of daily living
Secondary prevention
Life-style interventions
Medical interventions
Antiplatelet agents
Anticoagulants
Surgical interventions
Community care
Quality of life for patients and caregivers

Table 1–3. **Helsingborg Declaration: Basic Principles for Good Stroke Care**

The interests and needs of patients with stroke and their families should remain paramount.
Acute stroke should be considered to be a medical emergency.
Patients with stroke should receive immediate evaluation and treatment.
Treatment in an acute stroke care unit is desirable.
Selection of treatments of patients with stroke should be based on the scientific evidence.
Treatments of unproved value should not be used routinely.
Management of disability should be planned with the patient and family.
An interdisciplinary team should provide rehabilitation services.
Patients should have access to appropriate measures to prevent recurrent stroke.

Stroke Advocacy

Because of the inherent nature of the disease and the population affected, stroke has not received as much attention as it should. Spending on stroke research has been limited. In some situations, support for health services may not be optimal. Professional and governmental groups have approached stroke with a sense of nihilism. Persons with stroke and their families have not been forceful in advocating the importance of stroke research or in supporting strategies to optimize care. Thus, advocates for stroke, especially physicians and other health care providers, must continue their efforts aimed at increasing the visibility of the disease in the health care–planning activities of countries around the world. In addition, these groups must support programs that sponsor both basic and clinical research in stroke.

Future Trends

Beginning about 1960, the frequency of stroke in the United States, Canada, Australia, New Zealand, and many countries in Western Europe declined largely from the control of risk factors such as hypertension.[4,11,48–52] The decline was greater among women than among men.[51,53,54] However, these declines stopped during the early 1990s, and the incidence of stroke is now rising.[55,56] An estimated 50% increase in the incidence of stroke is predicted by 2050 largely due to the aging of populations in many industrialized societies.[3] In the United States, the incidence of stroke could exceed 1 million new cases annually by 2050. Some of the increase is from improved recognition of minor strokes.[57] In addition, better treatment of heart disease permits survival of a group of persons with advanced vascular disease who are at great risk for stroke.[57] The increase in the number of persons with stroke, combined with secondary human and economic costs, means that effectively managing ischemic stroke will grow in importance.[28] Thus, administration of interventions to prevent or treat stroke, and rehabilitation after stroke, will increase in importance as a public health issue.

TERMINOLOGY AND CLASSIFICATION OF ISCHEMIC STROKE

General Terms

Ischemic cerebrovascular disease encompasses a broad spectrum of clinical events based on the type and duration of the neurological symptoms, the area of brain affected, the involved artery, and the presumed cause. This classification is important in establishing a patient's prognosis and making decisions about evaluation and treatment. Although the term *cerebrovascular accident* (*CVA*) is used widely by physicians and other health care professionals, it is an appalling pseudoscientific characterization of stroke that substitutes labeling for understanding. The term should be abandoned because many strokes are not accidents, but preventable catastrophes.

Although the *cerebrovascular* component of this term accurately describes most strokes, these acute brain illnesses do not occur by accident. Stroke is secondary to disorders that affect the blood vessels of the brain. The term *stroke* conveys the precipitant nature and potential for devastation that occur with vascular disease; it accurately labels a sudden neurological deficit of presumed vascular origin.

The term *ischemic stroke* encompasses all cerebrovascular events secondary to a vascular occlusion that deprives parts of the brain of adequate blood flow. Most occlusions are the result of a blood clot that develops in either an intracranial or extracranial artery (*thrombosis*) or a clot that originates somewhere else in the body, most commonly the heart, and then migrates to obstruct an intracranial vessel (*embolus*). Less commonly, ischemic stroke can be secondary to venous occlusions or to nonthrombotic embolism. Types of ischemic cerebrovascular disease can be divided into subgroups based on the area of brain involved, the time course of the event, and the severity of neurological impairment (see Table 1–4).

Table 1–4. **Categorization of Ischemic Stroke**

Time Course
Transient ischemic attacks
  Amaurosis fugax
Cerebral infarction with transient symptoms
Reversible and partially reversible ischemic neurological deficits
Minor ischemic stroke
Acute ischemic stroke
Stroke-in-evolution
Completed stroke
Vascular dementia

Area of Brain—Vascular Infrastructure
Vertebral artery
  Posterior inferior cerebellar artery
Basilar artery
  Anterior inferior cerebellar artery
  Internal auditory artery
  Superior cerebellar artery
Posterior cerebral artery
Internal carotid artery
Anterior cerebral artery
Middle cerebral artery
Cortical branch arteries
Watershed (borderzone) infarction
Vascular centrencephalon
Lacunar infarction

Types of Ischemic Events

Ischemic events span a spectrum from relatively brief events, resolving spontaneously and completely, to events involving major brain injury that leads to death or disability. The priorities in care vary among patients depending on the type of vascular event. Prevention of recurrence may be the most important issue for treatment of a patient with a minor or transient event, whereas control of complications and rehabilitation take precedence in management of a patient with a multilobar brain injury.

The term *transient ischemic attack* (*TIA*) describes a brief episode of transient focal neurological impairment that is of vascular origin. The original definition of TIA included a time limit or neurological symptoms that could extend to 24 hours, but this time window is far too long. Episodes of TIA usually last only a few minutes and almost all resolve within 20 minutes.[58] In fact, most patients whose neurological symptoms persist more than 1 hour have a hypodense lesion found on CT of the brain.[58–61] These events are relatively common. Dennis et al[62] reported that the incidence of TIA is approximately 0.35/1000. The incidence of TIA has not changed since the 1970s.[63] Brown et al[63] recently reported that the incidences of hemi-spheric TIA and amaurosis fugax in a largely white population in Rochester, Minnesota, were 38/100,000 and 13/100,000 respectively. The latter figure may be higher, as it is underestimated because of under-reporting. The incidence of TIA in the vertebrobasilar circulation is estimated to be 14/100,000.[63] The rates of TIA likely differ in other populations. Occasionally, a patient will have a TIA in the presence of a physician, but most events occur when a physician is not in attendance. Thus, an event in a patient who has neurological signs when being examined should not be considered to be a TIA. A TIA is at the mildest end of the spectrum of symptomatic ischemic cerebrovascular disease. It should not be considered as a separate illness distinct from ischemic stroke; any differences are quantitative rather than qualitative.[64,65] Rather than being a risk factor for stroke, a TIA is a warning sign and a marker of instability for the underlying disease causing a stroke.[66] The occurrence of a TIA should lead to prompt evaluation and initiation of therapies to prevent stroke.

An episode of painless, transient monocular visual loss, or *amaurosis fugax* (transient monocular blindness), predicts ischemic stroke and is a warning for either retinal or cerebral ischemia. Its importance as an omen for stroke derives from the common blood supply (internal carotid artery) to the eye and the ipsilateral cerebral hemisphere. The incidence of amaurosis fugax is uncertain because physicians and patients often ignore these visual symptoms. Although the frequency of amaurosis fugax may be higher than the rate of hemisphere events, the risk of stroke after an ocular event is roughly half that following a TIA. Still, patients with amaurosis fugax should receive the same attention as persons with TIA. The treatment of patients with TIA or other warning symptoms of stroke is discussed in Chapters 10 and 11.

A diagnosis of a *cerebral infarction with transient symptoms* (*CITS*) is made when a patient clinically has a TIA but a subsequent brain imaging study demonstrates an infarction. In most cases, these patients will have symptoms that last 1 hour or longer. Terms such as *reversible ischemic neurological deficit* (*RIND*) and *partially reversible ischemic neurological deficit* (*PRIND*) previously were applied to events that lasted longer than 24 hours or cases in which the neurological signs did not completely disappear.[60] These terms have outlived their usefulness and have been supplanted by the term *minor ischemic stroke*.[65] Still, some differentiation is important. The risks of recurrent stroke or death are higher among persons who have had a minor stroke than among those who have had a TIA.[67] A *clinically silent infarction* (silent stroke) also may be found on brain imaging.[68–70] In this situation, the study demonstrates a small infarction most commonly located in the basal ganglia on CT or magnetic resonance imaging (MRI), although the patient does not have any symptoms of stroke or TIA. These strokes can be detected in up to 20% of patients who are seen with signs of an acute stroke.[68,69]

Ischemic stroke involves a series of changes in circulation, coagulation, endothelial cells, blood brain–barrier function, cellular metabolism, and release of neurotransmitters, all of which occur following arterial occlusion.[71] The end result is an area of necrosis in the brain. The first hours after stroke are dynamic, and the patient has the potential for either improvement or worsening. This time is critical for treatment success.[72] To emphasize the importance of management during the first few hours or days after onset, the term *acute (hyperacute) ischemic stroke* has been coined. The term *brain attack* is being used to describe stroke to the public.[73–76] This term emphasizes the urgent nature of acute stroke.[77] The goal is for persons to arrive in an emergency department as quickly as possible.[78–80] A patient who has neurological impairments on arrival in the emergency department should be considered to be having a stroke even if the symptoms have been present for only a few hours. The goal of modern treatment of acute stroke is to ameliorate ischemic brain injury. Thus, treatment should not be withheld for 24 hours while the potential diagnosis of a TIA is being excluded. The upper time limit for acute ischemic stroke has not been defined, but 24 hours probably is the maximal duration. A better time limit might be the first 3–12 hours. The entire health care system is adjusting to the emphasis on early stroke care.[80–82] Unfortunately, the changes are coming slowly. The diagnosis and treatment of acute ischemic stroke are discussed in Chapter 12.

The diagnosis of *stroke-in-evolution* (progressing stroke) is made when a patient's neurological signs are worsening.[83,84] As many as one-third of patients can deteriorate during the first few days after stroke.

This occurrence should prompt evaluation for the cause of the worsening.[85–87] Progression is more likely to occur in younger patients, those with events in the posterior circulation, and those with severe extracranial atherosclerosis.[84] However, neurological worsening might also occur among patients with stroke due to any cause, including lacunar strokes.[85] The causes of neurological deterioration are diverse. Deterioration during the first few hours after stroke may be secondary to progression of the brain illness, including metabolic effects, recurrent embolism, progression of thrombosis, or failure of flow in collateral channels. Specific interventions to reverse or halt these phenomena are the key of modern acute stroke care. Deterioration after the first 24 hours following stroke is usually due to neurological complications, such as brain edema, hydrocephalus, the effects of excitatory amino acids, or medical complications such as cardiac disorders and pneumonia.[88,89] Not surprisingly, outcomes after stroke are worse among those who had neurological deterioration than among those whose neurological status remained stable.[86] Thus, identification of features that forecast which patients will worsen and the causes for their deterioration are critical components of early care. See Chapter 13 for a discussion of the causes of neurological deterioration after acute ischemic stroke.

A patient whose neurological signs persist for at least 24 hours is considered to have had a *completed stroke*. The spectrum of neurological impairments is broad after stroke and reflects the size and location of the ischemic injury as well as the presumed cause. Whereas some patients may have minimal deficits, others can have a severe brain injury that could prove fatal. Priorities in management change following a completed stroke. Emphasis is placed on rehabilitation, control of medical and neurological complications, and prevention of recurrent stroke rather than initiation of therapies to limit the biological effects of the ischemic process. Management after admission to the hospital and rehabilitation are reviewed in Chapters 13 and 14.

Whereas a single stroke causes focal neurological impairments that reflect the area of the brain injury, the effects of recurrent strokes are more pervasive. In particular, resulting declines in cognition and intellect lead to *vascular dementia*.[90–97] A history of stroke is associated with greatly increased risk of dementia.[93] Stroke accounts for up to one-third of the cases of dementia, which can complicate approximately one-fourth of strokes.[93,94,98,99] Vascular dementia also is more likely in the elderly and patients with diabetes mellitus.[98,100]

Vascular dementia can be the result of multiple, bilateral infarctions, particularly in the basal ganglia.[94,101] Stepwise mental deterioration occurring in conjunction with other neurological signs is the hallmark for a variety of vascular dementia called *multi-infarct(ion) dementia*.[90,98,102] Vascular dementia can be heterogenous, and its course can be static, remitting, or progressive.[92,94,101,103] (See Table 1–5.) In addition to cognitive impairments in several domains, gait disturbances, incontinence, and mood disorders are common.[92]

Table 1–5. **Hachinski Scale to Differentiate Vascular and Degenerative Dementias**

Finding	Points
Abrupt onset of neurological symptoms	2
Stepwise deterioration	1
Fluctuating course of symptoms	2
Nocturnal confusion	1
Relative preservation of personality	1
Depression	1
Prominent somatic complaints	1
Emotional incontinence (pseudobulbar affect)	1
History of hypertension	1
History of stroke	2
Evidence of associated atherosclerosis	1
History of focal neurological symptoms	2
Evidence of focal neurological signs	2

Adapted from Hachinski et al.[104]

7 or more points—suggests multi-infarction dementia.

4 or fewer points—suggests degenerative dementia.

The identification of these patients is speeded by the application of the scale outlined in Table 1-5.[104–107] Additional information about vascular dementia is found in Chapter 13.

Modern brain imaging studies (CT and MRI) permit identification of diffuse white matter changes in the cerebral hemispheres (*leukoaraiosis*) in persons with dementia, including those with Alzheimer's disease.[92] The white matter abnormalities are most commonly found in persons who have a history of hypertension or hypercholesterolemia.[108] These findings may be of vascular origin and would prompt inclusion within the diagnosis of vascular dementia. The white matter findings on brain imaging also have led to the popularization of the diagnosis of *Binswanger's disease*, which is another presumed cause of vascular dementia.[94,109,110] The diagnosis of Binswanger's disease remains elusive, and the diagnosis is controversial.[111] The significance of the leukoaraiosis remains debatable, although its presence increases the risk of vascular deaths or stroke in persons with high-risk carotid artery lesions.

VASCULAR INFRASTRUCTURE

The clinical findings of ischemic stroke reflect the involved vessel and the location and extent of brain injury (see Table 1–6). These findings also reflect the marked variations in the vascular anatomy that can exist among patients.[112] In general, events are localized to either the vertebrobasilar or the carotid circulation. The vertebral and basilar arteries perfuse the brain stem, the cerebellum, and the posterior portions of the cerebral hemisphere (Fig. 1–1). The vertebral arteries arise from the subclavian arteries and pass through the lateral processes of the sixth through the second cervical vertebrae. Then, they traverse the dura mater to enter the cranial vault through the foramen magnum. The two vertebral arteries unite at approximately the pontomedullary junction to form the basilar artery. Clinically important branches of the vertebral arteries are the anterior spinal artery, the short circumferential arteries to the dorsolateral medulla, and the posterior inferior cerebellar artery. The basilar artery is situated anterior to the brain stem in the pre-pontine and interpeduncular cisterns. It then divides into its terminal branches, the posterior cerebral arteries. Its other major branches are the anterior inferior cerebellar, the superior cerebellar, and the internal auditory arteries. The posterior inferior cerebellar artery supplies the inferior and lateral aspect of the cerebellar hemisphere. The superior cerebellar artery perfuses the rostral cerebellum, and the anterior inferior cerebellar artery provides blood to the medial and the anterior cerebellum. Because of anatomic variations, the vascular territories of the cerebellum can differ considerably among patients. Congenital absence or hypoplasia

Table 1–6. **Categorization of Ischemic Stroke by the Bascular Infrastructure and the Area of the Brain**

Vertebral artery
- Anterior spinal artery
- Posterior inferior cerebellar artery

Basilar artery
- Anterioinferior cerebellar artery
- Internal auditory artery
- Superior cerebellar artery

Posterior cerebral artery
- Thalamic arteries
  - Tuberothalamic (polar) artery
  - Thalamogeniculate artery
  - Thalamoperforating (interpeduncular thalamic) artery
  - Posterior choroidal artery
- Branch cortical arteries

Internal carotid artery
- Ophthalmic artery
- Anterior choroidal artery

Anterior cerebral artery
- Recurrent artery of Huebner
- Branch cortical arteries

Middle cerebral artery
- Lenticulostriate arteries
- Branch cortical arteries

Watershed (borderzone) infarction

Lacunar infarction

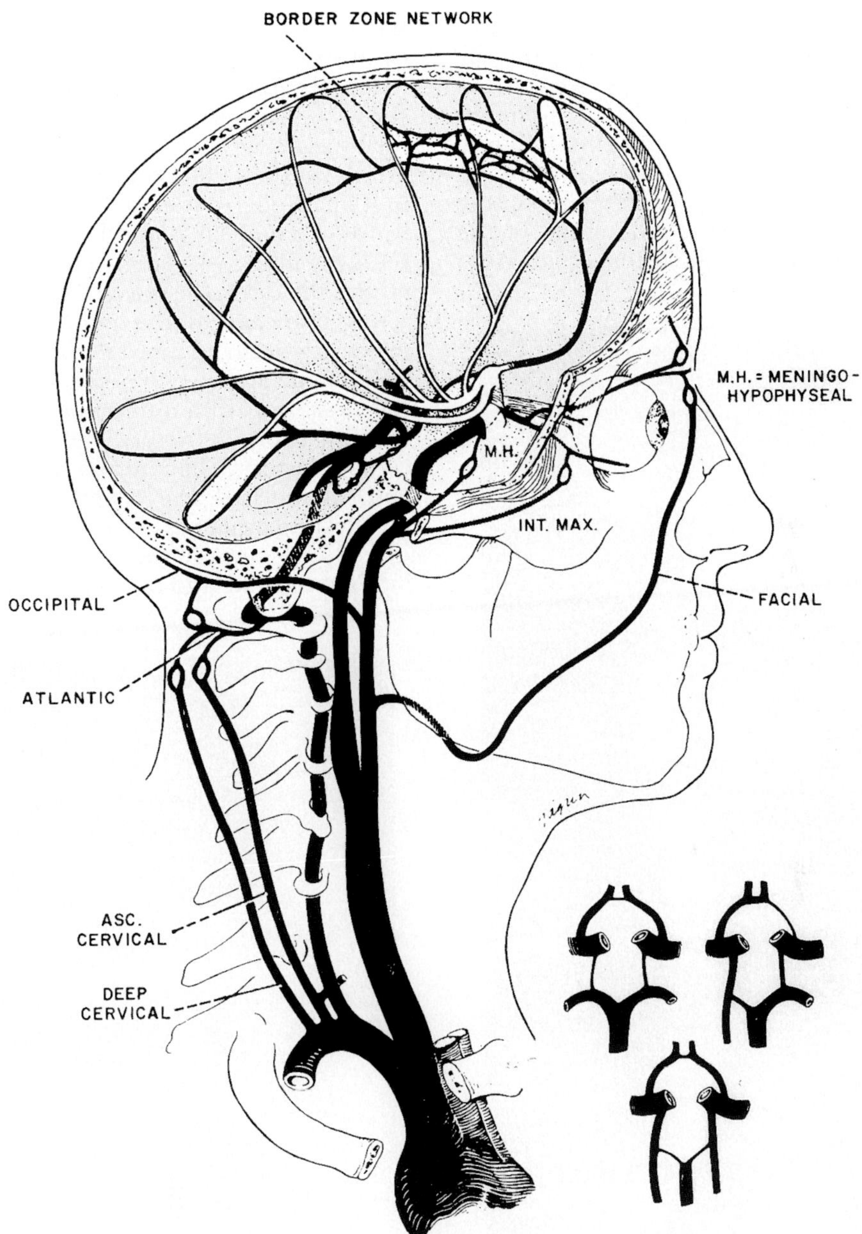

Figure 1–1. Collateral circulations of the brain. (Courtesy of Dr. C.M. Fisher.)

of one of the cerebellar arteries is common. The vascular beds also often differ between the right and the left cerebellar hemispheres.

The basilar artery also gives rise to numerous, small, short penetrating and circumferential arteries that perfuse the pons and the midbrain. The vascular beds of the brain stem are divided into ventral-medial, lateral, and dorsolateral territories.[113,114] The bifurcation of the basilar artery is also the site of the origin for small arteries that provide blood to the diencephalon. The posterior cerebral arteries also send small branches to the thalamus and adjacent deep structures and the larger pial branches to the medial temporal lobe, medial and superior parietal lobe, and the occipital lobe.

In most persons, the right common carotid artery rises from the brachiocephalic artery while the left common carotid artery is a branch of the arch of the aorta. Approximately at the angle of the jaw, the common carotid artery divides into the internal carotid artery and the external carotid artery (Figs. 1–2 and 1–3). The external carotid artery perfuses the soft tissues of the face, the scalp, and the meninges (Fig. 1–4). The internal carotid artery supplies the ipsilateral eye and cerebral hemisphere. It enters the cranial vault via the carotid canal and lies lateral to the pituitary in the cavernous sinus. As it penetrates the dura, the internal carotid artery sends branches to the pituitary. Its first major, clinically important branch is the ophthalmic artery. Other branches include the posterior communicating artery, the anterior choroidal artery, and the anterior cerebral artery. The internal carotid artery ends as the middle cerebral artery. Deep penetrating branches of the major intracranial arteries supply the basal ganglia, the internal capsule, and the deep hemispheric

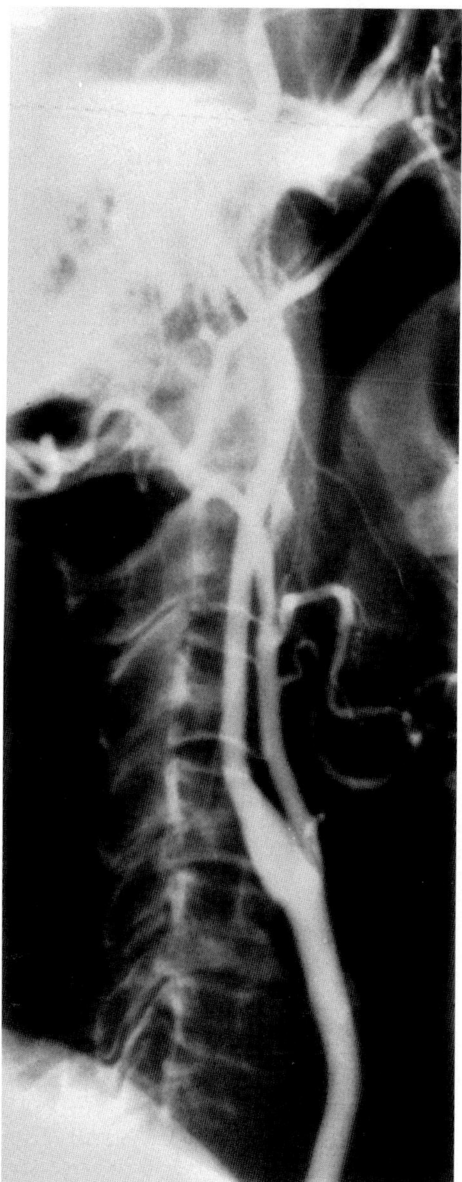

Figure 1–2. Left carotid arteriogram shows the normal extracranial circulation. Both the internal and external carotid arteries and the bifurcation are visualized.

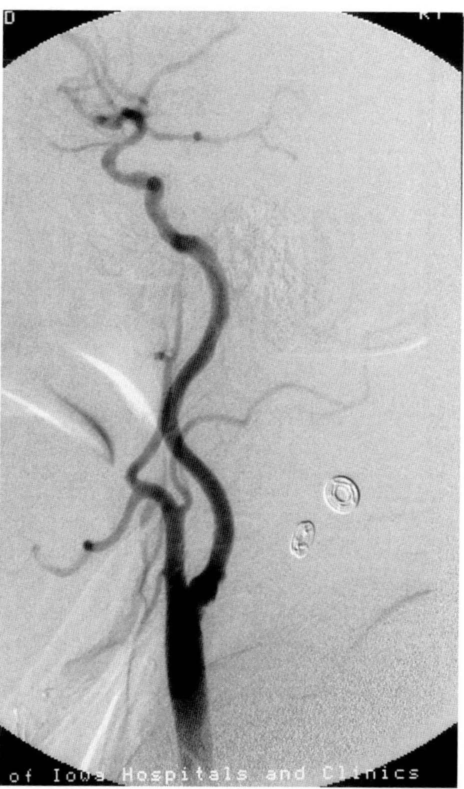

Figure 1–3. Lateral view of a right carotid arteriogram using subtraction techniques shows a mild area of ulceration of the origin of the internal carotid artery. The visualized vessels include the anterior, middle, and posterior cerebral arteries. The external carotid artery and its branches also are seen.

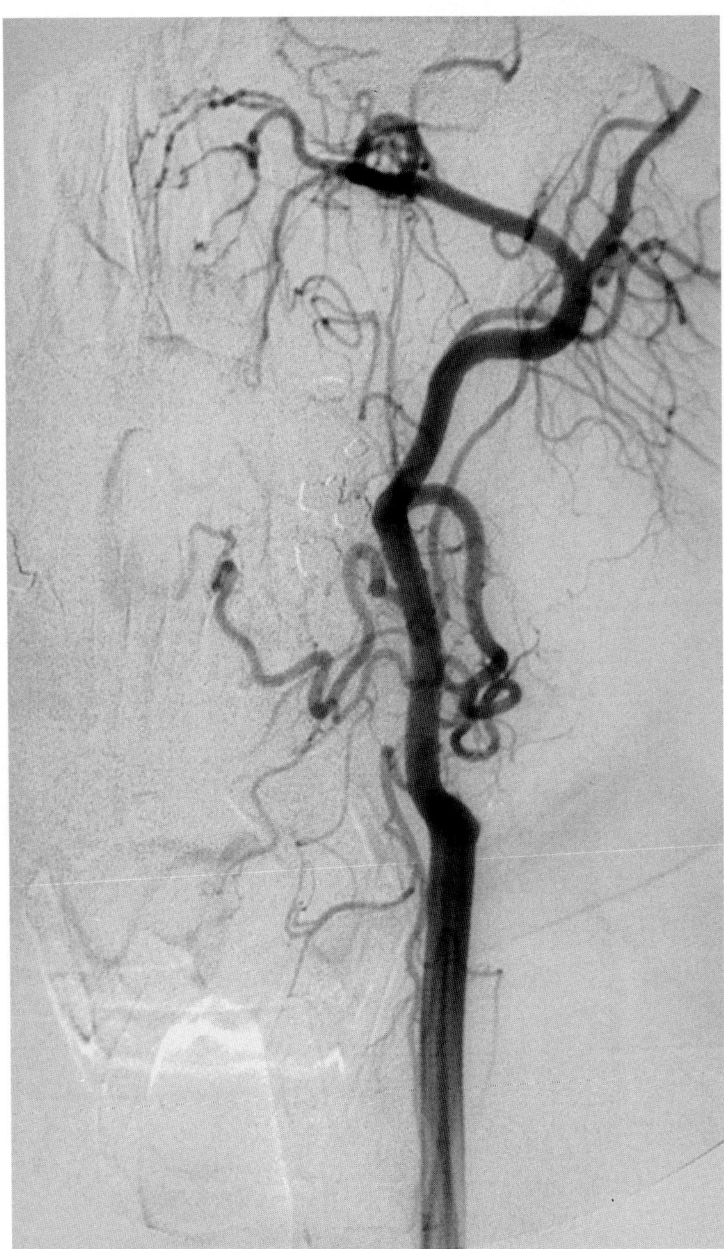

Figure 1–4. A lateral view of a left carotid arteriogram using subtraction techniques shows an occlusion of the internal carotid artery. The external carotid artery and several branches are visualized.

white matter.[113,115] Superficial branches perfuse the insula and the frontal, superior temporal, and lateral parietal lobes. A candelabra of the superficial branches of individual pial arteries are aligned from the frontal to the occipital poles.[116,117] The areas of perfusion form a series of wedges that extend from the cortex to deeper in the cerebral hemispheres. The long pial circumferential arteries have rich anastomoses. Vascular territories of the anterior, middle, and posterior cerebral arteries vary considerably among patients.[115]

Three systems of potential collateral circulation can limit the ischemic consequences of an arterial occlusion. Anastomoses between branches of the external carotid artery and the internal carotid artery can dampen the hemodynamic effects of an internal carotid artery occlusion. Important

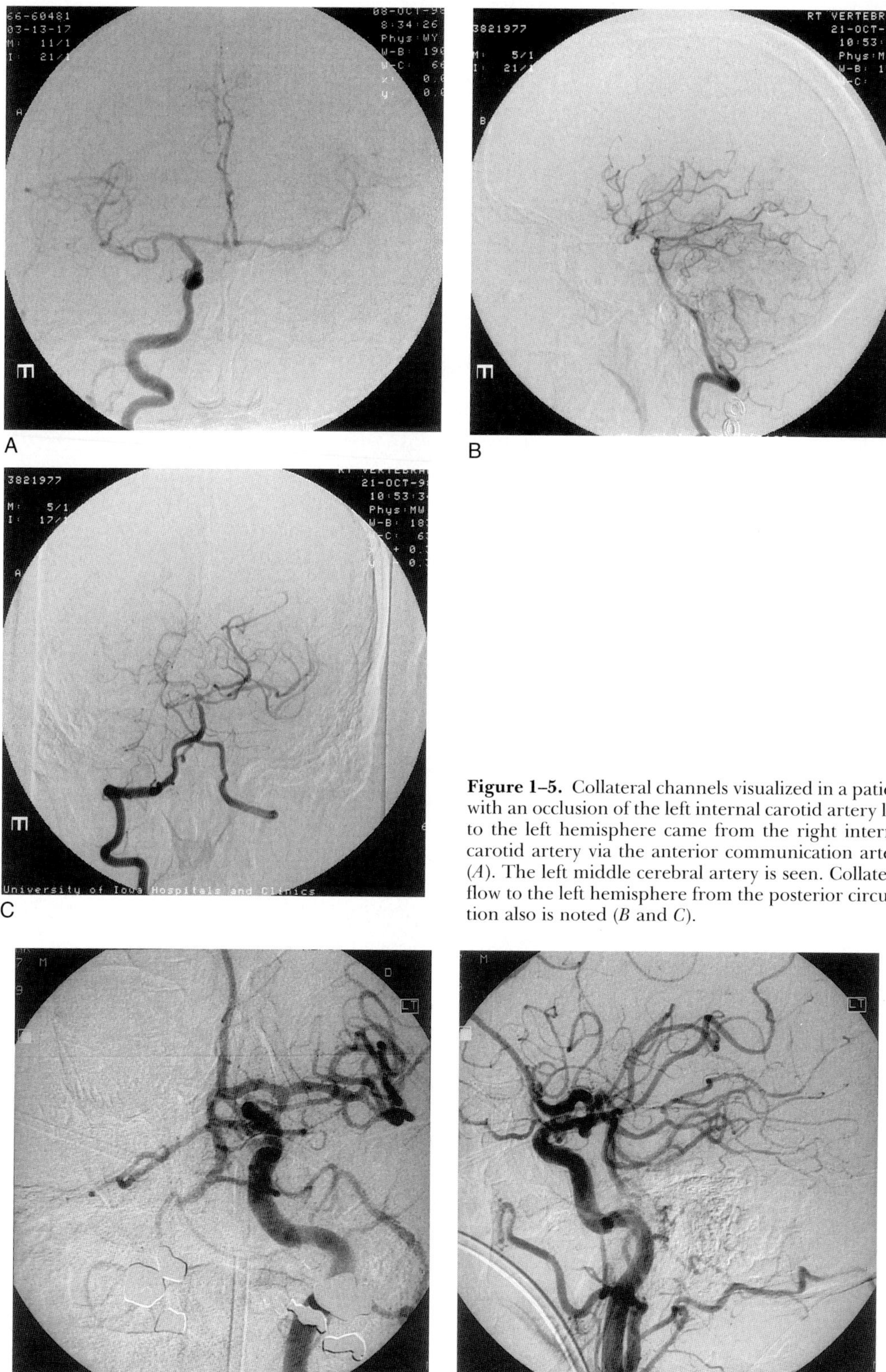

Figure 1–5. Collateral channels visualized in a patient with an occlusion of the left internal carotid artery low to the left hemisphere came from the right internal carotid artery via the anterior communication artery (*A*). The left middle cerebral artery is seen. Collateral flow to the left hemisphere from the posterior circulation also is noted (*B* and *C*).

Figure 1–6. Anterior–posterior (*A*) and lateral (*B*) views of a left carotid arteriogram using subtraction technique done in a patient with an occlusion of the basilar artery. Retrograde flow into the distal basilar artery is achieved via the posterior communicating artery.

collaterals include the internal maxillary artery, the ophthalmic artery, and the ethmoidal arteries. The circle of Willis permits diversion of blood from one carotid territory to the other or to the posterior circulation (Fig. 1–5). The anatomic integrity of the circle of Willis varies considerably; in particular, the anterior or posterior communicating arteries may be atretic, and one carotid circulation may be relatively isolated. In approximately 20% patients, at least one posterior cerebral artery will arise from the internal carotid artery (Fig. 1–6). Pial anastomoses permit diversion of flow from the distal branches of the anterior or the posterior cerebral arteries to those of the middle cerebral artery or vice versa. These anastomoses are at the border of the major vessels, and these borderzones are particularly vulnerable to hypotension because their arteries lie farthest from the parent vessel (Fig 1–7). Focal areas of

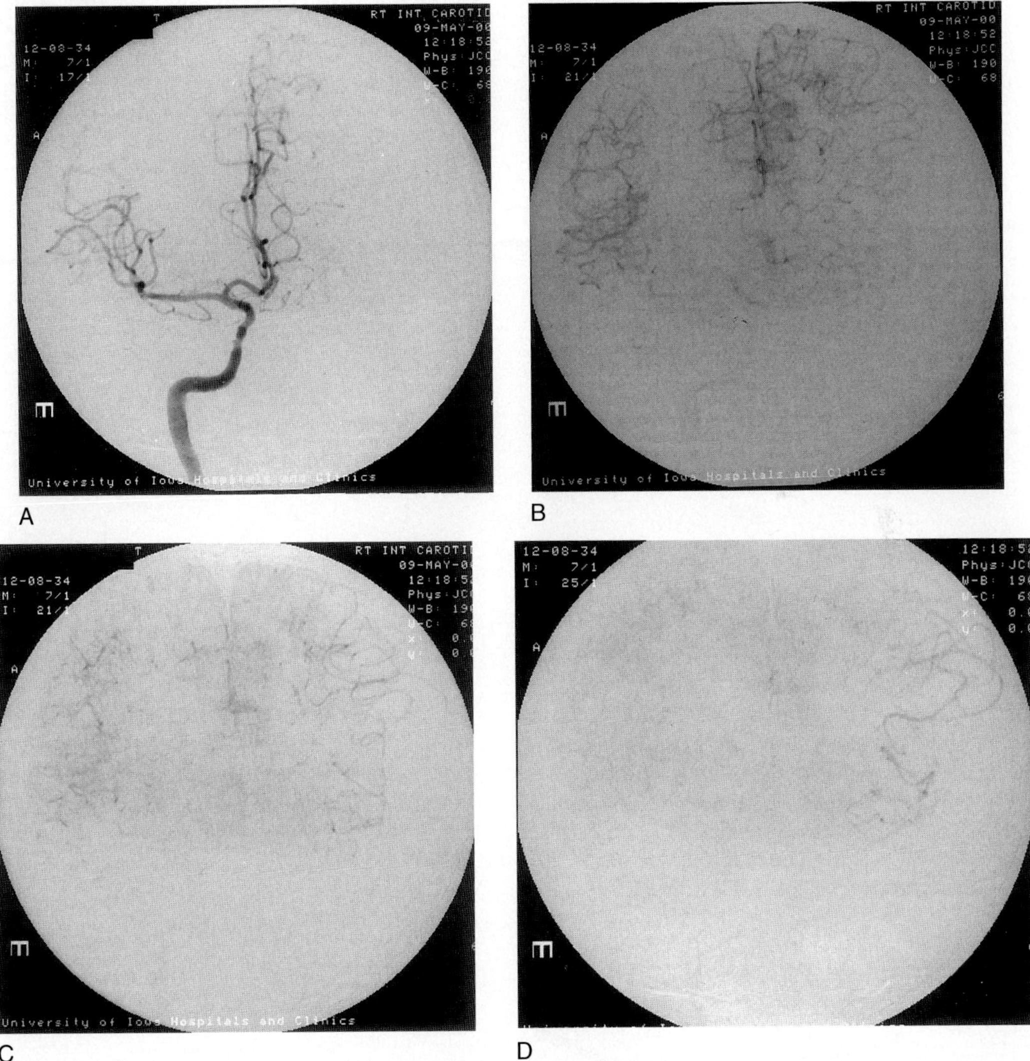

Figure 1–7. Collateral circulation via the circle of Willis and pial vessels. Anterior–posterior views of a right internal carotid artery arteriogram using subtraction techniques obtained in a patient with an occlusion of the distal portion of the left internal carotid artery. (*A*) The study demonstrates flow in both anterior cerebral arteries. (*B*) Visualization of distal branches of the left middle cerebral arteries is seen in conjunction with those on the right. (*C*) Retrograde flow into proximal portions of the left middle cerebral artery branches is noted. (*D*) The proximal (Sylvian) portions of the left middle cerebral artery are seen while the branches of the right middle cerebral artery are no longer visualized.

ischemia in these locations lead to *watershed (borderzone) infarctions*, which can involve either or both of the cerebral hemispheres. Watershed infarctions involve both the cerebral cortex and the deep white matter of the hemisphere. They usually are aligned from front to back in the hemisphere.

The *centrencephalon* is a term used in epilepsy to describe the sites in the upper brain stem and diencephalon that were thought to be the origin of generalized seizure disorders (Fig. 1–8). This term also is useful in understanding the vasculature of the brain and the pathogenesis of strokes that occur deep in the cerebral hemispheres and the brain stem (see Fig 1–7). Relatively short arteries that penetrate the brain in a basal–dorsal direction supply the medial and basal portions of the cerebral hemispheres and the brain stem. The penetrating arteries to the hemisphere include the recurrent artery of Huebner arising from the anterior cerebral artery, the lenticulostriate arteries from the proximal portion of the middle cerebral artery, and the anterior choroidal artery from the internal carotid artery. In addition, a series of vessels (interpeduncular-thalamic, posterior choroidal, thalamoperforating, thalamogeniculate arteries) from the distal basilar artery, proximal posterior cerebral artery, or the posterior communicating

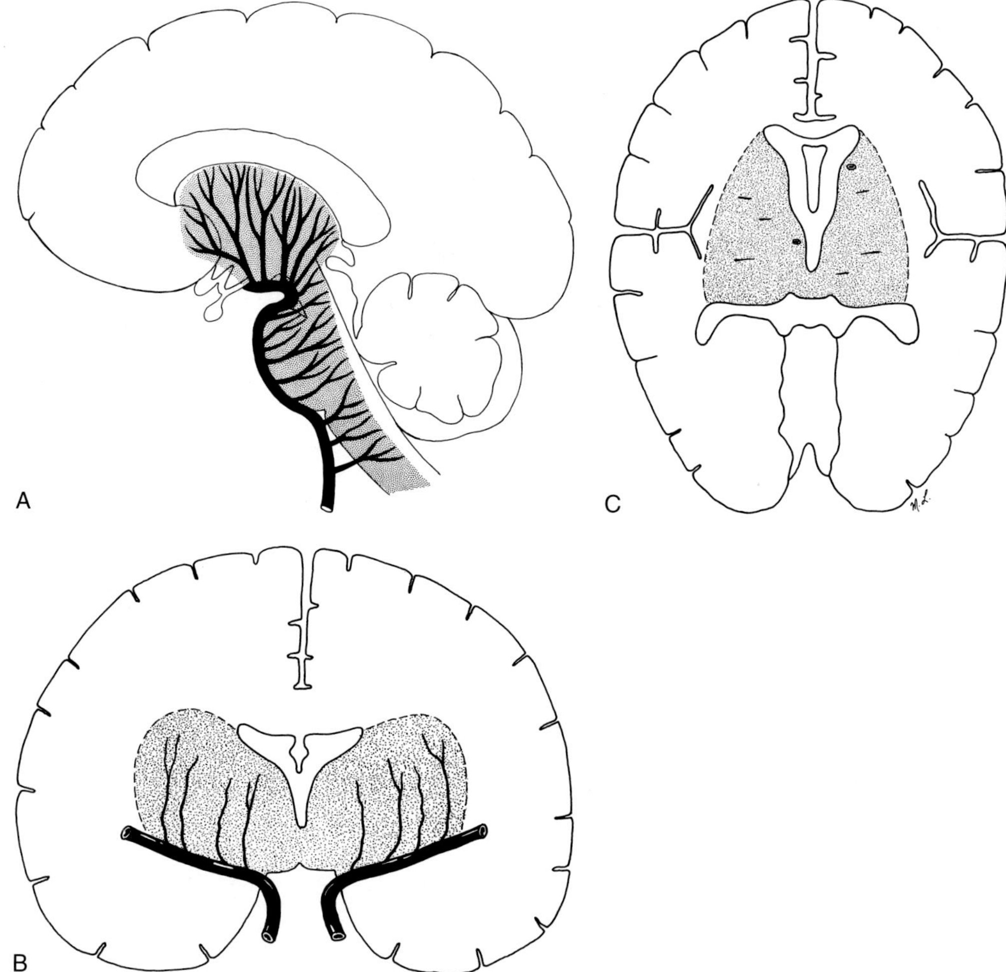

Figure 1–8. The vascular centrencephalon, the system of arteries arising from the basal arterial trunks and supplying central phylogenetically older parts of the brain. (Sagittal [A], coronal [B], and horizontal [C] sections.)

artery supply the thalamus and the posterior limb of the internal capsule. The vascular beds of these arteries form a series of triangular-shape wedges that encompass the basal ganglia, the thalamus, and the adjacent white matter structures.

Functionally, arteries within the vascular centrencephalon are end-arteries without major collateral connections from adjacent vessels. Because these arteries arise from large basal trunks, gradation between arterial and capillary pressure occurs over a relatively short distance, requiring these penetrating vessels to withstand high pressures, particularly in the presence of arterial hypertension. The *vascular centrencephalon* encompasses the areas of the brain that are the major sites for lacunar infarction and hypertensive hemorrhage. Hemorrhages tend to occur in small arteries that have undergone fibrinoid degeneration and the formation of microaneurysms that are noted in hypertensive persons, particularly those older than 65 years. Occlusion of a centrencephalic artery usually results in a small infarct because it supplies a limited cylinder of tissue. Hypertrophy and hyaline degeneration also predispose to occlusion of the penetrating arteries, creating small (*lacunar*) infarctions. Lacunar infarctions also can result from atherosclerotic occlusion of the lenticulostriate arteries or the paramedian branches of the basilar artery. These occlusions also can be due to local thrombosis of the parent artery or embolism from the heart or proximal arterial sources.

ISCHEMIC STROKE AS A SYMPTOM

Ischemic stroke is a symptom of an underlying vascular disease. The causes of stroke are grouped into several large categories (see Table 1–7 and Fig. 1–9). Determination of the most likely etiology is a critical part of stroke management because the cause influences prognosis and decisions for treatment. Regretfully, the accuracy in identifying a patient's type of ischemic cerebrovascular disease is poor.[45] Although several vascular diseases lead to an ischemic stroke, the differential diagnosis of the cause of stroke usually can be limited by the patient's clinical presentation. Still, even with an extensive battery of ancillary diagnostic tests, the diagnosis of stroke subtype can be difficult.[118–120]

Atherosclerosis is a leading cause of ischemic stroke, particularly among persons older than 50 years. As the name implies, *large artery atherosclerosis* affects major extracranial and intracranial arteries supplying the brain. Advanced atherosclerotic disease of the arch of the aorta also is increasingly recognized as a cause of embolization to the brain. The atherosclerotic plaque serves as a nidus for thrombosis or artery-to-artery embolism. It also can be the source of atherosclerotic debris (cholesterol embolism). Hypertensive or diabetic patients can have occlusion of the small penetrating arteries leading to *lacunar infarction*. These strokes produce discrete stroke syndromes involving the deep structures of the cerebral hemispheres and the brain stem.

A large number of non-atherosclerotic vascular diseases lead to stroke in all age groups. The *non-atherosclerotic vasculopathies* include both inflammatory and noninflammatory diseases of the intracranial or the extracranial arteries supplying the brain. The inflammatory arterial diseases

Table 1–7. General Categories for Causes of Ischemic Stroke

Large artery atherosclerosis
Arterial thrombosis
Artery-to-artery embolism
Small artery occlusion—Lacunar
Non-atherosclerotic vasculopathies
Inflammatory
Multisystem
Isolated
Infectious
Non-inflammatory
Cardioembolism
Hypercoagulable (pro-thrombotic) states
Inherited
Acquired
Undetermined cause
Non-thrombotic embolism

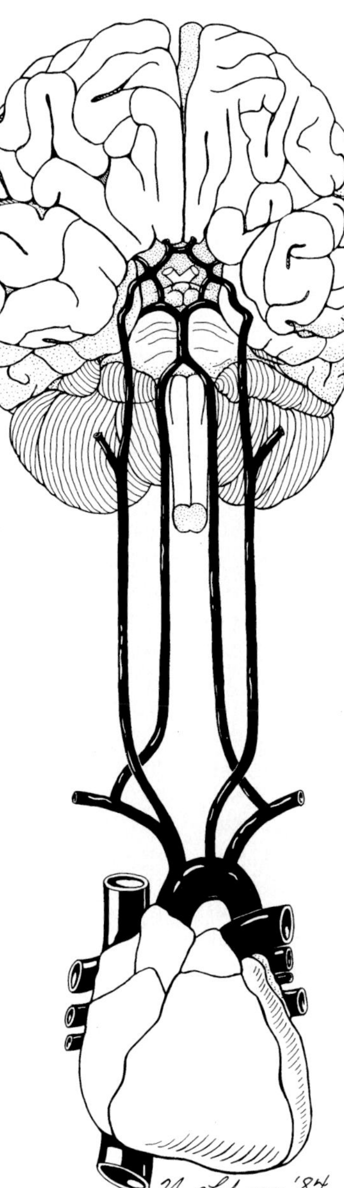

Figure 1–9. Causes of stroke.

(*vasculitis*) are divided into infectious or non-infectious vasculitides. The latter conditions are divided into multisystem vasculitis or isolated central nervous system vasculitis.

Approximately 20%–25% of ischemic strokes are secondary to embolism arising in the heart. *Cardioembolism* can cause stroke in any age group and usually results from thrombi complicating structural diseases of the heart. A persistent right-to-left shunt in the heart or the lung also can serve as a route for paradoxical embolism. Ischemic stroke can be a complication of cardiovascular operations.

Several inherited or acquired disorders of coagulation (*prothrombotic or hypercoagulable states*) can predispose to arterial thrombosis or embolization. These hypercoagulable states can result from disorders of red blood cells, platelets, viscosity, levels of clotting factors, or levels of thrombolytic factors. In addition, changes in coagulation due to pregnancy, malignancy, surgery, trauma, or infections can lead to ischemic stroke.

Rarely, ischemic stroke can result from embolization of air, amniotic fluid, fat, tumor tissue, or foreign bodies.

PATHOPHYSIOLOGY OF ISCHEMIC STROKE

Acute ischemic stroke involves a rapidly evolving, complex series of events, which include intravascular, endothelial, neuronal, glial, and inflammatory changes that either progress to cell death or resolve with the survival of a functioning neuron.[121] Whereas some cells may die immediately, other dysfunctional neurons may survive if interventions to improve perfusion and maintain cell function are prescribed rapidly. Time truly is a critical component of the course of acute ischemic stroke.[72,122,123] The understanding of the sequence of events that leads to neuronal death following the thromboembolic occlusion of a brain artery continues to evolve rapidly. Research advances are providing new insights into a number of cellular phenomena that develop during ischemia. Although the gap between the knowledge of the underpinning of the ischemic process and the patient is wide, these advances mean that strategies to treat acute ischemic stroke will continue to evolve.

The theory of the *ischemic penumbra* forms a critical underpinning for the current approach to acute ischemic stroke.[72,122,124,125] (See Fig. 1–10.) Following arterial occlusion, a core of brain may have an irreversible neuronal injury because of profound hypoperfusion and cell dysfunction.[126] (See Fig. 1–11.) This core of brain tissue rapidly becomes necrotic and unsalvageable. Although the core of completely ischemic tissue has markedly reduced cerebral blood flow and metabolic activity,

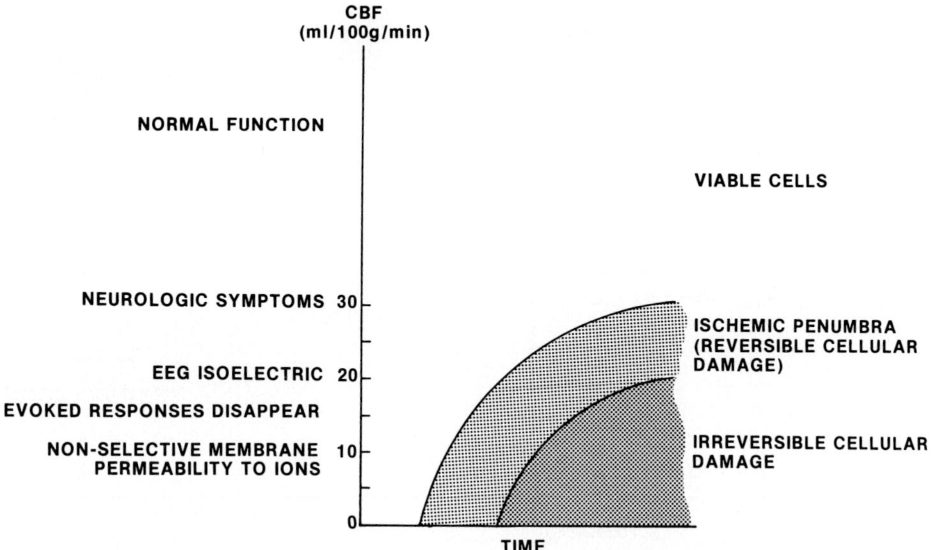

Figure 1–10. The ischemia penumbra. (Adapted from Astrup J, et al. Energy-requiring cell functions in the ischemic brain—their critical supply and possible inhibition in protective therapy. *J Neurosurg* 1982;56:482.)

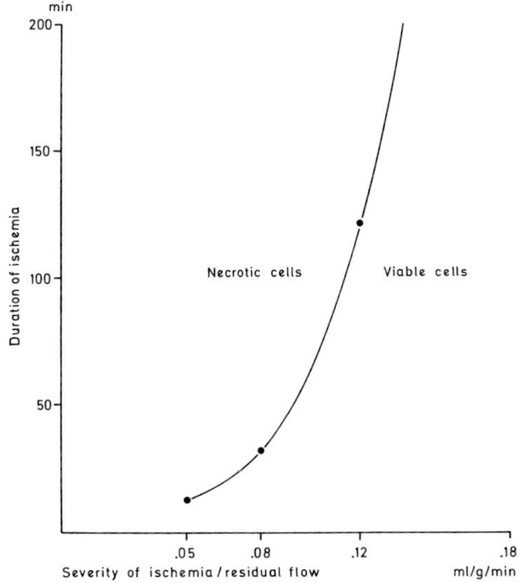

Figure 1–11. Relationship of cell survival to duration and severity of cerebral ischemia. (Courtesy of Professor W.D. Heiss.)

adjacent, partially ischemic tissue (penumbra) has borderline levels of blood flow and metabolic function.[127] Fortunately, the area of dysfunctional but not dead brain tissue may be relatively large in the setting of acute ischemic stroke. Potentially, the majority of the affected area of the brain may encompass the penumbra. Dysfunctional borderline areas have the potential for recovery with restitution of adequate perfusion or institution of measures to halt the metabolic consequences of ischemia. Conversely, these tissues could progress to cell death if flow is not restored or if the metabolic effects of ischemia cannot be reversed.[122] The ischemic penumbra appears to be more than a theory. Karonen et al[128] used perfusion- and diffusion-weighted MRI to help define the penumbra among patients with acute

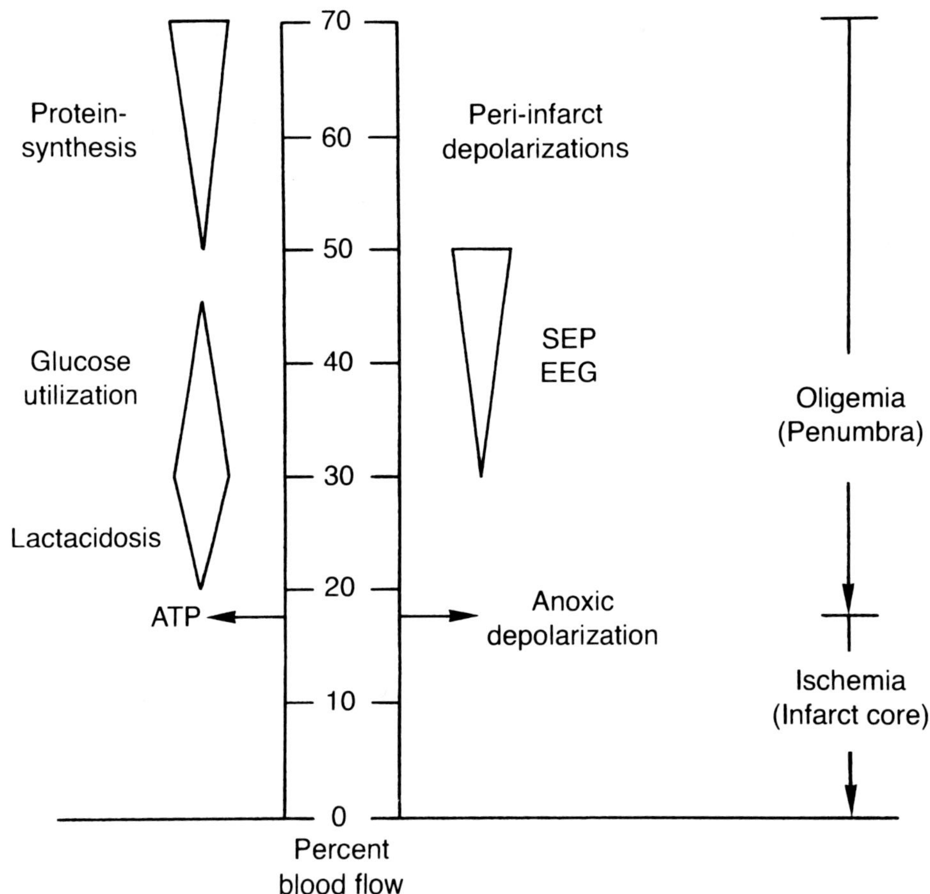

Figure 1–12. Thresholds of ischemia. (Courtesy of K. Hossmann, Max Planck Institute, Cologne.)

ischemic stroke. The tests were able to predict evolution of the illness.

Normally, cerebral blood flow is approximately 50–55 ML/100 g/min. A sophisticated autoregulatory mechanism maintains relatively constant flow despite a wide range of changes in arterial blood pressure.[124,127] Among patients with ischemic stroke, autoregulation is lost, and flow becomes pressure-dependent (Fig. 1–12.) Drops in pressure, vascular narrowing, and changes in the blood's rheological characteristics contribute to a decline in blood flow. With reductions in flow, neuronal electrical activity is disturbed. As flow declines to a rate of approximately 20–30 mL/100 g/min, metabolic activity slows and intracellular acidosis occurs.[71] At lower levels, neuronal metabolic function and intracellular water and ion homeostasis become disordered, neurotransmitters are released, and structural changes appear within the cell (Figs. 1–13, 1–14, 1–15, and 1–16.) The result is neuronal death.

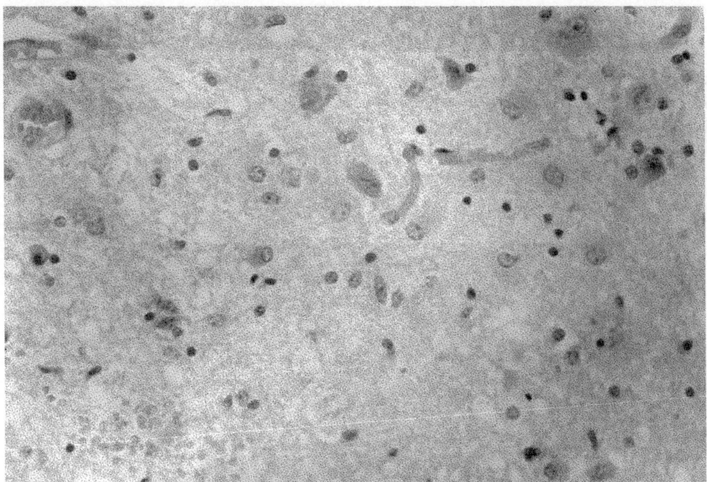

Figure 1–13. Microscopic findings of a subacute infarction. Neuronal loss and astrocytic proliferation are noted. (Courtesy of Dr. Robert Hammond, University of Western Ontario, London, Ontario.)

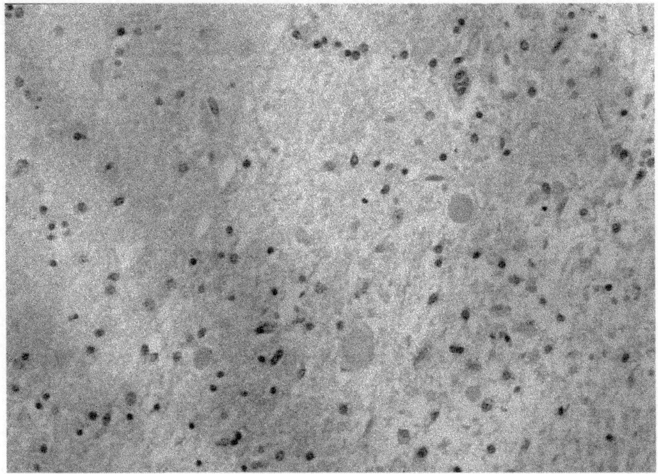

Figure 1-14. Microscopic findings of a subacute infarction. Astrocytic proliferation and the appearance of spheroids are present. (Courtesy of Dr. Robert Hammond, University of Western Ontario, London, Ontario.)

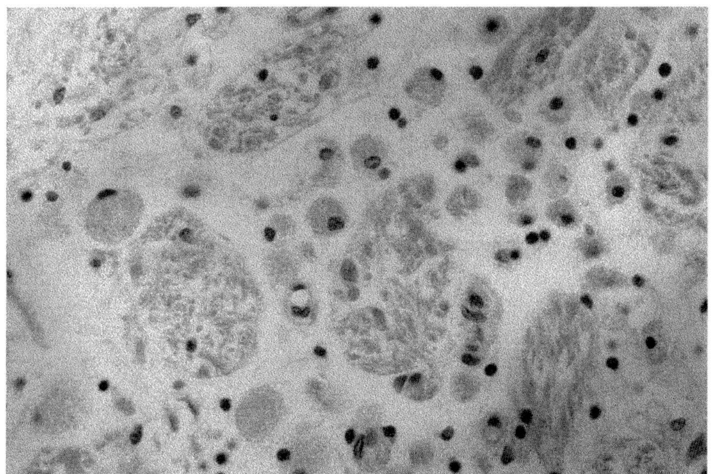

Figure 1–15. Microscopic findings of an old infarction. Numerous macrophages are detected. (Courtesy of Dr. Robert Hammond, University of Western Ontario, London, Ontario.)

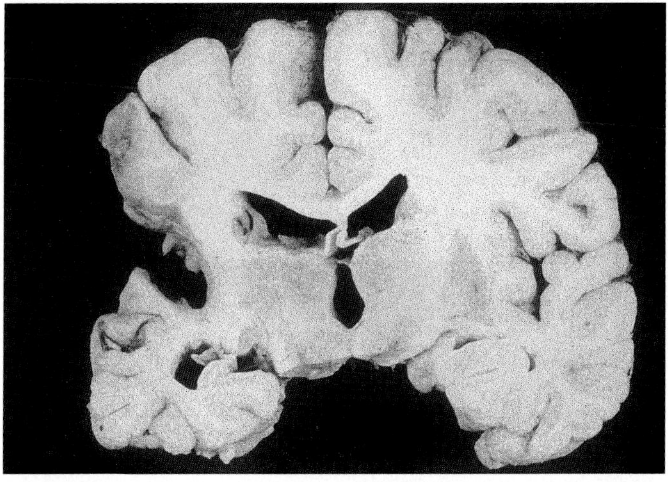

Figure 1–16. Pathological findings of an old infarction of the right hemisphere in the distribution of the middle cerebral artery. The infarction involves the frontal lobe, insular cortex, superior position of the temporal lobe and the putamen. The infarction likely was due to an embolus to the middle cerebral artery. Enlargement of the ipsilateral lateral ventricle is present. (Courtesy of Dr. Robert Hammond, University of Western Ontario, London, Ontario.)

Research is increasing our understanding of the cellular consequences of acute neuronal ischemia. Ischemia leads to anaerobic glycolysis and a resultant decline in the production of energy adenosine triphosphate; (ATP).[71,125,129] This decline in intracellular ATP limits the cell's ability to maintain energy-dependent mechanisms, such as stabilization of the cell membrane, to protect the homeostasis of the cell. Depolarization of the cell membrane allows transmembrane fluxes of sodium, potassium, chloride, and calcium. The depolarization of both ionotropic and metabotropic receptors by the release of excitatory amino acids further increases trans-membrane influxes of calcium.[88,124,129,132] Rises in intracellular calcium are critical to the synthesis of nitric oxide and the activation of phospholipidases, proteases, and endonucleases.[71,121,124,125,129] These enzymes destroy vital components of the cell. Calcium combined with metabolic acidosis stimulates a release of free radicals that compound the actions of other factors in leading to irreversible neuronal injury.[133] In addition, ischemia leads to the activation of genes that prompt apoptosis and cell death.[125,130,132,134] Inflammatory responses also may play a role in the course of acute brain ischemia.[132,135]

PROGNOSIS

Asymptomatic patients with evidence of arterial disease have a higher risk for ischemic stroke than that seen in persons who are of the same age and gender but who do not have findings of arterial disease. Annually, the risk of stroke in persons with asymptomatic stenosis of the internal carotid artery is approximately 1.3%–3%.[136,137] The likelihood of a stroke is higher in persons who have severely stenotic asymptomatic disease.[138,139] The risk of stroke is still higher in patients who have had neurological symptoms.[138] The risk of stroke is highest in persons who already have had an ischemic stroke. A TIA or an episode of amaurosis fugax conveys an intermediate risk.[137] A recent episode of TIA or amaurosis fugax should be considered a medical emergency because it identifies a person who has a very high risk for stroke. Approximately 10% of patients with ischemic stroke will have had premonitory symptoms. The risk of a stroke is highest in the first days after a TIA and declines rapidly thereafter.[140] Approximate risks of a stroke are 2%–5% during the first month, 10% during the first year, and 20% during the next 5 years.[138,141] Older patients and those with diabetes mellitus or congestive heart failure have a reduced survival after TIA.[142] Patients with more than one TIA per month and diabetes mellitus have a heightened risk of stroke.[143] Subgroups of patients at highest risk of stroke following a TIA also can be identified by the severity of the arterial disease or the presumed cause. Patients with a severe narrowing of the internal carotid artery have a very high risk of stroke (approximately 10%/year).[144] A similarly high rate is found among patients with an internal carotid occlusion and borderline blood flow to the brain.[145]

Stroke recurrence within 30 days of a stroke is seen in approximately 2% of cases.[146] Data from recent clinical trials demonstrate that the risk of recurrent stroke is approximately 1.5% in 1 week, 2%–3% vin 2 weeks, and 2%–5% in 1 month.[147–149] The risk of a second stroke is 13% at 1 year and 30% at 5 years.[150] Most recurrent strokes are in the same vascular territory as the first event.[151] Stroke recurrence is more frequent in African Americans and Hispanic Americans. The likelihood of a second stroke also is associated with elevated levels of blood pressure, congestive heart failure, or valvular heart disease.[146,152] The likelihood of early recurrent stroke does not seem to be affected by the presumed cause of the stroke.[149]

After stroke, prognoses vary considerably among patients (Table 1–8). Some patients recover completely; others die as a

Table 1–8. **Predictors of a High Mortality Following Acute Ischemic Stroke**

Advanced age
Severe co-morbid disease
Diabetes mellitus and hyperglycemia
Heart disease
Lung disease
Dementia
Clinical features of stroke
Decreased consciousness
Multiple severe deficits—motor, sensory, vision, cognition
High score on National Institutes of Health Stroke Scale
Seizures
Brain imaging findings
Multilobar infarction
Dense artery sign
Vascular imaging findings
Occlusion of basilar artery
Occlusion of internal carotid artery
Occlusion of middle cerebral artery

result of the stroke or its complications. Approximately 10%–20% of patients die within 1 month of stroke, with the highest mortality noted among patients with a major hemispheric stroke secondary to cardioembolism.[146,153–157] Rather than the cause, the site and the size of the brain injury are the major forecasters of outcomes. Deaths within 1 month are similar in men and women and among persons whose strokes occurred in the cerebral hemisphere or the brain stem.[7,158] Mortality at 1 year is approximately 20%.[155,159,160] The patient's neurological signs on admission, particularly a decline in consciousness, give an accurate estimate of the likelihood for survival.[161] Deaths after stroke also are associated with advanced age, seizures, and severe concomitant diseases.[153,155,171] The 30-day mortality is approximately 20% among persons older than 75 and one-half that rate among younger patients.[162] Most deaths within the first few days after stroke are the result of neurological injury and acute neurological complications, especially brain edema and increased intracranial pressure.[163] (See Table 1–9). Subsequent deaths largely are the result of medical complications, including infections, myocardial infarction, and pulmonary embolism.[163] When compared with age-matched healthy persons, a higher risk of death among persons with cerebrovascular disease persists up to 20 years after stroke.[164]

Table 1–9. **Leading Causes of Death Following Ischemic Stroke**

- Neurological
  - Brain destruction
  - Brain edema
    - Increased intracranial pressure
    - Herniation
  - Hemorrhagic transformation
- Non-neurological
  - Infection
    - Pneumonia
    - Sepsis
  - Myocardial infarction
  - Cardiac arrhythmias
  - Congestive heart failure
  - Pulmonary embolism
- Complications of therapies

By 3 months after stroke, approximately 30%–40% of patients make an almost complete recovery. By 1 year, approximately 65% of survivors are independent, and the rate is highest among persons with lacunar or brain stem strokes.[158,159,165] Younger patients are more likely to recover than older persons.[166] The remaining patients have varying degrees of disability. Cognitive or language impairments, motor deficits, sensory or visual loss, and poor balance are the leading causes of long-term disability.[167] The likelihood of cognitive declines and disability increases considerably with recurrent stroke.

Factors that affect a patient's prognosis after stroke include the severity of neurological deficits, age, cause of stroke, history of prior stroke, and presence of concomitant disease.[153] The most important factor is the severity of neurological impairments, as these signs reflect the extent of brain injury. Patients with multilobar infarctions generally have extensive impairments. The results of brain imaging also forecast recovery or the risk of complications with treatment of agents such as tissue plasminogen activator. Early demonstration of hypodensity of more than one-third of the hemisphere, early effacement of sulci, obliteration of the insular margin, prominent hypodensity in the basal ganglia (striatocapsular), or a dense artery sign are recognized as important prognostic clues.[168,169] Still, these findings also reflect the severity of neurological impairments. Subtype of ischemic stroke also portends outcome. In general, patients with lacunar strokes have a better early prognosis than do persons who have strokes secondary to other causes.[153,154,157] Patients with diabetes mellitus or an elevated blood glucose level also have poorer prognoses than do normoglycemic patients.[170]

SUMMARY

Stroke poses a global challenge. The growth and aging of the population will worsen the problem of ischemic stroke, particularly in populous developing countries. Stroke already is the second most common cause of death in the world and the leading cause of long-term disability. The economic and human costs are staggering. In the past, stroke terminology has hampered rather than helped our understanding of stroke, but the terminology is becoming simplified, standardized, and more precise. The brain has a unique vascular infrastructure, with the phylogenetically older parts being more prone to small vessel disease. The collateral circulation salvages brain when it functions and leads to watershed infarctions when it fails. The varied pathophysiology of ischemic stroke results in a range of clinical manifestations and in a spectrum of prognostic possibilities.

REFERENCES

1. American Heart Association. *2000 Heart and Stroke Statistical Update.*
2. Broderick J, Brott T, Kothari R, et al. The Greater Cincinnati/Northern Kentucky Stroke Study: preliminary first-ever and total incidence rates of stroke among blacks. *Stroke* 1998; 29:415–421.
3. Sudlow CL, Warlow CP. Comparing stroke incidence worldwide: what makes studies comparable? *Stroke* 1996;27:550–558.
4. Bonita R, Anderson CS, Broad JB, Jamrozik KD, Stewart-Wynne EG, Anderson NE. Stroke incidence and case fatality in Australasia. A comparison of the Auckland and Perth population-based stroke registers. *Stroke* 1994;25: 552-557.
5. Cheng XM, Ziegler DK, Lai YH, et al. Stroke in China, 1986 through 1990. *Stroke* 1995; 26:1990–1994.
6. Stegmayr B, Asplund K, Kuulasmaa K, Rajakangas AM, Thorvaldsen P, Tuomilehto J. Stroke incidence and mortality correlated to stroke risk factors in the WHO MONICA Project. An ecological study of 18 populations. *Stroke* 1997;28:1367–1374.
7. Thorvaldsen P, Asplund K, Kuulasmaa K, Rajakangas AM, Schroll M. Stroke incidence, case fatality, and mortality in the WHO MONICA project. World Health Organization Monitoring Trends and Determinants in Cardiovascular Disease. *Stroke* 1995;26: 361–367.
8. Feigin VL, Wiebers DO, Nikitin YP, O'Fallon WM, Whisnant JP. Risk factors for ischemic stroke in a Russian community: a population-based case-control study. *Stroke* 1998;29:34–39.
9. Eastern Stroke and Coronary Heart Disease Collaborative Research Group. Blood pressure, cholesterol, and stroke in eastern Asia. *Lancet* 1998;352:1801–1807.
10. Asplund K. Stroke in Europe. Widening gap between East and West. *Cerebrovasc Dis* 1996;6:3–6.
11. Numminen H, Kotila M, Waltimo O, Aho K, Kaste M. Declining incidence and mortality rates of stroke in Finland from 1972 to 1991. Results of three population-based stroke registers. *Stroke* 1996;27:1487–1491.
12. Thom TJ, Epstein FH. Heart disease, cancer, and stroke mortality trends and their interrelations. An international perspective. *Circulation* 1994;90:574–582.
13. Lanska DJ, Mi X. Decline in US stroke mortality in the era before antihypertensive therapy. *Stroke* 1993;24:1382–1388.
14. Wolfe CD, Tilling K, Beech R, Rudd AG. Variations in case fatality and dependency from stroke in western and central Europe. The European BIOMED Study of Stroke Care Group. *Stroke* 1999;30:350–356.
15. Bergen DC. The world-wide burden of neurologic disease. *Neurology* 1996;47:21–25.
16. Murray CJ, Lopez AD. Mortality by cause for eight regions of the world: Global Burden of Disease Study. *Lancet* 1997;349:1269–1276.
17. Al Rajeh S, Larbi EB, Bademosi O, et al. Stroke register. Experience from the Eastern Province of Saudia Arabia. *Cerebrovasc Dis* 1998;8:86–89.
18. Poungvarin N. Stroke in the developing world. *Lancet* 1998;352(Suppl 3):SIII19–SIII22
19. American Heart Association. *Heart Stroke Facts.* 1996.
20. May DS, Casper ML, Croft JB, Giles WH. Trends in survival after stroke among Medicare beneficiaries. *Stroke* 1994;25:1617–1622.
21. Shahar E, McGovern PG, Sprafka JM, et al. Improved survival of stroke patients during the 1980s. The Minnesota Stroke Survey. *Stroke* 1995;26:1–6.
22. Potts DC, Gilliam F, Gomez CR, Marsh EE, Mitchell VL, Sherrill R. Intraregional decline in case-fatality and hospital use afer occlusive stroke in the Southeastern United States. *J Stroke Cerebrovasc Dis* 1999;8:344–348.
23. Bots ML, Looman SJ, Koudstaal PJ, Hofman A, Hoes AW, Grobbee DE. Prevalence of stroke in the general population. The Rottendam Study. *Stroke* 1996;27:1499–1501.
24. Addington-Hall J, Lay M, Altmann D, McCarthy M. Symptom control, communication with health professionals, and hospital care of stroke patients in the last year of life as reported by surviving family, friends, and officials. *Stroke* 1995;26:2242–2248.
25. Lawrence L, Christie D. Quality of life after stroke: a three-year follow-up. *Ageing* 1979; 8:167–172.
26. Leibson CL, Ransom JE, Brown RD, O'Fallon WM, Hass SL, Whisnant JP. Stroke-attributable nursing home use: a population-based study. *Neurology* 1998;51:163–168.

27. Terent A, Marke LA, Asplund K, Norrving B, Jonsson E, Wester PO. Costs of stroke in Sweden. A national perspective. *Stroke* 1994;25: 2363–2369.
28. Murray CJ, Lopez AD. Alternative projections of mortality and disability by cause 1990–2020: Global Burden of Disease Study. *Lancet* 1997;349:1498–1504.
29. Evers SM, Engel GL, Ament AJ. Cost of stroke in The Netherlands from a societal perspective. *Stroke* 1997;28:1375–1381.
30. Smurawska LT, Alexandrov AV, Bladin CF, Norris JW. Cost of acute stroke care in Toronto, Canada. *Stroke* 1994;25:1628–1631.
31. Matchar DB. The value of stroke prevention and treatment. *Neurology* 1998;51:S31–S35
32. Taylor TN, Davis PH, Torner JC, Holmes J, Meyer JW, Jacobson MF. Lifetime cost of stroke in the United States. *Stroke* 1996;27:1459–1466.
33. Dobkin B. The economic impact of stroke. *Neurology* 1995;45:S6–S9.
34. Holloway RG, Witter DMJ, Lawton KB, Lipscomb J, Samsa G. Inpatient costs of specific cerebrovascular events at five academic medical centers. *Neurology* 1996;46:854–860.
35. Bergman L, van der Meulen JHP, Limburg M, Habbema JDF. Costs of medical care after first-ever stroke in the Netherlands. *Stroke* 1995; 26:1830–1836.
36. Leibson CL, Hu T, Brown RD, Hass SL, O'Fallon WM, Whisnant JP. Utilization of acute care services in the year before and after first stroke: a population-based study. *Neurology* 1996;46:861–869.
37. Beech R, Ratcliffe M, Tilling K, Wolfe C, on behalf of the participants of the European Study on Stroke Care. Hospital services for stroke care. *Stroke* 1996;27:1958–1964.
38. Adams HP, Jr. The importance of the Helsingborg declaration on stroke management in Europe. *J Intern Med* 1996;240:169–171.
39. Aboderin I, Venables G. Stroke management in Europe. Pan European Consensus Meeting on Stroke Management. *J Intern Med* 1996; 240:173–180.
40. European Ad Hoc Consensus Group. Optimizing intensive care in stroke. A European perspective. *Cerebrovasc Dis* 1997;7:113–128.
41. Lindley RI, Amayo EO, Marshall J, Sandercock PA, Dennis M, Warlow CP. Hospital services for patients with acute stroke in the United Kingdom: the Stroke Association Survey of consultant opinion. *Ageing* 1995;24:525–532.
42. Retchin SM, Brown RS, Yeh SC, Chu D, Moreno L. Outcomes of stroke patients in Medicare fee for service and managed care. *JAMA* 1997; 278:119–124.
43. Webster JRJ, Feinglass J. Stroke patients, "managed care," and distributive justice. *JAMA* 1997;278:161–162.
44. Neely KW, Norton RL. Survey of health maintenance organization instructions to members concerning emergency department and 911 use. *Ann Emerg Med* 1999;34:19–24.
45. Benesch C, Witter DMJ, Wilder AL, Duncan PW, Samsa GP, Matchar DB. Inaccuracy of the International Classification of Diseases (ICD-9-CM) in identifying the diagnosis of ischemic cerebrovascular disease. *Neurology* 1997;49: 660–664.
46. Leibson CL, Naessens JM, Brown RD, Whisnant JP. Accuracy of hospital discharge abstracts for identifying stroke. *Stroke* 1994;25:2348–2355.
47. Liu L, Reeder B, Shuaib A, Mazagri R. Validity of stroke diagnosis on hospital discharge records in Saskatchewan, Canada: implications for stroke surveillance. *Cerebrovasc Dis* 1999; 9:224–230.
48. Mayo NE, Neville D, Kirkland S, et al. Hospitalization and case-fatality rates for stroke in Canada from 1982 through 1991. The Canadian Collaborative Study Group of Stroke Hospitalizations. *Stroke* 1996;27:1215–1220.
49. May DS, Kittner SJ. Use of Medicare claims data to estimate national trends in stroke incidence, 1985-1991. *Stroke* 1994;25:2343–2347.
50. Kagan A, Popper J, Reed DM, MacLean CJ, Grove JS. Trends in stroke incidence and mortality in Hawaiian Japanese men. *Stroke* 1994;25:1170–1175.
51. Bonita R, Stewart A, Beaglehole R. International trends in stroke mortality: 1970–1985. *Stroke* 1990;21:989–992.
52. Truelsen T, Prescott E, Gronbaek M, Schnohr P, Boysen G. Trends in stroke incidence. The Copenhagen City Heart Study. *Stroke* 1997; 28:1903–1907.
53. Falkeborn M, Persson I, Terent A, Bergstrom R, Lithell H, Naessen T. Long-term trends in incidence of and mortality from acute myocardial infarction and stroke in women: analyses of total first events and of deaths in the Uppsala Health Care Region, Sweden. *Epidemiology* 1996; 7:67–74.
54. Zhang XH, Sasaki S, Kesteloot H. Changes in the sex ratio of stroke mortality in the period of 1955 through 1990. *Stroke* 1995;26: 1774–1780.
55. Cooper R, Sempos C, Hsieh SC, Kovar MG. Slowdown in the decline of stroke mortality in the United States, 1978-1986. *Stroke* 1990; 21:1274–1279.
56. Bonita R, Beaglehole R. The enigma of the decline in stroke deaths in the United States: the search for an explanation. *Stroke* 1996; 27:370–372.
57. Brown RD, Jr., Whisnant JP, Sicks JD, O'Fallon WM, Wiebers DO. Stroke incidence, prevalence, and survival. Secular trends in Rochester, Minnesota, through 1989. *Stroke* 1996; 27:373–380.
58. Bogousslavsky J, Regli F. Cerebral infarct in apparent transient ischemic attacks. *Neurology* 1985;35:1501–1503.
59. Koudstaal PJ, van Gijn J, Lodder J, et al. Transient ischemic attacks with and without a relevant infarct on computed tomographic scans cannot be distinguished clinically. Dutch Transient Ischemic Attack Study Group. *Arch Neurol* 1991;48:916–920.
60. Koudstaal PJ, van Gijn J, Frenken CW, et al. TIA, RIND, minor stroke: a continuum, or

different subgroups? Dutch TIA Study Group. *J Neurol Neurosurg Psychiatry* 1992;55:95–97.
61. Evans GW, Howard G, Murros KE, Rose LA, Toole JF. Cerebral infarction verified by cranial computed tomography and prognosis for survival following transient ischemic attack. *Stroke* 1991;22:431–436.
62. Dennis MS, Bamford JM, Sandercock PA, Warlow CP. Incidence of transient ischemic attacks in Oxfordshire, England. *Stroke* 1989; 20:333–339.
63. Brown RD, Jr., Petty GW, O'Fallon WM, Wiebers DO, Whisnant JP. Incidence of transient ischemic attack in Rochester, Minnesota, 1985–1989. *Stroke* 1998;29:2109–2113.
64. Dennis MS, Bamford JM, Sandercock PA, Warlow CP. A comparison of risk factors and prognosis for transient ischemic attacks and minor ischemic strokes. The Oxfordshire Community Stroke Project. *Stroke* 1989; 20:1494–1499.
65. Caplan LR. Are terms such as completed stroke or RIND of continued usefulness? *Stroke* 1983;14:431–433.
66. Hornig CR, Lammers C, Buttner T, Hoffmann O, Dorndorf W. Long-term prognosis of infratentorial transient ischemic attacks and minor strokes. *Stroke* 1992;23:199–204.
67. Eriksson SE. Differences in the outcome of patients with TIA versus minor stroke. *Acta Neurol Scand* 1992;85:208–211.
68. Davis PH, Clarke WR, Bendixen BH, Adams HP, Jr., Woolson RF, Culebras A. Silent cerebral infarction in patients enrolled in the TOAST Study. *Neurology* 1996;46:942–948.
69. Brainin M, McShane LM, Steiner M, Dachenhausen A, Seiser A. Silent brain infarcts and transient ischemic attacks. *Stroke* 1995; 26:1348–1352.
70. Siebler M, Sitzer M, Rose G, Bendfeldt D, Steinmetz H. Silent cerebral embolism caused by neurologically symptomatic high-grade carotid stenosis. Event rates before and after carotid endarterectomy. *Brain* 1993;116: 1005–1015.
71. Pulsinelli W. Pathophysiology of acute ischaemic stroke. *Lancet* 1992;339:533–536.
72. Fisher M, Bogousslavsky J. Further evolution toward effective therapy for acute ischemic stroke. *JAMA* 1998;279:1298–1303.
73. Camarata PJ, Heros PC, Latchaw RE. "Brain attack." The rationale for treating stroke as a medical emergency. *Neurosurgery* 1994; 34:144–158.
74. Adams HP, Jr. Treating ischemic stroke as an emergency. *Arch Neurol* 1998;55:457–461.
75. Heros RC, Camarata PJ, Latchaw RE. Brain attack. Introduction. *Neurosurg Clin N Am* 1997;8:135–144.
76. Hill MD, Hachinski V. Stroke treatment: time is brain. *Lancet* 1998;352(Suppl 3):SIII10–SIII14.
77. Petit, C. Victims of stroke much more likely to live through it. San Francisco Chronicle, 1991.
78. Smith MA, Doliszny KM, Shahar E, McGovern PG, Arnett DK, Luepker RV. Delayed hospital arrival for acute stroke: the Minnesota Stroke Survey. *Ann Intern Med* 1998;129:190–196.
79. Goldstein LB, Gradison M. Stroke-related knowledge among patients with access to medical care in the stroke belt. *J Stroke Cerebrovasc Dis* 1999;8:349–352.
80. Fuster V, Smaha L. AHA's new strategic impact goal designed to curb epidemic of cardiovascular disease and stroke. *Circulation* 1999; 99:2360.
81. Crocco TJ, Kothari RU, Sayre MR, Liu T. A nationwide prehospital stroke survey. *Prehospital Emergency Care* 1999;3:201–206.
82. Fuster V. Epidemic of cardiovascular disease and stroke: the three main challenges. Presented at the 71st Scientific Sessions of the American Heart Association. Dallas, Texas. *Circulation* 1999;99:1132–1137.
83. Toni D, Fiorelli M, Gentile M, et al. Progressing neurological deficit secondary to acute ischemic stroke. A study on predictability, pathogenesis, and prognosis. *Arch Neurol* 1995;52:670–675.
84. Yamamoto H, Bogousslavsky J, Van Melle G. Different predictors of neurological worsening in different causes of stroke. *Arch Neurol* 1998; 55:481–486.
85. Nakamura K, Saku Y, Ibayashi S, Fijishima M. Progressive motor deficits in lacunar infarction. *Stroke* 1999;52:29–33.
86. Roden-Jullig A. Progressing stroke. Epidemiology. *Cerebrovasc Dis* 1997;7(Suppl 5):2–5.
87. van der Worp HB, Kappelle LJ. Complications of acute ischaemic stroke. *Cerebrovasc Dis* 1998; 8:124–132.
88. Castillo J, Davalos A, Noya M. Progression of ischaemic stroke and excitotoxic aminoacids. *Lancet* 1997;349:79–83.
89. Castillo J. Deteriorating stroke: diagnostic criteria, predictors, mechanisms and treatment. *Cerebrovasc Dis* 1999;9(Suppl 3):1–8.
90. Hachinski VC. Multi-infarct dementia: a reappraisal. *Alzheimer Dis Assoc Disord* 1991;5:64–68.
91. Kase CS, Wolf PA, Kelly-Hayes M, Kannel WB, Beiser A, D'Agostino RB. Intellectual decline after stroke: the Framingham Study. *Stroke* 1998;29:805–812.
92. Roman GC, Tatemichi TK, Erkinjuntti T, et al. Vascular dementia: diagnostic criteria for research studies. Report of the NINDS-AIREN International Workshop. *Neurology* 1993; 43:250–260.
93. Kokmen E, Whisnant JP, O'Fallon WM, Chu CP, Beard CM. Dementia after ischemic stroke: a population-based study in Rochester, Minnesota (1960–1984). *Neurology* 1996;46:154–159.
94. Erkinjuntti T, Hachinski V. Rethinking vascular dementia. *Cerebrovasc Dis* 1993;3:3–23.
95. Censori B, Manara O, Agostinis C, et al. Dementia after first stroke. *Stroke* 1996; 27:1205–1210.
96. Bowler JV, Eliasziw M, Steenhuis R, et al. Comparative evolution of Alzheimer disease, vascular dementia, and mixed dementia. *Arch Neurol* 1997;54:697–703.

97. Chui HC, Victoroff JI, Margolin D, Jagust W, Shankle R, Katzman R. Criteria for the diagnosis of ischemic vascular dementia proposed by the State of California Alzheimer's Disease Diagnostic and Treatment Centers. *Neurology* 1992;42:473–480.
98. Tatemichi TK, Desmond DW, Paik M, et al. Clinical determinants of dementia related to stroke. *Ann Neurol* 1993;33:568–575.
99. Tatemichi TK, Desmond DW, Mayeux R, et al. Dementia after stroke: baseline frequency, risks, and clinical features in a hospitalized cohort. *Neurology* 1992;42:1185–1193.
100. Gorelick PB. Status of risk factors for dementia associated with stroke. *Stroke* 1997;28:459–463.
101. Ross GW, Petrovitch H, White LR, et al. Characterization of risk factors for vascular dementia. *Neurology* 1999;53:337–343.
102. Hachinski VC, Lassen NA, Marshall J. Multi-infarct dementia. A cause of mental deterioration in the elderly. *Lancet* 1974;2:207–210.
103. Bowler JV, Hachinski V. Criteria for vascular dementia: replacing dogma with data. *Arch Neurol* 2000;57:170–171.
104. Hachinski VC, Iliff LD, Zilhka E, et al. Cerebral blood flow in dementia. *Arch Neurol* 1975; 32:632–637.
105. Moroney JT, Bagiella E, Desmond DW, et al. Meta-analysis of the Hachinski Ischemic Score in pathologically verified dementias. *Neurology* 1997;49:1096–1105.
106. Moroney JT, Bagiella E, Hachinski VC, et al. Misclassification of dementia subtype using the Hachinski Ischemic Score: results of a meta-analysis of patients with pathologically verified dementias. *Ann N Y Acad Sci* 1997;826: 490–492.
107. Moroney JT, Bagiella E, Desmond DW, et al. Meta-analysis of the Hachinski Ischemic Score in pathologically verified dementias. *Neurology* 1997;49:1096–1105.
108. Breteler MM, van Swieten JC, Bots ML, et al. Cerebral white matter lesions, vascular risk factors, and cognitive function in a population-based study: the Rotterdam Study. *Neurology* 1994;44:1246–1252.
109. Caplan L, Schoene WC. Clinical features of subcortical arteriosclerotic encephalopathy (Binswanger disease). *Neurology* 1978;28: 1206–1215.
110. Roman GC. From UBOs to Binswanger's disease. Impact of magnetic resonance imaging on vascular dementia research. *Stroke* 1996;27: 1269–1273.
111. Hachinski V. Binswanger's disease: neither Binswanger's nor a disease. *J Neurol Sci* 1991; 103:1.
112. Chaturvedi S, Lukovits TG, Chen W, Gorelick PB. Ischemia in the territory of a hypoplastic vertebrobasilar system. *Neurology* 1999;52: 980–983.
113. Tatu L, Moulin T, Bogousslavsky J, Duvernoy H. Arterial territories of the human brain: cerebral hemispheres. *Neurology* 1998;50:1699–1708.
114. Vuilleumier P, Bogousslavsky J, Regli F. Infarction of the lower brainstem. Clinical, aetiological and MRI-topographical correlations. *Brain* 1995;118:1013–1025.
115. van der Zwan A, Hillen B. Review of the variability of the territories of the major cerebral arteries. *Stroke* 1991;22:1078–1084.
116. Damasio H. A computed tomographic guide to the identification of cerebral vascular territories. *Arch Neurol* 1983;40:138–142.
117. Damasio H, Frank R. Three-dimensional in vivo mapping of brain lesions in humans. *Arch Neurol* 1992;49:137–143.
118. Gordon DL, Bendixen BH, Adams HP, Jr., et al. Interphysician agreement in the diagnosis of subtypes of acute ischemic stroke: implications for clinical trials. The TOAST Investigators. *Neurology* 1993;43:1021–1027.
119. Madden KP, Karanjia PN, Adams HP, Jr., Clarke WR. Accuracy of initial stroke subtype diagnosis in the TOAST study. Trial of ORG 10172 in Acute Stroke Treatment. *Neurology* 1995;45: 1975–1979.
120. Johnson CJ, Kittner SJ, McCarter RJ, et al. Interrater reliability of an etiologic classification of ischemic stroke. *Stroke* 1995;26:46–51.
121. Fisher M. Clinical pharmacology of cerebral ischemia. Old controversies and new approaches. *Cerebrovasc Dis* 1991;1 (Suppl 1): 112–119.
122. Ginsberg MD, Pulsinelli WA. The ischemic penumbra, injury thresholds, and the therapeutic window for acute stroke. *Ann Neurol* 1994;36: 553–554.
123. Pulsinelli WA, Jacewicz M, Levy DE, Petito CK, Plum F. Ischemic brain injury and the therapeutic window. *Ann N Y Acad Sci* 1997;835:187–193.
124. Heiss WD, Graf R. The ischemic penumbra. *Curr Opin Neurol* 1994;7:11–19.
125. Lee JM, Zipfel GJ, Choi DW. The changing landscape of ischaemic brain injury mechanisms. *Nature* 1999;399:A7–14.
126. Kaufmann AM, Firlik AD, Fukui MB, Wechsler LR, Jungries CA, Yonas H. Ischemic care and penumbra in human stroke. *Stroke* 1999; 30:93–99.
127. Hakim AM. The cerebral ischemic penumbra. *Can J Neurol Sci* 1987;14:557–559.
128. Karonen JO, Ostergaard L, Liu Y, et al. Combined diffiusion and perfusion MRI with correlation to single-photon emission CT in acute ischemic stroke. Ischemic penumbra predicts infarct growth. *Stroke* 1999;30:1583–1590.
129. Morgenstern LB, Pettigrew LC. Brain protection—human data and potential new therapies. *New Horizons* 1997;5:397–405.
130. Chen J, Simon R. Ischemic tolerance in the brain. *Neurology* 1997;48:306–311.
131. Read SJ, Hirano T, Davis SM, Donnan GA. Limiting neurological damage after stroke: a review of pharmacological treatment options. *Drugs Aging* 1999;14:11–39.
132. Dirnagl U, Iadecola C, Moskowitz MA. Pathobiology of ischaemic stroke: an integrated view. *Trends in Neurosciences* 1999;22:391–397.
133. Zivin JA. Factors determining the therapeutic window for stroke. *Neurology* 1998;50:599–603.

134. Pulera MR, Adams LM, Liu H, et al. Apoptosis in a neonatal rat model of cerebral hypoxia-ischemia. *Stroke* 1998;29:2622–2630.
135. Barone FC, Feuerstein GZ. Inflammatory mediators and stroke: new opportunities for novel therapeutics. *J Cereb Blood Flow Metab* 1999; 19:819–834.
136. Bock RW, Gray-Weale AC, Mock PA, Robinson DA, Irwig L, Lusby RJ. The natural history of asymptomatic carotid artery disease. *J Vasc Surg* 1993;17:160–171.
137. Wilterdink JL, Easton JD. Vascular event rates in patients with atherosclerotic cerebrovascular disease. *Arch Neurol* 1992;49:857–863.
138. Norris JW. Risk of cerebral infarction, myocardial infarction and vascular death in patients with asymptomatic carotid disease, transient ischemic attack and stroke. *Cerebrovasc Dis* 1992;2(Suppl):2–5.
139. Norris JW, Zhu CZ, Bornstein NM, Chambers BR. Vascular risks of asymptomatic carotid stenosis. *Stroke* 1991;22:1485–1490.
140. Carolei A, Candelise L, Fiorelli M, Francucci BM, Motolese M, Fieschi C. Long-term prognosis of transient ischemic attacks and reversible ischemic neurologic deficits: a hospital-based study. *Cerebrovasc Dis* 1992;2:266–272.
141. Dennis M, Bamford J, Sandercock P, Warlow C. Prognosis of transient ischemic attacks in the Oxfordshire Community Stroke Project. *Stroke* 1990;21:848–853.
142. Evans BA, Sicks JD, Whisnant JP. Factors affecting survival and occurrence of stroke in patients with transient ischemic attacks. *Mayo Clin Proc* 1994;69:416–421.
143. Bruno A, Jeffries L, Lakind E, Qualls C. Predictors of cerebral infarction following transient ischemic attack. *J Stroke Cerebrovasc Dis* 1993;3:23–28.
144. North American Symptomatic Carotid Endarterectomy Trial Collaborators. Beneficial effect of carotid endarterectomy in symptomatic patients with high-grade carotid stenosis. *N Engl J Med* 1991;325:445–453.
145. Grubb RL, Jr., Derdeyn CP, Fritsch SM, et al. Importance of hemodynamic factors in the prognosis of symptomatic carotid occlusion. *JAMA* 1998;280:1055–1060.
146. Broderick JP, Phillips SJ, O'Fallon WM, Frye RL, Whisnant JP. Relationship of cardiac disease to stroke occurrence, recurrence, and mortality. *Stroke* 1992;23:1250–1256.
147. CAST (Chinese Acute Stroke Trial) Collaborative Group. CAST: randomised placebo-controlled trial of early aspirin use in 20,000 patients with acute ischaemic stroke. *Lancet* 1997;349: 1641–1649.
148. International Stroke Trial Collaborative Group. The International Stroke Trial (IST): a randomised trial of aspirin, subcutaneous heparin, both, or neither among 19435 patients with acute ischaemic stroke. *Lancet* 1997;349: 1569–1581.
149. The Publications Committee for the Trial of ORG 10172 in Acute Stroke Treatment (TOAST) Investigators. Low molecular weight heparinoid, ORG 10172 (danaparoid), and outcome after acute ischemic stroke: a randomized controlled trial. *JAMA* 1998; 279:1265–1272.
150. Burn J, Dennis M, Bamford J, Sandercock P, Wade D, Warlow C. Long-term risk of recurrent stroke after a first-ever stroke. The Oxfordshire Community Stroke Project. *Stroke* 1994;25: 333–337.
151. Cillessen JP, Kappelle LJ, van Swieten JC, Algra A, van Gijn J. Does cerebral infarction after a previous warning occur in the same vascular territory? *Stroke* 1993;24:351–354.
152. Alter M, Friday G, Lai SM, O'Connell JB, Sobel E. Hypertension and risk of stroke recurrence. *Stroke* 1994;25:1605–1610.
153. Arboix A, Garcia-Eroles L, Massons J, Oliveres M. Predictive factors of in-hospital mortality in 986 consecutive patients with first-ever stroke. *Cerebrovasc Dis* 1996;6:161–165.
154. Bamford J, Sandercock P, Dennis M, Burn J, Warlow C. Classification and natural history of clinically identifiable subtypes of cerebral infarction. *Lancet* 1991;337:1521–1526.
155. Petty GW, Brown RD, Jr., Whisnant JP, et al. Survival and recurrence after first cerebral infarction: a population-based study in Rochester, Minnesota, 1975 through 1989. *Neurology* 1998;50:208–216.
156. Chambers BR, Norris JW, Shurvell BL, Hachinski VC. Prognosis of acute stroke. *Neurology* 1987;37:221–225.
157. Anderson CS, Jamrozik KD, Broadhuest RJ, Stewart-Wynne EG. Predicting survival for one year among different subtypes of stroke. *Stroke* 1994;25:1935–1944.
158. Turney TM, Garraway WM, Whisnant JP. The natural history of hemispheric and brainstem infarction in Rochester, Minnesota. *Stroke* 1984;15:790–794.
159. Bamford J, Sandercock P, Dennis M, Burn J, Warlow C. A prospective study of acute cerebrovascular disease in the community. The Oxfordshire Community Stroke Project 1981–86. 2. Incidence, case fatality rates and overall outcome at one year of cerebral infarction, primary intracerebral and subarachnoid haemorrhage. *J Neurol Neurosurg Psychiatry* 1990;53:16–22.
160. Kaste M, Waltimo O. Prognosis of patients with middle cerebral artery occlusion. *Stroke* 1976; 7:482–485.
161. Bonita R, Ford MA, Steward AW. Predicting survival after stroke: a three-year follow-up. *Stroke* 1988;19:669–673.
162. Al Rajeh S. Stroke in the elderly aged 75 years and above. *Cerebrovasc Dis* 1994;4:402–406.
163. Silver FL, Norris JW, Lewis AJ, Hachinski VC. Early mortality following stroke: a prospective review. *Stroke* 1984;15:492–496.
164. Gresham GE, Kelly-Hayes M, Wolf PA, et al. Survival and functional status 20 or more years after first stroke: the Framingham Study. *Stroke* 1998;29:793–797.
165. Clavier I, Hommel M, Besson G, Noelle B, Perret JE. Long-term prognosis of symptomatic

lacunar infarcts. A hospital-based study. *Stroke* 1994;25:2005–2009.
166. Adunsky A, Hershkowitz M, Rabbi R, Asher-Sivron L, Ohry A. Functional recovery in young stroke patients. *Arch Phys Med Rehabil* 1992;73:859–862.
167. Ahlsio B, Britton M, Murray V, Theorell T. Disablement and quality of life after stroke. *Stroke* 1984;15:886–890.
168. von Kummer R, Holle R, Gizyska U, et al. Interobserver agreement in assessing early CT signs of middle cerebral artery infarction. *Am J Neuroradiol* 1996;17:1743–1748.
169. von Kummer R, Meyding-Lamade U, Forsting M, et al. Sensitivity and prognostic value of early CT in occlusion of the middle cerebral artery trunk. *Am J Neuroradiol* 1994;15: 9–15.
170. Bruno A, Biller J, Adams HP, Jr., et al. Acute blood glucose level and outcome from ischemic stroke. Trial of ORG 10172 in Acute Stroke Treatment (TOAST) Investigators. *Neurology* 1999;52:280–284.
171. Steiger H-J. Outcome of acute supratentorial cerebral infarction in patients under 60. *Acta Neurochir* 1991;111:73–79.

Chapter 2

EPIDEMIOLOGY OF ISCHEMIC STROKE

Although ischemic stroke can affect men and women of any age, some patient populations are at higher risk. Several conditions or factors can be used to identify these individuals. Some risk factors are modifiable, and others are not (Table 2–1.) In reality, many risk factors predispose to stroke because of their influence on the evolution of atherosclerosis. The relationships between some risk factors and ischemic stroke may not be as strong as are those for coronary artery disease because stroke can be secondary to conditions, such as trauma or infection, that are independent of traditional atherosclerotic risk factors. Some physicians consider transient ischemic attack (TIA) to be a risk factor for stroke, but it is not included in this chapter. In reality, TIA is an expression of symptomatic cerebrovascular disease and a consequence of an underlying illness, rather than a cause of stroke.

NON-MODIFIABLE RISK FACTORS

Age

Stroke can affect a person at any age. Still, advancing age is the single most important factor that predicts an increased likelihood of ischemic stroke.[1–4] Risks increase rapidly after the age of 55 in both men and women of all ethnic groups (Fig. 2–1). The risks of stroke approximately double with every 10-year increase in age. Ischemic stroke is a leading cause of acute-onset neurological impairments among persons older than 55, and stroke should be a leading consideration to explain new neurological symptoms in this population. Atherosclerosis and ischemic heart disease are the primary substrates for ischemic stroke in this age group. The formation of atherosclerotic plaques and the development of arterial stenoses

Table 2–1. **Risk Factors for Ischemic Stroke**

Non-modifiable risk factors
Advancing age
Gender (men > women)
Ethnicity (African Americans > Asian Americans, > Hispanic Americans or whites)
Social and economic status
Family history of vascular disease
Environmental factors
Leading modifiable risk factors
Arterial hypertension
Diabetes mellitus
Hyperlipidemia
Obesity
Physical inactivity
Hyperhomocystinemia
Tobacco use
Other modifiable, less common risk factors
Alcohol abuse
Drug abuse
Post-menopausal use of estrogens
Oral contraceptive use
Pregnancy and peripartum state
Migraine
Infections
Sleep apnea
Symptomatic disease in other arterial circulations
Heart disease
Coronary artery disease
Sources of embolism

increase with advancing age.[5,6] Still, the influence of well-recognized risk factors (hypertension, smoking, etc.) on the development of advanced atherosclerotic lesions is not as great in the elderly as among young persons.[5] Some of the lack of an association between the traditional atherosclerotic risk factors and stroke in older persons may be due to premature mortality from coronary artery disease in those persons with the highest risks. After the age of 75, atrial fibrillation appears to be the primary risk factor for ischemic stroke. The risk of stroke in persons older than 75 with atrial fibrillation is approximately four times that noted in younger patients. Atrial fibrillation now is recognized as the leading cause of ischemic stroke in women older than 75 (See Chapter 6). Because atrial fibrillation among persons older than 65 is usually a complication of structural heart disease, a relationship between atrial fibrillation and coronary artery disease is likely to be found.

Approximately 3%–5% of all ischemic strokes occur in children, adolescents, and young adults. Stroke is among the ten most common causes of death in childhood. The incidence of stroke is estimated to be 0.58–2.6/100,000 in children ages 1–14.[7,8] The incidence is higher in African American children; the rate is 3.1/100,000.[8] Among young women, the likelihood of stroke is greater than that of myocardial infarction. The risk of ischemic stroke in women rises from 0.6/100,000 at ages 15–19 to 16.2/100,000 at ages 40–44. Similar increases are noted among young

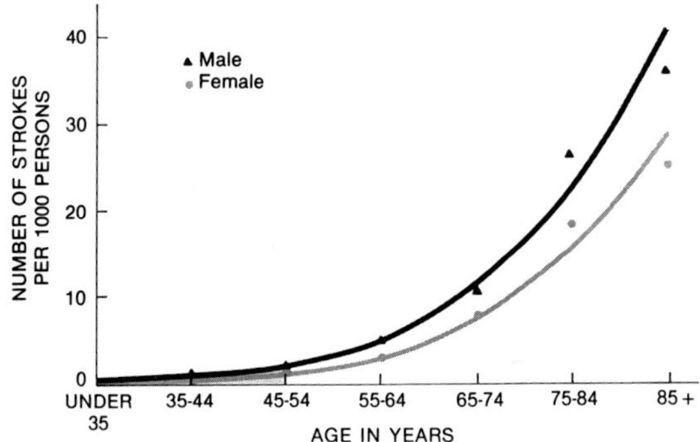

Figure 2–1. Incidence of strokes among men and women as affected by advancing age. (Reprinted from U.S. Dept. of Health, Education and Welfare, National Survey of Stroke, NIH Pub. No. 80-2069.)

men. The causes of stroke are much more diverse in younger persons.[9] Because it evolves over a person's lifetime, advanced atherosclerotic disease is uncommon in children and young adults.[10] Nonatherosclerotic vasculopathies, heart diseases, and disorders of coagulation are important causes of stroke in this population.[10] In children, disorders such as sickle cell disease, moyamoya disease, congenital heart disease, and traumatic arterial occlusions can lead to ischemic brain injury. Thus, ischemic stroke should be in the differential diagnosis for acute focal neurological impairments in children and young adults, especially if a predisposing factor is identified. See Chapter 9 for a discussion of the causes of ischemic stroke in children and young adults.

A person's age also influences prognosis. Elderly patients die more often and recover less from stroke than do persons under the age of 65.[11–16] (See Fig. 2–2.) Some of the increase in mortality and morbidity may be secondary to concomitant diseases. Other age-related physiological variables, such as stamina and plasticity of the nervous system, may also be important. Medical interventions or changes in behavior do not alter the effects of advancing age. As a result, age also influences responses to treatment. For example, carotid endarterectomy may be more dangerous in persons older than 80 years, but this same age group may benefit more because of their higher risk of having a stroke if untreated. Persons older than 75 have an increased risk of bleeding complications with acutely administered recombinant tissue plasminogen activator (rt-PA) for treatment of stroke. Persons older than 75 also have a higher risk of brain hemorrhage as a complication of long-term oral anticoagulant treatment used to prevent embolism among patients with atrial fibrillation.

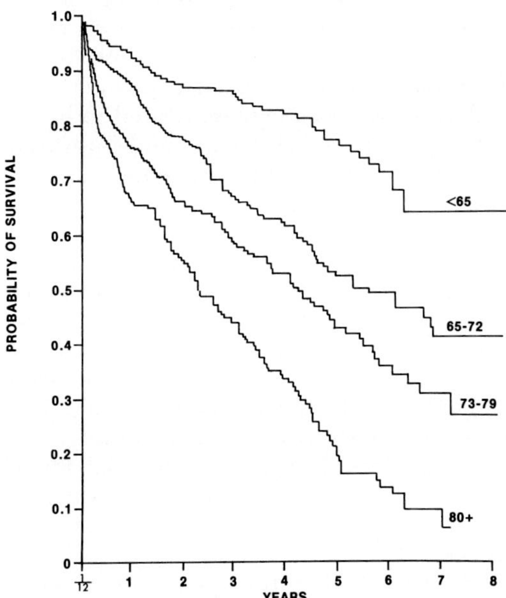

Figure 2–2. Effect of age on survival after cerebral infarction. (Reprinted from Chambers BR et al. Prognosis of acute stroke. *Neurology* 1987;37:224, with permission.)

Sex

Stroke is an important cause of death and disability in men and women of all age and ethnic groups.[17] In almost all age groups, ischemic stroke is more common in men than in women except for a slightly higher risk of stroke among women ages 15–30 because cerebrovascular events occur as a complication of pregnancy and the puerperium.[1,18] Because women generally live longer than men do and because age is such a potent risk factor for stroke, the overall incidence of stroke is higher in women. A sizeable proportion of deaths from stroke among women is in the age group of 80 or greater. Since the 1970s, the decline in frequency of and mortality from stroke has been greater in women than in men.[19] (See Fig. 2–3.) In the United States,

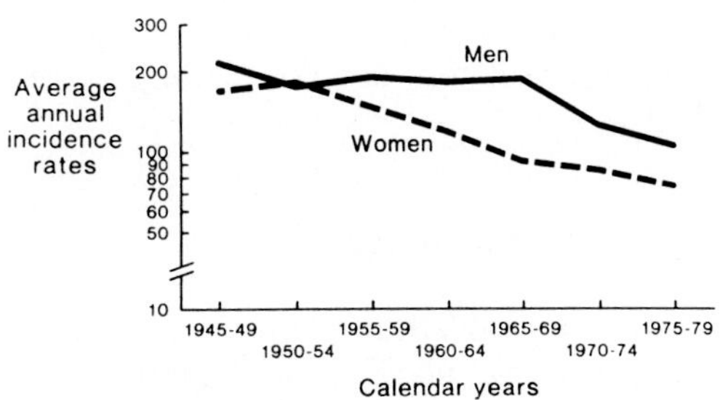

Figure 2–3. Differential decline of stroke incidence between men and women from 1945 to 1980. (Reprinted from Whisnant JP. The decline of stroke. *Stroke* 1984;15:160, with permission.)

approximately 60% of the persons who die from stroke are women but, when this statistic is adjusted for other factors, such as age and cause of stroke, no discernible differences in mortality from ischemic stroke are noted among men and women.

Although the causes of stroke generally occur at equal frequencies in both men and women, some differences are noted between the sexes. Accelerated atherosclerosis occurs at a younger age in men, and symptomatic atherosclerotic disease is seen more commonly in men than in women under the age of 50. The rates of ischemic stroke secondary to large artery atherosclerosis remain higher among men regardless of age. Because coronary artery disease becomes symptomatic at earlier ages among men, a skew showing higher rates of myocardial infarction–related cardioembolic stroke among men also may be present. Abuse of drugs and craniocerebral trauma leading to stroke also are more common among men. In addition, some rare causes of stroke, such as Fabry-Anderson disease, have an X-linked recessive inheritance. Conversely, other conditions that predispose to stroke occur more commonly in women. Ischemic stroke is a potential complication of pregnancy and the puerperium.[20] Although early studies suggested that oral contraceptives may incur an increased risk of stoke, there is no such evidence in current low-dose preparations.[21] These factors, and the potential for migraine-related brain ischemia, may be leading reasons for stroke in young women. The causes of stroke among postmenopausal women parallel those that occur in men of similar ages. In both sexes, atherosclerotic large artery or small artery disease and cardioembolism secondary to atrial fibrillation are the leading causes of stroke.

Ethnicity and Geography

Stroke affects all ethnic groups and races in the world. No geographic region of the world is protected from ischemic stroke. Although stroke occurs around the world, its incidence varies considerably among countries and ethnic groups. Rates of stroke are much higher in eastern Asia and Eastern Europe than in Western Europe, Australia, the United States, or Canada.[22–24] Epidemiological data are sketchy for estimating accurate rates in most of the Middle East, Africa, South Asia, or Latin America.[312] The likelihood is great that stroke is an important public health problem as life expectancy increases in these developing countries.[25]

The relative importance of different risk factors and causes of stroke vary with ethnicity.[26,27] The types of stroke also vary among ethnic groups; for example, lacunar infarctions are more common in Chinese than other populations.[28] An association of arterial hypertension and ischemic stroke is stronger in eastern Asian populations, where cholesterol concentrations are very low.[29] Western and Asian diets differ greatly. For example, a high-fat diet and hypercholesterolemia probably are leading risk factors for premature atherosclerosis and ischemic stroke in western cultures. The rates of smoking also vary considerably around the world. These differences likely contribute to differences in the rate of stroke, especially in younger populations.

The rates of stroke are lower in Canada and the United States than most other industrialized countries. The reasons for the lower rates have not been explained. The difference in rates may be related to better management of risk factors and improved treatment of acute ischemic stroke. Although the incidence of ischemic stroke has dropped considerably since the 1970s in the United States and Canada, similar declines have not be reported in many other countries. In fact, the rate of stroke has increased dramatically since 1970 in parts of Eastern Europe.[30] Some of the increase might be ascribed to the poor state of health care in these countries, including the absence of specialists, the non-availability of modern diagnostic equipment, and the lack of modern medications. The rates in Western Europe vary; for example, rates in Britain are higher than most other countries. Besides variances in health care, differences in risk factors (diet, smoking, alcohol abuse, etc) also may partially explain the geographic variations.

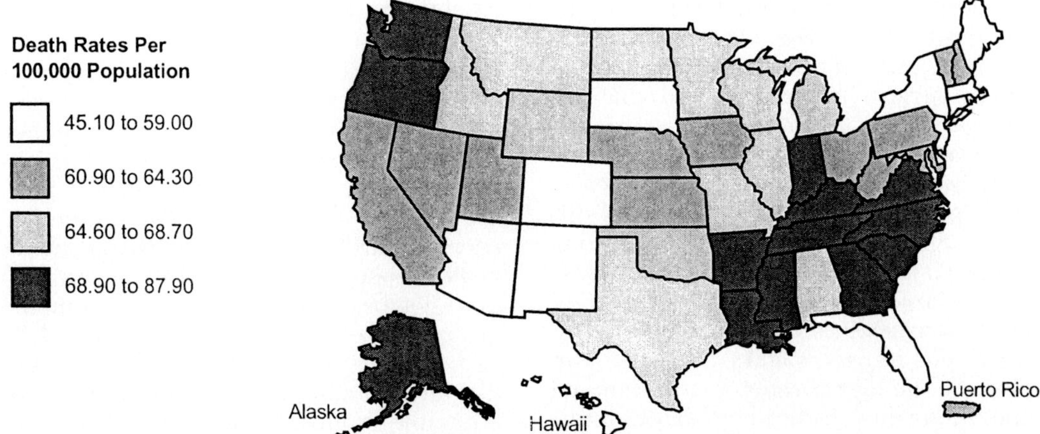

Figure 2–4. 1994–1996 stroke age-adjusted death rates (2000 standard) by state. (Reprinted from American Heart Association. *2000 Heart and Stroke Statistical Update*. Dallas, Texas, with permission.)

The incidence of stroke is considerably higher in the southeastern United States (the Stroke Belt) than in other parts of the country.[31–33] (See Fig. 2–4.) Risk factors such as hypertension, differences in diet, habits such as smoking, or migratory shifts may explain some of the geographic variations.[34] Some changes in the patterns of stroke in the southeastern United States are being reported, and the geographic region of the Stroke Belt may be shrinking or changing.[35] Some of the changes may be secondary to the movement of persons from the northern United States to the "Sun Belt." Changes in life-style and diet reflecting the age of mass communication and blending of cultures within sections of the United States also may explain the decline in the regional differences in stroke rates.

In the United States, stroke is a major public health problem among African Americans. Based on a population study in Cincinnati, Ohio, Broderick et al[36] estimated that the incidence of first or recurrent stroke in African Americans is 411/100,000; this rate is approximately twice that of white Americans. In comparison to whites, the differences are most marked in younger age groups and men. In these groups, the risk of stroke in African Americans is increased approximately two to four times.[4,37–41] African Americans also appear to have more severe strokes than whites, and their mortality rate from stroke in all age groups is almost twice as high as among whites.[38,42,43] In adults under the age of 45, the increase in stroke mortality in African Americans approaches a factor of 4.[39] Despite an overall decline in deaths from stroke, mortality from stroke in African Americans appears to be increasing.[44]

Although rates are higher in Hispanic Americans than in non-Hispanic white Americans younger than 65, the incidence of stroke is similar in the two groups in older persons.[39,41,43,45–48,313] Stroke recurrences are more frequent in African Americans and Hispanic Americans than among whites.[41] Over the age of 65, Native Americans have a slightly lower rate of stroke than whites. In younger age groups, the rates are similar.[49] Lanska[50] reported that the rates of stroke in immigrants to the United States were lower than in native-born Americans. Although the rates of stroke in persons living in Asia appear to be higher than in the United States, the frequency of stroke in Asian Americans appears not to be markedly different from the rate in non-Hispanic white Americans.

Further research is needed to understand the differences in the rates of stroke, mortality, and risk of recurrences in Americans of different ethnic groups. Some of the differences may be secondary to differences in the prevalence of important risk factors. For example, arterial hypertension and obesity are very prevalent in African Americans, and diabetes mellitus is very common in Hispanic Americans.[40,45,51] In addition, some causes of stroke are largely restricted to a specific ethnic group; for example, sickle cell disease is a leading cause of stroke among African American children.[52] In addition, issues such as access to health care, financial resources, and knowledge about stroke and its risk factors probably contribute to the higher rates of stroke among some minorities. Differences among ethic groups within a single country are not unique to the United States. Similar data have been reported in Canada.[314] In New Zealand, the rates of stroke are higher in Maori and Pacific Islanders than in persons with European ancestry.[53] Recently, Stewart et al[54] reported that the rate of stroke was higher in blacks than whites living in London, United Kingdom. The differences in rates could not be explained by other factors, including age, sex, or social class.

Sites of atherosclerosis also differ among ethnic groups. Intracranial disease is more common in persons of Asian or African heritage, and extracranial atherosclerosis is more common and more severe in persons of European heritage.[55–57] The differences in severity and locations of cerebrovascular atherosclerosis may not be on a genetic basis. Rather, differences in diet or other behavior may be important. Since World War II a radical change in diet has occurred in some parts of eastern Asia. The low-fat diet high in sodium and fish-based proteins is being replaced with meals that include more meat and animal fats. In the future, the medical community will learn whether the patterns of atherosclerosis subsequently change in Japan, Taiwan, and China.

The ethnicity of a patient remains important in the evaluation of the risk for stroke. It also is consequential in the determination of the cause of ischemic stroke and for treatment plans. As a result, research will continue to focus on the ethnic and geographic issues related to ischemic stroke.

Social and Economic Status

Persons in lower socio-economic groups have a higher risk of stroke than those who are more educated or who have higher incomes.[58] (See Table 2–2.) This issue has not received much attention in the past. The factors that lead to this difference probably are multiple. Knowledge about health-related issues and advances in care may not be prevalent in lower economic groups. Access to information may be limited. The prevalence of heart disease, obesity, and smoking is higher in lower socio-economic groups. Some of the increase in risk of stroke among African Americans may be secondary to socio-economic factors, such as a low income, non-use of medications because of financial concerns, or poor access to medical services.[59] These issues are not unique to African Americans or the United States. Similar socio-economic relationships have been reported in other countries, including those that have well-developed national health services.[60] Strategies to provide services and education to high-risk persons in lower socio-economic groups will need to be refined. Other socio-economic relationships to stroke also have been reported; for example, work-related stresses among men with jobs that have high demands and low rewards also may be associated with increased risk of stroke.[61] Some of these

Table 2–2. **Social Factors Associated With an Increased Risk of Ischemic Stroke**

- Low socio-economic class
  - Decreased health knowledge
  - Limited access to health information
  - Limited access to health care
  - Poor diet
  - Obesity
  - Alcohol and drug abuse
  - Smoking
  - High prevalence of heart disease
- Work-related stress
- Living alone
- Depression or anger

factors probably relate to the development of potent risk factors, including hypertension. Work-related stresses also may be associated with an increased likelihood of alcohol, tobacco, or drug abuse.

A person's marital status is important and, regardless of age, married persons have a lower risk of stroke than do single people.[1] Living alone also affects an individual's likelihood of reaching medical attention quickly after stroke and his or her outcomes after rehabilitation. One of the problems for elderly women is that many are widows who live alone. A reduced sense of well-being or psychiatric disease also play roles.[62] The incidence of stroke is higher among persons with depression than age-matched, non-depressed people.[1,63] People with a sense of anger have a doubled risk of stroke than persons who do not have such an anger profile.[64]

Family History of Vascular Disease

Ischemic stroke results from a number of inherited disorders of coagulation or of genetic disorders that predispose to arterial disease (see Chapters 8 and 9 and Table 2–3).[65–71] The number of genetic diseases recognized as leading to arterial or cardiac abnormalities likely will grow in the future, including genetic subtypes of several of the currently described inherited disorders that cause stroke. In addition, hereditary disorders, such as diseases of lipid metabolism, can promote premature development of atherosclerosis.[67,70,72–76] Familial predisposition to diabetes mellitus or migraine also may play a role in the development of stroke.[77] A family history of deep vein thrombosis, pulmonary embolism, or spontaneous abortions points to the possibility of a hereditary prothrombotic state.

With the high prevalence of atherosclerosis, coronary artery disease, and stroke around the world, most patients have at least one family member who has had a vascular event. Kiely et al[78] found that the relative risk for stroke increases with either a paternal or a maternal history of TIA or stroke, but the presence of symptoms in a sibling is less telling. The history of an ischemic vascular event, including stroke, in an elderly relative probably is not a potent risk factor for stroke, whereas myocardial infarction or stroke in multiple relatives may be important.[77] Ischemic events occurring before age 60 are considered premature and may portend a familial predisposition to vascular disease. Some of the familial predisposition to stroke is not due to a genetic basis but is environmental, due to diet, use of tobacco, or access to medical care.[71]

Table 2–3. **Familial Relationships: Vascular Disease and Ischemic Stroke**

Family history of vascular disease
Stroke or myocardial infarction, < age 60
Vascular death, < age 60
Vascular operations, < age 60
Deep vein thrombosis or pulmonary embolism—any age
Multiple miscarriages—female relatives
Inherited diseases
Prothrombotic diseases
Arterial diseases
Lipid metabolism diseases
Familial predisposition
Diabetes mellitus
Migraine
Common environmental factors
Diet
Socioeconomic status
Life-style
Access to health care

Environmental Factors

Epidemiological studies report a relationship between the incidence of stroke and factors as diverse as changes in the weather, time of day, day of week, or season of year.[79–88] (See Table 2–4.) In general, the rates of stroke are higher in winter than in other seasons and during colder weather than during times of more moderate temperatures. Although ischemic stroke also appears to be higher on Monday than on other days of the week, another peak of stroke among young adults occurring on

Table 2–4. **Environmental Factors Associated with An Increased Occurrence of Ischemic Stroke**

Season of the year—winter
Environmental temperature—cold weather
Day of the week—Monday
Weekends (stroke in young adults)
Time of day—at night or early morning

weekends may be 7secondary to heavy alcohol use. Ischemic stroke also appears to peak in the first hours after awakening in the morning. This rise may be secondary to changes in blood pressure or coagulation. These associations and potential responses require further clarification.[89,90]

COMMON POTENTIALLY CONTROLLABLE RISK FACTORS

Several very prevalent conditions potentiate the development of atherosclerosis. These conditions can affect almost all persons. The risk of stroke can be reduced if these factors are identified and controlled (See Table 2–1.)[3,91,92,315] Because these conditions are found in all segments of society, their treatment is crucial for an overall reduction in the incidence in stroke. Public health measures to screen and treat these risk factors can be applied to large segments of the general population. Although the impact of each of these interventions might be small for an individual patient, the overall implications for society are huge when large numbers of persons are treated. For example, vigorous control of hypertension and smoking cessation can be translated into a major reduction in the incidence of stroke. Because it is possible to detect some risk factors years before the development of symptomatic atherosclerosis, the effects of education to control risk factors will be greatest when applied to younger asymptomatic persons. Aggressive measures to control the risk factors do have an impact; for example, some of the decline in stroke in Canada and the United States is attributed to improved treatment of arterial hypertension.[92] However, one must remain cognizant of the fact that stroke will continue to be a public health problem even if these risk factors are treated successfully. Other conditions, such as advancing age, will continue to make a considerable contribution to the development of ischemic cerebrovascular disease.

The presence of multiple risk factors greatly increases the likelihood of stroke or generalized atherosclerosis.[93] Thus, all common risk factors should be sought and addressed. Control of risk factors is as important for asymptomatic patients in the general population as it is for persons with overt vascular disease. Although management after the development of ischemic symptoms focuses on medical or surgical measures to more directly prevent or treat the stroke, control of these risk factors to forestall the evolution of atherosclerosis remains a fundamental component of the overall care of these high-risk patients.

Arterial Hypertension

Arterial hypertension is the leading underlying, potentially treatable condition that promotes stroke.[94] The prevalence of hypertension has not declined since the 1970s.[3,95] In the United States, the prevalence of hypertension among African Americans (32% of the population) is higher than among whites or Hispanics.[96,97] Hypertension is calculated to be a factor in 70% of strokes and among survivors, it identifies a patient as having an increased risk of a second event[98–101] (See Fig. 2–5.) The risk of stroke increases 10–12 times if diastolic blood pressure is 105 mm Hg in comparison to a normal diastolic blood pressure of approximately 76 mm Hg.[102] Either a repeatedly measured diastolic blood pressure >95 mm Hg or a systolic blood pressure >160 mm Hg identifies a person as hypertensive. A diastolic blood pressure of 80–95 mm Hg is considered a borderline elevation. Overall, arterial hypertension increases the likelihood of stroke. The risk rises rapidly with higher levels of blood pressure.[103] The impact of an increase in diastolic blood pressure is much greater in young adults than in the

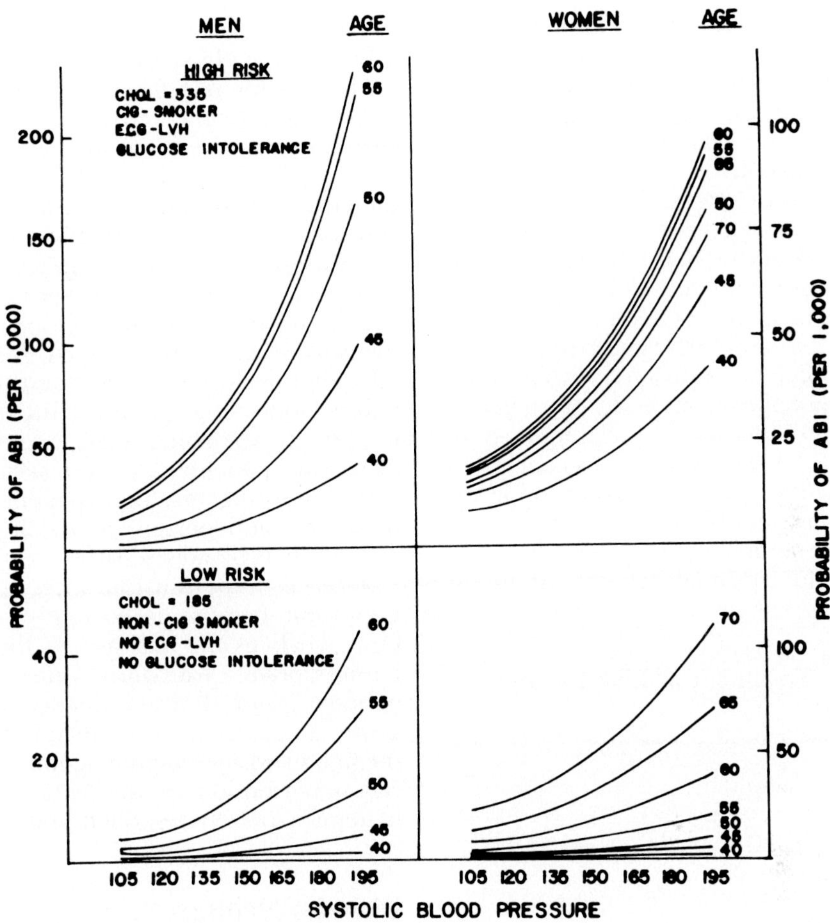

Figure 2–5. Risk of atherothrombotic brain infarction in 8 years, according to systolic blood pressure in each sex. (Framingham Study: 18-year follow up) (Reprinted from Kannel WB. Epidemiology of cerebrovascular disease. In: *Cerebral Arterial Disease*. Russell WR, ed. Edinburgh: Churchill-Lexington, 1976, with permission.)

elderly.[102,104] Although elevated diastolic blood pressure is a usual marker for hypertension, isolated systolic hypertension also predicts stroke in elderly persons.[2,16,103,105] Isolated systolic hypertension also is correlated with increased thickness and plaque formation of the internal carotid artery.[106] Both elevated diastolic and systolic blood pressures are associated with increased concentrations of hemoglobin, which is a risk factor for ischemic stroke.[107]

Chronic hypertension promotes the development of both large- and medium-caliber artery atherosclerosis and the lipohyalinosis of small penetrating arteries of the brain.[6,108] The vascular endothelium is the central focus of the effects of hypertension that promotes turbulence at the site of an atherosclerotic plaque.[109,110] Thus, hypertension can promote either major arterial occlusion and multilobar infarctions, or small artery occlusions that cause subcortical, lacunar infarctions.[111] The relationship between arterial hypertension and small vessel occlusive disease is so strong that the diagnosis of a lacunar infarction is questioned if the patient does not have a history of hypertension.[112] Because hypertension leads to coronary artery disease, cardiomyopathy, and atrial fibrillation, it is an indirect risk factor for stroke secondary to cardioembolism.

Because hypertension is asymptomatic, it is unrecognized in a sizable proportion of persons.[113] In addition, many patients with arterial hypertension are not treated adequately. Approximately 80% of Americans with hypertension are unaware of the medical problem or do not have hypertension controlled.[113] Under-treatment of arterial hypertension is an important problem; efforts to increase adherence to current guidelines to manage hypertension can greatly reduce the risk of stroke.[114] Reducing diastolic blood pressure by approximately 5 mm Hg can reduce the incidence of and mortality from stroke by 42% and 30% respectively.[115–117] In elderly patients, a drop of systolic blood pressure by approximately 11 mm Hg can lead to a 30% decline in the frequency of stroke.[116,118] A report from Asia concluded that a population-wide reduction of 3 mm Hg in diastolic blood pressure could reduce the number of strokes by one-third.[29] The optimal levels for blood pressure are 80–85 mm Hg diastolic and 130–140 mm Hg systolic.[119]

Options for treatments include changes in behavior, weight control, increased exercise, dietary modifications, and medications.[95,120–123] (See Table 2–5.) Most patients with sustained arterial hypertension require medications that are selected on a case-by-case basis. Some patients with extensive intracranial or extracranial arterial disease may need higher levels of blood pressure than usually desired to maintain adequate perfusion to the brain. Diuretics and beta-blocking agents are the usual first choices. In particular, elderly and African American patients are best treated first with diuretic agents. Many patients require multiple antihypertensive medications to control their blood pressure.

Arterial hypertension after stroke is important because it portends complications, such as an increase in the risk of hemorrhagic transformation of the ischemic lesion. It also influences decisions about acute treatment, including use of thrombolytic agents. Management of arterial hypertension in the setting of acute ischemic stroke is described in Chapter 12.

Table 2–5. **Treatment of Risk Factors for Stroke**

Arterial Hypertension
- Diet
- Anti-hypertensive medications
  - Diuretics
  - Beta-blockers
  - Alpha-1-adrenergic antagonists
  - Calcium channel blockers
  - Angiotensin converting enzyme inhibitors
  - Clonidine
  - Hydralazine
  - Methyldopa
  - Minoxidil

Diabetes Mellitus
- Diet
- Glucose-lowering medications
  - Insulin
  - Oral agents

Hyperlipidemia
- Diet
- Antilipemic medications
  - Niacin
  - Cholestyramine
  - Gemfibrozil
  - Colestipol
  - HMG-Co A reductase inhibitors (statins)

Diabetes Mellitus

Persons with either type I or type II diabetes mellitus have an increased susceptibility for large artery atherosclerosis and small artery occlusive disease.[16,94,124–127] In one large epidemiological study involving 3776 patients with type II diabetes mellitus, 99 (2.6%) patients had stroke.[128] Although glucose intolerance is accompanied by arterial disease, it may not be associated with an increased risk of stroke.[129–131] In contrast, diabetic patients often have elevated levels of triglycerides or high-density lipoproteins that persist even with control of the hyperglycemia.[132] Diabetes mellitus also leads to renal or cardiac disease, which indirectly promote arterial hypertension and stroke. Autonomic disturbances secondary to diabetic neuropathy also may play a role by causing hypotension. Diabetes also increases levels of fibrinogen; and clotting factors increase platelet aggregation, which in turn promotes arterial thrombosis.[131]

Approximately 2%–5% of strokes are attributed to diabetes mellitus, and approximately 16% of men and 30% of women with stroke also have diabetes mellitus.[101,133] When compared to non-diabetic persons, the risk of stroke doubles. The relative likelihood increases in proportion to increases in levels of blood glucose, especially in young adults.[100,104,112,134–137] A history of diabetes is associated with an approximately 11 times increase in the risk of stroke in persons ages 15–55.[138] Diabetic patients with stroke are typically younger than patients with stroke who do not have diabetes mellitus.[139] The severity of and mortality after stroke also are higher among patients with diabetes.[124,125,133,139–141] Some of the association between an elevated serum glucose levels and poor outcome might be secondary to the stress of a severe, acute stroke leading to hyperglycemia.

It is not evident that vigorous control of hyperglycemia alone is effective in lessening the risk of ischemic stroke, but the identification and management of diabetes improves a patient's overall health.[52,142] (See Table 2–5.) Any reduction in the rate of stroke may be secondary to an improvement in overall health. Although some patients can be treated for diabetes with diet and weight control, oral agents or insulin usually are needed to return the patient's blood glucose to normoglycemic levels. Adjustment of medical measures usually is needed during the course of treatment to maintain normoglycemic levels.[143] The control of blood sugar should be in concert with efforts to treat other risk factors. The presence of diabetic retinopathy can affect decisions about medications used to lower the risk of stroke in higher-risk patients. Oral anticoagulants may increase the risk of retinal hemorrhage and blindness. Antiplatelet agents, in particular ticlopidine, are often prescribed to prevent retinal ischemia.

A markedly elevated level of blood glucose can cause neurological deficits associated with alterations in consciousness. Usually focal signs are not prominent among patients with hyperglycemia. Conversely, hypoglycemia is more common than hyperglycemia in mimicking the symptoms and signs of acute ischemic stroke.[144] Prolonged periods of hypoglycemia can lead to neurological sequelae, including cognitive impairments. Thus, prompt treatment of a low serum glucose level is a critical component of urgent care in cases of suspected stroke. Treating abnormal blood glucose in the setting of acute ischemic stroke is described in Chapter 12.

Elevated Blood Lipids

In the past, the role of elevated blood lipids in the development of ischemic cerebrovascular disease was unclear largely because advancing age lessened the impact of the condition as a predisposing factor for stroke. In addition, sizeable proportions of strokes that are hemorrhagic or that are not secondary to atherosclerosis were included in the analyses.[102,145] In fact, the proper analysis is to study the relationship of hyperlipidemia to stroke secondary to atherosclerosis. This analysis could include or exclude cardioembolic strokes secondary to myocardial infarction or ischemic heart disease. The incidence of coronary artery disease and atherosclerosis of major intracranial or extracranial arteries increases with rising levels of serum cholesterol.[2,146–149] Recent data show that hypercholesterolemia is a key risk factor for ischemic stroke, especially in men under the age of 60. Hyperlipidemia causes a modest increase in risk of stroke in persons older than 62.[150] Some of the risk may be indirect, due to the potent effects of hyperlipidemia on coronary artery disease, leading to myocardial infarction and cardioembolism.

Sequential duplex ultrasound studies of the carotid arteries demonstrate that hypercholesterolemia accelerates the course of early atherosclerotic lesions (intimal-medial thickness [IMT]).[151] Although elevated lipids occur in men and women of any age, only a fraction will have familial hypercholesterolemia.[74] A family history of premature (age <60) atherosclerosis (myocardial infarction, lower extremity claudication, aortic aneurysm, or ischemic stroke) should prompt screening for elevated blood lipids even in asymptomatic persons.[152]

The data on the relationships between stroke of any type and dietary fat or hypercholesterolemia have been conflicting. For example, Gillman et al[153] noted that the risk of stroke was inversely related to the dietary consumption of fat. Several studies showed that total serum cholesterol, low-density lipoprotein (LDL) fraction, and triglycerides increase the risk of atherosclerosis.[99,145,154–157] High-density lipoprotein (HDL) fraction of cholesterol is associated with a lower risk of vascular disease, including ischemic stroke.[6,145,146,156–159] The desired levels of total cholesterol, LDL cholesterol, and HDL cholesterol are <200 mg/dL (5.20 mmol/L), <130 mg/dL (3.36 mmol/L), and >35 mg/dL (0.9 mmol/L), respectively. Wannamethee et al[316] reported that the risk of stroke is lowest among men with the highest HDL cholesterol levels. Elevated serum apolipoprotein A1 and B concentrations are found in young adults with stroke.[96,113,160] The significance of elevated apolipoproteins and stroke is uncertain. The influence of hypertriglyceridemia has not been determined on the course of atherosclerosis.

Patients with vascular events should have their lipids assessed. Unfortunately, a sizeable proportion of patients does not have their lipids checked.[161] The timing of lipid testing is important. The results of a fasting lipid profile can be affected by the cerebrovascular event, and delaying the tests until several weeks after the stroke may be prudent.

This evidence strongly supports cholesterol-lowering therapies, in particular the efficacy of the HMG-Co A reductase inhibitors (statins) in halting the progression or even promoting regression of IMT of the internal carotid artery in patients with hypercholesterolemia. More recently, data from clinical trials show the benefit of these drugs in reducing the risk of myocardial infarction and ischemic stroke.[162–169] (See Table 2–5 and Table 10–1). The benefits are especially prominent in diabetic patients.[170] The statins also may exert their benefit by direct action on the endothelium. Clofibrate use shows no benefit in preventing ischemic events, and it appears to increase the risk of stroke.[171] Identification and management of elevated lipids should begin at early ages.[91] Although low serum concentrations of total cholesterol have been correlated with an increased risk of intracranial hemorrhage, the benefit of the statins in lowering cholesterol among persons at high risk for ischemic stroke is not negated by a rise in the risk of bleeding. With treatment, very few patients likely will reach the low levels of cholesterol that are associated with intracranial hemorrhage. Treatment of high-normal serum cholesterol has been recommended as part of the management of patients with symptomatic atherosclerosis.[92,172] Although some patients can be treated solely with a low-fat diet, most affected persons will require medications.[161,168,172] (See Table 2–5.)

Obesity

Because obesity is very prevalent in North America, its impact on the public's health is great. Overweight men have approximately twice the risk of stroke than thin men.[146,173,174] Obesity increases the risk of stroke by a factor of 1.5–2.[100] However, obesity is not identified as a primary risk factor for stroke, though an elevated body weight predisposes to vascular disease via its aggravation of arterial hypertension, diabetes mellitus, and heart disease.[175] The risk from obesity appears to be separate from the risk associated with elevated serum cholesterol levels. Thus, obesity should be considered as a contributing factor for stroke. Weight reduction remains a component of general public health activities to lessen the likelihood of ischemic stroke.[91,92] Nevertheless, weight loss is difficult to achieve, and many patients will show little success in these efforts.[176]

Other Dietary Factors

A diet high in dietary fiber, potassium, vitamin C, fruits, or vegetables appears to decrease the risk of stroke.[146,177–184] The effects of caffeine on stroke risk are uncertain. Orencia et al[185] reported that a diet high in fish can lead to an overall increase in the risk of stroke. This association is not clear and may be related to a diet high in salt and low in potassium. Conversely, Keli et al[186] reported that eating fish at least once a week can reduce the incidence of ischemic stroke. A diet high in linoleic acid can reduce the risk of stroke, but high iron stores may be associated with an increased risk of atherosclerosis.[187,188] Liu et al[317] report that a diet high in whole grain foods is associated with a lower risk of ischemic stroke.

Physical Inactivity

Although physical inactivity is a well-known risk factor for coronary artery disease, its relationship to ischemic stroke is not as apparent.[175,189,190] Gillum et al[191] found the strongest relationship between a high risk of stroke and a low level of exercise among younger persons. Agnarsson et al[192] found that vigorous leisure time activity could reduce the risk of ischemic stroke by an odds ratio of 0.62. Lee et al[193] reported that vigorous exercise could lower the likelihood of stroke by reducing hypertension, glucose, cholesterol levels, and overall body weight. In addition, exercise can lower the risk of ischemic stroke in men and women by reducing platelet aggregation and increasing insulin utilization.[177] Moderate physical exercise also indirectly influences other risk factors, including diet and smoking. In general, persons are encouraged to maintain an active life-style to lessen the likelihood of a myocardial infarction and, as a consequence, the chances of a stroke.[91,189] The patient's overall health and the presence of other diseases, including musculoskeletal disorders that might limit activity, might modify such a recommendation.

Hyperhomocystinemia

Homocysteine is recognized increasingly as an important risk factor for premature vascular disease and stroke. Homocysteine is a metabolite of methionine that is methylated in the presence of the following vitamins: folate, pyridoxine, and vitamin B12.[194–202] Elevated serum levels of homocysteine are associated with an increased risk of atherosclerosis, aortic disease, ischemic heart disease, and stroke.[203–208] Eikelboom et al[318] found a strong correlation between homocysteine levels and stroke due to large artery atherosclerosis and, to a lesser extent, to small artery disease. Although increased homocysteine potentiates the course of atherosclerosis, a genetic mutation of methylene tetrahydrofolate reductase does not appear to be important in leading to vascular disease.[209] Homocysteine can lead to endothelial dysfunction, smooth muscle proliferation, changes in the extracellular matrix, and lipoprotein oxidation in the arterial wall.[210] Homocysteine appears to accelerate atherosclerosis and potentiates other risk factors, such as tobacco use or hypertension. Elevations of homocysteine are associated with arterial hypertension, an elevated uric acid level, an elevated hematocrit, and a possible hypercoagulable state.[157,203] Tobacco use, impaired renal function, diabetes mellitus, malignancy, systemic lupus erythematosus, and hypothyroidism appear to increase concentrations of homocysteine.[206] Penix[211] reported two cases of stroke among young persons with hyperhomocysteinemia secondary to a deficiency of vitamin B12. Abnormal blood levels of homocysteine are found in 5%–10% of the population.[194] Levels of homocysteine change with age and gender.[194] In all age groups, the levels of homocysteine are higher in men than in women.[198] The changes in homocysteine concentration may be particularly prominent among post-menopausal women.[212] The effects of an elevated homocysteine concentration are most pronounced in younger persons, and they are independent of the presence of other factors that predispose to atherosclerosis.[197,198,213] A Dutch study found that moderate hyperhomocysteinemia was a risk factor for ischemic stroke in children; it increased the risk of stroke in childhood by a factor of

4.4.[214] The degree of elevation is important, and the risk of stroke among persons with a homocysteine level >15.4 μmol/L is more than four times that of persons whose values are <10.3 μmol/L.[215] Another Dutch study found that the risk of vascular events increased approximately 6%–7% for every 1 μmol/L increase in homocysteine levels.[216] The Framingham Study also found an increase in stroke risk in elderly persons with elevated homocysteine levels.[217] A normal fasting level of homocysteine may not exclude the presence of this risk factor for accelerated atherosclerosis. Some patients with a normal fasting homocysteine level may have abnormal responses to a methionine challenge. The addition of a folic acid supplement to the diet lowers plasma homocysteine levels, but the usefulness of the vitamin in preventing ischemic events remains to be determined.[198,204,206,218,219,319]

Tobacco Use

Cigarette smoking is a potent risk factor for advanced atherosclerosis, myocardial infarction, and ischemic stroke.[2,6,52,94,127,175,220,221] It appears to be the primary life-style factor associated with a high risk of ischemic stroke.[222] The risk of stroke is increased by 1.9–6.1 times by smoking. Even environmental tobacco smoke may convey some risk.[99,104,137,190,223–227] Smoking is associated with an increase in the risk of intracranial or extracranial atherosclerosis.[228] Persons who smoke account for approximately 40% of patients enrolled in clinical trials testing therapies to prevent or treat stroke. This frequency is greater than the prevalence of smoking in the general population. Smoking particularly affects the frequency of ischemic stroke in younger adults.[138,154,227,229] Few non-smokers are among those under the age of 50 with strokes from extracranial large artery atherosclerosis. In the United States, the impact of smoking on an increased risk of ischemic stroke is greater in whites than in African Americans.[230]

Smoking damages the endothelium, accelerates atherosclerosis, and increases the immune response and cholesterol concentration in arterial walls and decreases endothelial function.[231–236] It also increases hemoglobin, serum fibrinogen, platelet aggregation, LDL cholesterol, and the hematocrit as it decreases HDL cholesterol levels.[100,107,232,237] Smoking promotes the progression of atherosclerotic plaques of the carotid artery. Similar findings are noted in studying the coronary arteries and the thoracic aorta.[220,238] Smoking can lead to stroke by aggravating coronary artery disease.[225] Advanced intracranial occlusive disease, causing moyamoya syndrome, also has been associated with smoking, particularly in young women using oral contraceptives.[239] A dosage effect is present; the longer and greater the use of cigarettes, the higher the likelihood for stroke.[224,230,234,235,238,240] Although cigarette smoking is most commonly implicated, the use of cigars, pipes, or chewing tobacco also probably increases the risk of atherosclerosis.[221] Chewing tobacco also can be a risk factor for stroke. The salt-cured product can induce hypertension, and some tobacco juice is inevitably swallowed. Passive exposure to smoke also appears to be a risk factor for stroke. Recently, You et al[241] found that spouses of smokers had twice the likelihood of stroke than persons whose spouses did not smoke. This secondary effect increases the importance of measures to control smoking in public places.

Halting the use of tobacco is a very effective strategy to reduce the incidence of stroke.[117] Adolescents and young adults should be encouraged not to start smoking or to stop smoking.[91] Within 2–5 years of halting tobacco consumption, a smoker's risk declines to that of a non-smoker.[224,235] Smoking cessation is difficult, and patients need assistance in stopping this addictive habit. A number of strategies, including medications and educational programs, are available.[176,242]

Alcohol Use

Mild-to-moderate alcohol consumption lessens the risk of ischemic heart disease and stroke, possibly by increasing the concentration of HDL cholesterol.[177,243–249,320] The definition of *mild-to-moderate consumption* of alcohol is amorphous but probably is less than 100 gm/week. One drink a week is sufficient to lower the likelihood of ischemic stroke.[250] Modest alcohol consumption appears beneficial regardless of the person's age, sex, or race.[247] The reduction correlates better with consumption of wine than with the use of either spirits or beer.[251]

Although modest alcohol consumption appears to be helpful in lowering the risk of stroke, other health problems associated with alcohol should prompt caution about using alcohol as a stroke-prevention strategy. Drinking a glass of wine is not an antidote to other dietary indiscretions. Alcohol abuse and acute alcohol intoxication can lead to ischemic stroke due to alcohol-induced cardiomyopathy, changes in viscosity, and disturbances in coagulation and fibrinolytic factors.[136,252–254] Bouts of heavy alcohol consumption on weekends and holidays are associated with a high risk of stroke, especially in young persons.[138,255–257] Young adults and adolescents should be warned about the increased likelihood of stroke that can occur with heavy alcohol consumption.[91] The impact of alcohol consumption on the frequency of stroke among young adults is discussed in Chapter 9.

Drug Abuse

The role of drug abuse in the etiology of stroke needs additional definition. Some of the perceived or real increase of stroke in young adults might be secondary to drug abuse. Abuse of drugs, in particular cocaine and stimulants, can cause stroke.[258–261] Persons abusing parenterally administered drugs also have a risk for infective endocarditis that leads to embolism to the brain. Drug abuse is most commonly implicated in stroke in young adults. However, the finding of recent drug abuse does not automatically lead to the diagnosis of a drug abuse–related stroke. Patients who abuse drugs may have other causes for stroke, and the illegal substances may be contributing factors (see Chapter 9).

Post-menopausal Use of Estrogens

Information is limited about the influence of the use of estrogens or estrogen/progesterone medications on the rate of ischemic stroke in post-menopausal women. In general, the data available suggest that women might lower their risk of both myocardial infarction and ischemic stroke by using post-menopausal estrogens.[262–264] This opinion is supported by clinical data that show that estrogens may slow the progression of atherosclerosis and lower cholesterol levels.[157] However, Fung et al[265] concluded that there is no evidence that hormonal replacement therapy can prevent ischemic stroke. Considerable additional research is needed to determine how post-menopausal estrogens affect the course of vascular disease. At present, the evidence suggests that post-menopausal estrogen supplementation may be helpful. Conversely, there is no evidence that post-menopausal use of estrogens increases the likelihood of ischemic stroke.

Oral Contraceptives

Shortly after the introduction of oral contraceptives, epidemiological studies noted that these medications increased the risk of stroke in young women. Because the occurrence of stroke in young women is still relatively rare, oral contraceptives often are implicated when an ischemic event occurs. This cause-and-effect association may not be valid. Some young women using oral contraceptives may have an increased risk for stroke. The risks seem to be lower in younger women (under age 35) and in those who do not smoke or have hypertension.[266,267] The relative risk of stroke as influenced by the generation of oral contraceptive medications has not been determined.[268,269] Use of oral contraceptives has been associated with advanced intracranial occlusive disease (moyamoya syndrome).[239] Recent studies have suggested that oral contraceptives may be a contributing factor for stroke but that their impact may be marginal.[21,266,270,271] At present, there is no evidence that oral contraceptive use is a major risk factor for stroke in young women; however, there is a clearly increased risk of cerebral venous thrombosis among users of oral contraceptives who also are carriers of a prothrombin gene mutation.[272] The issue of risk of stroke with oral contraceptive use should be examined in the light of the potential risk for stroke during and following pregnancy. The importance of oral contraceptives as a cause of stroke in young women is discussed in Chapter 9.

Migraine

Both migraine and ischemic stroke are common neurological illnesses. In the United States, approximately 10%–20% of women and about 5%–10% of men have a history of migraine headaches. Thus, stroke in a patient with a history of migraine should not be surprising. Migraine is associated with an increase in the risk of stroke, especially if the migraine is associated with an aura.[273,274] Migraine may be a contributing factor to the increase in stroke risk associated with the use of oral contraceptives or smoking.[273] Migraine is most commonly implicated as a cause of stroke in young adults.[229,270,275] Still, a "migrainous" stroke often is due to another vascular illness, especially arterial dissection.[276] In general, migraine appears to be a minor risk factor for stroke. Its contributions to the incidence of stroke seem to be modest. The interactions between migraine and stroke are discussed in more detail in Chapter 9.

OTHER RISK FACTORS

Infections

The role of infection in the course of atherosclerosis and stroke is evolving. In the past, the primary relationship between infection and stroke was assumed to be on the basis of a vasculitis secondary to an infectious illness or embolism secondary to infective endocarditis. The relationships between acute or subacute infections and stroke may be more complex. Grau et al[277] reported an increased risk of ischemic stroke in persons who had recurrent dental or otolaryngologic infections. This association needs additional study. Recent dental or otolaryngologic infection also could trigger dissection of a cervical artery.[278] However, the periodontal disease and recurrent infections could be a marker for poor health. The relationship between infection and stroke is not due to changes in levels of activity of coagulation factors.[279] Other infections, including Lyme disease, also may initiate stroke.[280]

New evidence suggests that subacute or recurrent infections affect the development and evolution of atherosclerosis and, by implication, the occurrence of stroke.[281] The early stages of atherosclerosis often involve an inflammatory process, and the presence of an infection could influence the initial development of an atherosclerotic plaque. Recent information has suggested that infection by *Chlamydia pneumoniae* can stimulate the evolution of atherosclerosis.[282–285] Markus and Mendall[286] concluded that infection with *Helicobacter pylori* also portends an increased risk of carotid atherosclerosis. Stroke also has been associated with a history of human immunodeficiency virus infection.[287] In contrast, elevations of titers of herpes simplex virus and cytomegalovirus are not associated with an increase in the risk of stroke.[288] These relationships need clarification, but a potential cause-and-effect association suggests that the infection prompts arteriopathic changes or stimulates an acute stroke. In the future, studies likely will evaluate the utility of antibiotics in forestalling the course of atherosclerosis.[289]

Snoring, Sleep Apnea, and Pulmonary Disease

A sizeable proportion of strokes occurs during sleep.[89] (See Table 2–1.) Palomaki[290] pointed out the relationship between excessive snoring and sleep apnea, and stroke in men. The calculated relative risk was approximately 2. The risk of stroke was correlated with the severity of snoring and the relative risk was estimated to be as high as 10 among persons with habitual snoring.[291] Stroke in persons with sleep apnea and snoring may be secondary to hypoxia and hemodynamic changes.[292–295] Sleep disorders also are more common after stroke.[292,293,296] Persons with poor pulmonary function also have a modest increase in the risk of stroke.[297] Information is needed about the usefulness of treating sleep apnea and pulmonary disease to reduce the chances of stroke.

SYMPTOMATIC DISEASE IN OTHER ARTERIAL TERRITORIES

Persons with symptomatic atherosclerotic disease in other vascular territories are at high risk for ischemic stroke (Table 2–6). Although atherosclerosis involves arteries throughout the body, its course can vary among vascular beds. Coronary artery atherosclerosis usually becomes symptomatic at a younger age than extracranial carotid artery atherosclerosis; the incidence of myocardial infarction among men ages 55–65 is higher that the rate of ischemic stroke in the same group. Thus, a history of angina pectoris, myocardial infarction, coronary artery angioplasty, or coronary artery bypass grafting marks a patient as being at high risk for stroke.[127] Similarly, patients who have intermittent claudication, peripheral vascular reconstructive operations, or abdominal aortic aneurysm also have an increased risk of ischemic stroke secondary to intracranial or extracranial atherosclerosis. In particular, advanced atherosclerosis of the lower extremities is strongly associated with severe carotid artery disease.[298,299] Alexandrova et al[300] found greater than 60% stenoses of the extracranial internal carotid artery in approximately 20% of patients with symptomatic peripheral vascular disease. The presence of symptomatic atherosclerosis elsewhere in the body is an important sign that points toward atherosclerosis as a cause of stroke. Conversely, patients with ischemic stroke secondary to atherosclerosis also have a high risk for advanced atherosclerosis in other circulations, including the presence of abdominal aortic aneurysms.[301]

Table 2–6. **Symptomatic Atherosclerosis**

Coronary artery disease
Myocardial infarction
Angina pectoris
Coronary artery angioplasty
Coronary artery bypass grafting
Peripheral vascular disease
Intermittent claudication
Digital ischemia
Arterial angioplasty
Arterial reconstruction operation
Abdominal aortic aneurysm
Bowel ischemia
Renal artery stenosis

HEART DISEASE

There is a strong interaction between cardiovascular and cerebrovascular diseases. Symptomatic coronary artery disease immediately identifies a person as being at high risk for stroke.[52,101,229,302–306] (See Fig. 2–6.) It also affects survival after stroke. A stroke also denotes a person who has a high risk for myocardial infarction or cardiac death. The rate of stroke in persons with a history of ischemic heart disease, congestive heart failure, or left ventricular hypertrophy is approximately two to four times that reported in persons without cardiac symptoms.[136,137,307,308] Although atherosclerotic heart disease earmarks a patient as being at high risk for cerebrovascular atherosclerosis, a large number of cardiac diseases can lead to embolism to the brain.[136,137] A sizeable proportion of ischemic strokes will be secondary to cardiogenic embolism.[309] Atrial fibrillation is the premier cardiac condition associated with embolism to the brain.[308,310] In many circumstances, the arrhythmia complicates a structural heart lesion.[311] Among persons older than 80,

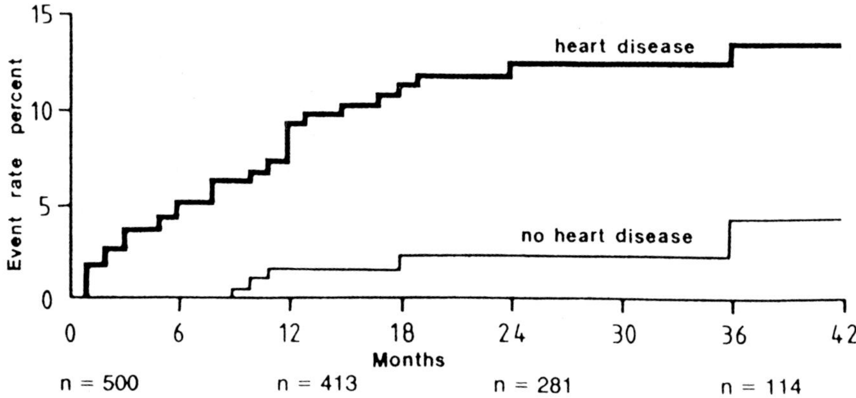

Figure 2–6. Incidence of cerebral ischemic events among persons with an asymptomatic cervical bruit as influenced by a history of heart disease. Patients with a history of heart disease had a significantly higher risk of stroke or transient ischemic attack than those without such a history ($p < 0.0005$). (Reprinted from Chambers B, Norris J. Outcome in patients with asymptomatic neck bruits. *N Engl J Med* 1986;315:860–865, with permission of publisher.)

atrial fibrillation is the main cardiac condition that is associated with stroke.[311] Cardioembolic stroke is described in more detail in Chapter 6.

SUMMARY

Everyone's risk for stroke is not alike. Advancing age, male gender, non-Caucasian origins, lower socio-economic status, and a family history of vascular disease increase this risk. Although these factors cannot be changed, there are also potentially modifiable risk factors, such as arterial hypertension, elevated lipids, physical inactivity, hyperhomocystinemia, and tobacco use. In addition, a diet rich in fruits and vegetables, modest-to-moderate alcohol intake, and estrogen replacement appear to play a protective role.

Atherosclerosis often affects simultaneously the coronary, cervical, and cerebral vessels, putting stroke patients at risk for heart attacks and patients with heart attacks at risk for stroke. The heart itself can be the source of mischief. Akinetic myocardial segments and valvular heart disease represent recognized causes of cerebral embolism. Atria fibrillation represents a particular problem because of its steeply climbing prevalence with increasing age. It fosters clots, which then can be hurled at the brain by the irregular contractions of the fibrillating heart.

REFERENCES

1. Simons LA, McCallum J, Friedlander Y, Simons J. Risk factors for ischemic stroke: Dubbo Study of the Elderly. *Stroke* 1998;29:1341–1346.
2. Fine-Edelstein JS, Wolf PA, O'Leary DH, et al. Precursors of extracranial carotid atherosclerosis in the Framingham Study. *Neurology* 1994;44:1046–1050.
3. Gorelick PB. Stroke prevention. *Arch Neurol* 1995;52:347–355.
4. Rosamond WD, Folsom AR, Chambless L, et al. Stroke incidence and survival among middle-aged adults. *Stroke* 1999;30:736–743.
5. Fabris F, Zanocchi M, Bo M, et al. Carotid plaque, aging, and risk factors. A study of 457 subjects. *Stroke* 1994;25:1133–1140.
6. Prati P, Vanuzzo D, Casaroli M, et al. Prevalence and determinants of carotid atherosclerosis in a general population. *Stroke* 1992;23:1705–1711.
7. Earley CJ, Kittner SJ, Feeser BR, et al. Stroke in children and sickle-cell disease: Baltimore-Washington Cooperative Young Stroke Study. *Neurology* 1998;51:169–176.
8. Broderick J, Talbot GT, Prenger E, Leach A, Brott T. Stroke in children within a major metropolitan area: the surprising importance of intracerebral hemorrhage. *J Child Neurol* 1993; 8:250–255.
9. Ganesan V, McShane MA, Liesner R, Cookson J, Hann I, Kirkham FJ. Inherited prothrombotic states and ischaemic stroke in childhood. *J Neurol Neurosurg Psychiatry* 1998;65:508–511.
10. Giovannoni G, Fritz VU. Transient ischemic attacks in younger and older patients. A comparative study of 798 patients in South Africa. *Stroke* 1993;24:947–953.
11. Al Rajeh S. Stroke in the elderly aged 75 years and above. *Cerebrovasc Dis* 1994;4:402–406.
12. Evans BA, Sicks JD, Whisnant JP. Factors affecting survival and occurrence of stroke in patients

with transient ischemic attacks. *Mayo Clin Proc* 1994;69:416–421.
13. Mayo NE, Neville D, Kirkland S, et al. Hospitalization and case-fatality rates for stroke in Canada from 1982 through 1991. The Canadian Collaborative Study Group of Stroke Hospitalizations. *Stroke* 1996;27:1215–1220.
14. Henon H, Godefroy O, Leys D, et al. Early predictors of death and disability after acute cerebral ischemic event. *Stroke* 1995;26:392–398.
15. Kalra L. Does age affect benefits of stroke unit rehabilitation? *Stroke* 1994;25:346–351.
16. Tanne D, Yaari S, Goldbourt U. Risk profile and prediction of long-term ischemic stroke mortality: a 21-year follow-up in the Israeli Ischemic Heart Disease (IIHD) Project. *Circulation* 1998;98: 1365–1371.
17. Hershey LA. Gender differences in cerebrovascular disease. *Neurology* 1993;3:1–4.
18. Wiebers DO. Ischemic cerebrovascular complications of pregnancy. *Arch Neurol* 1985; 42: 1106–1113.
19. Falkeborn M, Persson I, Terent A, Bergstrom R, Lithell H, Naessen T. Long-term trends in incidence of and mortality from acute myocardial infarction and stroke in women: analyses of total first events and of deaths in the Uppsala Health Care Region, Sweden. *Epidemiology* 1996; 7:67–74.
20. Kittner SJ, Stern BJ, Feeser BR, et al. Pregnancy and the risk of stroke. *N Engl J Med* 1996; 335:768–774.
21. Schwartz SM, Petitti DB, Siscovick DS, et al. Stroke and use of low-dose oral contraceptives in young women: a pooled analysis of two US studies. *Stroke* 1998;29:2277–2284.
22. Bonita R, Anderson CS, Broad JB, Jamrozik KD, Stewart-Wynne EG, Anderson NE. Stroke incidence and case fatality in Australasia. A comparison of the Auckland and Perth population-based stroke registers. *Stroke* 1994;25:552–557.
23. Cheng XM, Ziegler DK, Lai YH, et al. Stroke in China, 1986 through 1990. *Stroke* 1995; 26:1990–1994.
24. Feigin VL, Wiebers DO, Nikitin YP, O'Fallon WM, Whisnant JP. Risk factors for ischemic stroke in a Russian community: a population-based case-control study. *Stroke* 1998;29:34–39.
25. Poungvarin N. Stroke in the developing world. *Lancet* 1998;352 (Suppl 3):SIII19–SIII22.
26. Huang CY, Chan FL, Yu YL, Woo E, Chin D. Cerebrovascular disease in Hong Kong Chinese. *Stroke* 1990;21:230–235.
27. Jeng JS, Chung MY, Yip PK, Hwang BS, Chang YC. Extracranial carotid atherosclerosis and vascular risk factors in different types of ischemic stroke in Taiwan. *Stroke* 1994; 25:1989–1993.
28. Yip PK, Jeng JS, Lee TK, et al. Subtypes of ischemic stroke. A hospital-based stroke registry in Taiwan (SCAN-IV). *Stroke* 1997; 28:2507–2512.
29. Eastern Stroke and Coronary Heart Disease Collaborative Research Group. Blood pressure, cholesterol, and stroke in eastern Asia. *Lancet* 1998;352:1801–1807.
30. Asplund K. Stroke in Europe. Widening gap between East and West. *Cerebrovasc Dis* 1996; 6:3–6.
31. Casper ML, Wing S, Anda RF, Knowles M, Pollard RA. The shifting stroke belt. Changes in the geographic pattern of stroke mortality in the United States, 1962 to 1988. *Stroke* 1995; 26:755–760.
32. Howard G, Evans GW, Pearce K, et al. Is the stroke belt disappearing? An analysis of racial, temporal, and age effects. *Stroke* 1995; 26:1153–1158.
33. Lanska DJ, Peterson PM. Geographic variation in reporting of stroke deaths to underlying or contributing causes in the United States. *Stroke* 1995;26:1999–2003.
34. Lanska DJ, Kuller LH. The geography of stroke mortality in the United States and the concept of a stroke belt. *Stroke* 1995;26:1145–1149.
35. Lanska DJ, Peterson PM. Geographic variation in the decline of stroke mortality in the United States. *Stroke* 1995;26:1159–1165.
36. Broderick J, Brott T, Kothari R, et al. The Greater Cincinnati/Northern Kentucky Stroke Study: preliminary first-ever and total incidence rates of stroke among blacks. *Stroke* 1998; 29:415–421.
37. Kittner SJ, McCarter RJ, Sherwin RW, et al. Black-white differences in stroke risk among young adults. *Stroke* 1993;24 (Suppl):I13–I15.
38. Gorelick PB. Cerebrovascular disease in African Americans. *Stroke* 1998;29:2656–2664.
39. Morgenstern LB, Spears WD, Goff DCJ, Grotta JC, Nichaman MZ. African Americans and women have the highest stroke mortality in Texas. *Stroke* 1997;28:15–18.
40. Giles WH, Kittner SJ, Hebel JR, Losonczy KG, Sherwin RW. Determinants of black-white differences in the risk of cerebral infarction. The National Health and Nutrition Examination Survey Epidemiologic Follow-up Study. *Arch Intern Med* 1995;155:1319–1324.
41. Sheinart KF, Tuhrim S, Horowitz DR, et al. Stroke recurrence is more frequent in Blacks and Hispanics. *Neuroepidemiology* 1998; 17:188–198.
42. Kuhlemeier KV, Stiens SA. Racial disparities in severity of cerebrovascular events. *Stroke* 1994; 25:2126–2131.
43. Howard G, Anderson R, Sorlie P, Andrews V, Backlund E, Burke GL. Ethnic differences in stroke mortality between non-Hispanic whites, Hispanic whites, and blacks. The National Longitudinal Mortality Study. *Stroke* 1994; 25:2120–2125.
44. Gillum RF. Stroke mortality in blacks. Disturbing trends. *Stroke* 1999;30:1711–1715.
45. Sacco RL, Kargman DE, Zamanillo MC. Race-ethnic differences in stroke risk factors among hospitalized patients with cerebral infarction: the Northern Manhattan Stroke Study. *Neurology* 1995;45:659–663.
46. Worley KL, Lalonde DR, Kerr DR, Benavente O, Hart RG. Survey of the causes of stroke among Mexican Americans in South Texas. *Tex Med* 1998;94:62–67.

47. Gillum RF. Epidemiology of stroke in Hispanic Americans. *Stroke* 1995;26:1707–1712.
48. Kattapong VJ, Longstreth WT, Jr., Kukull WA, et al. Stroke risk factor knowledge in Hispanic and non-Hispanic white women in New Mexico: implications for targeted prevention strategies. *Health Care for Women International* 1998; 19:313–325.
49. Gillum RF. The epidemiology of stroke in Native Americans. *Stroke* 1995;26:514–521.
50. Lanska DJ. Geographic distribution of stroke mortality among immigrants to the United States. *Stroke* 1997;28:53–57.
51. Qureshi AI, Safdar K, Patel M, Janssen RS, Frankel MR. Stroke in young black patients. Risk factors, subtypes, and prognosis. *Stroke* 1995;26:1995–1998.
52. Wolf PA. Prevention of stroke. *Lancet* 1998;352 (Suppl 3):SIII15–SIII18.
53. Bonita R, Broad JB, Beaglehole R. Ethnic differences in stroke incidence and case fatality in Auckland, New Zealand. *Stroke* 1997; 28:758–761.
54. Stewart JA, Dundas R, Howard RS, Rudd AG, Wolfe CD. Ethnic differences in incidence of stroke: prospective study with stroke register. *BMJ* 1999;318:967–971.
55. Wityk RJ, Lehman D, Klag M, Coresh J, Ahn H, Litt B. Race and sex differences in the distribution of cerebral atherosclerosis. *Stroke* 1996; 27:1974–1980.
56. Bogousslavsky J, Barnett HJM, Fox AJ, Hachinski VC, Taylor W. Atherosclerotic disease of the middle cerebral artery. *Stroke* 1986; 17:1112–1120.
57. Feldmann E, Daneault N, Kwan E, et al. Chinese-white differences in the distribution of occlusive cerebrovascular disease. *Neurology* 1990;40:1541–1545.
58. Lynch J, Kaplan GA, Salonen R, Cohen RD, Salonen JT. Socioeconomic status and carotid atherosclerosis. *Circulation* 1995;92:1786–1792.
59. Howard G, Russell GB, Anderson R, et al. Role of social class in excess black stroke mortality. *Stroke* 1995;26:1759–1763.
60. van Rossum CTM, van de Mheen H, Breteler MMB, Grobbee DE, Mackenbach JP. Socioeconomic differences in stroke among Dutch elderly women. The Rotterdam Study. *Stroke* 1999;30:357–362.
61. Lynch J, Krause N, Kaplan GA, Salonen R, Salonen JT. Workplace demands, economic reward, and progression of carotid atherosclerosis. *Circulation* 1997;96:302–307.
62. Agewall S, Wikstrand J, Fagerberg B. Stroke was predicted by dimensions of quality of life in treated hypertensive men. *Stroke* 1998;29:2329–2333.
63. Everson SA, Roberts RE, Goldberg DE, Kaplan GA. Depressive symptoms and increased risk of stroke mortality over a 29-year period. *Arch Intern Med* 1998;158:1133–1138.
64. Everson SA, Kaplan GA, Goldberg DE, Lakka TA, Sivenius J, Salonen JT. Anger expression and incident Stroke. *Stroke* 1999;30:523–528.
65. Martin JB. Molecular genetics in neurology. *Ann Neurol* 1993;34:757–773.
66. Pfohl M, Fetter M, Koch M, Barth CM, Rudiger W, Haring HU. Association between angiotensin I-converting enzyme genotypes, extracranial artery stenosis, and stroke. *Atherosclerosis* 1998; 140:161–166.
67. Graffagnino C, Gasecki AP, Doig GS, Hachinski VC. The importance of family history in cerebrovascular disease. *Stroke* 1994;25:1599–1604.
68. Joutel A, Corpechot C, Ducros A, et al. Notch3 mutations in CADASIL, a hereditary adult-onset condition causing stroke and dementia. *Nature* 1996;383:707–710.
69. Natowicz M, Kelley RI. Mendelian etiologies of stroke. Ann Neurol 1987;22:175–192.
70. Rastenyte D, Tuomilehto J, Sarti C. Genetics of stroke—a review. *J Neurol Sci* 1998;153:132–145.
71. Kubota M, Yamaura A, Ono J, et al. Is family history an independent risk factor for stroke? *J Neurol Neurosurg Psychiatry* 1997;62:66–70.
72. Goldbourt U, Neufeld HN. Genetic aspects of arteriosclerosis. *Arteriosclerosis* 1986;6:357–377.
73. Couderc R, Mahieux F, Bailleul S, Fenelon G, Mary R, Fermanian J. Prevalence of apolipoprotein E phenotypes in ischemic cerebrovascular disease. A case-control study. *Stroke* 1993; 24:661–664.
74. Rubba P, Mercuri M, Faccenda F, et al. Premature carotid atherosclerosis: does it occur in both familial hypercholesterolemia and homocystinuria? Ultrasound assessment of arterial intima-media thickness and blood flow velocity. *Stroke* 1994;25:943–950.
75. McCarron MO, Delong D, Alberts MA. APOE genotype as a risk factor for ischemic cerebrovascular disease. A meta-analysis. *Neurology* 1999;53:1308–1311.
76. McCarron MO, Muir KW, Weir CJ, et al. The apolipoprotein E epsilon4 allele and outcome in cerebrovascular disease. *Stroke* 1998; 29:1882–1887.
77. Wannamethee SG, Shaper AG, Ebrahim S. History of parental death from stroke or heart trouble and the risk of stroke in middle-aged men. *Stroke* 1996;27:1492–1498.
78. Kiely DK, Wolf PA, Cupples LA, Beiser AS, Myers RH. Familial aggregation of stroke. The Framingham Study. *Stroke* 1993;24:1366–1371.
79. Korpelainen JT, Sotaniemi KA, Huikuri HV, Myllyla VV. Circadian rhythm of heart rate variability is reversibly abolished in ischemic Stroke. *Stroke* 1997;28:2150–2154.
80. Kelly-Hayes M, Wolf PA, Kase CS, Brand FN, McGuirk JM, D'Agostino RB. Temporal patterns of stroke onset. The Framingham Study. *Stroke* 1995;26:1343–1347.
81. Heyman A, Wilkinson WE, Hurwitz BJ, et al. Risk of ischemic heart disease in patients with TIA. *Neurology* 1984;34:626–630.
82. Schievink WI, Wijdicks EF, Kuiper JD. Seasonal pattern of spontaneous cervical artery dissection. *J Neurosurg* 1998;89:101–103.
83. Biller J, Jones MP, Bruno A, Adams HP, Jr., Banwart K. Seasonal variation of stroke—does it exist? *Neuroepidemiology* 1988;7:89–98.
84. Rothwell PM, Wroe SJ, Slattery J, Warlow CP. Is stroke incidence related to season or

temperature? The Oxfordshire Community Stroke Project. *Lancet* 1996;347:934–936.
85. Chaturvedi S, Adams HP, Jr., Woolson RF. Circadian variation in ischemic stroke subtypes. *Stroke* 1999;30:1972–1975.
86. Lanska DJ, Hoffmann RG. Seasonal variation in stroke mortality rates. *Neurology* 1999;52: 984–990.
87. Marler JR, Price TR, Clark GL, et al. Morning increase in onset of ischemic stroke. *Stroke* 1989; 20:473–476.
88. Marsh EE, Biller J, Adams HP, Jr., et al. Circadian variation in onset of acute ischemic stroke. *Arch Neurol* 1990;47:1178–1180.
89. Wroe SJ, Sandercock P, Bamford J, Dennis M, Slattery J, Warlow C. Diurnal variation in incidence of stroke: Oxfordshire community stroke project. *BMJ* 1992;304:155–157.
90. Smits MG, van den Berg JS, van Dijken A, Algra A, Otten H, van Gijn J. Type of weather and cerebral ischemic events: a relationship in moderate climates? *Cerebrovasc Dis* 1994;4:373–374.
91. Gorelick PB. Stroke prevention: windows of opportunity and failed expectations? A discussion of modifiable cardiovascular risk factors and a prevention proposal. *Neuroepidemiology* 1997; 16:163–173.
92. Gorelick PB, Sacco RL, Smith DB, et al. Prevention of a first stroke: a review of guidelines and a multidisciplinary consensus statement from the National Stroke Association. *JAMA* 1999;281:1112–1120.
93. Wolf PA, D'Agostino RB, Belanger AJ, Kannel WB. Probability of stroke: a risk profile from the Framingham Study. *Stroke* 1991;22:312–318.
94. Sacco RL. Risk factors and outcomes for ischemic stroke. *Neurology* 1995;45:S10–S14.
95. Kannel WB. Blood pressure as a cardiovascular risk factor: prevention and treatment. *JAMA* 1996;275:1571–1576.
96. Christopher R, Kailasanatha KM, Nagaraja D, Tripathi M. Case-control study of serum lipoprotein(a) and apolipoproteins A-I and B in stroke in the young. *Acta Neurol Scand* 1996;94: 127–130.
97. Burt VL, Whelton P, Roccella EJ, et al. Prevalence of hypertension in the U.S. adult population. *Hypertension* 1995;25:305–313.
98. Alter M, Friday G, Lai SM, O'Connell JB, Sobel E. Hypertension and risk of stroke recurrence. *Stroke* 1994;25:1605–1610.
99. Wilson PW, Hoeg JM, D'Agostino RB, et al. Cumulative effects of high cholesterol levels, high blood pressure, and cigarette smoking on carotid stenosis. *N Engl J Med* 1997;337: 516–522.
100. Bronner LL, Kanter DS, Manson JE. Primary prevention of stroke. *N Engl J Med* 1995; 333:1392–1400.
101. Bornstein NM, Aronovich BD, Karepov VG, et al. The Tel Aviv stroke registry: 3600 consecutive cases. *Stroke* 1996;27:1770–1773.
102. Prospective studies collaboration. Cholesterol, diastolic blood pressure, and stroke: 13,000 strokes in 450,000 people in 45 prospective cohorts. *Lancet* 1995;346:1647–1653.
103. Lindenstrom E, Boysen G, Nyboe J. Influence of systolic and diastolic blood pressure on stroke risk: a prospective observational study. Am J *Epidemiol* 1995;142:1279–1290.
104. Papademetriou V, Narayan P, Rubins H, Collins D, Robins S. Influence of risk factors on peripheral and cerebrovascular disease in men with coronary artery disease, low high-density lipoprotein cholesterol levels, and desirable low-density lipoprotein cholesterol levels. HIT Investigators. Department of Veterans Affairs HDL Intervention Trial. *Am Heart J* 1998; 136:734–740.
105. Davis BR, Vogt T, Frost PH, et al. Risk factors for stroke and type of stroke in persons with isolated systolic hypertension. Systolic Hypertension in the Elderly Program Cooperative Research Group. *Stroke* 1998; 29:1333–1340.
106. Bots ML, Hofman A, de Bruyn AM, de Jong PT, Grobbee DE. Isolated systolic hypertension and vessel wall thickness of the carotid artery. The Rotterdam Elderly Study. *Arterioscler Thromb* 1993;13:64–69.
107. Shimakawa T, Bild DE. Relationship between hemoglobin and cardiovascular risk factors in young adults. *J Clin Epidemiol* 1993;46: 1257–1266.
108. Bogousslavsky J, Castillo V, Kumral E, Henriques I, Van Melle G. Stroke subtypes and hypertension. *Arch Neurol* 1996;53:265–269.
109. Alexander RW. Hypertension and the pathogenesis of atherosclerosis. *Hypertension* 1995; 25:155–161.
110. Delcker A, Diener HC, Wilhelm H. Influence of vascular risk factors for atherosclerotic carotid artery plaque progression. *Stroke* 1995;26: 2016–2022.
111. Mast H, Thompson JL, Lee SH, Mohr JP, Sacco RL. Hypertension and diabetes mellitus as determinants of multiple lacunar infarcts. *Stroke* 1995;26:30–33.
112. Ferro JM, Crespo M, Ferro H. Role of vascular risk factors in lacunar and unexplained stokes in young adults: a case-control study. *Cerebrovasc Dis* 1995;5:188–193.
113. Wolf PA, Clagett P, Easton JD, et al. Preventing ischemic stroke in patients with prior stroke and transient ischemic attack. A statement for healthcare professionals from the Stroke Council of the American Heart Association. *Stroke* 1999; 30:1991–1994.
114. Klungel OH, Stricker BHC, Paes AHP, et al. Excess stroke among hypertensive men and women attributable to undertreatment of hypertension. *Stroke* 1999;30:1312–1318.
115. MacMahon S, Peto R, Cutler J, et al. Blood pressure, stroke, and coronary heart disease. Part 1, Prolonged differences in blood pressure: prospective observational studies corrected for the regression dilution bias. *Lancet* 1990; 335:765–774.
116. Phillips SJ, Whisnant JP. Hypertension and the brain. The National High Blood Pressure Education Program. *Arch Intern Med* 1992; 152:938–945.

117. Hart CL, Hole DJ, Smith GD. Risk factors and 20-year stroke mortality in men and women in the Renfrew/Paisley Study in Scotland. *Stroke* 1999;30:1999–2007.
118. Staessen JA, Thijs L, Gasowski J, Cells H, Fagard RH. Treatment of isolated systolic hypertension in the elderly: further evidence from the systolic hypertension in Europe (Syst-Eur) trial. *Am J Cardio* 1998;82:20R–22R.
119. Hansson L. The Hypertension Optimal Treatment Study and the importance of lowering blood pressure. *J Hypertension* 1999; 17(Suppl):S9–13.
120. Pickering TG. Advances in the treatment of hypertension. *JAMA* 1999;281:114–116.
121. Kaplan NM, Gifford RW, Jr. Choice of initial therapy for hypertension. *JAMA* 1996; 275:1577–1580.
122. Luscher TF, Cosentino F. The classification of calcium antagonists and their selection in the treatment of hypertension. A reappraisal. *Drugs* 1998;55:509–517.
123. Whisnant JP. Effectiveness versus efficacy of treatment of hypertension for stroke prevention. *Neurology* 1996;46:301–307.
124. Caplan LR. Diabetes and brain ischemia. *Diabetes* 1996;45 (Suppl 3):S95–S97.
125. Mankovsky BN, Metzger BE, Molitch ME, Biller J. Cerebrovascular disorders in patients with diabetes mellitus. *J Diabetes Complications* 1996; 10:228–242.
126. Savage PJ. Cardiovascular complications of diabetes mellitus: what we know and what we need to know about their prevention. *Ann Intern Med* 1996;124:123–126.
127. Whisnant JP, Brown RD, Petty GW, O'Fallon WM, Sicks JD, Wiebers DO. Comparison of population-based models of risk factors for TIA and ischemic stroke. *Neurology* 1999; 53:532–536.
128. Davis TM, Millns H, Stratton IM, Holman RR, Turner RC. Risk factors for stroke in type 2 diabetes mellitus: United Kingdom Prospective Diabetes Study (UKPDS) 29. *Arch Intern Med* 1999;159:1097–1103.
129. Brand FN, Kannel WB, Evans J, Larson MG, Wolf PA. Glucose intolerance, physical signs of peripheral artery disease, and risk of cardiovascular events: the Framingham Study. *Am Heart J* 1998;136:919–927.
130. Qureshi AI, Giles WH, Croft JB. Impaired glucose tolerance and the likelihood of nonfatal stroke and myocardial infarction: the Third National Health and Nutrition Examination Survey. *Stroke* 1998;29:1329–1332.
131. Lukovits TG, Mazzone TM, Gorelick TM. Diabetes mellitus and cerebrovascular disease. *Neuroepidemiology* 1999;18:1–14.
132. O'Brien T, Nguyen TT, Zimmerman BR. Hyperlipidemia and diabetes mellitus. *Mayo Clin Proc* 1998;73:969–976.
133. Tuomilehto J, Rastenyte D, Jousilahti P, Sarti C, Vartiainen E. Diabetes mellitus as a risk factor for death from stroke. Prospective study of the middle-aged Finnish population. *Stroke* 1996;27:210–215.
134. Barrett-Connor E, Khaw KT. Diabetes mellitus. An independent risk factor for stroke? *Am J Epidemiol* 1988;128:116–123.
135. Nathan DM. Long-term complications of diabetes mellitus. *N Engl J Med* 1993;328: 1676–1685.
136. Saito I, Segawa H, Shiokawa Y, Taniguchi M, Tsutsumi K. Middle cerebral artery occlusion: correlation of computed tomography and angiography with clinical outcome. *Stroke* 1987; 18:863–868.
137. Whisnant JP. Modeling of risk factors for ischemic stroke. The Willis Lecture. *Stroke* 1997; 28:1840–1844.
138. You RX, McNeil JJ, O'Malley HM, Davis SM, Thrift AG, Donnan GA. Risk factors for stroke due to cerebral infarction in young adults. *Stroke* 1997;28:1913–1918.
139. Jorgensen H, Nakayama H, Raaschou HO, Olsen TS. Stroke in patients with diabetes. The Copenhagen Stroke Study. *Stroke* 1994;25: 1977–1984.
140. Bruno A, Biller J, Adams HP, Jr., et al. Acute blood glucose level and outcome from ischemic stroke. Trial of ORG 10172 in Acute Stroke Treatment (TOAST) Investigators. *Neurology* 1999;52:280–284.
141. Murros K, Fogelholm R, Kettunen S, Vuorela AL, Valve J. Blood glucose, glycosylated haemoglobin, and outcome of ischemic brain infarction. *J Neurol Sci* 1992;111:59–64.
142. Alter M, Lai SM, Friday G, Singh V, Kumar VM, Sobel E. Stroke recurrence in diabetics. Does control of blood glucose reduce risk? *Stroke* 1997;28:1153–1157.
143. Turner RC, Cull CA, Frighi V, Holman RR. Glycemic control with diet, sulfonylurea, metformin, or insulin in patients with type 2 diabetes mellitus: progressive requirement for multiple therapies (UKPDS 49). UK Prospective Diabetes Study (UKPDS) Group. *JAMA* 1999; 281:2005–2012.
144. Wallis WE, Donaldson I, Scott RS, Wilson J. Hypoglycemia masquerading as cerebrovascular disease (hypoglycemic hemiplegia). Ann Neurol 1985;18:510–512.
145. Hachinski V, Graffagnino C, Beaudry M, et al. Lipids and stroke: a paradox resolved. *Arch Neurol* 1996;53:303–308.
146. Joensuu T, Salonen R, Winblad I, Korpela H, Salonen JT. Determinants of femoral and carotid artery atherosclerosis. *J Intern Med* 1994; 236:79–84.
147. Qizilbash N, Jones L, Warlow C, Mann J. Fibrinogen and lipid concentrations as risk factors for transient ischaemic attacks and minor ischaemic strokes. *BMJ* 1991;303:605–609.
148. Qizilbash N, Duffy SW, Warlow C, Mann J. Lipids are risk factors for ischaemic stroke. Overview and review. *Cerebrovasc Dis* 1992; 2:127–136.
149. Harjai KJ. Potential new cardiovascular risk factors: left ventricular hypertrophy, homocysteine, lipoprotein(a), triglycerides, oxidative stress, and fibrinogen. *Ann Intern Med* 1999; 131:376–386.

150. Aronow WS, Ahn C. Correlation of serum lipids with the presence or absence of atherothrombotic brain infarction and peripheral arterial disease in 1834 men and women aged ≥ 62 years. *Am J Cardiol* 1994;73:995–997.
151. O'Leary DH, Polak JF, Kronmal RA, et al. Carotid-artery intima and media thickness as a risk factor for myocardial infarction and stroke in older adults. Cardiovascular Health Study Collaborative Research Group. *N Engl J Med* 1999;340:14–22.
152. Dyker AG, Weir CJ, Lees KR. Influence of cholesterol on survival after stroke: retrospective study. *BMJ* 1997;314:1584–1588.
153. Gillman MW, Cupples LA, Millen BE, Ellison RC, Wolf PA. Inverse association of dietary fat with development of ischemic stroke in men. *JAMA* 1997;278:2145–2150.
154. McGill HCJ, McMahan CA, Malcom GT, Oalmann MC, Strong JP. Effects of serum lipoproteins and smoking on atherosclerosis in young men and women. The PDAY Research Group. Pathobiological Determinants of Atherosclerosis in Youth. *Arterioscler Thromb Vasc Biol* 1997;17:95–106.
155. Yatsu FM, Kataoka S. Pathogenesis of atherothrombotic brain infarctions. Role of lipids. *Cerebrovasc Dis* 1993;3:338–342.
156. Kwakkel G, Wagenaar RC, Kollen BJ, Lankhorst GJ. Predicting disability in stroke—a critical review of the literature. *Ageing* 1996; 25:479–489.
157. Espeland MA, Applegate W, Furberg CD, Lefkowitz D, Rice L, Hunninghake D. Estrogen replacement therapy and progression of intimal-medial thickness in the carotid arteries of postmenopausal women. ACAPS Investigators. Asymptomatic Carotid Atherosclerosis Progression Study. *Am J Epidemiol* 1995; 142:1011–1019.
158. Tanne D, Yaari S, Goldbourt U. High-density lipoprotein cholesterol and risk of ischemic stroke mortality. A 21-year follow-up of 8586 men from the Israeli Ischemic Heart Disease Study. *Stroke* 1997;28:83–87.
159. Wilt TJ, Rubins HB, Robins SJ, et al. Carotid atherosclerosis in men with low levels of HDL cholesterol. *Stroke* 1997;28:1919–1925.
160. Peynet J, Beaudeux JL, Woimant F, et al. Apolipoprotein(a) size polymorphism in young adults with ischemic stroke. *Atherosclerosis* 1999;142:233–239.
161. The Clinical Quality Improvement Network (CQIN) Investigators. Low incidence of assessment and modification of risk factors in acute care patients at high risk for cardiovascular events, particularly among females and the elderly. *Am J Cardiol* 1995;76:570–573.
162. Plehn JF, Davis BR, Sacks FM, et al. Reduction of stroke incidence after myocardial infarction with pravastatin: the Cholesterol and Recurrent Events (CARE) study. The Care Investigators. *Circulation* 1999;99:216–223.
163. Blauw GJ, Lagaay AM, Smelt AHM, Westendorp RGJ. Stroke, statins, and cholesterol. *Stroke* 1997;28:946–950.
164. Byington RP, Jukema JW, Salonen JT, et al. Reduction in cardiovascular events during pravastatin therapy. Pooled analysis of clinical events of the Pravastatin Atherosclerosis Intervention Program. *Circulation* 1995; 922:2419–2425.
165. Hebert PR, Gaziano JM, Chan KS, Hennekens CH. Cholesterol lowering with statin drugs, risk of stroke, and total mortality. An overview of randomized trials. *JAMA* 1997;278:313–321.
166. Hebert PR, Gaziano JM, Hennekens CH. An overview of trials of cholesterol lowering and risk of stroke. *Arch Intern Med* 1995;155:50–55.
167. Lewis SJ, Moye LA, Sacks FM, et al. Effect of pravastatin on cardiovascular events in older patients with myocardial infarction and cholesterol levels in the average range. Results of the Cholesterol and Recurrent Events (CARE) trial. *Ann Intern Med* 1998;12:681–689.
168. The Scandinavian Simvastatin Survival Study Group. Randomised trial of cholesterol lowering in 4444 patients with coronary heart disease: the Scandinavian Simvastatin Survival Study (4S). *Lancet* 1994;344:1383–1389.
169. Furberg CD, Adams HP, Jr., Applegate WB, et al. Effect of lovastatin on early carotid atherosclerosis and cardiovascular events. Asymptomatic Carotid Artery Progression Study (ACAPS) Research Group. *Circulation* 1994; 90:1679–1687.
170. Ansell BJ, Watson KE, Fogelman AM. An evidence-based assessment of the NCEP Adult Treatment Panel II Guidelines. *JAMA* 1999; 282:2051–2057.
171. Atkins D, Psaty BM, Koepsell TD, Longstreth WT, Jr., Larson EB. Cholesterol reduction and the risk for stroke in men. *Ann Intern Med* 1993;119:136–145.
172. Cleeman JI, Lenfant C. The National Cholesterol Education Program: progress and prospects. *JAMA* 1998;280:2099–2104.
173. Abbott RD, Behrens GR, Sharp DS, et al. Body mass index and thromboembolic stroke in nonsmoking men in older middle age. *Stroke* 1994;25:2370–2376.
174. Rexrode KM, Hennekens CH, Willett WC, et al. A prospective study of body mass index, weight change, and risk of stroke in women. *JAMA* 1997;277:1539–1545.
175. Wannamethee SG, Shaper AG, Walker M, Ebrahim S. Lifestyle and 15-year survival free of heart attack, stroke, and diabetes in middle-aged British men. *Arch Intern Med* 1998; 158:2433–2440.
176. Joseph LN, Babikian VL, Allen NC, Winter MR. Risk factor modification in stroke prevention: the experience of a stroke clinic. *Stroke* 1999; 30:16–20.
177. Bornstein NM. Lifestyle changes: smoking, alcohol, diet, and exercise. *Cerebrovasc Dis* 1994; 4:59–65.
178. Sasaki S, Zhang XH, Kesteloot H. Dietary sodium, potassium, saturated fat, alcohol, and stroke mortality. *Stroke* 1995;26:783–789.
179. Gale CR, Martyn CN, Winter PD, Cooper C. Vitamin C and risk of death from stroke and

coronary heart disease in cohort of elderly people. *BMJ* 1995;310:1563–1566.
180. Khaw KT, Woodhouse P. Interrelation of vitamin C, infection, haemostatic factors, and cardiovascular disease. *BMJ* 1995;310:1559–1563.
181. Gillman MW, Cupples LA, Gagnon D, et al. Protective effect of fruits and vegetables on development of stroke in men. *JAMA* 1995; 273:1113–1117.
182. Bulpitt CJ. Vitamin C and vascular disease. *BMJ* 1995;310:1548–1549.
183. Joshipura KJ, Ascherio A, Manson JE, et al. Fruit and vegetable intake in relation to risk of ischemic stroke. *JAMA* 1999;282:1233–1239.
184. Wolk A, Manson JE, Stampfer MJ, et al. Long-term intake of dietary fiber and decreased risk of coronary heart disease among women. *JAMA* 1999;281:1998–2004.
185. Orencia AJ, Daviglus ML, Dyer AR, Shekelle RB, Stamler J. Fish consumption and stroke in men. 30-year findings of the Chicago Western Electric Study. *Stroke* 1996;27:204–209.
186. Keli SO, Feskens EJ, Kromhout D. Fish consumption and risk of stroke. The Zutphen Study. *Stroke* 1994;328–332.
187. Simon JA, Fong J, Bernert JTJ, Browner WS. Serum fatty acids and the risk of stroke. *Stroke* 1995;26:778–782.
188. Kiechl S, Aichner F, Gerstenbrand F, et al. Body iron stores and presence of carotid atherosclerosis. Results from the Bruneck Study. *Arterioscler Thromb* 1994;14:1625–1630.
189. Kiely DK, Wolf PA, Cupples LA, Beiser AS, Kannel WB. Physical activity and stroke risk: the Framingham Study. *Am J Epidemiol* 1994; 140:608–620.
190. Lindenstrom E, Boysen G, Nyboe J. Lifestyle factors and risk of cerebrovascular disease in women. The Copenhagen City Heart Study. *Stroke* 1993;24:1468–1472.
191. Gillum RF, Mussolino ME, Ingram DD. Physical activity and stroke incidence in women and men. The NHANES I Epidemiologic Follow-up Study. *Am J Epidemiol* 1996;143:860–869.
192. Agnarsson U, Thorgeirsson G, Sigvaldason H, Sigfusson N. Effects of leisure-time physical activity and ventilatory function on risk for stroke in men: The Reykjavik Study. *Ann Intern Med* 1999;130:987–990.
193. Lee IM, Hennekens CH, Berger K. Exercise and risk of stroke in male physicians. *Stroke* 1999;30:1–6.
194. Sacco RL, Roberts JK, Jacobs BS. Homocysteine as a risk factor for ischemic stroke: an epidemiological story in evolution. *Neuroepidemiology* 1998;17:167–173.
195. Boushey CJ, Beresford SA, Omenn GS, Motulsky AG. A quantitative assessment of plasma homocysteine as a risk factor for vascular disease. Probable benefits of increasing folic acid intakes. *JAMA* 1995;274:1049–1057.
196. Markus HS, Ali N, Swaminathan R, Sankaralingam A, Molloy J, Powell J. A common polymorphism in the methylenetetrahydrofolate reductase gene, homocysteine, and ischemic cerebrovascular disease. *Stroke* 1997;28:1739–1743.
197. Selhub J, Jacques PF, Bostom AG, et al. Relationship between plasma homocysteine, vitamin status and extracranial carotid-artery stenosis in the Framingham Study population. *J Nutr* 1996;126:1258S–1265S.
198. Malinow MR, Nieto FJ, Szklo M, Chambless LE, Bond G. Carotid artery intimal-medial wall thickening and plasma homocyst(e)ine in asymptomatic adults. The Atherosclerosis Risk in Communities Study. *Circulation* 1993; 87:1107–1113.
199. Malinow MR. Homocyst(e)ine and arterial occlusive diseases. *J Intern Med* 1994;236:603–617.
200. Selhub J, Jacques PF, Rosenberg IH, et al. Serum total homocysteine concentrations in the third national health and nutrition examination survey (1991-1994): population reference ranges and contribution of vitamin status to high serum concentrations. *Ann Intern Med* 1999; 131:331–339.
201. Yoo JH, Chung CS, Kang SS. Relation of plasma homocyst(e)ine to cerebral infarction and cerebral atherosclerosis. *Stroke* 1998;29:2478–2483.
202. Taylor LMJ, Moneta GL, Sexton GJ, Schuff RA, Porter JM. Prospective blinded study of the relationship between plasma homocysteine and progression of symptomatic peripheral arterial disease. *J Vasc Surg* 1999;29:8–21.
203. Evers S, Koch HG, Grotemeyer KH, Lange B, Deufel T, Ringelstein EB. Features, symptoms, and neurophysiological findings in stroke associated with hyperhomocysteinemia. *Arch Neurol* 1997;54:1276–1282.
204. Graham IM, Daly LE, Refsum HM, et al. Plasma homocysteine as a risk factor for vascular disease. The European Concerted Action Project. *JAMA* 1997;277:1775–1781.
205. Selhub J, Jacques PF, Bostom AG, et al. Association between plasma homocysteine concentrations and extracranial carotid-artery stenosis. *N Engl J Med* 1995;332:286–291.
206. Eikelboom JW, Lonn E, Genest J, Jr., Hankey G, Yusuf S. Homocyst(e)ine and cardiovascular disease: a critical review of the epidemiologic evidence. *Ann Intern Med* 1999;131:363–375.
207. Kark JD, Selhub J, Adler B, et al. Nonfasting plasma total homocysteine level and mortality in middle-aged and elderly men and women in Jerusalem. *Ann Intern Med* 1999;131:321–330.
208. Konecky N, Malinow MR, Tunick PA, et al. Correlation between plasma homocyst(e)ine and aortic atherosclerosis. *Am Heart J* 1997; 133:534–540.
209. McQuillan BM, Beilby JP, Nidorf M, Thompson PL, Hung J. Hyperhomocysteinemia but not the C677T mutation of methylenetetrahydrofolate reductase is an independent risk determinant of carotid wall thickening. The Perth Carotid Ultrasound Disease Assessment Study (CUDAS). *Circulation* 1999;99:2383–2388.
210. Bellamy MF, McDowell IF. Putative mechanisms for vascular damage by homocysteine. *J Inherited Metab Dis* 1997;20:307–315.
211. Penix LP. Ischemic strokes secondary to vitamin B12 deficiency-induced hyperhomocystinemia. *Neurology* 1998;51:622–624.

212. Ridker PM, Manson JE, Buring JE, Shih J, Matias M, Hennekens CH. Homocysteine and risk of cardiovascular disease among postmenopausal women. *JAMA* 1999;281: 1817–1821.
213. Perry IJ, Refsum H, Morris RW, Ebrahim SB, Ueland PM, Shaper AG. Prospective study of serum total homocysteine concentration and risk of stroke in middle-aged British men. *Lancet* 1995;346:1395–1398.
214. van Beynum I, Smeitink JA, den Heijer M, te Poele Pothoff MT, Blom HJ. Hyperhomocysteinemia: a risk factor for ischemic stroke in children. *Circulation* 1999; 99:2070–2072.
215. Verhoef P, Hennekens CH, Malinow MR, Kok FJ, Willett WC, Stampfer MJ. A prospective study of plasma homocyst(e)ine and risk of ischemic stroke. *Stroke* 1994;25:1924–1930.
216. Bots ML, Launer LJ, Lindemans J, et al. Homocysteine and short-term risk of myocardial infarction and stroke in the elderly: the Rotterdam Study. *Arch Intern Med* 1999; 159:38–44.
217. Bostom AG, Rosenberg IH, Silbershatz H, et al. Nonfasting plasma total homocysteine levels and stroke incidence in elderly persons: the Framingham Study. *Ann Intern Med* 1999; 131:352–355.
218. Stampfer MJ, Malinow MR. Can lowering homocysteine levels reduce cardiovascular risk? *N Engl J Med* 1995;332:328–329.
219. Graham I. Homocysteine in health and disease. *Ann Intern Med* 1999;131:387–388.
220. Inoue T, Oku K, Kimoto K, et al. Relationship of cigarette smoking to the severity of coronary and thoracic aortic atherosclerosis. *Cardiology* 1995;86:374–379.
221. Haheim LL, Holme I, Hjermann I, Leren P. Smoking habits and risk of fatal stroke: 18 years follow up of the Oslo Study. *J Epidemiol Community Health* 1996;50:621–624.
222. Ellekjaer EF, Wyller TB, Sverre JM, Holmen J. Lifestyle factors and risk of cerebral infarction. *Stroke* 1992;23:829–834.
223. Howard G, Wagenknecht LE, Cai J, Cooper L, Kraut MA, Toole JF. Cigarette smoking and other risk factors for silent cerebral infarction in the general population. *Stroke* 1998; 29:913–917.
224. Wannamethee SG, Shaper AG, Whincup PH, Walker M. Smoking cessation and the risk of stroke in middle-aged men. *JAMA* 1995; 274:155–160.
225. Donnan GA, McNeil JJ, Adena MA, Doyle AE, O'Malley HM, Neill GC. Smoking as a risk factor for cerebral ischaemia. *Lancet* 1989;2:643–647.
226. Whisnant JP, Homer D, Ingall TJ, et al. Duration of cigarette smoking is the strongest predictor of severe extracranial carotid artery atherosclerosis. *Stroke* 1990;21:707–714.
227. Love BB, Biller J, Jones MP, Adams HP, Jr., Bruno A. Cigarette smoking. A risk factor for cerebral infarction in young adults. *Arch Neurol* 1990;47:693–698.
228. Ingall TJ, Homer D, Baker HLJ, Kottke BA, O'Fallon WM, Whisnant JP. Predictors of intracranial carotid artery atherosclerosis. Duration of cigarette smoking and hypertension are more powerful than serum lipid levels. *Arch Neurol* 1991;48:687–691.
229. Haapaniemi H, Hillbom M, Juvela S. Lifestyle-associated risk factors for acute brain infarction among persons of working age. *Stroke* 1997; 28:26–30.
230. Mast H, Thompson JL, Lin IF, et al. Cigarette smoking as a determinant of high-grade carotid artery stenosis in Hispanic, black, and white patients with stroke or transient ischemic attack. *Stroke* 1998;29:908–912.
231. Law MM, Gelabert HA, Moore WS, et al. Cigarette smoking increases the development of initial hyperplasia after vascular injury. *J Vasc Surg* 1996;23:401–409.
232. Donnan GA, You R, Thrift A, McNeil JJ. Smoking as a risk factor for stroke. *Cerebrovasc Dis* 1993;3:129–138.
233. McVeigh GE, Lemay L, Morgan D, Cohn JN. Effects of long-term cigarette smoking on endothelium-dependent responses in humans. *AM J Cardiol* 1996;78:668–672.
234. Petrik PV, Gelabert HA, Moore WS, Quinones-Baldrich W, Law MM. Cigarette smoking accelerates carotid artery intimal hyperplasia in a dose-dependent manner. *Stroke* 1995;26: 1409–1414.
235. Tell GS, Polak JF, Ward BJ, Kittner SJ, Savage PJ, Robbins J. Relation of smoking with carotid artery wall thickness and stenosis in older adults. The Cardiovascular Health Study. The Cardiovascular Health Study (CHS) Collaborative Research Group. *Circulation* 1994; 90:2905–2908.
236. Blann AD, McCollum CN. Adverse influence of cigarette smoking on the endothelium. *Thromb Haemost* 1993;70:707–711.
237. Sharp DS, Benowitz NC, Bath PMW, Martin JF, Beswick AD, Elwood PC. Cigarette smoking sensitizes and desensitizes impedances measured ADP- induced platelet aggregation in whole blood. *Thromb Haemost* 1993;74:730–737.
238. Witteman JC, Grobbee DE, Valkenburg HA, van Hemert AM, Stijnen T, Hofman A. Cigarette smoking and the development and progression of aortic atherosclerosis. A 9-year population-based follow-up study in women. *Circulation* 1993;88:2156–2162.
239. Levine SR, Fagan SC, Pessin MS, et al. Accelerated intracranial occlusive disease, oral contraceptives, and cigarette use. *Neurology* 1991;41:1893–1901.
240. You RX, McNeil JJ, Hurley SF, et al. Smoking as a risk factor for cortical ischaemia presumably due to carotid occlusive disease. *Neuroepidemiology* 1993;12:141–147.
241. You RX, Thrift AG, McNeil JJ, Davis SM, Donnan GA. Ischemic stroke risk and passive exposure to spouses' cigarette smoking. Melbourne Stroke Risk Factor Study (MERFS) Group. *Amer J Public Health* 1999;89:572–575.
242. Hughes JR, Goldstein MG, Hurt RD, Shiffman S. Recent advances in the pharmacotherapy of smoking. *JAMA* 1999;281:72–76.

243. Kiechl S, Willeit J, Egger G, Oberhollenzer M, Aichner F. Alcohol consumption and carotid atherosclerosis: evidence of dose-dependent atherogenic and antiatherogenic effects. Results from the Bruneck Study. *Stroke* 1994; 25:1593–1598.
244. Kiechl S, Willeit J, Rungger G, Egger G, Oberhollenzer F, Bonora E. Alcohol consumption and atherosclerosis: what is the relation? Prospective results from the Bruneck Study. *Stroke* 1998;29:900–907.
245. Steinberg D, Pearson TA, Kuller LH. Alcohol and atherosclerosis. *Ann Intern Med* 1991; 114:967–976.
246. Shinton R, Sagar G, Beevers G. The relation of alcohol consumption to cardiovascular risk factors and stroke. The West Birmingham Stroke Project. *J Neurol Neurosurg Psychiatry* 1993; 56:458–462.
247. Sacco RL, Eikind M, Boden-Albala B, et al. The potential effect of moderate alcohol consumption on ischemic stroke. *JAMA* 1999;281:53–60.
248. Hansagi H, Romelsjo A, Gerhardsson DV, Andreasson S, Leifman BA. Alcohol consumption and stroke mortality. 20-year follow-up of 15,077 men and women. *Stroke* 1995; 26:1768–1773.
249. Hommel M, Jaillard A. Alcohol for stroke prevention? *N Engl J Med* 1999;341:1605–1606.
250. Berger K, Ajani UA, Kase CS, et al. Light-to-moderate alcohol consumption and the risk of stroke among U.S. male physicians. *N Engl J Med* 1999;341:1557–1564.
251. Truelsen T, Gronbaek M, Schnohr P, Boysen G. Intake of beer, wine, and spirits and risk of stroke. *Stroke* 1998;29:2467–2472.
252. Hendriks HF, Veenstra J, Velthuis-te WE, Schaafsma G, Kluft C. Effect of moderate dose of alcohol with evening meal on fibrinolytic factors. *BMJ* 1994;308:1003–1006.
253. Rodgers H, Aitken PD, French JM, Curless RH, Bates D, James OF. Alcohol and stroke. A case-control study of drinking habits past and present. *Stroke* 1993;24:1473–1477.
254. Wannamethee SG, Shaper AG. Patterns of alcohol intake and risk of stroke in middle-aged British men. *Stroke* 1996;27:1033–1039.
255. Kilpatrick TJ, Matkovic Z, Davis SM, McGrath CM, Dauer RJ. Hematologic abnormalities occur in both cortical and lacunar infarction. *Stroke* 1993;24:1945–1950.
256. Haapaniemi H, Hillbom M, Juvela S. Weekend and holiday increase in the onset of ischemic stroke in young women. *Stroke* 1996;27: 1023–1027.
257. Hillbom M, Haapaniemi H, Juvela S, Palomaki H, Numminen H, Kaste M. Recent alcohol consumption, cigarette smoking, and cerebral infarction in young adults. *Stroke* 1995;26: 40–45.
258. Kaku DA, Lowenstein DH. Emergence of recreational drug abuse as a major risk factor for stroke in young adults. *Ann Intern Med* 1990; 113:821-827.
259. Levine SR, Brust JC, Futrell N, et al. Cerebrovascular complications of the use of the "crack" form of alkaloidal cocaine. *N Engl J Med* 1990;323:699–704.
260. Daras M, Tuchman AJ, Marks S. Central nervous system infarction related to cocaine abuse. *Stroke* 1991;22:1320–1325.
261. Brust JCM, Richter RW. Stroke associated with addiction to heroin. *J Neurol Neurosurg Psychiatry* 1976;39:194–199.
262. Grodstein F, Stampfer MJ, Manson JE, et al. Postmenopausal estrogen and progestin use and the risk of cardiovascular disease. *N Engl J Med* 1996;335:453–461.
263. Sourander L, Rajala T, Raiha I, Makinen J, Erkkola R, Helenius H. Cardiovascular and cancer morbidity and mortality and sudden cardiac death in postmenopausal women on oestrogen replacement therapy (ERT). *Lancet* 1998; 352:1965–1969.
264. Mendelsohn ME, Karas RH. The protective effects of estrogen on the cardiovascular system. *N Engl J Med* 1999;340:1801–1811.
265. Fung MM, Barrett-Connor E, Bettencourt RR. Hormone replacement therapy and stroke risk in older women. *J Women's Health* 1999;8: 359–364.
266. WHO Collaborative Study of Cardiovascular Disease and Steroid Hormone Contraception. Ischaemic stroke and combined oral contraceptives: results of an international, multicentre, case-control study. *Lancet* 1996;348:498–505.
267. Chasan-Taber L, Stampfer MJ. Epidemiology of oral contraceptives and cardiovascular disease. *Ann Intern Med* 1998;128:467–477.
268. Lidegaard O, Kreiner S. Cerebral thrombosis and oral contraceptives. A case-control study. *Contraception* 1998;57:303–314.
269. Heinemann LA, Lewis MA, Thorogood M, Spitzer WO, Guggenmoos H, Bruppacher R. Case-control study of oral contraceptives and risk of thromboembolic stroke: results from International Study on Oral Contraceptives and Health of Young Women. *BMJ* 1997; 315:1502–1504.
270. Carolei A, Marini C, De Matteis G. History of migraine and risk of cerebral ischaemia in young adults. The Italian National Research Council Study Group on Stroke in the Young. *Lancet* 1996;347:1503–1506.
271. Schwartz SM, Siscovick DS, Longstreth WT, Jr., et al. Use of low-dose oral contraceptives and stroke in young women. *Ann Intern Med* 1997;127:596–603.
272. Martinelli I, Sacchi E, Landi G, Taioli E, Duca F, Mannucci PM. High risk of cerebral-vein thrombosis in carriers of a prothrombin-gene mutation and in users of oral contraceptives. *N Engl J Med* 1998;338:1793–1797.
273. Tzourio C, Tehindrazanarivelo A, Iglesias S, et al. Case-control study of migraine and risk of ischaemic stroke in young women. *BMJ* 1995;310:830–833.
274. Merikangas KR, Fenton BT, Cheng SH, Stolar MJ, Risch N. Association between migraine and stroke in a large-scale epidemiological study of the United States. *Arch Neurol* 1997; 54:362–368.

275. Bogousslavsky J, Regli F, Van Melle G, Payot M, Uske A. Migraine stroke. *Neurology* 1988; 38:223–227.
276. Shuaib A. Stroke from other etiologies masquerading as migraine-stroke. *Stroke* 1991; 22:1068–1074.
277. Grau AJ, Buggle F, Ziegler C, et al. Association between acute cerebrovascular ischemia and chronic and recurrent infection. *Stroke* 1997; 28:1724–1729.
278. Grau AJ, Brandt T, Forsting M, Winter R, Hacke W. Infection-associated cervical artery dissection. Three cases. *Stroke* 1997;28:453–455.
279. Grau AJ, Buggle F, Becher H, et al. Recent bacterial and viral infection is a risk factor for cerebrovascular ischemia: clinical and biochemical studies. *Neurology* 1998;50:196–203.
280. Hammers-Berggren S, Grondahl A, Karlsson M, von Arbin M, Carlsson A, Stiernstedt G. Screening for neuroborreliosis in patients with Stroke. *Stroke* 1993;24:1393–1396.
281. Bova IY, Bornstein NM, Korczyn AD. Acute infection as a risk factor for ischemic stroke. *Stroke* 1996;27:2204–2206.
282. Yamashita K, Ouchi K, Shirai M, Gondo T, Nakazawa T, Ito H. Distribution of *Chlamydia pneumoniae* infection in the athersclerotic carotid artery. *Stroke* 1998;29:773–778.
283. Fagerberg B, Gnarpe J, Gnarpe H, Agewall S, Wikstrand J. *Chlamydia pneumoniae* but not cytomegalovirus antibodies are associated with future risk of stroke and cardiovascular disease. A prospective study in middle-aged to elderly men with treated hypertension. *Stroke* 1999;30:299–305.
284. Cook PJ, Honeybourne D, Lip GY, Beevers DG, Wise R, Davies P. *Chlamydia pneumoniae* antibody titers are significantly associated with acute stroke and transient cerebral ischemia: the West Birmingham Stroke Project. *Stroke* 1998;29: 404–410.
285. Shor A, Phillips JI *Chlamydia pneumoniae* and atherosclerosis. *JAMA* 1999;282:2071–2073.
286. Markus HS, Mendall MA. Helicobacter pylori infection: a risk factor for ischaemic cerebrovascular disease and carotid atheroma. *J Neurol Neurosurg Psychiatry* 1998;64:104–107.
287. Qureshi AI, Janssen RS, Karon JM, et al. Human immunodeficiency virus infection and stroke in young patients. *Arch Neurol* 1997; 54:1150–1153.
288. Ridker PM, Hennekens CH, Stampfer MJ, Wang F. Prospective study of herpes simplex virus, cytomegalovirus, and the risk of future myocardial infarction and stroke. *Circulation* 1998;98: 2796–2799.
289. Schussheim AE, Fuster V. Antibiotics for myocardial infarction? A possible role of infection in atherogenesis and acute coronary syndromes. *Drugs* 1999;57:283–291.
290. Palomaki H. Snoring and the risk of ischemic brain infarction. *Stroke* 1991;22:1021–1025.
291. Partinen M, Palomaki H. Snoring and cerebral infarction. *Lancet* 1985;2:1325–1326.
292. Dyken ME, Somers VK, Yamada T, Ren ZY, Zimmerman MB. Investigating the relationship between stroke and obstructive sleep apnea. *Stroke* 1996;27:401–407.
293. Bassetti C, Aldrich MS, Chervin RD, Quint D. Sleep apnea in patients with transient ischemic attack and stroke: a prospective study of 59 patients. *Neurology* 1996;47:1167–1173.
294. Qureshi AI, Giles WH, Croft JB, Bliwise DL. Habitual sleep patterns and risk for stroke and coronary heart disease: a 10-year follow-up from NHANES I. *Neurology* 1997;48:904–911.
295. Pressman MR, Schetman WR, Figueroa WG, Van Uitert B, Caplan HJ, Peterson DD. Transient ischemic attacks and minor stroke during sleep. Relationship to obstructive sleep apnea syndrome. *Stroke* 1995;26:2361–2365.
296. Good DC, Henkle JQ, Gelber D, Welsh J, Verhulst S. Sleep-disordered breathing and poor functional outcome after stroke. *Stroke* 1996;27:252–259.
297. Wannamethee SG, Shaper AG, Ebrahim S. Respiratory function and risk of stroke. *Stroke* 1995;26:2004–2010.
298. Ogren M, Hedblad B, Isacsson SO, Janzon L, Jungquist G, Lindell SE. Non-invasively detected carotid stenosis and ischaemic heart disease in men with leg arteriosclerosis. *Lancet* 1993; 342:1138–1141.
299. Smith FB, Rumley A, Lee AJ, Leng GC, Fowkes FG, Lowe GD. Haemostatic factors and prediction of ischaemic heart disease and stroke in claudicants. *Brit J Haematol* 1998;100:758–763.
300. Alexandrova NA, Gibson WC, Norris JW, Maggisano R. Carotid artery stenosis in peripheral vascular disease. *J Vasc Surg* 1996; 23:645–649.
301. Karanjia PN, Madden KP, Lobner S. Coexistence of abdominal aortic aneurysm in patients with carotid stenosis. *Stroke* 1994; 25:627–630.
302. Bogousslavsky J, Cachin C, Regli F, Despland PA, Van Melle G, Kappenberger L. Cardiac sources of embolism and cerebral infarction—clinical consequences and vascular concomitants. *Neurology* 1991;41:855–859.
303. Maggioni AP, Franzosi MG, Farina ML, et al. Cerebrovascular events after myocardial infarction: analysis of the GISSI trial. Gruppo Italiano per lo Studio della Streptochinasi nell'Infarto Miocardico (GISSI). *BMJ* 1991;302:1428–1431.
304. Maggioni AP, Franzosi MG, Santoro E, White H, Van de Werf F, Tognoni. The risk of stroke in patients with acute myocardial infarction after thrombolytic and antithrombotic treatment. Gruppo Italiano per lo Studio della Sopravvivenza nell'Infarto Miocardico II (GISSI-2), and the International Study Group. *N Engl J Med* 1992;327:1–6.
305. Broderick JP, Phillips SJ, O'Fallon WM, Frye RL, Whisnant JP. Relationship of cardiac disease to stroke occurrence, recurrence, and mortality. *Stroke* 1992;23:1250–1256.
306. Kallikazaros I, Tsioufis C, Sideris S, Stefanadis C, Toutouzas P. Carotid artery disease as a marker for the presence of severe coronary artery disease in patients evaluated for chest pain. *Stroke* 1999;30:1002–1007.

307. Brass LM, Hartigan PM, Page WF, Concato J. Importance of cerebrovascular disease in studies of myocardial infarction. *Stroke* 1996;27: 1173–1176.
308. Whisnant JP, Wiebers DO, O'Fallon WM, Sicks JD, Frye RL. A population-based model of risk factors for ischemic stroke: Rochester, Minnesota. *Neurology* 1996;47:1420–1428.
309. Martin R, Bogousslavsky J. Mechanism of late stroke after myocardial infarct: the Lausanne Stroke Registry. *J Neurol Neurosurg Psychiatry* 1993;56:760–764.
310. Wolf PA, Mitchell JB, Baker CS, Kannel WB, D'Agostino RB. Impact of atrial fibrillation on mortality, stroke, and medical costs. *Arch Intern Med* 1998;158:229–234.
311. Wolf PA, Abbott RD, Kannel WB. Atrial fibrillation as an independent risk factor for stroke: the Framingham Study. *Stroke* 1991;22:983–988.
312. Walker RW, McLarty GD, Kitange HM, et al. Stroke mortality in urban and rural Tanzania. *Lancet* 2000;355:1684–1687.
313. Morgenstern LB, Wein TH, Smith MA, Moye LA, Pandey DK, Labauge P. Comparison of stroke hospitalization rates among Mexican-Americans and non-Hispanic whites. *Neurology* 2000;54:2000–2002.
314. Anand SS, Yusuf S, Vuksan V, et al. Differences in risk factors, atherosclerosis, and cardiovascular disease between ethnic groups in Canada: the Study of Health Assessment and Risk in Ethnic groups (SHARE) *Lancet* 2000;356:279–284.
315. Bogousslavsky J, Kaste M, Olsen TS, Hacke W, Orgogozo JM, for the EUSI Executive Committee. Risk factors and stroke prevention. *Cerebrovasc Dis* 2000;10(suppl3):12–21.
316. Wannamethee SG, Shaper AG, Ebrahim S. HDL-cholesterol, total cholesterol, and the risk of stroke in middle-aged British men. *Stroke* 2000;31:1882–1888.
317. Liu S, Manson JE, Stampfer MJ, et al. Whole grain consumption and risk of ischemic stroke in women. A prospective study. *Jama* 2000; 284:1534–1540.
318. Eikelboom JW, Hankey GJ, Anand SS, Lofthouse E, Staples N, Baker RI. Association between high hymocyst(e)ine and ischemic stroke due to large-and small-artery disease but not other etiologic subtypes of ischemic stroke. *Stroke* 2000;31:1069–1075.
319. Vermeulen EGJ, Stehouwer CDA, Twisk JWR, et al. Effect of homocysteine-lowering treatment with folic acid plus vitamin B6 on progression of subclinical atherosclerosis: a randomised, placebo-controlled trial. *Lancet* 2000; 355:517–522.
320. Gronbaek M, Becker U, Johansen D, et al. Type of alcohol consumed and mortality from all causes, coronary heart disease, and cancer. *Ann Intern Med* 2000;133:411–419.

Chapter 3

PRESENTATIONS OF ISCHEMIC STROKE AND TRANSIENT ISCHEMIC ATTACK

The diagnosis of ischemic stroke remains clinical; it is based on the findings of the history and physical examination. In particular, the nuances of the history are critical because many of the examination findings are not specific for stroke.

The spectrum of clinical presentations of patients with ischemic cerebrovascular disease is broad (See Table 1–4). A patient may have no neurological symptoms, a transient or minor episode of neurological dysfunction, or a disabling or life-threatening stroke. Although presentations can differ, clinicians should remember that these events are variations on a common, underlying cerebrovascular process. Priorities in treatment vary, but most of the management of patients with ischemic cerebrovascular disease is similar, regardless of the clinical presentation. As a rule of thumb, prevention is the focus of management for a patient who has either a normal neurological examination or minimal neurological impairments; a transient ischemic attack (TIA) serves as the model for this situation. Historical features of the event are critical because the patient's examination usually is normal. Conversely, a patient who has moderate-to-severe neurological deficits on examination prompts a different approach; care emphasizes rehabilitation and prevention of medical or neurological complications. In this situation, the interval from the neurological symptoms greatly influences decisions. A recent onset of symptoms represents a neurological emergency necessitating urgent evaluation and treatment in an inpatient setting. Conversely, a patient who is asymptomatic or whose neurological symptoms occurred several days before presentation probably is not acutely ill.

The differentiation of the types of ischemic cerebrovascular disease is described in Chapter 1. The most important variables in separating the categories of stroke are the time course, the areas of the brain affected, the presumed vascular territory, and the most likely cause of stroke. For the purposes of this chapter, patients with ephemeral neurological symptoms are included in the group with TIA, and those with more sustained neurological impairments are presumed to have had an ischemic stroke. A simple differentiation involves the neurological examination; if no abnormalities are detected, then the working diagnosis is TIA. If the neurological examination is abnormal, then the assumption is that the patient has had a stroke.

TRANSIENT ISCHEMIC ATTACK

A TIA in itself is not a serious event. The symptoms last a few minutes and then completely resolve. Unless it occurs during an activity that is dangerous if neurological impairments develop transiently (eg, driving, operating equipment), there are no sequelae. The importance of a TIA is that it serves as an omen of an impending stroke.[1] Although a TIA is a warning of a stroke, it should not be considered as a risk factor for stroke. Rather, it is a neurological manifestation of the vascular disease that is not different from a more disabling stroke. The patient has had a thomboembolic stroke that becomes a TIA because of recovery of adequate perfusion to the affected area of the brain. Approximately two-thirds of strokes occur in the same vascular territory as a prior TIA because it represents a change in the underlying vascular disease.[2] For example, an intramural hematoma within an atherosclerotic plaque or loss of the endothelial surface over an arterial lesion can lead to a decline in blood flow or intraluminal thrombosis. Overall, the risk of ischemic stroke within 5 years is approximately 20%.[3] In addition to being a warning for possible stroke, a TIA also portends a high risk for myocardial infarction or vascular death.[1–3]

Although any patient who has had a TIA is vulnerable for a stroke, some patients are at higher risk. Episodes of amaurosis fugax are not as ominous as a TIA or a minor stroke.[3] Severe neurological impariments (eg, weakness of an entire half of the body) during the TIA or prolonged events (ie, duration longer than 1 hour) are associated with a higher likelihood of a stroke than brief or minor neurological attacks. Events lasting longer than 1 hour generally are associated with severe cardiac or extracranial atherosclerotic disease.[4] An event that is present on arising in the morning also appears to convey an unusually high risk. In crescendo TIA, several events occur in a cluster over the previous few days and may result from any cause.[5,6] A working definition for the diagnosis of crescendo TIA is at least three events in a period of 48 hours. In this situation, the chance of stroke may be as high as approximately 20% during the next few days.[5] Crescendo TIA should be considered an emergency that prompts urgent evaluation and treatment.

Keys to Diagnosis of Transient Ischemic Attack

Very few patients will have a TIA in the presence of a physician, so the diagnosis usually is based entirely on the history obtained from the patient and any observers.[7] An episode of transient neurological impairment may not represent a TIA, even in a patient who has other risk factors for cerebrovascular disease.[8] Several conditions that can cause transient neurological symptoms are included in the differential diagnosis.[8–11](See Table 3–1.) The diagnosis of TIA can be difficult; in one large series, approximately one-third of patients were not recognized properly and misdiagnoses are fairly high among physicians who have limited experience dealing with patients with TIA or stroke.[12] Agreement in the diagnosis of TIA if fairly high among neurologists, but they have difficulty in differentiating carotid from vertebrobasilar symptoms.[13,14] Approximately one-half to one-third of patients with TIA may be mislabeled and either over-diagnosis or under-diagnosis of TIA can be dangerous.[9] Problems in appreciating the nuances of a history are the chief reason for misdiagnosis.

TIME COURSE

A TIA should be a discrete event with a defined onset and resolution (Table 3–2). An amorphous event, or one with waxing and waning symptoms, is atypical. Similarly, a gradual increase in symptoms over a few days is not compatible with TIA. Such a history is more compatible with an intracranial mass, such as a tumor or subdural hematoma (Table 3–3). A TIA usually lasts a few minutes; an event that is only a few seconds in duration usually is not a TIA. A brief episode of posturally induced symptoms, such as lightheadedness, usually is not a TIA. Conversely, if an event that lasts several hours, then it probably is not a TIA.[4] As a rule of thumb, the

Table 3–1. **Differential Diagnosis of Transient Ischemic Attacks**

- Migraine and migraine equivalents
- Focal or generalized epilepsy
  - Todd's paralysis
- Syncope and presyncope
- Mass lesion with waxing and waning symptoms
  - Subdural hematoma
  - Tumor
  - Arteriovenous malformation
- Metabolic disturbance
  - Hypoglycemia
  - Hyponatremia
- Primary ear/labyrinthine disease
  - Meniere's disease
  - Glaucoma
  - Papilledema
- Hysteria

Table 3–2. **General Clinical Features of Transient Ischemic Attack**

- Discrete events with defined onset and resolution
  - Usually sudden onset
  - Can resolve slowly
  - Usually not provoked
- Duration usually 5–20 minutes
- Dysfunction of one portion of the brain
  - Vascular territory of one artery
  - Usually no loss of consciousness or confusion
  - Usually no lightheadedness or wooziness
- Loss of neurological function
  - Weakness or heaviness of limb or side of face
  - Numbness of limb or side of face
  - Incoordination or clumsiness of limbs
  - Visual loss in one or both eyes
  - Slurred speech
  - Trouble understanding or producing words
  - Maximal at onset
  - Should not spread from one body part to another
- Can be associated with headache

Table 3–3. **Key Features in Differentiating Non-Ischemic Causes of Transient Neurological Impairments**

- Migraine or migraine equivalents
  - Sudden onset of neurological symptoms
  - March of symptoms from one body part to another
    - Sensory—tingling more than numbness
    - Motor—weakness not prominent
    - Visual—peripheral to central, right to left fields
  - Binocular visual symptoms common
  - Positive symptoms—scintillating scotoma, fortification spectra
  - Prominent headache, which usually is unilateral and intense
  - Headache lasts longer than neurological symptoms
  - Headache usually follows the neurological symptoms
  - Associated nausea, vomiting, photophobia, phonophobia
  - Can have neurological symptoms without headache (migraine equivalent)
- Seizures
  - Sudden onset of neurological symptoms
  - May have an aura (focal neurological symptoms)
  - March of symptoms from one body part to another
    - Sensory—tingling more than numbness
    - Motor—involuntary movements or jerking more than weakness
  - Positive symptoms—involuntary movements or jerking
  - Loss of consciousness, confusion, or agitation
  - Incontinence, tongue bites, or sore muscles
  - Residual weakness (Todd's paralysis) or mental status changes
  - Can have headache after episode
- Syncope
  - Can occur spontaneously or be provoked by activity, such as posture change
  - Visual blurring, lightheadedness, dizziness, or woozziness common
  - Brief loss of consciousness
  - Collapse without jerking or involuntary movements
  - Focal neurological impairments (weakness, sensory loss, etc.) uncommon
  - May have chest pain or palpitations
- Intracranial mass—tumor or subdural hematoma
  - Symptoms associated with waxing and waning
  - Slow progression or stuttering course
  - Discrete events of sudden onset atypical
  - Gradual increase in focal neurological impairments over time
  - Confusion, mental status changes, or behavioral symptoms
  - Headaches gradually increasing and not associated with events
- Hypoglycemia
  - Occurs primarily in diabetic patients taking insulin
  - Can have focal neurological impairments
  - Usually does not have a distinct onset—rather, events gradually evolve
  - Confusion or decreased alertness may be subtle

neurological symptoms last 5–20 minutes. Because of the relatively short duration of the symptoms, the presence of neurological impairments at the time the patient reaches an emergency department usually precludes the diagnosis of TIA. Waiting 24 hours for the symptoms to resolve to exclude the diagnosis of TIA cannot be defended.

NATURE OF NEUROLOGICAL SYMPTOMS

During a TIA, neurological impairments reflect dysfunction of one portion of the brain (Table 3–2). Neurological symptoms that suggest multiple areas of brain disturbance or that are global or non-specific, such as dizziness, lightheadedness, confusion, or loss of consciousness usually are not secondary to TIA. They are more likely secondary to seizures or syncope.[8,15,16] In particular, posturally related symptoms are likely to be secondary to syncope or pre-syncope. Although these symptoms are not consistent with TIA, elderly patients with these complaints have a high risk for vascular complications, especially cardiac events.[17] Thus, these patients warrant careful cardiovascular evaluation and treatment even if the diagnosis of TIA is refuted.

The symptoms of TIA usually involve a loss of neurological function; these "negative" phenomena include weakness, numbness, visual loss, or clumsiness. "Positive" phenomena, such as bright visual disturbances (i.e., sparkles, shimmering, or lightning) or involuntary movements usually are not secondary to TIA; a seizure or migraine is more likely. Occasionally, brief, involuntary, coarse, irregular trembling of an arm, hand, or leg can occur in association with flow-related TIA in the carotid circulation.[18–21] Neurological impairments usually are maximal at the time of onset. The spread from one body part to another is unusual. Occasionally, a patient may not recognize all of the simultaneous neurological symptoms during a TIA. As a result, the history may suggest a march. Care should be taken in differentiating a pseudo-march of symptoms from a stepwise progression of symptoms from one body part to another. A seizure or migraine is more likely if a patient clearly describes symptoms migrating from one part of the body to another over an interval of seconds or minutes.

ASSOCIATED SYMPTOMS

Although headache is a paramount symptom in migraine, approximately 20% of patients will have a headache as part of a TIA.[22] Headaches are more likely with posterior circulation and cortical events. The headache usually is mild. It can be unilateral with a carotid TIA. Usually the headaches are occipital and nuchal with a vertebrobasilar TIA. Nausea, vomiting, photophobia, and phonophobia are unusual with TIA, and their presence suggests the diagnosis of migraine. Thus, the presence of a headache does not exclude a diagnosis of TIA; however, if the headache is the primary complaint, then the diagnosis of TIA is less likely.

PROVOCATION OF EVENTS

Because embolism is the most common cause of TIA, most events occur without any obvious provocation. The high metabolic activity of the brain means that even patients with borderline perfusion usually do not have symptoms secondary to activity. Rarely, postural changes, exercise, or a heavy meal can induce a TIA. External compression of the vertebral artery in the neck can cause symptoms in the posterior circulation that occur with head turning or extension of the neck. Occasionally, a TIA can be provoked by postural changes. Included in this category of events is the limb-shaking TIA. However, as a rule, events that stereotypically happen with postural changes are more likely due to global hypoperfusion than to a TIA. Intermittent vertigo that is exacerbated by postural changes, turning, or rolling over in bed usually is due to a non-vascular labyrinthine process or benign positional vertigo.

Differentiating Symptoms in Carotid or Vertebrobasilar Circulations

Symptoms of TIA in the carotid circulation differ from events that happen in the posterior circulation.[15] (See Table 3–4.) Localizing symptoms to the appropriate vascular territory is important because doing so influences subsequent evaluation and treatment options. At times, differentiation can be difficult. For example, patients with slurring of speech could have symptoms in either circulation, and patients can have difficulty delineating a monocular visual disturbance from a homonymous visual field defect. Overall, the problem in physician recognition of carotid circulation events appears less than in diagnosis of vertebrobasilar events. In part, this distinction probably reflects the symptoms of lightheadedness, ill-described visual problems, and vertigo that could be a TIA or some other neurological symptom.

Table 3–4. **Symptoms of Transient Ischemic Attack: Carotid or Vertebrobasilar Circulation**

Carotid Circulation
- Ipsilateral transient monocular blindness (amaurosis fugax)
- Contralateral homonymous hemianopia
- Contralateral paresis or sensory loss
- Aphasia (dominant hemisphere)
- Dysarthria

Vertebrobasilar Circulation
- Binocular visual loss
- Vertigo
- Unilateral, bilateral, or crossed paresis
- Unilateral, bilateral, or crossed sensory loss
- Dysarthria
- Limb or gait ataxia
- Diplopia
- Dysphagia

Symptoms of Carotid Arterial Circulation

Symptoms of carotid artery TIA can refer to the ipsilateral eye or cerebral hemisphere (Table 3–4). Although a patient can have both ocular and cerebral symptoms, the events rarely occur simultaneously. A patient who presents with neurological symptoms suggestive of a carotid circulation TIA should be quizzed about the occurrence of ipsilateral monocular visual symptoms. Patients seem to ignore a brief visual event, particularly if it does not involve complete visual loss. The occurrence of several stereotypical spells does not portend the likely cause of the TIA.

AMAUROSIS FUGAX

Amaurosis fugax (transient monocular blindness) is a painless, relatively brief episode of loss of vision in one eye. It is an important presentation of extracranial carotid atherosclerosis and an ulcerated atherosclerotic plaque in particular.[23–25] However, the patient's age and ethnicity affect the relationship between amaurosis fugax and stenosis of the internal carotid artery. Young patients may have other causes of the visual loss, including migraine. African Americans with amaurosis fugax are much less likely to have atherosclerosis of the carotid artery than are whites. Ahuja et al[26] found severe stenosis of the artery in only 1 of 29 African American patients with transient monocular blindness. Patients with retinal artery infarction and amaurosis fugax have the same high risk for either myocardial infarction or ischemic stroke, as do patients with TIA.[27]

In general, the symptoms of amaurosis fugax are stereotyped. The attack occurs suddenly. Although a descending or ascending curtain is a textbook description, most patients' visual complaints are less precise.[28] They describe scum, haze, fog, or grayness in the vision of one eye. Complete blindness or a quadrantic visual field defect also occurs with embolic occlusion of a branch retinal artery.[28,29]

Occasionally, vision will decline from the periphery with a progressive constriction of the visual field. Some patients may describe brief episodes of positive visual phenomena (sparkles) in the eye. The attacks usually last from a few seconds to a few minutes.[29] Permanent monocular blindness can result from a central retinal artery occlusion, but a cilioretinal artery occlusion secondary to giant cell arteritis also should be considered.[30] In exceptional circumstances, positive phenomena (sparkles) are seen. Rarely, patients with borderline perfusion to the eye have visual loss induced by sudden exposure to bright light.[31,32] Patients with severe extracranial arterial disease can have progressive visual loss due to venous stasis retinopathy. Severe arterial disease leading to poor venous drainage can cause increased intraocular pressure (glaucoma) and visual loss.

SYMPTOMS OF HEMISPHERIC ISCHEMIA

Contralateral weakness or numbness of the hand is the most common neurological symptom of TIA of the carotid circulation. Rather than reporting paralysis, the patient usually describes the hand as being numb, heavy, or clumsy. The hand does not work correctly, and the patient may complain of dropping an object or not being able to do a complex act, such as eating or dialing a telephone. An observer may report clumsiness or limpness of the hand. A physician should not try to distinguish a historical report of transient sensory loss from motor dysfunction. Differentiating numbness or weakness by history can be difficult; many patients will use the terms interchangeably.[7] In addition, separation of motor or sensory loss is not critical in this situation.

Localization of the neurological problem can be difficult if the symptoms are restricted to the hand or upper limb. Occasionally, a root or peripheral nerve lesion can cause intermittent hand dysfunction. As a rule, the entire hand will be affected during a TIA. Weakness or numbness restricted to one or two digits usually is not due to a TIA. A needles and pins sensation (paresthesia) usually is not a symptom of TIA; it is more likely due to a neuropathic process. If the patient describes prominent limb pain, then the condition probably is not a TIA. The combination of numbness or weakness of the hand and the same side of the face is relatively common with a carotid circulation TIA. The presence of upper limb and face symptoms excludes a peripheral or cervical process and increases the likelihood of a cerebrovascular cause for intermittent or transient symptoms. In addition to the numbness or weakness reported by the patient, an observer may note sagging or drooping of the lower part of one side of the face and lips. Numbness of the tongue or buccal regions can occur. These symptoms should be restricted to one side of the face, tongue, and mouth. The occurrence of a cheiro-oral syndrome (numbness of the lips and ipsilateral hand) could represent a migraine rather than a TIA.

Numbness or weakness of the lower limb alone or in combination with upper limb or face symptoms is infrequent. If a patient has a TIA while walking, the patient or an observer may describe a gait disturbance, such as dragging the leg. While unilateral weakness or numbness can occur with a TIA in the posterior circulation, these symptoms usually are ascribed to carotid circulation ischemia. In exceptional circumstances, ipsilateral or bilateral leg weakness can happen with a carotid circulation TIA when the contralateral anterior cerebral artery arises from the affected carotid.[33] Paraparesis rarely occurs with TIA in either the carotid or vertebrobasilar circulation.

A language disturbance can occur with a TIA in the dominant hemisphere, and disorders of articulation can occur with a carotid event in either hemisphere. If the patient is alone, no history of speech or language disturbance usually is reported. Thus, the symptoms usually are recognized if a patient is talking to someone else and that other person reports the language or articulation problem. A potential scenario is a listener recognizing the language impairment during a telephone conversation. Although differentiating aphasia from dysarthria is important because articulatory symptoms also occur with TIA in the vertebrobasilar circulation, the historical subtleties that differentiate the abnormalities can be hard to elicit. A report of speech that is incoherent or nonsensical points to aphasia, whereas speech described as thick or slurred points to dysarthria. Usually, the speech abnormality accompanies motor dysfunction, and the pattern of weakness can help clarify whether the patient has dysarthria or aphasia. Theoretically, a patient with a TIA affecting the non-dominant hemisphere could have neglect or other cognitive impairments. Still, the subtle nature of these impairments means that most patients and observers do not recognize the symptoms.

A contralateral homonymous visual field defect can occur with a TIA in the carotid circulation, but such visual symptoms more commonly develop with vertebrobasilar ischemia. The patient usually will describe an inability to see off to one side, and this symptom could be confused with an episode of monocular visual loss.

Vertebrobasilar Arterial Circulation

The symptoms of TIA in the vertebrobasilar circulation can produce ischemia of the brain stem, ear, cerebellum, diencephalon, or posterior cerebral hemispheres. Transient events in the vertebrobasilar circulation are more common in elderly than in young persons.[34] Because of the overlap of the symptoms of posterior circulation TIA with those of global ischemia or pre-syncope that also develop in the elderly, the diagnosis of these events can be difficult. In addition, the variety of symptoms that occur alone or in combination can lead physicians to miss the diagnosis of TIA in the vertebrobasilar circulation. Usually a combination of the symptoms listed in Table 3–4 is reported.

The two most common symptoms are binocular visual disturbances and vertigo. The visual symptoms include a one-sided or bilateral blurring of vision that is described as a distortion in the clarity of vision—a sensation of vision being out of focus. Less commonly, complete loss of vision can happen in either or both the right and left fields. Patients with double vision but without other symptoms usually have a non-vascular cause but, in the presence of other complaints, double vision buttresses the diagnosis of posterior circulation TIA. Many patients have a sense of spinning or whirling (vertigo). Vertigo should be separated from dizziness, dysequilibrium, or lightheadedness.[35,36] Rarely, stroke or TIA can cause isolated vertigo, but in most cases vertigo accompanies other symptoms.[35] It can be accompanied by hearing loss or tinnitus in exceptional circumstances. Because vertigo often is secondary to a number of acute labyrinthine disorders, isolated episodic vertigo usually should not be ascribed to TIA until other causes are excluded.

Motor or sensory symptoms (weakness, numbness, or clumsiness) can be unilateral or bilateral.[37] Localization to the posterior circulation can be difficult if the symptoms are unilateral. Although paresis or sensory loss affecting one side of the body can be confused with ischemia in the carotid circulation, a transient hemiparesis also can be a presentation of an impending basilar artery occlusion.[38] Posterior circulation TIA causing ischemia in the basis pontis may cause recurrent attacks with either right- or left-sided weakness (alternating hemiparesis). Weakness, visual symptoms, or vertigo can be associated with incoordination of the limbs, poor balance, a staggering gait, or dysarthria. A circumoral pattern of numbness can point to pontine ischemia.[37] Numbness of the buccal mucosa, lips, throat, or tongue can occur. Poor balance (ataxia) is a relatively common symptom that patients may describe as dizziness, imbalance, or incoordination. A sudden collapse with weakness of all four limbs (drop attack) has been described as a symptom of vertebrobasilar TIA. These events presumably are due to bilateral ischemia of the basis pontis but are very rare.[39] Distinguishing a drop attack or a seizure from a syncopal attack can be difficult and needs careful review of the event.

The subclavian steal syndrome can induce transient symptoms in the vertebrobasilar circulation and classically is provoked by recurrent arm activities.[40] Blood from the posterior circulation of the brain is diverted to the limb during the activity. Because of the longer length of the left subclavian artery, its occlusion is more commonly associated with subclavian steal syndrome than the right subclavian artery. However, true clinical subclavian steal syndrome is relatively rare in comparison to the number of patients with reversed vertebral flow identified radiologically.[41–43]

Examination of Patients with Suspected Transient Ischemic Attack

The physical examination focuses on the neurological and vascular systems. The general medical examination, including vital signs, provides information about the patient's general health and the presence of risk factors for stroke, such as hypertension. It may provide clues of a non-vascular cause for the patient's symptoms. Assessment of the eyes or ears may provide an alternative explanation for visual symptoms or vertigo. Diabetic or hypertensive changes can be seen on ophthalmoscopic examination.

OCULAR FINDINGS

Detection of a retinal embolus (fibrin-platelet or cholesterol) in a patient with amaurosis fugax is important.[24,44] (Table 3–5.) A fibrin-platelet embolus is seen rarely because it usually disappears quickly, but cholesterol embolus (Hollenhorst plaque) is found more frequently.[45] (See Fig. 3–1.) These highly refractile lesions, located at the bifurcation of retinal arterioles, may persist for days or weeks after the visual symptoms. A cholesterol embolus usually is composed of atherosclerotic debris most commonly arising from an ulcerated plaque of the internal carotid artery or the aorta.[46] Occasionally, a cholesterol embolus can be found in a patient without visual complaints.[44] An asymptomatic or symptomatic cholesterol embolus portends an increased risk for stroke, myocardial infarction, or vascular death, and its incidental discovery should invoke the same response as in a symptomatic patient.[47,48]

Table 3–5. **Ocular Findings of Ischemic Cerebrovascular Disease**

Visual loss
Partial visual field loss
Blindness
Anterior ischemic optic neuropathy
Central retinal artery occlusion
Branch retinal artery occlusion
Retinal pallor
Optic disk atrophy
Hypertensive or diabetic retinopathy
Intra-arterial retinal artery embolus
Fibrin-platelet
Cholesterol debris (Hollenhorst plaque)
Venous stasis retinopathy
Ocular ischemia
Retinal microaneurysms
Retinal hemorrhages
Optic disk edema
Chemosis and conjunctival hyperemia
Glaucoma
Corneal edema
Rubeosis iridis

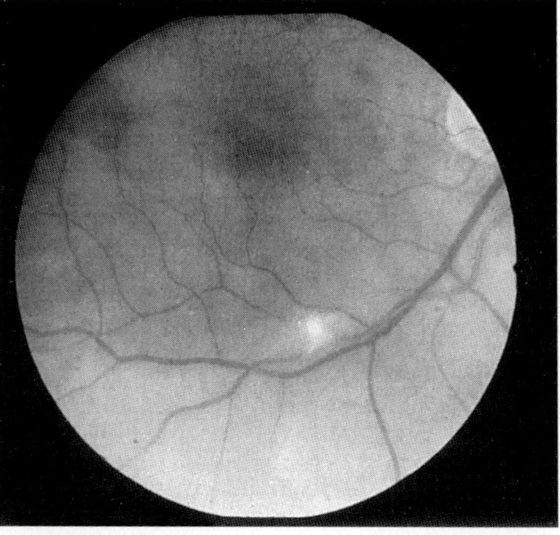

Figure 3–1. Retinal embolus in the optic fundus seen in a patient following an episode of amaurosis fugax.

Venous stasis retinopathy or retinal pallor also can be found. Other ocular abnormalities seen among patients with severe vascular disease include dot/blot microaneurysms; intraretinal hemorrhages; dark, dilated veins; retinal clouding; conjunctival hyperemia; chemosis; glaucoma; rubeosis iridis; corneal edema; and a swollen disk.[29] Anterior ischemic optic neuropathy usually is due to vasculitis rather than carotid artery disease.[49]

VASCULAR EXAMINATION

Asymmetry in blood pressure values or differences in the strength of pulses by palpation between the arms could provide a clue about subclavian steal syndrome as a cause of posterior circulation TIA.[40] Detection of an irregular cardiac rhythm, cardiac murmur, or cardiomegaly can provide support for a cardioembolic cause for TIA. Auscultation of a bruit over the neck or calvarium suggests an arterial cause for a TIA. Although the neurological examination should be normal in a patient with a history of TIA, mild impairments can be found among patients who have had a minor stroke.

A cervical bruit is a marker of generalized atherosclerosis, and it is often heard when examining a patient with a TIA or an ischemic stroke (Table 3–6). The most common location is inferior to the angle of the jaw and just anterior to the sternocleidomastoid muscle. Less common locations for bruits are the supraclavicular region, the posterior aspect of the neck, the tip of the mastoid process, the temple, or the orbit.[50] A diffuse sound over the neck also can be auscultated.[51] Issues related to a carotid artery bruit are described in Chapter 5.

NEUROLOGICAL EXAMINATION

The patient's neurological examination usually is normal. No neurological impairments should be present that could be attributed to the recent cerebrovascular event. If a patient is seen during a TIA, the neurological signs should mimic those found during an acute ischemic stroke. Dissociation between the patient's symptoms and examination findings can occur. For example, the patient may complain of only weakness while sensory loss also is detected on examination.

Table 3–6. **Differential Diagnosis of an Asymptomatic Cervical Bruit**

Atherosclerotic stenosis
Internal carotid artery
External carotid artery
Common carotid artery
Subclavian artery
Augmentation bruit (contralateral carotid occlusion)
Fibromuscular dysplasia
Arterial kink or loop
Transmitted cardiac murmur
Venous hum
High-flow states
Hyperthyroidism
Anemia
Intracranial arteriovenous malformation
Carotid-cavernous fistula
Vascular fistula in the arm (hemodialysis)

DIAGNOSIS OF ISCHEMIC STROKE

A diagnosis of ischemic stroke is based on the patient's history and the findings detected on neurological examination. Occasionally, neurological signs can improve or worsen as the patient is being examined. Because similar neurological abnormalities are found on examining patients with several brain diseases, the history of the illness is critical (Table 3–7). The overall approach to a patient with a suspected ischemic stroke parallels that used for the diagnosis of a patient with a possible TIA.

Clinical Features of Ischemic Stroke

TIME COURSE

The time course of ischemic stroke is usually relatively short. In most instances,

Table 3–7. **Clinical Features of Acute Ischemic Stroke**

Sudden onset of focal neurological signs
- Course of evolution usually <24 hours
- Maximal severity at onset
- Awakening in the morning with signs
- Waxing and waning
- Stepwise or gradual worsening

Neurological signs reflect vascular territory of one artery
- Patterns of individual arteries
- Rarely multifocal or bilateral signs

Consciousness usually preserved
- Coma uncommon
- Can be groggy or drowsy

Can be accompanied by seizures

Can be associated with headache

Can be associated with nausea and vomiting (posterior fossa)

patients seek medical attention within the first hours or days after onset of symptoms. A neurological illness that has evolved over several days or weeks probably is not a stroke. As suggested by the term *stroke,* the symptoms usually begin suddenly. Because many strokes are secondary to acute embolic occlusion, the focal neurological symptoms usually are of maximum severity almost immediately. Still, many patients can have waxing and waning of symptoms, or stepwise or progressive worsening of neurological symptoms, during the first few hours. A stroke can occur at any time during the day and with any activity. However, approximately one-third of patients will have symptoms present on awakening in the morning or shortly thereafter. Because most ischemic strokes do not cause pain, the actual time of onset may not be known if the event occurs during sleep.

CONSCIOUSNESS

With the exception of acute basilar occlusion leading to a massive brain stem infarction, severe disturbances in consciousness are uncommon in the first hours after ischemic stroke. Patients with multilobar hemispheric infarctions can have decreased alertness or act stunned. Patients with non-dominant hemisphere lesions may not comprehend what has happened to them. Confusion, agitation, or restlessness is uncommon. After admission to the hospital, a patient with a severe multilobar infarction can have a decline in consciousness secondary to brain edema or other complications. Neurological worsening after stroke is discussed in Chapter 13.

SEIZURES

Approximately 5% of patients with ischemic stroke will have a seizure at the onset of stroke, but recurrent seizures are uncommon.[52] Status epilepticus is exceptional. Seizures most commonly complicate a cortical infarction secondary to embolism, and they usually occur with cortical or watershed lesions.[53–55] A post-ictal state following a generalized seizure may cause depression in consciousness. Early seizures are not a benign complication.[56] They warrant treatment.

HEADACHE

Headaches are present in approximately 15%–25% of cases and are more common with ischemic events in the posterior circulation.[57–59] (See Fig. 3–2). Although headache is present, it usually is not a primary complaint. The headache usually is unilateral or focal, and it can be severe.[60] Headaches are more common with thrombotic or cardioembolic stroke than with lacunes and are more frequent in women, younger patients, and in those with a past history of stroke.[57,59] Prominent headache, face pain, or nuchal pain also may point to an arterial dissection as the cause of the acute stroke.[61,62] Rarely, facial pain or paresthesias occurs with acute ischemia affecting the spinal nucleus of the trigeminal nerve in the medulla. Allodynia or pain syndromes secondary to the stroke itself usually do not occur during the first hours after the event.

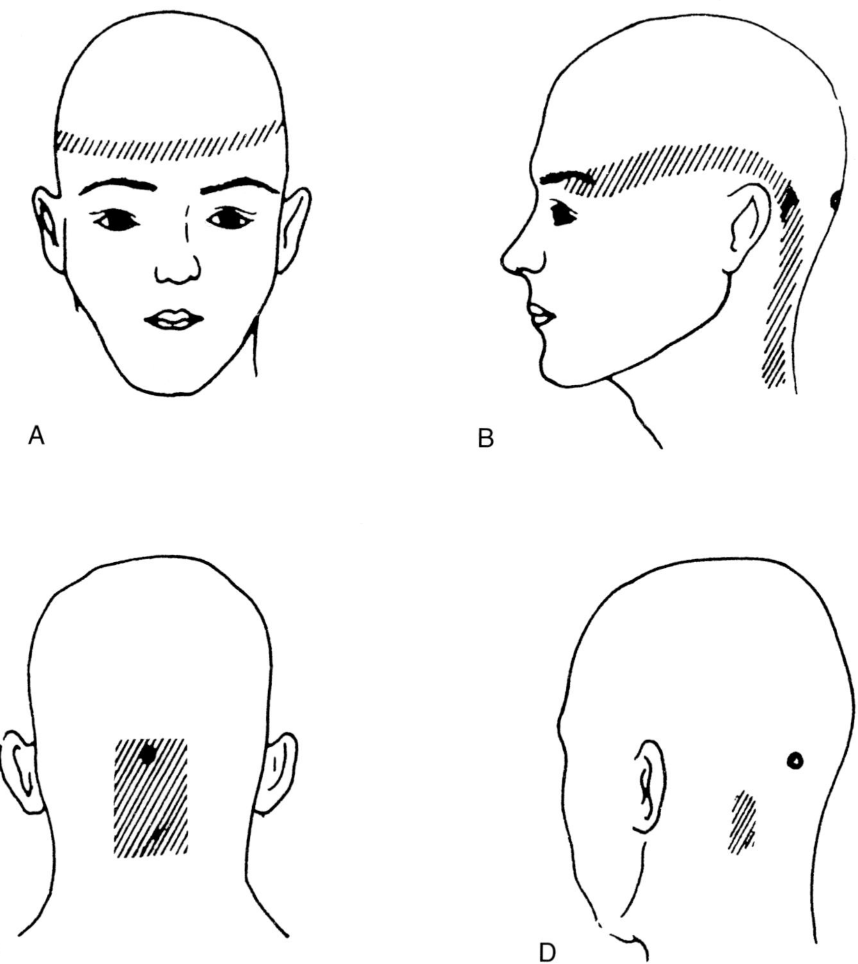

Figure 3–2. Patterns of headache with occlusion of the internal carotid artery (*A*), middle cerebral artery (*B*), basilar artery (*C*), and posterior cerebral artery (*D*). (Reprinted from Fisher, CM. Headache in cerebrovascular disease. In: Vinken PJ, Bruya GW, eds. *Handbook of Clinical Neurology, Vol. 5. Headaches and Cranial Neuralgias.* Amsterdam: North Holland, 1968;124, with permission.)

OTHER SYMPTOMS

Nausea and vomiting are prominent in many patients with ischemic strokes of the brain stem and cerebellum, but these symptoms are distinctly unusual with events in the cerebral hemispheres. The presence of nausea and vomiting in a patient whose focal neurological signs reflect hemispheric dysfunction points to an intracerebral hemorrhage rather than an infarction.

The focal neurological signs reflect the site and size of the ischemic stroke (see Table 3–7). The spectrum of neurological impairments is broad and usually involves a combination of motor, sensory, and cognitive signs. The neurological impairments also mirror the caliber of the occluded intracranial vessel.

Differential Diagnosis of Ischemic Stroke

The differential diagnosis of ischemic stroke is not extensive (Table 3–8). Although 5%–15% of patients first thought to have a stroke subsequently are diagnosed with

Table 3–8. **Differential Diagnosis of Ischemic Stroke**

Hemorrhagic stroke
Intracerebral hemorrhage
Subarachnoid hemorrhage
Intraventricular hemorrhage
Intracranial mass
Subdural hematoma
Brain tumor
Brain abscess
Craniocerebral trauma
Encephalitis
Metabolic disturbances
Hypoglycemia
Seizures with post-ictal neurological impairments

other conditions, most of the other alternatives are neurological diseases that would profit from prompt attention.[63,64] Hemorrhagic stroke is the most important alternative diagnosis because many of the symptoms overlap (Table 3–9). In particular, both illnesses present with sudden development of focal neurological signs that prompt a patient to seek medical attention during the first hours after onset. Differentiating ischemic from hemorrhagic stroke is critical because management of the two diseases contrasts markedly. In general, headache and early depression in consciousness are more likely with hemorrhage.[65] Nausea and vomiting in association with signs that suggest involvement of the cerebral hemisphere also predict bleeding. In contrast, patients with small intraparenchymal hematomas will have no specific clinical findings that would distinguish the bleeding nature of the stroke. The presentations of intraventricular and subarachnoid hemorrhage differ markedly from ischemic stroke; patients with the former have prominent headache and little, if any, focal neurological impairment. The features of both illnesses, including the presence of risk factors, overlap. Imaging of the brain remains the most effective way to differentiate hemorrhagic stroke from ischemic stroke.

Table 3–9. **Clinical Findings Pointing Toward Intracranial Hemorrhage**

Prominent depression in consciousness appears early
Coma
Delirium
Focal neurological signs do not fit one vascular territory pattern
Headache can be chief complaint
Severe nausea and vomiting—particularly if other signs suggest involvement of a cerebral hemisphere
Nuchal rigidity
Unstable vital signs
Marked arterial hypertension

The other components of the differential diagnosis usually can be excluded by a patient's history. For example, the tempo of developing neurological impairments is slower for brain tumors than for stroke. Central nervous system infections usually have prodromal symptoms, and the course of the illness usually evolves over hours to a few days. Hypoglycemia can mimic an ischemic stroke, and it should be considered as an alternative diagnosis in any diabetic patient with acute neurological impairments.[66] Confusion or a disturbance in alertness provides clues for the diagnosis of hypoglycemia. The differential diagnosis of acute ischemic stroke is discussed further in Chapter 12.

Examination of Patients with Ischemic Stroke

Examination of a patient with a suspected stroke is similar to assessing a patient with a TIA, emphasizing evaluation of the heart and the blood vessels. Detection of an asymmetry in pulses or arterial blood pressure, or auscultation of cervical or cranial bruits, is included. The findings on neurological examination are critical for localizing the stroke, which influences prognosis, decisions about the likely cause, acute treatment, rehabilitation, and strategies to prevent recurrent stroke. The components of the emergent examination of a patient

Table 3–10. **General Aspects of the Clinical Findings of Ischemic Strokes of the Cerebral Hemisphere**

Finding	Isolated Subcortical	Branch Cortical	Multilobar
Consciousness	Usually normal	Usually normal	Normal to coma
Cognitive impairments (aphasia, neglect, etc.)	Usually absent	Present	Prominent
Dysarthria	Usually present	Absent	Prominent
Visual field defect	Usually absent	Present	Prominent
Conjugate gaze paresis	Absent	Present	Prominent
Contralateral motor impairments	Arm, leg, and face equal	Arm, leg, and face unequal	Arm, leg, and face equal
Contralateral sensory loss	Same pattern as motor	Same pattern as motor	Same pattern as motor
Motor and sensory loss	Motor without sensory or vice versa	Motor and sensory equal	Motor and sensory equal

with a suspected acute ischemic stroke are discussed in more detail in Chapter 12.

Neurological signs reflect the size and location of the stroke (Table 3–10, Fig. 3–3). Cerebral infarctions are differentiated into lesions that affect the left (dominant), right (non-dominant), or both hemispheres. Hemispheric infarctions also are divided into multilobar, branch cortical, or isolated subcortical lesions. Watershed (border-zone) infarctions at the terminal beds of the anterior, middle, and posterior cerebral arteries can affect one or both hemispheres. Ischemic strokes also affect the brain stem and/or cerebellum. The impairments also mirror the size and vascular territory of the occluded artery. The presence of decreased consciousness, a cranial nerve palsy, nystagmus, prominent ataxia, bilateral motor or sensory signs, prominent dysarthria, or dysphagia points toward an infarction in the vertebrobasilar circulation. Conversely, cognitive or language impairments, visual field defects, or unilateral motor or sensory abnormalities usually are secondary to an infarction of the cerebral hemisphere. Features that differentiate isolated subcortical, branch cortical,

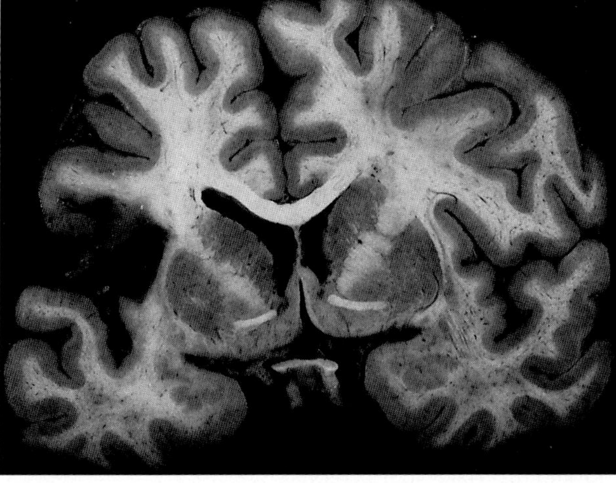

Figure 3–3. Old infarct in the territory of the cortical branches of the left middle cerebral artery. A wedge-shaped area involving the frontal operculum and the insula has been replaced by a cavity transversed by gliovascular strands. (Courtesy of Dr. David Munoz, London Health Sciences Centre)

or multilobar infarctions of the cerebral hemispheres are outlined in Table 3–10.

Stroke Scales

Clinical scales have been developed to help differentiate a hemorrhagic from an ischemic stroke. Unfortunately, these scales have neither the specificity nor the sensitivity to make them useful during the emergent assessment of a patient with an acute ischemic stroke and cannot substitute for brain imaging.[67,68] These scales should not be used as a substitute for computed tomography when deciding about emergent treatment with any agent that affects coagulation. Although these scales might be employed in a situation in which brain imaging cannot be obtained, in general the best strategy is not to use these rating instruments.

Other scales are used to quantify the types and the severity of neurological impairments with ischemic stroke.[69] Most scales involve the addition of scores obtained from individually tested items that are then added to form a total score. The total scores on these scales generally correlate with the severity of the stroke, the size of stroke seen on brain imaging studies, and prognosis. They can be used to influence decisions about treatment.

The most widely used tool is the National Institutes of Health Stroke Scale (NIHSS) (see Table 3–11). The NIHSS has been tested extensively and can be performed successfully by neurologists, other physicians, and other health care professionals.[70–72] The score on the NIHSS correlates with the size of the lesion seen on brain imaging studies.[73] Methods to ensure its reliable use are available.[74] It can be used to predict outcomes and responses to rehabilitation.[70,75–77] A patient with an NIHSS score under 4 has a very high likelihood of an excellent outcome, whereas a patient with a score greater than 20 has less than a 5% probability of making a recovery.[77] The NIHSS score also can be used to influence decisions about treatment. For example, caution is advised when considering administration of tissue plasminogen activator to patients with an NIHSS score greater than 22.[78]

Table 3–11. **Components of the National Institutes of Health Stroke Scale (NIHSS)**

Level of consciousness
- 0—Alert
- 1—Drowsy
- 2—Stuporous
- 3—Comatose

Questions—level of consciousness
- 0—Knows age and month
- 1—Answers one correctly
- 2—Cannot answer either

Commands—level of consciousness
- 0—Follows two commands
- 1—Follows one command
- 2—Cannot follow either command

Best gaze
- 0—Normal eye movements
- 1—Partial gaze palsy
- 2—Forced deviation of eyes

Visual fields
- 0—No visual loss
- 1—Partial hemianopia
- 2—Complete hemianopia
- 3—Bilateral visual field loss

Facial weakness
- 0—Normal symmetrical movement
- 1—Minor unilateral facial weakness
- 2—Partial unilateral facial weakness
- 3—Complete paralysis of one or both sides

Left Arm—motor
- 0—No drift/normal
- 1—Drift of limb
- 2—Some effort against gravity
- 3—No effort against gravity
- 4—No movement

Right Arm—motor
- 0—No drift / normal
- 1—Drift of limb
- 2—Some effort against gravity
- 3—No effort against gravity
- 4—No movement

(Continued on following page)

Table 3–11—*continued*

Left Leg—motor
- 0—No drift / normal
- 1—Drift of limb
- 2—Some effort against gravity
- 3—No effort against gravity
- 4—No movement

Right Leg—motor
- 0—No drift / normal
- 1—Drift of limb
- 2—Some effort against gravity
- 3—No effort against gravity
- 4—No movement

Limb ataxia
- 0—No limb ataxia
- 1—Present in one limb
- 2—Present in two limbs

Sensory examination
- 0—Normal sensation
- 1—Mild-to-moderate sensory loss
- 2—Severe-to-total sensory loss

Best language
- 0—No language impairment
- 1—Mild-to-severe aphasia
- 2—Severe aphasia
- 3—Mute or global aphasia

Dysarthria
- 0—Normal articulation
- 1—Mild-to-moderate dysarthria
- 2—Severe dysarthria

Extinction and inattention
- 0—No abnormality
- 1—Visual or auditory inattention or extinction
- 2—Profound hemi-inattention

MANIFESTATIONS OF ISCHEMIC STROKE OF THE CEREBRAL HEMISPHERES

Internal Carotid Artery Occlusion

Depending on the presence and patency of collateral channels, *occlusion of the internal carotid artery* causes a wide spectrum of clinical presentations. Some patients may have no neurological sequelae, whereas others may have a life-threatening multilobar infarction. Thrombosis at the site of a high-grade atherosclerotic plaque at the origin of the internal carotid artery is the most common cause of an occlusion. Secondary artery-to-artery embolism can occlude distal branches. An infarction usually involves both deep structures in the hemisphere and cortical representation of the anterior choroidal and middle cerebral arteries. In some patients, flow also is diminished in the anterior cerebral and posterior cerebral arteries. The clinical features of an occlusion of the internal carotid artery mimic those of a large stroke in the territory of the middle cerebral artery. Patients with occlusion of the internal carotid artery usually have depressed alertness; contralateral hemiplegia and sensory loss; a conjugate gaze palsy with the eyes deviated toward the affected hemisphere; a contralateral homonymous hemianopia; and prominent behavioral or cognitive impairments, such as neglect or aphasia (Table 3–12).

Table 3–12. **Findings of Multilobar Infarction Secondary to Occlusion of the Internal Carotid Artery or the Proximal Portion of the Middle Cerebral Artery**

- Decreased level of consciousness (drowsiness, stunned, inattentive)
- Contralateral hemiparesis (affecting primarily upper limb and face)
- Contralateral hemisensory loss (affecting primarily upper limb and face)
- Contralateral homonymous hemianopia
- Dysarthria
- Gaze preference away from paresis (toward lesion)
- Global aphasia (dominant)
- Contralateral neglect (either hemisphere but more prominent with non-dominant)
- Apraxia of the non-paralyzed limbs (dominant)
- Construction apraxia, visuospatial disturbances, and topographic disorientation (non-dominant)
- Loss of melody of speech (non-dominant)
- Anosognosia and asomatognosia (non-dominant)

Their NIHSS score likely will be greater than 15. The prognosis of patients with a major stroke following occlusion of the internal carotid artery usually is guarded. They have a high risk for serious brain edema that leads to an increase in intracranial pressure and herniation. These patients also likely will have serious sequelae from their stroke if they survive. In addition, the success of medical therapies is relatively low.

Proximal Middle Cerebral Artery Occlusion

Embolism arising from the heart or proximal extracranial arteries leads to *occlusion of the proximal middle cerebral artery.*[79] (See Fig. 3–4.) Because the middle cerebral artery is the terminal branch of the internal carotid artery, it is the recipient of most emboli in the carotid circulation (Fig. 3–5). Thus, ischemic stroke in the middle cerebral artery territory is the most common clinical stroke syndrome. Although much less common than embolism, thrombosis secondary to a high-grade stenosis of the involved segment also can occur.[80,81] Occlusion before the origin of the lenticulostriate arteries can lead to infarction of both the basal ganglia and the cortex. The findings of a major stroke secondary to occlusion of the proximal portion of the middle cerebral artery mimic those of an internal carotid artery occlusion.[82] Most patients have a combination of motor, sensory, and behavioral abnormalities (see Table 3–12). Patients with major stroke secondary to middle cerebral artery occlusion also have a very poor prognosis.[82] The issues described with occlusions of the internal carotid artery also occur with occlusions of the proximal portion of the middle cerebral artery.

Striatocapsular and Subcortical Lacunar Infarction

Depending on the extent and patency of the pial collaterals, infarction secondary to

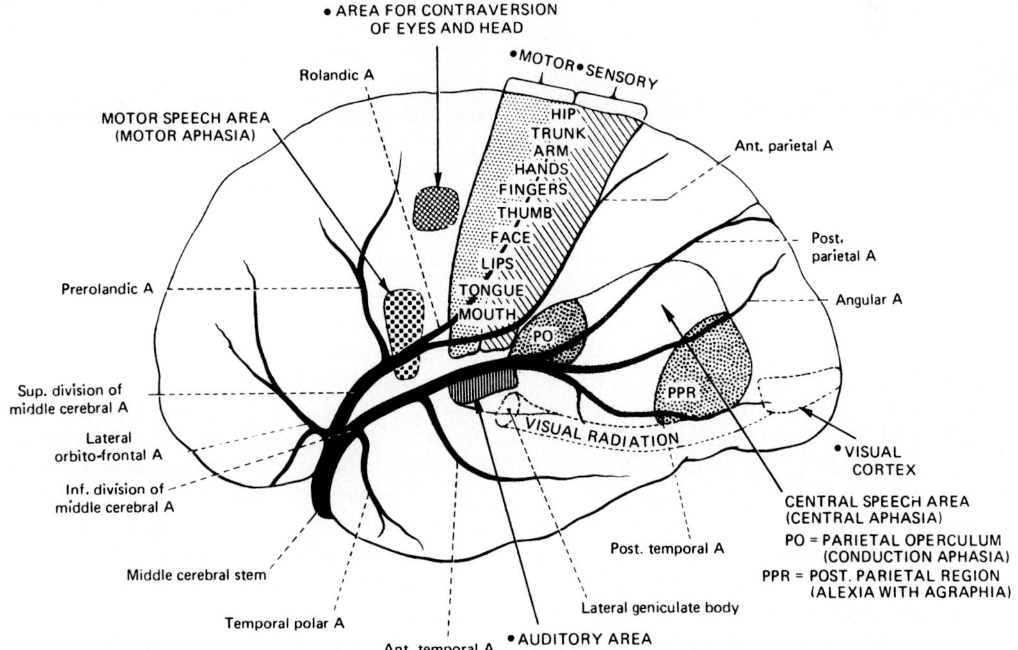

Figure 3–4. Lateral view of the cerebral hemisphere, showing the middle cerebral artery distribution with its corresponding areas of functional localization. (Courtesy of Dr. C.M. Fisher.)

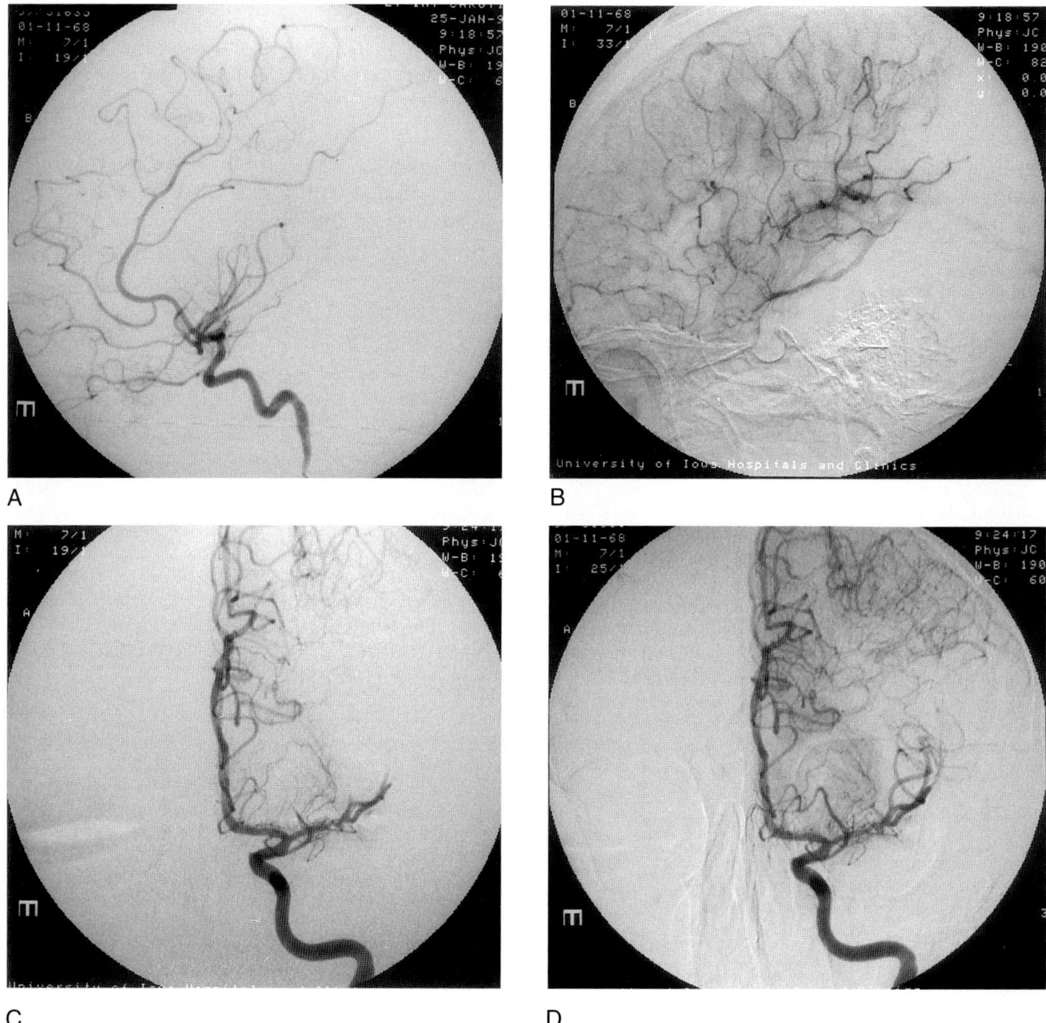

Figure 3–5. Two images of lateral (*A & B*) and anterior-posterior views (*C & D*) using subtraction techniques of a left carotid arteriogram. The middle cerebral artery is occluded at its bifurcation by an embolus (*A & C*). The second film (*B & D*) shows retrograde perfusion of the cortical branches via pial collaterals from the anterior cerebral artery. This patient had an infarction restricted to the insular cortex.

a proximal occlusion of the middle cerebral artery can be restricted to the head of the caudate, the anterior limb of the internal capsule, and the putamen (*striatocapsular infarction*).[83–88] (See Fig. 3–6.) These infarctions account for approximately 1% of all ischemic strokes.[87] This infarction is larger than that seen with occlusion of a single lenticulostriate artery. Most of these strokes are secondary to embolism to that segment of the middle cerebral artery. Patients with striatocapsular infarctions usually have a contralateral hemiparesis involving the arm, leg, and face, and dysarthria, but isolated sensorimotor stroke or hemichorea also may occur.[87,89–92] (See Table 3–13.) A striatocapsular infarction of the dominant hemisphere may cause an atypical aphasia; in the non-dominant hemisphere, a subtle neglect can occur.[93,94] Some patients with large lenticulostriate infarctions likely have associated cortical infarctions, particularly in the insula, that cannot be detected by imaging but that may partially explain behavioral symptoms.[95] The prognosis of

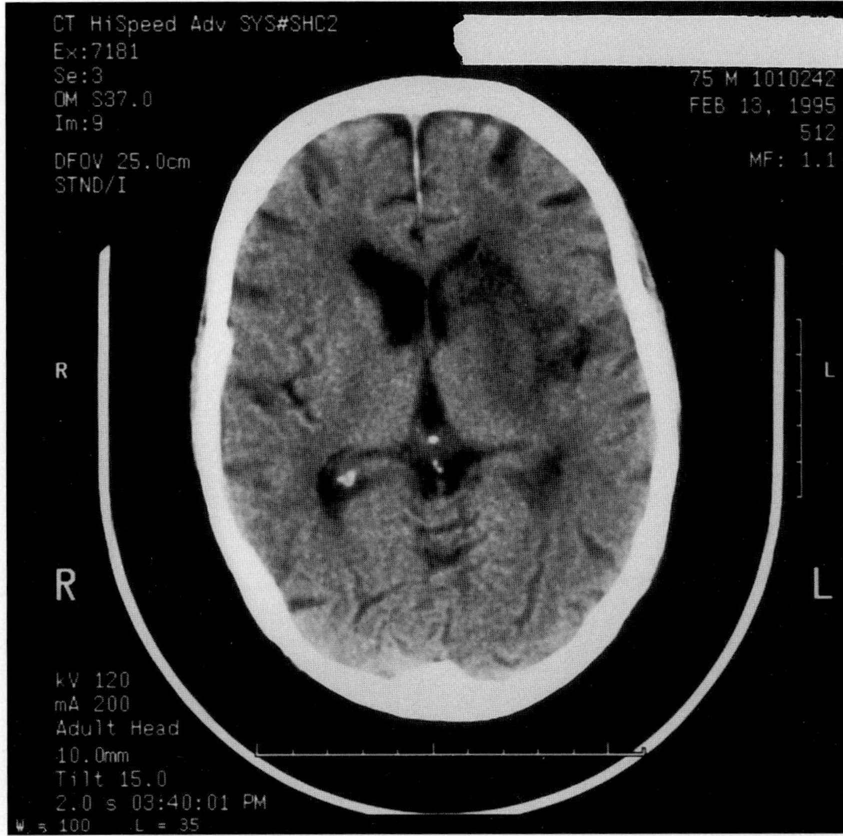

Figure 3–6. A computed tomographic scan is from a patient with a left hemisphere stroke. A large (striatocapsular) infarction is present in the head of the caudate, the anterior limb of the internal capsule, and the putamen.

Table 3–13. **Striatocapsular, Insular, and Watershed Infarctions**

Striatocapsular	*Watershed*
Contralateral hemiparesis (with or without sensory loss)	Contralateral hemiparesis (hand and face relatively spared)
Contralateral sensory loss (usually with motor loss)	Contralateral hemisensory loss (hand and face relatively spared)
Dysarthria	Transcortical motor aphasia (dominant)
Hemichorea	Transcortical sensory aphasia (dominant)
Apathy	Mutism, apathy, abulia (dominant)
Atypical aphasia (dominant)	Anosognosia (non-dominant)
Hemisensory neglect (non-dominant)	*Bilateral Watershed*
Insular	Man-in-the-barrel syndrome
Contralateral weakness of face and hand	Dementia
Conduction aphasia (dominant)	Cortical blindness
Vertigo and contralateral ataxia	

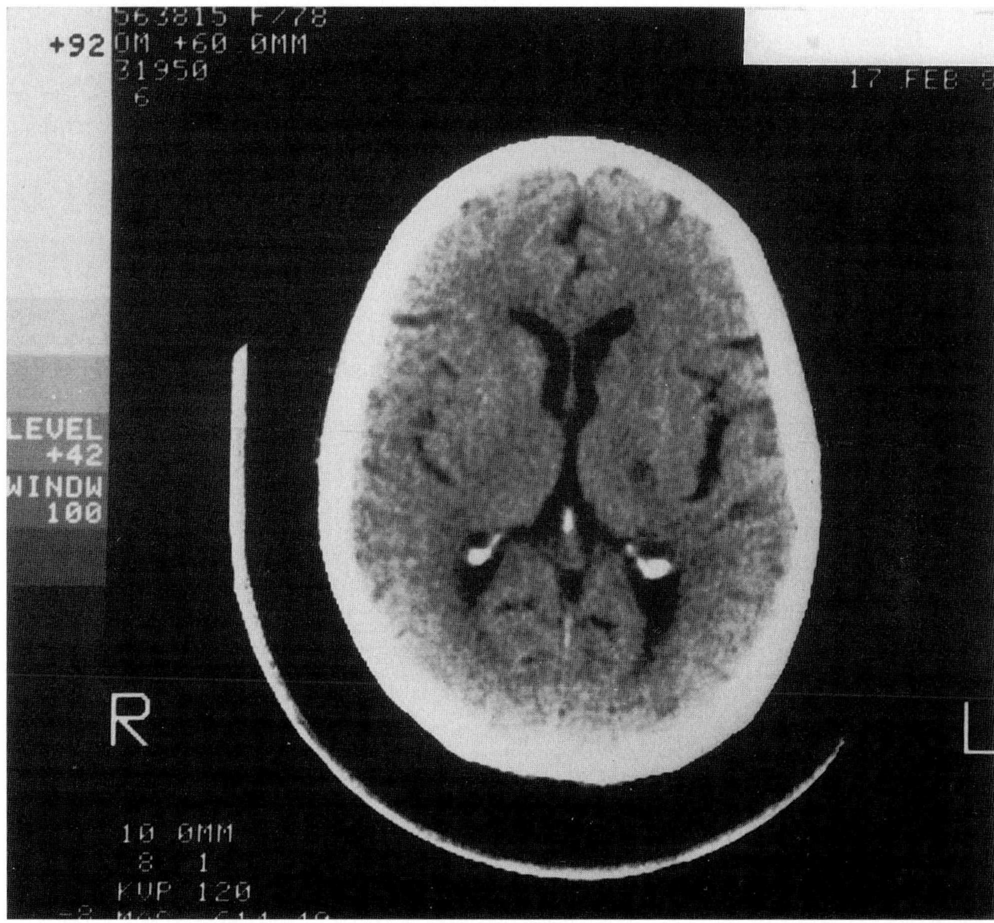

Figure 3–7. A lacunal infarction in the posterior limb of the internal capsule within the territory of the anterior choroidal artery.

patients with striatocapsular infarctions generally is good. In particular, the behavioral and cognitive impairments improve. The presence of a striatocapsular infarction should prompt a search for a source of embolism.

Occlusion of a lenticulostriate branch produces a relatively small *lacunar infarction* in the internal capsule or the basal ganglia (Fig. 3–7). These are leading locations for strokes that produce lacunar syndromes. Patients can present with a contralateral hemiparesis that equally affects the face, upper limb, and lower limb (*pure motor hemiparesis*).[96,97] (See Table 3–14.) Differentiating a pure motor hemiparesis due to a capsular infarction or pontine stroke is not easy.[97] There may be a prominent disturbance in articulation with

Table 3–14. **Infarction Secondary to Occlusion of the Anterior Choroidal Artery**

Contralateral hemiparesis (can occur with or without sensory loss)
Contralateral hemisensory loss (can occur with or without motor loss)
Lacunar syndromes—pure motor hemiparesis, pure sensory stroke, sensorimotor stroke, ataxia-hemiparesis
Contralateral visual field defect
Atypical aphasia, apraxia, or amnesia—dominant
Contralateral neglect—non-dominant

contralateral limb weakness and incoordination (*dysarthria-clumsy hand syndrome*).[98] Less commonly, a contralateral hemiparesis that is more severe in the lower limb and incoordination (*ataxic hemiparesis*) can be detected.[99–101] A lesion of the capsular genu can cause contralateral facial and lingual paresis.[102] A small infarction in the distribution of a lenticulostriate artery also can produce hemichorea.[103]

Occlusion of the Bifurcation of the Middle Cerebral Artery

Occlusion at the *bifurcation of the middle cerebral artery* causes ischemia in the cortex while deep hemispheric structures are preserved (see Fig. 3–7). Embolism is the most common cause for occlusion at this site. An intra-arterial clot in this location is the origin of the "dense middle cerebral artery sign." Ischemic signs include a contralateral hemiparesis and sensory loss with relative preservation of the lower limb. Associated sensorimotor stroke with involvement of the face and arm occurs with cortical lesions.[90] A contralateral homonymous hemianopia or an ipsilateral conjugate paresis can be detected. Language impairments (most often a global aphasia) occur with dominant hemisphere lesions, whereas contralateral neglect, anosognosia, and asomatognosia are found with non-dominant hemisphere strokes.

Insular Infarction

Prominent pial collateral channels can preserve most of the cortex, and the infarction is restricted to the insular cortex. The insular cortex is perfused by short penetrating arterioles that arise from the proximal portions of the major branches. Because the distal territories of the branches receive retrograde perfusion, the proximal vessels become the new "watershed" with impaired perfusion. Patients with an *isolated insular infarction* have motor impairments of the contralateral hand and side of the face. A dominant hemisphere lesion can cause conduction aphasia. Insular cortex lesions also can cause vertigo, nausea, and ataxia.[104] (See Table 3–13.)

Occlusion of Branches of the Middle Cerebral Artery

The superficial (pial) branches of the middle cerebral artery supply most of the lateral surface of the cerebral hemisphere (Fig. 3–8).

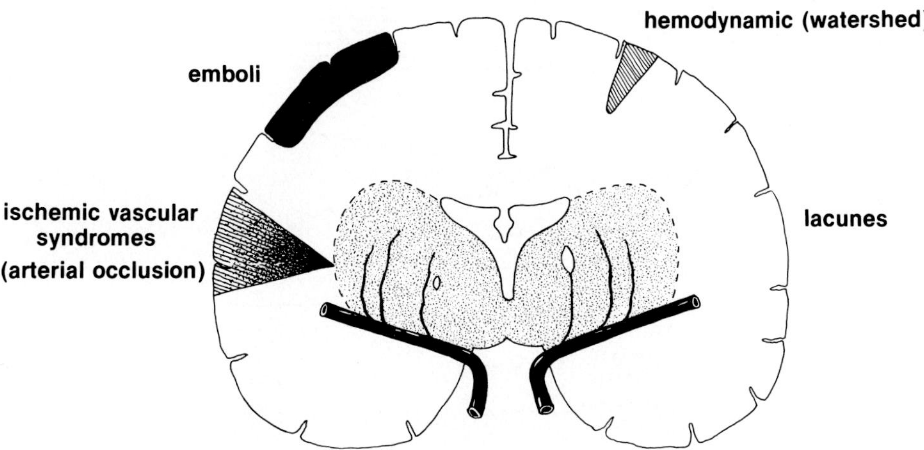

Figure 3–8. Typical locations of types of infarctions of the cerebral hemisphere.

Branch cortical infarctions usually are secondary to embolic occlusion of one or more of these vessels.[105] Clinical manifestations vary according to the number and location of the occluded vessels.[106] Vascular syndromes in the cortical territory of the middle cerebral artery generally are divided into anterior/superior and inferior/posterior territories. In general, anterior/superior strokes involve the frontal lobe, and inferior/posterior strokes involve the parietal and temporal lobes.[107] The presence of a monoparesis usually suggests a cortical infarction.[108] Motor and sensory loss affecting the upper limb and face more than the lower limb without visual field loss are prominent with anterior/superior strokes.[109–111] However, Mohr et al[112] found a relatively poor correlation between cortical convexity localization of the stroke and pattern of limb or facial weakness. Anterior lesions also can produce a conjugate gaze palsy.[110,113] A lesion of the parietal operculum can produce isolated numbness of the face and hand.[114]

Language disturbances (mutism, aphemia, or non-fluent [Broca] aphasia) and buccolingual apraxia occur with dominant hemisphere strokes, whereas neglect is found with strokes in the non-dominant hemisphere (Fig. 3–9). Although contralateral motor and sensory impairments occur with posterior/inferior infarctions, the motor deficits are milder than with the anterior lesions.[107,109] Conversely, the contralateral visual field defect is conspicuous. Fluent aphasia (Wernicke) is found with dominant hemisphere infarctions, whereas neglect, anosognosia, asomatognosia, and constructional apraxia develop among patients with non-dominant lesions.[115]

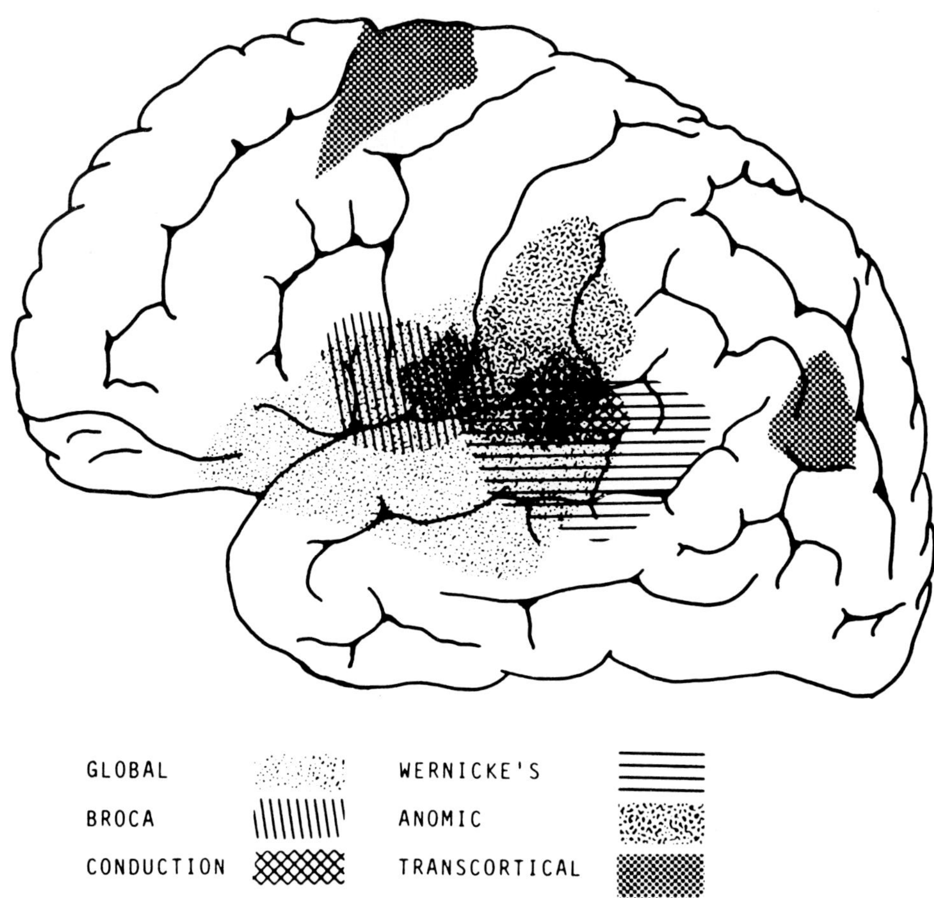

Figure 3–9. Usual sites of lesions producing the different aphasias. (Reprinted from Kertesz A. *Aphasia and Associated Disorders*. New York: Grune and Stratton, 1979;161, with permission.)

Specific neurological impairments correlate with occlusions in discrete cortical branches of the middle cerebral artery.[116] Occlusion of the orbitofrontal branch can produce a frontal lobe syndrome with behavioral and emotional disturbances, forced grasping, and a conjugate deviation of the eyes. Infarction in the distribution of the precentral artery causes weakness of the tongue and lower half of the face and motor aphasia or aphemia. Occlusion of the central branch can produce brachial monoplegia and sensory ataxia. Infarctions in the territory of the posterior parietal, posterior temporal, or angular arteries can cause left–right disorientation, alexia, agraphia, aphasia, acalculia, and sensory loss (Fig. 3–10).

Two areas of cortical infarction can occur in the more anterior and posterior aspects of the vascular territory of the middle cerebral artery.[117] Multiple superficial and/or subcortical infarctions also occur.[118,119] The presumed scenario involves an embolic occlusion of the middle cerebral artery followed by lysis of the clot and secondary distal embolism in two different cortical branches.[119,105] Global aphasia without hemiparesis can result from two areas of infarction in posterior and anterior language areas, with relative preservation of the primary motor cortex.[120]

Borderzone Infarction

Infarctions at the junctions of the terminal branches of the anterior, middle, and posterior cerebral arteries generally are secondary to the combined effects of severe disease of the proximal vessels, microembolism, and hypotension.[121–128,255] (See Figs. 3–11, 3–12.) A unilateral infarction usually is due to a combination of decreased perfusion and embolization.[126] Patients with severe arterial disease have hypoperfusion that hampers the circulation's ability to clear microemboli.[129] Although the infarctions mostly occur in persons with severe stenosis of the internal carotid artery, they also develop in persons with mild-to-moderate

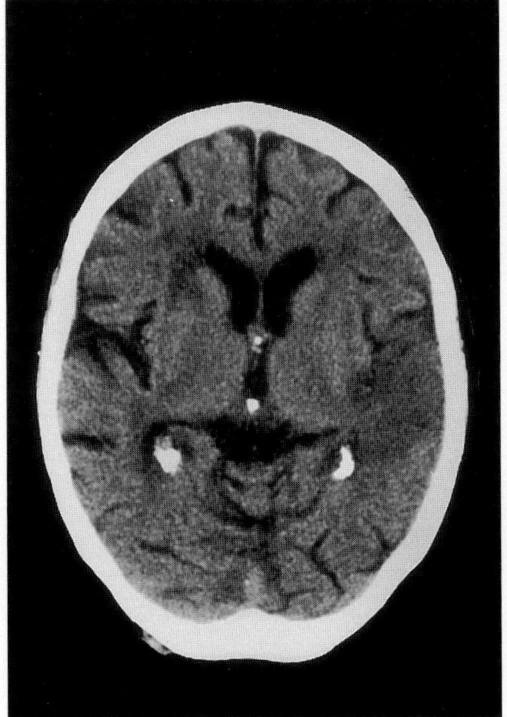
A

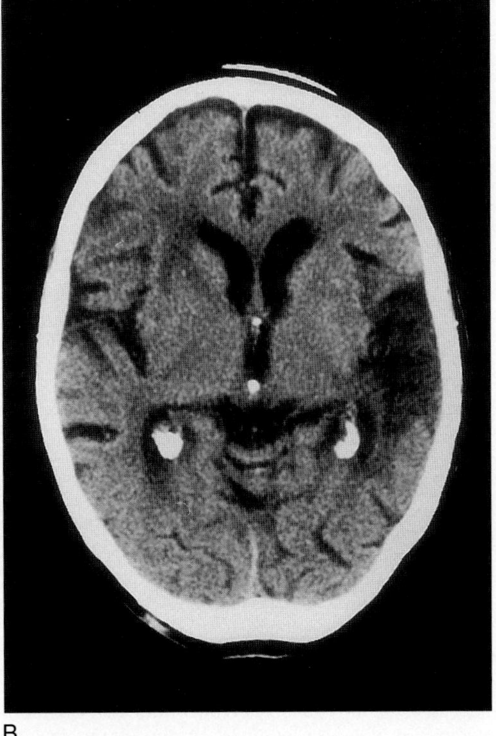
B

Figure 3–10. Evolution of ischemic infarct on CT scan. CT scan showing hypodensity of the left temporal lobe, consistent with an acute infarct (*A*). One year later, the CT scan shows encephalomalacia of the left temporal lobe (*B*). (Courtesy of Dr. D. Lee.)

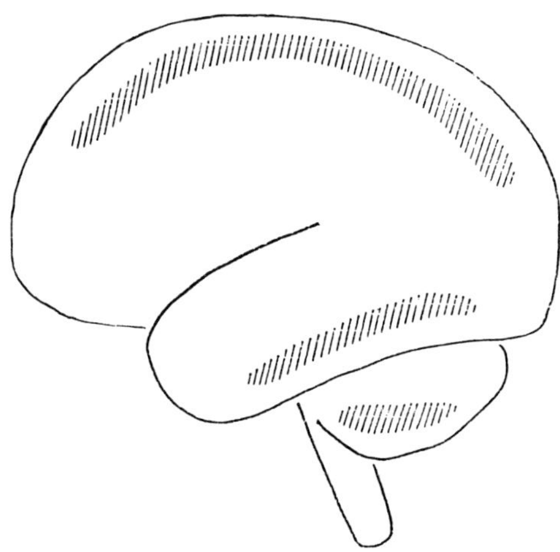

Figure 3–11. Usual locations of borderzone (watershed) infarctions in the cerebral hemisphere or cerebellar hemisphere.

Figure 3–12. FLAIR magnetic resonance imaging shows bilateral watershed infarctions in the border between the anterior and middle cerebral arteries.

narrowing.[124,130] An important factor inducing these strokes is anatomic variations of the circle of Willis, which thus hampers collateral flow.[123] The resulting *borderzone (watershed) infarctions* occur slightly lateral to the mid-sagittal plane in the frontal and parietal lobes.[123] (See Fig. 3–13.) Multiple small infarctions can be scattered in the

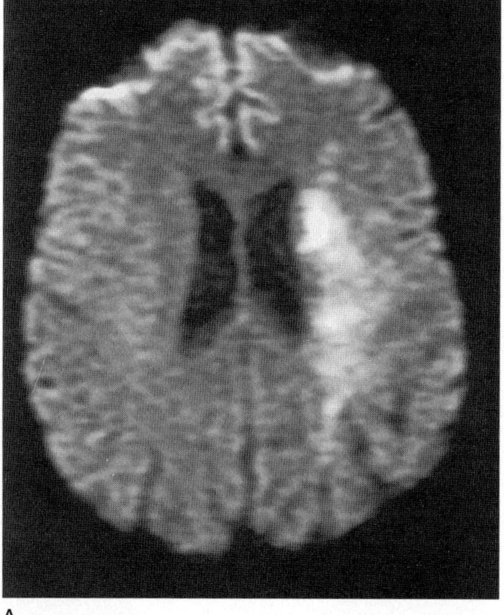

A

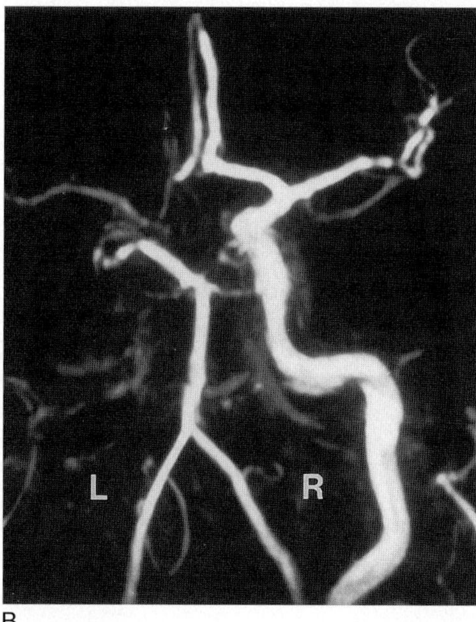

B

Figure 3–13. Left internal carotid artery occlusion and internal borderzone/watershed infarct. This 70-year-old woman with hypertension had fluctuating right hemiparesis and dysphasia. The DWI magnetic resonance image shows an acute internal borderzone/watershed infarct in the left paraventricular region (*A*). On magnetic resonance angiography, there is no signal from the left internal carotid artery suggesting an occlusion or severe stenosis of the artery (*B*). The left middle cerebral is not visualized, whereas the left anterior cerebral artery is probably predominantly supplied by the right anterior cerebral artery and anterior communicating artery. (Courtesy of Dr. B. Silver.)

watershed region.[131] The most common clinical features are contralateral motor and sensory loss sparing the face, with the hand usually less affected less than the shoulder (see Table 3–13). The *man-in-the-barrel syndrome* is caused by bilateral watershed infarctions that result in paralysis of both shoulders with relative preservation of the lower limbs and hands.[132] Bilateral lesions also can cause weakness of the tongue and limbs with relative sparing of the face.[133] Anterior lesions produce motor defects, sensory loss, aphasia, and behavioral signs, whereas posterior lesions cause visual field defects, fluent aphasia, and sensory loss.[94,121,122] Dominant hemisphere watershed infarctions can produce a transcortical motor or sensory aphasia sometimes accompanied by encephalopathy, mutism, or apathy.[134] Bilateral borderzone infarctions usually occur in the setting of severe hypotension.[126] Bilateral infarctions can complicate a major cardiovascular operation during which the patient is treated with extracorporeal circulatory device. Dementia, cortical blindness, prominent motor signs, and pseudobulbar palsy mark bilateral superficial or deep hemispheric infarctions.[126,135]

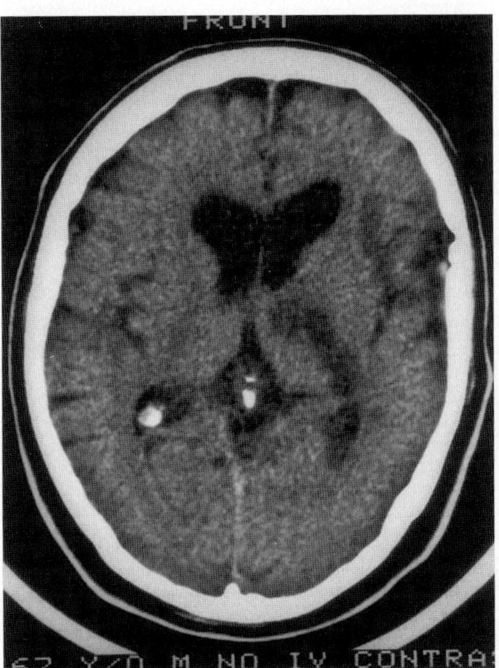

Figure 3–14. Computed tomogram of the brain obtained from a patient with a remote left hemisphere stroke. An area of hypodensity in the posterior limb and genu of the internal capsule and adjacent area of the thalamus. The infarction is compatible with a proximal occlusion of the anterior choroidal artery.

Centrum Semiovale Infarction

Large infarctions restricted to the *centrum semiovale* produce neurological signs that are similar to a multilobar infarction of the middle cerebral artery. In contrast, a small infarction in the centrum semiovale can produce a lacunar syndrome, such as an isolated hemiparesis or hemisensory loss.[136,137] Behavioral signs can be present. Non-dominant hemisphere lesions can produce the symptom of denial of paralysis.[138] In contrast to lesions in the striatum, capsule, and the adjacent portion of the corona radiata that usually are due to disease of the middle cerebral artery, large strokes in the centrum semiovale usually are seen in persons with severe disease of the internal carotid artery.[139–141]

Anterior Choroidal Artery Occlusion

Occlusions of the *anterior choroidal artery* can be secondary to embolism or local artery disease.[85,142–144] (See Fig. 3–14.) The artery perfuses the optic tract, the posterior limb of the internal capsule, the lateral aspects of the thalamus, the medial aspects of the basal ganglia, and the inferior portions of the optic radiations.[145,146] Both small artery disease and embolization can lead to occlusions of the anterior choroidal artery (Fig. 3–15). Infarctions in the territory of the anterior choroidal artery are relatively common, presenting as a lacunar syndrome or a more severe neurological syndrome (Table 3–14). Signs include a contralateral hemiparesis, sensory loss, dysarthria, a visual field defect, and behavioral abnormalities.[89] The combination of moderate motor and sensory impairments that affect the face and the limbs without causing cognitive or behavioral abnormalities should point to an infarction involving the posterior limb of the internal capsule and adjacent thalamus in the vascular territory of the

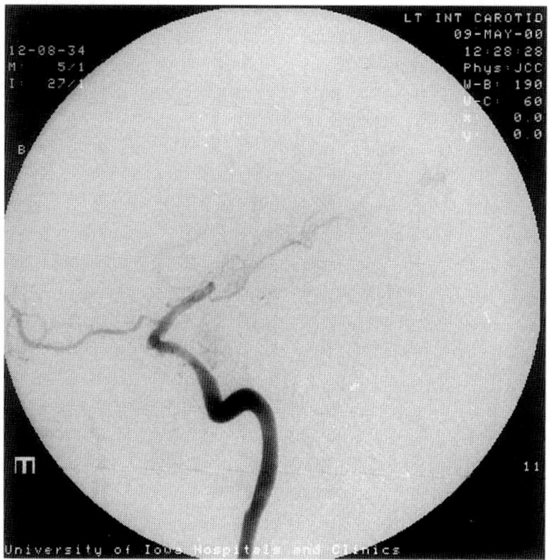

Figure 3–15. A lateral view of a left internal carotid arteriogram shows distal occlusion of the internal carotid artery. Both the ophthalmic artery (anterior) and the anterior choroidal artery (posterior) are well visualized.

anterior choroidal artery. Infarction of the lateral geniculate nucleus can cause loss of vision in the contralateral upper and lower fields with relative preservation of vision at the horizon.[144] This visual disturbance, which is called a *homonymous sectoranopsia,* is very uncommon. The lacunar syndromes include isolated motor deficits, a marked dysarthria, a combination of a mild hemiparesis and sensory loss (*motor/sensory stroke*), or an ataxic hemiparesis due to involvement of the caudal portion of the posterior limb of the internal capsule and adjacent parts of the corona radiata.[92,147,148] (See Table 3–15.) Presumably, the ataxic motor deficits are secondary to a loss of positional sense. The visual impairments include a homonymous hemianopia, a quadrantic field defect, or a sector visual field loss. Language impairments can accompany dominant hemisphere lesions, whereas visuospatial impairments, neglect, and constructional apraxia can be found with infarctions in the non-dominant hemisphere.

Anterior Cerebral Artery Occlusion

Infarctions in the distribution of the *anterior cerebral artery* are much less common than in the middle cerebral artery territory (Fig. 3–16). Stenotic disease of the proximal anterior cerebral artery or its branches occurs in patients with generalized intracranial atherosclerosis, but occlusions are more

Table 3–15. **Lacunar Syndromes**

Syndrome	Impairments	Localization
Pure motor hemiparesis	Contralateral hemiparesis	Internal capsule
	Arm, leg, face affected	Pons
	Dysarthria	Pyramid–medulla
	No sensory loss	Corona radiata
Pure sensory stroke	Contralateral hemisensory loss	Lateral thalamus
	Arm, leg, face affected	
	No motor loss	
Sensorimotor stroke	Contralateral hemiparesis	Posterior limb of internal capsule
	Contralateral hemisensory loss	Adjacent thalamus
Dysarthria-clumsy hand	Prominent dysarthria	Pons
	Mild facial weakness	Genu of internal capsule
	Clumsiness of the hand	
Hemiparesis—homolateral ataxia	Arm and leg ataxia	Pons
	Leg weakness—ankle	

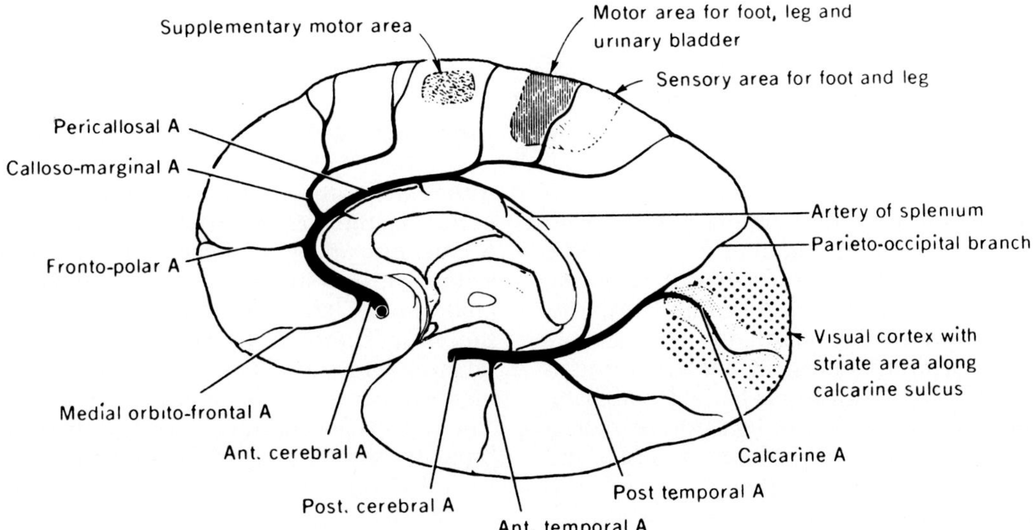

Figure 3–16. Medial view of the cerebral hemisphere, showing the distributions of the anterior and posterior cerebral arteries with their corresponding areas of functional localization. (Courtesy of Dr. C.M. Fisher.)

commonly secondary to embolism. Vasospasm following rupture of an anterior communicating artery aneurysm and subarachnoid hemorrhage is a relatively common cause of unilateral or bilateral infarctions in the anterior cerebral artery circulation. The anterior cerebral artery perfuses the medial and inferior aspects of the frontal lobe, most of the corpus callosum, the anterior diencephalon, a portion of the caudate nucleus, part of the anterior limb of the internal capsule, and the parasagittal surface of the parietal lobe.[149,150] The deep structures are largely perfused from the *recurrent artery of Huebner*, which arises from the first portion of the anterior cerebral artery. Small branches of the anterior cerebral artery and the anterior communicating artery also supply blood to the anterior hypothalamus, basal forebrain, fornix, and lamina terminalis.[83] An occlusion of the recurrent artery of Huebner causes a lacunar stroke that leads to a hemiparesis and dysarthria or the combination of paresis and limb ataxia.[151] In addition, abulia, agitation, or hyperactivity can complicate infarctions in the caudate nucleus.[13,149] (See Table 3–16.) The neurological findings of occlusion of the proximal portion of the anterior cerebral artery include a hemiparesis and sensory loss that

Table 3–16. **Infarction Secondary to Occlusion of the Anterior Cerebral Artery**

Unilateral

- Contralateral hemiparesis (affecting primarily the lower limb)
- Contralateral hemisensory loss (affecting primarily the lower limb)
- Ipsilateral limb apraxia
- Impairment in bowel or bladder control
- Transcortical motor aphasia (dominant)
- Contralateral spatial neglect (non-dominant)
- Abulia or apathy (dominant or non-dominant)
- Euphoria or disinhibition (dominant or non-dominant)
- Impaired executive function (dominant or non-dominant)

Bilateral

- Bilateral hemiparesis (affecting primarily the lower limbs)
- Bilateral hemisensory loss (affecting primarily the lower limbs) (the motor and sensory signs can mimic a paraparesis, or “spinal” sensory level)
- Severe impairment of bowel or bladder control
- Akinetic mutism
- Prominent disturbances in affect

involves the lower limb more often than the upper.[152,153] In general, the leg is affected more than the arm, which, in turn, is impaired more than the face and tongue.[154,155] A paraparesis can be seen in association with bilateral anterior cerebral artery strokes. Urinary and fecal incontinence also are found among patients with large infarctions. Dominant hemisphere strokes produce transcortical aphasia, apraxia, mutism, abulia, and apathy, whereas non–dominant hemisphere lesions cause neglect, confusion, abulia, and apathy.[94,152,153,155] Bilateral frontal and basal forebrain ischemia produce severe behavioral disorders, including amnesia and akinetic mutism.[156] (See Table 3–16.) Infarctions of the corpus callosum, secondary to occlusion of distal branches of the anterior cerebral artery, lead to a disconnection syndrome of apraxia, agraphia, and alien hand.[157]

Posterior Cerebral Artery Occlusion

Although localized atherosclerotic disease occurs in the *posterior cerebral artery*, most occlusions of the posterior cerebral artery or its branches are secondary to embolism.[158] (See Fig. 3–17.) Because the posterior cerebral arteries serve as the terminal vessels of the basilar artery, involvement of both vessels is common. The posterior cerebral artery and its deep branches supply most of the thalamus, the rostral brain stem, the occipital lobe, and the medial aspects of the temporal and parietal lobes (see Figs. 3–16 and 3–18). Clinical findings vary depending on the

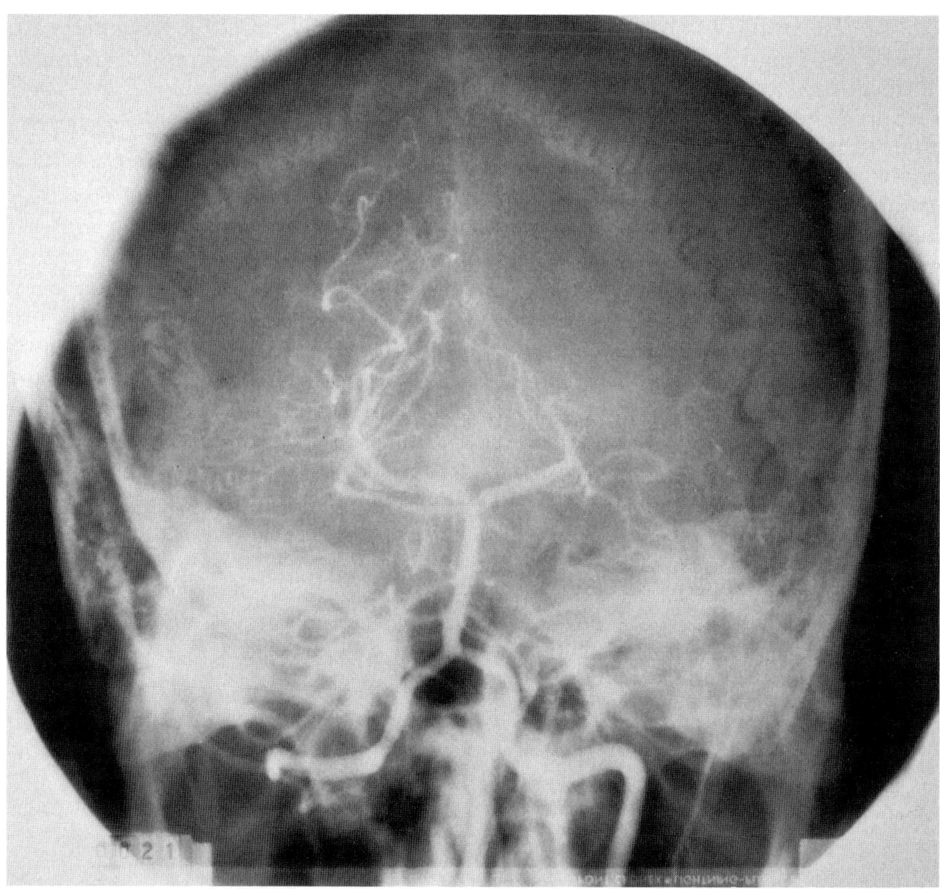

Figure 3–17. Distal occlusion of the left posterior cerebral artery.

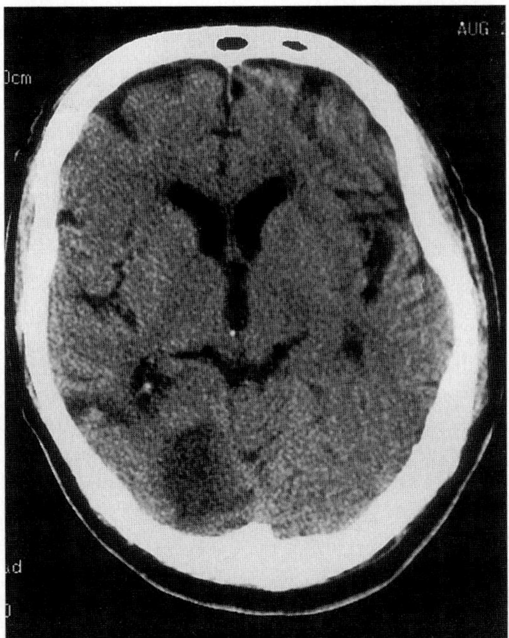

Figure 3–18. A computed tomographic scan of the brain done without contrast reveals a right occipital lobe infarction in the distribution of the cortical branches of the posterior cerebral artery. (Courtesy of AJ Fox, MD, London Health Sciences Center, London, Ontario.)

Table 3–17. **Infarction Secondary to Occlusion of the Posterior Cerebral Artery**

Unilateral—Distal
- Contralateral homonymous hemianopia
- Visual hallucinations or metamorphopsias
- Alexia (dominant)
- Transcortical sensory aphasia (dominant)
- Hemiachromatopsia (dominant)
- Memory disturbances (dominant or non-dominant)
- Visual hemineglect (non-dominant)

Unilateral—Proximal
- The above findings
- Contralateral hemiparesis
- Contralateral hemisensory loss

Bilateral
- Bilateral visual loss
- Cortical blindness
- Anton's syndrome
- Balint's syndrome
- Prosopagnosia
- Severe amnesia

location of the occlusion. With a proximal occlusion of the posterior cerebral artery, behavioral disturbances, contralateral motor and sensory impairments, and a visual field abnormality are found.[159–161] (See Table 3–17.) Neurological impairments can appear similar to those seen with a proximal middle cerebral artery occlusion.[162] Visual dysfunction without other complaints is prominent with more distal occlusion of the posterior cerebral artery or its branches. Headaches, dizziness, nausea, and vomiting are common symptoms.

A contralateral homonymous hemianopia is the most common finding in patients with a superficial infarction in the territory of the posterior cerebral artery. Occasionally, sparing of central (macular) vision is found. A contralateral inferior or superior quadrantanopia is detected when the infarction is restricted to the supra- or infracalcarine cortex. Achromatopsia, which can be a quadrantic or hemi-field defect, is found if the lingual and fusiform gyri are infarcted. Visual neglect is found with large infarctions of the non-dominant occipital lobe and adjacent aspects of the parietal and temporal lobes. A large dominant hemisphere posterior cerebral infarction that extends into the splenium of the corpus callosum can produce the syndrome of alexia without agraphia in combination with a contralateral homonymous hemianopia. Visual hallucinations, visual perseverations, and visual distortions also can occur. Bilateral superficial infarctions can cause complex visual-behavioral disturbances, including cortical blindness, Anton's syndrome, prosopagnosia, and Balint's syndrome.[163] The hallmark of Anton's syndrome is the patient's assertion that he or she can still see despite obvious blindness. An inability to see a full field of vision at one time (simultanagnosia), poor hand–eye coordination (optic ataxia), and an inability to fixate the eyes on an object (apraxia of gaze) mark

Balint's syndrome. Bilateral temporal lobe ischemia can cause an agitated delirium. Occasionally, patients with a superficial posterior cerebral artery infarction in the dominant hemisphere can have a transcortical aphasia. A visual agnosia can been found with a non-dominant hemisphere stroke.

Thalamic Infarction and Top-of-the-Basilar Occlusion

The proximal portion of the posterior cerebral artery gives rise to several small vessels that provide blood to the thalamus and the rostral brain stem.[85] Isolated thalamic infarctions result from occlusion of the thalamogeniculate or posterior choroidal arteries arising from the posterior cerebral artery, the tuberothalamic branches of the posterior communicating artery, and the interpeduncular-thalamic artery, that usually arises from the distal basilar artery.[164] Strokes in the distribution of these vessels produce distinct clinical findings that mimic some of the features of the lacunar syndromes, including pain, pure sensory stroke, or ataxia-hypesthesia (Table 3–18).[106,136,164–170] (See Fig. 3–19.) Paramedian thalamic strokes can cause hypersomnolence with prolonged periods of sleeping, but sensory and motor deficits are less pronounced.[171] Paramedian

Table 3–18. **Vascular Syndromes of the Thalamus**

Artery	Areas Affected	Clinical Findings
Thalamogeniculate	Inferolateral thalamus	Contralateral hemisensory loss Limb incoordination or hemiataxia Dystonic posturing Involuntary movements Thalamic pain syndrome
Interpeduncular-thalamic Unilateral infarction	Paramedian thalamus	Decreased consciousness Disorientation Memory loss Impaired vertical gaze Dystonia or tremor Aphasia (dominant) Neglect (non-dominant)
Bilateral infarctions	Paramedian thalamus	Coma Amnesia Loss of sleep-wake cycle Aphasia Neglect Vertical gaze palsy Ataxia
Posterior choroidal	Pulvinar lateral geniculate	Contralateral hemisensory loss Contralateral mild hemiparesis Contralateral visual field defect Sector or quadrantic visual fields
Tuberothalamic or polar	Ventral anterior thalamus	Abulia and amnesia Aphasia (dominant) Mild contralateral hemiparesis Mild contralateral hemisensory loss

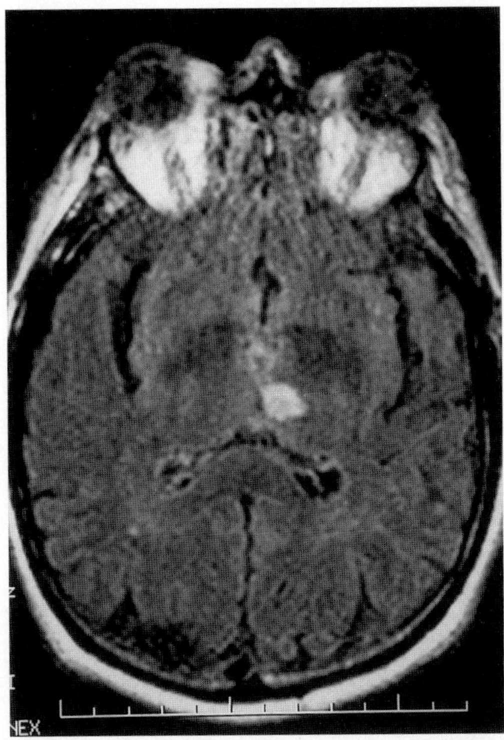

Figure 3–19. FLAIR Magnetic Resonance Image demonstrates an infarction of the medial aspect of the thalamus in the distribution of the interpeduncular thalamic artery.

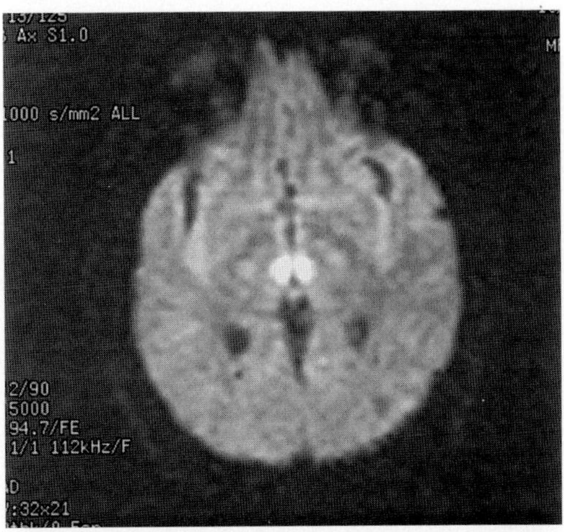

Figure 3–20. Diffusion weighted magnetic resonance imaging demonstrates mirror lesions in the medial aspects of the thalamus bilaterally. The findings are compatible with an occlusion of the interpedincular thalamic artery (thalamoperforating). This patient had symptoms described in Table 3–18.

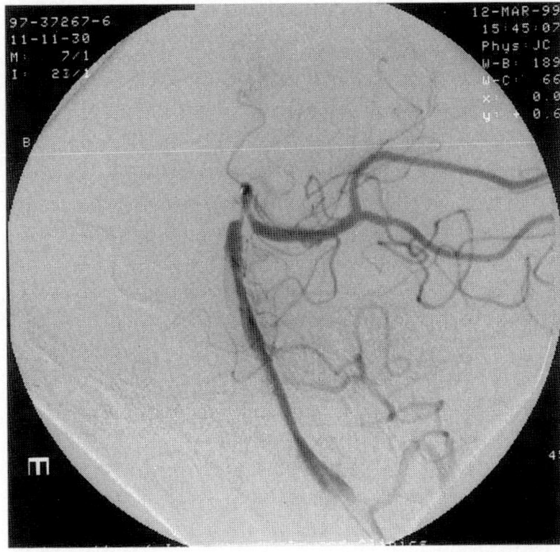

Figure 3–21. Lateral view of a left vertebral arteriogram demonstrates embolic occlusion of the distal basilar artery.

thalamic infarctions can cause disinhibition and exaggerated responses to stimuli—findings that mimic a frontal lobe lesion.[172] (See Fig. 3–20.) Astasia and an inability to sit in the presence of little motor or sensory loss also occur in association with thalamic infarctions.[173] Infarctions in the dominant thalamus can produce an aphasia that is marked by anomia, verbal paraphasias, perseveration, jargon speech, and decreased comprehension.[174] Some of the behavioral signs may be secondary to deafferentation of the cortex.[175] Anterior thalamic infarctions also cause prominent behavioural signs including severe perseveration, memory problems, naming problems, and apathy.[256]

Combined deep and superficial infarctions in the territories of both posterior cerebral arteries can be secondary to embolism of the distal basilar artery (*top-of-the-basilar syndrome*).[176] (See Fig. 3–21 and Table 3–19.) Most patients have a decline in consciousness with waxing and waning alertness, monotonous speech, memory impairments, disturbed vertical eye movements, pupillary abnormalities, and visual field defects.[176–182] The memory and learning impairments persist.[183] Bilateral involvement produces more profound behavioral deficits than unilateral infarctions.[179,180,182]

Table 3–19. **Infarctions of the Mesencephalon and the Top-of-the-Basilar Syndrome**

Abnormalities in consciousness
Memory disturbances
Akinetic mutism
Ipsilateral oculomotor nerve paralysis
Bilateral weakness of the levator palpebrae and superior rectus
Impaired vertical gaze
Contralateral hemiparesis
Contralateral sensory loss
Ipsilateral or contralateral limb ataxia
Flapping tremor

Posterior Choroidal Artery Occlusion

The posterior choroidal artery supplies the lateral geniculate nucleus, pulvinar, posterior portions of the thalamus, and the hippocampus. It can be occluded secondary to small artery disease or embolism that affects the basilar or posterior cerebral arteries. The most common abnormalities include a sectoranopsia, quadrantic visual field defect, aphasia, and memory loss.[184] Some of the findings mimic those found with occlusions of the anterior choroidal artery.

MANIFESTATIONS OF ISCHEMIC STROKE IN THE BRAIN STEM AND CEREBELLUM

The manifestations of ischemic stroke in the vertebrobasilar circulation reflect the affected level of the brain stem and the extent of cerebellar involvement (Table 3–20 and Fig. 3–22). Occlusion of the vertebral artery and its branches secondary to a local arterial process, such as a dissection or atherosclerosis, usually causes infarction in the medulla or inferior cerebellum.[185–187] Bilateral distal vertebral occlusions cause low flow in the posterior circulation, leading to a stepwise deterioration reflecting ischemia in the brain stem and the cerebellum.[188] Thrombotic or embolic occlusion of the basilar artery or its major branches can lead to ischemia of the pons, the midbrain, and the cerebellum.[185] Occlusion of a small penetrating artery from the basilar artery can lead to a lacunar syndrome. Multiple areas of infarction can occur simultaneously in the posterior circulation.[189]

Medullary Infarction and Posterior Inferior Cerebellar Artery Occlusion

A common brain stem stroke is caused by infarction of the dorsolateral medulla (*Wallenberg's syndrome*), which usually is secondary to occlusion of the vertebral artery. The dorsolateral medulla receives most of its blood supply from small penetrating arteries arising from the vertebral artery rather than from the posterior inferior cerebellar artery (PICA). In contrast, infarction of the inferior cerebellum

Table 3–20. **Infarctions in the Medial and Dorsolateral Medulla**

Lateral Medullary Syndrome of Wallenberg
Ipsilateral facial pain and numbness
Ipsilateral palatal paresis
Ipsilateral vocal cord paralysis with hoarseness of voice
Ipsilateral Horner's syndrome
Contralateral body sensory loss to pain and temperature
Skew deviation
Ipsilateral tonic deviation of eyes
Ipsilateral horizontal, gaze-evoked nystagmus
Gait ataxia with ipsilateral lateropulsion
Ipsilateral dysmetria, dyssynergia, dysdiadokinesia
Hiccups
Medial Medullary Infarction
Ipsilateral tongue weakness
Contralateral hemiparesis
Contralateral sensory loss to fine touch and proprioception
Bilateral Medullary Infarction
Quadriparesis
Bilateral tongue paralysis

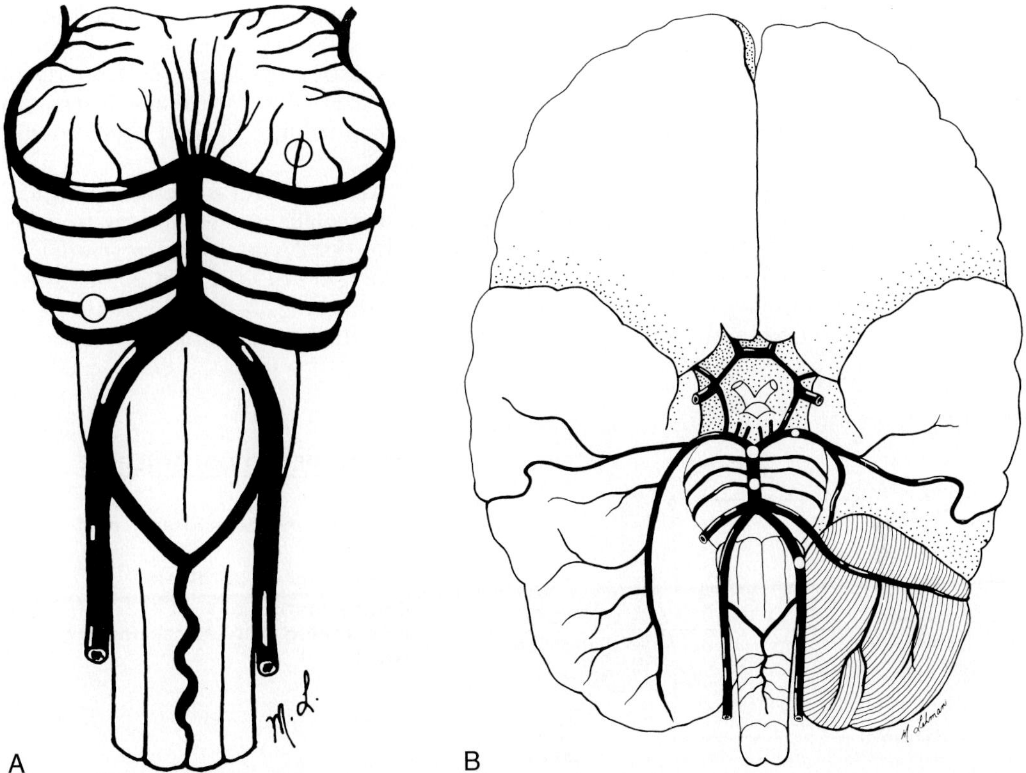

Figure 3–22. The segmental vascular supply to the brainstem (*A, B*). Open circles indicate sites of thromboembolism in the vertebrobasilar system.

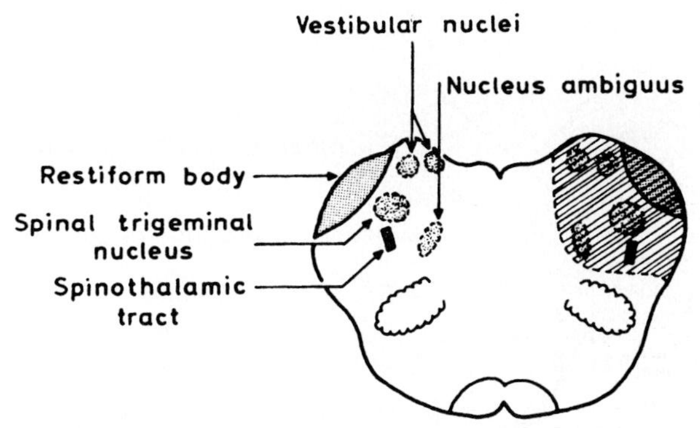

LATERAL MEDULLARY SYNDROME

1. Loss of pain and temperature sensations over the ipsilateral face and contralateral half of the body
2. Ataxia (loss of coordination)
3. Vertigo
4. Loss of gag reflex, difficulty in swallowing and difficulty in articulation
5. Ipsilateral Horner's syndrome
6. Vomiting

Figure 3–23. Structures involved in a dorsolateral medullary infarction. (Reprinted from Afifi AK, Bergman RA. *Basic Neuroscience*. Baltimore: Urban & Schwarzenberg, 1980;133–134, with permission.)

secondary to occlusion of the PICA often accompanies ischemia of the dorsolateral medulla.[190–192] (See Fig. 3–23.) In exceptional cases, the caudal pons also is affected.[193] On examination, patients have ipsilateral vocal and palatal paralysis, ipsilateral facial sensory loss, an ipsilateral Horner' syndrome, and sensory loss to pain and temperature on the opposite side of the body (Table 3–20). Occasionally, patients can exhibit a loss of vibratory and position sense due to involvement of the posterior columns or crossing fibers.[194] Headache, nausea, vomiting, vertigo, hiccups, facial pain, and facial weakness can occur.[190,195,196] Eye movement abnormalities include a skew deviation, horizontal gaze-evoked nystagmus, hypermetric saccades to the affected side and tonic deviation of the eyes toward the involved side.[197,198] Incoordination of the ipsilateral limbs, truncal and gait ataxia, and horizontal nystagmus are secondary to cerebellar ischemia in the PICA territory.[199] Isolated cerebellar infarction in the PICA territory presents with imbalance; dysmetria, dyssynergia, and dysdiadochokinesia of the ipsilateral arm and leg; lateropulsion; vertigo; and nystagmus.[190,200]

Unilateral or bilateral medial medullary infarctions usually are secondary to occlusion of the distal vertebral artery adjacent to the origin of the anterior spinal artery.[201] (See Fig. 3–24 and Table 3–20.) The classic abnormalities of this uncommon

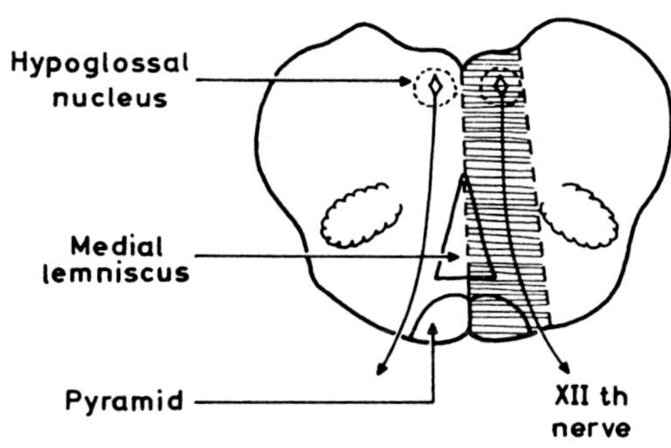

Figure 3–24. Structures involved in a medical medullary infarction. (Reprinted from Afifi AK, Bergman RA. *Basic Neuroscience.* Baltimore: Urban & Schwarzenberg, 1980;133–134, with permission.)

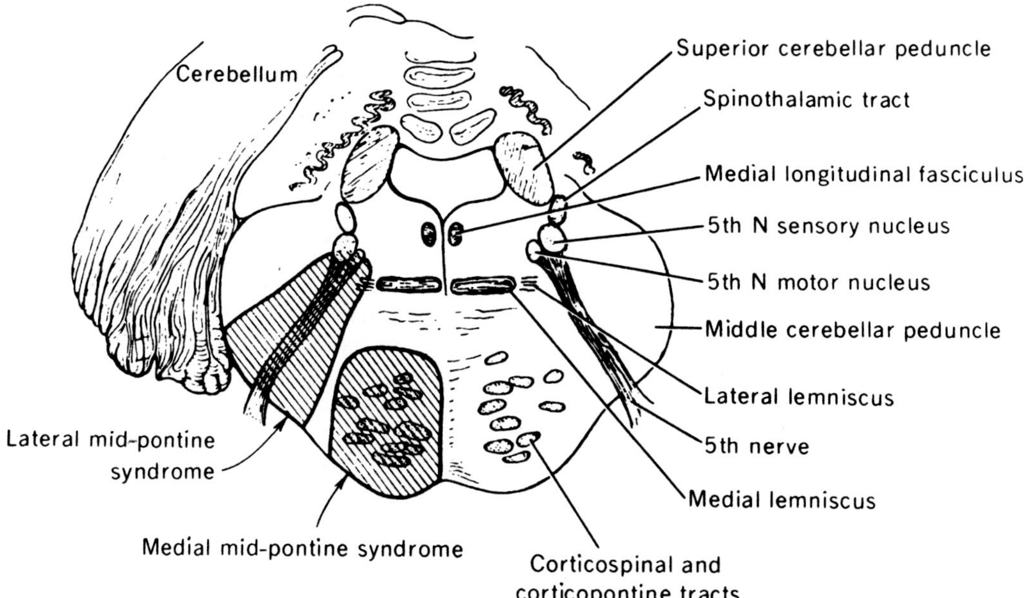

Figure 3–25. Structures involved in a medial medpontine and lateral midpontine infarction. (Courtesy of Dr. C.M. Fisher.)

location of stroke include gaze-evoked nystagmus, contralateral loss of vibratory and position sense, and contralateral hemiparesis combined with ipsilateral hypoglossal nerve palsy.[201–203] A unilateral pure motor hemiplegia can result from a pyramidal infarction.[204] With bilateral infarction, the patient has quadriplegia and complete tongue paralysis. Because corticospinal fibers that innervate the upper and lower limbs cross at different levels in the pyramidal decussation, an infarction can result in paralysis of the ipsilateral arm and the contralateral leg.

Pontine Infarction and Anterior Inferior Cerebellar Artery Occlusion

The size and location of pontine infarctions correlate with the likely cause; a lesion extending the surface of the base of the pons to the tegmentum usually is due to large artery disease, whereas small, deep lesions usually are lacunes.[205] Small pontine infarctions usually are due to occlusion of a short penetrating branch arising from the basilar artery.[206,207] (See Fig. 3–25.) These infarctions, which can be located in the tegmentum or the base, usually are secondary to primary small artery disease. They lead to lacunar syndromes, including pure motor hemiparesis, dysarthria-clumsy hand, ataxia-hemiparesis, pure sensory stroke, or a sensorimotor stroke.[96,98–100,154,166,207–211] (See Table 3–14.) A patient with a pure motor paresis secondary to a pontine infarction is more likely to have dysarthria, gait instability, and vertigo than a patient with a capsular stroke.[97,212] Surprisingly, anosognosia for the paralysis has been described among patients with pontine infarctions.[213] Small pontine strokes also can cause a disorder of ocular rotation, including conjugate palsy, an internuclear ophthalmoplegia, the one-and-a-half syndrome, or a sixth nerve palsy.[207,212] (See Table 3–21.) Other signs include ataxia, nystagmus, facial weakness, and a dissociated sensory loss.[196,206,209] In particular, loss of vibratory and position senses with preservation of pain and temperature occur with midline pontine lesions that affect the medial lemniscus.[209,212]

A number of classic neurological syndromes have been described in association with pontine infarctions. These include *Millard-Gubler syndrome* (ipsilateral facial weakness and contralateral hemiparesis), *Foville syndrome* (ipsilateral conjugate gaze palsy and contralateral hemiparesis), *Landry syndrome* (ipsilateral abducens palsy and contralateral hemiparesis), and *Raymond-Cestan syndrome* (ipsilateral conjugate gaze palsy and contralateral sensory and motor deficits).[214]

Table 3–21. **Infarctions in the Pons and with Occlusion of the Basilar Artery**

Unilateral or Partial Pontine Infarctions
- Ipsilateral facial weakness
- Ipsilateral eye abduction weakness
- Ipsilateral conjugate gaze weakness
- Internuclear ophthalmoplegia
- "One-and-a-half" syndrome
- Contralateral hemisensory loss
- Contralateral hemiparesis

Locked-in Syndrome
- Quadriparesis
- Bilateral facial paresis
- Lingual and pharyngeal paresis
- Anarthria
- Horizontal gaze paresis
- Retained vertical gaze
- Retained consciousness

Massive Pontine Infarction
- Coma
- Quadriparesis
- Extensor posturing
- Bilateral facial weakness
- Lingual and pharyngeal paresis
- Anarthria
- Ocular bobbing
- Small, unreactive pupils
- Skew deviation

Basilar Artery Occlusion

Basilar artery thrombosis often leads to a major infarction of the pons (Fig. 3–26). The most common cause of basilar artery thrombosis is extensive atherosclerosis, although embolism or a dolichoectatic basilar artery are other potential causes.[215,216] The leading sources of emboli are the vertebral artery and the heart.[217] The patient usually has headache, vertigo, dysarthria, numbness and hemiparesis that can evolve into a severe dysarthria, and weakness of all four limbs.[218] (See Table 3–21.) Consciousness varies from normal alertness to stupor or coma.[219] Sudden bilateral hearing loss can occur.[220,221] Prominent dysarthria is secondary to the interruption of corticolingual pathways.[222,223] A transient state of mutism or anarthria can evolve into the severe articulatory distrubance.[223] Abnormal horizontal eye movements, ocular bobbing, nystagmus, skew deviation, and small, unreactive pupils are present.[219] *Locked-in syndrome* can result from a major pontine stroke.[224] On examination, the patient has quadriplegia, sensory impairments in all four limbs, bulbar palsy, facial diplegia, and bilateral conjugate gaze palsies. Alertness is preserved, and the patient can communicate through blinking and vertical eye movements (see Table 3–21). Basilar artery occlusion or rupture of a basilar artery plaque can be

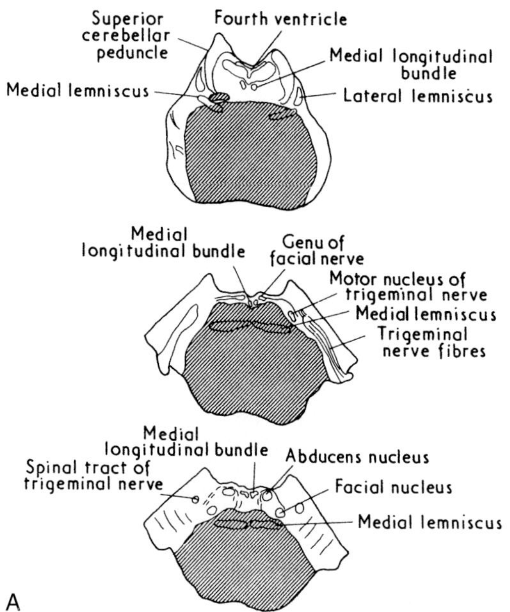

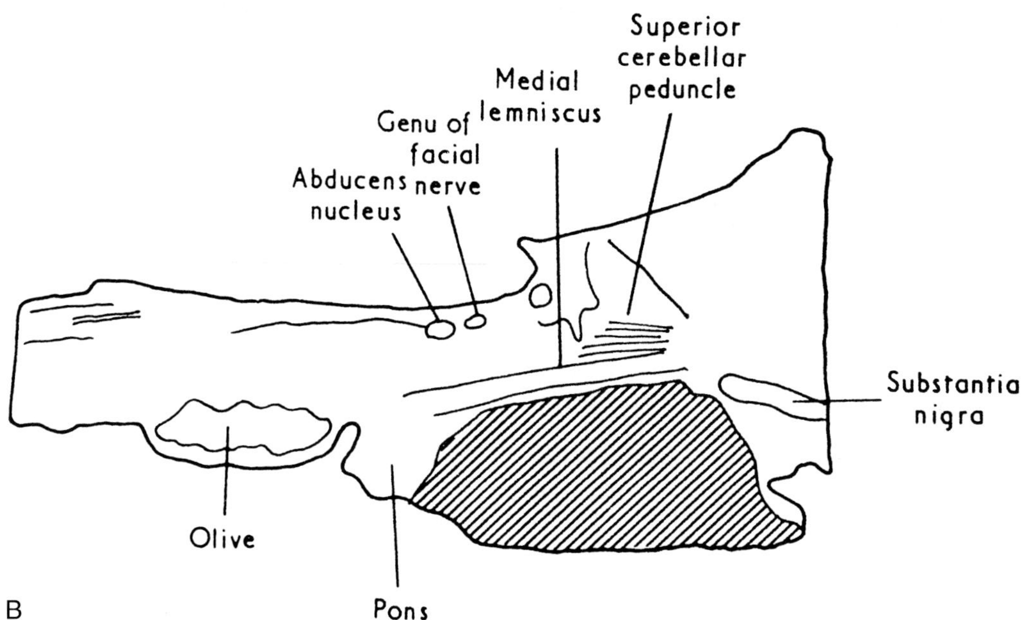

Figure 3–26. Axial (*A*) and coronal (*B*) diagrams of a ventral pontine infarction in a patient with "locked-in" syndrome secondary to occlusion of the basilar artery. (Reprinted from Hawkes CH. "Locked in" syndrome: report of seven cases. BMJ, 1974;4:379, with permission.)

associated with secondary involvement of the anterior inferior cerebellar artery (AICA).[225] Infarction of both the dorsolateral pons and the medial aspect of the cerebellum results. In addition, ipsilateral auditory and vestibular dysfunction develops because the internal auditory artery often is a branch of the AICA. Clinical features of an infarction secondary to an AICA occlusion include ipsilateral facial paralysis, ipsilateral facial sensory loss, ipsilateral deafness, ipsilateral Horner's syndrome, ipsilateral limb ataxia, and contralateral sensory loss to pain and temperature on the body.[226–228]

Mesencephalic Infarction and Superior Cerebellar Artery Occlusion

The distal basilar artery perfuses the caudal midbrain via its short penetrating branches and the superior cerebellar artery. Infarctions of the midbrain usually are secondary to embolism of the distal basilar artery. Patients with infarctions in the midbrain usually have a combination of limb weakness, ataxia, involuntary movements, sensory impairments, disorders of ocular movements, visual hallucinations, and decreased alertness.[229–231] (See Table 3–19.) Small mesencephalic infarctions can produce isolated disturbances of the oculomotor or trochlear nerves or limb movements. An infarction in the oculomotor complex can cause bilateral ptosis, bilateral internuclear ophthalmoplegia, or convergence or retraction nystagmus.[232] Among the discrete ischemic stroke syndromes of the mesencephalon are *Weber syndrome* (ipsilateral oculomotor nerve palsy and contralateral hemiparesis), *Benedikt syndrome* (ipsilateral oculomotor nerve palsy and contralateral tremor, chorea, or athetosis), and *Claude syndrome* (ipsilateral oculomotor palsy and contralateral limb ataxia). Unilateral or bilateral ptosis, and supranuclear disorders of ocular rotation, including paralysis of upgaze, upbeat nystagmus, skew deviation, or convergence–retraction nystagmus, can be found.

A stroke restricted to the vascular territory of the superior cerebellar artery (SCA) is relatively rare; most patients have a cerebellar infarction in conjunction with other areas of brain ischemia.[190,196] The SCA perfuses the dorsolateral midbrain and superior cerebellum; it causes ipsilateral limb ataxia, ipsilateral Horner's syndrome, ipsilateral trochlear nerve palsy, and contralateral loss of sensation to pain and temperature on the body.[226,233–235]

Cerebellar Infarction

Small infarctions in the cerebellar hemisphere usually are not associated with evidence of brain stem dysfunction (Fig. 3–27). The neurological signs are ipsilateral to the stroke, and include dysmetria,

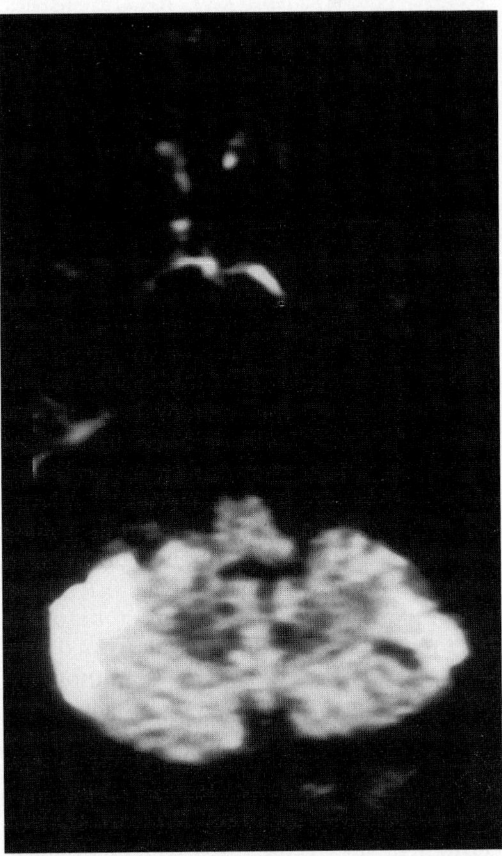

Figure 3–27. Diffusion-weighted magnetic resonance imaging th rough the posterior fossa. Diffusion defects are seen as high signal zones in both cerebellar hemispheres, especially on the right. (Courtesy of AJ Fox, MD, London Health Sciences Center, London, Ontario.)

Table 3–22. **Infarctions of the Cerebellum**

Ipsilateral limb ataxia, dysmetria, dyssynergia
Truncal and gait ataxia
Dysarthria
Ipsilateral vertical and rotatory nystagmus
Mass-producing Cerebellar Infarctions
The above findings
Decreased consciousness
Ipsilateral facial weakness and sensory loss
Ipsilateral hearing loss and tinnitus
Ipsilateral conjugate gaze paresis
Quadriparesis

dyssynergia, and dysdiadochokinesia that usually is most marked in the upper limb.[234] Truncal and gait ataxia, nystagmus, and dysarthria also can be detected (Table 3–22). These strokes usually are secondary to small artery occlusions.

Occlusions of the proximal portions of the PICA, the AICA, or the SCA that lead to infarctions confined to the cerebellum usually cause vertigo, gait instability, headache, and limb ataxia, whereas more distal occlusions cause dysarthria, limb ataxia, and gait instability.[200,236] The large cerebellar infarctions usually are secondary to cardioembolism, atherosclerosis of the basilar artery, or dissection of the vertebral or basilar artery.[200,215,237,238] Borderzone infarctions in the cerebellum also result from occlusion of the vertebral or basilar arteries.[238] A large cerebellar infarction may present as a mass with secondary hydrocephalus, brain stem compression, or tonsillar herniation. These strokes, which usually are larger than 2.5 cm. in diameter, primarily result from occlusion of the SCA or the PICA. In addition to exhibiting the symptoms of the smaller cerebellar infarctions, these lesions can cause secondary brain stem or cranial nerve dysfunction secondary to compression, and decreased consciousness due to hydrocephalus (see Table 3–22). Initial signs include truncal and appendicular ataxia, nystagmus, dysarthria, nausea, and vomiting. These findings usually are present upon being admitted to the hospital, and the other neurological signs and decline in consciousness evolve subsequently. Initially, signs of pontine dysfunction, such as a gaze palsy, facial nerve palsy, or hemiparesis, appear.[239] Late in the course of the illness, consciousness is impaired, respiratory and cardiac rhythm disturbances develop, ocular bobbing is present, and pupillary abnormalities are detected. The clinical findings of mass-producing cerebellar infarctions are described in more detail in Chapter 13.

LACUNAR SYNDROMES

Lacunar strokes were first described by Dechambre and Marie approximately 100 years ago.[240] In a series of papers, Fisher and colleagues[96,98,99,166,241] popularized the concept of the lacune that was associated with discrete clinical findings. Still, the concept of a lacunar infarction is a source of controversy.[242] Lacunes are small infarctions located deep in the cerebral hemispheres, brain stem, or cerebellum. They are most commonly found among persons with diabetes mellitus or hypertension.[243] Lacunes can be secondary to occlusion of small penetrating branches of the internal carotid artery, middle cerebral artery, posterior cerebral artery, anterior cerebral artery, or basilar artery.[244] Lacunar infarctions also can be secondary to a mural thrombosis of the parent artery, atherosclerosis at the origin of the penetrating arteries with secondary thrombosis, lipohyalinosis, microaneurysm formation, or embolism.[245] Lacunar infarctions are described in more detail in Chapter 5.

Lacunar syndromes are not synonymous with lacunar strokes.[246] (See Table 3–14.) Differentiating a lacunar syndrome from a lacunar infarction is critical because the prognoses differ, and the likelihood of death is lower in patients with lacunes than in persons with strokes of other causes.[247–250] Lacunar syndromes due to non–small artery occlusions are more common in non-hypertensive and younger patients and those who have headache, nausea, or vomiting with the event.[246] Some lacunar syndromes are poor predictors of lacunar infarction.[246,251] Infarctions in the basal ganglia, thalamus, internal capsule, brain stem, lobar white matter, or brain stem produce restricted neurological signs that are called *lacunar syndromes.*[210] These syndromes, which are described in Table 3–15, also can be found among patients with large artery disease or cardioembolic events.

Pure motor hemiparesis is the most common lacunar syndrome. Patterns of involvement of the face, arm, and leg vary considerably among patients with pure motor hemiparesis. Melo et al[252] reported that the face, arm, and leg are equally involved in 50% of cases. Still, weakness can be restricted to one limb and many patients will have dysarthria. The sensorimotor stroke is the next most common lacunar syndrome. It usually is due to a lesion of the posterior limb of the internal capsule and the adjacent thalamus secondary to occlusion of the anterior choroidal artery.[147] Pure sensory stroke that most commonly results from a thalamic infarction usually is due to small artery occlusions (lacunar infarction).[253] The pattern of sensory loss can be partial or dense, and it can be dissociated with preservation of some sensory modalities.[253,254] Sensory loss may not equally affect the face, arm, and leg; pain or dysesthesias can accompany it.

SUMMARY

Although the range of clinical presentations of patients with ischemic cerebrovascular disease is ample and varied, pragmatically they fall into two categories. Patients with no or minimal neurological impairments and patients with moderate-to-severe neurological deficits. The primary goal in the first category is prevention of a major stroke. The goals in the second are acute treatment, rehabilitation, and avoidance of complications. The more recent the event the greater the urgency of intervention. Sudden neurological deficits, whether transient or permanent, have a differential diagnosis, including intracerebral hemorrhage, seizures, and an array of acute medical conditions. These conditions profit from prompt medical attention.

Ischemic cerebrovascular disease can manifest with a bewildering variety of eponymous combinations but, for management purposes, most patients can be classified into those with carotid, vertebrobasilar, or lacunar syndromes. A correct diagnosis is the necessary prelude to appropriate treatment, particularly for prevention of recurrent events.

REFERENCES

1. Hankey GJ, Slattery JM, Warlow CP. Transient ischaemic attacks: which patients are at high (and low) risk of serious vascular events? *J Neurol Neurosurg Psychiatry* 1992;55:640–652.
2. Hankey GJ, Slattery JM, Warlow CP. The prognosis of hospital-referred transient ischaemic attacks. *J Neurol Neurosurg Psychiatry* 1991; 54:793–802.
3. Hornig CR, Lammers C, Buttner T, Hoffmann O, Dorndorf W. Long-term prognosis of infratentorial transient ischemic attacks and minor strokes. *Storke* 1992;23:199–204.
4. Kimura K, Minematsu K, Yasaka M, Wada K, Yamaguchi T. The duration of symptoms in transient ischemic attack. *Neurology* 1999; 52:976–980.
5. Crespo M, Melo TP, Oliveira V, Ferro JM. Clustering transient ischemic attacks. *Cerebrovasc Dis* 1993;3:213–220.
6. Rothrock JF, Lyden PD, Yee J, Wiederholt WC. 'Crescendo' transient ischemic attacks: clinical and angiographic correlations. *Neurology* 1988; 38:198–201.
7. Price TR, Gotshall RA, Poskanzer DC, et al. Cooperative study of hospital frequency and character of transient ischemic attacks. VI. Patients examined during an attack. *JAMA* 1977; 238:2512–2515.
8. Landi G. Clinical diagnosis of transient ischaemic attacks. *Lancet* 1992;339:402–405.
9. Ferro JM, Falcao I, Rodrigues G, et al. Diagnosis of transient ischemic attack by the nonneurologist. A validation study. *Stroke* 1996;27: 2225–2229.
10. Lee H, Lerner A. Transient inhibitory seizures mimicking crescendo TIAs. *Neurology* 1990; 40:165–166.
11. Kaplan PW. Focal seizures resembling transient ischemic attacks due to subclinical ischemia. *Cerebrovasc Dis* 1993;3:241–243.
12. Martin PJ, Young G, Enevoldson TP, Humphrey PR. Overdiagnosis of TIA and minor stroke: experience at a regional neurovascular clinic. *Q J Med* 1997;90:759–763.
13. Kumral E, Evyapan D, Balkir K. Acute caudate vascular lesions. *Stroke* 1999;30:100–108.
14. Kraaijeveld CL, van Gijn J, Schouten HJ, Staal A. Interobserver agreement for the diagnosis of transient ischemic attacks. *Stroke* 1984;15: 723–725.
15. Futty DE, Conneally M, Dyken ML, et al. Cooperative study of hospital frequency and

character of transient ischemic attacks. V. Symptom analysis. *JAMA* 1977;238:2386–2390.
16. Hanson PA, Chodos R. Hemiparetic seizures. *Neurology* 1978;28:920–923.
17. Koudstaal PJ, Algra A, Pop GA, Kappelle LJ, van Latum JC, van Gijn J. Risk of cardiac events in atypical transient ischaemic attack or minor stroke. The Dutch TIA Study Group. *Lancet* 1992;340:630–633.
18. Baquis GD, Pessin MS, Scott RM. Limb-shaking. A carotid TIA. *Stroke* 1985;16:444–448.
19. Leira EC, Ajax T, Adams HP, Jr. Limb-shaking carotid transient ischemic attacks successfully treated with modification of the antihypertensive regimen. *Arch Neurol* 1997;54:904–905.
20. Hess DC, Nichols FT, III, Sethi KD, Adams RJ. Transient cerebral ischemia masquerading as paroxysmal dyskinesia. *Cerebrovasc Dis* 1991; 1:54–57.
21. Tatemichi TK, Young WL, Prohovnik I, et al. Perfusion insufficiency in limb-shaking transient ischemic attacks. *Stroke* 1990;21:341–347.
22. Koudstaal PJ, van Gijn J, Kappelle LJ. Headache in transient or permanent cerebral ischemia. Dutch TIA Study Group. *Stroke* 1991; 22:754–759.
23. Adams HP, Jr., Putman SF, Corbett JJ, Sires BP, Thompson HS. Amaurosis fugax: the results of arteriography in 59 patients. *Stroke* 1983; 14:742–744.
24. Bull DA, Fante RG, Hunter GC, et al. Correlation of ophthalmic findings with carotid artery stenosis. *J Cardiovasc Surg* 1992;33:401–406.
25. Perez-Burkhardt JL, Gonzalez-Fajardo JA, Rodriguez E, Mateo AM. Amaurosis fugax as a symptom of carotid artery stenosis. Its relationship with ulcerated plaque. *J Cardiovasc Surg* 1994;35:15–18.
26. Ahuja RM, Chaturvedi S, Eliott D, Joshi N, Puklin JE, Abrams GW. Mechanisms of retinal arterial occlusive disease in African American and Caucasian patients. *Stroke* 1999;30: 1506–1509.
27. Hankey GJ, Slattery JM, Warlow CP. Prognosis and prognostic factors of retinal infarction: a prospective cohort study. *BMJ* 1991;302: 499–504.
28. Bruno A, Corbett JJ, Biller J, Adams HP, Jr., Qualls C. Transient monocular visual loss patterns and associated vascular abnormalities. *Stroke* 1990;21:34–39.
29. Burde RM. Amaurosis fugax. *J Clin Neuro-Ophthalmol* 1989;9:185–189.
30. Bogousslavsky J, Regli F, Despland PA, Zografos L. Optic nerve head infarction. *Cerebrovasc Dis* 1991;1:341–344.
31. Furlan AJ, Whisnant JP, Kearns TP. Unilateral visual loss in bright light. An unusual symptom of carotid artery occlusive disease. *Arch Neurol* 1979;36:675–676.
32. Wiebers DO, Swanson JW, Cascino TL, Whisnant JP. Bilateral loss of vision in bright light. *Stroke* 1989;20:554–558.
33. Chimowitz MI, Lafranchise EF, Furlan AJ, Awad IA. Ipsilateral leg weakness associated with carotid stenosis. *Stroke* 1990;21:1362–1364.
34. Giovannoni G, Fritz VU. Transient ischemic attacks in younger and older patients. A comparative study of 798 patients in South Africa. *Stroke* 1993;24:947–953.
35. Baloh RW. Stroke and vertigo. *Cerebrovasc Dis* 1992;2:3–10.
36. Gomez CR, Cruz-Flores S, Malkoff MD, Sauer CM, Burch CM. Isolated vertigo as a manifestation of vertebrobasilar ischemia. *Neurology* 1996;47:94–97.
37. Pessin MS, Gorelick PB, Kwan ES, Caplan LR. Basilar artery stenosis: middle and distal segments. *Neurology* 1987;37:1742–1746.
38. Fisher CM. The 'herald hemiparesis' of basilar artery occlusion. *Arch Neurol* 1988;45: 1301–1303.
39. Brust JCM, Plank CR, Healton EB, Sanchez GF. The pathology of drop attacks. A case report. *Neurology* 1979;29:786–790.
40. Fields WS, Lemak NA. Joint study of extracranial arterial occlusion. VII. Subclavian steal—a review of 168 cases. *JAMA* 1972;222:1139–1143.
41. Hennerici M, Klemm C, Rautenberg W. The subclavian steal phenomenon: a common vascular disorder with rare neurologic deficits. *Neurology* 1988;38:669–673.
42. Yip PK, Liu HM, Hwang BS, Chen RC. Subclavian steal phenomenon: a correlation between duplex sonographic and angiographic findings. *Neuroradiology* 1992;34:279–282.
43. Zelenock GB, Cronenwett JL, Graham LM, et al. Brachiocephalic arterial occlusions and stenoses. Manifestations and management of complex lesions. *Arch Surg* 1985;120:370–376.
44. Bruno A, Russell PW, Jones WL, Austin JK, Weinstein ES, Steel SR. Concomitants of asymptomatic retinal cholesterol emboli. *Stroke* 1992; 23:900–902.
45. Hollenhorst RW. The ocular manifestations of internal carotid artery thrombosis. *Med Clin N Am* 1960;44:897–908.
46. Howard RS, Russell RW. Prognosis of patients with retinal embolism. *J Neurol Neurosurg Psychiatry* 1987;50:1142–1147.
47. Bruno A, Jones WL, Austin JK, Carter S, Qualls C. Vascular outcome in men with asymptomatic retinal cholesterol emboli. *Ann Intern Med* 1995; 122:249–253.
48. Klein R, Klein BE, Jensen SC, Moss SE, Meuer SM. Retinal emboli and stroke: the Beaver Dam Eye Study. *Archives of Ophthalmology* 1999;117: 1063–1068.
49. Fry CL, Carter JE, Kanter MC, Tegeler CH, Tuley MR. Anterior ischemic optic neuropathy is not associated with carotid artery atherosclerosis. *Stroke* 1993;24:539–542.
50. Chambers BR, Norris JW. Clinical significance of asymptomatic neck bruits. *Neurology* 1985;35: 742–745.
51. Besson G, Bogousslavsky J, Hommel M, Stauffer JC, Siche JP. Patent foramen ovale in young stroke patients with mitral valve prolapse. *Acta Neurol Scand* 1994;89:23–26.
52. Kilpatrick CJ, Davis SM, Tress BM, Rossiter SC, Hopper JL, Vandendriesen ML. Epileptic seizures in acute stroke. *Arch Neurol* 1990;47: 157–160.

53. Davalos A, de Cendra E, Molins A, Ferrandiz M, Lopez-Pousa S, Genis D. Epileptic seizures at the onset of stroke. *Cerebrovasc Dis* 1992;2:327–331.
54. Daniele O, Mattaliano A, Tassinari CA, Natale E. Epileptic seizures and cerebrovascular disease. *Acta Neurol Scand* 1989;80:17–22.
55. Pohlmann-Eden B, Cochius JI, Hoch DB, Hennerici M. Stroke and epilepsy: critical review of the literature. *Cerebrovasc Dis* 1997;7:2–9.
56. Kilpatrick CJ, Davis SM, Hopper JL, Rossiter SC. Early seizures after acute stroke. Risk of late seizures. *Arch Neurol* 1992;49:509–511.
57. Arboix A, Massons J, Oliveres M, Arribas MP, Titus F. Headache in acute cerebrovascular disease. A prospective clinical study in 240 patients. *Cephalalgia* 1994;14:37–40.
58. Ferro JM, Melo TP, Oliveira V, et al. A multivariate study of headache associated with ischemic stroke. *Headache* 1995;35:315–319.
59. Jorgensen HS, Jespersen HF, Nakayama H, Raaschou HO, Olsen TS. Headache in stroke: the Copenhagen Stroke Study. *Neurology* 1994;44:1793–1797.
60. Gorelick PB, Hier DB, Caplan LR, Langenberg P. Headache in acute cerebrovascular disease. *Neurology* 1986;36:1445–1450.
61. Fisher CM. The headache and pain of spontaneous carotid dissection. *Headache* 1982;22:60–65.
62. Silbert PL, Mokri B, Schievink WI. Headache and neck pain in spontaneous internal carotid and vertebral artery dissections. *Neurology* 1995; 45:1517–1522.
63. Norris JW, Hachinski VC. Misdiagnosis of stroke. *Lancet* 1982;1:328–331.
64. The Members of the Lille Stroke Program. Misdiagnoses in 1,250 consecutive patients admitted to an acute stroke unit. *Cerebrovasc Dis* 1997;7:284–288.
65. Harrison MJ. Clinical distinction of cerebral haemorrhage and cerebral infarction. *Postgrad Med J* 1980;56:629–632.
66. Wallis WE, Donaldson I, Scott RS, Wilson J. Hypoglycemia masquerading as cerebrovascular disease (hypoglycemic hemiplegia). *Ann Neurol* 1985;18:510–512.
67. Weir CJ, Murray GD, Adams FG, Muir KW, Grosset DG, Lees KR. Poor accuracy of stroke scoring systems for differential clinical diagnosis of intracranial haemorrhage and infarction. *Lancet* 1994;344:999–1002.
68. Besson G, Robert C, Hommel M, Perret J. Is it clinically possible to distinguish nonhemorrhagic infarct from hemorrhagic stroke? *Stroke* 1995;26:1205–1209.
69. Sacco RL, VanGool R, Mohr JP, Hauser WA. Nontraumatic coma. Glasgow Coma Score and coma etiology as predictors of 2–week outcome. *Arch Neurol* 1990;47:1181–1184.
70. Muir KW, Weir CJ, Murray GD, Povey C, Lees KR. Comparison of neurological scales and scoring systems for acute stroke prognosis. *Stroke* 1996;27:1817–1820.
71. Brott T, Adams HP, Jr., Olinger CP, et al. Measurements of acute cerebral infarction: a clinical examination scale. *Stroke* 1989;20: 864–870.
72. Lyden P, Brott T, Tilley B, et al. Improved reliability of the NIH Stroke Scale using video training. NINDS TPA Stroke Study Group. *Stroke* 1994;25:2220–2226.
73. Brott T, Marler JR, Olinger CP, et al. Measurements of acute cerebral infarction: lesion size by computed tomography. *Stroke* 1989;20:871–875.
74. Albanese MA, Clarke WR, Adams HP, Jr., Woolson RF. Ensuring reliability of outcome measures in multicenter clinical trials of treatments for acute ischemic stroke. The program developed for the Trial of Org 10172 in Acute Stroke Treatment (TOAST). *Stroke* 1994;25: 1746–1751.
75. Pallicino P, Snyder W, Granger C. The NIH Stroke Scale and the FIM in stroke rehabilitation. *Stroke* 1992;23:919.
76. DeGraba TJ, Hallenbeck JM, Pettigrew KD, Dutka AJ, Kelly BJ. Progression in acute stroke: value of the initial NIH stroke scale score on patient stratification in future trials. *Stroke* 1999; 30:1208–1212.
77. Adams HP, Jr., Davis PH, Leira EC, et al. Baseline NIH Stroke Scale score strongly predicts outcome after stroke. *Neurology* 1999;53: 126–131.
78. Adams HP, Jr., Brott TG, Furlan AJ, et al. Guidelines for thrombolytic therapy for acute stroke: a supplement to the guidelines for the management of patients with acute ischemic stroke. A statement for healthcare professionals from a Special Writing Group of the Stroke Council, American Heart Association. *Circulation* 1996;94:1167–1174.
79. Lhermitte F, Gautier JC, Derouesne C. Nature of occlusions of the middle cerebral artery. *Neurology* 1970;20:82–88.
80. Caplan L, Babikian V, Helgason C, et al. Occlusive disease of the middle cerebral artery. *Neurology* 1985;35:975–982.
81. Lyrer PA, Engelter S, Radu EW, Steck AJ. Cerebral infarcts related to isolated middle cerebral artery stenosis. *Stroke* 1997;28: 1022–1027.
82. Heinsius T, Bogousslavsky J, Van Melle G. Large infarcts in the middle cerebral artery territory. Etiology and outcome patterns. *Neurology* 1998; 50:341–350.
83. Ghika JA, Bogousslavsky J, Regli F. Deep perforators from the carotid system. Template of the vascular territories. *Arch Neurol* 1990;47: 1097–1100.
84. Donnan GA, Bladin PF, Berkovic SF, Longley WA, Saling MM. The stroke syndrome of striatocapsular infarction. *Brain* 1991;114:51–70.
85. Donnan GA, Norrving B, Bamford J, Bogousslavsky J. Subcortical infarction: classification and terminology. *Cerebrovasc Dis* 1993;3: 248–251.
86. Bladin PF, Berkovic SF. Striatocapsular infarction. *Neurology* 1984;34:1423–1430.
87. Levine RL, Lagreze HL, Dobkin JA, Turski PA. Large subcortical hemispheric infarctions. Presentation and prognosis. *Arch Neurol* 1988; 45:1074–1077.

88. Donnan GA, O'Malley HM, Quang C, Hurley S. The capsular warning syndrome. The high risk of early stroke. *Cerebrovasc Dis* 1996;6:202–207.
89. Ghika J, Bogousslavsky J, Regli F. Infarcts in the territory of lenticulostriate branches from the middle cerebral artery. Etiological factors and clinical features in 65 cases. *Schweiz Arch Neurol Psychiatr* 1991;142:5–18.
90. Blecic SA, Bogousslavsky J, Van Melle G, Regli F. Isolated sensarimotor stroke. A reevaluation of clinical, topographic, and etiological patterns. *Cerebrovasc Dis* 1993;3:357–363.
91. Goldblatt D, Markesbery W, Reeves AG. Recurrent hemichorea following striatal lesions. *Arch Neurol* 1974;31:51–54.
92. Landi G, Anzalone N, Cella E, Boccardi E, Musicco M. Are sensorimotor strokes lacunar strokes? A case-control study of lacunar and non-lacunar infarcts. *J Neurol Neurosurg Psychiatry* 1991;54:1063–1068.
93. Fromm D, Holland AL, Swindell CS, Reinmuth OM. Various consequences of subcortical stroke. Prospective study of 16 consecutive cases. *Arch Neurol* 1985;42:943–950.
94. Mega MS, Alexander MP. Subcortical aphasia: the core profile of capsulostriatal infarction. *Neurology* 1994;44:1824–1829.
95. Godefroy O, Rousseaux M, Pruvo JP, Cabaret M, Leys D. Neuropsychological changes related to unilateral lenticulostriate infarcts. *J Neurol Neurosurg Psychiatry* 1994;57:480–485.
96. Fisher CM, Curry HB. Pure motor hemiplegia. *Trans Am Neurol Assoc* 1964;89:94–97.
97. Nighoghossian N, Ryvlin P, Trouillas P, Laharotte JC, Froment JC. Pontine versus capsular pure motor hemiparesis. *Neurology* 1993; 43:2197–2201.
98. Fisher CM. A lacunar stroke. The dysarthria-clumsy hand syndrome. *Neurology* 1967;17: 614–617.
99. Fisher CM, Cole M. Homolateral ataxia and rural paresis. A vascular syndrome. *J Neurol Neurosurg Psychiatry* 1965;28:48–55.
100. Fisher CM. Ataxic hemiparesis. A pathologic study. *Arch Neurol* 1978;35:126–128.
101. Sage JI, Lepore FE. Ataxic hemiparesis from lesions of the corona radiata. *Arch Neurol* 1983;40:449–450.
102. Bogousslavsky J, Regli F. Capsular genu syndrome. *Neurology* 1990;40:1499–1502.
103. Kase CS, Maulsby GO, deJuan E, Mohr JP. Hemichorea-hemiballism and lacunar infarction in the basal ganglia. *Neurology* 1981;31:452–455.
104. Brandt T, Botzel K, Yousry T, Dieterich M, Schulze S. Rotational vertigo in embolic stroke of the vestibular and auditory cortices. *Neurology* 1995;45:42–44.
105. Babikian VL, Caplan LR. Brain embolism is a dynamic process with variable characteristics. *Neurology* 2000;54:797–801.
106. Bogousslavsky J. Topographic patterns of cerebral infarcts. *Cerebrovasc Dis* 1991;1:61–68.
107. Bogousslavsky J, Van Melle G, Regli F. Middle cerebral artery pial territory infarcts: a study of the Lausanne Stroke Registry. *Ann Neurol* 1989; 25:555–560.
108. Boiten J, Kappelle LJ, for the Dutch TIA Trial Study Group. A history of monoparesis does not differentiate between superficial and small deep (lacunar) infarction. *Cerebrovasc Dis* 1995;5: 204–207.
109. Kunesch E, Binkofski F, Steinmetz H, Freund HJ. The pattern of motor deficits in relation to the site of stroke lesions. *Eur Neurol* 1995;35: 20–26.
110. Sindermann F, Dichgans J, Bergleiter R. Occlusion of the middle cerebral artery and its branches: angiographic and clinical correlates. *Brain* 1969;92:607–620.
111. Bogousslavsky J. Frontal stroke syndromes. *Eur Neurol* 1994;34:306–315.
112. Mohr JP, Foulkes MA, Polis AT, et al. Infarct topography and hemiparesis profiles with cerebral convexity infarction: the Stroke Data Bank. *J Neurol Neurosurg Psychiatry* 1993;56:344–351.
113. Tijssen CC, van Gisbergen JA, Schulte BP. Conjugate eye deviation: side, site, and size of the hemispheric lesion. *Neurology* 1991;41: 846–850.
114. Bogousslavsky J, Dizerens K, Regli F, Despland PA. Opercular cheiro-oral syndrome. *Arch Neurol* 1991;48:658–661.
115. Caplan LR, Kelly M, Kase CS, et al. Infarcts of the inferior division of the right middle cerebral artery. Mirror image of Wernicke's aphasia. *Neurology* 1986;36:1015–1020.
116. Waddington MM, Ring BA. Syndromes of occlusions of middle cerebral artery branches. *Brain* 1968;91:685–696.
117. Bogousslavsky J. Double infarction in one cerebral hemisphere. *Ann Neurol* 1991;30:12–18.
118. Bogousslavsky J, Bernasconi A. Acute multiple infarction involving the anterior circulation. *Arch Neurol* 1996;53:50–57.
119. Baird AE, Lovblad KO, Schlaug G, Edelman RR, Warach S. Multiple acute stroke syndrome. Marker of embolic disease? *Neurology* 2000;54: 674–678.
120. Legatt AD, Rubin MJ, Kaplan LR, Healton EB, Brust JC. Global aphasia without hemiparesis: multiple etiologies. *Neurology* 1987;37:201–205.
121. Bogousslavsky J, Regli F. Borderzone infarctions distal to internal carotid artery occlusions: prognostic implications. *Ann Neurol* 1986;20: 346–350.
122. Weiller C, Ringelstein EB, Reiche W, Buell U. Clinical and hemodynamic aspects of low-flow infarcts. *Stroke* 1991;22:1117–1123.
123. Mull M, Schwarz M, Thron A. Cerebral hemispheric low-flow infarcts in arterial occlusive disease. Lesion patterns and angiomorphological conditions. *Stroke* 1997;28:118–123.
124. Leblanc R, Yamamoto YL, Tyler JL, Diksic M, Hakim A. Borderzone ischemia. *Ann Neurol* 1987;22:707–713.
125. Baird AE, Donnan GA, Saling M. Mechanisms and clinical features of internal watershed infarction. *Clin Exp Neurol* 1991;28:50–55.
126. Belden JR, Caplan LR, Pessin MS, Kwan E. Mechanisms and clinical features of posterior border-zone infarcts. *Neurology* 1999;53: 1312–1318.

127. Bladin CF, Chambers BR. Clinical features, pathogenesis, and computed tomographic characteristics of internal watershed infarctions. *Stroke* 1993;24:1925–1932.
128. Sloan MA, Haley EC, Jr. The syndrome of bilateral hemispheric border zone ischemia. *Stroke* 1990;21:1668–1673.
129. Caplan LR, Hennerici M. Impaired clearance of emboli (washout) is an important link between hypoperfusion, embolism, and ischemic stroke. *Arch Neurol* 1998;55:1475–1482.
130. Hupperts RM, Warlow CP, Slattery J, Rothwell PM. Severe stenosis of the internal carotid artery is not associated with borderzone infarcts in patients randomised in the European Carotid Surgery Trial. *J Neurol* 1997;244:45–50.
131. Hopperts RMM, Lodder J, Hoets-Van Raak L, Kessels F. Borderzone small deep infarcts. *Cerebrovasc Dis* 1997;7:280–283.
132. Sage JI, Van Uitert RL. Man-in-the-barrel syndrome. *Neurology* 1986;1102–1103.
133. Fisher M, McQuillen JB. Bilateral cortical border-zone infarction. A pseudobrainstem stroke. *Arch Neurol* 1981;38:62–63.
134. Bogousslavsky J, Regli F. Unilateral watershed cerebral infarcts. *Neurology* 1986;36:373–377.
135. Caplan L, Schoene WC. Clinical features of subcortical arteriosclerotic encephalopathy (Binswanger disease). *Neurology* 1978;28: 1206–1215.
136. Kim JS. Pure sensory stroke. Clinical-radiological correlates of 21 cases. *Stroke* 1992;23:983–987.
137. Leys D, Mounier-Vehier F, Rondepierre P, et al. Small infarcts in the centrum ovale: study of predisposing factors. *Cerebrovasc Dis* 1994;4:83–87.
138. Ellis S, Small M. Localization of lesion in denial of hemiplegia after acute stroke. *Stroke* 1997;28:67–71.
139. Nakano S, Yokogami K, Ohta H, Goya T, Wakisaka S. CT-defined large subcortical infarcts: correlation of location with site of cerebrovascular occlusive disease. *Am J Neuroradiol* 1995;16:1581–1585.
140. Lammie GA, Wardlaw JM. Small centrum ovale infarcts—a pathological study. *Cerebrovasc Dis* 1999;9:82–90.
141. Boiten J, Rothwell PM, Slattery J, Warlow C. Frequency and degree of carotid stenosis in small centrum ovale infarcts as compared to lacunar infarcts. *Cerebrovasc Dis* 1997;7:138–143.
142. Bruno A, Graff-Radfor NR, Biller J, Adams HP, Jr. Anterior choroidal artery territory infarction: a small vessel disease. *Stroke* 1999;20:616–619.
143. Leys D, Mounier-Vehier F, Lavenu I, Rondepierre P, Pruvo JP. Anterior choroidal artery territory infarcts. Study of presumed mechanisms. *Stroke* 1994;25:837–842.
144. Helgason C, Caplan LR, Goodwin J, Hedges T. Anterior choroidal artery-territory infarction. Report of cases and review. *Arch Neurol* 1986; 43:681–686.
145. Abrahams JM, Hurst RW, Bagley LJ, Zager EL. Anterior choroidal artery supply to the posterior cerebral artery distribution: embryological basisi and clinical implications. *Neurosurgery* 1999;44: 1308–1314.
146. Paroni SG, Agatiello LM, Stocchi A, Solivetti FM. CT of ischemic infarctions in the territory of the anterior choroidal artery: a review of 28 cases. *Am J Neuroradiol* 1987;8:229–232.
147. Mohr JP, Kase CS, Meckler RJ, Fisher CM. Sensorimotor stroke due to thalamocapsular ischemia. *Arch Neurol* 1977;34:739–741.
148. Ichikawa K, Tsutsumishita A, Fujioka A. Capsular ataxic hemiparesis. A case report. *Arch Neurol* 1982;39:585–586.
149. Caplan LR, Schmakmann JD, Kase CS, et al. Caudate infarcts. *Arch Neurol* 1990;47: 133–143.
150. Kubis N, Guichara J, France Woimant Departments of Neurology and Neuroradiology HLPF. Isolated anterior cerebral artery infarcts: a series of 16 patients. *Cerebrovasc Dis* 1999; 9:185–187.
151. Bogousslavsky J, Martin R, Moulin T. Homolateral ataxia and crural paresis: a syndrome of anterior cerebral artery territory infarction. *J Neurol Neurosurg Psychiatry* 1992; 55:1146–1149.
152. Bogousslavsky J, Regli F. Anterior cerebral artery territory infarction in the Lausanne Stroke Registry. *Arch Neurol* 1990;47:144–150.
153. Klatka LA, Depper MH, Marini AM. Infarction in the territory of the anterior cerebral artery. *Neurology* 1998;51:620–622.
154. Schneider R, Gautier JC. Leg weakness due to stroke. Site of lesions, weakness patterns and causes. *Brain* 1994;117:347–354.
155. Webster JE, Gurjian ES, Lindner DW, Hardy WG. proximal occlusion of the anterior cerebral artery. *Arch Neurol* 1960;2:19–26.
156. Minagar A, David NJ. Bilateral infarction in the territory of the anterior cerebral arteries. *Neurology* 1999;52:886–888.
157. Giroud M, Dumas R. Clinical and topographical range of callosal infarction: a clinical and radiological correlation study. *J Neurol Neurosurg Psychiatry* 1995;59:238–242.
158. Pessin MS, Lathi ES, Cohen MB, Kwan ES, Hedges TR, Caplan LR. Clinical features and mechanism of occipital infarction. *Ann Neurol* 1987;21:290–299.
159. Fisher CM. Unusual vascular events in the territory of the posterior cerebral artery. *Can J Neurol Sci* 1986;13:1–7.
160. Hommel M, Besson G, Pollak P, Kahane P, Le Bas JF, Perret J. Hemiplegia in posterior cerebral artery occlusion. *Neurology* 1990;40: 1496–1499.
161. Georgiadis AL, Yamamoto Y, Kwan ES, Pessin MS, Caplan LR. Anatomy of sensory findings in patients with posterior cerebralartery territory infarction. *Arch Neurol* 1999;56:835–838.
162. Chambers BR, Brooder RJ, Donnan GA. Proximal posterior cerebral artery occlusion simulating middle cerebral artery occlusion. *Neurology* 1991;41:385–390.
163. Aldrich MS, Alessi AG, Beck RW, Gilman S. Cortical blindness. Etiology, diagnosis, and prognosis. *Ann Neurol* 1987;21:149–158.
164. Bogousslavsky J, Caplan LR. Vertebrobasilar occlusive disease. Review of selected aspects. 3

thalamic infarcts. *Cerebrovasc Dis* 1993;3: 193–205.

165. Bogousslavsky J, Regli F, Uske A. Thalamic infarcts: clinical syndromes, etiology, and prognosis. *Neurology* 1988;38:837–848.
166. Fisher CM. Pure sensory stroke involving face, arm and leg. *Neurology* 1965;15:76–80.
167. Solomon DH, Barohn RJ, Bazan C, Grissom J. The thalamic ataxia syndrome. *Neurology* 1994;44:810–814.
168. Melo TP, Bogousslavsky J, Moulin T, Nader J, Regli F. Thalamic ataxia. *J Neurol* 1992;239: 331–337.
169. Graff-Radford NR, Eslinger PJ, Damasio AR, Yamada T. Nonhemorrhagic infarction of the thalamus: behavioral, anatomic, and physiologic correlates. *Neurology* 1984;34:14–23.
170. Caplan LR, DeWitt LD, Pessin MS, Gorelick PB, Adelman LS. Lateral thalamic infarcts. *Arch Neurol* 1988;45:959–964.
171. Bassetti C, Mathis J, Gugger M, Lovblad KO, Hess CW. Hypersomnia following paramedian thalamic stroke: a report of 12 patients. *Ann Neurol* 1996;39:471–480.
172. Eslinger PJ, Warner GC, Grattan LM, Easton JD. "Frontal lobe" utilization behavior associated with paramedian thalamic infarction. *Neurology* 1991;41:450–452.
173. Masdeu JC, Gorelick PB. Thalamic astasia: inability to stand after unilateral thalamic lesions. *Ann Neurol* 1988;23:596–603.
174. Gorelick PB, Hier DB, Benevento L, Levitt S, Tan W. Aphasia after left thalamic infarction. *Arch Neurol* 1984;41:1296–1298.
175. Levasseur M, Baron JC, Sette G, et al. Brain energy metabolism in bilateral paramedian thalamic infarcts. A positron emission tomography study. *Brain* 1992;115:795–807.
176. Caplan LR. "Top of the basilar" syndrome. *Neurology* 1980;30:72–79.
177. Biller J, Sand JJ, Corbett JJ, Adams HP, Jr., Dunn V. Syndrome of the paramedian thalamic arteries. Clinical and neuroimaging correlation. *J Clin Neuro-Ophthalmol* 1985;5:217–223.
178. Gentilini M, De Renzi E, Crisi G. Bilateral paramedian thalamic artery infarcts: report of eight cases. *J Neurol Neurosurg Psychiatry* 1987;50: 900–909.
179. Castaigne P, Lhermitte F, Buge A, Escourolle R, Hauw JJ, Lyon-Caen O. Paramedian thalamic and midbrain infarct: clinical and neuropathological study. *Ann Neurol* 1981;10:127–148.
180. Guberman A, Stuss D. The syndrome of bilateral paramedian thalamic infarction. *Neurology* 1983;33:540–546.
181. Kobari M, Ishihara N, Yunoki K. Bilateral thalamic infarction associated with selective downward gaze paralysis. *Eur Neurol* 1987;26:246–251.
182. Tatemichi TK, Steinke W, Duncan C, et al. Paramedian thalamopeduncular infarction: clinical syndromes and magnetic resonance imaging. *Ann Neurol* 1992;32:162–171.
183. Kotila M, Hokkanen L, Laaksonen R, Valanne L. Long-term prognosis after left tuberothalamic infarction. A study of 7 cases. *Cerebrovasc Dis* 1994;4:44–50.
184. Neau JP, Bogousslavsky J. The syndrome of posterior choroidal artery territory infarction. *Ann Neurol* 1996;39:779–788.
185. Caplan LR, Tettenborn B. Vertebrobasilar occlusive disease. Review of selected aspects. *Cerebrovasc Dis* 1992;2:320–326.
186. Fisher CM. Occlusion of the vertebral arteries. Causing transient basilar symptoms. *Arch Neurol* 1970;22:13–19.
187. Vuilleumier P, Bogousslavsky J, Regli F. Infarction of the lower brainstem. Clinical, aetiological and MRI-topographical correlations. *Brain* 1995;118:1013–1025.
188. Caplan LR. Bilateral distal vertebral artery occlusion. *Neurology* 1983;33:552–558.
189. Bernasconi A, Bogousslavsky J, Bassetti C, Regli F. Multiple acute infarcts in the posterior circulation. *J Neurol Neurosurg Psychiatry* 1996;60: 289–296.
190. Kase CS, Norrving B, Levine SR, et al. Cerebellar infarction. Clinical and anatomic observations in 66 cases. *Stroke* 1993;24:76–83.
191. Graf KJ, Pessin MS, DeWitt LD, Caplan LR. Proximal intracranial territory posterior circulation infarcts in the New England Medical Center Posterior Circulation Registry. *Eur Neurol* 1997;37:157–168.
192. Sacco RL, Freddo L, Bello JA, Odel JG, Onesti ST, Mohr JP. Wallenberg's lateral medullary syndrome. Clinical-magnetic resonance imaging correlations. *Arch Neurol* 1993;50:609–614.
193. Fisher CM, Tapia J. Lateral medullary infarction extending to the lower pons. *J Neurol Neurosurg Psychiatry* 1987;50:620–624.
194. Kim JS, Lee JH, Lee MC. Sensory changes in the ipsilateral extremity. A clinical variant of lateral medullary infarction. *Stroke* 1995;26: 1956–1958.
195. Barth A, Bogousslavsky J, Regli F. Infarcts in the territory of the lateral branch of the posterior inferior cerebellar artery. *J Neurol Neurosurg Psychiatry* 1994;57:1073–1076.
196. Barth A, Bogousslavsky J, Regli F. The clinical and topographic spectrum of cerebellar infarcts: a clinical-magnetic resonance imaging correlation study. *Ann Neurol* 1993;33:451–456.
197. Brazis PW. Ocular motor abnormalities in Wallenberg's lateral medullary syndrome. *Mayo Clin Proc* 1992;67:365–368.
198. Dieterich M, Brandt T. Wallenberg's syndrome: lateropulsion, cyclorotation, and subjective visual vertical in thirty-six patients. *Ann Neurol* 1992;31:399–408.
199. Duncan GW, Parker SW, Fisher CM. Acute cerebellar infarction in the PICA territory. *Arch Neurol* 1975;32:364–368.
200. Malm J, Kristensen B, Carlberg B, Fagerlund M, Olsson T. Clinical features and prognosis in young adults with infratentorial infarcts. *Cerebrovasc Dis* 1999;9:282–289.
201. Toyoda K, Imamura T, Saku Y, et al. Medial medullary infarction: analyses of eleven patients. *Neurology* 1996;47:1141–1147.
202. Kim JS, Kim HG, Chung CS. Medial medullary syndrome. Report of 18 new patients and a review of the literature. *Stroke* 1995;26:1548–1552.

203. Bassetti C, Bogousslavsky J, Mattle H, Bernasconi A. Medial medullary Stroke: report of seven patients and review of the literature. *Neurology* 1997;48:882–890.
204. Chokroverty S, Rubino FA, Haller C. Pure motor hemiplegia due to pyramidal infarction. *Arch Neurol* 1975;32:647–648.
205. Toyoda K, Saku Y, Ibayashi S, Sadoshima S, Ogasawara T, Fujishima M. Pontine infarction extending to the basal surface. *Stroke* 1994;25: 2171–2178.
206. Fisher CM, Caplan LR. Basilar artery branch occlusion: a cause of pontine infarction. *Neurology* 1971;21:900–905.
207. Kataoka S, Hori A, Shirakawa T, Hirose G. Paramedian pontine infarction. Neurological/ topographical correlation. *Stroke* 1997;28: 809–815.
208. Kim JS, Lee JH, Im JH, Lee MC. Syndromes of pontine base infarction. A clinical-radiological correlation study. *Stroke* 1995;26:950–955.
209. Shintani S, Tsuruoka S, Shiigai T. Pure sensory stroke caused by a pontine infarct. Clinical, radiological, and physiological features in four patients. *Stroke* 1994;25:1512–1515.
210. Gorman MJ, Dafer R, Levine SR. Ataxic hemiparesis: critical appraisal of a lacunar syndrome. *Stroke* 1998;29:2549–2555.
211. Stiller J, Shanzer S, Yang W. Brainstem lesions with pure motor hemiparesis. Computed tomographic demonstration. *Arch Neurol* 1982;39: 660–661.
212. Bassetti C, Bogousslavsky J, Barth A, Regli F. Isolated infarcts of the pons. *Neurology* 1996;46: 165–175.
213. Evyapan D, Kumral E. Pontine anosognosia for hemiplegia. *Neurology* 1999;53:647–649.
214. Silverman IE, Liu GT, Volpe NJ, Galetta SL. The crossed paralyses. The original brain-stem syndromes of Millard-Gubler, Foville, Weber, and Raymond-Cestan. *Arch Neurol* 1995;52:635–638.
215. Amarenco P, Hauw JJ, Gautier JC. Arterial pathology in cerebellar infarction. *Stroke* 1990;21:1299–1305.
216. Bogousslavsky J, Regli F, Maeder P, Meuli R, Nader J. The etiology of posterior circulation infarcts. A prospective study using magnetic resonance imaging and magnetic resonance angiography. *Neurology* 1993;43:1528–1533.
217. Schwarz S, Egelhof T, Schwab S, Hacke W. Basilar artery embolism. Clinical syndrome and neuroradiologic patterns in patients without permanent occlusion of the basilar artery. *Neurology* 1997;49:1346–1352.
218. Patterson JR, Grabois M. Locked-in syndrome: a review of 139 cases. *Stroke* 1986;17:758–764.
219. Ferbert A, Bruckmann H, Drummen R. Clinical features of proven basilar artery occlusion. *Stroke* 1990;21:1135–1142.
220. Huang MH, Huang CC, Ryu SJ, Chu NS. Sudden bilateral hearing impairment in vertebrobasilar occlusive disease. *Stroke* 1993;24: 132–137.
221. Khurana RK, O'Donnell PP, Suter CM, Inayatullah M. Bilateral deafness of vascular origin. *Stroke* 1981;12:521–523.
222. Urban PP, Hopf HC, Zorowka PG, Fleischer S, Andreas J. Dysarthria and lacunar stroke: pathophysiologic aspects. *Neurology* 1996;47: 1135–1141.
223. Orefice G, Fragassi NA, Lanzillo R, Castellano A, Grossi D. Transient muteness followed by dysarthria in patients with pontomesencephalic stroke. Report of two cases. *Cerebrovasc Dis* 1999; 9:124–126.
224. Fisher CM. Bilateral occlusion of basilar artery branches. *J Neurol Neurosurg Psychiatry* 1977;40: 1182–1189.
225. Amarenco P, Rosengart A, DeWitt LD, Pessin MS, Caplan LR. Anterior inferior cerebellar artery territory infarcts. Mechanisms and clinical features. *Arch Neurol* 1993;50:154–161.
226. Amarenco P. The spectrum of cerebellar infarctions. *Neurology* 1991;41:973–979.
227. Amarenco P, Hauw JJ. Cerebellar infarction in the territory of the anterior and inferior cerebellar artery. *Brain* 1990;113:139–155.
228. Hankey GJ, Dunne JW. Five cases of sudden hearing loss of presumed vascular origin. *Med J Aust* 1987;147:188–190.
229. Bogousslavsky J, Maeder P, Regli F, Meuli R. Pure midbrain infarction: clinical syndromes, MRI, and etiologic patterns. *Neurology* 1994; 44:2032–2040.
230. Hommel M, Bogousslavsky J. The spectrum of vertical gaze palsy following unilateral brainstem stroke. *Neurology* 1991;41:1229–1234.
231. Martin PJ, Chang HM, Wityk R, Caplan LR. Midbrain infarction: associations and aetiologies in the New England Medical Center Posterior Circulation Registry. *J Neurol Neurosurg Psychiatry* 1998;64:392–395.
232. Biller J, Shapiro R, Evans LS, Haag JR, Fine M. Oculomotor nuclear complex infarction. *Arch Neurol* 1984;41:985–987.
233. Amarenco P, Roullet E, Govjoa C, Cheron F, Hauw JJ, Bousser MG. Infarction in the anterior rostral cerebellum (the territory of the lateral branch of the superior cerebellar artery). *Neurology* 1991;41:253–258.
234. Amarenco P, Hauw JJ. Cerebellar infarction in the territory of the superior cerebellar artery. *Neurology* 1990;40:1383–1390.
235. Erdemoglu AK, Duman T. Superior cerebellar artery territory stroke. *Acta Neurol Scand* 1998; 98:283–287.
236. Chaves CJ, Caplan LR, Chung CS, et al. Cerebellar infarcts in the New England Medical Center Posterior Circulation Stroke Registry. *Neurology* 1994;44:1385–1390.
237. Amarenco P, Levy C, Cohen A, Toubouc PJ, Roullet E, Bousser MG. Causes and mechanisms of territorial and nonterritorial cerebellar infarcts in 115 consecutive patients. *Stroke* 1994; 25:105–112.
238. Amarenco P, Caplan LR. Vertebrovasilar occlusive disease. Review of selected aspects. 3 mechanisms of cerebellar infarctions. *Cerebrovasc Dis* 1993;3:66–73.
239. Kanis KB, Ropper AH, Adelman LS. Homolateral hemiparesis as an early sign of cerebellar mass effect. *Neurology* 1994;44:2194–2197.

240. Besson G, Hommel M, Perret J. Historical aspects of the lacunar concept. *Cerebrovasc Dis* 1991;1:306–310.
241. Fisher CM. Lacunar strokes and infarcts: a review. *Neurology* 1982;32:871–876.
242. Landau WM. Clinical neuromythology VI. Au clair de lacune: holy, wholly, holey logic. *Neurology* 1989;39:725–730.
243. You R, McNeil JJ, O'Malley HM, Davis SM, Donnan GA. Risk factors for lacunar infarction syndromes. *Neurology* 1995;45: 1483–1487.
244. Mohr JP. Lacunes. *Stroke* 1982;13:3–11.
245. Carter BS, Ogilvy CS, Candia GJ, Rosas HD, Buonanno F. One-year outcome after decompressive surgery for massive nondominant hemispheric infarction. *Neurosurgery* 1997;40: 1168–1175.
246. Arboix A, Marti-Vilalta JL. Lacunar sydromes not due to lacunar infarcts. *Cerebrovasc Dis* 1992; 2:287–292.
247. Landi G, Cella E, Boccardi E, Musicco M. Lacunar versus non-lacunar infarcts: pathogenetic and prognostic differences. *J Neurol Neurosurg Psychiatry* 1992;55:441–445.
248. Boiten J, Lodder J. Lacunar infarcts: pathogenesis and validity of the clinical syndromes. *Stroke* 1991;22:1374–1378.
249. Boiten J, Lodder J. Prognosis for survival, handicap, and recurrence of stroke in lacunar and superficial infarction. *Cerebrovasc Dis* 1993;3: 221–226.
250. Toni D, Fiorelli M, De Michele M, et al. Clinical and prognostic correlates of stroke subtype misdiagnosis within 12 hours from onset. *Stroke* 1995;26:1837–1840.
251. Toni D, Del Duca R, Fiorelli M, et al. Pure motor hemiparesis and sensorimotor stroke. Accuracy of very early clinical diagnosis of lacunar strokes. *Stroke* 1994;25:92–96.
252. Melo TP, Bogousslavsky J, Van Melle G, Regli F. Pure motor stroke: a reappraisal. *Neurology* 1992;42:789–795.
253. Shintani S. Clinical-radiologic correlations in pure sensory stroke. *Neurology* 1998;51: 297–302.
254. Paciaroni M, Bogousslavsky J. Pure sensory syndromes in thalamic stroke. *Eur Neurol* 1998;39: 211–217.
255. Chaves CJ, Silver B, Schlaug G, Dashe J, Caplan LR, Warach S. Diffusion- and perfusion-weighted MRI patterns in borderzone infarcts. *Stroke* 2000;31:1090–1096.
256. Ghika-Schmid F, Bogousslavsky J. The acute behavioral syndrome of anterior thalamic infarction: A prospective study of 12 cases. *Ann Neurol* 2000;48:220–227.

Chapter 4

EVALUATION OF THE PATIENT WITH A TRANSIENT ISCHEMIC ATTACK OR AN ISCHEMIC STROKE

GENERAL PRINCIPLES

The purposes of evaluating a patient with a suspected transient ischemic attack (TIA) or ischemic stroke are multiple. Studies are performed to determine whether neurological symptoms are due to ischemia. They also detect the presence of medical or neurological complications or serious comorbid diseases. In addition, tests are used to screen for the presence of risk factors that would predispose to stroke and to search for the most likely cause of the ischemic

Table 4–1. **Emergent Diagnostic Tests for the Evaluation of a Patient with Recent Transient Ischemic Attack or Ischemic Stroke**

Computed tomography of the brain
12-lead electrocardiogram
Chest roentgenogram
Complete blood count
Platelet count
Prothrombin time and international normalized ratio
Activated partial thromboplastin time
Blood glucose
Serum electrolytes and chemistries
Electroencephalogram (if seizures suspected)
Cerebrospinal fluid examination (if subarachnoid hemorrhage suspected)

Table 4–2. **Non-emergent Evaluation of a Patient With a Transient Ischemic Attack or Ischemic Stroke**

Magnetic resonance imaging of the brain
T_1- and T_2-weighted images
FLAIR images
Diffusion and perfusion images
Positron emission tomography
Single photon emission tomography
Electroencephalogram and evoked potentials
Cerebrospinal fluid examination
Arteriography
Digital subtraction arteriography
Carotid duplex
Transcranial Doppler ultrasonography
Magnetic resonance angiography
Computed tomographic angiography
Echocardiography
Transthoracic
Transesophageal
Contrast-enhanced
Color-coded Doppler
Gated magnetic resonance imaging of the heart
Cine computed tomography of the heart
Fasting lipid profile

symptoms. Results of the diagnostic evaluation influence decisions about acute and long-term care (Tables 4–1 and 4–2). In general, tests are divided into those needed on an emergent basis and those obtained after the patient's condition has stabilized. Both are ordered on a case-by-case basis.

Because the differential diagnosis of TIA or ischemic stroke is not very extensive (see Tables 3–1 and 3–6), the evaluation required to confirm a diagnosis is relatively limited.[1–4] Emergent tests generally include those needed to exclude other acute neurological diseases and those that look for acute complications. These tests help guide decisions about urgent care (see Table 4–1). Imaging of the brain (computed tomography [CT] or magnetic resonance imaging [MRI]) is a key immediate diagnostic test. In exceptional cases, electroencephalography (EEG) may be needed if a seizure disorder is an alternative diagnosis for the cause of transient symptoms or if a patient is unconscious. Rarely, examination of the cerebrospinal fluid (CSF) is necessary if subarachnoid hemorrhage is suspected and brain imaging does not show blood or if a central nervous system infection is an alternative diagnosis. Blood tests are done to rule out a metabolic disorder, such as hypoglycemia, that can mimic a TIA or stroke. Occasionally, consultation from an ophthalmologist or an otolaryngologist is sought to help dismiss primary eye or ear diseases that can be confused with a TIA or stroke. Studies used to screen for acute medical or neurological complications or comorbid diseases include brain imaging, chest x-ray, electrocardiogram, and blood tests.[2,3] The results of these tests can influence decisions about emergent care, such as the prescription of recombinant tissue plasminagen activator (rt-PA).

IMAGING OF THE BRAIN

With the exception of patients who have amaurosis fugax, almost all patients with a suspected TIA or stroke should have a brain imaging test. Brain imaging is helpful in distinguishing an ischemic stroke from a brain tumor, a subdural hematoma, or another intracranial mass. Because of the poor sensitivity and specificity of clinical scales in differentiating hemorrhagic from ischemic stroke, brain imaging remains the best way to exclude an intracranial hemorrhage as the cause of the acute neurological impairments.[5,6] In addition to excluding other causes of the neurological symptoms, the brain imaging test provides information about the acute ischemic stroke itself. The size and location of the ischemic stroke provide clues about prognosis and clues about the likely cause of the vascular event. Acute complications identified by brain imaging include hydrocephalus, brain edema, mass effect and herniation, and hemorrhagic transformation of the infarction.

Computed Tomography

EMERGENT COMPUTED TOMOGRAPHY

General Comments

Computed tomography of the brain is the most widely used emergent brain imaging study in the management of persons with stroke. Computed tomography is readily available in most countries, and it is noninvasive and relatively inexpensive. The required radiation exposure is relatively low. Methods to shield a fetus can be used so that the test can be performed in pregnant women. Because CT can be done in a few minutes, it can be performed in critically ill patients, including those who are comatose, agitated, or intubated. The rapid speed of data acquisition avoids most movement artifacts. If a brain tumor or a vascular malformation is a serious consideration, then a contrast-enhanced scan may help but, in most other instances, a non-enhanced scan is sufficient. Computed tomography has disadvantages, and it can miss a lesion in the brain stem or the cerebellum because of bone-induced artifacts. It also may not detect a small ischemic stroke in either the cerebral cortex or deep in the cerebral hemisphere.

Computed tomography is particularly useful in the urgent evaluation of patients with suspected acute ischemic stroke because the most important alternative diagnosis is hemorrhagic stroke.[1,2,7,8] During the first hours after onset of stroke, the yield of CT in detecting intracerebral hemorrhage approaches 100%.[9] Its ability to detect subarachnoid hemorrhage (SAH) is approximately 95% during the first 1–2 days after aneurysmal rupture. Computed tomography may not discover a small, focal collection of blood in the subarachnoid space that occurs following a minor SAH; fortunately, however, the presentation of a minor SAH differs sufficiently from ischemic stroke so that the possibility of a minor subarachnoid collection is not great. In general, the absence of hemorrhage or a normal CT supports the diagnosis of ischemic stroke as the cause of neurological symptoms. A potential problem with CT is the ability of physicians to differentiate the important findings among patients with acute stroke.[10] The CT test is only as effective as the physicians' ability to interpret the results.

Computed Tomography Findings of Acute Ischemic Stroke

Although a CT study performed shortly after the onset of stroke can be normal, most examinations during the first 6 hours detect an ischemic locus.[11–13] In cases of acute stroke, the lesion often is observed as a restricted area of hypodensity (Figs. 4–1

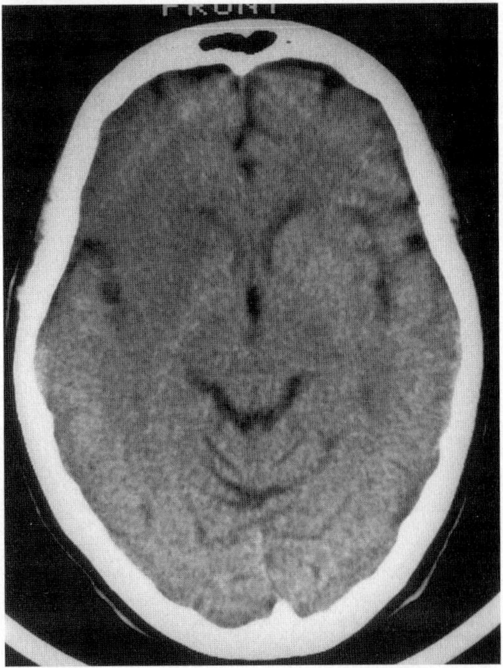

Figure 4–1. Computed tomogram of the brain obtained from a patient with a recent hemisphere infarction. An infarction is noted in the right frontal lobe and insular region.

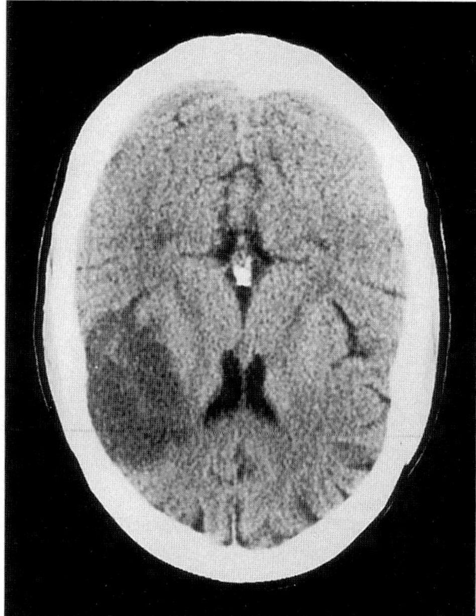

A

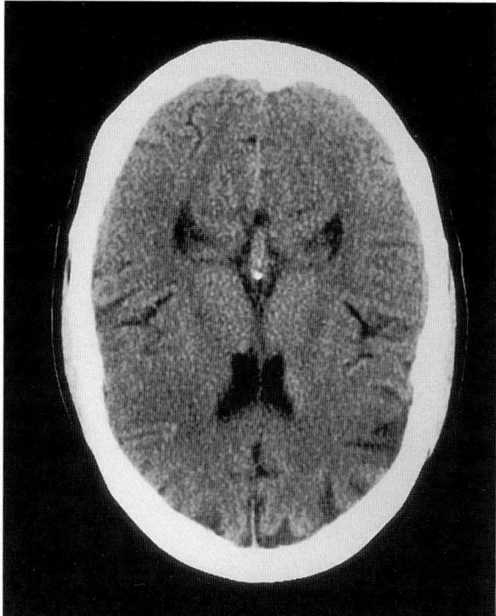

B

Figure 4–2. Fogging phenomenon. Computed tomographic scan (*A*) shows a well-circumscribed hypodense infarct involving the left frontal operculum and insula. On a follow-up CT scan performed on day 12 (*B*), the infarct is nearly isodense to the surrounding normal brain parenchyma, presumably due to petechial hemorrhage. However, the normal grey matter/cortical ribbon is absent in the infarct. (Courtesy of Dr. B. Silver.)

and 4–2). Still, a normal test does not preclude the diagnosis of ischemic stroke. The yield of CT in detecting ischemic lesions increases during the first 24 hours. The size of the stroke affects the likelihood of early detection by CT; a small subcortical infarction often is not seen, whereas a large cortical infarction usually is visualized. Patients with a history of previous stroke usually have abnormalities. Dark areas of hypodensity reflect the region of brain affected by the prior stroke (Fig. 4–3). Approximately 20% of patients with acute stroke have CT evidence of a previous stroke even when the event was clinically silent.[14,15] These strokes often are multiple, small, and located in the basal ganglia. Most patients with a TIA have a normal CT study. Patients who have had a "prolonged" TIA might have a small ischemic lesion found by CT, which is consistent with the diagnosis of cerebral infarction with transient symptoms.[16,17] These strokes usually are small and subcortical in location. As in the scenario of an acute stroke, the CT may show evidence of prior brain events.

Several CT findings found in the first hours after ischemic stroke influence decisions about treatment, in particular, those con-

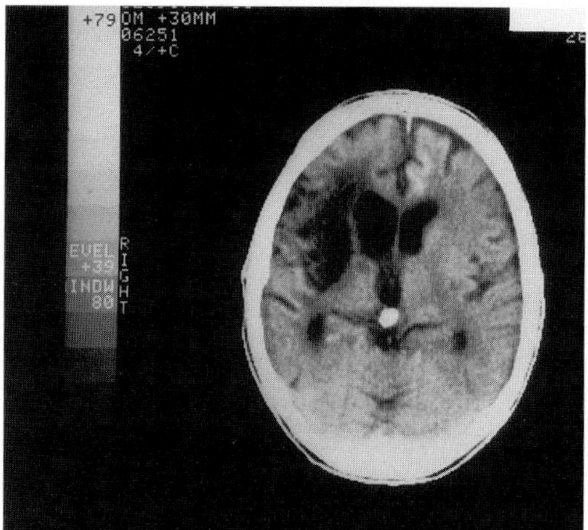

Figure 4–3. Old infarction of the right hemisphere seen on computed tomography. The infarction shows an area of marked hypodensity. The ipsilateral lateral ventricle is dilated secondary to atrophy of the hemisphere.

Table 4–3. **Computed Tomographic Findings that Influence Decisions About Emergent Treatment of Ischemic Stroke**

Intracranial hemorrhage or hemorrhagic transformation
Age of infarction (hypodensity)
Brain edema with mass effect or shift of midline structures
Dense artery sign
Hypodensity involving more than one-third of hemisphere
Obliteration of sulci
Loss of insular ribbon
Prominent hypodensity in the lenticulostriate territory

traindicating thrombolytic therapy.[13,18–21] (See Table 4–3.) A relatively dark, hypodense lesion suggests that the "acute" stroke may be older than 3 hours. In such a situation, the physician should again query the patient or observers about the time of onset of stroke. A dense artery sign, most commonly secondary to an embolus of cardiac origin, can be found in the first portion of the middle cerebral artery in approximately 10%–40% of patients with a major stroke in that vascular territory.[22–24] (See Figs. 4–4 and 4–5.) Although the sensitivity of the dense artery sign is low, its presence during the first days after stroke is very specific for an occlusion of the middle cerebral artery.[22] Because the presence of the dense artery sign is associated with an occlusion of the proximal portion of the middle cerebral artery, it generally forecasts a multilobar infarction and a poor prognosis.[25–28] This finding can be subtle, and occasionally calcification of the middle cerebral artery may be mislabeled as a dense artery sign. Von Kummer et al[29] found high agreement among radiologists in recognizing this sign. Computed tomography also can visualize calcification of the basilar artery and large dolichoectatic aneurysms of the basilar artery. These findings provide evidence to support a diagnosis of ischemia as the cause of a patient's symptoms of brain stem or cerebellar dysfunction.

Early hypodensity in the basal ganglia (lenticulostriate territory) and the insular cortex also predict a major hemispheric infarction.[13,30,31] Other early signs of a multilobar infarction include a large area of obliteration of the cortex-adjacent

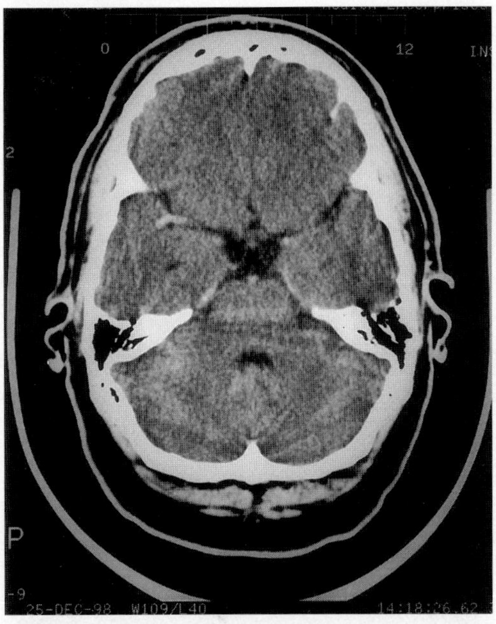

Figure 4–4. An embolus in the right middle cerebral artery (dense artery sign) found in a patient with an acute right hemisphere stroke.

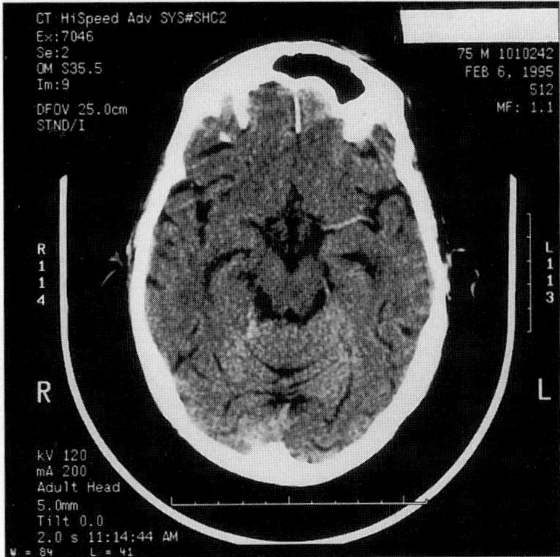

Figure 4–5. An emergent computed tomographic scan obtained from a patient with an acute left hemisphere stroke. The dense artery sign (embolus of the middle cerebral artery) is noted.

white matter junction or multiple sulci in the cerebral hemisphere. The tissue hypodensity reflects the area of decreased perfusion and non-viable brain.[13] Von Kummer et al[18,24] concluded that such findings involving more than one-third of the cerebral hemisphere predicted a poor outcome and an increased risk of hemorrhage secondary to thrombolytic therapy. These CT abnormalities generally are seen among patients with clinical evidence of a severe stroke.[32] In a recent study, radiologists' interpretation of the early CT findings of an infarction in greater than one-third of the cerebral hemisphere had a sensitivity of 60%–85% and a specificity of 86%–97%.[32] Although CT can detect many of these changes and most neuroradiologists usually agree about their presence, physicians may have difficulty in recognizing more subtle abnormalities; in particular, areas of hypodensity and sulcal effacement can be overlooked.[10,29] In one trial that tested emergent administration of thrombolytic therapy, approximately one-sixth of enrolled patients were subsequently judged to be ineligible, after treatment largely because the physicians did not recognize CT findings that would have contraindicated treatment.[33] Sequential CT studies display enlargement of the volume of the infarction during the first week after stroke in approximately one-third of patients.[34] Outcomes among patients with increases in volume size are poorer than among those without this change.[34]

The pattern and size of infarction seen on CT corresponds to the location of arterial occlusion (Figs. 4–6 and 4–7). Several groups have provided detailed templates that describe the most common patterns of vascular territories in the cerebral hemispheres, brain stem, and cerebellum.[21,35–37]

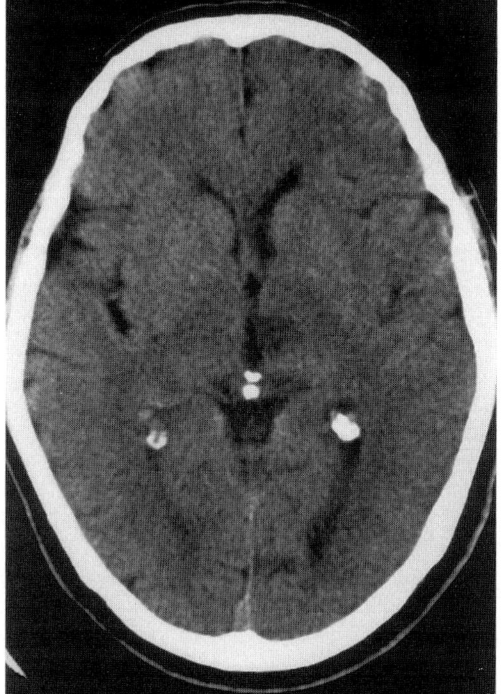

Figure 4–6. Computed tomogram of the brain demonstrates an infarction in the left median thalamus (thalamoperforating artery).

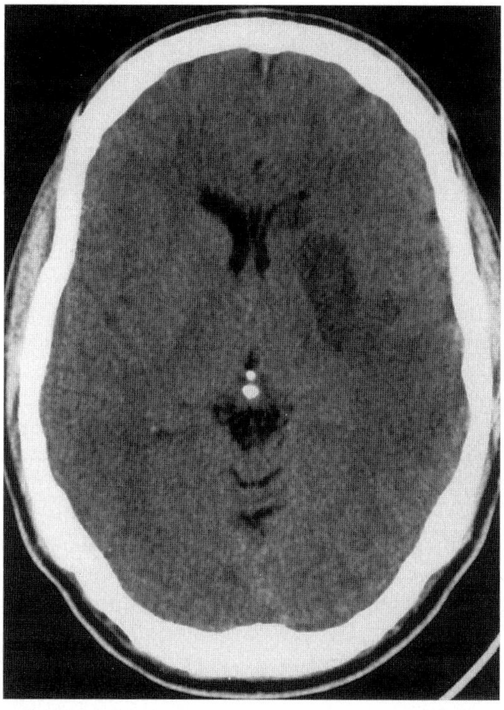

Figure 4–7. Computed tomogram of the brain shows infarctions in the left head of the caudate, left putamen and left temporal lobe.

The size and location of infarction on CT also provide information about the likely cause of stroke.[38] Physicians usually agree about the size of infarction seen on CT, particularly when it is either very large or very small.[39] As a rule, the volume of the infarction correlates with the severity of neurological impairments and the score on the National Institutes of Health Stroke Scale (NIHSS).[40] In general, lacunar infarctions are less than 1 cm. in size and oval in shape. A small (< 1 cm.) lesion restricted to a basal ganglion, the thalamus, or the internal capsule usually suggests a lacunar infarction secondary to occlusion of a small penetrating artery. An infarction that involves the cerebellar or hemispheric cortex usually is secondary to an embolus occluding a superficial artery.[41] These strokes result from cardioembolism or atherosclerotic disease of the proximal portion of the internal carotid artery or vertebral artery. Other acute proximal artery lesions, such as arterial dissections, also cause these strokes. These lesions usually are wedge-shaped with the point aimed centrally. They affect the cortex and adjacent white matter structures and correspond to the mapped territory of an occluded branch cortical artery. Occasionally, infarctions in two different areas of the same vascular territory can occur with a proximal arterial occlusion, with lysis and consequent distal migration of the embolus. A multilobar hemispheric lesion on CT usually is due to artery-to-artery or cardiogenic embolism, and it predicts a major stroke.[42,43] In one series of 44 patients with large infarctions found on CT, 25 had > 50% stenosis and 17 had an occlusion of the ipsilateral internal carotid artery.[44]

A subcortical infarction larger than 1.5 cm. usually is not a lacune. In particular, large lenticulostriate infarctions usually are secondary to occlusion of the proximal portion of the middle cerebral artery. For example, Steinke et al[45] noted that the CT findings among persons who had stroke secondary to a dissection of the internal carotid artery included large lenticulostriate infarctions. Multiple cortical and white matter ischemic lesions (watershed infarctions) seen at the junction of terminal perfusion areas of the major cortical arteries (middle, anterior, and posterior cerebral) usually occur in the setting of hypotension or microembolism compounding a severe narrowing of an extracranial or intracranial artery. Subcortical or cortical borderzone lesions can be due to either carotid atherosclerosis or cardioembolism.[46] Acute bilateral lesions often are precipitated by a major cardiovascular operation associated with profound hypotension. In this setting, atherosclerotic disease of the internal carotid artery is often mild. Infarctions of similar age in multiple vascular territories suggest cardioembolism as the cause of stroke. Two or more isolated areas of infarction in the same vascular territory may be secondary to a proximal embolus that breaks into pieces and occludes distal arteries.

Follow-Up Computed Tomography

Subsequent CT studies reflect a patient's prognosis and influence decisions about acute management, including hydrocephalus, brain edema, or mass effect, which prompt medical or surgical therapies to control increased intracranial pressure (Table 4–4). Approximately one-third of patients will have enlargement of the stroke found on sequential CT studies.[34] These patients have poorer outcomes than do patients whose infarctions do not enlarge on follow-up studies. Early temporal lobe involvement found on CT usually is associated with a poor prognosis and a very large infarction.[47] Sequential CT studies provide help in the management of multilobar infarction of the cerebral hemisphere; brain edema evolves during the first 4–5 days following the stroke. The edema, which appears isodense on CT, usually arises adjacent to the area of necrotic tissue and spreads to adjacent white matter regions. Sulci of the ipsilateral hemisphere become effaced as the brain swells.[48] Subsequently, the ipsilateral lateral ventricle and Sylvian fissure are compressed, and the contralateral

Table 4–4. **Potential Findings on Subsequent Computed Tomography Scans Performed After Acute Ischemic Stroke**

Delineation of the infarction
- Increased hypodensity
- Anatomic definition

Subarachnoid or intraventricular hemorrhage
Hemorrhagic transformation of infarction
- Patterns
  - Small areas of petechia
  - Confluent areas of petechia
  - Small hematoma
  - Hematoma producing mass effect

Brain edema and mass effect
- Stages with multilobar hemispheric infarction
  - Obliteration of ipsilateral sulci
  - Compression of ipsilateral third ventricle
  - Compression of ipsilateral Sylvian fissure
  - Contralateral ventricular dilation
  - Compression of basal cisterns
  - Contralateral displacement (shift)
    - Cingulate gyrus
    - Third ventricle
    - Medial temporal lobe (uncus)
    - Pineal

Mass-producing lobar cerebellar infarction
- Swollen cerebellar hemisphere
- Compression and distortion of brain stem
- Obliteration of prepontine cistern
- Obliteration of fourth ventricle
- Dilated third and lateral ventricles

ventricle dilates secondary to obstruction of CSF flow in the third ventricle or the foramen of Munro. With severe hemispheric brain edema, the basal cisterns become obliterated.[48] Displacement of midline structures (cingulate gyrus, third ventricle, and the pineal) toward the contralateral side corresponds to the volume of the necrotic mass. This lateral shift usually coincides with the appearance of clinical findings of uncal herniation. The CT findings develop in concert with neurological worsening, including a decline in consciousness. Because serious brain edema, which will lead to neurological deterioration, is unlikely among patients with lacunar infarctions, striatocapsular infarctions, or branch cortical infarctions, subsequent CT studies are not as critical in managing these persons as in those with multilobar infarctions.

A follow-up CT may be especially important in management of patients with acute cerebellar infarction. A cerebellar lesion greater than 2.5 cm. often is associated with a secondary mass effect causing compression of the brain stem, the fourth ventricle, or the aqueduct of Sylvius (see Table 4–4). Loss of the basal cisterns, in particular the pre-pontine cistern, suggests compression by a cerebellar mass. In addition, the swollen cerebellum compresses the fourth ventricle and distorts the aqueduct of Sylvius, which leads to acute dilation of the third and lateral ventricles. These CT findings, associated with the development of multiple cranial nerve palsies, motor impairments, and a decline in consciousness, can prompt emergent surgical treatment.

A CT study done in the first few days after stroke also can detect hemorrhagic transformation of an infarction in approximately 10%–40% of patients. In most cases, this bleeding is minor and is not associated with neurological worsening.[11] Hemorrhagic changes are most likely in association with cortical infarctions secondary to cardioembolism. Multilobar infarctions in persons with moderate-to-severe neurological impairments also are more likely to be accompanied by bleeding than smaller lesions. Hemorrhagic changes have a propensity to develop in the subcortical nuclei (lenticulostriate region) among patients with large strokes. The severity of CT-detected hemorrhagic changes within the area of infarction has been categorized as (*1*) small petechiae areas (hemorrhagic infarction—grade 1), (*2*) small confluent hemorrhagic area (hemorrhagic infarction–grade 2), (*3*) small hematoma (cerebral hemorrhage—grade 1), and (*4*) large hematoma (cerebral hemorrhage—grade 2). The hematomas usually can be divided by size (≥ 2 cm. would be considered large) or by neurological worsening as ascribed to the hemorrhagic lesion.[48] Intracranial bleeding associated with neurological worsening usually suggests a large, mass-producing hematoma within the ischemic area or a hematoma complicated by intraventricular or subarachnoid bleeding.

Magnetic Resonance Imaging

Magnetic resonance imaging is less readily available and more expensive than CT. Although MRI does not involve an exposure to radiation, it often takes 30–40 minutes to complete a study.[49] (See Fig. 4–8 and Table 4–5.) Some acutely ill patients may be too unstable medically for transfer to an MRI facility.[49] Monitoring the patient's neurological, cardiovascular, and pulmonary status also can be difficult during the test. Agitated or confused patients may not tolerate MRI, and resultant movement artifacts may ruin the images. Patients with cardiac pacemakers or other electronic devices cannot have MRI.[49] An important advantage of MRI is that it gives axial, sagittal, and coronal views that allow a detailed assessment of the size and location of any ischemic lesion. In addition, the test can incorporate T_1-weighted, T_2-weighted, balanced, and FLAIR techniques. Each of these techniques provides information that might be useful in

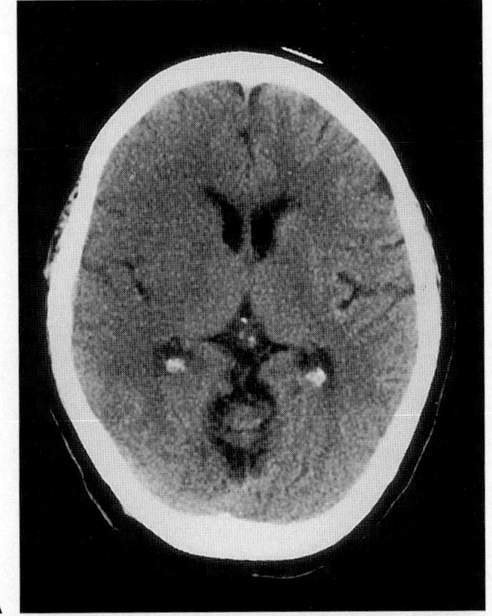

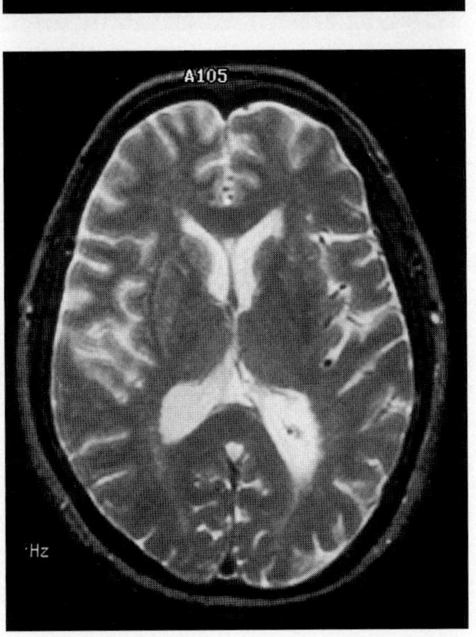

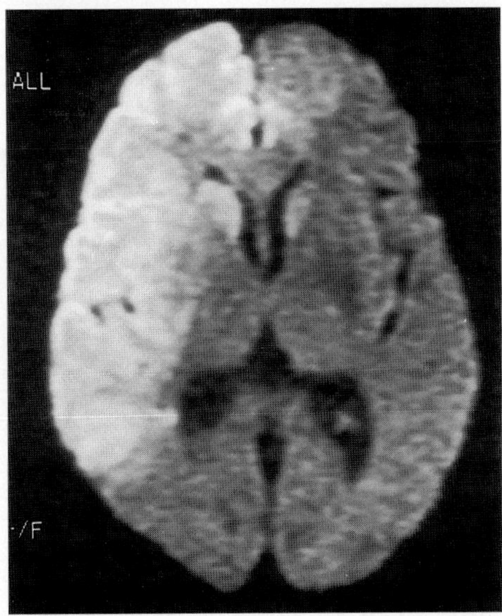

Figure 4–8. Acute ischemic infarct on CT and MRI. This 77-year-old woman with atrial fibrillation was found unconscious in her chair. She spontaneously moved only her left arm. The CT scan (*A*) shows hypodensity of the basal ganglia, loss of the cortical ribbon, and effacement of sulci over the frontal, parietal, temporal, and insular lobes on the right side. On the T_2-weighted MRI (*B*), the flow void signals of the right middle cerebral artery and its branches are absent suggesting absent or reduced flow in these arteries. There are no definite signal changes in the brain parenchyma. In contrast, the DWI MRI (*C*) shows markedly increased signal intensity in the right middle cerebral artery and both anterior cerebral artery territories. (Courtesy of Dr. E. Wong.)

Table 4–5. **Advantages, and Disadvantages of Magnetic Resonance Imaging in Acute Ischemic Stroke**

Advantages
Several sequences of studies
- T1, T2, balanced, FLAIR
- Perfusion and diffusion
- Contrast enhanced

Several views
- Axial
- Sagittal
- Coronal

Findings
- Early detection of ischemic lesions
- Poor perfusion
- Mis-match of diffusion and perfusion scans
- Detect small infaractions
- Detect infarctions in brain stem and cerebellum

Absence of flow void—occlusion or poor flow
Detect arterial pathology—dissection

Disadvantages
Not readily available
More expensive than CT
Can take 30–45 minutes
May miss subarachnoid blood
Patient isolated during procedure
Patient need sedation
Claustrophobia
Cannot be done if metallic fragments or pacemaker present in patient

treating patients with acute ischemic stroke. In general, T_2-weighted imaging is the usual way to detect an ischemic lesion. FLAIR images can demonstrate cortical infarctions that are not visualized by other MRI techniques.[50] Three-dimensional MRI can define the anatomy of an infarction.[51] (See Fig. 4–9.)

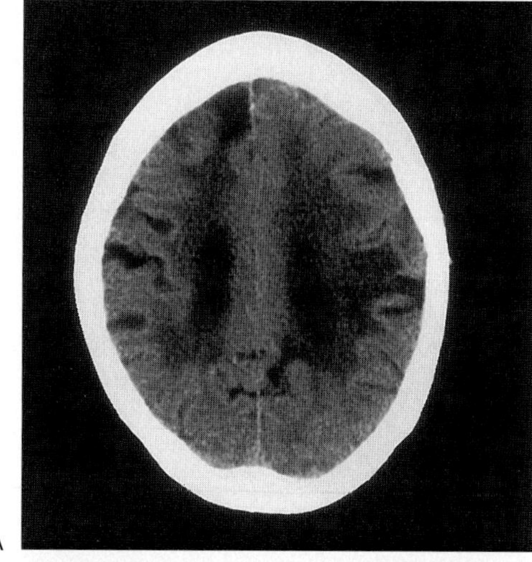
A

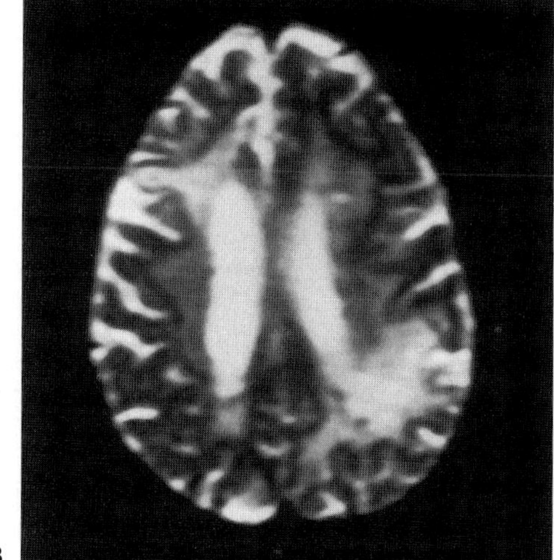
B

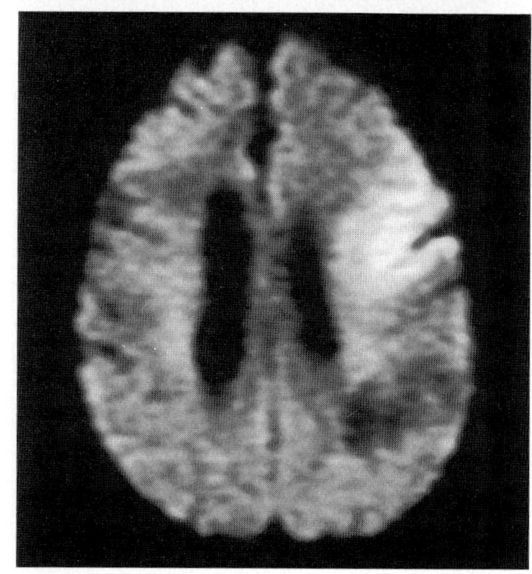
C

Figure 4–9. Acute and chronic infarct appearances on MRI and DWI. The CT scan (*A*) shows old infarcts in the right frontal and left fronto-parietal lobes. The T_2-weighted MRI (*B*) shows increased signal in the right frontal and left fronto-parietal lobes. The DWI MRI (*C*) shows increased signal in the left frontal lobe, indicating a recent infarct. The remote infarcts appear as areas of decreased signal. (Courtesy of Dr. B. Silver.)

Because MRI is not distorted by adjacent bone, the test is particularly useful in assessing ischemic lesions in the brain stem and the cerebellum, which might not be visualized by CT.[52–55] Magnetic resonance imaging also can show small subcortical ischemic lesions in the cerebral hemispheres.[52,56,57] Mohr et al[58] found that MRI and CT generally were equal in visualizing larger infarctions within the first few hours after stroke. Bryan et al[59] found that MRI was more sensitive than CT in detecting stroke within the first 24 hours. T_1- and T_2-weighted MRI may not be sufficiently sensitive to demonstrate an infarction in the first few hours after ischemic stroke and yield results to guide management.[58,60] Saunders et al[61] found a strong correlation between the volume of the ischemic lesion found on MRI and outcomes; fatal lesions were, on average, five times larger than those among patients who recovered from their strokes. Most of these abnormalities likely were detected more than 6 hours after the onset of stroke. Magnetic resonance imaging also detects multiple abnormalities usually restricted to the deep lobar white matter in elderly patients.[62–64] It can also find abnormalities among elderly patients who have had a TIA.[65] Some of these lesions, often clinically silent strokes, are more common among persons with chronic hypertension. In addition, MRI often detects abundant white matter changes in the cerebral hemispheres (Fig. 4–10). These abnormalities have been correlated with vascular dementia, such as Binswanger's disease. They create confusion for a physician who is trying to determine the exact location or size of a new stroke. Magnetic resonance imaging often reveals symptomatic or asymptomatic brain lesions that complicate cardiovascular operations, including brain stem or lacunar infarctions.[66]

Magnetic resonance imaging is an efficient way to define an intracranial hemorrhage or to consider non-vascular causes for a patient's acute neurological impairments. It is more sensitive than CT in defining the location and severity of acute complications of ischemic stroke, including brain edema, mass effect, and herniation.[60] Magnetic resonance imaging also is more sensitive than CT in detecting minor areas of hemorrhagic transformation. Because of changes in the breakdown products of a hematoma detected

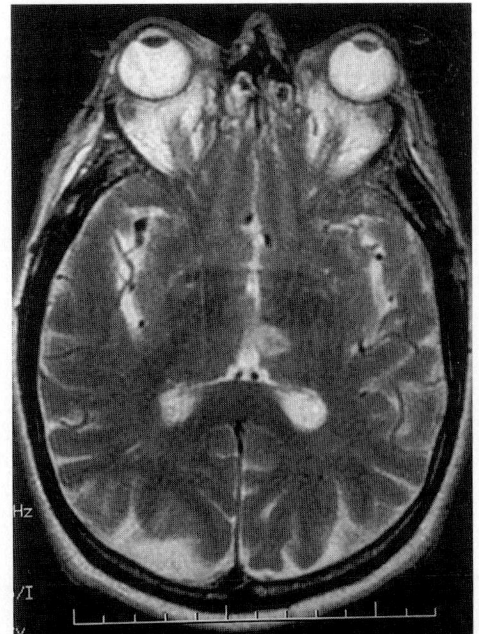

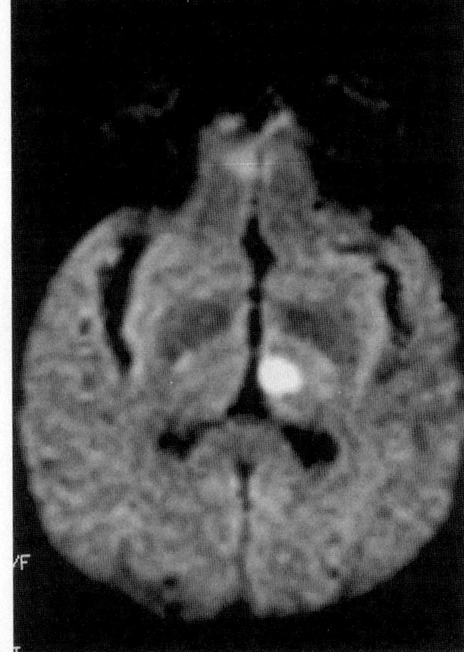

Figure 4–10. T_2-weighted (*A*) and diffusion- (*B*) magnetic resonance imaging reveal an infarction in the medial aspect of the left thalamus.

Table 4–6. **Changes in Magnetic Resonance Imaging Signals in Patients with Recent Intraparenchymal Hemorrhage**

Interval from Time Comparison of Hemorrhage	Blood Degradation Product	T-1 Signal in Comparison to Normal Brain	T-2 Signal in Comparison to Normal Brain
4–6 hours	Oxyhemoglobin	Isointense	Isointense
1–3 days	Deoxyhemoglobin	Isointense	Hyperintense or hypointense
4–7 days	Intracellular methemoglobin	Hyperintense	Hypointense
1–4 weeks	Extracelluar methemoglobin	Hyperintense	Hyperintense
>4 weeks	Hemosiderin	Hypointense	Hypointense

by in T_1- and T_2-weighted MRI, the age of any bleeding lesion also can be estimated by MRI. The time-linked changes in MRI findings of hemorrhage are outlined in Table 4–6.

Magnetic resonance imaging can detect flow voids in the major intracranial arteries at the base of the brain. Absence of a flow void marks an area of arterial occlusion.[67] (See Figs. 4–11, 4–12, and 4–13.) In particular, occlusion of the proximal portion of the middle cerebral artery or internal carotid artery is visualized by the MRI finding of an absent flow void.[68] A midline sagittal MRI view can show a lesion in the pre-pontine cistern consistent with basilar artery thrombosis.[69] An MRI also can display a large flow void in a dolichoectatic basilar artery.[70,71] The absence of flow voids in both internal carotid arteries and proximal portions of the anterior and middle cerebral arteries

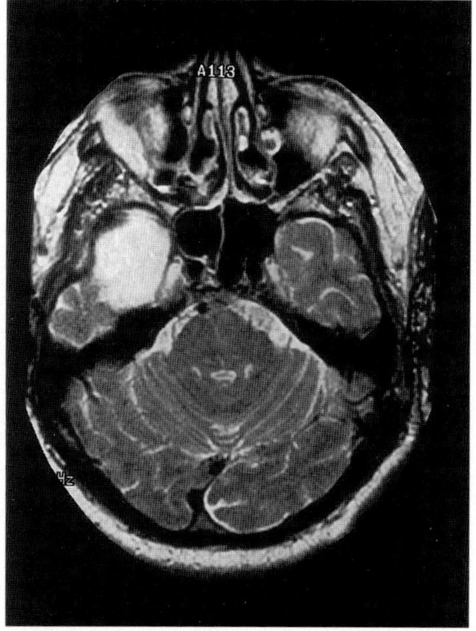

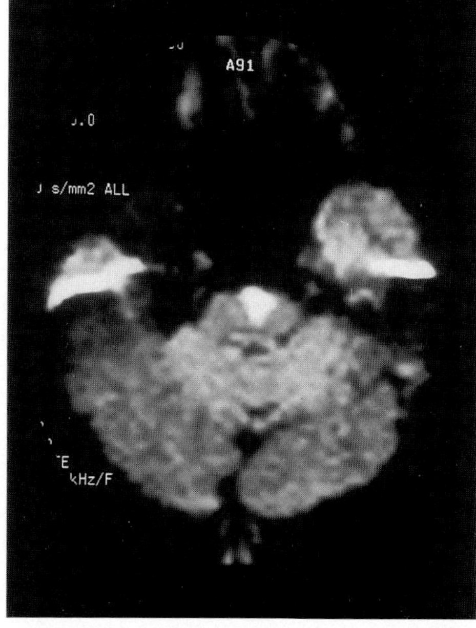

Figure 4–11. Diffusion weighted imaging in acute brainstem stroke. T_2-weighted MRI (*A*) shows slightly increased signal in the left paramedian pons and an incidental arachnoid cyst in the right middle cranial fossa. The acute infarct is clearly demonstrated on the DWI MRI (*B*). (Courtesy of Dr. E. Wong.)

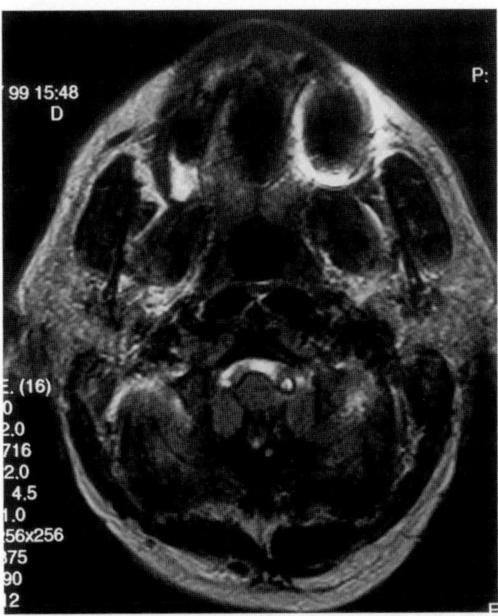

Figure 4–12. T_2-weighted MRI in a patient with a brain stem stroke demonstrates a thrombus in the left vertebral artery.

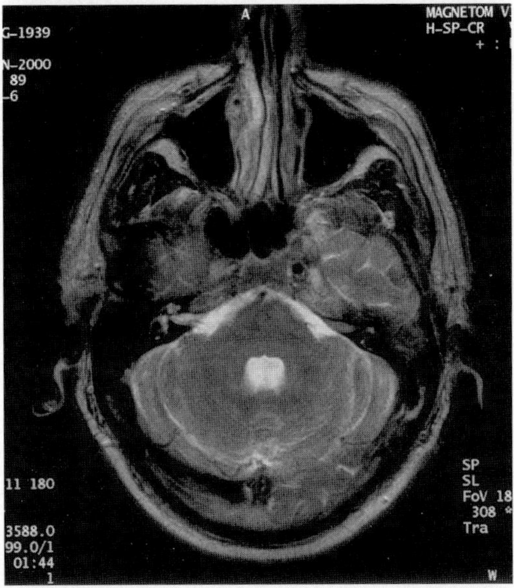

Figure 4–13. A T_2-weighted MRI of the brain shows an absent flow void in the right internal carotid artery in a patient with a carotid artery occlusion.

points toward moyamoya disease as the cause of stroke in a child or young adult.[72] In a person with a dissection of an intracranial or extracranial artery, MRI can show an eccentric curvilinear, band-like, bamboo-cut, or crescent-shaped area of hyperintensity adjacent to a flow void of reduced caliber.[73–75] The yield of MRI in detecting dissections is higher with carotid than with vertebral artery lesions.[76] An abnormal flow void can be the hallmark of other vascular lesions, including an intracranial aneurysm or vascular malformation. Magnetic resonance imaging also provides information on the structure of atherosclerotic plaques, including the presence of hemorrhages or fibrotic changes.[77]

CONTRAST-ENHANCED MAGNETIC RESONANCE IMAGING

Contrast-enhanced MRI can be used to screen for an inflammatory or meningeal process that is the cause of stroke. The meninges and the ventricular surface may show increased uptake secondary to local increases in vascularity. Contrast-enhanced MRI can show a slow-flow state in cortical arteries consistent with proximal occlusion of a major intracranial artery.[67,78,79] The sluggish flow permits contrast to stagnate in the pial vessels. At normal pressures, rapid flow does not allow for the contrast to be seen in the pial arteries. With low flow leading to vasodilation, the MRI can detect contrast in the dilated vessels. This arterial enhancement precedes changes in T_2-weighted images and subsequently resolves.[80] Rother et al[81] noted that contrast-enhanced MRI performed within 6 hours after stroke detects a reduction in regional cerebral blood volume before ischemic changes are found. Using contrast enhancement, Kluytmans et al[82] showed that MRI can detect increased mean transit time and peak time in white and gray matter, and increased cerebral blood volume in white matter, in the first hours after stroke.

PERFUSION AND DIFFUSION MAGNETIC RESONANCE IMAGING

Newer MRI methods, including perfusion and diffusion scanning, are useful in rapidly identifying an area of acute brain

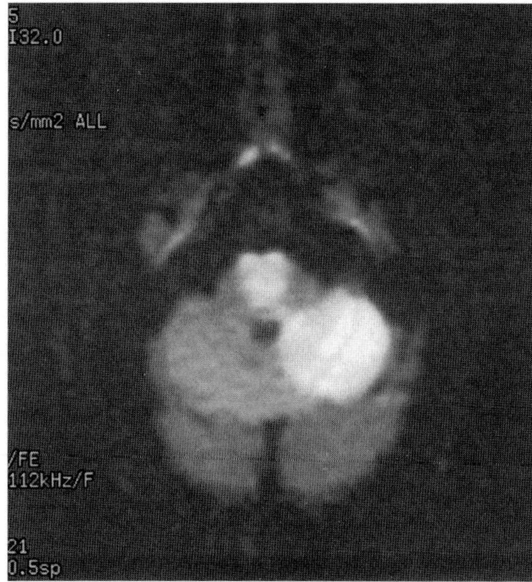

Figure 4–14. Diffusion-weighted MRI study obtained in a patient with presumed basilar thrombosis. Areas of changes in diffusion are noted in the left cerebellar hemisphere and pons.

ischemia.[60,83–96,413] (See Fig. 4–14.) These techniques rapidly define the size and site of an ischemic brain lesion within the first few hours after stroke. They also can be used to predict subtype of ischemic stroke.[96] These tests can detect structural brain changes following a TIA.[97] The combination of diffusion- and perfusion-weighted imaging can predict enlargement of the stroke and can help define the ischemic penumbra.[98] Sequential studies can ascertain responses to treatment.[86,88,99–103] The abnormalities on MRI, which are related to increases in tissue water, are seen before the development of abnormalities seen on T_2-weighted images.[104] Lovblad[87] found that the volume of stroke measured by diffusion-weighted MRI could be correlated with clinical outcomes. Early changes detected on diffusion-weighted MRI have high correlations with subsequent images detected on conventional MRI; the sensitivity and specificity of the test are 100% and 86%–94%, respectively, when performed within 6 hours of stroke.[105,106] The differences in perfusion- and diffusion-weighted images might identify patients at risk for progression of the ischemic penumbra.[100,107] Baird et al[108] noted that sequential diffusion-weighted MRI studies could assess changes in the ischemic focus (Fig. 4–15). Burdette et al[109] described a

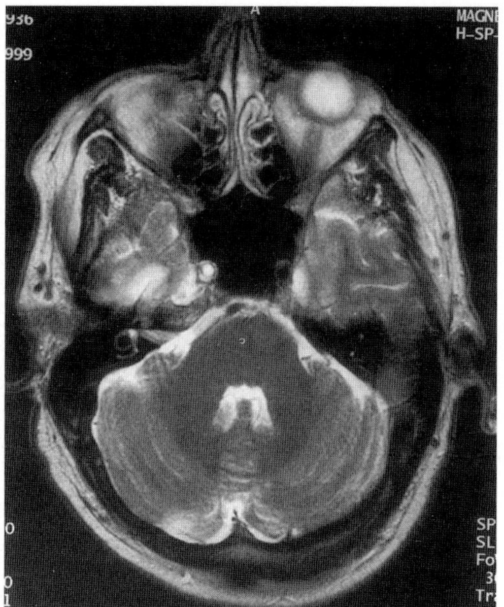
A

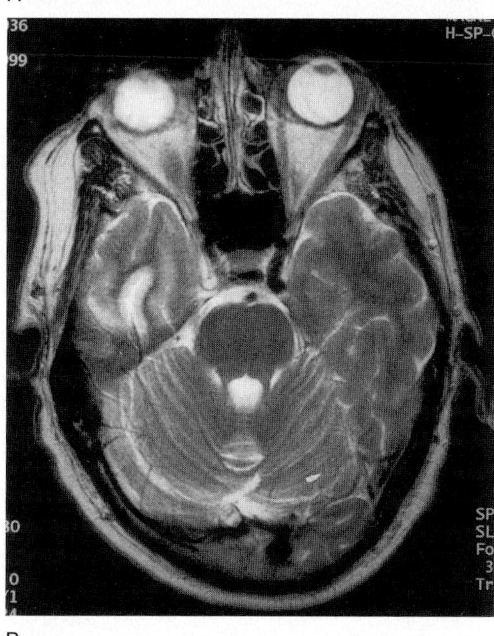
B

Figure 4–15. Adjacent T_2-weighted MRI scan (*A* and *B*) show a normal flow void in the left internal carotid artery and a thrombus in the right internal carotid artery.

time relationship pertaining to the ability of diffusion-weighted MRI to detect an ischemic stroke. The yield was approximately 100% within 24 hours, 96% on days 1–4, and less than 60% by days 10–14. Studies were negative when performed more than 2 weeks after the ictus or very soon after the onset of ischemia. Diffusion MRI can help distinguish old lesions that appear acute on conventional MRI.[93] This differentiation is critical in acute settings and a particularly important attribute of the new MRI technology. Lansberg et al[94] found that diffusion MRI was more sensitive and accurate in detecting acute stroke than CT. Diffusion-weighted MRI can miss lacunes. This test can show positive results after seizures and among patients with non-stroke causes of cell death, such as brain abscess. In contrast, a normal MRI study in a patient with "stroke-like" deficits should prompt an evaluation for another diagnosis.[110] Thus, the usefulness of these MRI studies has not been established and their role in patient care remains controversial. The role of MRI (including diffusion-weighted MRI) in management of patients with acute ischemic cerebrovascular disease is in flux.[111–113,95] At present, MRI has not replaced CT as the desired emergent diagnostic procedure to image the brain in most patients. If diffusion and/or perfusion MRI is found to be useful in the initial evaluation, then extensive efforts will be needed to validate these techniques. Educational programs will be needed so physicians can learn the nuances of interpreting findings provided by this technology.

OTHER NEUROLOGICAL DIAGNOSTIC TESTS

Electroencephalography

The role of EEG is limited in the evaluation of patients with a suspected TIA or stroke. The test may be helpful in differentiating a seizure from a TIA. Following stroke, EEG findings include generalized slow activity, a focal area of slow (delta) activity, and periodic lateralized epileptiform discharges (PLED).[114,115] Electro-encephalography can evaluate the extent of hemispheric injury or signs of global brain dysfunction, differentiating patients with good or poor prognoseis.[116] Extensive abnormalities on EEG, which usually reflect multilobar or bilateral infarction, predict a poor outcome. Because approximately 5% of patients with acute ischemic stroke have seizures with the event, an EEG may help if seizures are a consideration (Fig. 4–16).

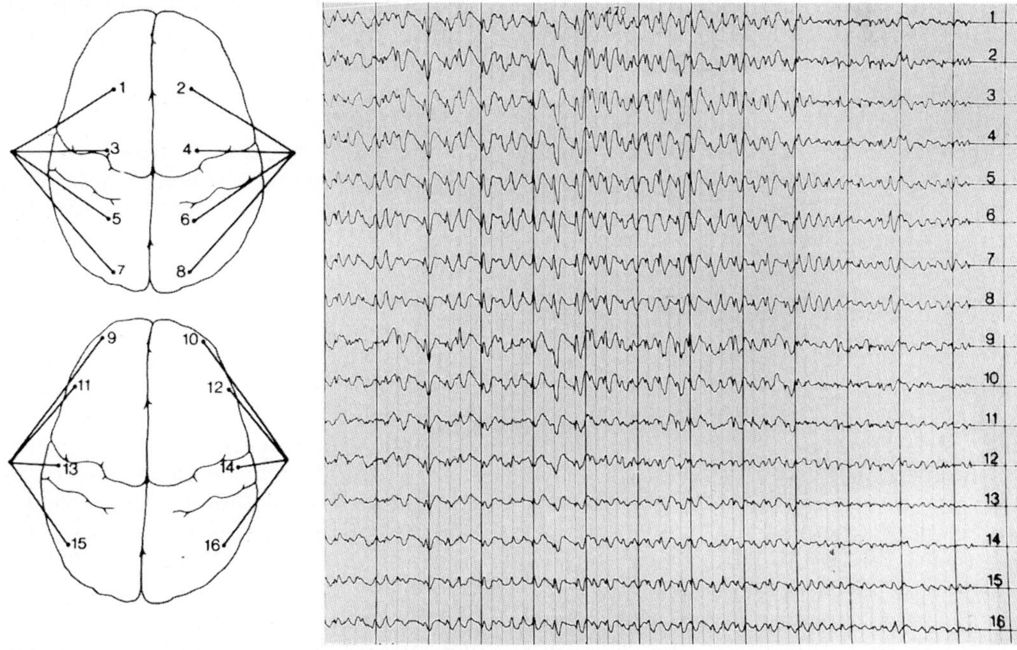

Figure 4–16. An 80-year-old man was admitted with acute onset of confusion and a mild right hemiparesis. The EEG showed 3 HZ spike and wave activity. Following treatment with diazepam, the EEG normalized and the patient's symptoms resolved. (Reprinted from Norris JW, Hachinski VC. Misdiagnosis of stroke. *Lancet* 1982;1:328, by permission.)

The EEG might detect intermittent epileptiform activity in a patient without clinically overt seizure activity. An EEG is not indicated to screen for a potential epileptogenic focus in a patient who has not had seizures following stroke. Electroencephalography frequently is ordered as an ancillary way to assess brain function in patients having carotid endarterectomy or cardiac surgery.[117,118] The monitoring is started before the part of the procedure that is associated with a decline in perfusion. A slowing of the EEG correlates with the development of ischemia, and this change in brain activity can prompt changes in the surgical procedure.[117] Still, most complications of carotid endarterectomy are of ischemic origin and cannot be predicted by EEG. Thus, the role of EEG monitoring may decline in the future. A preoperative EEG does not predict the likelihood of ischemic events during carotid or cardiac surgery.[119]

Cerebrospinal Fluid Examination

Examination of the CSF is necessary to screen for blood in a patient with a suspected SAH but whose CT does not show blood.[9,120] Because the clinical features of an SAH differ considerably from those of ischemic stroke, the former rarely is part of the differential diagnosis. Lumbar puncture is not needed for the initial evaluation of most patients. A mild rise in white blood cell count and total protein are the usual CSF findings after ischemic stroke. The major indication for examination of the CSF after ischemic stroke is to screen for an infectious and inflammatory cause. In particular, CSF leucocytosis and an abnormal CSF protein, including elevated globulins, may be detected in a patient with meningovascular syphilis, another infectious arteritis, granulomatous angiitis, or a multisystem vasculitis.[121] An elevation of the CSF levels of the BB fraction of creatine kinase or lactic acid dehydrogenase can be found in stroke.[122–124] The importance of these findings in predicting outcomes or responses to treatment is not clear.

ASSESSMENT OF CEREBRAL BLOOD FLOW AND BRAIN METABOLISM

Positron Emission Tomography

Positron emission tomography (PET) is a research tool that is critical for research on the pathophysiology of stroke in humans.[125,126] Its results provide important information about changes in cerebral blood flow, cerebral blood volume, cerebral tissue oxygenation, and brain metabolism, all of which evolve in the days following acute ischemic stroke.[125] A key finding of acute stroke is dissociation between cerebral blood flow, blood volume, and brain metabolic activity. For example, "luxury perfusion" involves normal or increased blood flow in comparison to brain metabolism, whereas "misery perfusion" reflects reduced blood flow in comparison to brain metabolic activity.[125,127] During the autoregulation stage of ischemia, cerebral blood volume is increased. Later, during the oligemic phase, cerebral blood flow is decreased, oxygen extraction fraction is increased, and the cerebral metabolic rate for oxygen is normal. The results of PET provide critical data supporting the concepts of the ischemic penumbra and the evolving or progressing stroke (see Chapter 1).[126,128] Although PET has been invaluable in research, its usefulness is less clear in a clinical setting. Its role in influencing decisions about acute care has not been defined. The technology is not widely available, and it involves exposure to a radioisotope that often must be created on site. Costs have decreased, but the study remains expensive. Positron emission tomography also has limitations in its ability to define small areas of pathology or anatomic correlates with areas of abnormal perfusion or metabolism. The oxygen extraction fraction can measure compensatory flow among patients with occlusions of the internal carotid artery.[129] Recently, Grubb et al[130] used PET to screen patients with symptomatic occlusions of the internal carotid artery. A group of patients with a decreased metabolic response to provocative tests are at very high risk for recurrent stroke and thus might benefit from reconstructive operations.[131] Other studies confirm these Findings.[414,415] The results of these studies may rekindle interest in extracranial–intracranial bypass operations.[130,414,415] If these results are substantiated, then the role of PET in selecting patients for surgery, including carotid endarterectomy, could expand.

Single Photon Emission Computed Tomography

Single photon emission computed tomography (SPECT) also can be used to assess cerebral blood flow and possibly cerebral metabolism in patients with ischemic cerebrovascular disease.[4,125,132–135] This technology is more widely available than PET. It is also less expensive than PET and uses commercially prepared radioisotopes. Stimulating blood flow with agents such as acetazolamide or adenosine can highlight the areas of borderline flow or metabolism among patients with severe extracranial occlusive disease.[136,137] Single photon emission computed tomography also can define areas of hypoperfusion in persons with extensive intracranial or extracranial arterial disease, such as moyamoya disease, which could influence decisions about surgical management. Single photon emission computed tomography changes correlate with a patient's age, the cause of stroke, and the severity of neurological impairments.[138–140] It also can differentiate stroke from other causes of focal neurological impairments, such as seizures leading to a Todd's paralysis.[136] The early changes detected by SPECT correlate with the NIHSS score and with neurological outcomes.[140–142] Local hyperperfusion can be seen during the first hours after stroke.[143,144] Baird et al[145] and Brass et al[146] found that SPECT perfusion measurements during the first 48 hours after stroke have a sensitivity of 79%–86% and a specificity of 95%–98% in detecting a cortical ischemic lesion. Although SPECT is more sensitive than CT, it can miss small lacunar or subcortical infarctions. Using SPECT, Ueda et al[147] found that a comparison between blood flow in the cerebral hemisphere and the cerebellum could predict the presence of salvageable tissue and the risk of hemorrhage. The brain tissue might be salvageable if flow to the ischemic tissue in the cerebral hemisphere is greater than 55% that of the cerebellum (used as a reference). In such a situation, treatment to restore circulation could be started up to 6 hours after stroke. If flow to the ischemic hemisphere is less than 35% that of the control flow in the cerebellum, then the likelihood of success is low and the risk of bleeding is great. Alexandrov et al[134] also reported that the results of SPECT could help identify patients at highest risk for bleeding complications following thrombolytic therapy. The usefulness of SPECT as an ancillary tool to help select patients for treatment with either intravenous or intra-arterial thrombolysis must be tested.

Functional Computed Tomography

Several methods using CT have been developed to assess brain metabolism and cerebral blood flow. Hunter et al[148] correlated findings on three-dimensional, functional CT with the perfused cerebral blood volume in patients with acute ischemic neurological impairments. Contrast-enhanced, high-resolution CT also can assess cerebrovascular physiology.[149] Cerebral blood flow studies using radiolabeled xenon were performed for a number of years. This technology, which involved use of several cortical probes to measure superficial flow, has largely been abandoned. Computed tomography measurement of blood flow using non-radiolabeled xenon also can quantify localized cerebral blood flow, but this technology has not gained widespread acceptance.[150–152]

Magnetic Resonance Imaging Spectroscopy

Magnetic resonance imaging spectroscopy detects metabolic abnormalities and biochemical markers within the first hours after stroke.[153,154,413]. It can measure declines in levels of choline and creatine, and rises in lactate with stroke and its spatial resolution is reasonable.[155,156] These changes evolve rapidly and persist for weeks. A localized area of increased lactate is a good surrogate for ischemia when differentiating a stroke from a non-vascular lesion found on brain imaging.[83,155] This test could be used as a supplement to traditional MRI.

IMAGING OF EXTRACRANIAL AND INTRACRANIAL ARTERIES

Arteriography and Digital Subtraction Angiography

Arteriography and digital subtraction angiography (DSA) are traditional ways to evaluate the anatomy and the presence of any pathology in the intracranial and extracranial vasculature (Table 4–7). Arteriography has been used since the 1930s, and DSA is a refinement of this angiographic technique. Arteriography and DSA are the standards against which other studies to evaluate vessels are compared.[157] Inter-rater agreement is relatively good in defining the DSA findings.[158] These tests visualize the lumen and detect the presence of a stenosis or an occlusion secondary to atherosclerosis of the subclavian, vertebral, basilar, or internal carotid arteries. Although arteriography defines the presence of extracranial or intracranial vascular disease in patients with cortical, brain stem, cerebellar, or subcortical infarctions, the size and the location of the stroke do not correlate with these findings. For example, Kappelle et al[159] demonstrated stenosis of the internal carotid artery in 14 of 45 patients with capsular infarctions. Arteriography is highly accurate in detecting severe atherosclerotic disease in patients with a TIA or amaurosis fugax.[160] Arteriography is the standard way to define the severity of a stenosis of the internal carotid artery as a prelude to carotid endarterectomy. When DSA is compared with surgical findings, the agreement rate is approximately 93%, which is higher than with other imaging methods.[161] As a result, the sensitivity and the specificity of other vascular imaging technologies are compared to the yield of arteriography or DSA.

Table 4–7. **Indication and Adverse Experiences with Arteriography and Digital Subtraction Angiography**

Indications
- Prepare for operation or arterial intervention
  - Define location and extent of lesion
    - Stenosis
    - Ulceration
    - Intraluminal thrombus
    - Intraluminal embolus
  - Assess collateral circulation
- Differentiate high-grade stenosis from occlusion
- Screen for presence or extent of non-atherosclerotic lesions
  - Dissection
  - Fibromuscular dysplasia
  - Moyamoya disease
  - Vasculitis
  - Aneurysm
  - Vascular malformation

Adverse Experiences
- Stroke
  - Embolism
    - Thrombi at tip of catheter
    - Atherosclerotic debris
  - Arterial occlusion
  - Spasm of artery
- Contrast agent neurotoxicity
  - Encephalopathy
  - Visual loss
  - Seizures
- Local bleeding—arterial puncture
- Myocardial ischemia
- Allergic reaction

Investigators in the North American Symptomatic Carotid Endarterectomy Trial (NASCET) and the European Carotid Surgery Trial (ECST) developed different methods to calculate the severity of arterial narrowing as found by arteriography.[162]

CALCULATION OF SEVERITY OF STENOSIS
ORIGIN OF INTERNAL CAROTID ARTERY

$$\% \text{ STENOSIS} \quad \frac{\text{DIAMETER AT LEVEL OF MOST SEVERE NARROWING}}{\text{DIAMETER OF ARTERY} - 2 \text{ CM ABOVE STENOSIS}} \quad \text{X } 100$$

Figure 4–17. Calculation of severity of stenosis, origin of internal carotid artery.

(See Fig. 4–17.) The NASCET criteria involve estimation of the diameter at the point of most severe narrowing in comparison with the diameter of the internal carotid artery approximately 2 cm. above the carotid bifurcation.[163] Despite this relatively straightforward criterion, many physicians have difficulty in calculating degree of stenosis, and the narrowing often is either over- or under-estimated.[163,164] A major over- or under-estimation of the stenosis is a problem when deciding about carotid endarterectomy.[165] A minor discrepancy (approximately 10%) in the calculation of the narrowing probably should be anticipated. The ECST criteria are more problematic than those used by NASCET. The diameter at the point of greatest narrowing is calculated against the presumed normal arterial lumen. In general, the degree of stenosis is calculated to be greater using the ECST criteria than with the NASCET method; for example, a 50% narrowing using the NASCET criteria is approximately equal to a 70% narrowing using the ECST method.[166,167] A string-sign (a long segment of severe narrowing) can be found with a large and severe atherosclerotic plaque.[168]

A number of arteriographic findings besides the severity of narrowing predict the risk of stroke.[169] Arteriography and DSA also can detect ulceration of a plaque and an intraluminal clot.[170–172] The intraluminal thrombus usually arises at the carotid bifurcation and has a tail that extends cephalically. Ulcers range from a shallow roughening of the luminal surface to large, deep pits in the plaque. Still, one study found that arteriography's ability to detect ulceration found at surgery resulted in a sensitivity of 74% and a specificity of only 46%.[173] Arteriography does not provide information about the nature of the plaque within the arterial wall.

Arteriography and DSA can demonstrate fibromuscular dysplasia their findings usually include a section of narrowing and dilation, a string sign, or a false aneurysm. Arteriographic findings of an arterial dissection are a string sign, a double lumen, or a false aneurysm. Both usually are located approximately 2 cm. above the carotid bifurcation.

Arteriography and DSA give information about the vascular anatomy of the intracranial arteries, including the collateral channels. (Figs. 4–18 and 4–19). These tests are particularly useful in detecting intracranial arterial disease, including embolic occlusions of branch cortical vessels. Because of their ability to visualize medium-caliber intracranial arteries, arteriography and DSA are used to search for intracranial vasculitis, moyamoya disease, or an intracranial arterial stenosis. The findings of moyamoya disease usually are bilateral with occlusion of the distal internal carotid artery and proximal middle and anterior cerebral arteries. Its hallmark is a mesh of tiny vessels in the base of the brain. Arteriography and DSA remains the key diagnostic tests. Arteriography also is used to detect segmental areas of smooth narrowing and dilations (sausage-like appearance) in multiple, medium-caliber intracranial arteries in persons with vasculitis.[174]

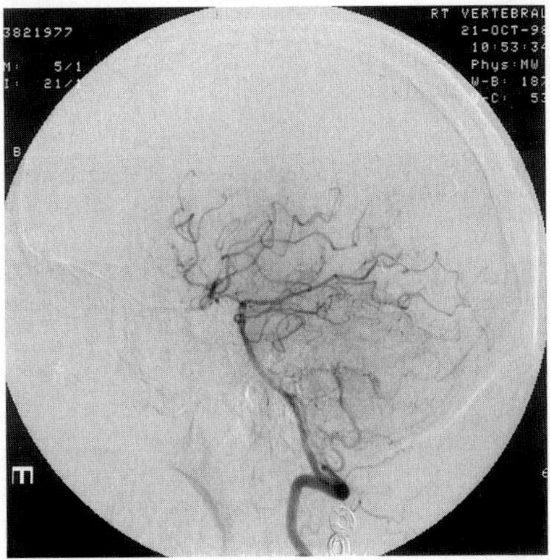

Figure 4–18. A left vertebral arteriogram using subtraction techniques obtained in a patient with an occlusion of the internal carotid artery. The anterior and middle cerebral arteries are receiving flow via an anterior–posterior and posterior communicating artery view posterior communicating artery.

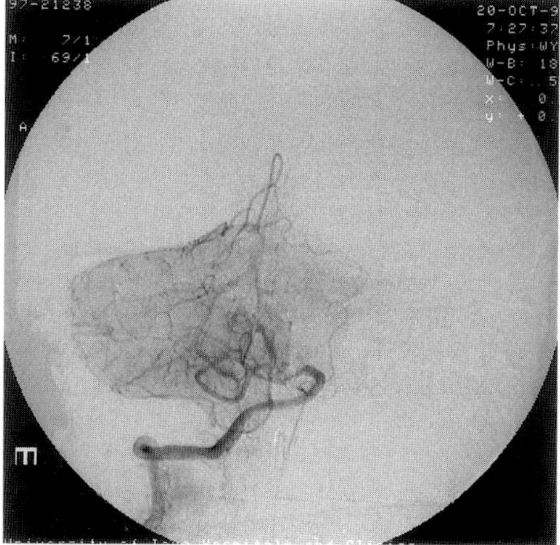

A

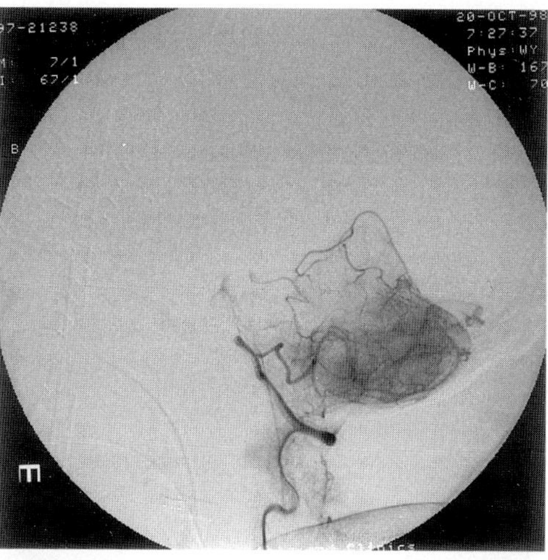

B

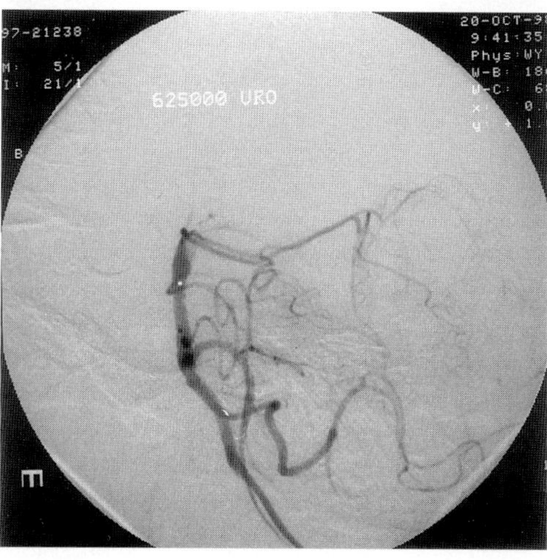

C

Figure 4–19. Two lateral views of a vertebral arteriogram, using subtraction techniques, in a patient with basilar artery thrombosis. The basilar artery is noted to be occluded at its proximal portion (*A* and *B*). The posterior inferior cerebellar artery is the source of collateral flow to the branches of the superior cerebellar artery. (*C*) The patient has received intra-arterial treatment with urokinase patency of the basilar artery and its branches is advised.

Still, arteriography gives a false-negative result in almost 50% of these patients. Sequential studies can show evolution of the changes, including occlusions, development of collateral channels, and prolonged circulation time.[174] Arteriography and DSA also are the usual tests to assess for intracranial aneurysms or vascular malformations.

Arteriography and DSA have limitations (See Table 4–7). They are invasive and may be accompanied by serious complications, including stroke, myocardial infarction, or death.[175–177] Hankey et al[178] reported major complications among 13 of 382 patients (3.4%) undergoing arteriography. Investigators of the Asymptomatic Carotid Atherosclerosis Study (ACAS) reported that the frequency of serious complications of arteriography exceeded those of carotid endarterectomy.[179] Manipulation of the catheter during the procedure might cause embolism of clots arising from the catheter tip or the endothelial surface of the artery or embolizaton of atherosclerotic debris from an ulcerated plaque. The contrast agent can induce an allergic reaction or transient neurological symptoms, including an encephalopathy or seizures.[180] Whereas, in the past, physicians expressed concern about an increased likelihood of side effects in patients with migraine, more recent data suggest that the risks are not high in this situation.[181] Migraine should not be considered a contraindication for an arteriogram or DSA.

Arteriography and DSA usually involve a puncture of the femoral artery, and a local hematoma or a false aneurysm can develop. Patients with prolonged coagulation times, thrombocytopenia, or renal failure often cannot undergo arteriography. With the development of new devices that permit placement of microsutures to close the arterial puncture site, however, patients with bleeding disorders can have arteriography without a major risk of hemorrhage. Because of the invasive nature of arteriography and DSA, the indications for these tests should be clear, and the timing of the procedures is critical. These tests should not be performed unless no other test can adequately define the vascular pathology or the cause of stroke. If arteriography and DSA are done in preparation for carotid endarterectomy or another reconstructive operation, the timing should be in close proximity to the surgery.

Digital Intravenous Subtraction Angiography

Because of the side effects of arteriography and DSA described previously, many physicians and surgeons prefer to use other diagnostic studies to examine the arterial tree.[182–187] *Digital intravenous subtraction angiography* was developed as a substitute for intra-arterial studies because it avoided the potential morbidity of an arterial puncture and intra-arterial manipulation of a catheter. High rates of adverse experiences related to the needed large volumes of contrast- and movement-related artifacts limited the use of this technique. In addition, inter-rater agreement in reading the findings of tests was poor.[158] Digital intravenous subtraction angiography has been abandoned in favor of DSA and other non-invasive methods to image the extracranial or intracranial vasculature.

Carotid Artery Duplex

Ultrasonography of the extracranial portion of the internal carotid artery (carotid duplex) is a widely used diagnostic tool for evaluating patients with either a TIA or an ischemic stroke. Carotid duplex is readily available, relatively inexpensive, and easily performed.[188] (See Fig. 4–20.) Because it is non-invasive, it is not associated with major morbidity. Carotid duplex provides key information about the anatomy and the pathology of the bifurcation of the common carotid artery and the origins of the

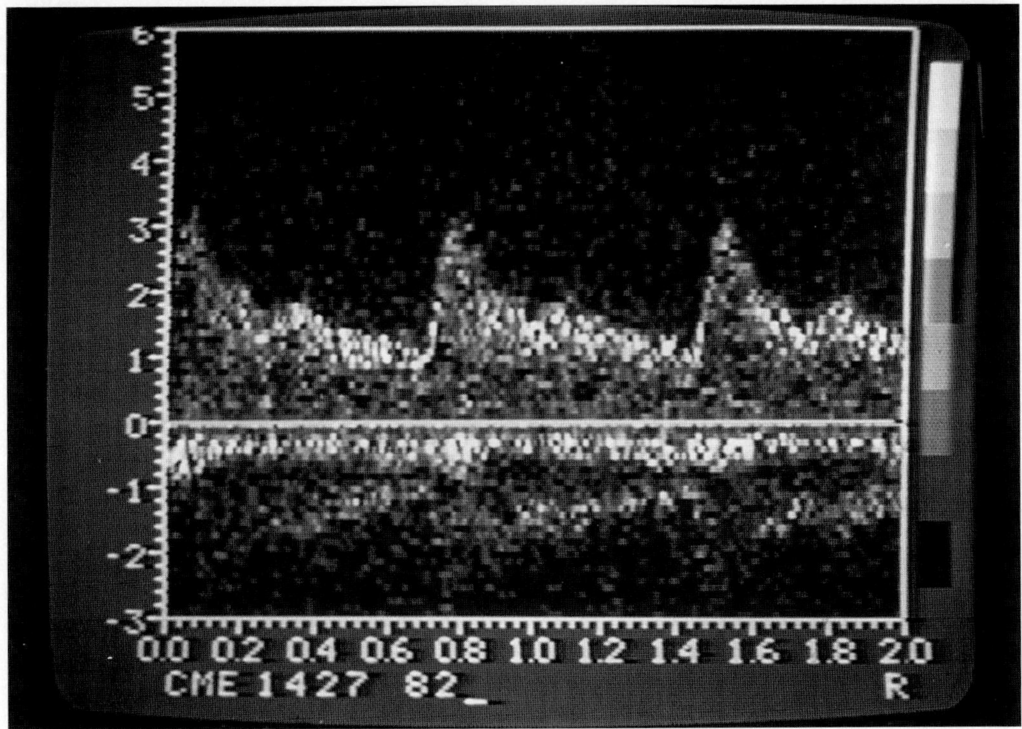

Figure 4–20. Normal Doppler sonogram. (Reprinted from D'Alton JG, Norris JW. Carotid Doppler evaluation in cerebrovascular disease. *Can Med Assoc J* 1983;129:1184, by permission.)

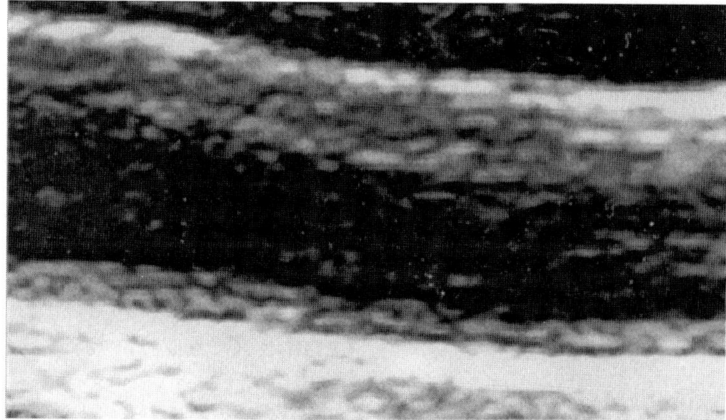

Figure 4–21. Intimal-medial thickening of the common carotid artery in a patient with severe atherosclerosis.

internal and external carotid arteries. A ratio between the arterial lumen of the internal carotid and common carotid arteries can be used to calculate the severity of narrowing.[189, 190]

Duplex imaging can be used to measure *intimal-medial thickness*. (*IMT*)[191,192] (See Fig. 4–21.) Changes in IMT correlate with the presence of risk factors for accelerated atherosclerosis.[192–195] In particular, early growth in IMT has been correlated with elevated blood lipid concentrations. An increase in the thickness of the arterial wall is correlated with early atherosclerotic changes, which in turn are associated with a heightened risk of coronary artery disease.[191,192,196–201] Changes in IMT also predict the finding of coronary artery calcification that in turn predicts myocardial infarction.[202] Sequential testing of IMT can be used to monitor responses to treatment of risk factors, such as the administration of agents to lower serum cholesterol concentration.

Carotid duplex is used to assay the integrity of an atherosclerotic plaque. Complications including intra-plaque hemorrhage, calcification, fibrosis, and ulceration can be visualized because of differences in densities.[157,188,203–207] A hypo-echoic plaque is associated with an increased stroke risk in asymptomatic persons.[208] Park et al[209] found that ulcerations were more common in patients with a TIA or a stroke than in asymptomatic persons. They also detected intra-plaque hemorrhage in 202 of 289 patients (68%) in patients with stenoses greater than 90%. This finding was detected in only 97 of 299 patients (32%) with milder narrowing. Plaque ulceration and the presence of an intraluminal clot are associated with embolism, but plaque hemorrhages and fissures are not.[210] (See Fig. 4–22.) Carotid duplex also can detect an intraluminal clot in a patient with an acute occlusion of the internal carotid artery or a thrombus arising from an ulcerated plaque.

Carotid duplex also measures changes in blood flow that equate with the severity of the arterial narrowing and residual lumen. An occlusion or severe narrowing of the distal internal carotid artery or the middle cerebral artery may produce slow flow and a secondary exaggeration of the degree of narrowing of the arterial lumen at the

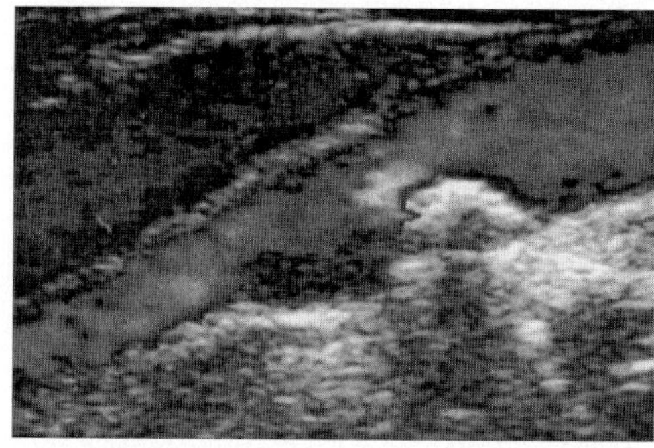

Figure 4–22. Color Doppler picture of flow changes in a medium size plaque with distal ulceration.

carotid bifurcation.[211] Similarly, the presence of a contralateral severe stenosis or occlusion may cause an increase in peak systolic velocity that leads to an overestimation of the degree of narrowing in the insonated vessel.[212,213] The results of carotid duplex generally correspond to the pathological findings of specimens removed during carotid endarterectomy. [214] Using digital angiography as a standard, numerous groups have examined the sensitivity and specificity of carotid duplex in detecting arterial narrowing of varying severity. For stenoses of approximately 50%–70%, carotid duplex has a sensitivity of 74%–96%, specificity of 68%–98%, positive predictive value of approximately 90%, and a negative predictive value of 95%.[215,216] Ultrasound may be least accurate in patients with high-grade stenoses, as it over-estimates the narrowing and mislabels high-grade stenoses as occlusions.[217] In persons with severe stenosis (70%–99%), carotid duplex's sensitivity, specificity, positive predictive value, and negative predictive value are approximately 83%–96%, 60%–91%, 68%–90%, and 90%–100%, respectively[168,217–221] For occlusions, duplex has a sensitivity of 80%, specificity of 95%, positive predictive value of 70%, and a negative predictive value of 95%.[219] (See Fig. 4–23.) Performing color-coded carotid duplex provides information about changes in the direction of blood flow and turbulence; it also adds to the sensitivity of the test when assessing patients with severe atherosclerotic disease.

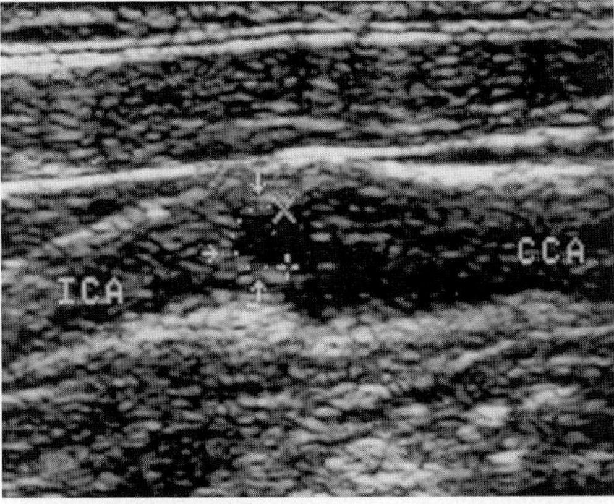

Figure 4–23. Occlusion at the origin of internal carotid artery visible on B-mode scanning. This should correspond to absence of Doppler signal on pulsed-wave analysis.

The results of carotid duplex greatly influence decisions about management. Results can be used as a screening measure for either asymptomatic or symptomatic patients and also to assess progression of carotid disease.[222–226] If a carotid duplex is normal, then an arteriogram often can be avoided. If the carotid duplex shows moderate-to-severe stenosis, then the results may prompt consideration of carotid endarterectomy. Although, in many instances, the results of carotid duplex lead to cerebral arteriography in preparation for surgery, some physicians and surgeons will proceed with surgery based solely on the results of the non-invasive test.[227] The presence of a severe narrowing or occlusion of the origin of the internal carotid artery provides important data to support the diagnosis of large artery atherosclerosis. This information may be useful in the emergent evaluation of a patient with an acute ischemic stroke. Detection of an occlusion of the internal carotid artery portends a multilobar infarction with a high risk of mortality or disability. One recent study suggested that the results of carotid duplex imaging as a component of urgent evaluation of a patient with an acute hemispheric stroke can influence treatment with intravenous anticoagulation.[228]

The results of the carotid duplex can be buttressed by the use of magnetic resonance angiography (MRA).[221] Guzman[229] concluded that the combination of carotid duplex and MRA are equal to arteriography in screening the carotid arteries before endarterectomy. Arteriography could be reserved for when the results of the duplex and MRA disagree.[224,227,230] Collier[231] estimated that up to 90% of arteriograms could be avoided if carotid duplex were performed with care. Some physicians disagree with the approach of substituting carotid duplex and MRA for a traditional arteriogram.[232–234] For example, Bain et al[233] believe that arteriography still is required to obtain the necessary detail about the vascular pathology to make accurate decisions about carotid endarterectomy.

Although carotid duplex ultrasonography is an important part of the evaluation of most patients with a TIA or an ischemic stroke, it does have limitations. Carotid duplex does not provide information about the entire extent of the internal carotid artery; a tandem intracranial stenosis can be missed. It may not differentiate a high-grade stenosis from an occlusion of the internal carotid artery. Most important, it is vulnerable to errors in technique that can lead to over- or under-estimation of the degree of arterial narrowing.[235] Devices can vary considerably among laboratories.[236] In the wrong hands, the test may not provide sufficient sensitivity and specificity to be useful clinically. Tests can be misinterpreted as showing a high-grade stenosis, and surgery might be recommended inappropriately. Conversely, a poorly done duplex may mislead a physician to the conclusion that a narrowed segment is not as severe as it actually is. An ultrasonography laboratory should have strong quality-control efforts correlated with the degree of stenosis found by DSA or arteriography.[236,237] If the laboratory cannot provide assurance that its carotid duplex results are reliable, then the test should be avoided.

Ultrasonography of the Vertebral and Cervical Arteries

Ultrasonography of the neck can be used to measure vertebral artery flow velocities and the direction of flow. The test can detect vertebral occlusion or dissection in patients with posterior circulation TIA or stroke.[238–240] The test can provide information about flow, but it does not give sufficient detail to determine the location or severity of a stenosis of the vertebral artery. Directional Doppler ultrasonography can be used to measure the direction of flow of the vertebral arteries. Reversal of flow in one artery can be detected in a case of subclavian steal syndrome, and the absence of flow is consistent with an occlusion or absence of the vertebral artery. Because the caliber of the vertebral arteries often varies considerably, information about absent or low flow secondary to an acquired pathology should be viewed with caution. The artery may be atretic. Ultrasonography of the neck also can assess the patency of the major cervical and supraclavicular vessels in patients with diseases such as Takayasu's arteritis.[241]

Other Non-invasive Studies of the Carotid Circulation

In the past, *retinal artery pressure* measurements, bidirectional supraorbital *Doppler ultrasonography,* and *oculoplethysmography (OPG)* were widely used as non-invasive tools to assess patients with suspected extracranial stenosis of the internal carotid artery. These tests depended on recording changes in flow or pressure from one carotid circulation to the other. With the advent of carotid duplex studies, these tests have been largely abandoned.

Transcranial Doppler Ultrasonography

Transcranial Doppler ultrasonography (TCD) is a non-invasive method to assess flow of the major intracranial arteries, including the basilar artery, the distal portions of the vertebral arteries, and the proximal portions of the anterior, middle, and posterior cerebral arteries.[242–245] Blood flow can be measured before and after administration of acetazolamide to detect areas of borderline flow.[246] Color-coded TCD studies also can be used to image the intracranial arteries.[247–251] Muller et al[252] reported that the sensitivity and specificity of TCD in detecting severe disease of major arteries are 87% and 95%, respectively. Contrast-enhanced TCD has been used to screen for occlusion of intracranial arteries.[251]

The role of TCD is evolving. It can be used to assess for occlusion of the distal internal carotid artery or to assess hemodynamic changes secondary to a major artery occlusion.[253–256] It also has been used to screen the intracranial vasculature of children with sickle cell disease and to assess for vascular changes in patients with systemic lupus erythematosus.[257–259] Transcranial Doppler Ultrasonography also can assess patency of an extracranial-to-intracranial arterial anastomosis or moyamoya disease.[260] The technique has been used to sequentially assess patients with recent aneurysmal SAH.[261] Changes in velocities correlate with cerebral arterial vasospasm, appearing well before the development of signs of brain ischemia (Fig. 4–24). Sequential studies might be helpful in monitoring

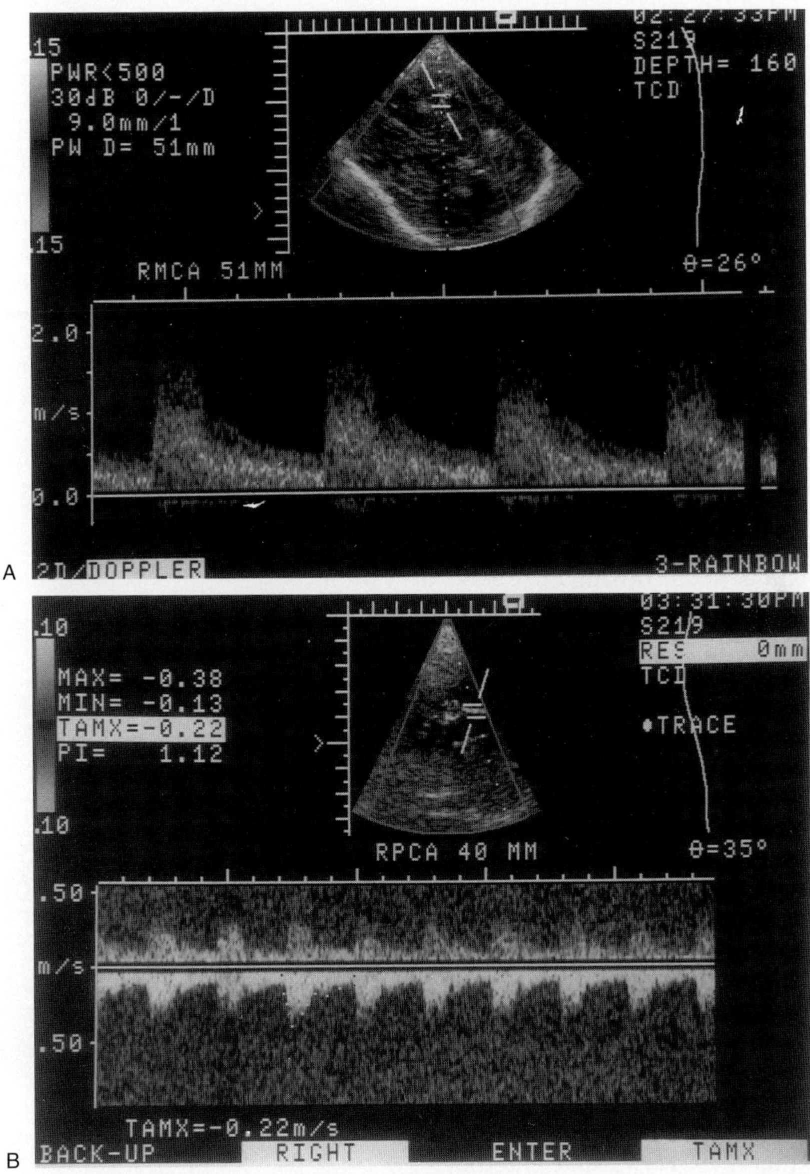

Figure 4–24. Transcranial Doppler ultrasongraphic study obtained in a patient with a recent subarachnoid hemorrhage. The first study reveals normal velocities and waves in the middle cerebral artery (*A*). A second study shows abnormal velocity and flow in the posterior cerebral artery, which is attributed to vasospasm after subarachnoid hemorrhage(*B*).

responses to treatment with thrombolytic or antithrombotic agents.

The frequency of microemboli detected by TCD may portend the risk of stroke among persons with arterial or cardiac diseases. A high number of signals is correlated with high-risk situations and a high probability of embolic stroke.[262–270] Grosset et al[271] concluded that TCD could help differentiate embolic from non-embolic causes of occlusion of the middle cerebral artery. Contrast-enhanced echocardiography can be complemented by TCD to detect paradoxical emboli in a patient with a right-to-left shunt.[248,268] In patients with carotid stenosis, microembolization is detected more commonly in those with a TIA than in patients with asymptomatic disease.[264] Microemboli also can be detected by TCD monitoring in persons with disease in the vertebrobasilar circulation.[272]

Transcranial Doppler Ultrasonography has been used to monitor for embolization in patients undergoing cardiovascular or carotid operations.[273] Stendel et al[274] found that TCD could be used to help monitor patients having carotid endarterectomy. A decline in flow or an increase in the rate of microembolization could portend the development of ischemia during the operation. Conversely, Cao et al[275] found that TCD was not useful in monitoring patient responses to carotid operations.

The usefulness of TCD in evaluation after stroke is not clear. Although absence of flow in an intracranial artery may forecast a proximal occlusion, technical problems could give false-positive results. In particular, TCD can be non-diagnostic in women, older persons, and African Americans.[276] Issues related to the angle of insonation and placement of the probe can be difficult to overcome. In addition, the thickness of the patient's skull may alter the yield of TCD.[250] This failure of insonation can be largely overcome by intravenous injection of a contrast agent such as galactose. Mauer et al[277] used TCD to help decide treatment with thrombolytic agents and to monitor responses to therapies. However, Comerota et al[276] did not recommend TCD as part of emergent evaluation because they concluded that the results of the test did not clearly change treatment plans. Additional research is needed to define the role of TCD in management of most patients with ischemic cerebrovascular disease.

Magnetic Resonance Angiography

Magnetic resonance angiography is used increasingly to assess patients with ischemic cerebrovascular disease (Fig. 4–25). It has several advantages. It is non-invasive, and it can be done in conjunction with MRI. The test examines supra-aortic vessels and the extracranial and intracranial components of both carotid arteries and the vertebrobasilar circulation.[278,279] It also can provide information about the anatomy of the circle of Willis and major collateral vessels.[230,280] It has been used to define the vascular pathology among patients with acute stroke.[96] Still, MRA has limitations, and its role in patient care is not settled.

Several techniques are used, but either two- or three-dimensional time-of-flight methods are reported to have the best sensitivity and specificity.[281–284] Kallmes et al[285] reported that spectrum bias can

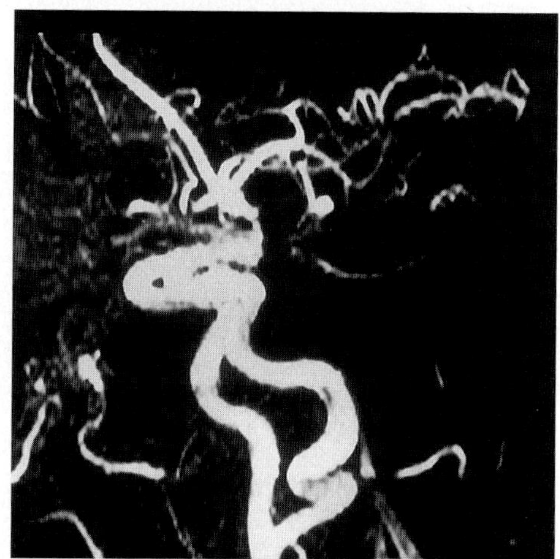

Figure 4–25. Magnetic resonance angiography in a sagittal projection shows both carotid arteries filling well and absence of filling in the basilar artery between the vertebral junction region and the distal basilar. (Courtesy of A J Fox, MD, London Health Sciences Center, London Ontario.)

limit the specificity of MRA. Gadolinium enhancement may improve the ability of MRA to elucidate the vascular anatomy of the major cerebral and cerebellar arteries.[286] Magnetic resonance angiography is relatively expensive, and it can be a time-consuming, which is a potential problem in an acute situation. It also is vulnerable to artifacts; in particular, movement can produce images that mimic a stenosis of an extracranial vessel. It usually is not helpful in visualizing medium- to small-caliber vessels.[287]

Magnetic resonance angiography is particularly effective in evaluating for the presence of a severe stenosis or an occlusion of the proximal portion of a major intracranial artery.[279,282,288–290] (See Fig. 4–26.) It is becoming an alternative to DSA and conventional arteriography in evaluating patients with a suspected intracranial occlusion. Korogi et al[291] assessed the value of MRA in detecting a stenosis or an occlusion of the proximal portion of the middle cerebral artery or the distal segment of the internal carotid artery. They found that MRA had a sensitivity of 88% and a specificity of 97% in detecting lesions of the middle cerebral artery and a sensitivity of 85% and a specificity of 96% in evaluating abnormalities of the internal carotid artery (Fig. 4–27). Kenton et al[249] concluded that the results of TCD and MRA agree closely. Magnetic resonance angiography can screen for abnormalities of the basilar artery, including stenosis, occlusion, or fusiform aneurysm.[71,292] Rother et al[293] reported that MRA has a sensitivity of 97% and a specificity of 99% in detecting either a stenosis or an occlusion of the basilar artery. The test does less well in rating the severity of basilar narrowing. In general, MRA can detect a stenosis or an occlusion of the major branches of the basilar artery, including the superior, anterior inferior, and posterior inferior cerebellar arteries.[292]

Magnetic resonance angiography can be used to monitor the patency of an extracranial–intracranial arterial anastomosis.[294] It also can detect moyamoya disease.[295] Magnetic resonance angiography appears to be superior to MRI in detecting disease (ie, dissection) of the distal vertebral artery.[76,239,296] However, Zuber et al[297] noted that MRA is less reliable in detecting dissections of the vertebral artery than of the carotid artery. Kanser et al[298] reported that sequential MRA studies are an effective way to monitor the course of vertebral dissections. In addition, MRA can be used to assess the patency of

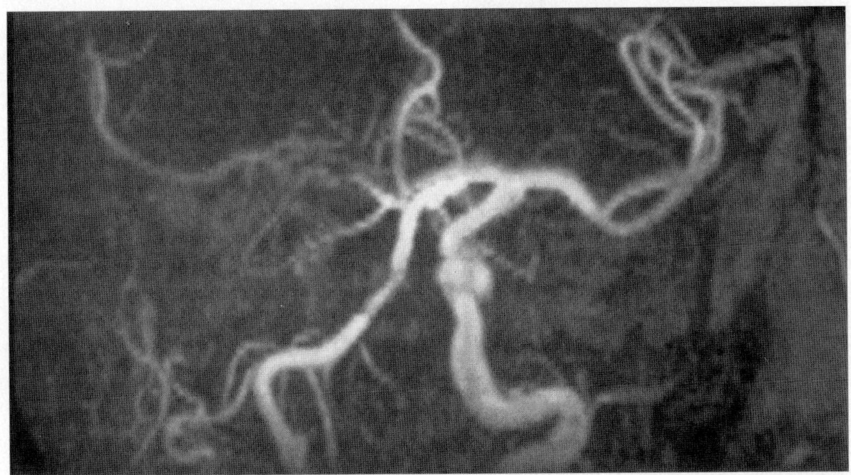

Figure 4–26. Anterior–posterior view of an intracranial magnetic resonance angiogram. The right internal carotid artery is not visualized, and the right middle cerebral artery is seen less intensely than the left middle cerebral artery.

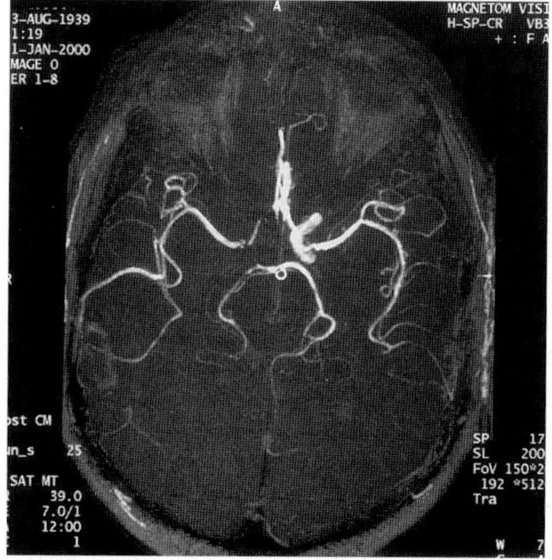

A

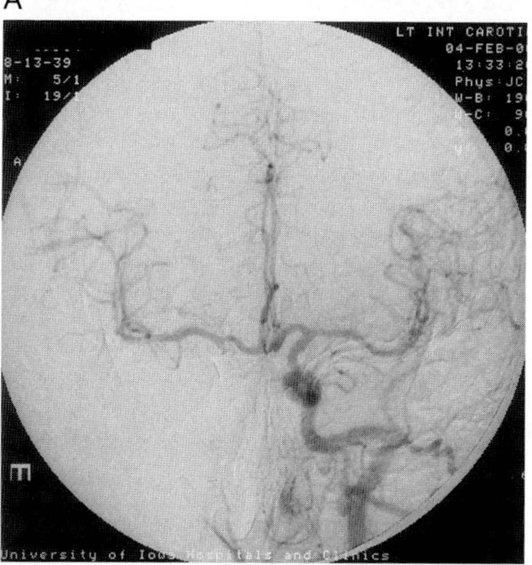

B

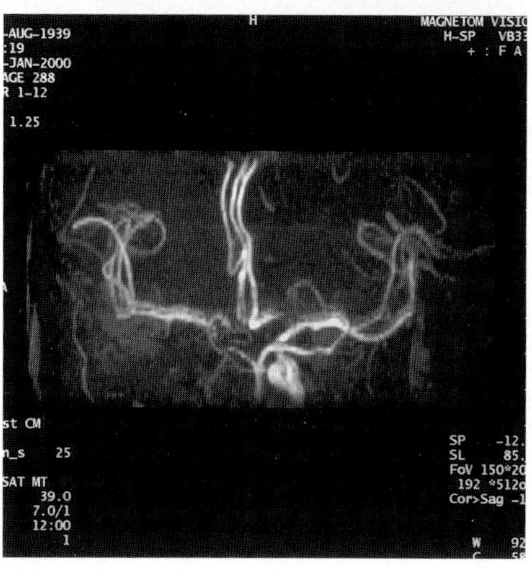

C

Figure 4–27. Comparison of the results of magnetic resonance angiography and intra-arterial digital subtraction angiography in a patient with a right internal carotid arteriogram. The carotid occlusion is demonstrated on anterior–posterior views of both studies (*A* and *B*). A basal view of the magnetic resonance angiogram also shows occlusion of the internal carotid artery and the status of the circle of Willis (*C*).

surgical extracranial-to-intracranial anastomoses. The test also can evaluate the location and size of an intracranial aneurysm or a vascular malformation.

Considerable research has focused on the role of MRA, alone or in conjunction with duplex ultrasound, for characterization of the severity of carotid artery disease.[299,279] Magnetic resonance angiography can be used for patients with heavily calcified carotid plaques that are resistant to imaging by duplex ultrasound. The sensitivity and specificity of MRA in detecting moderate-to-severe stenosis or occlusion are reported to be 84%–100% and 76%–100%, respectively.[215,221,230,267,278,284,299–301] The positive and negative predictive values of MRA results range from 53% to 100% and 72% to 100%.[215,218,219] Magarelli, et al.[300] reported that MRA generally over-estimates the severity of stenosis by approximately 5%. Still, MRA can differentiate a pseudo-occlusion (very severe stenosis) from a true occlusion. Atlas[219] found MRA was better in detecting occlusions than stenoses. It also can define carotid artery dissections.[302] Because of the limitations of spatial resolution, MRA likely cannot detect an ulceration of a plaque, nor does it give information about the composition of an arterial wall. Fortunately, duplex ultrasound can give this information. In contrast, MRA can visualize a tandem lesion of the distal internal carotid artery.

The combination of duplex ultrasound and MRA appears to be superior to MRA alone. When the two tests show complementary results, their yield seems to replicate the findings of arteriography.[215] Thus, it appears that the combination of MRA and duplex ultrasound can be used as a pre-operative screening tool to select persons for carotid endarterectomy. However, meticulous technique and interpretation are required for the effective use of MRA.

Computed Tomography Angiography

Dynamic, spiral computed tomography angiography (CTA) can be used to examine the extracranial or intracranial vasculature (Fig. 4–28). This test involves first injecting a non-ionic contrast agent and then rapidly collecting a series of images. computed tomography angiography appears to be better than TCD in evaluating the basilar artery. It detects dissections of the vertebral or carotid arteries. Shrier et al[303] found a high agreement between CTA and DSA. Wildermuth et al[304] detected

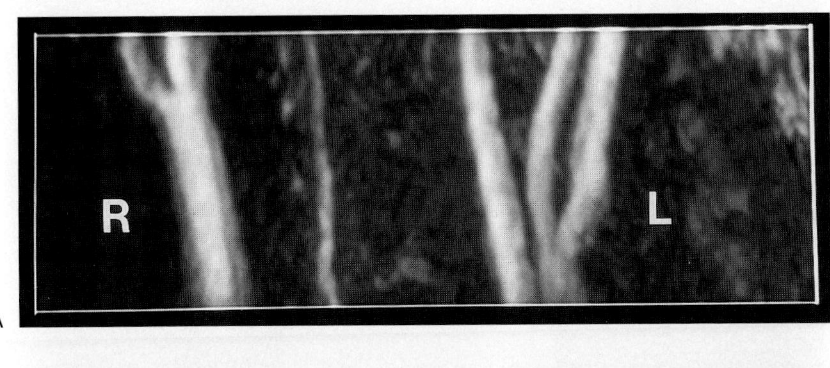

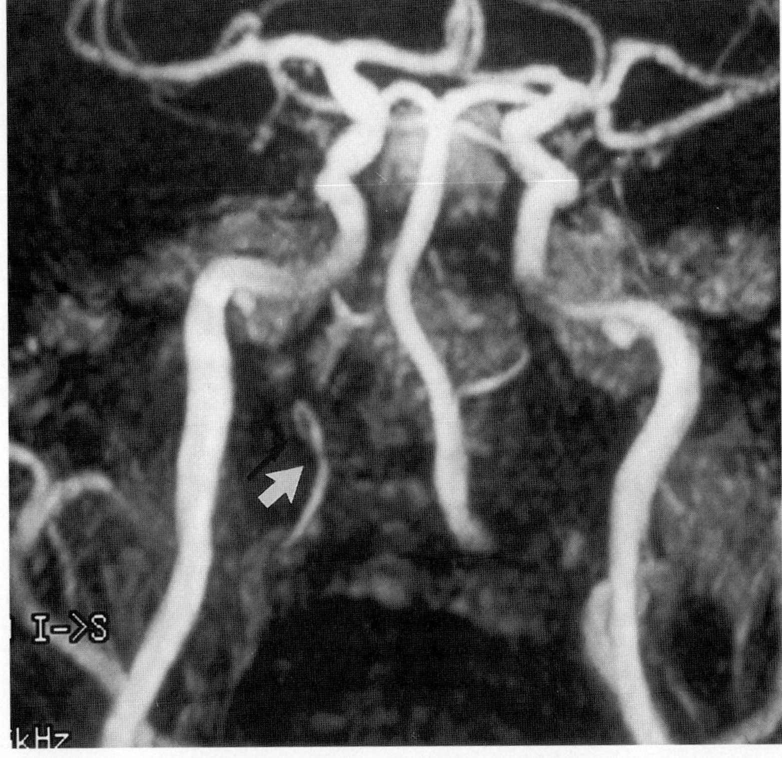

Figure 4–28. Magnetic resonance and CT angiography. This 59-year-old smoker presented with recurrent episodes of dysphasia, right hemiparesis and sensory loss with complete recovery between episodes. Magnetic resonance angiography of the carotid bifurcations (*A*) shows a moderate (~50%) stenosis of the origin of the left internal carotid artery at its origin. Magnetic resonance angiography of the vertebrobasilar system (*B*) shows that the right vertebral artery is hypoplastic and ends at the right posterior inferior cerebellar artery (arrow), whereas the basilar artery is formed solely by the left vertebral artery. The patient proceeded to have a carotid endarterectomy.

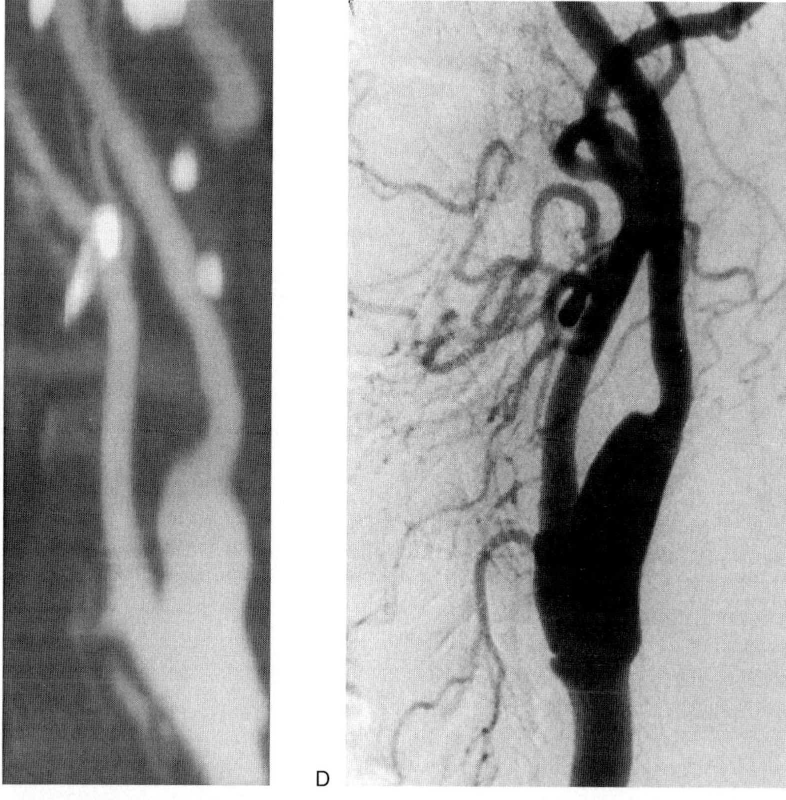

Figure 4–28. Computed tomography angiography (*C*) performed postoperatively shows a widely patent left internal carotid artery at its origin. The cerebral angiogram (*D*) is shown for comparison. (Courtesy of Dr. B. Demaerschalk.)

thromboembolic occlusion of the middle cerebral artery using CTA in 34 of 40 patients with moderate-to-severe hemispheric strokes. Computed tomography angiography also can assess the status of collateral channels and look for the presence of an internal carotid artery thrombosis. The sensitivity and specificity of CTA in detecting disease of the extracranial portion of the internal carotid artery are not as high as MRA.[300] Still, Leclerc et al[305] found that CTA correctly classified the degree of stenosis of the internal carotid artery in 96% of vessels. Computed tomography angiography also can visualize the severity of the stenosis and the presence of calcification, but it may miss ulceration.[306] As with MRA, CTA complements carotid duplex. The combination may be an alternative to conventional arteriography.[307,308] Brandt et al[309] found that CTA was superior to TCD in diagnosing basilar artery occlusion. The role of CTA should be defined further.

EVALUATION OF THE HEART

Examination of the heart is a key component of the assessment of patients with ischemic cerebrovascular disease because of the strong relationship between cardiac disease and stroke.[310] Cardiac diagnostic tests, which are done during both the emergent and subsequent evaluation of patients with a TIA or a stroke, are listed in Table 4–2. They screen for the cause of stroke, look for serious comorbid heart disease, and detect cardiac complications of the stroke.

Electrocardiogram and Chest X-ray

A clinical evaluation of the heart and vasculature should be part of the assessment of all patients with a TIA or a stroke. Results of the clinical examination influence decisions about the subsequent evaluation of the

Table 4–8. **Electrocardiographic Changes and Cardiac Arrhythmias Following Ischemic Stroke**

Pathological Q waves	ST segment depression
Negative T waves	U waves
QT prolongation	Sinus bradycardia
Unifocal ventricular premature beats	Bigeminy/trigeminy
Multifocal ventricular premature beats	Asytolic intervals
Ventricular tachycardia	Atrial fibrillation
Ventricular fibrillation	Torsades de pointes
Sinoatrial block	Atrioventricular block

heart. In addition, almost all patients should have an electrocardiogram (ECG) and a chest x-ray. These tests are relatively inexpensive, non-invasive, rapidly performed, and readily available at most hospitals. They provide important information that can influence acute care and long-term management. The resting 12-lead ECG can demonstrate changes of ischemic heart disease, other structural heart diseases, conduction defects, or sustained cardiac arrhythmias (Table 4–8) and (Fig. 4–29). A stroke can be the presentation of a recent, otherwise clinically silent, myocardial infarction; and ECG findings may be the first hint leading to diagnosis of an acute cardiac lesion. Abnormalities on the ECG also might point to an underlying cardiac condition that leads to embolism, such as atrial fibrillation or a recent myocardial infarction. Acute cardiac complications of stroke include myocardial ischemia or life-threatening arrhythmias.

Electrocardiogram findings of acute stroke can include depression or elevation of

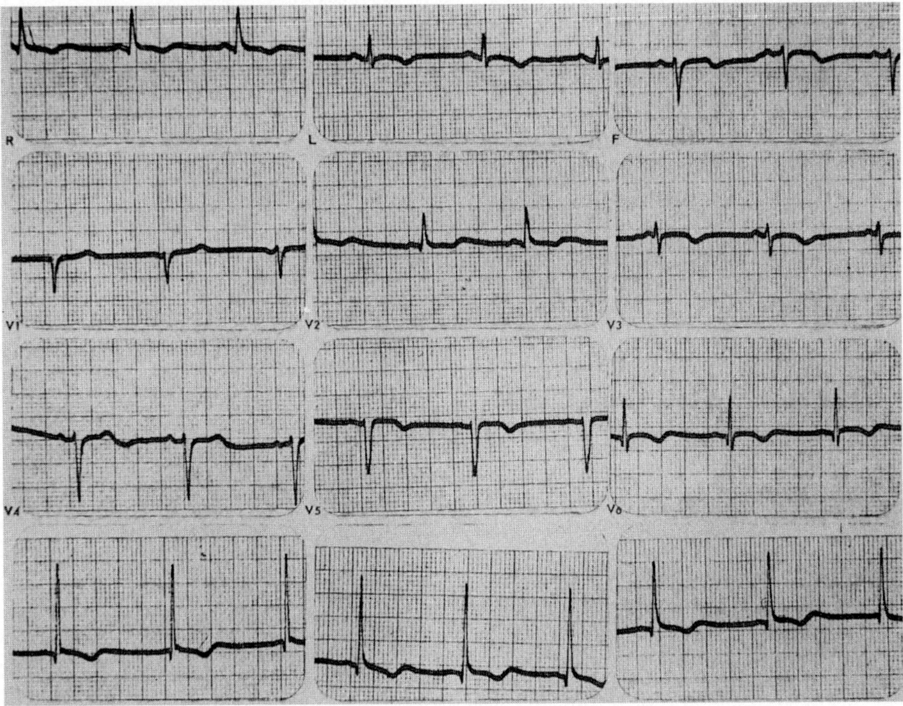

Figure 4–29. Electrocardiogram shows bradycardia, prolonged QT interval, and inverted T waves in a patient with an acute stroke.

the ST segment, inversion of T waves, or prominent U waves.[311,312] Electrocardiogram changes are more common with intracranial hemorrhages or increased intracranial pressure, and they may be secondary to myocardial ischemia or damage to myocardial fibers.[313] Still, McDermott[314] noted ST segment depression in 29% of patients who had an ECG within 5 days of a TIA or stroke. Some of the cardiac abnormalities may be secondary to a recent, clinically silent myocardial infarction. In addition, the cardiac ischemia can be the result of coronary artery vasospasm or direct toxicity of catecholamines that are elevated secondary to the stress of the neurological event. Both ventricular and atrial arrhythmias are detected during the first 48 hours after stroke in approximately 50% of patients (Table 4–8). Sinus bradycardia and ventricular ectopy are the most common rhythm disturbances.[315] The frequency of cardiac arrhythmias after stroke is increased in elderly patients or those who have a history of congestive heart failure or previous myocardial infarction.[315,316] Cardiac complications also appear to be more common when ischemic strokes are located in the insular region or the subcortical structures of the right hemisphere.[311,317–320]

A chest x-ray can reveal enlargement of the heart, changes in the contour of the aorta, evidence of vascular congestion, or pulmonary disease. It may show pulmonary complications of stroke, including pneumonia. Because persons with brain stem strokes may have paralysis of the bulbar musculature, they are at particularly high risk for aspiration and pneumonia. In addition, seriously ill, bedridden patients are at risk for pulmonary sequelae. Repeated radiologic assessments of the lungs may be needed during hospitalization of seriously ill patients.

Cardiac Rhythm Monitoring

Although cardiac monitoring (including *bedside, Holter,* and *King-of-Hearts monitoring*) is an important part of the emergent care of patients with acute ischemic stroke, prolonged cardiac monitoring is of limited usefulness in the investigation of most patients with episodic symptoms suggestive of TIA.[321,322] Ambulatory electrocardiography has been used to detect intermittent atrial fibrillation.[322] In one series, only 12 of 184 patients with TIA had a cardiac arrhythmia detected by prolonged monitoring; intermittent atrial fibrillation, occurring in 6 patients, was the most common arrhythmia.[321] However, patients with recurrent syncope, pre-syncope symptoms, lightheadedness, or loss of consciousness may have an underlying cardiac arrhythmia. Although these symptoms are atypical for TIA, they have importance in elderly persons because the symptoms of global ischemia of the brain often are due to an intermittent cardiac arrhythmia. The most common intermittent cardiac arrhythmias are sick sinus syndrome (bradycardia–tachycardia syndrome) or intermittent heart block (third degree atrioventricular block).[323] Cardiac monitoring can be helpful in detecting a cardiac arrhythmia as a cause of these complaints.

Studies to Screen for Coronary Artery Disease

A strong relationship exists between atherosclerotic cerebrovascular disease and coronary artery disease.[324] A sizeable proportion of patients with a TIA or stroke has a history of symptomatic coronary artery disease.[314,325] Myocardial infarction or severe arrhythmias (sudden death) are the leading causes of death in persons who have a stroke or a TIA, including those who have not had any prior symptoms of cardiac ischemia. The risk of myocardial ischemia in patients with TIA is approximately the same as among persons with known three-vessel coronary artery disease.[326] Chimowitz et al[327] found a strong relationship between coronary artery disease and the subtype of ischemic stroke. Fifteen of 30 patients with large artery atherosclerosis had evidence of myocardial ischemia, whereas only 9 of 39 patients with strokes of other causes had ischemic heart disease. Myocardial infarction is a common cause of perioperative death following carotid endarterectomy.[328] It also is the leading long-term cause of death among persons who have had the carotid operation; the risk of cardiac death is higher among persons who have clinically overt heart disease.[329] In a study of patients without cardiac symptoms that included coronary artery arteriography, Hertzer et al[330] found severe coronary artery disease in 37% of 506 patients scheduled for carotid endarterectomy. Thus, evaluation of the heart for the presence of co-existing, although asymptomatic, coronary artery disease is an important part of the evaluation of patients with ischemic cerebrovascular disease. *Coronary artery angiography* is an invasive procedure that involves some morbidity including the possibility of stroke.[331] Although angiography remains the ultimate diagnostic study to assess the presence and extent of atherosclerotic disease of the coronary arteries, other diagnostic tests, which have sufficient specificity and sensitivity, can be performed to screen patients. The two most common cardiac stress tests are *graded exercise testing* (treadmill testing) and *radioisotope thallium cardiac scanning*, which usually involves the use of dipyridamole to cause coronary artery vasodilation.[327,331,332] Exercise tests often need to be modified for patients who have residual neurological impairments.[333] *Dobutamine stress echocardiography* also can be done to assess the extent of the coronary artery disease.[334] Results of the stress testing are useful in helping to formulate plans for treatment of the heart disease, including medical therapies, coronary artery angioplasty, or coronary artery bypass surgery.

CARDIAC IMAGING FOR A SOURCE OF EMBOLI

A key component of cardiac evaluation is imaging the heart to look for a source for embolization to the brain. Results of the clinical examination, chest x-ray and ECG can produce enough data to support the diagnosis of cardioembolism. For example, a cardiac murmur, an enlarged heart, atrial fibrillation, or a history of rheumatic fever provides compelling evidence for the diagnosis of cardioembolic stroke in a young adult. Similarly, the absence of abnormalities of other vascular lesions in an elderly woman with atrial fibrillation can suggest a diagnosis of cardioembolism. In contrast, in many circumstances, the diagnosis of cardioembolic stroke is uncertain, and ancillary diagnostic tests are needed to image the heart.

Cardiac imaging studies are performed to examine the function of the left ventricle, left atrium, mitral valve, and aortic valve to search for the presence of masses on the endocardial surface or the valves and to discover any congenital or structural abnormalities of the heart.[310] The most commonly performed tests are *transthoracic echocardiography* (*TTE*) and *transesophageal echocardiography* (*TEE*) (Table 4–9). These tests can be done with contrast enhancement using an injection of agitated saline that contains microbubbles and with or without *color Doppler* images. *Gated magnetic resonance imaging* and *contrast-enhanced rapid computed tomography* also can be used.[335] Each test has limitations, and all are expensive. A decision to order one or more of these tests is made on a case-by-case basis and is needed only if the results will alter management. Although the results of cardiac imaging tests might influence treatment of underlying heart disease in some patients, in general, treatment decisions

Table 4–9. **Echocardiographic Findings that Are Correlated with Risk of Embolism**

Left ventricular thrombus	Left atrial thrombus
Left atrial appendage thrombus	Left atrial enlargement
Akinetic segment	Venticular aneurysm
Left atrial turbulence	Valvular vegetations
Valvular strands	Lambl's excrescences
Left atrial myxoma	Patent foramen ovale
Atrial septal aneurysm	Mitral valve prolapse
Mitral annulus calcification	Calcific aortic stenosis
Plaque of the aortic arch	

revolve around the use of long-term oral anticoagulants to prevent embolism. If a patient has contraindications for treatment with an oral anticoagulant and the medication cannot be prescribed regardless of the results of the cardiac evaluation, one could argue that the tests are not needed. Conversely, if the clinical features and cardiac diagnostic tests, including ECG, provide compelling evidence for the diagnosis of cardioembolism and a decision supporting long-term treatment with anticoagulants already has been made, then imaging tests might be superfluous.

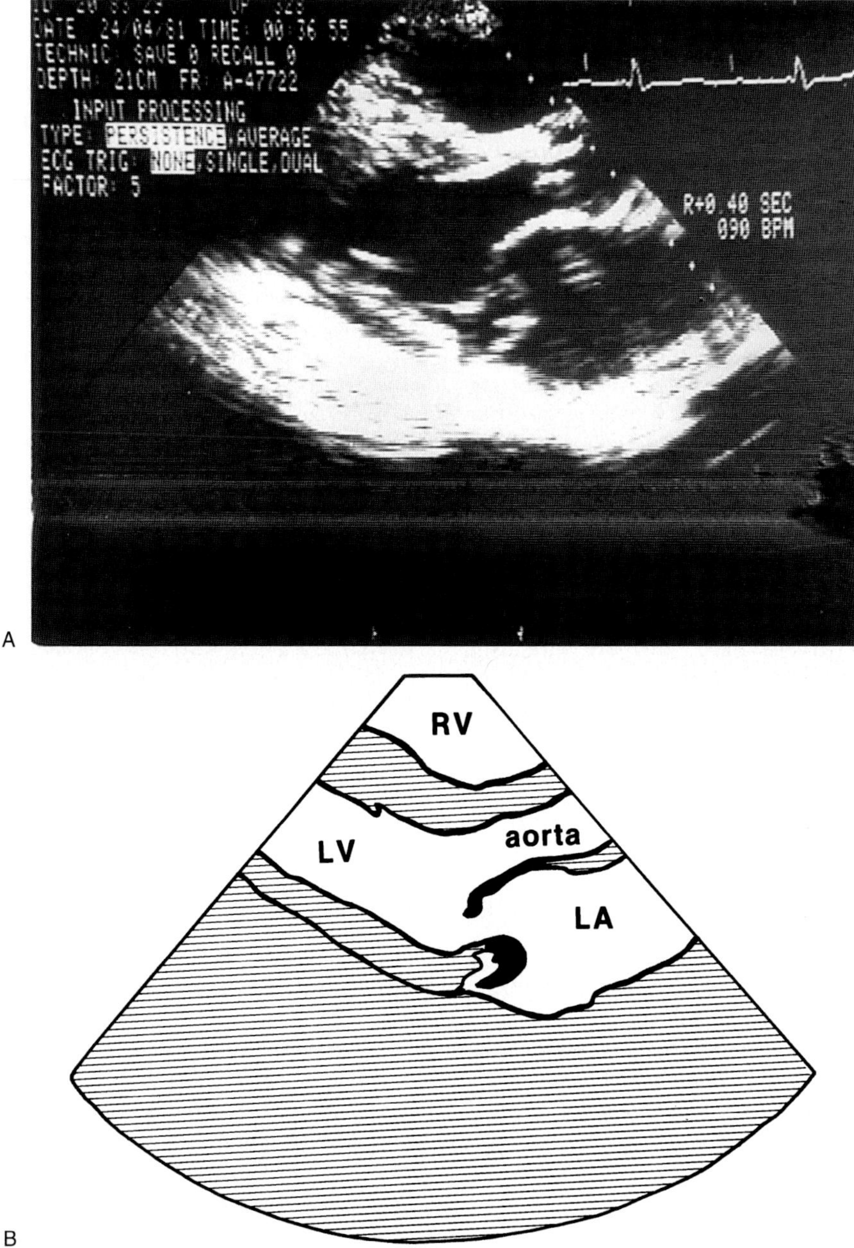

Figure 4–30. Two-dimensional transthoracic echocardiogram (and diagrams) in a patient with marked mitral valve prolapse using long axis (*A* and *B*) and apical four-chamber (*C* and *D*) views. (Courtesy of D.R. Boughner, MD, University of Western Ontario.)

Transthoracic Echocardiography

M-mode or two-dimensional TTE was the first ancillary cardiac imaging study developed. It is non-invasive, safe, and easy to perform (Figs. 4–30 and 4–31). The test is available at most hospitals. Technically, TTE can be performed satisfactorily except on people with obesity, large chests, or severe lung disease where cardiac structures are difficult to insonate from the anterior surface of the chest wall. Because the left ventricle is the most anterior part of the heart, it is most easily evaluated by TTE. Transthoracic echocardiography can assess the integrity of the left ventricular wall, the

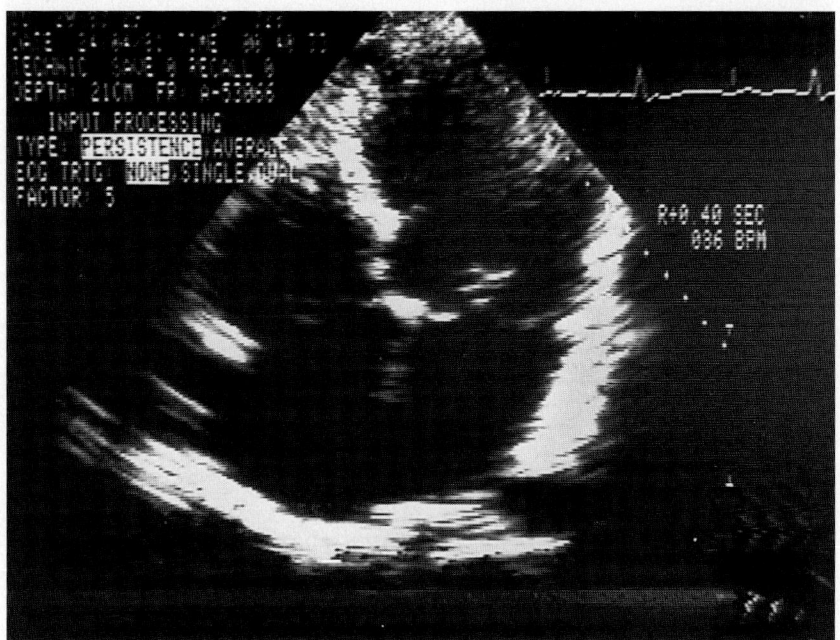

C

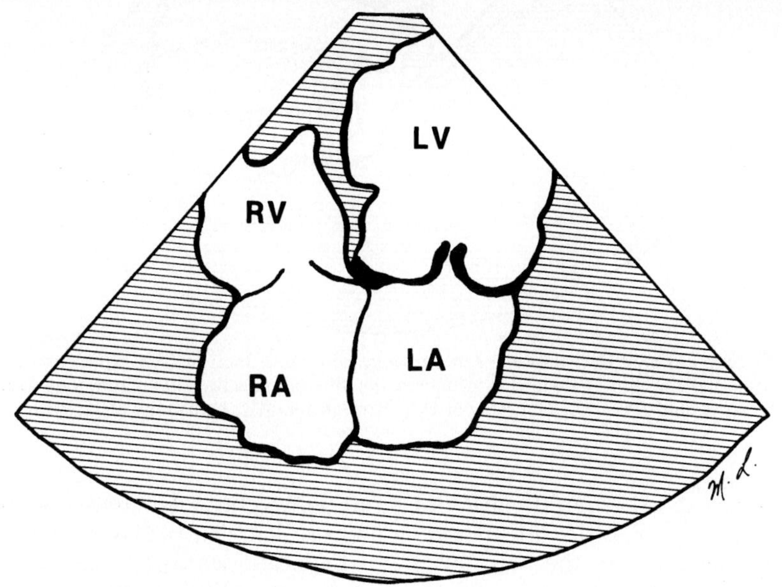

D

Figure 4–30. (*continued*)

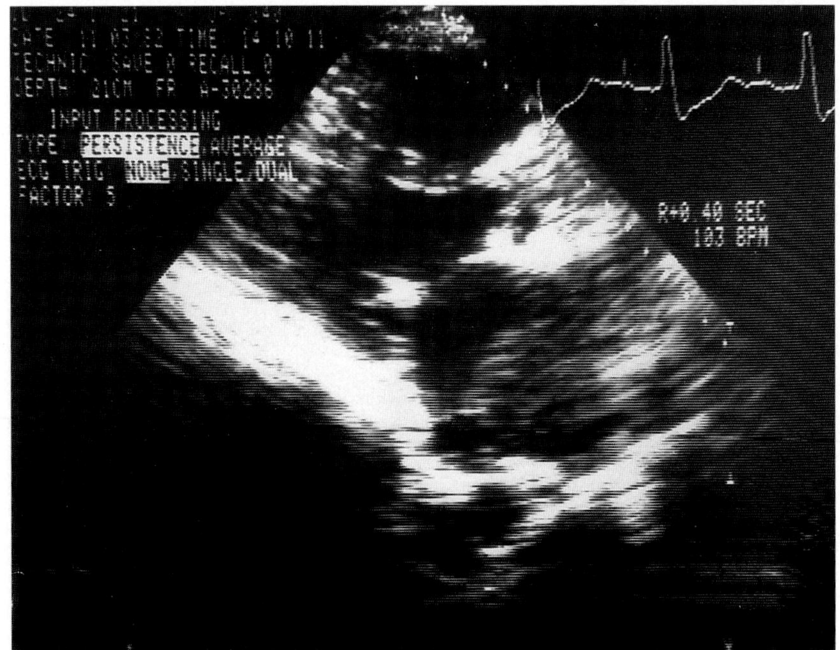

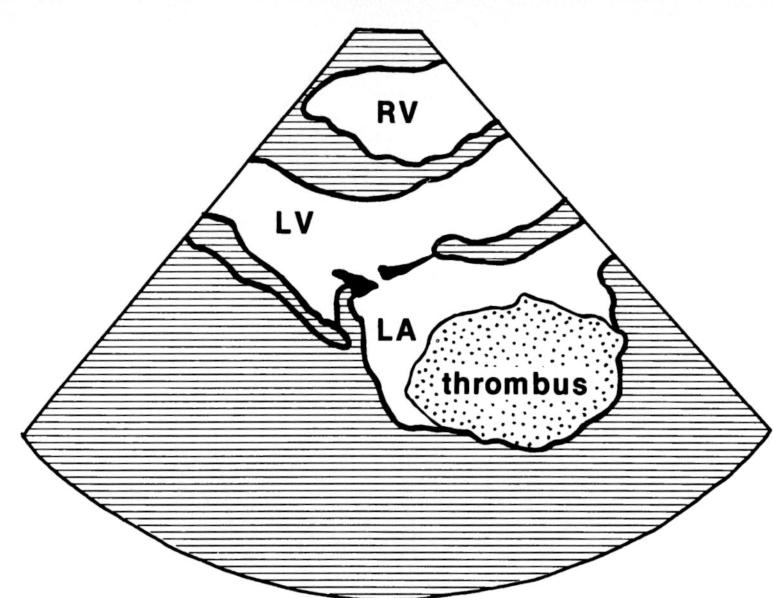

Figure 4–31. Two-dimensional transthoracic echocardiography (and diagrams) in a patient with severe mitral stenosis due to rheumatic heart disease and showing a major thrombus in the left atrium, long-axis (*A* and *B*) and apical four-chamber (*C* and *D*) views. (Courtesy of D.R. Broughner, MD, University of Western Ontario.)

ventricular cavity, and the mitral valve, but it does not reliably provide information about the left atrium or the left atrial appendage.[336] Transthoracic echocardiography also can be used to assess an increase in left ventricular mass or moderate-to-severe left ventricular systolic dysfunction, which can identify a patient as being at high risk for a TIA or stroke.[337,338] Although TTE has been used widely, numerous

C

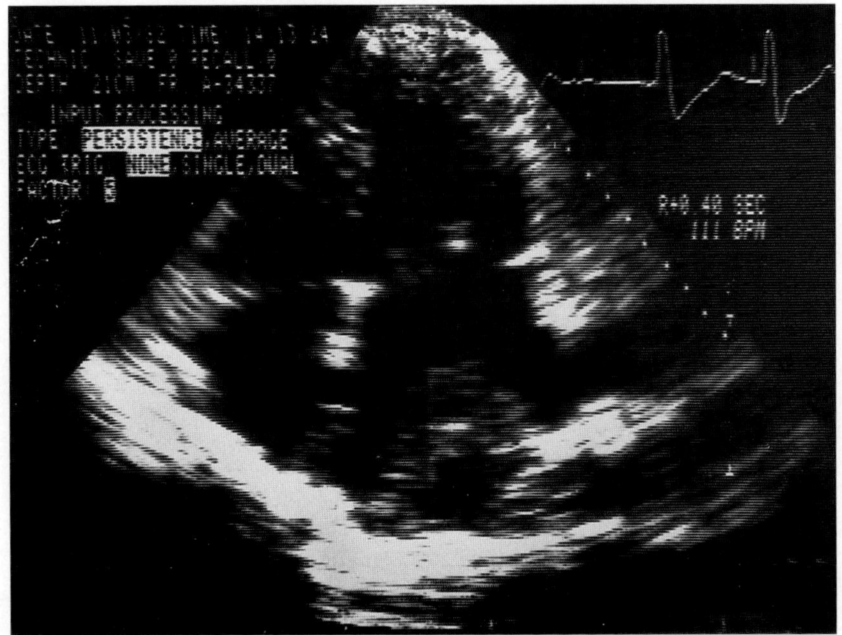

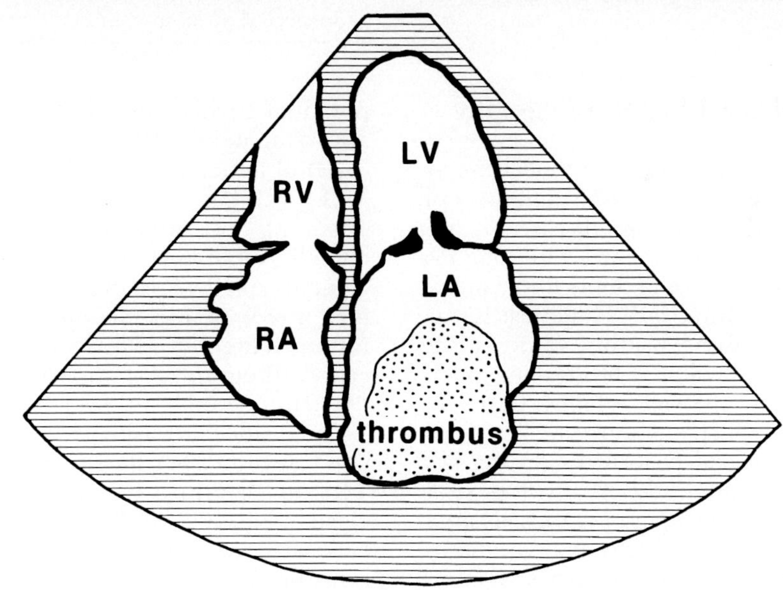

D

Figure 4–31. (*continued*)

studies show that it is not a very effective tool to search for cardiac lesions leading to embolic stroke. The yield of TTE in detecting a likely source for emboli (eg, intraluminal thrombus, akinetic segment, atrial myxoma, valvular abnormality) is relatively low. Sansoy et al[339] found a highly probable source for embolization in less than 3% of 1010 patients with stroke who had TTE. Most patients with stroke screened with TTE will have a normal study. The likelihood of finding an important cardiac abnormality is greater in persons younger than 45.[336,340,341] Hart[342] concluded that TTE is primarily indicated to screen for a left ventricular thrombus, mitral valve prolapse, mitral stenosis, aortic stenosis, aortic valve vegetations, or left ventricular abnormalities. Because the left ventricle often is the source of emboli following acute myocardial infarction and because TTE is a non-invasive test that adequately screens the left ventricle in most patients, it may be particularly useful in assessing for the risk of stroke in this situation.

Transthoracic echocardiography has been overused in the evaluation of patients with ischemic stroke; most patients do not need this test. The chance of detection of an important cardiac disease that is an occult cause of stroke is very low in patient who has another obvious etiology already diagnosed. The likelihood of TTE finding a cardiac abnormality in a patient older than 45 who does not have a history of heart disease is extraordinarily low.[343,344] The use of TTE should be restricted to patients with cryptogenic stroke who have other evidence suggesting disease of the left ventricle.

Table 4–10. **Indications for Transesophageal or Transthoracic Echocardiography**

Transesophageal Echocardiography Preferred
Suspected left atrial or valvular lesion
Unexplained stroke—especially in a young person
Patients with—
- Atrial fibrillation
- Prosthetic cardiac valve
- Possible right-to-left shunt
- Suspected endocarditis
- Suspected aortic atherosclerosis

Transthoracic Echocardiography Preferred
Suspected left ventricular lesion
Patients with—
- Acute anterior myocardial infarction
- Ventricular aneurysm
- Dilated cardiomyopathy
- Suspected atrial myxoma

Transesophageal Echocardiography

The development of TEE was a major advance in the evaluation of patients with ischemic cerebrovascular disease. It has become the single most important diagnostic test to screen most patients for a cardiac source of embolism.[345–348] The test is particularly helpful in assessing young adults with a TIA or stroke.[349] Multiplanar techniques increase the yield of TEE in detecting potential sources of emboli.[350]

Transesophageal echocardiography is a moderately invasive test. It involves swallowing a probe, and patients with dysphagia following stroke might not be able to perform this task. In one series of more than 10,000 procedures, approximately 200 patients could not tolerate the test.[351] Patients with constrictive disease of the esophagus, including esophageal malignancies, cannot have the test. Because the test is invasive, it is associated with the potential for pulmonary, bleeding, or cardiac complications. Still, the risk of major adverse experiences is relatively low.[351]

The yield of TEE is relatively high. In several series, TEE found at least one potential cardiac source for embolism in approximately 35%–45% of patients with cerebral ischemia.[352–361] In comparison to TTE, TEE has a much higher likelihood of detecting potential cardiac sources of emboli (Table 4–10). In one head-to-head comparison, TTE found cardiac abnormalities in 8% of 145 patients, whereas TEE found changes in 46%.[362] Transesophageal echocardiography is superior to TTE in detecting thrombi in the left atrium.[363,364] The specificity, sensitivity, positive predictive value, and negative predictive value of TEE in detecting left atrial thrombi are close to 100%.[357,365] Transesophageal echocardiography also can visualize vegetations or thickening of the mitral or aortic valves among patients with infective endocarditis.[366] In addition, it provides information about the size of the left atrium. Benjamin et al[367] demonstrated that the risk of stroke among men increased by a factor of 2.4 with every 10-mm. increase in left atrial size. Among women, the ratio was 1.4. Transesophageal echocardiography also can demonstrate reduced function of the left atrial appendage, which appears to be a risk factor for stroke.[368]

Abnormalities detected by TEE can be correlated with the presence of hypertension and atrial fibrillation.[353,355,369] Warner and Momah[353] found abnormal studies in 53% of patients with atrial fibrillation and 28% of patients with sinus rhythm. Transesophageal echocardiography is used to categorize the risk of embolization in patients with atrial fibrillation. The most commonly detected high-risk abnormalities are thrombi in the left atrium or the left at-rial appendage, or increased size of the left atrium.[370–373] Decreased left atrial appendage flow or spontaneous echocardiographic contrast in the left atrium also identify higher-risk persons with atrial fibrillation.[371,374–377] (See Fig. 4–32.) The appearance of spontaneous echocardiographic contrast appears to be associated with increased fibrinogen levels and increased viscosity of the blood.[378] The results of TEE can guide decisions about treatment with anticoagulants or antiplatelet aggregating agents to prevent stroke in persons with atrial fibrillation who have not had a TIA or stroke.[379,380] Hata et al[381] found that the results of TEE changed management decisions about anticoagulant treatment in approximately 10% of patients evaluated for a potential embolic stroke. McNamara et al[382] concluded that TEE was cost-effective in selecting patients for treatment with oral anticoagulants. Findings on TEE also can guide decisions about cardioversion in patients with atrial fibrillation.[383]

A potential limitation of TEE is its sensitivity. It detects a large number of findings of questionable significance, such as spontaneous echocardiographic contrast in the left atrium, patent foramen ovale, strands on the mitral valve, and an atrial septal aneurysm.[349] Zabalgoitia et al[369] evaluated the potential risk of embolism to the brain associated with abnormalities detected by TEE. They noted that the relative risk was increased by a factor of 2.5 with an appendage thrombus, a factor of 3.7 with dense spontaneous contrast in the left atrium, and a factor of 1.7 if the peak flow velocity was diminished in the left atrial appendage. Conversely, Huber et al[384] concluded that TEE does not help define

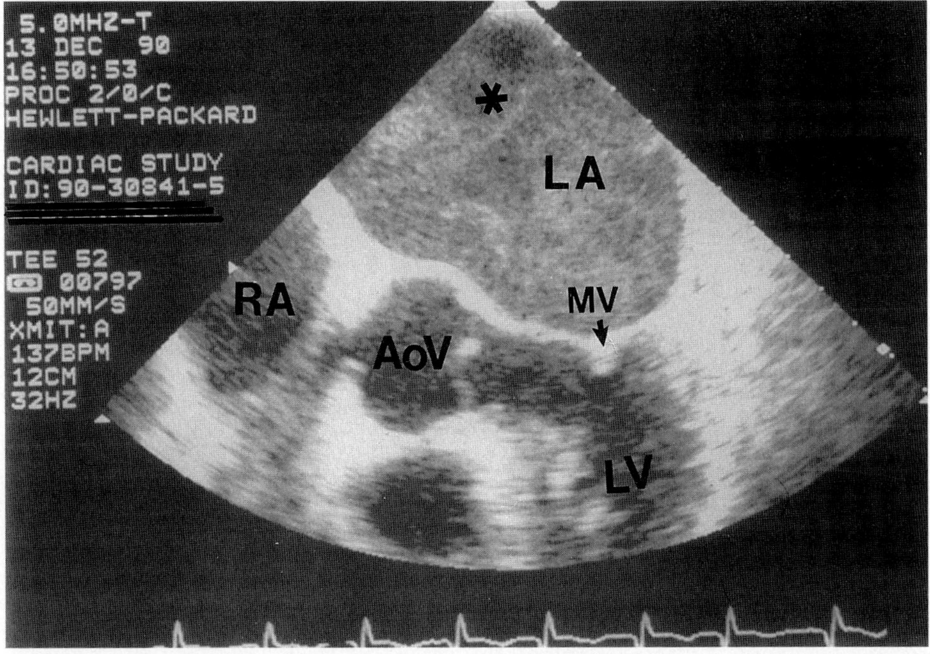

Figure 4–32. A transesophageal echocardiographic view of the base of the heart. Spontaneous ultrasound contrast is seen in the left atrium. This finding is an echocardiographic marker of low flow states associated with thromboembolism. (LA = left atrium; MV = mitral valve.) (Courtesy of Richard E. Kerber, MD, Department of Medicine, University of Iowa, Iowa City.)

higher- and lower-risk groups for recurrent stroke. Some of the lack of correlation might be due to the high rates of abnormalities found by TEE.

Strands on either native or prosthetic mitral or aortic valves can be identified on TEE. These abnormalities are small and thread-like, and they are attached to the valve. They are more common with mechanical than bioprosthetic valves.[385] Freedberg et al[386] found mitral or aortic strands in approximately 10% of patients who had TEE performed after an embolic event. These changes appear to be more important in persons under the age 60.[387]

Contrast-enhanced TEE is used widely to assess for the presence of an intracardiac right-to-left shunt, most commonly a patent foramen ovale (PFO).[358,388] A small amount of saline that has been shaken to create microbubbles is injected intravenously during TEE. Early detection of these bubbles in the left atrium correlates with an abnormal right-to-left shunt. Contrast TEE has a sensitivity of 89%–92% and a specificity of 94%–100% in detecting a PFO.[389,390] Color Doppler contrast-enhanced TEE has a sensitivity and specificity of nearly 100%.[389] A PFO is found most commonly in young adults with cryptogenic stroke.[391] The size of the PFO as documented by the number of bubbles detected by TEE is associated with the risk of embolization. A large shunt or a large PFO is associated with an increased risk of embolic stroke.[392] Stone et al[393] noted that embolization occurred in 5 of 16 patients with large shunts, whereas no embolic events were reported in 18 patients with smaller shunts.

TEE also has become the standard way to evaluate the ascending, arch, and descending portions of the thoracic aorta.[355,356,364] The yield of TEE in detecting plaques in older patients with cryptogenic stroke is high.[394] (See Table 4–10.) No other diagnostic study, including arteriography, appears to be equal to TEE in evaluating the presence or severity of atherosclerotic plaques of the ascending portion or the arch of the aorta.[394] A thick, complex, mobile, or friable plaque, or a plaque with superimposed thrombus, is rated as a high-risk lesion.[395] Conversely, a plaque less than 4 mm. in thickness is not correlated with a high rate of embolism. The thickness of the aortic plaque formation can guide management during major cardiovascular operations.[396,397] Very thick plaques are associated with a high risk of embolization of atherosclerotic debris; thus, the location of severe plaque formation detected by TEE influences placement of the aortic clamp.[396,398]

Ultrafast Computed Tomography Imaging of the Heart

Ultrafast CT imaging of the heart and the aorta is an alternative to TEE. It will visualize lesions in the left ventricle, left atrium, and aorta and it can detect intracardiac thrombi and protruding aortic atheromas or thrombi. Tenenbaum et al[399] found that ultrafast CT had a sensitivity of 87% and a specificity of 82% in detecting protruding aortic atheromas. Another study noted that ultrafast CT could give a false-positive result if stagnant blood is present in the left atrium; it could be confused with a left atrial thrombus.[400] Love et al[401] also reported that ultrafast CT might not visualize left ventricular clots. This technique can be done to assess the coronary arteries and the function of native or prosthetic cardiac valves.

Ultrafast CT requires the use of intravenous contrast agent, and technical problems can limit its use.[401] Although the role of the test is limited because of the widespread availability of TEE, ultrafast CT can be done if a cardioembolic cause of stroke is possible but the patient cannot tolerate TEE.

Magnetic Resonance Imaging of the Heart

Cine MRI of the heart is another alternative study for assessing patients at risk for cardioembolic stroke.[402] Indications for cine MRI of the heart are the same as those for ultrafast CT.

OTHER DIAGNOSTIC TESTS

Virtually all patients with a TIA or an ischemic stroke should have a complete blood count taken (see Table 4–1). A low hematocrit or hemoglobin value may point to an underlying malignancy or to a hematologic disorder, such as sickle cell disease or thalassemia. Polycythemia (usually defined as a hematocrit value greater than 50%) is an important risk factor for ischemic stroke. The total white blood cell count, especially leucocytosis, may point to an infectious cause of stroke, including infective endocarditis. The platelet count also is important; both thrombocytosis and thrombocytopenia are associated with increased risk for ischemic stroke. Thrombocytosis may be isolated, or it may be a component of a myeloproliferative disease; whereas a low platelet count is a feature of thrombotic thrombocytopenic purpura. A low platelet count does influence decisions about treatment or prevention of ischemic stroke because thrombocytopenia can increase bleeding risks. A complete blood count and platelet count can be done rapidly and, because the results influence treatment decisions, they should be part of the initial, emergent evaluation. Furthermore, monitoring the complete blood count and platelet count is part of the subsequent management of persons at risk for stroke. In particular, potential declines in the platelet count or the white blood cell count (neutrophil count) mandate monitoring these parameters during the first 3 months of treatment with ticlopidine. Occasionally, microscopic examination of the cellular elements of the blood may provide clues to the cause of stroke.

Measurements of the prothrombin time (international normalized ratio) and activated partial thromboplastin time (aPTT) are parts of the emergent evaluation of patients with acute ischemic stroke or TIA. Abnormalities of these tests suggest a prothrombotic state. In particular, a prolonged aPTT is a marker of the lupus anticoagulant or an elevated antiphospholipid antibody. Abnormalities of the prothrombin time or aPTT also are associated with an increased risk of bleeding following acute treatment with an antithrombotic or thrombolytic agent. Results of initial studies can be used for subsequent comparisons of the level of anticoagulation with oral anticoagulants or heparin.

Additional tests of coagulation can be ordered on a case-by-case basis (Table 4–11). In general, these tests are obtained if a patient has an atypical stroke or if either clinical or initial laboratory tests point to a hypercoagulable state. Disorders of coagulation, which can be inherited or secondary to a disease or medications, are described in more detail in Chapter 8. The timing of some of these tests is critical, as results can be affected by the acute neurological event and should be interpreted with caution if they are obtained within the first weeks after stroke. For example, an elevated serum

Table 4–11. **Coagulation and Serological Tests for Evaluation of Patients with Transient Ischemic Attack or Ischemic Stroke**

Sickle cell study	Hemoglobin electrophoresis
Fibrinogen	Fibrin degradation products
D—dimer	Thrombin time
Alpha–2 antiplasmin	Antithrombin III
Protein C	Protein S
Factor II	Factor V
Factor VII	Factor VIII
Factor IX	Factor X
Factor XI	Factor XII
Factor V-Leiden	Russel venom time
Erythrocyte sedimentation rate	C-reactive protein
Serum protein electrophoresis	Rheumatoid factor
Complement	Antinuclear antibody
Serologic test for syphilis	

fibrinogen value is common following ischemic stroke. Abnormally low concentrations of protein C, protein S, and antithrombin III can follow stroke. These tests should not be ordered until at least 6 weeks after the neurological event and are not reliable when a patient is taking warfarin on a long-term basis. Assessments for a Factor V-Leiden deficiency (activated protein C resistance) can be done during the first days after a stroke. Similarly, tests for the presence of a hemoglobinopathy should be performed if sickle cell disease is suspected as a cause of stroke. Because sickle cell disease is an important cause of ischemic stroke in young persons of African or Middle Eastern ancestry and, because the illness complicates acute management, screening for the disease should be part of emergent evaluation in these patients.

The presence of a prolonged aPTT at baseline should prompt additional testing, including mixing tests, kaolin clotting, or measurement of Russell viper venom time to confirm the presence of a lupus anticoagulant.[403] Assessments of the blood fibrinogen, D-dimer, fibrinogen degradation products, plasminogen, and alpha-2-antiplasmin, and thrombin time are done as part of a consumption profile if disseminated intravascular coagulation is suspected. Several of these tests also are performed in patients with cryptogenic stroke.[404,405] The thrombin time and plasma concentrations of factors II, V, VII, VIII, IX, X, XI and XII, also can be measured, but the usefulness of these studies is unknown when evaluating a patient with a TIA or an ischemic stroke.[406,407] Measurement of activated factor X can be used to monitor responses to treatment with low molecular weight heparins or danaparoid. It also is an alternative way to assess levels of anticoagulation with heparin in patients with a lupus anticoagulant.

Assessment for IgG and IgM antiphospholipid antibodies also can be done if the patient has an atypical stroke, if clinical findings suggest the presence of antiphospholipid antibodies, or in the presence of an unexplained prolongation of the aPTT.[408,409] Although most patients do not require measurement of the erythrocyte sedimentation rate, it is a reasonable screening tool to look for an inflammatory or infectious cause of stroke. The test can be supplemented by measurement of the C-reactive protein. A recent study showed that an elevation in C-reactive protein strongly predicts an increased risk of death after stroke.[410] Other tests for a multisystem inflammatory process, including antinuclear antibody, rheumatoid factor, complement, or serum protein electrophoresis, can be obtained on a case-by-case basis. The yield of these tests is relatively low. Serum measurements of the syphilis serology can be used to screen for meningovascular syphilis as a cause of stroke. In addition, abnormal syphilis serology reactions can be found in patients with multisystem vasculitides, including lupus.

If infective endocarditis is suspected, then sequential blood for cultures for aerobic and anaerobic organisms should be obtained. Usually, a minimum of six samples is required. Cultures of the urine, sputum, and blood should be obtained if a patient develops a fever after stroke.

Measurements of serum chemistries should be included in the emergent evaluation. In particular, concentrations of blood glucose and serum electrolytes can influence decisions about emergent care. An elevated blood glucose concentration points to underlying diabetes, thus predicting outcomes after stroke because it is associated with more severe neurological impairments.[411] An abnormally low glucose concentration can confirm hypoglycemia as the cause of acute neurological symptoms. Severe hypoglycemia can lead to major neurological sequelae, including stroke and cortical blindness.[412] The presence of kidney or liver disease also should be sought using relevant blood tests, including measurements of the concentrations of urea nitrogen, creatinine, bilirubin, alkaline phosphatase, and aspartate aminotransferase. The presence of hepatic or renal dysfunction can influence both acute and long-term care. Analysis of the urine also provides clues about the presence of renal disease or diabetes.

Measurements of concentrations of serum lipids should be part of the evaluation of most patients with an ischemic stroke or a TIA. In addition, total cholesterol concentration, measurements of triglycerides, HDL, and LDL cholesterol levels should be obtained. The patient should have fasted for at least 12 hours before this testing. Timing also is critical; a sample obtained more than 48 hours after onset or less than 6 weeks following stroke may give unreliable (low) results. Thus, assessment of serum lipids likely will be delayed until several weeks after the stroke.

SUMMARY

The clinician's ability to diagnose is amplified continuously by developing technology. But, unless investigations are guided by clinical hypotheses and judgment, information overload, contradictions, and confusion can derail good management. In most cases of possible stroke, the evaluation consists of imaging the brain, assessing the blood vessels, testing the heart, and screening the blood.

Timing of testing can be crucial. For example, early imaging dictates decision making in thrombolytic therapy, but early testing may miss a lipid disorder. If the initial investigations do not yield the expected results, then the simple act of retaking the history usually proves more fruitful than ordering another array of expensive tests.

REFERENCES

1. Adams HP, Jr. Investigation of the patient with ischemic Stroke. *Cerebrovasc Dis* 1991;1:50–54.
2. Adams HP, Jr., Brott TG, Crowell RM, et al. Guidelines for the management of patients with acute ischemic stroke. A statement for healthcare professionals from a special writing group of the Stroke Council, American Heart Association. *Circulation* 1994;90:1588–1601.
3. Adams HP, Jr. Management of patients with acute ischaemic stroke. *Drugs* 1997;54 (Suppl 3): 60–69.
4. Donnan GA. Investigation of patients with stroke and transient ischaemic attacks. *Lancet* 1992;339:473–477.
5. Weir CJ, Murray GD, Adams FG, Muir KW, Grosset DG, Lees KR. Poor accuracy of stroke scoring systems for differential clinical diagnosis of intracranial haemorrhage and infarction. *Lancet* 1994;344:999–1002.
6. Besson G, Robert C, Hommel M, Perret J. Is it clinically possible to distinguish nonhemorrhagic infarct from hemorrhagic stroke? *Stroke* 1995;26: 1205–1209.
7. Abrams HL, McNeil BJ. Medical implications of computed tomography ("CAT scanning"). *N Engl J Med* 1978;298:310–318.
8. Marik PE, Rakusin A, Sandhu SS. The impact of the accessibility of cranial CT scans on patient evaluation and management decisions. *J Intern Med* 1997;241:237–243.
9. Ruff RL, Dougherty JH, Jr. Evaluation of acute cerebral ischemia for anticoagulant therapy: computed tomography or lumbar puncture. *Neurology* 1981;31:736–740.
10. Schriger DL, Kalafut M, Starkman S, Krueger M, Saver JL. Cranial computed tomography interpretation in acute stroke: physician accuracy in determining eligibility for thrombolytic therapy. *JAMA* 1998;279:1293–1297.
11. Horowitz SH, Zito JL, Donnarumma R, Patel M, Alvir J. Computed tomographic-angiographic findings within the first five hours of cerebral infarction. *Stroke* 1991;22:1245–1253.
12. von Kummer R, Nolte PN, Schnittger H, Thron A, Ringelstein EB. Detectability of cerebral hemisphere ischaemic infarcts by CT within 6 h of stroke. *Neuroradiology* 1996;38:31–33.
13. Grond M, von Kummer R, Sobesky J, Schmulling S, Heiss WD. Early computed-tomography abnormalities in acute stroke. *Lancet* 1997;350:1595–1596.
14. Brainin M, McShane LM, Steiner M, Dachenhausen A, Seiser A. Silent brain infarcts and transient ischemic attacks. *Stroke* 1995;26:1348–1352.
15. Davis PH, Clarke WR, Bendixen BH, Adams HP, Jr., Woolson RF, Culebras A. Silent cerebral infarction in patients enrolled in the TOAST Study. *Neurology* 1996;46:942–948.
16. Bogousslavsky J, Regli F. Cerebral infarct in apparent transient ischemic attacks. *Neurology* 1985;35:1501–1503.
17. Dennis M, Bamford J, Sandercock P, Molyneux A, Warlow C. Computed tomography in patients with transient ischaemic attacks: when is a transient ischaemic attack not a transient ischaemic attack but a stroke? *J Neurol* 1990;237:257–261.
18. von Kummer R, Allen KL, Holle R, et al. Acute stroke: usefulness of early CT findings before thrombolytic therapy. *Radiology* 1997;205: 327–333.
19. Marks MP. CT in ischemic stroke. *Neuroimaging Clinics of North America* 1998;8:515–523.
20. Adams HP, Jr., Brott TG, Furlan AJ, et al. Guidelines for thrombolytic therapy for acute stroke: a supplement to the guidelines for the management of patients with acute ischemic stroke. A statement for healthcare professionals from a Special Writing Group of the Stroke Council, American Heart Association. *Circulation* 1996;94:1167–1174.
21. Barber PA, Demchuk AM, Zhang J, Buchan AM, for the ASPECTS Study Group. Validity and reliability of a quantitive computed tomography score in predicting outcome of hyperacute stroke before thrombolytic therapy. *Lancet* 2000;355:1670–1674.

22. Leys D, Pruvo JP, Godefroy O, Rondepierre P, Leclerc X. Prevalence and significance of hyperdense middle cerebral artery in acute stroke. *Stroke* 1992;23:317–324.
23. Tomsick T, Brott T, Barsan W, Broderick J, Haley EC, Spilker J. Thrombus localization with emergency cerebral CT. *Am J Neuroradiol* 1992;13:257–263.
24. von Kummer R, Meyding-Lamade U, Forsting M, et al. Sensitivity and prognostic value of early CT in occlusion of the middle cerebral artery trunk. *Am J Neuroradiol* 1994;15:9–15.
25. Giroud M, Beuriat P, Becker F, Binnert D, Dumas R. Dense middle cerebral artery: etiologic significance and prognosis. *Rev Neurol* 1990; 146:224–227.
26. Launes J, Ketonen L. Dense middle cerebral artery sign: an indicator of poor outcome in middle cerebral artery area infarction. *J Neurol Neurosurg Psychiatry* 1987;50:1550–1552.
27. Tomsick T, Brott T, Barsan W, et al. Prognostic value of the hyperdense middle cerebral artery sign and stroke scale score before ultraearly thrombolytic therapy. *Am J Neuroradiol* 1996; 17:79–85.
28. Manelfe C, Larrue V, von Kummer R, et al. Association of hyperdense middle cerebral artery sign with clinical outcome in patients treated with tissue plasminogen activator. *Stroke* 1999;30:769–772.
29. von Kummer R, Holle R, Gizyska U, et al. Interobserver agreement in assessing early CT signs of middle cerebral artery infarction. *Am J Neuroradiol* 1996;17:1743–1748.
30. Tomura N, Uemura K, Inugami A, Fujita H, Higano S, Shishido F. Early CT finding in cerebral infarction: obscuration of the lentiform nucleus. *Radiology* 1988;168:463–467.
31. Truwit CL, Barkovich AJ, Gean-Marton A, Hibri N, Norman D. Loss of the insular ribbon: another early CT sign of acute middle cerebral artery infarction. *Radiology* 1990;176:801–806.
32. Marks MP, Holmgren EB, Fox AJ, Patel S, von Kummer R, Froehlich J. Evaluation of early computed tomographic findings in acute ischemic stroke. *Stroke* 1999;30:389–392.
33. Hacke W, Kaste M, Fieschi C, et al. Intravenous thrombolysis with recombinant tissue plasminogen activator for acute hemispheric stroke. The European Cooperative Acute Stroke Study (ECASS). *JAMA* 1995;274:1017–1025.
34. Pantano P, Caramia F, Bozzao L, Dieler C, von Kummer R. Delayed increase in infarct volume after cerebral ischemia. *Stroke* 1999;30:502–507.
35. Damasio H. A computed tomographic guide to the identification of cerebral vascular territories. *Arch Neurol* 1983;40:138–142.
36. Greenberg JO, Smolen A, Cosio L. Computerized tomography in infarctions of the vertebral–basilar system. *Comput Radiol* 1982;6:149–153.
37. Tatu L, Moulin T, Bogousslavsky J, Duvernoy H. Arterial territories of human brain: brainstem and cerebellum. *Neurology* 1996;47:1125–1135.
38. Tomura N, Inugami A, Kanno I, et al. Differentiation between cerebral embolism and thrombosis on sequential CT scans. *J Comput Assist Tomogr* 1990;14:26–31.
39. Pullicino P, Snyder W, Munschauer F, Pordell R, Greiner F. Interrater agreement of computed tomography infarct measurement. *J Neuroimaging* 1996;6:16–19.
40. Saver JL, Johnson KC, Homer D, et al. Infarct volume as a surrogate or auxillary outcome measure in ischemic stroke clinical trials. *Stroke* 1999;30:293–298.
41. Ringelstein EB, Koschorke S, Holling A, Thron A, Lambertz H, Minale. Computed tomographic patterns of proven embolic brain infarctions. *Ann Neurol* 1989;26:759–765.
42. Kittner SJ, Sharkness CM, Sloan MA, et al. Features on initial computed tomography scan of infarcts with a cardiac source of embolism in the NINDS Stroke Data Bank. *Stroke* 1992;23:1748–1751.
43. Saito I, Segawa H, Shiokawa Y, Taniguchi M, Tsutsumi K. Middle cerebral artery occlusion: correlation of computed tomography and angiography with clinical outcome. *Stroke* 1987; 18:863–868.
44. Lodder J, Hupperts R, Boreas A, Kessels F. The size of territorial brain infarction on CT relates to the degree of internal carotid artery obstruction. *J Neurol* 1996;243:345–349.
45. Steinke W, Schwartz A, Hennerici M. Topography of cerebral infarction associated with carotid artery dissection. *J Neurol* 1996; 243:323–328.
46. Hennerici M, Daffertshofer M, Jakobs L. Failure to identify cerebral infarct mechanisms from topography of vascular territory lesions. *Am J Neuroradiol* 1998;1067–1074.
47. Rasmussen D, Kohler O, Worm-Petersen S, et al. Computed tomography in prognostic stroke evaluation. *Stroke* 1992;23:506–510.
48. Wardlaw JM, Sellar R. A simple practical classification of cerebral infarcts on CT and its interobserver reliability. *Am J Neuroradiol* 1994;15: 1933–1939.
49. von Kummer R, Patel S. Neuroimaging in acute stroke. *J Stroke Cerebrovasc Dis* 1999;8:127–138.
50. Brant-Zawadzki M, Atkinson D, Detrick M, Bradley WG, Scidmore G. Fluid-attenuated inversion recovery (FLAIR) for assessment of cerebral infarction. Initial clinical experience in 50 patients. *Stroke* 1996;27:1187–1191.
51. Damasio H, Frank R. Three-dimensional in vivo mapping of brain lesions in humans. *Arch Neurol* 1992;49:137–143.
52. Shuaib A, Lee D, Pelz D, Fox A, Hachinski VC. The impact of magnetic resonance imaging on the management of acute ischemic stroke. *Neurology* 1992;42:816–818.
53. Chabriate H, Mrissa R, Levy C, et al. Brain stem MRI signal abnormalities in CADASIL. *Stroke* 1999;30:457–459.
54. Davis SM, Tress BM, Dowling R, Donnan GA, Kiers L, Rossiter SC. Magnetic resonance imaging in posterior circulation infarction: impact on diagnosis and management. *Aust N Z J Med* 1989;19:219–225.
55. Simmons Z, Biller J, Adams HP, Jr., Dunn V, Jacoby CG. Cerebellar infarction: comparison of computed tomography and magnetic resonance imaging. *Ann Neurol* 1986;19:291–293.

56. Bruno A, Yuh WT, Biller J, Adams HP, Jr., Cornell SH. Magnetic resonance imaging in young adults with cerebral infarction due to moyamoya. *Arch Neurol* 1988;45:303–306.
57. Chimowitz MI, Estes ML, Furlan AJ, Awad IA. Further observations on the pathology of subcortical lesions identified on magnetic resonance imaging. *Arch Neurol* 1992;49:747–752.
58. Mohr JP, Biller J, Hilal SK, et al. Magnetic resonance versus computed tomographic imaging in acute stroke. *Stroke* 1995;26:807–812.
59. Bryan RN, Levy LM, Whitlow WD, Killian JM, Preziosi TJ, Rosario JA. Diagnosis of acute cerebral infarction: comparison of CT and MR imaging. *Am J Neuroradiol* 1991;12:611–620.
60. Fisher M, Prichard JW, Warach S. New magnetic resonance techniques for acute ischemic stroke. *JAMA* 1995;274:908–911.
61. Saunders DE, Clifton AG, Brown MM. Measurement of infarct size using MRI predicts prognosis in middle cerebral artery infarction. *Stroke* 1995;26:2272–2276.
62. Longstreth WT, Jr., Manolio TA, Arnold A, et al. Clinical correlates of white matter findings on cranial magnetic resonance imaging of 3301 elderly people. The Cardiovascular Health Study. *Stroke* 1996;27:1274–1282.
63. Price TR, Manolio TA, Kronmal RA, et al. Silent brain infarction on magnetic resonance imaging and neurological abnormalities in community-dwelling older adults. The Cardiovascular Health Study. CHS Collaborative Research Group. *Stroke* 1997;28:1158–1164.
64. van Swieten JC, van den Hout JH, van Ketel BA, Hijdra A, Wokke JH, van Gijn J. Periventricular lesions in the white matter on magnetic resonance imaging in the elderly. A morphometric correlation with arteriolosclerosis and dilated perivascular spaces. *Brain* 1991;114:761–774.
65. Bhadelia RA, Anderson M, Polak JF, et al. Prevalence and associations of MRI-demonstrated brain infarcts in elderly subjects with a history of transient ischemic attack. The Cardiovascular Health Study. *Stroke* 1999;30: 383–388.
66. Schmidt R, Fazekas F, Offenbacher H, et al. Brain magnetic resonance imaging in coronary artery bypass grafts: a pre- and postoperative assessment. *Neurology* 1993;43:775–778.
67. Yuh WT, Crain MR, Loes DJ, Greene GM, Ryals TJ, Sato Y. MR imaging of cerebral ischemia: findings in the first 24 hours. *Am J Neuroradiol* 1991;12:621–629.
68. Mead GE, Wardlaw JM. Detection of intraluminal thrombus in acute stroke by proton density MR imaging. *Cerebrovasc Dis* 1998;8:133–134.
69. Knepper L, Biller J, Adams HP, Jr., Yuh W, Ryals T, Godersky J. MR imaging of basilar artery occlusion. *J Comput Assist Tomogr* 1990;14:32–35.
70. Salbeck R, Busse O, Reinbold WD. MRI findings in megadolicho–basilar artery. *Cerebrovasc Dis* 1993;3:309–312.
71. Aichner FT, Felber SR, Birbamer GG, Posch A. Magnetic resonance imaging and magnetic resonance angiography of vertebrobasilar dolichoectasia. *Cerebrovasc Dis* 1993;3:280–284.
72. Fujisawa I, Asato R, Nishimura K, et al. Moyamoya disease: MR imaging. *Radiology* 1987; 164:103–105.
73. Kitanaka C, Tanaka J, Kuwahara M, Teraoka A. Magnetic resonance imaging study of intracranial vertebrobasilar artery dissections. *Stroke* 1994;25:571–575.
74. Mullges W, Ringelstein EB, Leibold M. Noninvasive diagnosis of internal carotid artery dissections. *J Neurol Neurosurg Psychiatry* 1992;55: 98–104.
75. Sue DE, Brant-Zawadzki MN, Chance J. Dissection of cranial arteries in the neck: correlation of MRI and arteriography. *Neuroradiology* 1992;34:273–278.
76. Levy C, Laissy JP, Raveau V, et al. Carotid and vertebral artery dissections: three-dimensional time-of-flight MR angiography and MR imaging versus conventional angiography. *Radiology* 1994;190:97–103.
77. Gortler M, Goldmann A, Mohr W, Widder B. Tissue characterisation of atherosclerotic carotid plaques by MRI. *Neuroradiology* 1995;37:631–635.
78. Mueller DP, Yuh WT, Fisher DJ, Chandran KB, Crain MR, Kim YH. Arterial enhancement in acute cerebral ischemia: clinical and angiographic correlation. *Am J Neuroradiol* 1993;14:661–668.
79. Cloft HJ, Murphy KJ, Prince MR, Brunberg JA. 3D gadolinium-enhanced MR angiography of the carotid arteries. *Magn Reson Imaging* 1996;14:593–600.
80. Crain MR, Yuh WT, Greene GM, et al. Cerebral ischemia: evaluation with contrast-enhanced MR imaging. *Am J Neuroradiol* 1991;12:631–639.
81. Rother J, Guckel F, Neff W, Schwartz A, Hennerici M. Assessment of regional cerebral blood volume in acute human stroke by use of single-slice dynamic susceptibility contrast-enhanced magnetic resonance imaging. *Stroke* 1996;27:1088–1093.
82. Kluytmans M, van der Grond J, Viergever MA. Gray matter and white matter perfusion imaging in patients with severe carotid artery lesions. *Radiology* 1998;209:675–682.
83. Hommel M, Grand S, Devoulon P, Le Bas JF. New directions in magnetic resonance in acute cerebral ischemia. *Cerebrovasc Dis* 1994;4:3–11.
84. Koroshetz WJ, Gonzalez G. Diffusion-weighted MRI: an ECG for "brain attack"? *Ann Neurol* 1997;41:565–566.
85. Lutsep HL, Albers GW, DeCrespigny A, Kamat GN, Marks MP, Moseley ME. Clinical utility of diffusion-weighted magnetic resonance imaging in the assessment of ischemic stroke. *Ann Neurol* 1997;41:574–580.
86. Warach S, Dashe JF, Edelman RR. Clinical outcome in ischemic stroke predicted by early diffusion-weighted and perfusion magnetic resonance imaging: a preliminary analysis. *J Cereb Blood Flow Metab* 1996;16:53–59.
87. Lovblad KO, Baird AE, Schlaug G, et al. Ischemic lesion volumes in acute stroke by diffusion-weighted magnetic resonance imaging correlate with clinical outcome. *Ann Neurol* 1997;42:164–170.
88. Baird AE, Warach S. Magnetic resonance imaging of acute stroke. *J Cereb Blood Flow Metab* 1998;18:583–609.

89. Sorensen AG, Buonanno FS, Gonzalez RG, et al. Hyperacute stroke: evaluation with combined multisection diffusion-weighted and hemodynamically weighted echo-planar MR imaging. *Radiology* 1996;199:391–401.
90. Albers G. Expanding the window for thrombolytic therapy in acute stroke. The potential role of acute MRI for patient selection. *Stroke* 1999;30:2230–2237.
91. Barber PA, Darby DG, Desmond PM, et al. Identification of major ischemic change. Diffusion-weighted imaging versus computed tomography. *Stroke* 1999;30:2059–2065.
92. Chaves CJ, Silver B, Schlaug G, Dashe J, Caplan LR, Warach S. Diffusion- and perfusion-weighted MRI patterns in borderzone infarcts. *Stroke* 2000;31:1090–1096.
93. Albers GW, Lansberg MG, Norbash AM, et al. Yield of diffusion-weighted MRI for detection of potentially relevant findings in stroke patients. *Neurology* 2000;54:1562–1567.
94. Lansberg MG, Albers GW, Beaulieu C, Marks MP. Comparison of diffusion-weighted MRI and CT in acute stroke. *Neurology* 2000;54:1557–1561.
95. Hacke W, Warach S. Diffusion-weighted MRI as an evolving standard of care in acute stroke. *Neurology* 2000;54:1548–1549.
96. Lee LJ, Kidwell CS, Alger J, Starkman S, Saver JL. Impact on stroke subtype diagnosis of early diffusion-weighted magnetic resonance imaging and magnetic resonance angiography. *Stroke* 2000;31:1081–1089.
97. Kidwell CS, Alger JR, Di Salle F, et al. Diffusion MRI in patients with transient ischemic attacks. *Stroke* 1999;30:1174–1180.
98. Karonen JO, Ostergaard L, Liu Y, et al. Combined diffusion and perfusion MRI with correlation to sinlge-photon emission CT in acute ischemic stroke. Ischemic penumbra predicts infarct growth. *Stroke* 1999;30: 1583–1590.
99. Fisher M. Characterizing the target of acute stroke therapy. *Stroke* 1997;28:866–872.
100. Barber PA, Darby DG, Desmond PM, et al. Prediction of stroke outcome with echoplanar perfusion- and diffusion-weighted MRI. *Neurology* 1998;51:418–426.
101. Lansberg MG, Tong DC, Norbash AM, Yenari MA, Moseley ME. Intra-arterial rtPA treatment of stroke assessed by diffusion- and perfusion-weighted MRI. *Stroke* 1999;30:678–680.
102. Marks MP, Tong DC, Beaulieu C, Albers GW, de Crespigny A, Moseley ME. Evaluation of early reperfusion and IV tPA therapy using diffusion- and perfusion-weighted MRI. *Neurology* 1999;52:1792–1798.
103. Tong DC, Yenari MA, Albers GW, O'Brien M, Marks MP, Moseley ME. Correlation of perfusion- and diffusion-weighted MRI with NIHSS score in acute (<6.5 hour) ischemic stroke. *Neurology* 1998;50:864–870.
104. Warach S, Gaa J, Siewert B, Wielopolski P, Edelman RR. Acute human stroke studied by whole brain echo planar diffusion-weighted magnetic resonance imaging. *Ann Neurol* 1995;37:231–241.
105. Lovblad KO, Laubach HJ, Baird AE, et al. Clinical experience with diffusion-weighted MR in patients with acute stroke. *Am J Neuroradiol* 1998;19:1061–1066.
106. Gonzalez RG, Schaefer PW, Buonanno FS, et al. Diffusion-weighted MR imaging: diagnostic accuracy in patients imaged within 6 hours of stroke symptom onset. *Radiology* 1999;210:155–162.
107. Neumann-Haefelin T, Wittsack HJ, Wenserski F, et al. Diffussion- and perfusion- weighted MRI the DWI/PWI mismatch region in acute stroke. *Stroke* 1999;30:1591–1597.
108. Baird AE, Benfield A, Schlaug G, et al. Enlargement of human cerebral ischemic lesion volumes measured by diffusion-weighted magnetic resonance imaging. *Ann Neurol* 1997; 41:581–589.
109. Burdette JH, Ricci PE, Petitti N, Elster AD. Cerebral infarction: time course of signal intensity changes on diffusion-weighted MR images. *Am J Roentgenol* 1998;171:791–795.
110. Ay H, Buonanno FS, Rordorf G, et al. Normal diffusion-weighted MRI during stroke-like deficits. *Neurology* 1999;52:1784–1792.
111. Zivin JA. Diffusion-weighted MRI for diagnosis and treatment of ischemic stroke. *Ann Neurol* 1997;41:567–568.
112. Zivin JA, Holloway RG. Weighing the evidence on DWI. Caveat emptor. *Neurology* 2000; 54:1552.
113. Powers WJ. Testing a test. *Neurology* 2000; 54:1549–1551.
114. Petty GW, Labar DR, Fisch BJ, Pedley TA, Mohr JP, Khandji A. Electroencephalography in lacunar infarction. *J Neurol Sci* 1995;134:47–50.
115. Macdonell RA, Donnan GA, Bladin PF, Berkovic SF, Wriedt CH. The electroencephalogram and acute ischemic stroke. Distinguishing cortical from lacunar infarction. *Arch Neurol* 1988; 45:520–524.
116. Cillessen JP, van Huffelen AC, Kappelle LJ, Algra A, van Gijn J. Electroencephalography improves the prediction of functional outcome in the acute stage of cerebral ischemia. *Stroke* 1994;25:1968–1972.
117. Aron KV, Cohen DE, Strobl FT. Effect of intraoperative intervention on neurological outcome based on electroencephalographic monitoring during cardiopulmonary bypass. *Ann Thorac Surg* 1989;48:476–483.
118. Stoughton J, Nath RL, Abbott WM. Comparison of simultaneous electroencephalographic and mental status monitoring during carotid endarterectomy with regional anesthesia. *J Vasc Surg* 1998;28:1014–1021.
119. Illig KA, Burchfiel JL, Ouriel K, DeWeese JA, Shortell CK, Green RM. Value of preoperative EEG for carotid endarterectomy. *Cardiovasc Surg* 1998;6:490–495.
120. Caplan LR, Flamm ES, Mohr JP, et al. Lumbar puncture and stroke. A statement for physicians by a Committee of the Stroke Council, American Heart Association. *Circulation* 1987;75: 505A–07A.
121. Oliveira V, Povoa P, Costa A, Ducla-Soares J. Cerebrospinal fluid and therapy of isolated

angiitis of the central nervous system. *Stroke* 1994;25:1693–1695.
122. Lampl Y, Paniri Y, Eshel Y, Sarova-Pinhas I. Cerebrospinal fluid lactate dehydrogenase levels in early stroke and transient ischemic attacks. *Stroke* 1990;21:854–857.
123. Donnan GA, Zapf P, Doyle AE, Bladin PF. CSF enzymes in lacunar and cortical stroke. *Stroke* 1983;14:266–269.
124. Bell RD, Khan M. Cerebrospinal fluid creatine kinase-BB activity. *Arch Neurol* 1999; 56:1327–1328.
125. Heiss WD, Podreka I. Role of PET and SPECT in the assessment of ischemic cerebrovascular disease. *Cerebrovasc Brain Metab Rev* 1993; 5:235–263.
126. Baron JC. Mapping the ischaemic penumbra with PET: Implications for acute stroke treatment. *Cerebrovasc Dis* 1999;9:193–201.
127. Brooks DJ. The clinical role of PET in cerebrovascular disease. *Neurosurg Rev* 1991; 14:91–96.
128. Read SJ, Hirano T, Abbott DF, et al. Identifying hypoxic tissue after acute ischemic stroke using PET and 18F-fluoromisonidazole. *Neurology* 1998;51:1617–1621.
129. Derdeyn CP, Videen TO, Fritsch SM, Carpenter DA, Grubb RL, Jr., Powers WJ. Compensatory mechanisms for chronic cerebral hypoperfusion in patients with carotid occlusion. *Stroke* 1999;30:1019–1024.
130. Grubb RL, Jr., Derdeyn CP, Fritsch SM, et al. Importance of hemodynamic factors in the prognosis of symptomatic carotid occlusion. *JAMA* 1998;280:1055–1060.
131. Derdeyn CP, Grubb RL, Jr., Powers WJ. Cerebral hemodynamic impairment. *Neurology* 1999; 53:251–259.
132. Podreka I, Suess E, Goldenberg G, et al. Initial experience with technetium-99m HMPAO brain SPECT. *J Nucl Med* 1987;28:1657–1666.
133. Rango M, Candelise L, Perani D, et al. Cortical pathophysiology and clinical neurologic abnormalities in acute cerebral ischemia. A serial study with single photon emission computed tomography. *Arch Neurol* 1989;1318–1322.
134. Alexandrov AV, Masdeu JC, Devous MDS, Black SE, Grotta JC. Brain single-photon emission CT with HMPAO and safety of thrombolytic therapy in acute ischemic stroke. Proceedings of the meeting of the SPECT Safe Thrombolysis Study Collaborators and the members of the Brain Imaging Council of the Society of Nuclear Medicine. *Stroke* 1997;28:1830–1834.
135. Bowler JV, Wade JP, Jones BE, Nijran K, Steiner TJ. Single-photon emission computed tomography using hexamethylpropyleneamine oxime in the prognosis of acute cerebral infarction. *Stroke* 1996;27:82–86.
136. Masdeu JC, Brass LM. SPECT imaging of stroke. *J Neuroimaging* 1995;5 (Suppl 1):S14–S22.
137. Soricelli A, Postiglione A, Cuocolo A, et al. Effect of adenosine on cerebral blood flow as evaluated by single-photon emission computed tomography in normal subjects and in patients with occlusive carotid disease. A comparison with acetazolamide. *Stroke* 1995;26:1572–1576.
138. Baird AE, Austin MC, McKay WJ, Donnan GA. Changes in cerebral tissue perfusion during the first 48 hours of ischemic stroke. Relation to clinical outcome. *J Neurol Neurosurg Psychiatry* 1996; 61:26–29.
139. Alexandrov AV, Ehrlich LE, Bladin CF, Black SE. Clinical significance of increased uptake of HMPAO on brain SPECT scans in acute stroke. *J Neuroimaging* 1996;6:150–155.
140. Laloux P, Richelle F, Jamart J, De Coster P, Laterre C. Comparative correlations of HMPAO SPECT indices, neurological score, and stroke subtypes with clinical outcome in acute carotid infarcts. *Stroke* 1995;26:816–821.
141. Barber PA, Davis SM, Infeld B, et al. Spontaneous reperfusion after ischemic stroke is associated with improved outcome. *Stroke* 1998;29:2522–2528.
142. Hanson SK, Grotta JC, Rhoades H, et al. Value of single-photon emission-computed tomography in acute stroke therapeutic trials. *Stroke* 1993;24:1322–1329.
143. Shimosegawa E, Hatazawa J, Inugami A, et al. Cerebral infarction within six hours of onset: prediction of completed infarction with technetium-99m-HMPAO SPECT. *J Nucl Med* 1994;35:1097–1103.
144. Kim JH, Shin T, Park JH, Chung SH, Choi NC, Lim BH. Various patterns of perfusion-weighted MR imaging and MR angiographic findings in hyperacute ischemic stroke. *Am J Neuroradiol* 1999;20:613–620.
145. Baird AE, Austin MC, McKay WJ, Donnan GA. Sensitivity and specificity of 99mTc-HMPAO SPECT cerebral perfusion measurements during the first 48 hours for the localization of cerebral infarction. *Stroke* 1997;28:976–980.
146. Brass LM, Walovitch RC, Joseph JL, et al. The role of single photon emission computed tomography brain imaging with 99mTc-bicisate in the localization and definition of mechanism of ischemic stroke. *J Cereb Blood Flow Metab* 1994;14 (Suppl 1):S91–S98.
147. Ueda T, Sakaki S, Yuh WT, Nochide I, Ohta S. Outcome in acute stroke with successful intraarterial thrombolysis and predictive value of initial single-photon emission-computed tomography. *J Cereb Blood Flow Metab* 1999;19:99–108.
148. Hunter GJ, Hamberg LM, Ponzo JA, et al. Assessment of cerebral perfusion and arterial anatomy in hyperacute stroke with three-dimensional functional CT: early clinical results. *Am J Neuroradiol* 1998;19:29–37.
149. Hamberg LM, Hunter GJ, Halpern EF, Hoop B, Gazelle GS, Wolf GL. Quantitative high-resolution measurement of cerebrovascular physiology with slip-ring CT. *Am J Neuroradiol* 1996;17:639–650.
150. Beristain X, Dujovny M, Gaviria M. Xenon/CT quantitative local cerebral blood flow. *Surg Neurol* 1996;46:437–440.
151. Kaufmann AM, Firlik AD, Fukui MB, Wechsler LR, Jungries CA, Yonas H. Ischemic care and penumbra in human stroke. *Stroke* 1999; 30:93–99.

152. Firlik AD, Kaufmann AM, Wechsler LR, Firlik KS, Fukui MB, Yonas H. Quantitative cerebral blood flow determinations in acute ischemic stroke. Relationship to computed tomography and angiography. *Stroke* 1997;28:2208–2213.
153. Le Bihan D, Jezzard P, Haxby J, Sadato N, Rueckert L, Mattay V. Functional magnetic resonance imaging of the brain. *Ann Intern Med* 1995;122:296–303.
154. Detre JA, Alsop DC, Vives LR, Maccotta L, Teener JW, Raps EC. Noninvasive MRI evaluation of cerebral blood flow in cerebrovascular disease. *Neurology* 1998;50:633–641.
155. Lanfermann H, Kugel H, Heindel W, Herholz K, Heiss WD, Lackner K. Metabolic changes in acute and subacute cerebral infarctions: findings at proton MR spectroscopic imaging. *Radiology* 1995;196:203–210.
156. Rudkin TM, Arnold DL. Proton magnetic resonance spectroscopy for the diagnosis and management of cerebral disorders. *Arch Neurol* 1999;56:919–926.
157. Lord RS. Non-invasive testing for cerebrovascular disease. *Cardiovasc Surg* 1996;4:424–437.
158. Rothwell PM, Gibson RJ, Villagra R, Sellar R, Warlow CP. The effect of angiographic technique and image quality on the reproducibility of measurement of carotid stenosis and assessment of plaque surface morphology. *Clin Radiol* 1998;53:439–443.
159. Kappelle LJ, Koudstaal PJ, van Gijn J, Ramos LM, Keunen JE. Carotid angiography in patients with lacunar infarction. A prospective study. *Stroke* 1988;19:1093–1096.
160. Adams HP, Jr., Putman SF, Corbett JJ, Sires BP, Thompson HS. Amaurosis fugax: the results of arteriography in 59 patients. *Stroke* 1983; 14:742–744.
161. Liberopoulos K, Kaponis A, Kokkinis K, et al. Comparative study of magnetic resonance angiography, digital subtraction angiography, duplex ultrasound examination with surgical and histological findings of atherosclerotic carotid bifurcation disease. *Int Angiol* 1996;15:131–137.
162. Eliasziw M, Smith RF, Singh N, Holdsworth DW, Fox AJ, Barnett HJM. Further comments on the measurement of carotid stenosis from angiograms. North American Symptomatic Carotid Endarterectomy Trial (NASCET) Group. *Stroke* 1994;25:2445–2449.
163. Fox AJ. How to measure carotid stenosis. *Radiology* 1993;186:316–318.
164. Pelz DM, Fox AJ, Eliasziw M, Barnett HJM. Stenosis of the carotid bifurcation: subjective assessment compared with strict measurement guidelines. *Can Assoc Radiol J* 1993;44:247–252.
165. Chang YJ, Golby AJ, Albers GW. Detection of carotid stenosis. From NASCET results to clinical practice. *Stroke* 1995;26:1325–1328.
166. Read SJ, Jackson GD, Abbott DF, et al. Experience with diffusion-weighted imaging in an acute stroke unit. *Cerebrovasc Dis* 1998; 8:135–143.
167. Rothwell PM, Gibson RJ, Slattery J, Sellar RJ, Warlow CP. Equivalence of measurements of carotid stenosis. A comparison of three methods on 1001 angiograms. European Carotid Surgery Trialists' Collaborative Group. *Stroke* 1994;25: 2435–2439.
168. Fredericks RK, Thomas TD, Lefkowitz DS, Troost BT. Implications of the angiographic string sign in carotid atherosclerosis. *Stroke* 1990;21:476–479.
169. Rothwell PM, Salinas R, Ferrando LA, Slattery J, Warlow CP. Does the angiographic appearance of a carotid stenosis predict the risk of stroke independently of the degree of stenosis? *Clin Radiol* 1995;50:830–833.
170. Caplan L, Stein R, Patel D, Amico L, Cashman N, Gewertz B. Intraluminal clot of the carotid artery detected radiographically. *Neurology* 1984;34:1175–1181.
171. Pelz DM, Buchan A, Fox AJ, Barnett HJM, Vinuela F. Intraluminal thrombus of the internal carotid arteries: angiographic demonstration of resolution with anticoagulant therapy alone. *Radiology* 1986;160:369–373.
172. Buchan A, Gates P, Pelz D, Barnett HJM. Intraluminal thrombus in the cerebral circulation. Implications for surgical management. *Stroke* 1988;19:681–687.
173. Streifler JY, Eliasziw M, Fox AJ, et al. Angiographic detection of carotid plaque ulceration. Comparison with surgical observations in a multicenter study. North American Symptomatic Carotid Endarterectomy Trial. *Stroke* 1994;25: 1130–1132.
174. Alhalabi M, Moore PM. Serial angiography in isolated angiitis of the central nervous system. *Neurology* 1994;44:1221–1226.
175. Davies KN, Humphrey PR. Complications of cerebral angiography in patients with symptomatic carotid territory ischaemia screened by carotid ultrasound. *J Neurol Neurosurg Psychiatry* 1993;56:967–972.
176. Gerraty RP, Bowser DN, Infeld B, Mitchell PJ, Davis SM. Microemboli during carotid angiography. Association with stroke risk factors or subsequent magnetic resonance imaging changes? *Stroke* 1996;27:1543–1547.
177. Swanson PD, Calanchini PR, Dyken ML, et al. A cooperative study of hospital frequency and character of transient ischemic attacks. II. Performance of angiography among six centers. *JAMA* 1977;237:2202–2206.
178. Hankey GJ, Warlow CP, Molyneux AJ. Complications of cerebral angiography for patients with mild carotid territory ischaemia being considered for carotid endarterectomy. *J Neurol Neurosurg Psychiatry* 1990;53:542–548.
179. Executive Committee for the Asymptomatic Carotid Atherosclerosis Study. Endarterectomy for asymptomatic carotid artery stenosis. *JAMA* 1995;273:1421–1428.
180. Haley EC, Jr. Encephalopathy following arteriography: a possible toxic effect of contrast agents. *Ann Neurol* 1984;15:100–102.
181. Shuaib A, Hachinski VC. Migraine and the risks from angiography. *Arch Neurol* 1988;45:911–912.
182. Thiele BL, Jones AM, Hobson RW, et al. Standards in noninvasive cerebrovascular

testing. Report from the Committee on Standards for Noninvasive Vascular Testing of the Joint Council of the Society for Vascular Surgery and the North American Chapter of the Inter-national Society for Cardiovascular Surgery. *J Vasc Surg* 1992;15:495–503.

183. Polak JF, Kalina P, Donaldson MC, et al. Carotid endarterectomy: preoperative evaluation of candidates with combined Doppler sonography and MR angiography. Work in progress. *Radiology* 1993;186:333–338.
184. Strandness DE, Jr. Angiography before carotid endarterectomy—no. *Arch Neurol* 1995;52: 832–833.
185. Lustgarten JH, Solomon RA, Quest DO, Khanjdi AG, Mohr JP. Carotid endarterectomy after noninvasive evaluation by duplex ultrasonography and magnetic resonance angiography. *Neurosurgery* 1994;34:612–618.
186. Back MR, Harward TR, Huber TS, Carlton LM, Flynn TC, Seeger JM. Improving the cost-effectiveness of carotid endarterectomy. *J Vasc Surg* 1997;26:456–462.
187. Hankey GJ, Warlow CP. Symptomatic carotid ischaemic events: safest and most cost effective way of selecting patients for angiography, before carotid endarterectomy. *BMJ* 1990;300: 1485–1491.
188. Hankey GJ, Warlow CP. The role of imaging in the management of cerebral and ocular ischaemia. *Neuroradiology* 1991;33:381–390.
189. de Bray JM, Glatt B. Quantification of atheromatous stenosis in the extracranial internal carotid artery. *Cerebrovasc Dis* 1995;5:414–426.
190. Bladin CF, Alexandrov AV, Murphy J, Maggisano R, Norris JW. Carotid Stenosis Index. A new method of measuring internal carotid artery stenosis. *Stroke* 1995;26:230–234.
191. Niskanen L, Rauramaa R, Miettinen H, Haffner SM, Mercuri M, Uusitupa M. Carotid artery intima-media thickness in elderly patients with NIDDM and in nondiabetic subjects. *Stroke* 1996;27:1986–1992.
192. Sander D, Klingelhofer J. Early carotid atherosclerosis of the internal and external carotid artery related to twenty-four blood pressure variability. *Cerebrovasc Dis* 1997;7:338–344.
193. Espeland MA, Tang R, Terry JG, Davis DH, Mercuri M, Crouse JR, III. Associaion of risk factors with segement-specific intimal-medial thickness of the extracranial carotid artery. *Stroke* 1999;30:1047–1055.
194. Riley WA, Barnes RW, Applegate WB, et al. Reproducibility of noninvasive ultrasonic measurement of carotid atherosclerosis. The Asymptomatic Carotid Artery Plaque Study. *Stroke* 1992;23:1062–1068.
195. Tonstad S, Joakimsen O, Stensland-Bugge E, Ose L, Bonaa KH, Leren TP. Carotid intima-media thickness and plaque in patients with familial hypercholesterolaemia mutations and control subjects. *Eur J Clin Invest* 1998;28:971–979.
196. Bonithon-Kopp C, Touboul PJ, Berr C, Magne C, Ducimetiere P. Factors of carotid arterial enlargement in a population aged 59 to 71 years: the EVA study. *Stroke* 1996;27:654–660.
197. Bots ML, Hoes AW, Koudstaal PJ, Hofman A, Grobbee DE. Common carotid intima-media thickness and risk of stroke and myocardial infarction: the Rotterdam Study. *Circulation* 1997;96:1432–1437.
198. O'Leary DH, Polak JF, Kronmal RA, et al. Carotid artery intima and media thickness as a risk factor for myocardial infarction and stroke in older adults. *N Engl J Med* 1999;340:14–22.
199. Wong M, Edelstein J, Wollman J, Bond MG. Ultrasonic-pathological comparison of the human arterial wall. Verification of intima-media thickness. *Arterioscler Thromb* 1993;13:482–486.
200. Ebrahim S, Papacosta O, Whincup P, et al. Carotid plaque, intima media thickness, cardiovascular risk factors, and prevalent cardiovascular disease in men and women: the British Regional Heart Study. *Stroke* 1999;30: 841–850.
201. Bots ML, Hoes AW, Hofman A, Witteman JC, Grobbee DE. Cross-sectionally assessed carotid intima-media thickness relates to long-term risk of stroke, coronary heart disease and death as estimated by available risk functions. *J Intern Med* 1999;245:269–276.
202. Davis PH, Dawson JD, Mahoney LT, Lauer RM. Increased carotid intimal-medial thickness and coronary calcification are related in young and middle-aged adults. *Circulation* 1999;100: 838–842.
203. Beletsky VY, Kelley RE, Fowler M, Phifer T. Ultrasound densitometric analysis of carotid plaque composition. Pathoanatomic correlation. *Stroke* 1996;27:2173–2177.
204. Falke P, Matzsch T, Sternby NH, Bergqvist D, Stavenow L. Intraplaque haemorrhage at carotid artery surgery—a predictor of cardiovascular mortality. *J Intern Med* 1995;238:131–135.
205. Hatsukami TS, Ferguson MS, Beach KW, et al. Carotid plaque morphology and clinical events. *Stroke* 1997;28:95–100.
206. Salonen R, Tervahauta M, Salonen JT, et al. Ultrasonographic manifestations of common carotid atherosclerosis in elderly eastern Finnish men. Prevalence and associations with cardiovascular diseases and risk factors. *Arterioscler Thromb* 1994;14:1631–1640.
207. Kagawa R, Moritake K, Shima T, Okada Y. Validity of B-mode ultrasonographic findings in patients undergoing carotid endarterectomy in comparison with angiographic and clinicopathologic features. *Stroke* 1996;27:700–705.
208. Polak JF, Shemanski L, O'Leary DH, et al. Hypoechoic plaque at US of the carotid artery: an independent risk factor for incident stroke in adults aged 65 years or older. Cardiovascular Health Study. *Radiology* 1998;208:649–654.
209. Park AE, McCarthy WJ, Pearce WH, Matsumura JS, Yao JS. Carotid plaque morphology correlates with presenting symptomatology. *J Vasc Surg* 1998;27:872–878.
210. Sitzer M, Muller W, Siebler M, et al. Plaque ulceration and lumen thrombus are the main sources of cerebral microemboli in high-grade internal carotid artery stenosis. *Stroke* 1995;26: 1231–1233.

211. Eljamel MS, Humphrey PR, Shaw MD. Dissection of the cervical internal carotid artery. The role of Doppler/duplex studies and conservative management. *J Neurol Neurosurg Psychiatry* 1990;53:379–383.
212. Busuttil SJ, Franklin DP, Youkey JR, Elmore JR. Carotid duplex overestimation of stenosis due to severe contralateral disease. *Am J Surg* 1996;172: 144–147.
213. AbuRahma AF, Richmond BK, Robinson PA, Khan S, Pollack JA, Alberts S. Effect of contralateral severe stenosis or carotid occlusion on duplex criteria of ipsilateral stenoses: comparative study of various duplex parameters. *J Vasc Surg* 1995;22:751–761.
214. Suwanwela N, Can U, Furie KL, et al. Carotid Doppler ultrasound criteria for internal carotid artery stenosis based on residual lumen diameter calculated from en bloc carotid endarterectomy specimens. *Stroke* 1996;27:1965–1969.
215. Jackson MR, Chang AS, Robles HA, et al. Determination of 60% or greater carotid stenosis: a prospective comparison of magnetic resonance angiography and duplex ultrasound with conventional angiography. *Ann Vasc Surg* 1998; 12:236–243.
216. Bray JM, Galland F, Lhoste P, et al. Colour Doppler and duplex sonography and angiography of the carotid artery bifurcations. Prospective, double-blind study. *Neuroradiology* 1995;37: 219–224.
217. Worthy SA, Henderson J, Griffiths PD, Oates CP, Gholkar A. The role of duplex sonography and angiography in the investigation of carotid artery disease. *Neuroradiology* 1997;39:122–126.
218. Huston J, Nichols DA, Luetmer PH, et al. MR angiographic and sonographic indications for endarterectomy. *Am J Neuroradiol* 1998;19: 309–315.
219. Atlas SW. MR angiography in neurologic disease. *Radiology* 1994;193:1–16.
220. Moneta GL, Edwards JM, Chitwood RW, et al. Correlation of North American Symptomatic Carotid Endarterectomy Trial (NASCET) angiographic definition of 70% to 99% internal carotid artery stenosis with duplex scanning. *J Vasc Surg* 1993;17:152–157.
221. Kuntz KM, Skillman JJ, Whittemore AD, Kent KC. Carotid endarterectomy in asymptomatic patients—is contrast angiography necessary? A morbidity analysis. *J Vasc Surg* 1995;22:706–714.
222. Lewis RF, Abrahamowicz M, Cote R, Battista RN. Predictive power of duplex ultrasonography in asymptomatic carotid disease. *Ann Intern Med* 1997;127:13–20.
223. Ogren M, Hedblad B, Isacsson SO, Janzon L, Jungquist G, Lindell SE. Non-invasively detected carotid stenosis and ischaemic heart disease in men with leg arteriosclerosis. *Lancet* 1993;342:1138–1141.
224. Vanninen R, Manninen H, Soimakallio S. Imaging of carotid artery stenosis: clinical efficacy and cost-effectiveness. *Am J Neuroradiol* 1995;16:1875–1883.
225. Wilterdink JL, Feldmann E, Easton JD, Ward R. Performance of carotid ultrasound in evaluating candidates for carotid endarterectomy is optimized by an approach based on clinical outcome rather than accuracy. *Stroke* 1996;27:1094–1098.
226. Olin JW, Fonseca C, Childs MB, Piedmonte MR, Hertzer NR, Young JR. The natural history of asymptomatic moderate internal carotid artery stenosis by duplex ultrasound. *Vasc Med* 1998; 3:101–108.
227. Kent KC, Kuntz KM, Patel MR, et al. Perioperative imaging strategies for carotid endarterectomy. An analysis of morbidity and cost-effectiveness in symptomatic patients. *JAMA* 1995;274:888–893.
228. Adams HP, Jr., Bendixen BH, Leira EC, et al. Antithrombotic treatment of ischemic Stroke among patients with occlusion or severe stenosis of the internal carotid artery. *Neurology* 1999;53:122–125.
229. Guzman RP. Appropriate imaging before carotid endarterectomy. *Can J Surg* 1998;41:218–223.
230. Saouaf R, Grassi CJ, Hartnell GG, Wheeler H, Suojanen JN. Complete MR angiography and Doppler ultrasound as the sole imaging modalities prior to carotid endarterectomy. *Clin Radiol* 1998;53:579–586.
231. Collier PE. Changing trends in the use of preoperative carotid arteriography: the community experience. *Cardiovasc Surg* 1998;6:485–489.
232. Barnett HJM, Eliasziw M, Meldrum HE. The identification by imaging methods of patients who might benefit from carotid endarterectomy. *Arch Neurol* 1995;52:827–831.
233. Bain DJ, Fergie N, Quin RO, Greene M. Role of arteriography in the selection of patients for carotid endarterectomy. *Br J Surg* 1998;85: 768–770.
234. Eliasziw M, Rankin RN, Fox AJ, Haynes RB, Barnett HJM. Accuracy and prognostic consequences of ultrasonography in identifying severe carotid artery stenosis. North American Symptomatic Carotid Endarterectomy Trial (NASCET) Group. *Stroke* 1995;26:1747–1752.
235. Markus HS, Ackerstaff R, Babikian V, et al. Intercenter agreement in reading Doppler embolic signals. A multicenter international study. *Stroke* 1997;28:1307–1310.
236. Howard G, Baker WH, Chambless LE, Howard VJ, Jones AM, Toole JF. An approach for the use of Doppler ultrasound as a screening tool for hemodynamically significant stenosis (despite heterogeneity of Doppler performance). A multicenter experience. Asymptomatic Carotid Atherosclerosis Study Investigators. *Stroke* 1996;27:1951–1957.
237. Sellar RJ. Imaging blood vessels of the head and neck. *J Neurol Neurosurg Psychiatry* 1995;59: 225–237.
238. Kimura K, Yasaka M, Moriyasu H, Tsuchiya T, Yamaguchi T. Ultrasonographic evaluation of vertebral artery to detect vertebrobasilar axis occlusion. *Stroke* 1994;25:1006–1009.
239. Auer A, Felber S, Schmidauer C, Waldenberger P, Aichner F. Magnetic resonance angiographic and clinical features of extracranial vertebral artery dissection. *J Neurol Neurosurg Psychiatry* 1998;64:474–481.

240. Hoffmann M, Sacco RL, Chan S, Mohr JP. Noninvasive detection of vertebral artery dissection. *Stroke* 1993;24:815–819.
241. Sun Y, Yip PK, Jeng JS, Hwang BS, Lin WH. Ultrasonographic study and long-term follow-up of Takayasu's arteritis. *Stroke* 1996;27:2178–2182.
242. Hennerici M, Rautenberg W, Schwartz A. Transcranial Doppler ultrasound for the assessment of intracranial arterial flow velocity—Part 2. Evaluation of intracranial arterial disease. *Surg Neurol* 1987;27:523–532.
243. Klotzsch C, Kuhne D, Berlit P. Diagnosis of giant fusiform basilar aneurysm by color-coded transcranial duplex sonography. *Cerebrovasc Dis* 1994;4:371–372.
244. Rother J, Schwartz A, Wentz KU, Rautenberg W, Hennerici M. Middle Cerebral Artery Stenoses: Assessment by Magnetic Resonance Angiography and Transcranial Doppler Ultrasound. *Cerebrovasc Dis* 1994;4:273–279.
245. Stolz E, Kaps M, Kern A, Dorndorf W. Frontal bone windows for transcranial color-coded duplex sonography. *Stroke* 1999;30:814–820.
246. Chimowitz MI, Furlan AJ, Jones SC, et al. Transcranial Doppler assessment of cerebral perfusion reserve in patients with carotid occlusive disease and no evidence of cerebral infarction. *Neurology* 1993;43:353–357.
247. Baumgartner RW, Mattle HP, Schroth G. Assessment of ≥ 50% and ≤ 50% intracranial stenoses by transcranial color-coded duplex sonography. *Stroke* 1999;30:87–92.
248. Gerriets T, Seidel G, Fiss I, Modrau B, Kaps M. Contrast-enhanced transcranial color-coded duplex sonography. *Neurology* 1999;52:1133–1137.
249. Kenton AR, Martin PJ, Abbott RJ, Moody AR. Comparison of transcranial color-coded sonography and magnetic resonance angiography in acute stroke. *Stroke* 1997;28:1601–1606.
250. Seidel G, Kaps M, Gerriets T. Potential and limitations of transcranial color-coded sonography in Stroke patients. *Stroke* 1995;26:2061–2066.
251. Posert T, Braun B, Meves S, et al. Cost-enhanced transcranial color-coded sonography in acute hemispheric brain infarction. *Stroke* 1999;30:1819–1826.
252. Muller M, Hermes M, Bruckmann H, Schimrigk K. Transcranial Doppler ultrasound in the evaluation of collateral blood flow in patients with internal carotid artery occlusion: correlation with cerebral angiography. *Am J Neuroradiol* 1995;16:195–202.
253. Goertler M, Kross R, Baeumer M, et al. Diagnostic impact and prognostic relevance of early contrast-enhanced transcranial color-coded duplex sonography in acute stroke. *Stroke* 1998;29:955–962.
254. Anzola GP, Gasparotti R, Magoni M, Prandini F. Transcranial Doppler sonography and magnetic resonance angiography in the assessment of collateral hemispheric flow in patients with carotid artery disease. *Stroke* 1995;26:214–217.
255. Vernieri F, Pasqualetti P, Passarelli F, Rossini PM, Silvestrini M. Outcome of carotid artery occlusion is predicted by cerebrovascular reactivity. *Stroke* 1999;30:593–598.
256. Alexandrov AV, Demchuk AM, Wein TH, Grotta JC. Yield of transcranial Doppler in acute cerebral ischemia. *Stroke* 1999;30:1604–1609.
257. Adams RJ, McKie VC, Nichols FT, et al. The use of transcranial untrasonography to predict stroke in sickle cell disease. *N Engl J Med* 1992;326:605–610.
258. Seibert JJ, Miller SF, Kirby RS, et al. Cerebrovascular disease in symptomatic and asymptomatic patients with sickle cell anemia: screening with duplex transcranial Doppler US—correlation with MR imaging and MR angiography. *Radiology* 1993;189:457–466.
259. Csepany T, Valikovics A, Fulesdi B, Kiss E, Szegedi G, Csiba L. Transcranial Doppler may reveal asymptomatic cerebral vasculopathy in systemic lupus erythematosus. *Cerebrovasc Dis* 1995;5:178–181.
260. Laborde G, Harders A, Klimek L, Hardenack M. Correlation between clinical, angiographic and transcranial Doppler sonographic findings in patients with moyamoya disease. *Neurol Res* 1993;15:87–92.
261. Mayberg MR, Batjer HH, Dacey R, et al. Guidelines for the management of aneurysmal subarachnoid hemorrhage. A statement for healthcare professionals from a special writing group of the Stroke Council, American Heart Association. *Stroke* 1994;25:2315–2328.
262. Silvestrini M, Troisi E, Matteis M, Cupini LM, Caltagirone C. Transcranial Doppler assessment of cerebrovascular reactivity in symptomatic and asymptomatic severe carotid stenosis. *Stroke* 1996;27:1970–1973.
263. Cullinane M, Wainwright R, Brown A, Monaghan M, Markus HS. Asymptomatic embolization in subjects with atrial fibrillation not taking anticoagulants: a prospective study. *Stroke* 1998;29:1810–1815.
264. Daffertshofer M, Ries S, Schminke U, Hennerici M. High-intensity transient signals in patients with cerebral ischemia. *Stroke* 1996;27:1844–1849.
265. Georgiadis D, Grosset DG, Kelman A, Faichney A, Lees KR. Prevalence and characteristics of intracranial microemboli signals in patients with different types of prosthetic cardiac valves. *Stroke* 1994;25:587–592.
266. Otis S, Rush M, Boyajian R. Contrast-enhanced transcranial imaging. Results of an American phase-two study. *Stroke* 1995;26:203–209.
267. Young GR, Humphrey PR, Shaw MD, Nixon TE, Smith ET. Comparison of magnetic resonance angiography, duplex ultrasound, and digital subtraction angiography in assessment of extracranial internal carotid artery stenosis. *J Neurol Neurosurg Psychiatry* 1994;57:1466–1478.
268. Devuyst G, Despland PA, Bogousslavsky J, Jeanrenaud X. Complementarity of contrast transcranial Doppler and contrast transesophageal echocardiography for the detection of patent foramen ovale in stroke patients. *Eur Neurol* 1997;38:21–25.
269. Koennecke HC, Trocio SH, Jr., Mast H, Mohr JP. Microemboli on transcranial Doppler in patients

with spontaneous carotid artery dissection. *J Neuroimaging* 1997;7:217–220.

270. Koennecke HC, Mast H, Trocio SH, Jr., et al. Frequency and determinants of microembolic signals on transcranial Doppler in unselected patients with acute carotid territory ischemia. A prospective study. *Cerebrovasc Dis* 1998;8:107–112.
271. Grosset DG, Georgiadis D, Abdullah I, Bone I, Lees KR. Doppler emboli signals vary according to stroke subtype. *Stroke* 1994;25:382–384.
272. Koennecke HC, Mast H, Trocio SS, Jr., Sacco RL, Thompson JL, Mohr JP. Microemboli in patients with vertebrobasilar ischemia: association with vertebrobasilar and cardiac lesions. *Stroke* 1997;28:593–596.
273. Gaunt ME. Transcranial Doppler: preventing stroke during carotid endarterectomy. *Annals of the Royal College of Surgeons of England* 1998;80: 377–387.
274. Stendel R, Hupp T, al Hassan AA, Brock M. The use of direct intra-operative Doppler ultrasonography in carotid thromboendarteriectomy. A prospective study. *Acta Neurochir* 1998;140: 925–931.
275. Cao P, Giordano G, Zannetti S, et al. Transcranial Doppler monitoring during carotid endarterectomy: is it appropriate for selecting patients in need of a shunt? *J Vasc Surg* 1997;26:973–979.
276. Comerota AJ, Katz ML, Hosking JD, Hashemi HA, Kerr RP, Carter AP. Is transcranial Doppler a worthwhile addition to screening tests for cerebrovascular disease? *J Vasc Surg* 1995;21:90–95.
277. Maurer M, Mullges W, Becker G. Diagnosis of MCA–occlusion and monitoring of systemic thrombolytic therapy with contrast enhanced transcranial duplex-sonography. *J Neuroimaging* 1999;9:99–101.
278. Fellner C, Strotzer M, Fraunhofer S, et al. MR angiography of the supra-aortic arteries using a dedicated head and neck coil: image quality and assessment of stenoses. *Neuroradiology* 1997; 39:763–771.
279. Yucel EK, Anderson CM, Edelman RR, et al. Magnetic resonance angiography. Update on applications for extracranial arteries. *Circulation* 1999;100:2284–2301.
280. Graves MJ. Magnetic resonance angiography. *Br J Radiol* 1997;70:6–28.
281. Oelerich M, Lentschig MG, Zunker P, Reimer P, Rummeny EJ, Schuierer. Intracranial vascular stenosis and occlusion: comparison of 3D time-of-flight and 3D phase-contrast MR angiography. *Neuroradiology* 1998;40:567–573.
282. Fujita N, Hirabuki N, Fujii K, et al. MR imaging of middle cerebral artery stenosis and occlusion: value of MR angiography. *Am J Neuroradiol* 1994;15:335–341.
283. Siewert B, Wielopolski PA, Schlaug G, Edelman RR, Warach S. STAR MR angiography for rapid detection of vascular abnormalities in patients with acute cerebrovascular disease. *Stroke* 1997;28:1211–1215.
284. Scarabino T, Carriero A, Magarelli N, et al. MR angiography in carotid stenosis: a comparison of three techniques. *Eur J Radiol* 1998;28:117–125.
285. Kallmes DF, Omary RA, Dix JE, Evans AJ, Hillman BJ. Specificity of MR angiography as a confirmatory test of carotid artery stenosis. *Am J Neuroradiol* 1996;17:1501–1506.
286. Enochs WS, Ackerman RH, Kaufman JA, Candia M. Gadolinium-enhanced MR angiography of the carotid arteries. *J Neuroimaging* 1998;8:185–190.
287. Tsuruda J, Saloner D, Norman D. Artifacts associated with MR neuroangiography. *Am J Neuroradiol* 1992;13:1411–1422.
288. Johnson BA, Heiserman JE, Drayer BP, Keller PJ. Intracranial MR angiography: its role in the integrated approach to brain infarction. *Am J Neuroradiol* 1994;15:901–908.
289. Barber PA, Davis SM, Darby DG, et al. Absent middle cerebral artery flow predicts the presence and evolution of the ischemic penumbra. *Neurology* 1999;52:1125–1132.
290. Remonda L, Heid O, Schroth G. Carotid artery stenosis, occlusion, and pseudo-occlusion: first-pass, gadolinium-enhanced, three-dimensional MR angiography—preliminary study. *Radiology* 1998;209:95–102.
291. Korogi Y, Takahashi M, Mabuchi N, et al. Intracranial vascular stenosis and occlusion: diagnostic accuracy of three-dimensional, Fourier transform, time-of-flight MR angiography. *Radiology* 1994;193:187–193.
292. Wentz KU, Rother J, Schwartz A, Mattle HP, Suchalla R, Edelman RR. Intracranial vertebrobasilar system: MR angiography. *Radiology* 1994;190:105–110.
293. Rother J, Wentz KU, Rautenberg W, Schwartz A, Hennerici M. Magnetic resonance angiography in vertebrobasilar ischemia. *Stroke* 1993;24: 1310–1315.
294. Kodama T, Ueda T, Suzuki Y, Yano T, Watanabe K. MRA in the evaluation of EC-IC bypass patency. *J Comput Assist Tomogr* 1993;17:922–926.
295. Barboriak DP, Provenzale JM. MR arteriography of intracranial circulation. AM *J Roentgenol.* 1998; 171:1469–1478.
296. Rother J, Schwartz A, Rautenberg W, Hennerici M. Magnetic resonance angiography of spontaneous vertebral artery dissection suspected on Doppler ultrasonography. *J Neurol* 1995;242: 430–436.
297. Zuber M, Meary E, Meder JF, Mas JL. Magnetic resonance imaging and dynamic CT scan in cervical artery dissections. *Stroke* 1994;25:576–581.
298. Kasner SE, Hankins LL, Bratina P, Morgenstern LB. Magnetic resonance angiography demonstrates vascular healing of carotid and vertebral artery dissections. *Stroke* 1997;28:1993–1997.
299. Laster REJ, Acker JD, Halford HH, Nauert TC. Assessment of MR angiography versus arteriography for evaluation of cervical carotid bifurcation disease. *Am J Neuroradiol* 1993;14:681–688.
300. Magarelli N, Scarabino T, Simeone AL, et al. Carotid stenosis: a comparison between MR and spiral CT angiography. *Neuroradiology* 1998;40: 367–373.
301. Huston J, Lewis BD, Wiebers DO, Meyer FB, Riederer SJ, Weaver AL. Carotid artery: prospective blinded comparison of two-dimensional

time-of-flight MR angiography with conventional angiography and duplex US. *Radiology* 1993;186:339–344.
302. van Putten MJ, Bloem BR, Smit VT, Aarts NJ, Lammers GJ. An uncommon cause of stroke in young adults. *Arch Neurol* 1999;56:1018–1020.
303. Shrier DA, Tanaka H, Numaguchi Y, Konno S, Patel U, Shibata D. CT angiography in the evaluation of acute stroke. *Am J Neuroradiol* 1997;18:1011–1020.
304. Wildermuth S, Knauth M, Brandt T, Winter R, Sartor K, Hacke W. Role of CT angiography in patient selection for thrombolytic therapy in acute hemispheric stroke. *Stroke* 1998;29: 935–938.
305. Leclerc X, Godefroy O, Pruvo JP, Leys D. Computed tomographic angiography for the evaluation of carotid artery stenosis. *Stroke* 1995;26:1577–1581.
306. Link J, Brossmann J, Grabener M, et al. Spiral CT angiography and selective digital subtraction angiography of internal carotid artery stenosis. *Am J Neuroradiol* 1996;17:89–94.
307. Bluemke DA, Chambers TP. Spiral CT angiography: an alternative to conventional angiography. *Radiology* 1995;195:317–319.
308. Lubezky N, Fajer S, Barmeir E, Karmeli R. Duplex scanning and CT angiography in the diagnosis of carotid artery occlusion: a prospective study. *Eur J Vasc Endovasc Surg* 1998;16:133–136.
309. Brandt T, Knauth M, Wildermuth S, et al. CT angiography and Doppler sonography for emergency assessment in acute basilar artery ischemia. *Stroke* 999;30:606–612.
310. Vandenberg B, Biller J. Cardiac evaulation of the patient with stroke. *Cerebrovasc Dis* 1991;1(Suppl 1):73–82.
311. Oppenheimer SM, Hachinski VC. The cardiac consequences of stroke. *Neurol Clin* 1992;10: 167–176.
312. Chua HC, Sen S, Cosgriff RF, Gerstenblith G, Beauchamp NJ, Jr., Oppenheimer SM. Neurogenic ST depression in stroke. *Clin Neurol Neurosurg* 1999;101:44–48.
313. Kolin A, Norris JW. Myocardial damage from acute cerebral lesions. *Stroke* 1984;15:990–993.
314. McDermott MM, Lefevre F, Arron M, Martin GJ, Biller J. ST segment depression detected by continuous electrocardiography in patients with acute ischemic stroke or transient ischemic attack. *Stroke* 1994;25:1820–1824.
315. Britton M, de Faire U, Helmers C, Miah K, Ryding C, Wester PO. Arrhythmias in patients with acute cerebrovascular disease. *Acta Med Scand* 1979;205:425–428.
316. Myers MG, Norris JW, Hachinski VC, Weingert ME, Sole MJ. Cardiac sequelae of acute stroke. *Stroke* 1982;13:838–842.
317. Oppenheimer SM. Neurogenic cardiac effects of cerebrovascular disease. Curr Opin *Neurol* 1994; 7:20–24.
318. Korpelainen JT, Sotaniemi KA, Huikuri HV, Myllya VV. Abnormal heart rate variability as a manifestation of autonomic dysfunction in hemispheric brain infarction. *Stroke* 1996;27: 2059–2063.
319. Lane RD, Wallace JD, Petrosky PP, Schwartz GE, Gradman AH. Supraventricular tachycardia in patients with right hemisphere strokes. *Stroke* 1992;23:362–366.
320. Svigelj V, Grad A, Tekavcic I, Kiauta T. Cardiac arrhythmia associated with reversible damage to insula in a patients with subarachnoid hemorrhage. *Stroke* 1994;25:1053–1055.
321. Rem JA, Hachinski VC, Boughner DR, Barnett HJM. Value of cardiac monitoring and echocardiography in TIA and stroke patients. *Stroke* 1985;16:950–956.
322. Bell C, Kapral M. Use of ambulatory electrocardiography for the detection of paroxysmal atrial fibrillation in patients with stroke. *Can J Neurol Sci* 2000;27:25–31.
323. Koudstaal PJ, van Gijn J, Klootwijk AP, van der Meche FG, Kappelle LJ. Holter monitoring in patients with transient and focal ischemic attacks of the brain. *Stroke* 1986;17:192–195.
324. Chimowitz MI, Mancini GB. Asymptomatic coronary artery disease in patients with stroke. Prevalence, prognosis, diagnosis, and treatment. *Stroke* 1992;23:433–436.
325. Bellersen L, Koudstaal PJ, Algra A, Tijssen JGP, Roelandt JRTC. Risk factors for cardiac death in patients with a transcient ischemic attack of ischemic stroke. *Cerebrovasc Dis* 1993;3:146–153.
326. Heyman A, Wilkinson WE, Hurwitz BJ, et al. Risk of ischemic heart disease in patients with TIA. *Neurology* 1984;34:626–630.
327. Chimowitz MI, Poole RM, Starling MR, Schwaiger M, Gross MD. Frequency and severity of asymptomatic coronary disease in patients with different causes of stroke. *Stroke* 1997;28: 941–945.
328. Estes JM, Guadagnoli E, Wolf R, LoGerfo FW, Whittemore AD. The impact of cardiac comorbidity after carotid endarterectomy. *J Vasc Surg* 1998;28:577–584.
329. Rihal CS, Gersh BJ, Whisnant JP, et al. Influence of coronary heart disease on morbidity and mortality after carotid endarterectomy: a population–based study in Olmsted County, Minnesota (1970–1988). *J Am Coll Cardiol* 1992;19: 1254–1260.
330. Hertzer NR, Young JR, Beven EG, et al. Coronary angiography in 506 patients with extracranial cerebrovascular disease. *Arch Intern Med* 1985;145:849–852.
331. Garber AM, Solomon NA. Cost-effectiveness of alternative test strategies for the diagnosis of coronary artery disease. *Ann Intern Med* 1999;130:719–728.
332. Urbinati S, Di Pasquale G, Andreoli A, et al. Heart-brain interactions in cerebral ischaemia: a non–invasive cardiologic study protocol. *Neurol Res* 1992;14:112–117.
333. Macko RF, DeSouza CA, Tretter LD, et al. Treadmill aerobic exercise training reduces the energy expenditure and cardiovascular demands of hemiparetic gait in chronic stroke patients. A preliminary report. *Stroke* 1997;28: 326–330.
334. Elhendy A, van Domburg RT, Bax JJ, Roelandt JR. Relation between the extent of coronary

artery disease and tachyarrhythmias during dobutamine stress echocardiography. *Am J Cardio* 1999;83:832–835.

335. Gross MF, Friedman MH. Dynamics of coronary artery curvature obtained from biplane cineangiograms. *J Biomechanics* 1998;31:479–484.
336. Urbinati S, Di Pasquale G, Andreoli A, et al. Role and indication of two-dimensional echocardiography in young adults with cerebral ishcemia: a prospective study in 125 patients. *Cerebrovasc Dis* 1992;2:14–21.
337. Bikkina M, Levy D, Evans JC, et al. Left ventricular mass and risk of stroke in an elderly cohort. *JAMA* 1994;272:33–36.
338. Atrial Fibrillation Investigators. Echocardiographic predictors of stroke in patients with atrial fibrillation: a prospective study of 1066 patients from 3 clinical trials. *Arch Intern Med* 1998;158:1316–1320.
339. Sansoy V, Abbott RD, Jayaweera AR, Kaul S. Low yield of transthoracic echocardiography for cardiac source of embolism. *Am J Cardiol* 1995;75:166–169.
340. Biller J, Johnson MR, Adams HP, Jr., Kerber RE, Toffol GJ, Butler MJ. Echocardiographic evaluation of young adults with nonhemorrhagic cerebral infarction. *Stroke* 1986;17:608–612.
341. Asinger RW, Mikell FL, Elsperger J, Hodges M. Incidence of left-ventricular thrombosis after acute transmural myocardial infarction. Serial evaluation by two-dimensional echocardiography. *N Engl J Med* 1981;305:297–302.
342. Hart RG. Cardiogenic embolism to the brain. *Lancet* 1992;339:589–594.
343. Beattie JR, Cohen DJ, Manning WJ, Douglas PS. Role of routine transthoracic echocardiography in evaluation and management of stroke. *J Intern Med* 1998;243:281–291.
344. Donaldson RM, Emanuel RW, Earl CJ. The role of two-dimensional echocardiography in the detection of potentially embolic intracardiac masses in patients with cerebral ischaemia. *J Neurol Neurosurg Psychiatry* 1981;44:803–809.
345. Cohen A, Chauvel C. Transesophageal echocardiography in the management of transient ischemic attack and ischemic stroke. *Cerebrovasc Dis* 1996;6(Suppl 1):15–25.
346. Censori B, Colombo F, Valsecchi MG, et al. Early transoesophageal echocardiography in cryptogenic and lacunar stroke and transient ischaemic attack. *J Neurol Neurosurg Psychiatry* 1998;64: 624–627.
347. Husain AM, Alter M. Transesophageal echocardiography in diagnosing cardioembolic stroke. *Clinical Cardiology* 1995;18:705–708.
348. Mendel T, Pasierski T, Szwed H, Baranska-Gieruszczak M, Czlonkowska A. Transesophageal echocardiographic findings in patients with anterior and posterior circulation infarcts. *Acta Neurol Scand* 1998;97:63–67.
349. DeRook FA, Comess KA, Albers GW, Popp RL. Transesophageal echocardiography in the evaluation of stroke. *Ann Intern Med* 1992;117: 922–932.
350. Autore C, Cartoni D, Piccininno M. Multiplane transesophageal echocardiography and stroke. *Am J Cardio* 1998;81:79G–81G.
351. Daniel WG, Erbel R, Kasper W, et al. Safety of transesophageal echocardiography. A multicenter survey of 10,419 examinations. *Circulation* 1991;83:817–821.
352. Comess KA, DeRook FA, Beach KW, Lytle NJ, Golby AJ, Albers GW. Transesophageal echocardiography and carotid ultrasound in patients with cerebral ischemia: prevalence of findings and recurrent stroke risk. *J Am Coll Cardiol* 1994;23:1598–1603.
353. Warner MF, Momah KI. Routine transesophageal echocardiography for cerebral ischemia. Is it really necessary? *Arch Intern Med* 1996;156:1719–1723.
354. Jones EF, Donnan GA, Calafiore P, Tonkin AM. Transoesophageal echocardiography in the investigation of stroke: experience in 135 patients with cerebral ischaemic events. *Aust N Z J Med* 1993;23:477–483.
355. Leung DY, Black IW, Cranney GB, et al. Selection of patients for transesophageal echocardiography after Stroke and systemic embolic events. Role of transthoracic echocardiography. *Stroke* 1995;26:1820–1824.
356. Rauh R, Fischereder M, Spengel FA. Transesophageal echocardiography in patients with focal cerebral ischemia of unknown cause. *Stroke* 1996;27:691–694.
357. Tegeler CH, Downes TR. Cardiac imaging in stroke. *Stroke* 1991;22:1206–1211.
358. Meissner I, Whisnant J, Khandheria BK, et al. Prevalence of potential risk factors for stroke assessed by transesophageal echocardiography and carotid ultrasonography: the SPARC Study. *Mayo Clin Proc* 1999;74:862–869.
359. O'Brien PJ, Thiemann DR, McNamara RL, et al. Usefulness of transesophageal echocardiography in predicting mortality and morbidity in stroke patients without clinically known cardiac sources of embolus. *Am J Cardio* 1998;81:1144–1151.
360. Roijer A, Lindgren A, Algotsson L, Norrving B, Olsson B, Eskilsson J. Cardiac changes in stroke patients and controls evaluated with transoesophageal echocardiography. *Scand Cardiovasc J* 1997;31:329–337.
361. Roijer A, Lindgren A, Rudling O, et al. Potential cardioembolic sources in an elderly population without stroke. A transthoracic and transoesophageal echocardiographic study in randomly selected volunteers. *Eur Heart J* 1996;17: 1103–1111.
362. Albers GW, Comess KA, DeRook FA, et al. Transesophageal echocardiographic findings in stroke subtypes. *Stroke* 1994;25:23–28.
363. Black IW, Hopkins AP, Lee LC, Jacobson BM, Walsh WF. Role of transoesophageal echocardiography in evaluation of cardiogenic embolism. *Br Heart J* 1991;66:302–307.
364. Grullon C, Alam M, Rosman HS, et al. Transesophageal echocardiography in unselected patients with focal cerebral ischemia: when is it useful? *Cerebrovasc Dis* 1994;4:139–145.
365. Manning WJ, Weintraub RM, Waksmonski CA, et al. Accuracy of transesophageal echocardiography for identifying left atrial thrombi. A prospective, intraoperative study. *Ann Intern Med* 1995;123:817–822.

366. Lopez JA, Fishbein MC, Siegel RJ. Echocardiographic features of nonbacterial thrombotic endocarditis. *Am J Cardio* 1987;59:478–480.
367. Benjamin EJ, D'Agostino RB, Belanger AJ, Wolf PA, Levy D. Left atrial size and the risk of stroke and death. *Circulation* 1995;92:835–841.
368. Kamalesh M, Copeland TB, Sawada S. Severely reduced left atrial appendage function: a cause of embolic stroke in patients in sinus rhythm? *J Am Soc Echocardiogr* 1998;11:902–904.
369. Zabalgoitia M, Halperin JL, Pearce LA, Blackshear JL, Asinger RW, Hart RG. Transesophageal echocardiographic correlates of clinical risk of thromboembolism in nonvalvular atrial fibrillation. Stroke Prevention in Atrial Fibrillation III Investigators. *J Am Coll Cardiol* 1998;31:1622–1626.
370. Stollberger C, Chnupa P, Kronik G, et al. Transesophageal echocardiography to assess embolic risk in patients with atrial fibrillation. ELAT Study Group. Embolism in left atrial thrombi. *Ann Intern Med* 1998;128:630–638.
371. Di Pasquale G, Urbinati S, Pinelli G. New echocardiographic markers of embolic rsik in atrial fibrillation. *Cerebrovasc Dis* 1995;5: 315–322.
372. Brickner ME, Friedman DB, Cigarroa CG, Grayburn PA. Relation of thrombus in the left atrial appendage by transesophageal echocardiography to clinical risk factors for thrombus formation. *Am J Cardio* 1994;74:391–393.
373. Gersh BJ, Gottdiener JS. Shadows on the cave wall: the role of transesophageal echocardiography in atrial fibrillation. *Ann Intern Med* 1995;123:882–884.
374. Panagiotopoulos K, Toumanidis S, Saridakis N, Vemmos K, Moulopoulos S. Left atrial and left atrial appendage functional abnormalities in patients with cardioembolic stroke in sinus rhythm and idiopathic atrial fibrillation. *J Am Soc Echocardiogr* 1998;11:711–719.
375. Jones EF, Calafiore P, McNeil JJ, Tonkin AM, Donnan GA. Atrial fibrillation with left atrial spontaneous contrast detected by transesophageal echocardiography is a potent risk factor for stroke. *Am J Cardiol* 1996;78:425–429.
376. Chimowitz MI, DeGeorgia MA, Poole RM, Hepner A, Armstrong WM. Left atrial spontaneous echo contrast is highly associated with previous stroke in patients with atrial fibrillation or mitral stenosis. *Stroke* 1993;24:1015–1019.
377. The Stroke Prevention in Atrial Fibrillation Investigators Committee on Echocardiography. Transesophageal echocardiographic correlates of thromboembolism in high-risk patients with nonvalvular atrial fibrillation. *Ann Intern Med* 1998;128:639–647.
378. Briley DP, Giraud GD, Beamer NB, et al. Spontaneous echo contrast and hemorheologic abnormalities in cerebrovascular disease. *Stroke* 1994;25:1564–1569.
379. Manning WJ, Douglas PS. Transesophageal echocardiography and atrial fibrillation: added value or expensive toy? *Ann Intern Med* 1998;128:685–687.
380. Stoddard MF, Dawkins PR, Prince CR, Ammash NM. Left atrial appendage thrombus is not uncommon in patients with acute atrial fibrillation and a recent embolic event: a transesophageal echocardiographic study. *J Am Coll Cardiol* 1995;25:452–459.
381. Hata JS, Ayres RW, Biller J, et al. Impact of transesophageal echocardiography on the anticoagulation management of patients admitted with focal cerebral ischemia. *Am J Cardiol* 1993;72:707–710.
382. McNamara RL, Lima JA, Whelton PK, Powe NR. Echocardiographic identification of cardiovascular sources of emboli to guide clinical management of stroke: a cost-effectiveness analysis. *Ann Intern Med* 1997;127:775–787.
383. Klein AL, Grimm RA, Black IW, et al. Cardio-version guided by transesophageal echocardiography: the ACUTE Pilot Study. A randomized, controlled trial. Assessment of Cardioversion Using Transesophageal Echocardiography. *Ann Intern Med* 1997;126:200–209.
384. Huber M, Curtius JM, Hojer C, Vogelsberg H. Transesophageal echocardiography does not improve clinical risk estimation in recurrent embolic stroke. *Cerebrovasc Dis* 1994;4:38–43.
385. Orsinelli DA, Pearson AC. Detection of prosthetic valve strands by transesophageal echocardiography: clinical significance in patients with suspected cardiac source of embolism. *J Am Coll Cardiol* 1995;26:1713–1718.
386. Freedberg RS, Goodkin GM, Perez JL, Tunick PA, Kronzon I. Valve strands are strongly associated with systemic embolization: a transesophageal echocardiographic study. *J Am Coll Cardiol* 1995;26:1709–1712.
387. Roberts JK, Omarali I, Di Tullio MR, Sciacca RR, Sacco RL, Homma S. Valvular strands and cerebral ischemia. Effect of demographics and strand characteristics. *Stroke* 1997;28: 2185–2188.
388. Tanus-Santos JE, Moreno JH. Pulmonary embolism and impending paradoxical embolism: a role for transesophageal echocardiography? *Clin Cardiol* 1999;22:158–159.
389. Schneider B, Zienkiewicz T, Jansen V, Hofmann T, Noltenius H, Meinertz T. Diagnosis of patent foramen ovale by transesophageal echocardiography and correlation with autopsy findings. *Am J Cardiol* 1996;77:1202–1209.
390. Klotzsch C, Janssen G, Berlit P. Transesophageal echocardiography and contrast-TCD in the detection of a patent foramen ovale: experiences with 111 patients. *Neurology* 1994;44:1603–1606.
391. Hausmann D, Mugge A, Becht I, Daniel WG. Diagnosis of patent foramen ovale by transesophageal echocardiography and association with cerebral and peripheral embolic events. *Am J Cardiol* 1992;70:668–672.
392. Serena J, Segura T, Perez-Ayuso MJ, Bassaganyas J, Molins A, Davalos. The need to quantify right-to-left shunt in acute ischemic stroke: a case-control study. *Stroke* 1998;29: 1322–1328.
393. Stone DA, Godard J, Corretti MC, et al. Patent foramen ovale: association between the degree of shunt by contrast transesophageal echocardiography and the risk of future ischemic neurologic events. *Am Heart J* 1996;131:158–161.

394. Toyoda K, Yasaka M, Nagata S, Yamaguchi T. Aortogenic embolic stroke: a transesophageal echocardiographic approach. *Stroke* 1992;23: 1056–1061.
395. Tunick PA, Kronzon I. Protruding atherosclerotic plaque in the aortic arch of patients with systemic embolization: a new finding seen by transesophageal echocardiography. *Am Heart J* 1990;120:658–660.
396. Marschall K, Kanchuger M, Kessler K, et al. Superiority of transesophageal echocardiography in detecting aortic arch atheromatous disease: identification of patients at increased risk of stroke during cardiac surgery. *J Cardiothorac Vasc Anesth* 1994;8:5–13.
397. Ribakove GH, Katz ES, Galloway AC, et al. Surgical implications of transesophageal echocardiography to grade the atheromatous aortic arch. *Ann Thorac Surg* 1992;53:758–761.
398. Choudhary SK, Bhan A, Sharma R, et al. Aortic atherosclerosis and perioperative stroke in patients undergoing coronary artery bypass: role of intra-operative transesophageal echocardiography. *International J Cardiol* 1997;61:31–38.
399. Tenenbaum A, Garniek A, Shemesh J, et al. Dual-helical CT for detecting aortic atheromas as a source of stroke: comparison with transesophageal echocardiography. *Radiology* 1998; 208:153–158.
400. Nakanishi T, Hamada S, Takamiya M, et al. A pitfall in ultrafast CT scanning for the detection of left atrial thrombi. *J Comput Assist Tomogr* 1993;17:42–45.
401. Love BB, Struck LK, Stanford W, Biller J, Kerber R, Marcus M. Comparison of two-dimensional echocardiography and ultrafast cardiac computed tomography for evaluating intracardiac thrombi in cerebral ischemia. *Stroke* 1990;21:1033–1038.
402. Drangova M, Zhu Y, Bowman B, Pelc NJ. In vitro verification of myocardial motion tracking from phase-contrast velocity data. *Magn Reson Imaging* 1998;16:863–870.
403. Exner T, Triplett DA, Taberner D, Machin SJ. Guidelines for testing and revised criteria for lupus anticoagulants. SSC Subcommittee for the Standardization of Lupus Anticoagulants. *Thromb Haemost* 1991;65:320–322.
404. Folsom AR, Wu KK, Shahar E, Davis CE. Association of hemostatic variables with prevalent cardiovascular disease and asymptomatic carotid artery atherosclerosis. The Atherosclerosis Risk in Communities (ARIC) Study Investigators. *Arterioscler Thromb* 1993;13: 1829–1836.
405. Ernst E, Resch KL. Fibrinogen as a cardiovascular risk factor: a meta-analysis and review of the literature. *Ann Intern Med* 1993;118:956–963.
406. Fon EA, Mackey A, Cote R, et al. Hemostatic markers in acute transient ischemic attacks. *Stroke* 1994;25:282–286.
407. Eby CS. A review of the hypercoagulable state. *Hematol Oncol Clin North Am* 1993;7:1121–1142.
408. D'Olhaberriague L, Levine SR, Salowich-Palm L, et al. Specificity, isotype, and titer distribution of anticardiolipin antibodies in CNS diseases. *Neurology* 1998;51:1376–1380.
409. Coull BM, Goodnight SH. Antiphospholipid antibodies, prethrombotic states, and stroke. *Stroke* 1990;21:1370–1374.
410. Muir KW, Weir CJ, Alwan W, Squire IB, Lees KR. C-reactive protein and outcome after ischemic stroke. *Stroke* 1999;30:981–985.
411. Bruno A, Biller J, Adams HP, Jr., et al. Acute blood glucose level and outcome from ischemic stroke. Trial of ORG 10172 in Acute Stroke Treatment (TOAST) Investigators. *Neurology* 1999;52:280–284.
412. Gold AE, Marshall SM. Cortical blindness and cerebral infarction associated with severe hypoglycemia. *Diabetes Care* 1996;19:1001–1003.
413. Parsons MW, Barber PA, Yang Q, et al. Combined 1H MR spectroscopy and diffusion-weighted MRI improves the prediction of stroke outcome. *Neurology* 2000;55:498–505.
414. Yamauchi H, Fukuyama H, Nagahama Y, et al. Significance of increased oxygen extraction fraction in five-year prognosis of major cerebral occlusive diseases. *J Nucl Med* 1999;40: 1992–1998.
415. Derdeyn CP, Videen TO, Simmons NR, et al. Count-based PET method for predicting ischemic stroke in patients with symptomatic carotid arterial occlusion. *Radiology* 1999;212: 499–506.

Chapter 5

ATHEROSCLEROTIC CEREBROVASCULAR DISEASE

Atherosclerosis is the leading cause of ischemic stroke in North America and most countries around the world.[1] It affects major intracranial and extracranial arteries and is a leading cause of occlusions of penetrating arteries that perfuse the deep portions of the brain. The most common locations for symptomatic cerebrovascular atherosclerosis are the origin of the internal carotid artery, the intracavernous portion of the internal carotid artery, the first segment of the middle cerebral artery, the origin of and the distal portion of the vertebral artery, and the mid portion of the basilar artery. Atherosclerosis also involves the aorta and major cervical arteries. The origin of the internal carotid artery is the most frequent site for severe atherosclerosis in persons of European ancestry, whereas intracranial arteries are more commonly affected among persons of African or Asian heritage.[2–4] Diabetic persons also have a high rate of intracranial atherosclerosis.

GENERAL FEATURES OF ATHEROSCLEROSIS

Atherosclerosis involves multiple arteries throughout the body, including the aorta, coronary arteries, arteries to other organs, and arteries to the lower limbs. Symptomatic atherosclerotic disease elsewhere in the body identifies a person as having a high risk for ischemic stroke. For example, persons with claudication in the lower limbs are known to have a propensity for stroke.[5] Atherosclerosis of the aorta and the major brachiocephalic arteries also is a potential direct cause for stroke. Atherosclerotic coronary artery disease indirectly leads to stroke through cerebral embolism as a complication of acute myocardial infarction. The risk is greatest among persons with anterior myocardial infarction. (See Chapter 6.) In general, coronary artery disease usually becomes symptomatic one decade before symptoms of cerebrovascular atherosclerosis develop. Thus, a sizeable proportion of patients with stroke have a past history of ischemic heart diseases. In addition to myocardial infarction, patients can have a history of angina pectoris, congestive heart failure, or cardiovascular procedures. Ischemic heart disease also is associated with atrial fibrillation, a well-established risk factor for stroke in the elderly. Long-standing ischemic heart disease leads to embolism to the brain from an intraventricular thrombus that develops on an akinetic segment or from a dilated cardiomyopathy. Stroke is also a leading complication of interventions to treat myocardial infarction or coronary artery disease. (See Chapter 6.) Conversely, atherosclerosis of the intracranial and extracranial arteries predicts symptomatic or asymptomatic coronary artery disease.[6] Severe atherosclerotic stenosis of the aorta and renal arteries can promote severe hypertension, which in turn causes cerebrovascular disease. Patients with a transient ischemic attack (TIA) or a stroke also have an increased risk of symptomatic peripheral artery disease or abdominal aortic aneurysm.

Course of Atherosclerosis

Atherosclerosis is a lifetime illness; it slowly evolves over many years.[7] (See Table 5–1.) Its course is accelerated by risk factors, including hypertension, diabetes mellitus, hyperlipidemia, and tobacco use, as discussed in Chapter 2. The cause of atherosclerosis is uncertain, but the course and maturation of the disease seem to be influenced by the elevated blood cholesterol, which accumulates in the endothelial cells of the arterial wall.[1] Endothelial injury from factors including mechanical shear stress, toxins, homocysteine, infections, or immunologic mediators also play a role.[1,8]

Pathologically, atherosclerotic lesions begin with an inflammatory reaction, smooth muscle proliferation, and thickening of the arterial wall (See Table 5–1). The first atherosclerotic change in the artery is called a *fatty streak*. It is characterized by the adhesion of monocytes to the endothelium and their migration to subendothelial portions of the arterial wall. In this location, they develop a foamy appearance micro-

Table 5–1. **Changes in Atherosclerotic Lesions**

Initial findings
Inflammatory infiltration
Smooth muscle proliferation
Thickening of the arterial wall
Subsequent stage—fatty streak
Inflammation
Accumulation of lipids
Formation of atherosclerotic plaque
Fibrous changes
Core of plaque
Cellular debris
Free lipids
Cholesterol crystals
Cap of plaque
Smooth muscle cells
Foam cells
Lymphocytes
Connective tissue
Complicated plaque
Stenosis of the lumen
Calcification of the plaque
Intraplaque hemorrhage
Ulceration of the plaque
Fracturing of the plaque
Thrombosis

scopically because they are accumulating lipids intracellularly.[9] Fatty streaks can be found in the aorta and the coronary arteries of adolescents and young adults. The most common locations for the development of fatty streaks are vascular bifurcations or other areas with turbulent blood flow. As a person ages, the fatty streak is transformed into a *fibrous plaque*. A plaque usually is found in middle-age or older adults. It consists of a *core* of cellular debris, free extracellular lipid, and cholesterol crystals covered by a *cap* that consists of foam cells, transformed smooth muscle cells, lymphocytes, and connective tissue.[9] The plaque grows insidiously over many years as a result of the elaboration of cytokines and factors released by endothelial cells, macrophages, platelets, and smooth muscle cells.[9] Areas of *calcification* or *hemorrhage* also can occur within the plaque.

A plaque gradually increases over years and slowly impinges on the vascular lumen and, as a result, blood flow becomes constricted [7] (See Table 5–1 and Fig. 5–1.) The narrowing leads to local turbulence of blood flow or sluggish perfusion. This turbulence and slow flow can activate platelets and clotting factors, which in turn promote thrombosis. An intra-plaque hemorrhage can cause sudden expansion of a plaque, leading to arterial occlusion.

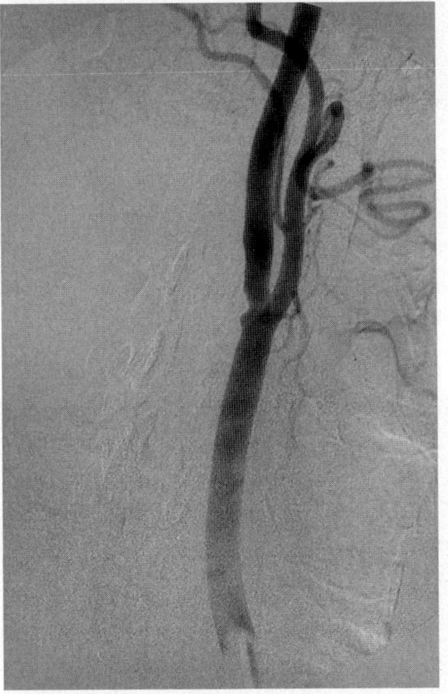

Figure 5–1. Lateral view of a carotid arteriogram using subtraction technique demonstrates a mildly ulcerated plaque at the origin of the internal carotid artery.

Fracturing of the Cap and Acute Thrombosis

Fracturing of the cap of the plaque disrupts the endothelial surface of the artery and leads to acute thrombosis (Table 5–2). Release of tissue factors promotes the development of a clot adjacent to the plaque.[10] Local occlusion and secondary artery-to-artery embolism can result.[11,12] Fracture of an atherosclerotic plaque now is perceived to be the leading cause of acute thrombosis of the coronary artery and myocardial infarction.[7,13,14] (See Fig. 5–2.) A similar scenario likely occurs with cerebrovascular atherosclerosis.[15] Carr et al[16] found that plaque rupture is common in patients having endarterectomy to treat symptomatic disease of the internal carotid

Table 5–2. **Causes of Ischemic Stroke Secondary to Intracranial or Extracranial Atherosclerosis**

Severe stenosis or occlusion
Hypoperfusion
Watershed (borderzone) infarctions
Steal syndromes
Fracturing of plaque
Acute arterial thrombosis and occlusion
Acute thrombosis with secondary distal embolism
Ulceration of plaque
Acute thrombosis with secondary distal embolism
Embolization of cholesterol debris

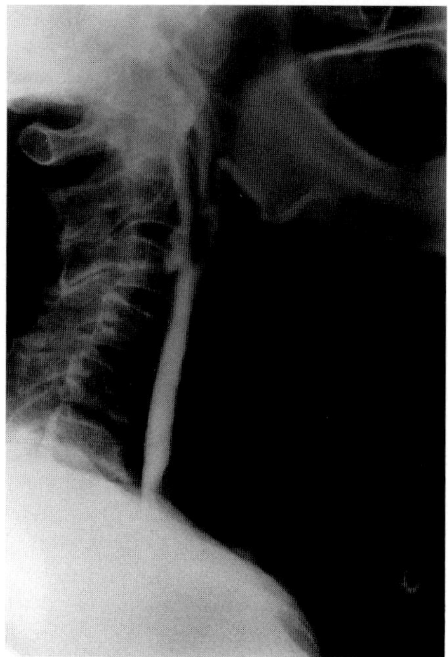

Figure 5–2. Deep ulcer in an atherosclerotic plaque located at the origin of the internal carotid artery.

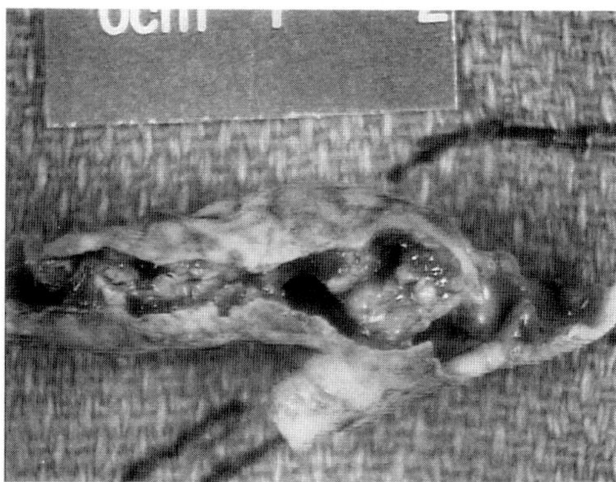

Figure 5–3. An advanced atherosclerotic plaque at the origin of the internal carotid artery removed at the carotid endarterectomy. The plaque shows multiple areas of ulceration and intraplaque hemorrhage. (Courtesy of Patrick Hitchon, MD, University of Iowa, Iowa City.)

artery. Patients with irregular plaques of the internal carotid artery are likely to have an increased risk of myocardial infarction and vascular death.[17] Plaque instability can be due to factors such as infections, autoimmunity, or genetic predisposition, and these conditions may be separate from the traditional risk factors for accelerated atherosclerosis.[17]

Ulceration of the surface of the plaque can be the source of atherosclerotic debris (cholesterol embolism) that migrates to occlude distal vessels (Figs. 5–3, 5–4, 5–5 and 5–6). The sites that most commonly give rise to cholesterol embolism to the brain or eye arise from the bifurcation of the internal carotid artery and the aorta. Although cholesterol embolism is most commonly recognized in the eye (Hollenhorst plaque), these emboli also go to the brain. The presence of cholesterol emboli in the eye usually is associated with extensive atherosclerosis and plaque formation.[18] Manipulation of an intra-arterial catheter may be an important cause of cholesterol embolization, producing "trash toes" following angiography.

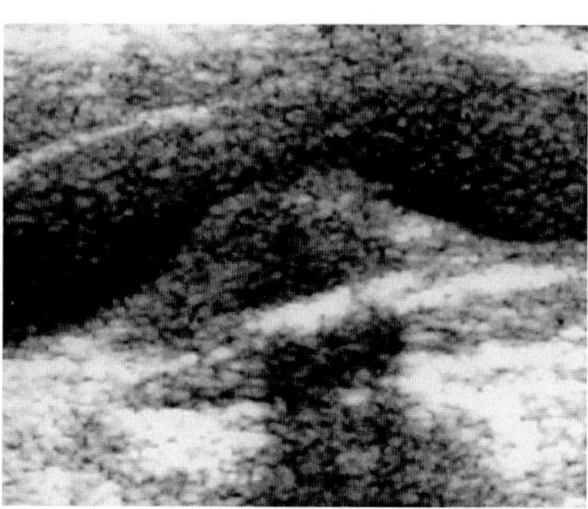

Figure 5–4. Large fibrotic plaque with hypodense core, indicating either hemorrhage or liquefied lipids.

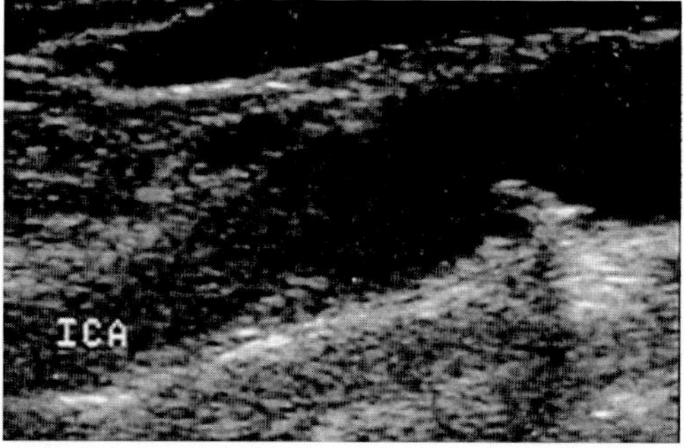

Figure 5–5. Large ulcer crater following rupture of unstable plaque. Previous Doppler examination showed moderately stenosing plaque with hypodense center.

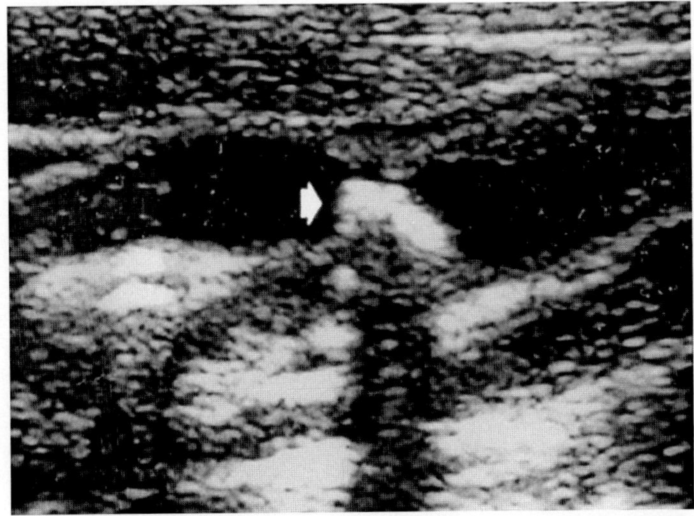

Figure 5–6. Large calcified atherosclerotic plaque protruding into the lumen of the internal carotid artery, producing high-grade stenosis. Note acoustic shadowing below the plaque.

Hypoperfusion

In addition to leading to thromboembolism, severe stenosis or occlusion secondary to intracranial or extracranial atherosclerosis potentiates the effects of hypotension leading to failure of perfusion to one or more portions of the brain (Table 5–2). A frequent clinical scenario is stroke following a major cardiovascular operation during which severe hypotension is present. The resultant infarctions usually occur in the watershed (borderzone) between the terminal perfusion beds of the anterior, middle, and posterior cerebral arteries. (See Chapter 3.) Both cortical areas and deep white matter structures are affected. In addition, atherosclerotic occlusion of a major extracranial artery may encourage diversion of blood from one vascular bed to another. The best known, albeit uncommon, example is in patients with subclavian steal syndrome, which complicates occlusion or stenosis of the proximal portion of the subclavian artery.

CLINICAL PRESENTATIONS OF CEREBROVASCULAR ATHEROSCLEROSIS

The clinical presentations of cerebrovascular atherosclerosis include ischemic stroke, TIA, amaurosis fugax, ischemic oculopathy, a cranial or cervical bruit, or an asymptomatic lesion. Descriptions of the clinical features are in Chapter 3. The details about the evaluation of patients with suspected atherosclerotic disease are included in Chapter 4. Decisions about treatment of atherosclerotic lesions to prevent stroke are described in Chapters 10 and 11. Although atherosclerosis does involve multiple intracranial or extracranial vessels, the anatomic locations of the lesions influence clinical findings, the results of evaluation, and decisions about treatment. Thus, a discussion about specific clinical relationships to anatomic locations of arterial pathology is relevant.

LARGE ARTERY ATHEROSCLEROSIS

Internal Carotid Artery Stenosis or Occlusion

The close proximity of the carotid artery to the surface of the neck permits physicians to assess the vessel for progressive changes of atherosclerosis (Table 5–3). Thickness of the arterial wall (intimal-medial thickness [IMT]) can be measured reliably and reproducibly. (See Chapter 4.) Increases in IMT can be detected in approximately 10% of asymptomatic adults with screening of the carotid artery.[19] The course of development

Table 5–3. **Differential Diagnosis of an Asymptomatic Cervical Bruit**

Atherosclerotic stenosis
Internal carotid artery
External carotid artery
Common carotid artery
Subclavian artery
Augmentation bruit (contralateral carotid occlusion)
Fibromuscular dysplasia
Arterial kink or loop
Transmitted cardiac murmur
Intracranial arteriovenous malformation
Carotid-cavernous fistula
Hyperthyroidism
Anemia
Vascular fistula in arm (hemodialysis)

of a plaque in the region of the carotid bifurcation is correlated with the presence of risk factors, such as hyperlipidemia and diabetes mellitus, and the likelihood of major cardiovascular events.[20,21] The presence of plaque in the carotid artery is strongly associated with the risk of vascular events, and the degree of risk is greater than with the early changes in IMT.[22]

Advanced atherosclerosis of the internal carotid artery can cause either a TIA or an ischemic stroke; the symptoms and signs are described in Chapter 3. Severe cases usually are associated with advancing age, cigarette smoking, hypertension, and hypercholesterolemia.[19,23–25] Still, a young man (< 35 year) who has several risk factors also can develop premature symptomatic atherosclerosis of the internal carotid artery. It is less common in persons of Asian or African heritage than in persons of European ancestry.

STENOSIS AT THE ORIGIN OF THE INTERNAL CAROTID ARTERY

The atherosclerotic plaque can form a high-grade stenosis that promotes thrombosis and occlusion of the internal carotid artery (Fig. 5–7). The development of carotid stenosis or occlusion can cause symptoms purely on the basis of diminished

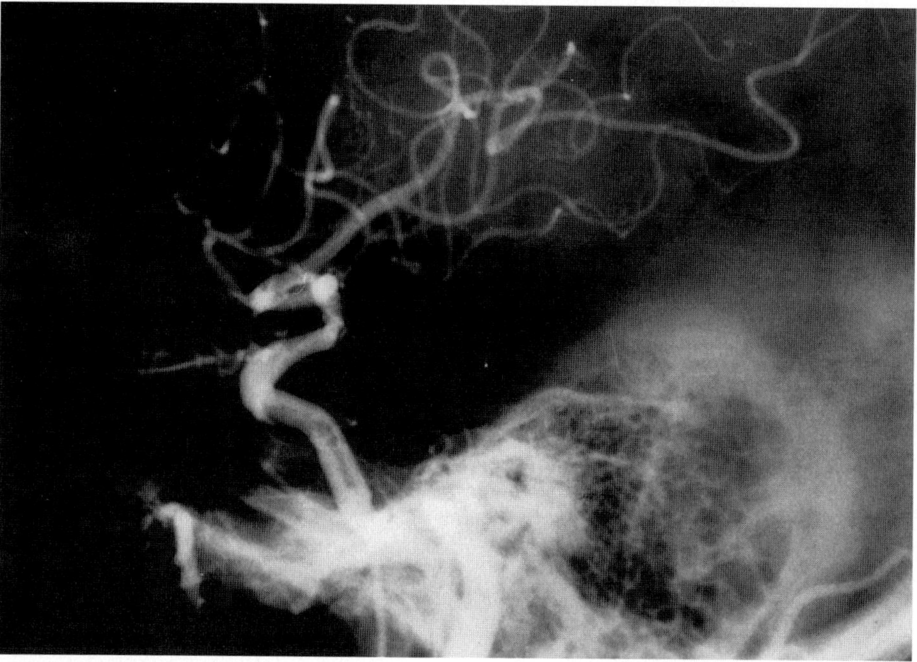

Figure 5–7. Embolus located in the carotid siphon that arose from a proximal thrombosis at the origin of the internal carotid artery.

flow. Still, the degree of carotid stenosis correlates poorly with hemodynamic status because collateral pathways can influence cerebral blood flow.[26] In general, both TIA and stroke are secondary to embolization that might be aggravated by a low flow situation. Presumably the emboli are the result of a thrombus that occurs at the fractured plaque (See Fig. 5–7). Recurrent events secondary to strokes in a watershed pattern can occur as the result of progressive stenosis of the internal carotid artery.[27] In general, narrowing greater than approximately 50% is associated with artery-to-artery embolism. The risk of stroke rises dramatically with increases in the severity of stenosis.

The appearance of neurological symptoms can be secondary to sudden worsening of the narrowing as a result of intraplaque hemorrhage.[28,29] The atheroscleortic plaques of symptomatic patients removed by carotid endarterectomy show intra-plaque hemorrhage, a necrotic lipid core, and calcification.[30] In general, the extent of stroke correlates with the severity of the narrowing of the internal carotid artery.[31] Ulceration of the surface of the plaque also is associated with neurological symptoms.[29] Fractures of the plaque can induce arterial thrombosis with secondary embolization. In addition, pieces of the atherosclerotic debris can migrate to the brain. The fracture of a plaque with secondary thrombosis is the most likely explanation for acute occlusion of the internal carotid artery.[15]

Occasionally, an atherosclerotic plaque can be detected approximately 1–2 cm. above the carotid bifurcation, extending to the base of the skull. This location is atypical of atherosclerosis, and a stenosis at this site is more likely due to a non-atherosclerotic vasculopathy, such a dissection or tubular fibromuscular dysplasia. A severe atherosclerotic stenosis at this location usually cannot be treated with traditional carotid operations; angioplasty and stenting might be the best choice.

TANDEM STENOSIS

The intracavernous portion is the second most common location of atherosclerosis on the internal carotid artery (Fig. 5–8). Severe disease in this location appears to be more common than has been widely assumed. Its presence can affect decisions about treatment, including a recommendation for carotid endarterectomy or angioplasty and stenting. Rouleau et al[32] found severe stenosis in the carotid siphon ipsilateral to severe stenosis at the origin of the internal carotid artery in 65 of 672 patients. The potential for a second stenotic lesion (*tandem stenosis*) is a primary reason that magnetic resonance angiography or conventional arteriography is needed to complement carotid duplex prior to carotid endarterectomy.

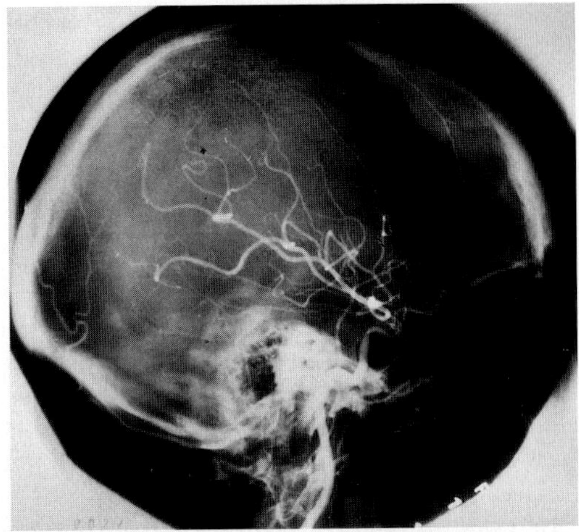

Figure 5–8. A left carotid arteriogram demonstrates a stenosis in the carotid siphon.

The usual evaluation of a patient with suspected atherosclerosis of the extracranial portion of the internal carotid artery includes non-invasive studies. (See Chapter 4.) In the past, they were usually considered as a prelude to arteriography but, with increased sensitivity and specificity, decisions about surgery now are made without subjecting the patient to the added risk. Arteriography usually is recommended only to evaluate the presence of a tandem (second intracranial) stenosis. Arteriography now can be combined with endovascular treatment.

Carotid endarterectomy has been established as a valuable tool in preventing stroke in persons with high-grade stenosis and recent ischemic symptoms.[33–37] The operation is not effective in treating occlusion of the internal carotid artery. Carotid endarterectomy is discussed in more detail in Chapter 11.

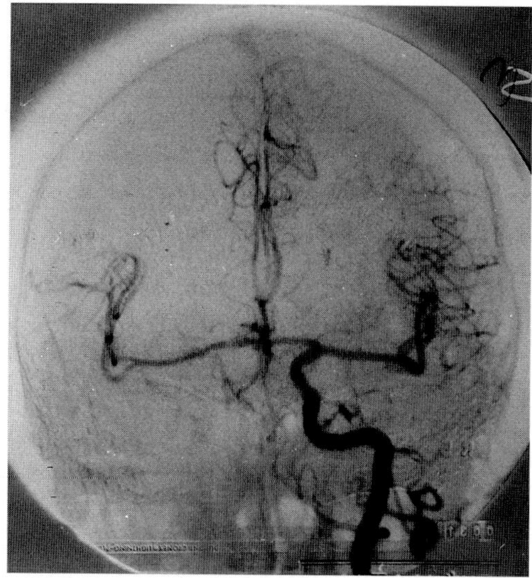

Figure 5–10. Cross-filling of blood to the right hemisphere from the left internal carotid artery in a patient with a right internal carotid artery occlusion.

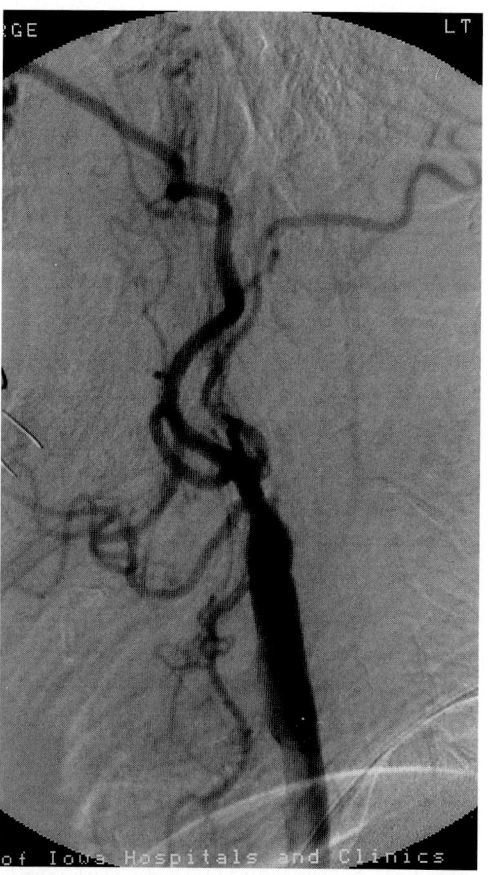

Figure 5–9. Lateral view. Left carotid arteriogram using subtraction techniques demonstrates occlusion of the origin of the internal carotid artery.

OCCLUSION OF THE INTERNAL CAROTID ARTERY

An occlusion of the internal carotid artery may cause no neurological sequelae, and a clinically silent occlusion is sometimes found during evaluation for other complaints. The prognosis in this situation is benign.[38] (See Fig. 5–9.) Collateral channels via the anterior cerebral artery, posterior communicating artery, or ophthalmic artery can preserve flow to the hemisphere despite occlusion of the internal carotid artery.[39] (See Fig. 5–10.) Conversely, symptomatic occlusion secondary to atherosclerosis of the internal carotid artery is not a benign illness.[31] A recent clinical trial demonstrated that non-invasive detection of a carotid occlusion in the setting of acute ischemic stroke is associated with severe neurological impairments and poor outcomes.[40] Hankey and Warlow[41] reported that the long-term risk of recurrent stroke was approximately 7% per year and that emboli could arise in a stump beginning at the origin of the internal carotid artery and reach the brain via collaterals.[42] This secondary hemodynamic compromise also can cause ischemia. Patients with poor metabolic and vascular reserve appear to have a high risk for stroke following occlusion of an internal carotid artery.[43,44] These patients can be identified using techniques such as PET and may benefit from revascularization procedures. The usefulness of extracranial–intracranial revascularization procedures might need to be tested in the future.

TORTUOSITY, KINKING, OR COILS

Tortuosity, kinking, or *coiling* of the internal carotid artery often is of atherosclerotic origin and is most common in elderly persons with hypertension.[45] The importance of these arterial changes has not been established, and the risk of stroke seems to be less than with stenosis or occlusion of the artery. Although these arterial lesions most often cause a cervical bruit, they cause other symptoms by compressing adjacent structures. These arterial changes are usually identified by arteriography. Most patients do not need local therapy, but surgical resection of the involved segment can be performed.

Asymptomatic Carotid Artery Bruit

A bruit usually is the result of a stenotic arterial lesion that causes turbulence in blood flow. A cervical bruit is a marker of generalized atherosclerosis. Persons with this finding are at increased risk for stroke, myocardial infarction, and vascular death.[46–48] Approximately 4%–5% of asymptomatic persons older than 65 have cervical bruits auscultated on physical examination.[49] The prevalence of a cervical bruit increases with advancing age and is more common in women.[49] (See Table 5–3.) Cervical bruits are heard in approximately 20% of patients with symptomatic peripheral artery disease and 10% of patients scheduled for coronary artery bypass surgery.[50]

Cervical bruits are most commonly located inferior to the angle of the jaw and anterior to the sternocleidomastoid muscle (Fig. 5–11). Less common locations for bruits are the supraclavicular region, the posterior aspect of the neck, the mastoid process, the temple, and the orbit.[51] A diffuse sound over the neck or head can be heard.

Most patients are unaware of the bruit. Occasionally, a patient can complain of hearing a sound in the head. It usually is described as low-pitched and swishing. Lying on the ear ipsilateral to the affected internal carotid artery may augment the sound. It will have a rhythmicity that is synchronous with the pulse. Some patients may recognize that pressure on the neck (specifically, the internal carotid artery) may diminish the intensity of the sound. The noise usually is heard by the ear on the side of the bruit and reflects transmission of the vibration (sound) along the distal portion of the internal carotid artery.

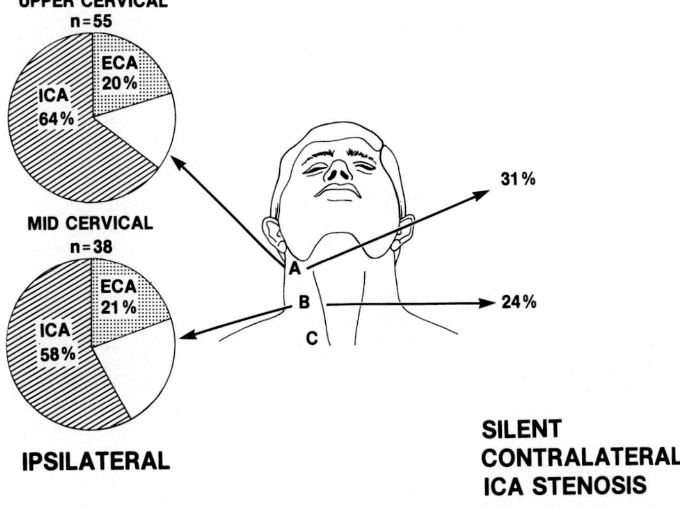

Figure 5–11. (*A*) The frequency of Doppler ultrasonography discovering a stenosis of at least 35% in patients with a unilateral carotid artery bruit. Upper cervical bruits (point A) were heard in 55 patients, and 64% of them had a stenosis of the internal carotid artery (ICA) and 20% had narrowing of the external carotid artery (ECA). The finding for a mid-cervical bruit (point B) in 38 patients was associated with an internal carotid artery stenosis or external carotid artery stenosis in 58% and 21% of cases, respectively. (*continued*)

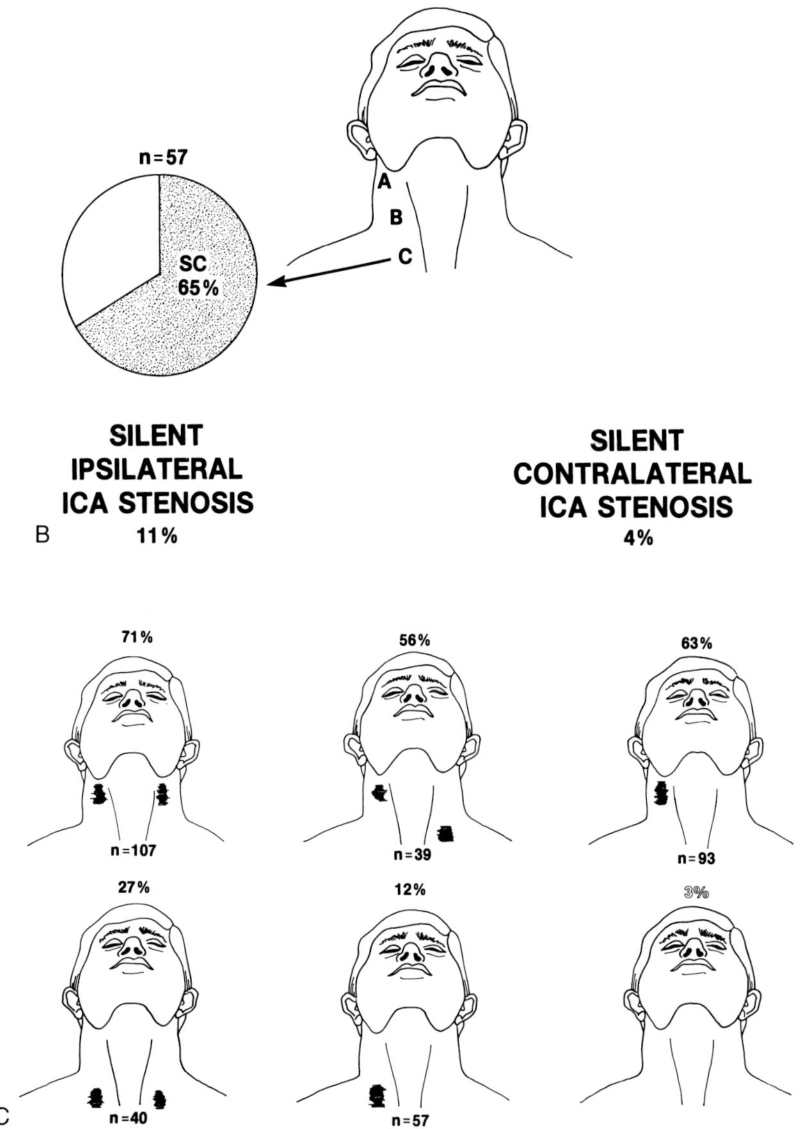

Figure 5–11. (*continued*) (*B*) The frequency of Doppler ultrasonography discovering a stenosis of at least 35% in 57 patients with a unilateral supraclavicular bruit (point C). Subclavian (SC) stenosis was detected in 65% of patients and 11% and ipsilateral stenosis of the internal carotid artery. (*C*) The frequency of Doppler ultrasonography discovering a stenosis of at least 35% of one or both internal carotid arteries among 336 patients with a cervical bruit. The bottom right figure represents the frequency of stenosis in a group of patients who did not have a cervical bruit auscultated. Stenosis of the internal carotid artery was found in 71% of patients with bilateral upper cervical bruits and 63% of patients with a unilateral cervical bruit. The frequency of stenosis was much lower when the bruits were mid-cervical or supraclavicular in location. (Figures reprinted from Chambers B, Norris J. Clinical significance of asymptomatic neck bruits. *Neurology* 1985;35:742–745, with permission of publisher.)

The finding of a cervical bruit does not necessarily correlate with the presence of severe narrowing of the internal carotid artery. A focal cervical bruit has a sensitivity of 63% and a specificity of 61% for predicting ipsilateral high-grade stenosis.[52] Often, no bruit is heard if the artery is occluded or if the stenosis is very severe. Occasionally, a cervical bruit is identified over an artery that has increased flow because the contralateral internal carotid artery is occluded.[51] Such an *augmentation bruit* may mislead the physician in determining the site of arterial pathology. A bruit may represent a high-grade stenosis of the external carotid artery. A cardiac murmur may be transmitted to the neck. Non-atherosclerotic conditions, such as fibromuscular dysplasia, or high-flow states, including severe anemia, hyperthyroidism, or an arteriovenous malformation, also can cause cervical or cranial bruits.[53] The quality, pitch, tone, and duration of the sound can differentiate a bruit secondary to stenosis from other conditions. A short, high-pitched, pistol-shot sound restricted to systole usually portends a stenosis of the internal carotid artery.

Asymptomatic Carotid Artery Plaque or Stenosis

Atherosclerotic plaques of the internal carotid artery can be detected by non-invasive testing in a sizeable proportion of men and women. Josse et al[49] found that asymptomatic plaques are more common in men than in women at most ages. By the age of 75, approximately 6% of healthy persons can have an asymptomatic stenosis greater than 50%. Detecting a severe but asymptomatic stenosis of the origin of the internal carotid artery can happen through a number of scenarios. The arterial lesion may be found on screening using a non-invasive test, such as the carotid duplex in the setting of a health fair or in the hospital as part of an evaluation in preparation for coronary artery bypass surgery. The stenosis also can be detected on evaluation of an asymptomatic bruit. Finally, arterial abnormalities might be found during evaluation of a patient who has had contralateral carotid or vertebrobasilar ischemic symptoms.

PROGNOSIS OF ASYMPTOMATIC BRUIT OR STENOSIS

Compared to healthy, age-matched controls, an asymptomatic stenosis or bruit forecasts an increased risk of stroke, myocardial infarction, or vascular death. The leading cause of death in this group of patients is myocardial infarction. Not surprisingly, the risk of stroke in persons with an asymptomatic internal carotid artery stenosis or bruit is lower than in persons who have had amaurosis fugax, TIA, or ischemic stroke (Figs. 5–12 and 5–13). The lower risk is probably because the underlying arterial disease has not

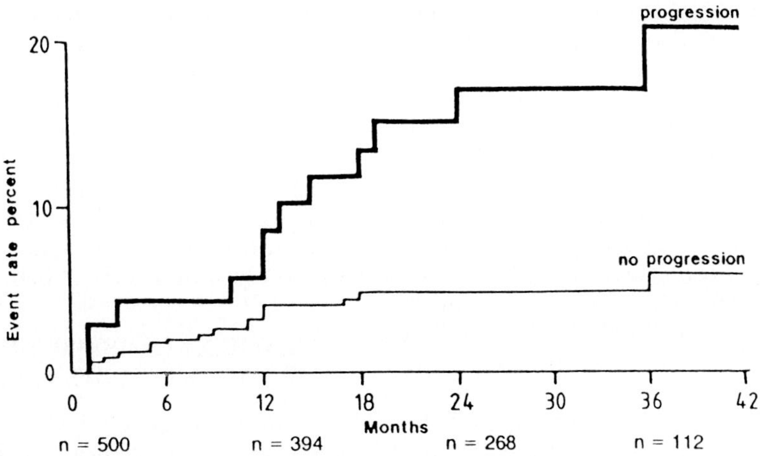

Figure 5–12. Incidence of cerebral ischemic events in persons who have an asymptomatic bruit as influenced by evidence of progression of the arterial narrowing (increased stenosis) detected by sequential non-invasive testing. Patients with increasing severity of stenosis had a significantly higher risk of ischemic events ($p < 0.0005$). (Reprinted from Chambers B, Norris J. Outcome in patients with asymptomatic neck bruits. *N Engl J Med* 1986;315:860–865, with permission of publisher.)

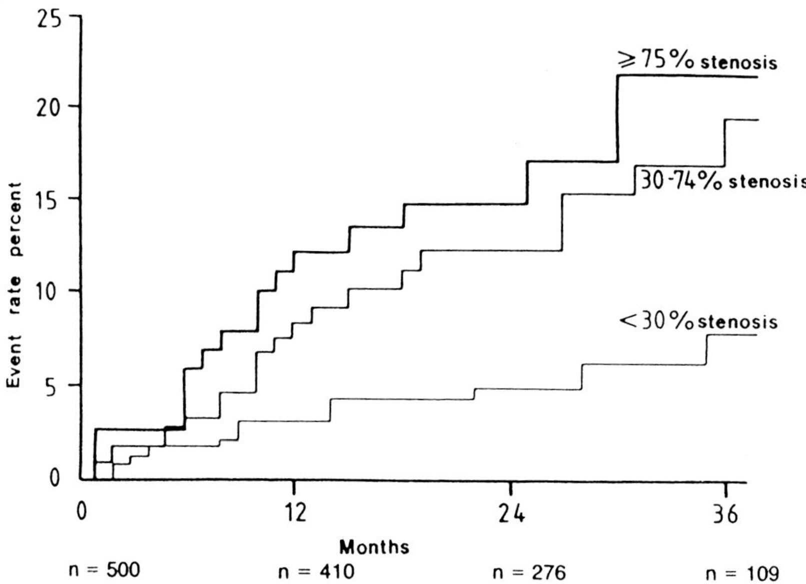

Figure 5–13. Incidence of cardiac ischemic events as influenced by the severity of carotid artery stenosis among patients with asymptomatic narrowing. Patients with severe (>75%) narrowing had a significantly higher risk of cardiac events than did those with mild (<30%) stenosis ($p < 0.0025$). (Reprinted from Chambers B, Norris J. Outcome in patients with asymptomatic neck bruits. *N Engl J Med* 1986;315:860–865, with permission of publisher.)

become sufficiently unstable to cause symptoms. For example, the cap of the plaque likely has not ruptured. Comparisons of specimens obtained by carotid endarterectomy report a lower rate of intra-plaque hemorrhage or fracture of the plaque in patients who are asymptomatic than in persons who have had neurological symptoms. Asymptomatic patients with severe extracranial stenosis often have brain-imaging evidence of silent stroke. Brott et al[54] reported that 15% of the patients enrolled in the Asymptomatic Carotid Atherosclerosis Study had lesions. The estimated annual risk for clinically obvious stroke in asymptomatic patients is approximately 2%–3%.[55–58] Events are higher in persons with more severe (80%–99%) narrowing.[47,55,56,59] The risk of ipsilateral stroke without warning TIA is less.[60] A European study found that the 3-year rate of stroke was 5.7% in persons with an asymptomatic 70%–99% narrowing of the internal carotid artery.[61] Mackey et al[59] noted that the annual risk of stroke without warning TIA was 4.2% in patients with a stenosis greater than 80%. Bogousslavsky et al[60] found that the risk of stroke without warning TIA was 1.7% per year among patients with a high-grade stenosis. Strokes are as likely to occur in other vascular territories as in areas of the brain supplied by the artery with the bruit.

The risk of stroke in patients with asymptomatic stenosis of the internal carotid artery is relatively low in patients who have coronary artery bypass surgery.[50,62] However, the risk of stroke is higher in patients with an asymptomatic stenosis than in those without the abnormality, and the presence of an asymptomatic stenosis increases the likelihood of mortality following cardiac surgery by a factor of 3.[63] The risk of stroke following non-cardiac operations is not increased by the presence of a cervical bruit.[64]

TREATMENT OF ASYMPTOMATIC CAROTID ARTERY STENOSIS

Carotid endarterectomy has been found to be effective in preventing stroke in asymptomatic persons with a stenosis greater than 60%.[57,65–68] However, the benefits from surgery are less than when the operation is performed after a TIA or a minor stroke, and the overall effects are modest.[57,68–70] Indications for carotid endarterectomy in an asymptomatic patient are controversial.[61,71–73] Some groups believe that surgery should be delayed until the patient has had neurological symptoms. This strategy can be questioned based on the experience of Castaldo et al.[74] They reported that patients in the Asymptomatic Carotid Atherosclerosis Study had intensive education about the symptoms of TIA and were instructed to contact the investigators immediately if they had a warning attack. Despite these efforts, a sizeable proportion of patients did not seek medical attention promptly. It is unlikely that patients in a general clinical setting would do better. Surgery probably should be avoided in the very elderly, if the stroke risk is low without surgery, or if the risk for perioperative events is high.[66] Carotid endarterectomy has not been established as a useful adjunctive procedure for coronary artery bypass grafting if the patient has had no neurological symptoms.[75] Percutaneous transluminal angioplasty may become an alternative to surgery for treatment of an asymptomatic carotid stenosis.[76,77] Surgical or endovascular management of severe disease of the internal carotid artery is discussed in more detail in Chapter 11.

Middle Cerebral Artery Stenosis

Atherosclerosis of the middle cerebral artery most commonly affects its first portion (*M-1 segment*), which extends from the origin of the artery to its bifurcation in the Sylvian fissure. The lenticulostriate vessels arise from this section, and the origins of these vessels can be affected by the development of an atherosclerotic plaque. Less commonly, the distal M-1 segment or the proximal portions of the first major branches of the middle cerebral artery (*M-2 segment*) can be involved.[78] Severe or symptomatic atherosclerosis of the middle cerebral artery appears to be more common in persons of Asian and African ancestry than in persons of European background. Advanced atherosclerosis of the middle cerebral artery also appears to be relatively common in diabetic patients.

Neurological symptoms range from a TIA to a multilobar infarction. Secondary ischemic lesions visualized by brain imaging include small lacunes, larger striatocapsular lesions, branch cortical strokes, or combined cortical and subcortical infarctions.[79,80] In the past, extracranial-to-intracranial revascularization procedures were attempted to lower the risk of stroke in patients with symptomatic stenosis of the middle cerebral artery. The results of an international study of superficial temporal artery to middle cerebral artery anastomoses did not demonstrate a benefit for patients with this arterial lesion.[81] Thus, management has emphasized medical interventions. Based on an uncontrolled comparison, Chimowitz et al[82] concluded that anticoagulants were superior to antiplatelet agents in preventing stroke in persons with stenotic intracranial lesions. Further study of anticoagulants in underway.[217,218] Preliminary data also suggest that angioplasty might be an option for treatment of a severe stenosis of the middle cerebral artery.[83,84] Further information is needed about the safety and efficacy of endovascular treatment for intracranial arterial stenoses.

Other Sites of Intracranial Arterial Stenosis

Intracranial atherosclerosis occurs in approximately one-third of patients with symptomatic stenosis of the extracranial portion of the internal carotid artery.[85] Disseminated atherosclerotic lesions (stenoses) can be detected in the proximal portion of the posterior cerebral arteries, the proximal portion of the anterior cerebral arteries, and surface (pial) branches of the major arteries supplying the cerebral hemispheres.

Disseminated intracranial atherosclerosis, often found in the branches of the anterior cerebral artery, most commonly occurs in patients with diabetes mellitus. The segmental areas of narrowing found on vascular imaging can be confused with intracranial vasculitis. The patient's clinical findings, examination of the CSF, and the absence of abnormalities suggestive of vasculitis support a diagnosis of intracranial atherosclerosis.

Binswanger Disease

Binswanger disease is a subcortical encephalopathy that probably is related to atherosclerosis.[86,87] It is more common in patients who have a history of hypertension or diabetes mellitus. The usual presentation is a slowly progressive dementia and gait disturbance that overlap with the symptoms of normal pressure hydrocephalus. It is among the causes of vascular dementia. (See Chapter 13.) The course is marked by a subacute onset of neurological symptoms evolving over weeks interspersed with long plateau periods of stability. Motor signs and a pseudobulbar palsy usually are seen. Acute ischemic stroke is part of the clinical course.[86,87] Brain imaging studies show multiple periventricular white matter lesions most prominent in the frontal lobes. Treatment is based on managing the cerebrovascular atherosclerosis.

Basilar Artery Stenosis

The middle portion of the basilar artery is the most common location for advanced atherosclerosis. Patients with severe *stenosis of the basilar artery* can have recurrent TIA of the posterior circulation, with symptoms of ischemia in the rostral brain stem and diencephalon resulting from hypoperfusion or distal embolization.[88] Ischemic symptoms also can be secondary to transient occlusion of a branch penetrating artery perfusing the pons. The most common symptoms are vertigo, perioral numbness, diplopia, dysphagia, and paresis.[89] (See Chapter 3.) Transient loss of consciousness and drop attacks also can occur.

Patients with high-grade stenosis of the basilar artery are at risk for a local thrombosis. Acute basilar artery thrombosis can present with a transient hemiparesis. The other signs of basilar artery occlusion are described in Chapter 3. Embolization arising from the clot in the basilar artery can migrate to the distal basilar artery, the proximal segment of the posterior cerebral artery, or penetrating arteries going to the diencephalon. Computed tomography (CT) may show calcification of the basilar artery. An area of absence of flow void or a decrease in the caliber of flow void in the prepontine cistern is a magnetic resonance imaging (MRI) hallmark of a high-grade stenosis or occlusion of the basilar artery (Fig. 5–14). Magnetic resonance angiography is very sensitive in detecting stenosis or occlusion in this region. Arteriography also can demonstrate arterial pathology.

Patients with severe disease often are treated with oral anticoagulants for long-

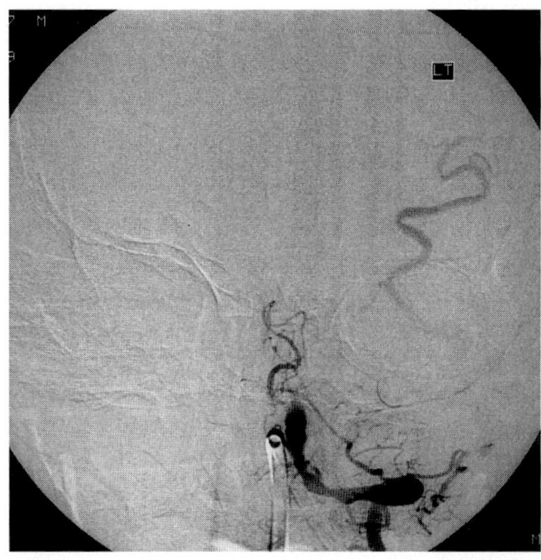

A

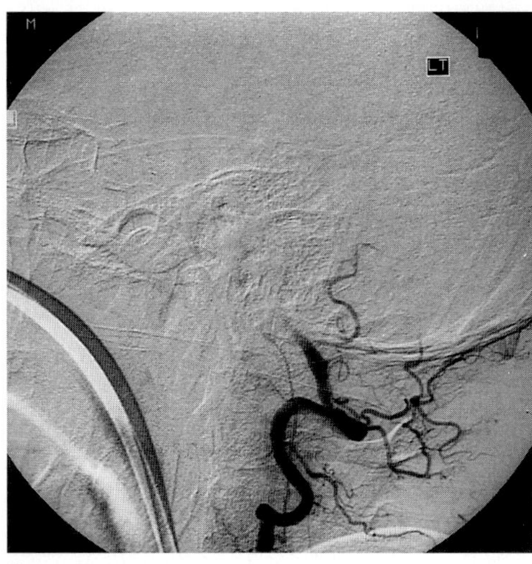

B

Figure 5–14. Thrombotic occlusion of the midportion of the basilar artery is demonstrated on anterior–posterior (*A*) and lateral (*B*) views of a left vertebral arteriogram.

term prophylaxis; the superiority of oral anticoagulants over antiplatelet agents in prevention of stroke has not been established in this situation. (See Chapter 10.) Intra-arterial administration of thrombolytic agents also is used to treat patients with acute basilar artery thrombosis. Angioplasty also is being prescribed for patients with high-grade stenosis.[90,91] (See Chapter 11.) Considerable research is needed to provide guidance about the best management of patients.

Dolichoectasia of the Basilar Artery

Dolichoectasia describes an elongated, enlarged, and tortuous vessel—most commonly the basilar artery (Table 5–4 and Figs. 5–15 and 5–16). Occasionally, the distal portion of the internal carotid artery and the proximal segment of the middle cerebral artery also can be affected.[92,93] The cause of dolichoectasia is uncertain, but atherosclerosis often is implicated because these arterial lesions have a pathologic resemblance to the findings of fusiform atherosclerotic aneurysms found elsewhere in the body. Nakatomi et al[93] concluded that these lesions start with fragmentation of the internal elastic lamina. Besides its relationship to *atherosclerosis,* dolichoectasia has been ascribed to *arterial dissection* or *Fabry-Anderson disease.*[92,94–96] Two types of

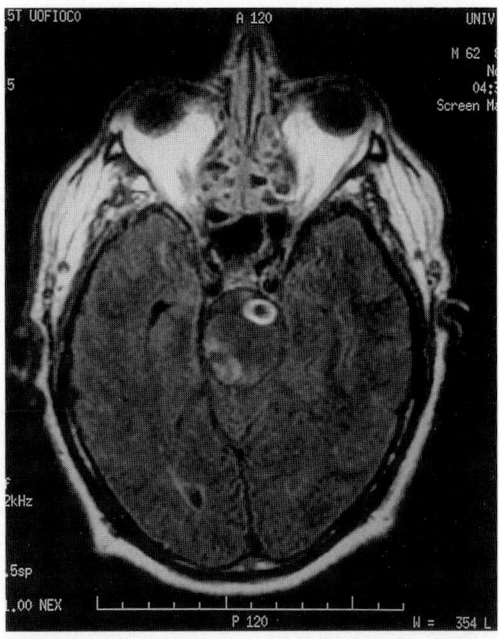

Figure 5–15. An axial FLAIR-magnetic resonance image demonstrates a large basilar artery (dolichoectatic) and a patchy area of ischemia in the dorsum of the right side of the pons.

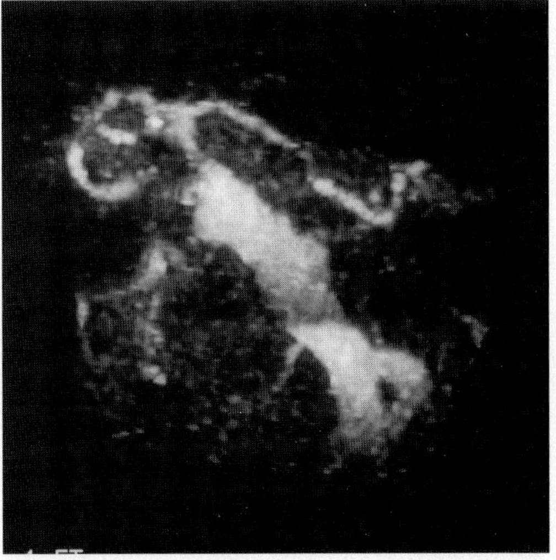

Figure 5–16. Magnetic resonance angiography demonstrates an enlarged basilar artery in a patient with a dolichoectatic basilar artery. The proximal and middle portions of the artery are affected.

Table 5–4. **Features of Dolichoectasia of the Basilar Artery**

- Basilar artery
  - Enlarged and elongated
  - Mass present in pre-pontine cistern
  - Serpentine course
  - Bifurcation elevated above brain stem
  - Distortion of course of branches
- Compression
  - Brain stem
  - Cranial nerves
- Subarachnoid hemorrhage
- Ischemic stroke
  - Occlusion of penetrating arteries
    - Distortion of origin and course
    - Thrombosis
  - Artery-to-artery embolism
  - Dissection

dolichoectasia may be present. In the *classic dissecting variety*, the internal elastic lamina is damaged but the intima is not thickened.[97] In the other form, a *segmental ectasia* involves abnormalities of both the internal elastic lamina and the intima.[97]

Dolichoectasia of the intracranial arteries is relatively common; in one registry of 387 patients with a first stroke, 12 had dolichoectasia.[98] In another series of 70 patients with stroke in the brain stem or the cerebellum, dolichoectasia was found in 12 (17%).[99] Patients with dolichoectasia do not differ from other patients with stroke with regard to age, gender, or the past history of diabetes mellitus, hypertension, or tobacco use.[98]

CLINICAL FEATURES

Ischemic stroke (often a lacune) results from proximal occlusion of the penetrating arteries that arise from the dolichoectatic parent vessel.[98,100–102] Less commonly, ischemic stroke can be secondary to occlusion of the basilar artery or to thrombosis with distal embolization.[100,101,103] Infarctions usually are located in the cerebellum, the brain stem, and the diencephalon.[101] Recurrent vertebrobasilar TIA also can occur.[104] Rarely, a dilated artery can rupture leading to an intracranial hemorrhage.

Intramural hemorrhage may be critical for a dolichoectatic lesion to enlarge and cause symptoms.[93] The enlarged, dolichoectatic artery can compress the brain stem or the cranial nerves as the lesion grows.[94,105] This presentation often involves the gradual development of multiple cranial nerve palsies or bilateral motor or sensory findings. Intramural hemorrhage can cause sudden enlargement of the lesion and rapid development of brain stem or cranial nerve compression.[94] Arterial compression of the trigeminal or facial nerve may cause unilateral facial pain, facial weakness, or hemifacial spasm. The mass effect of a very large aneurysm can cause recurrent headaches.

DIAGNOSTIC STUDIES

A CT or an MRI can detect a dolichoectatic basilar artery.[106–108] The usual finding is a large round lesion that appears to move from one side of the pre-pontine cistern to the other. A *serpentine course* of the enlarged artery is characteristic. The basilar artery usually extends above the brain stem, and the basilar bifurcation may impinge on the floor of the third ventricle. Enlarged internal carotid and middle cerebral arteries also can be visualized. Magnetic resonance angiography is also sufficient to confirm the presence of the aneurysmal basilar artery.[106] An eccentric, dilated signal void and an intraluminal thrombus may be detected.[109] The use of arteriography usually is not needed; however, it does have a characteristic appearance using this modality. The arteriogram shows an enlarged artery that has a tortuous course, and it can demonstrate intraluminal flaps, a clot, or a double lumen.[95] In addition, the long length of the artery means that major branches, such as the posterior cerebral artery, may have a prolonged course. Transcranial Doppler ultrasonography also can be used to assess a dolichoectatic basilar artery.[110]

TREATMENT

Because ischemic events often are secondary to occlusion of small penetrating arteries, the acute prognosis of patients with dolichoectasia is relatively good.[98] However, the long-term prognosis is poor.[103,105] Recurrent ischemic strokes are common, and the mass of the aneurysm can progressively impinge on the brain stem leading to increasing neurological deficits. Most patients are treated with antiplatelet agents or anticoagulants, although the efficacy of these medical therapies is uncertain. The likelihood of bleeding from a dolichoectatic basilar artery seems to be low, and this risk should not be a contraindication for long-term anticoagulation. Surgical procedures, including trapping or resection of a dilated segment have been attempted.[92] Preserving the small penetrating arteries that arise from the parent vessel is challenging for surgery.

Vertebral Artery Atherosclerosis

The vertebral artery is differentiated into four anatomic segments.[111] The first is from its origin at the subclavian artery to the vertebral artery's entry into the transverse process of the sixth cervical vertebra. The second segment corresponds to the rostral course of the vertebral artery in the lateral processes of the sixth to the second cervical vertebrae. The third extends from the second cervical vertebra to the vertebral artery's penetration of the dura. The final segment is intracranial and includes the artery's course in penetrating the dura to where it joins with the other vertebral artery to form the basilar artery. The most common location for *atherosclerosis of the vertebral artery* is the first segment. Patients with atherosclerotic stenosis or occlusion in this region have the familiar risk factors of hypertension, smoking, and coronary artery disease.[112] Ischemic symptoms can be secondary to artery-to-artery embolism or hemodynamic compromise.[112–117] Mural thrombosis in the proximal vertebral artery can lead to emboli that cause occlusion in the posterior cerebral artery, the posterior inferior cerebellar artery, or the basilar artery. An occlusion of the vertebral artery can present as an acute basilar artery thrombosis secondary to distal embolization.[113] Less commonly, atherosclerotic disease can cause stenosis of the second or third segments of the vertebral artery. The distal segment of the vertebral artery often can have stenosis adjacent to the origin of the posterior inferior cerebellar artery.[88,118] Rotational movements thus potentiate the effects of atherosclerosis.[119] Antiplatelet aggregating agents and anticoagulants often are prescribed to patients with vertebral artery stenosis. (See Chapter 10.) Revascularization operations and angioplasty are also prescribed.[111] (See Chapter 11.) In particular, the proximal portion of the vertebral artery can be treated with a local operative approach. No surgical intervention has been established as effective.

Atherosclerosis of the Great Vessels Arising from the Arch of the Aorta

Atherosclerotic disease often involves the great vessels arising from the arch of the aorta, producing neurological symptoms including TIA or stroke in the hemisphere or posterior circulation, visual symptoms, syncope, or arm ischemia.[120] It more commonly affects the origins and the first segment of the subclavian arteries than the common carotid arteries. In general, risk factors for subclavian atherosclerosis are the same as for atherosclerosis in other cervical vessels. Accelerated atherosclerosis may result from prolonged maintenance hemodialysis and renal failure.[121,122] The increased flow induced by the fistula in the arm leads to arterial changes in the proximal vessels in the upper arm. Recurrent ischemic symptoms in the posterior circulation can follow surgery on the subclavian or the brachial artery.[123] The neurological symptoms may be secondary to local thrombosis, injury to the vessels in the neck by excessive rotation of the head, dissection of vessels in the neck, or ligation of important collateral channels.

SUBCLAVIAN STEAL SYNDROME

A clinical presentation of disease of the brachiocephalic vessels is *subclavian steal syndrome*. It is a relatively uncommon cause of TIA in the vertebrobasilar circulation and is usually due to an atherosclerotic high-grade stenosis or an occlusion of the subclavian artery.[124,125] Because the left subclavian artery arises directly from the aorta and is longer than the right, the likelihood of subclavian steal syndrome is greater with lesions on the left. In this situation, blood ascends cephalically via the right vertebral artery and then descends down the neck via the left vertebral artery. It is thus diverted from the basilar artery and the brain to perfuse the affected upper limb. These changes in blood flow can produce a to-and-fro phenomenon detected by angiography or sonography.[126] Usually, this diversion is asymptomatic, but with classic subclavian steal syndrome the neurological symptoms are provoked by recurrent exercise of the arm.[125] In this situation, blood is diverted from the posterior circulation to meet the increased metabolic demands of the limb. True clinical subclavian steal syndrome is relatively rare in comparison to the number of patients who have reversed vertebral flow identified by radiologic or non-invasive methods.[120,126,127] The most common symptoms are lightheadedness, vertigo, and bilateral visual disturbances. Symptoms mimicking a basilar artery stenosis also can occur. Brachiocephalic arterial occlusions also can cause monocular visual symptoms and global ischemia, including lightheadedness, syncope, and arm ischemia.[120]

The diagnosis of subclavian steal syndrome should be considered for patients with TIA or ischemic stroke in the posterior circulation if a supraclavicular bruit is heard. In addition, differences in blood pressure readings or the strength of the pulses between the two upper limbs point to a subclavian stenosis or occlusion. As a rule of thumb, a severe stenosis of the subclavian artery is unlikely unless the differences in blood pressure readings are more than 25 mm Hg or are greater than 25% of the higher figure. The risk of stroke in patients with subclavian steal syndrome is not as high with atherosclerotic lesions elsewhere in the neck.[124] Most patients are treated medically. They should be advised to avoid activities that would promote the symptoms of steal. Endarterectomy of the stenotic segment can be performed. A revascularization operation often involves development of a new collateral channel from the internal carotid artery.[120,128] Because patients with subclavian steal syndrome often have concomitant moderate-to-severe stenosis of the internal carotid artery, care must be taken to avoid reducing perfusion to the ipsilateral cerebral hemisphere. Surgical treatment of both the carotid and subclavian lesions can be combined.[129] Endovascular treatment also can be an option.

Atherosclerosis of the Arch of the Aorta

Identification of severe atherosclerotic disease of the arch of the aorta as a cause of stroke has increased markedly with the advent of transesophageal echocardiography (TEE).[130–136] (See Figs. 5–17 and 5–18.) Because TEE assesses both the aortic wall and the lumen, it detects plaques and superimposed thrombus that cannot

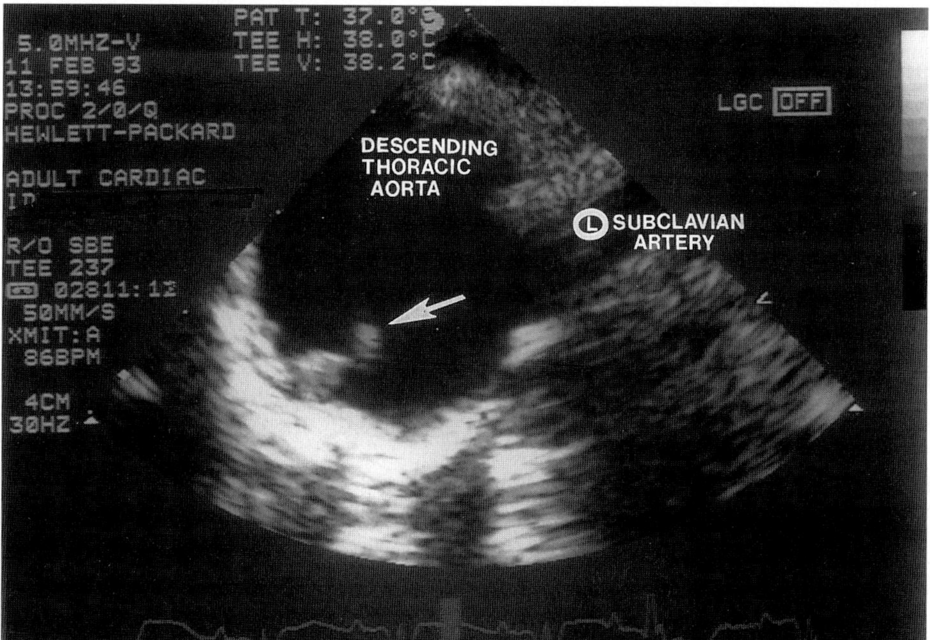

Figure 5–17. Transesophageal echocardiographic view of the descending thoracic aorta. The arrow indicates a mobile, protruding atheromatous plaque. The plaque is opposite to the origin of the left subclavian artery. (Courtesy of Richard E. Kerber, MD, Department of Medicine, University of Iowa, Iowa City.)

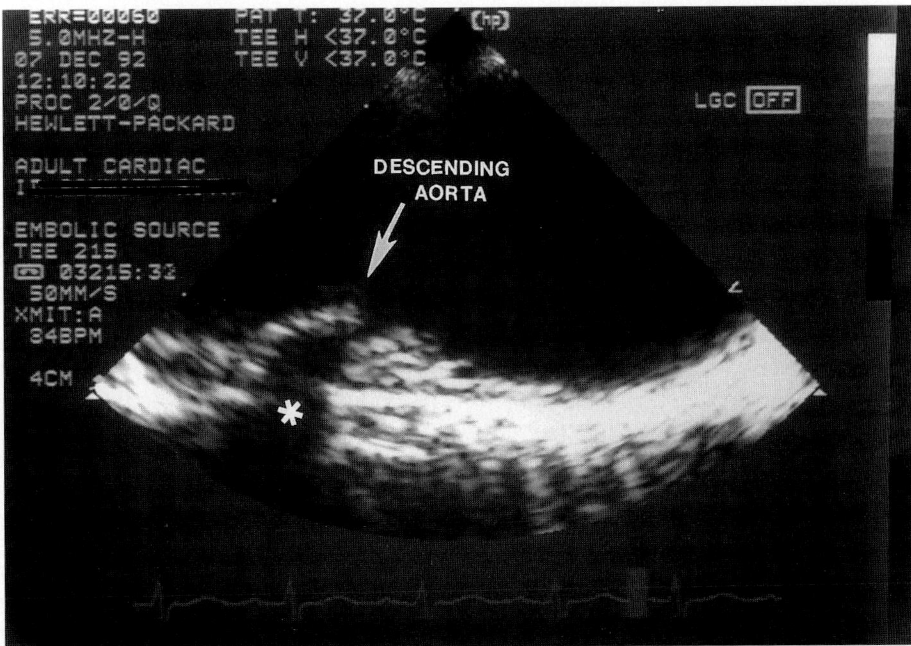

Figure 5–18. Transesophageal echocardiographic view of the descending thoracic aorta. The arrow denotes a protruding calcified plaque. The asterisk indicates an area of shadowing produced by the calcification in the protruding plaque. (Courtesy of Richard E. Kerber, MD, Department of Medicine, University of Iowa, Iowa City.)

be seen by aortography. Transesophageal echocardiography has become a key tool in assessing patients for disease of the aorta, in particular to detect the presence of advanced disease of the arch.[137] Besides TEE, dual helical CT also can be used to detect protruding aortic atheromas. Computed tomography can be performed when a patient cannot undergo TEE.

Aortic lesions, in particular advanced and friable plaques, can be the source of atherosclerotic debris.[138–141] Embolism also can occur from a complicating thrombus developing on a relatively small aortic plaque.[142] Advanced atherosclerotic disease can lead to a plaque that is mobile in the aortic lumen; this lesion has been called the *shagbark aorta* because the appearance is similar to the bark of the shagbark hickory tree. Proximal aortic atherosclerosis is an independent risk factor for stroke, especially among persons older than 60.[133,136–138,143,144] The presence of a simple aortic lesion increases the risk of stroke by a factor of 2.3, whereas a more complex atherosclerotic plaque increases the risk of stroke by a rate of 7.1.[145]

Extensive aortic plaque formation is a risk factor for stroke complicating heart surgery.[146–150] The presence of a protruding or mobile atheroma in the aortic arch portends a high risk for emboli during the operation, especially in persons older than 60.[151] Intraoperative placement of the aortic clamp can fracture the plaque leading to embolization of pieces of plaque or thrombi. Severe atherosclerotic disease of the aorta might be a risk factor for other intra-arterial interventions as well as arteriography.[130,152] Arteriography can be complicated by release of atherosclerotic debris from the aorta leading to focal areas of ischemia in the toes—*trash toes syndrome*. Severe atherosclerosis of the aorta also can be the substrate for a dissection that leads to stroke.[153] Patients with severe atherosclerosis of the thoracic aorta also have a high risk of vascular mortality, including deaths from myocardial infarction.[154]

The proximal (arch) aorta may be a relatively common but occult source of embolism to the brain and other organs.[132,155,156] In a series of 62 patients with embolic stroke, Toyoda et al[157] found atherosclerotic lesions of the aorta in 26 patients (42%). In another study, ulcerated, protruding aortic plaques were found in 9 of 23 patients with cryptogenic stroke, a rate that was much higher than in the group of patients with a known cause of stroke.[158] Another study of patients with cryptogenic stroke found that aortic atherosclerosis was the most common abnormality detected by TEE.[159] The severity of aortic atherosclerosis is associated with advancing age. Severe atherosclerosis of the aorta is more advanced in persons who smoke or have elevated plasma homocysteine levels.[160,161] Advanced atherosclerosis of the aorta can be detected in a sizeable proportion of patients with other risk factors for stroke. For example, Blackshear et al[162] reported that TEE detected aortic plaques in more than one-half of patients with atrial fibrillation. Still, most of these plaques were found in the descending aorta.

The severity of a plaque, as defined by TEE, is associated with its risk of embolization. An aortic plaque thicker than 4–5 mm. appears to be risky.[141,163–165] A French study concluded that a plaque 4 mm. thick or greater was associated with a risk of stroke that approaches a rate of 11.9/1000 patient-years.[166,167] Layered or immobile plaques appear to be associated with lower risk.[156] Advanced, pedunculated, mobile plaques have the greatest risk for embolization.[156] Ulceration of the plaque also identifies a high-risk aortic lesion.[168] Sequential studies show that most aortic plaques remain stable.[132]

Dissection of the Ascending Aorta

In the past, dissection of the aorta was often ascribed to *syphilic aortitis*, but this has largely disappeared with the availability of antibiotic treatment. Presently, although a dissection of the arch of the aorta can occur in patients with connective tissue diseases such as *Marfan's syndrome*, *atherosclerosis* is the most common underlying reason for the acute aortic process. Dissection of the aorta usually presents with severe chest and back pain. If the dissection occurs in the proximal portions of the arch, then the major arteries perfusing the brain also may be affected.[153,169] Stroke can be a complication. In some patients, signs of the acute thoracic event may be relatively subtle, and the findings of stroke predominate. Emergent thrombolytic therapy is dangerous in the setting of a patient with an acute dissection of the aorta.[170] Thus, the condition should be considered in patients who present with stroke, particularly if chest or back pain is present, if vital signs are unstable, if hypotension is noted, or if the pulses of the upper limbs are asymmetrical. The presence of widening of the aortic silhouette on chest x-ray is an important diagnostic clue.[170] A CT of the chest often is needed to confirm the aortic lesion. An aortic dissection also can be detected by TEE.[171,172] Because dissection of the aorta is a potential catastrophe, treatment is aimed at it rather than the neurological complications. Lowering blood pressure and surgical resection are among the treatment options.

The best treatment for severe atherosclerosis of the aortic arch has not yet been established. Antiplatelet aggregating agents can be prescribed.[138] Long-term oral anticoagulant therapy has been advised, although data supporting the efficacy of this approach are lacking.[173] Oral anticoagulants might increase the risk of cholesterol embolization to the limbs, causing small areas of digital ischemia, and elsewhere in the body—*purple toe syndrome*. (See Chapter 10.) Replacement of the ascending aorta for severe atherosclerosis has been attempted.[174,175] In one series of 17 operated patients, 4 died, stroke occurred in 3, and other major morbidity was noted in 9.[176] (See Chapter 11.) At present, the best medical and surgical treatment for patients with symptomatic severe atherosclerosis of the ascending aorta remains unsettled.

Other Atherosclerotic Disease of the Aorta

Atherosclerosis of the descending thoracic and abdominal aorta is relatively common in patients with cerebrovascular disease. Karanjia et al[177] found abdominal aortic aneurysms in 18 of 89 patients with carotid artery disease. Although advanced atherosclerosis of the descending thoracic aorta or the abdominal aorta likely will not cause symptoms of brain ischemia, it is an important cause of morbidity or mortality. It also could lead to ischemia of the spinal cord. Patients with cerebrovascular atherosclerosis should be evaluated clinically for the presence of aortic atherosclerosis, including the presence of an abdominal aortic aneurysm. Treatment of atherosclerosis of the descending thoracic or abdominal aorta is beyond the purview of this book.

SMALL VESSEL OCCLUSIVE (LACUNAR) DISEASE

The term *lacune* was coined by Dechambre approximately 100 years ago and, in 1901, Marie described the lacunar state as a series of strokes that led to a dementia.[178] Lacunes account for approximately 10% of all symptomatic strokes and are most commonly found in patients with a history of hypertension or diabetes mellitus.[179–181,25] These lesions also can occur in children.[182] The mechanism of lacunar infarction is hemodynamic impairment in the microcirculation in the perforating arteries of the brain.[194] The pathological hallmarks are 15–20 mm., irregular cavities deep in the cerebral hemisphere, brain stem, and cerebellum. These lesions can be secondary to either hemorrhagic or ischemic stroke. True lacunar infarctions usually are smaller than 0.5–1 cm. when they are detected by brain imaging studies (Fig. 5–19). If the lesion is larger than 1 cm., then the diagnosis of a lacunar infarction secondary to small artery should be questioned.

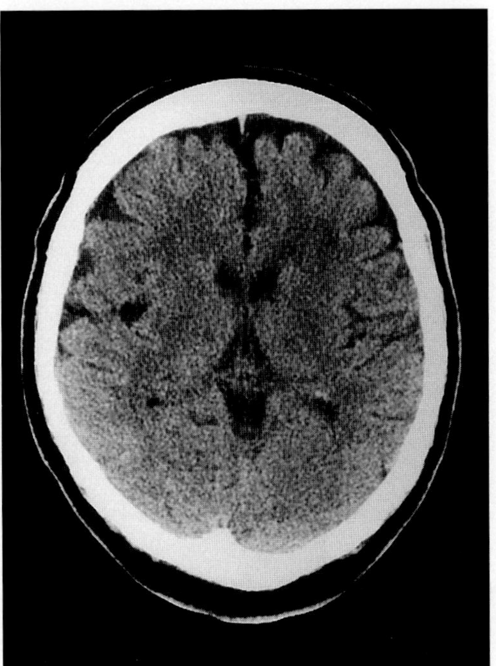

Figure 5–19. Lacunar infarcts. The computed tomographic scan shows lacunar infarcts in the thalami bilaterally. (Courtesy of Dr. E. Wong.)

Lacunar Syndromes

In a series of papers, Fisher and colleagues popularized the clinical–pathological relationships of lacunar strokes.[183–190] Several distinct clinical syndromes (*pure motor hemiparesis, isolated sensory stroke, dysarthria-clumsy hand, crural paresis and homolateral ataxia*, and *sensori-motor stroke*) reflect a restricted area of injury to subcortical motor or sensory structures.[191–194] (See Chapter 3.) Despite the large amount of information about small vessel occlusive disease, the concept of lacunar infarction has been questioned.[195] Despite these reservations, the concept of the lacunar stroke remains valid, and it should be recognized as an important part of the spectrum of ischemic cerebrovascular disease.

Since the advent of brain imaging studies, the physician's ability to diagnose lacunes has increased greatly (Fig. 5–20). Scans can detect small subcortical lesions that were either clinically silent or symptomatic. In addition, brain imaging studies help physicians to differentiate lacunar syndromes not due to small artery disease from true lacunes. Despite the advances in evaluating patients with stroke, inter-physician agreement in the diagnosis of lacunar stroke is low.[196] Clinical features of the lacunar syndromes can be imitated by cortical infarctions.[197] For example, in one study, less than 50% of cases of sensorimotor stroke could be ascribed to lacunar infarction.[198] A proportion of patients with

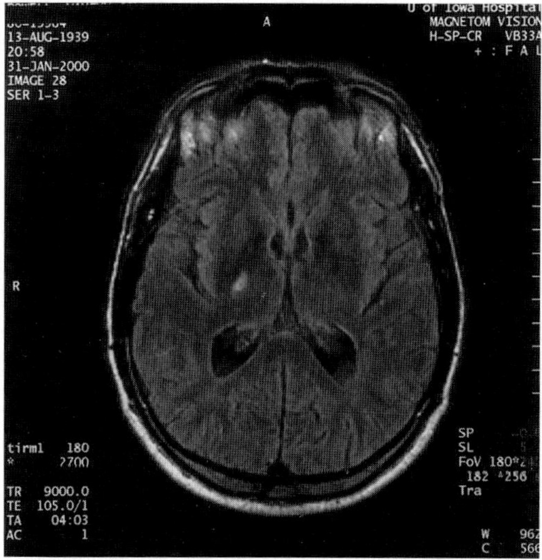

Figure 5–20. A small lacunar infarction in the territory of the anterior choroidal artery noted in a patient with chronic hypertension.

findings compatible with lacunar syndromes can have large subcortical infarctions. The size of subcortical infarction can influence clinical features.[199] Boiten and Lodder[200] concluded that lacunar syndromes had a sensitivity and a specificity of 95% and 93%, respectively, in predicting a lacune. The Dutch TIA Study Group reported that lacunar syndromes had a positive predictive value of 0.74 for a lacunar stroke.[201] In particular, pure motor hemiparesis may not be specific for a lacunar stroke.[202] The signs may be due to large striatocapsular infarctions secondary to embolic occlusions of the proximal segment of the middle cerebral artery.[25,203,204] Ghika et al[205] found a source for embolism in approximately 30% of patients with infarctions in deep perforating arteries in the cerebral hemisphere. Both cardiac and large artery sources of emboli can be identified in patients with large subcortical infarctions.[181,206] Kappelle et al[207] found stenosis of the internal carotid artery in 14 of 45 patients who had lacunar infarctions. Another report suggests that patients with lacunar infarctions have less extensive carotid atherosclerosis than among patients with cortical infractions.[194] Cardioembolism seems to be an uncommon cause of lacunar strokes.[208]

Lacunar Stroke

The decision to include small vessel occlusive disease in a chapter on atherosclerosis may be controversial. In the past, arterial pathology underlying lacunes is often ascribed to lipohyalinosis or fibrinoid necrosis.[209,210] However, the number of patients with lacunar infarctions who have had evaluation of the underlying arterial pathology is small. Most of the epidemiological risk factors, clinical features, findings on evaluation, and options for treatment of persons with lacunar infarctions overlap with those seen in patients with atherosclerotic disease in larger intracranial or extracranial arteries. In addition, pathological examination of the small arteries causing lacunar stroke often shows an atherosclerotic stenosis of the vessels with or without an overlying thrombosis.[210,211] In addition, mural atheroma of a major intracranial artery can lead to occlusion of the penetrating branch arteries that lead to lacunar infarction of the brain stem or subcortical hemispheric structures (Table 5–5).

Despite these overlying features between large and small artery occlusive disease, differentiating lacunar strokes is important because both acute and long-term prognoses differ. Recovery of neurological impairments may be so rapid in a patient with a minor subcortical infarction that a diagnosis of TIA is made instead of stroke.[201] In the Oxfordshire study, the 30-day and 1-year mortality rates with lacunes were 2% and 7%, respectively; these rates were lower than with other types of ischemic stroke.[212] Most deaths were due to cardiac disease or other complications rather than the neurological consequences of the stroke. Anderson et al[213] found that 1 year mortality after stroke was approximately 14% in persons with lacunes compared to 25% in persons with large artery atherosclerosis. Arboix et al[179] reported that more than 78% of patients with lacunes recovered completely. Two studies found that approximately 62% of patients with lacunes were independent at 30 days.[212,214] Boiten and Lodder[215] reported that survival was high and disability was low following a lacunar stroke, but the rate

Table 5–5. **Arteries Occluded in Lacunar Infarction**

Artery	Parent Artery	Primary Affected Area of the Brain
Recurrent artery of Huebner	Anterior cerebral	Head of caudate Anterior limb of internal capsule
Lenticulstriate	Middle cerebral	Anterior limb of internal capsule Putamen Globus pallidus
Anterior choroidal	Internal carotid	Genu and posterior limb of internal capsule Globus pallidus Lateral aspect of thalamus
Polar (tuberothalamic)	Posterior communicating Posterior cerebral	Anterior thalamus
Thalamoperforating (interpeduncular–thalamic)	Basilar Posterior cerebral	Medial thalamus
Thalamogeniculate	Posterior cerebral	Posterior and lateral thalamus
Posterior choroidal	Posterior cerebral	Pulvinar Posterior limb of internal capsule Lateral geniculate
Pontine	Basilar	Medial and ventral areas of brain stem

of recurrence was similar to that reported with strokes of other causes.

Treatment

The acute prognosis of persons with lacunar infarction is probably determined by the size of the brain lesion rather than the type of arterial pathology exhibited. Persons with lacunar infarction are at relatively high risk for recurrent stroke. In addition, recurrent stroke in persons with a history of lacunar stroke is as likely to be due to large artery atherosclerosis as to another lacune. In the Dutch TIA Trial Study, 107 recurrent strokes occurred among 1216 patients who were treated after a lacunar infarction; 39 were due to large artery atherosclerosis and 30 were ascribed to small artery occlusions.[201,216] Most clinical trials testing the usefulness of medical or surgical interventions in preventing recurrent stroke have included patients with lacunar infarctions. No data show a difference in responses to treatment with antiplatelet aggregating agents between persons with lacunar infarctions and those with stroke secondary to large artery atherosclerosis. (See Chapters 10 and 11.) Because of the potential relationship between hypertensive hemorrhage and lacunar infarction, the chronic use of anticoagulants might be problematic. Conversely, a lacunar infarction can be ipsilateral to a high-grade stenosis of the internal carotid artery, and risk of another stroke has not been differentiated from that seen among patients with cortical infarctions. At present, persons with lacunar infarction should receive the same medical and surgical measures, including carotid endarterectomy, as patients with cortical infarctions.

SUMMARY

Atherosclerosis causes the majority of strokes in developed countries and threatens to do the same in the rest of the world. It acts in several insidious ways—by producing myocardial infarction, or akinetic segments causing brain embolism, by encrusting the ascending aorta with friable plaques, by encroaching into the lumen of the cervical arteries, and by narrowing and obstructing the small cerebral arteries. Each of these manifestations has its own susceptible populations and creates its own distinctive syndromes, but both the causes and the treatment of atherosclerosis tend to be similar—management of risk factors and enhancement of protective factors for all cases, including antiplatelet aggregating agents for threatened and recurrent atherosclerotic stroke and removal of obstruction in selected cases by surgical or endovascular means.

REFERENCES

1. Yatsu FM, Fisher M. Atherosclerosis: current concepts on pathogenesis and interventional therapies. *Ann Neurol* 1989;26:3–12.
2. Bogousslavsky J, Barnett HJM, Fox AJ, Hachinski VC, Taylor W. Atherosclerotic disease of the middle cerebral artery. *Stroke* 1986; 17:1112–1120.
3. Feldmann E, Daneault N, Kwan E, et al. Chinese-white differences in the distribution of occlusive cerebrovascular disease. *Neurology* 1990;40:1541–1545.
4. Wityk RJ, Lehman D, Klag M, Coresh J, Ahn H, Litt B. Race and sex differences in the distribution of cerebral atherosclerosis. *Stroke* 1996;27:1974–1980.
5. Alexandrova NA, Gibson WC, Norris JW, Maggisano R. Carotid artery stenosis in peripheral vascular disease. *J Vasc Surg* 1996;23: 645–649.
6. Bogousslavsky J, Castillo V, Kumral E, Henriques I, Van Melle G. Stroke subtypes and hypertension. *Arch Neurol* 1996;53:265–269.
7. Fuster V, Badimon JJ, Chesebro JH. Atherothrombosis: mechanisms and clinical therapeutic approaches. *Vasc Med* 1998;3:231–239.
8. Malek AM, Alper SL, Izumo S. Hemodynamic shear stress and its role in atherosclerosis. *JAMA* 1999;282:2035–2042.
9. Navab M, Fogelman AM, Berliner JA, et al. Pathogenesis of atherosclerosis. *Am J Cardiol* 1995;76:18C–23C.
10. Badimon JJ, Lettino M, Toschi V, et al. Local inhibition of tissue factor reduces the thrombogenicity of disrupted human atherosclerotic plaques: effects of tissue factor pathway inhibitor on plaque thrombogenicity under flow conditions. *Circulation* 1999;99:1780–1787.
11. Lafont A, Libby P. The smooth muscle cell: sinner or saint in restenosis and the acute coronary syndromes? *J Am Coll Cardiol* 1998;32:283–285.
12. Sitzer M, Muller W, Siebler M, et al. Plaque ulceration and lumen thrombus are the main sources of cerebral microemboli in high-grade internal carotid artery stenosis. *Stroke* 1995;26:1231–1233.
13. Kullo IJ, Edwards WD, Schwartz RS. Vulnerable plaque: pathobiology and clinical implications. *Ann Intern Med* 1998;129:1050–1060.
14. Gutstein DE, Fuster V. Pathophysiology and clinical significance of atherosclerotic plaque rupture.*Cardiovas Res* 1999;41:323–333.
15. Lammie GA, Sandercock PAG, Dennis MS. Recently occluded intracranial and extracranial carotid arteries.*Stroke* 1999;30:1319–1325.
16. Carr S, Farb A, Pearce WH, Virmani R, Yao JS. Atherosclerotic plaque rupture in symptomatic carotid artery stenosis. *J Vasc Surg* 1996;23: 755–765.
17. Rothwell PM, Villagra R, Gibson R, Donders RC, Warlow CP, . Evidence of a chronic systemic cause of instability of atherosclerotic plaques. *Lancet* 2000;355:19–24.
18. Bruno A, Russell PW, Jones WL, Austin JK, Weinstein ES, Steel SR. Concomitants of asymptomatic retinal cholesterol emboli. *Stroke* 1992;23:900–902.
19. Prati P, Vanuzzo D, Casaroli M, et al. Prevalence and determinants of carotid atherosclerosis in a general population.*Stroke* 1992;23:1705–1711.
20. Niskanen L, Rauramaa R, Miettinen H, Haffner SM, Mercuri M, Uusitupa M. Carotid artery intima-media thickness in elderly patients with NIDDM and in nondiabetic subjects. *Stroke* 1996;27:1986–1992.
21. O'Leary DH, Polak JF, Kronmal RA, et al. Carotid-artery intima and media thickness as a risk factor for myocardial infarction and stroke in older adults. Cardiovascular Health Study Collaborative Research Group. *N Engl J Med* 1999;340:14–22.
22. Ebrahim S, Papacosta O, Whincup P, et al. Carotid plaque, intima media thickness, cardiovascular risk factors, and prevalent cardiovascular disease in men and women: the British Regional Heart Study. *Stroke* 1999;30:841–850.
23. Fine-Edelstein JS, Wolf PA, O'Leary DH, et al. Precursors of extracranial carotid atherosclerosis in the Framingham Study. *Neurology* 1994;44:1046–1050.
24. Ingall TJ, Homer D, Baker HLJ, Kottke BA, O'Fallon WM, Whisnant JP. Predictors of intracranial carotid artery atherosclerosis. Duration of cigarette smoking and hypertension are more powerful than serum lipid levels. *Arch Neurol* 1991;48:687–691.
25. Inzitari D. Risk factors and outcome of patients with carotid artery stenosis presenting with lacunar stroke. *Neurology* 2000;54:660–666.
26. Powers WJ. Cerebral hemodynamics in ischemic cerebrovascular disease. *Ann Neurol* 1991;29: 231–240.
27. Chollet F, Rolland Y, Albucher JF, Manelfe C, Marc-Vergnes JP, Guiraud-Chaumeil B. Recurrent right hemiplegia associated with progressive ipsilateral carotid artery stenosis. *Stroke* 1996;27:753–755.

28. Falke P, Matzsch T, Sternby NH, Bergqvist D, Stavenow L. Intraplaque haemorrhage at carotid artery surgery—a predictor of cardiovascular mortality. *J Intern Med* 1995;238:131–135.
29. Park AE, McCarthy WJ, Pearce WH, Matsumura JS, Yao JS. Carotid plaque morphology correlates with presenting symptomatology. *J Vasc Surg* 1998;27:872–878.
30. Hatsukami TS, Ferguson MS, Beach KW, et al. Carotid plaque morphology and clinical events. *Stroke* 1997;28:95–100.
31. Lodder J, Hupperts R, Boreas A, Kessels F. The size of territorial brain infarction on CT relates to the degree of internal carotid artery obstruction. *J Neurol* 1996;243:345–349.
32. Rouleau PA, Huston J, Gilbertson J, et al. Carotid artery tandem lesions: frequency of angiographic detection and consequences for endarterectomy. *Am J Neuroradiol* 1999;20:621–625.
33. Mayberg MR, Wilson SE, Yatsu F, et al. Carotid endarterectomy and prevention of cerebral ischemia in symptomatic carotid stenosis. Veterans Affairs Cooperative Studies Program 309 Trialist Group. *JAMA* 1991;266:3289–3294.
34. North American Symptomatic Carotid Endarterectomy Trial Collaborators. Beneficial effect of carotid endarterectomy in symptomatic patients with high-grade carotid stenosis. *N Engl J Med* 1991;325:445–453.
35. European Carotid Surgery Trialists' Collaborative Group. MRC European Carotid Surgery Trial: interim results for symptomatic patients with severe (70–99%) or with mild (0–29%) carotid stenosis. *Lancet* 1991;337:1235–1243.
36. European Carotid Surgery Trialists' Collaborative Group. Endarterectomy for moderate symptomatic carotid stenosis: interim results from the MRC European Carotid Surgery Trial. *Lancet* 1996;347:1591–1593.
37. Barnett HJM, Taylor DW, Eliasziw M, et al. Benefit of carotid endarterectomy in patients with symptomatic moderate or severe stenosis. North American Symptomatic Carotid Endarterectomy Trial Collaborators. *N Engl J Med* 1998;339: 1415–1425.
38. Powers WJ, Derdeyn CP, Fritsch SM, et al. Benign prognosis of never-symptomatic carotid occlusion. *Neurology* 2000;54:878–882.
39. van Everdingen KJ, Visser GH, Klijn CJ, Kappelle LJ, van der Grond J. Role of collateral flow on cerebral hemodynamics in patients with unilateral internal carotid artery occlusion. *Ann Neurol* 1998;44:167–176.
40. Adams HP, Jr., Bendixen BH, Leira EC, et al. Antithrombotic treatment of ischemic stroke among patients with occlusion or severe stenosis of the internal carotid artery. *Neurology* 1999;53:122–125.
41. Hankey GJ, Warlow CP. Prognosis of symptomatic carotid artery occlusion. *Cerebrovasc* Dis 1991;1:245–256.
42. Ryan PG, Day AL. Stump embolization from an occluded internal carotid artery. Case report. *J Neurosurg* 1987;67:609–611.
43. Grubb RL, Jr., Derdeyn CP, Fritsch SM, et al. Importance of hemodynamic factors in the prognosis of symptomatic carotid occlusion. *JAMA* 1998;280:1055–1060.
44. Klijn CJ, Kappelle LJ, Tulleken CA, van Gijn J. Symptomatic carotid artery occlusion. A reappraisal of hemodynamic factors. *Stroke* 1997; 28:2084–2093.
45. Del Corso L, Moruzzo D, Conte B, et al. Tortuosity, kinking, and coiling of the carotid artery: expression of atherosclerosis or aging? *Angiology* 1998;49:361–371.
46. Ingall TJ, Homer D, Whisnant JP, Baker HLJ, O'Fallon WM. Predictive value of carotid bruit for carotid atherosclerosis. *Arch Neurol* 1989; 46:418–422.
47. Norris JW, Zhu CZ, Bornstein NM, Chambers BR. Vascular risks of asymptomatic carotid stenosis. *Stroke* 1991;22:1485–1490.
48. Kuller LH, Sutton KC. Carotid artery bruit: is it safe and effective to auscultate the neck? *Stroke* 1984;15:944–947.
49. Josse MO, Touboul PJ, Mas JL, Laplane D, Bousser MG. Prevalence of asymptomatic internal carotid artery stenosis. *Neuroepidemiology* 1987;6:150–152.
50. Hart RG, Easton JD. Management of cervical bruits and carotid stenosis in preoperative patients. *Stroke* 1983;14:290–297.
51. Chambers BR, Norris JW. Clinical significance of asymptomatic neck bruits. *Neurology* 1985; 35:742–745.
52. Sauve JS, Thorpe KE, Sackett DL, et al. Can bruits distinguish high-grade from moderate symptomatic carotid stenosis? The North American Symptomatic Carotid Endarterectomy Trial. *Ann Intern Med* 1994;120:633–637.
53. Gareeboo H. Severe anaemia as a cause of cranial bruit in adults. *BMJ* 1968;1:294.
54. Brott T, Tomsick T, Feinberg W, et al. Baseline silent cerebral infarction in the Asymptomatic Carotid Atherosclerosis Study. *Stroke* 1994; 25:1122–1129.
55. Bock RW, Gray-Weale AC, Mock PA, Robinson DA, Irwig L, Lusby RJ. The natural history of asymptomatic carotid artery disease. *J Vasc Surg* 1993;17:160–171.
56. Norris JW. Risk of cerebral infarction, myocardial infarction and vascular death in patients with asymptomatic carotid disease, transient ischemic attack and stroke. *Cerebrovasc Dis* 1992;2(Suppl):2–5.
57. Executive Committee for the Asymptomatic Carotid Atherosclerosis Study. Endarterectomy for asymptomatic carotid artery stenosis. *JAMA* 1995;273:1421–1428.
58. Olin JW, Fonseca C, Childs MB, Piedmonte MR, Hertzer NR, Young JR. The natural history of asymptomatic moderate internal carotid artery stenosis by duplex ultrasound. *Vasc Med* 1998;3:101–108.
59. Mackey AE, Abrahamowicz M, Langlois Y, et al. Outcome of asymptomatic patients with carotid disease. Asymptomatic Cervical Bruit Study Group.*Neurology* 1997;48: 896–903.
60. Bogousslavsky J, Despland PA, Regli F. Asymptomatic tight stenosis of the internal

carotid artery: long-term prognosis. *Neurology* 1986;36:861–863.
61. The European Carotid Surgery Trialists Collaborative Group. Risk of stroke in the distribution of an asymptomatic carotid artery. *Lancet* 1995;345:209–212.
62. Gerraty RP, Gates PC, Doyle JC. Carotid stenosis and perioperative stroke risk in symptomatic and asymptomatic patients undergoing vascular or coronary surgery. *Stroke* 1993;24:1115–1118.
63. Brener BJ, Brief DK, Alpert J, Goldenkranz RJ, Parsonnet V. The risk of stroke in patients with asymptomatic carotid stenosis undergoing cardiac surgery. A followup study. *J Vasc Surg* 1987;5:269–279.
64. Ropper AH, Wechsler LR, Wilson LS. Carotid bruit and the risk of stroke in elective surgery. *N Engl J Med* 1982;307:1388–1390.
65. Brott T, Toole JF. Medical compared with surgical treatment of asymptomatic carotid artery stenosis. *Ann Intern Med* 1995;123:720–722.
66. Cronenwett JL, Birkmeyer JD, Nackman GB, et al. Cost-effectiveness of carotid endarterectomy in asymptomatic patients. *J Vasc Surg* 1997; 25:298–309.
67. Chaturvedi S, Halliday A. Is another clinical trial warranted regarding endarterectomy for asymptomatic carotid stenosis? *Cerebrovasc Dis* 1998;8:210–213.
68. Hobson RW, Weiss DG, Fields WS, et al. Efficacy of carotid endarterectomy for asymptomatic carotid stenosis. The Veterans Affairs Cooperative Study Group. *N Engl J Med* 1993;328:221–227.
69. Lee TT, Solomon NA, Heidenreich PA, Oehlert J, Garber AM. Cost-effectiveness of screening for carotid stenosis in asymptomatic persons. *Ann Intern Med* 1997;126:337–346.
70. Libman RB, Sacco RL, Shi T, Correll JW, Mohr JP. Outcome after carotid endarterectomy for asymptomatic carotid stenosis. *Surg Neurol* 1994;41:443–449.
71. Barnett HJM, Haines SJ. Carotid endarterectomy for asymptomatic carotid stenosis. *N Engl J Med* 1993;328:276–278.
72. Barnett HJM, Meldrum HE, Eliasziw M. The dilemma of surgical treatment for patients with asymptomatic carotid disease. *Ann Intern Med* 1995;123:723–725.
73. Perry JR, Szalai JP, Norris JW. Consensus against both endarterectomy and routine screening for asymptomatic carotid artery stenosis. Canadian Stroke Consortium. *Arch Neurol* 1997;54:25–28.
74. Castaldo JE, Nelson JJ, Reed JF, Longenecker JE, Toole JF. The delay in reporting symptoms of carotid artery stenosis in an at-risk population. The Asymptomatic Carotid Atherosclerosis Study experience: a statement of concern regarding watchful waiting. *Arch Neurol* 1997;54:1267–1271.
75. Ivey TD, Strandness E, Williams DB, Langlois Y, Misbach GA, Kruse AP. Management of patients with carotid bruit undergoing cardiopulmonary bypass. *J Thorac Cardiovasc Surg* 1984;87: 183–189.
76. Gil-Peralta A, Mayol A, Marcos JR, et al. Percutaneous transluminal angioplasty of the symptomatic atherosclerotic carotid arteries. Results, complications, and follow-up. *Stroke* 1996;27:2271–2273.
77. Jordan WDJ, Voellinger DC, Fisher WS, Redden D, McDowell HA. A comparison of carotid angioplasty with stenting versus endarterectomy with regional anesthesia. *J Vasc Surg* 1998;28: 397–402.
78. Ueda S, Fujitsu K, Inomori S, Kuwabara T. Thrombotic occlusion of the middle cerebral artery. *Stroke* 1992;23:1761–1766.
79. Lyrer PA, Engelter S, Radu EW, Steck AJ. Cerebral infarcts related to isolated middle cerebral artery stenosis. *Stroke* 1997;28:1022–1027.
80. Caplan L, Babikian V, Helgason C, et al. Occlusive disease of the middle cerebral artery.*Neurology* 1985;35:975–982.
81. The EC/IC Bypass Study Group. Failure of extracranial-intracranial arterial bypass to reduce the risk of ischemic stroke. Results of an international randomized trial. *N Engl J Med* 1985;313:1191–1200.
82. Chimowitz MI, Kokkinos J, Strong J, et al. The Warfarin-Aspirin Symptomatic Intracranial Disease Study. *Neurology* 1995;45:1488–1493.
83. McKenzie JD, Wallace RC, Dean BL, Flom RA, Khayata MH. Preliminary results of intracranial angioplasty for vascular stenosis caused by atherosclerosis and vasculitis. *Am J Neuroradiol* 1996;17:263–268.
84. Mori T, Mori K, Fukuoka M, Arisawa M, Honda S. Percutaneous transluminal cerebral angioplasty: serial angiographic follow-up after successful dilatation. *Neuroradiology* 1997;39:111–116.
85. Kappelle LJ, Eliaziw M, Fox AJ, Sharpe BL, Barnett HJM, for the North American Symptomatic Carotid Endarterectomy Trial (NASCET) Group. Importance of intracranial atherosclerotic disease in patients with symptomatic stenosis of the internal carotid artery. *Stroke* 1999;30:282–286.
86. Caplan L, Schoene WC. Clinical features of subcortical arteriosclerotic encephalopathy (Binswanger disease). *Neurology* 1978;28: 1206–1215.
87. Kinkel WR, Jacobs L, Polachini I, Bates V, Heffner RR, Jr. Subcortical arteriosclerotic encephalopathy (Binswanger's disease). Computed tomographic, nuclear magnetic resonance, and clinical correlations. *Arch Neurol* 1985;42:951–959.
88. Muller-Kuppers M, Graf KJ, Pessin MS, DeWitt LD, Caplan LR. Intracranial vertebral artery disease in the New England Medical Center Posterior Circulation Registry. *Eur Neurol* 1997;37:146–156.
89. Pessin MS, Gorelick PB, Kwan ES, Caplan LR. Basilar artery stenosis: middle and distal segments. *Neurology* 1987;37:1742–1746.
90. Nakayama T, Tanaka K, Kaneko M, Yokoyama T, Uemura K. Thrombolysis and angioplasty for acute occlusion of intracranial vertebrobasilar arteries. Report of three cases. *J Neurosurg* 1998;88:919–922.
91. Nakatsuka H, Ueda T, Ohta S, Sakaki S. Successful percutaneous transluminal angioplasty

for basilar artery stenosis: technical case report. *Neurosurgery* 1996;39:161–164.
92. Anson JA, Lawton MT, Spetzler RF. Characteristics and surgical treatment of dolichoectatic and fusiform aneurysms. *J Neurosurg* 1996;84:185–193.
93. Nakatomi H, Segawa H, Kurata A, et al. Clinicopathological study of intracranial fusiform and dolichoectatic aneurysms. Insight on the mechanism of growth. *Stroke* 2000;31:896–900.
94. Mizutani T. A fatal, chronically growing basilar artery: a new type of dissecting aneurysm. *J Neurosurg* 1996;84:962–971.
95. Mizutani T, Aruga T. "Dolichoectatic" intracranial vertebrobasilar dissecting aneurysm. *Neurosurgery* 1992;31:765–773.
96. Maisey DN, Cosh JA. Basilar artery aneurysm and Anderson-Fabry disease. *J Neurol Neurosurg Psychiatry* 1980;43:85–87.
97. Mizutani T, Miki Y, Kojima H, Suzuki H. Proposed classification of nonatherosclerotic cerebral fusiform and dissecting aneurysms. *Neurosurgery* 1999;45:253–260.
98. Ince B, Petty GW, Brown RD, Jr., Chu CP, Sicks JD, Whisnant JP. Dolichoectasia of the intracranial arteries in patients with first ischemic stroke: a population-based study. *Neurology* 1998; 50:1694–1698.
99. Bogousslavsky J, Regli F, Maeder P, Meuli R, Nader J. The etiology of posterior circulation infarcts. A prospective study using magnetic resonance imaging and magnetic resonance angiography. *Neurology* 1993;43:1528–1533.
100. Pessin MS, Chimowitz MI, Levine SR, et al. Stroke in patients with fusiform vertebrobasilar aneurysms. *Neurology* 1989;39:16–21.
101. Besson G, Bogousslavsky J, Moulin T, Hommel M. Vertebrobasilar infarcts in patients with dolichoectatic basilar artery. *Acta Neurol Scand* 1995;91:37–42.
102. Watanabe T, Sato K, Yoshimoto T. Basilar artery occlusion caused by thrombosis of atherosclerotic fusiform aneurysm of the basilar artery. *Stroke* 1994;25:1068–1070.
103. Schwartz A, Rautenberg W, Hennerici M. Dolichoectatic intracranial arteries: Review of selected aspects. *Cerebrovasc Dis* 1993;3:273–279.
104. Hirsh LF, Gonzalez CF. Fusiform basilar aneurysm simulating carotid transient ischemic attacks.*Stroke* 1979;10:598–601.
105. Echiverri HC, Rubino FA, Gupta SR, Gujrati M. Fusiform aneurysm of the vertebrobasilar arterial system. *Stroke* 1989;20:1741–1747.
106. Aichner FT, Felber SR, Birbamer GG, Posch A. Magnetic resonance imaging and magnetic resonance angiography of vertebrobasilar dolichoectasia. *Cerebrovasc Dis* 1993;3:280–284.
107. Salbeck R, Busse O, Reinbold WD. MRI findings in megadolicho-basilar artery. *Cerebrovasc Dis* 1993;3:309–312.
108. Vishteh AG, Spetzler RF. Evolution of a dolichoectatic aneurysm into a giant serpentine aneurysm during long-term follow up. *J Neurosurg* 1999;91:346–352.
109. Iwama T, Andoh T, Sakai N, Iwata T, Hirata T, Yamada H. Dissecting and fusiform aneurysms of vertebro-basilar systems. MR imaging. *Neuroradiology* 1990;32:272–279.
110. Klotzsch C, Kuhne D, Berlit P. Diagnosis of giant fusiform basilar aneurysm by color-coded transcranial duplex sonography. *Cerebrovasc Dis* 1994;4:371–372.
111. Molnar RG, Naslund TC. Vertebral artery surgery. *Surg Clin N Am* 1998;78:901–913.
112. Wityk RJ, Chang HM, Rosengart A, et al. Proximal extracranial vertebral artery disease in the New England Medical Center Posterior Circulation Registry. *Arch Neurol* 1998;55:470–478.
113. Pessin MS, Daneault N, Kwan ES, Eisengart MA, Caplan LR. Local embolism from vertebral artery occlusion. *Stroke* 1988;19:112–115.
114. Koroshetz WJ, Ropper AH. Artery-to-artery embolism causing stroke in the posterior circulation. *Neurology* 1987;37:292–295.
115. Caplan LR, Amarenco P, Rosengart A, et al. Embolism from vertebral artery origin occlusive disease. *Neurology* 1992;42:1505–1512.
116. Caplan LR. Brain embolism, revisited. *Neurology* 1993;43:1281–1287.
117. Levine SR, Quint DJ, Pessin MS, Boulos RS, Welch KM. Intraluminal clot in the vertebrobasilar circulation: clinical and radiologic features. *Neurology* 1989;39:515–522.
118. Shin HK, Yoo KM, Chang HM, Caplan LR. Bilateral intracranial vertebral artery disease in the New England Medical Center Posterior Circulation Registry. *Arch Neurol* 1999;56: 1353–1358.
119. Kuether TA, Nesbit GM, Clark WM, Barnwell SL. Rotational vertebral artery occlusion: a mechanism of vertebrobasilar insufficiency. *Neurosurgery* 1997;41:427–432.
120. Zelenock GB, Cronenwett JL, Graham LM, et al. Brachiocephalic arterial occlusions and stenoses. Manifestations and management of complex lesions. *Arch Surg* 1985;120:370–376.
121. Lindner A, Charra B, Sherrard DJ, Scribner BH. Accelerated atherosclerosis in prolonged maintenance hemodialysis. *N Engl J Med* 1974;290:697–701.
122. Jungers P, Massy ZA, Khoa TN, et al. Incidence and risk factors of atherosclerotic cardiovascular accidents in predialysis chronic renal failure patients: a prospective study. *Nephrology, Dialysis, Transplantation* 1997;12:2597–2602.
123. Amar AP, Levy ML, Giannotta SL. Iatrogenic vertebrobasilar insufficiency after surgery of the subclavian or brachial artery: review of three cases. *Neurosurgery* 1998;43:1450–1457.
124. Fields WS, Lemak NA. Joint Study of Extracranial Arterial Occlusion. VII. Subclavian steal—a review of 168 cases. *JAMA* 1972; 222:1139–1143.
125. de Bray JM, Zenglein JP, Laroche JP, et al. Effect of subclavian syndrome on the basilar artery. *Acta Neurol Scand* 1994;90:174–178.
126. Yip PK, Liu HM, Hwang BS, Chen RC. Subclavian steal phenomenon: a correlation between duplex sonographic and angiographic findings. *Neuroradiology* 1992;34:279–282.
127. Hennerici M, Klemm C, Rautenberg W. The subclavian steal phenomenon: a common vascular

disorder with rare neurologic deficits. *Neurology* 1988;38:669–673.

128. Law MM, Colburn MD, Moore WS, Quinones-Baldrich WJ, Machleder HI, Gelabert HA. Carotid-subclavian bypass for brachiocephalic occlusive disease. Choice of conduit and long-term follow-up. *Stroke* 1995;26:1565–1571.
129. Mingoli A, Feldhaus RJ, Farina C, Naspetti R, Schultz RD, Cavallaro. Concomitant subclavian and carotid artery disease: the need for a combined surgical correction. *J Cardiovasc Surg* 1992;33:593–598.
130. Tunick PA, Kronzon I. Protruding atherosclerotic plaque in the aortic arch of patients with systemic embolization: a new finding seen by transesophageal echocardiography. *Am Heart J* 1990;120:658–660.
131. Leung DY, Black IW, Cranney GB, et al. Selection of patients for transesophageal echocardiography after stroke and systemic embolic events. Role of transthoracic echocardiography. *Stroke* 1995;26:1820–1824.
132. Geraci A, Weinberger J. Natural history of aortic arch atherosclerotic plaque. *Neurology* 2000; 54:749–751.
133. Lehmann ED, Hopkins KD, Gosling RG. Atherosclerosis in the ascending aorta and risk of ischaemic stroke. *Lancet* 1995;346:589–590.
134. Kronzon I, Tunick PA. Atheromatous disease of the thoracic aorta: pathologic and clinical implications. *Ann Intern Med* 1997;126:629–637.
135. Devuyst G, Bogousslavsky J. Status of patent foramen ovale, atrial septal aneurysm, atrial septal defect and aortic arch atheroma as risk factors for stroke. *Neuroepidemiology* 1997;16: 217–223.
136. Di Tullio MR, Sacco RL, Homma S. Atherosclerotic disease of the aortic arch as a risk factor for recurrent ischemic stroke. *N Engl J Med* 1996;335:1464–1465.
137. Heinzlef O, Cohen A, Amarenco P. An update on aortic causes of ischemic stroke. *Curr Opin Neurol* 1997;10:64–72.
138. Donnan GA, Jones EF. Aortic arch atheroma and stroke. *Cerebrovasc Dis* 1995;5:10–13.
139. Mitusch R, Doherty C, Wucherpfennig H, et al. Vascular events during follow-up in patients with aortic arch atherosclerosis. *Stroke* 1997; 28:36–39.
140. Mitusch R, Stierle U, Tepe C, Kummer-Kloess D, Kessler C, Sheikhzadeh A. Systemic embolism in aortic arch atheromatosis. *Eur Heart J* 1994;15:1373–1380.
141. Tenenbaum A, Fisman EZ, Schneiderman J, et al. Disrupted mobile aortic plaques are a major risk factor for systemic embolism in the elderly. *Cardiology* 1998;89:246–251.
142. Laperche T, Laurian C, Roudaut R, Steg PG. Mobile thromboses of the aortic arch without aortic debris. A transesophageal echocardiographic finding associated with unexplained arterial embolism. The Filiale Echocardiographie de la Societe Francaise de Cardiologie. *Circulation* 1997;96:288–294.
143. Davila-Roman VG, Barzilai B, Wareing TH, Murphy SF, Schechtman KB, Kouchoukos NT. Atherosclerosis of the ascending aorta. Prevalence and role as an independent predictor of cerebrovascular events in cardiac patients. *Stroke* 1994;25:2010–2016.
144. Ferrari E, Vidal R, Chevallier T, Baudouy M. Atherosclerosis of the thoracic aorta and aortic debris as a marker of poor prognosis: benefit of oral anticoagulants. *J Am Coll Cardiol* 1999;33:1317–1322.
145. Jones EF, Kalman JM, Calafiore P, Tonkin AM, Donnan GA. Proximal aortic atheroma. An independent risk factor for cerebral ischemia. *Stroke* 1995;26:218–224.
146. Ricotta JJ, Faggioli GL, Castilone A, Hassett JM. Risk factors for stroke after cardiac surgery: Buffalo Cardiac-Cerebral Study Group. *J Vasc Surg* 1995;21:359–363.
147. Ribakove GH, Katz ES, Galloway AC, et al. Surgical implications of transesophageal echocardiography to grade the atheromatous aortic arch. *Ann Thorac Surg* 1992;53:758–761.
148. Masdeu JC, Gorelick PB. Thalamic astasia: inability to stand after unilateral thalamic lesions. *Ann Neurol* 1988;23:596–603.
149. Tomochika Y, Tanaka N, Ono S, et al. Assessment by transesophageal echography of atherosclerosis of the descending thoracic aorta in patients with hypercholesterolemia. *Am J Cardiol* 1999;83:703–709.
150. Barbut D, Lo YW, Hartman GS, et al. Aortic atheroma is related to outcome but not numbers of emboli during coronary bypass. *Ann Thorac Surg* 1997;64:454–459.
151. Choudhary SK, Bhan A, Sharma R, et al. Aortic atherosclerosis and perioperative stroke in patients undergoing coronary artery bypass: role of intra-operative transesophageal echocardiography. *International J Cardiol* 1997;61:31–38.
152. Tunick PA, Culliford AT, Lamparello PJ, Kronzon I. Atheromatosis of the aortic arch as an occult source of multiple systemic emboli. *Ann Intern Med* 1991;114:391–392.
153. Crawford ES. The diagnosis and management of aortic dissection. *JAMA* 1990;264:2537–2541.
154. Montgomery DH, Ververis JJ, McGorisk G, et al. Natural history of severe atheromatous disease of the thoracic aorta: a transesophageal echocardiographic study. *J Am Coll Cardiol* 1996;27: 95–101.
155. Tunick PA, Perez JL, Kronzon I. Protruding atheromas in the thoracic aorta and systemic embolization. *Ann Intern Med* 1991;115: 423–427.
156. Karalis DG, Chandrasekaran K, Victor MF, Ross JJJ, Mintz GS. Recognition and embolic potential of intraaortic atherosclerotic debris. *J Am Coll Cardiol* 1991;17:73–78.
157. Toyoda K, Yasaka M, Nagata S, Yamaguchi T. Aortogenic embolic stroke: a transesophageal echocardiographic approach. *Stroke* 1992; 23:1056–1061.
158. Stone DA, Hawke MW, LaMonte M, et al. Ulcerated atherosclerotic plaques in the thoracic aorta are associated with cryptogenic stroke: a multiplane transesophageal echocardiographic study. *Am Heart J* 1995;130:105–108.

159. Rauh R, Fischereder M, Spengel FA. Transesophageal echocardiography in patients with focal cerebral ischemia of unknown cause. *Stroke* 1996;27:691–694.
160. Inoue T, Oku K, Kimoto K, et al. Relationship of cigarette smoking to the severity of coronary and thoracic aortic atherosclerosis. *Cardiology* 1995;86:374–379.
161. Konecky N, Malinow MR, Tunick PA, et al. Correlation between plasma homocyst(e)ine and aortic atherosclerosis. *Am Heart J* 1997;133:534–540.
162. Blackshear JL, Pearce LA, Hart RG, et al. Aortic plaque in atrial fibrillation: prevalence, predictors, and thromboembolic implications. *Stroke* 1999;30:834–840.
163. Kistler JP. The risk of embolic stroke. Another piece of the puzzle. *N Engl J Med* 1994;331: 1517–1519.
164. Jones EF, Donnan GA. The proximal aorta: a source of stroke. *Baillieres Clin Neurol* 1995;4: 207–220.
165. Amarenco P, Cohen A, Tzourio C, et al. Atherosclerotic disease of the aortic arch and the risk of ischemic stroke. *N Engl J Med* 1994;331:1474–1479.
166. Cohen A, Tzourio C, Bertrand B, Chauvel C, Bousser MG, Amarenco P. Aortic plaque morphology and vascular events: a follow-up study in patients with ischemic stroke. FAPS Investigators. French Study of Aortic Plaques in Stroke. *Circulation* 1997;96:3838–3841.
167. The French Study of Aortic Plaques in Stroke Group. Atherosclerotic disease of the aortic arch as a risk factor for recurrent ischemic stroke. *N Engl J Med* 1999;334:1216–1221.
168. Di Tullio MR, Sacco RL, Gersony D, et al. Aortic atheromas and acute ischemic stroke: a transesophageal echocardiographic study in an ethnically mixed population. *Neurology* 1996;46: 1560–1566.
169. Spittell PC, Spittell JAJ, Joyce JW, et al. Clinical features and differential diagnosis of aortic dissection: experience with 236 cases (1980 through 1990). *Mayo Clin Proc* 1993;68:642–651.
170. Flemming KD, Brown RD, Jr. Acute cerebral infarction caused by aortic dissection. Caution in the thrombolytic era. *Stroke* 1999;30:477–478.
171. Khan IA, Vasavada BC, Sacchi TJ. Asymptomatic dissection of the ascending aorta: diagnosis by transesophageal echocardiography. *Am J Emerg Med* 1999;17:172–173.
172. Kimura BJ, Phan JN, Housman LB. Utility of contrast echocardiography in the diagnosis of aortic dissection. *J Am Soc Echocardiogr* 1999;12:155–159.
173. Dressler FA, Craig WR, Castello R, Labovitz AJ. Mobile aortic atheroma and systemic emboli: efficacy of anticoagulation and influence of plaque morphology on recurrent stroke. *J Am Coll Cardiol* 1998;31:134–138.
174. Bojar RM, Payne DD, Murphy RE, et al. Surgical treatment of systemic atheroembolism from the thoracic aorta. *Ann Thorac Surg* 1996;61: 1389–1393.
175. Belden JR, Caplan LR, Bojar RM, Payne DD, Blachman P. Treatment of multiple cerebral emboli from an ulcerated, thrombogenic ascending aorta with aortectomy and graft replacement. *Neurology* 1997;49:621–622.
176. King RC, Kanithanon RC, Shockey KS, Spotnitz WD, Tribble CG, Kron IL. Replacing the atherosclerotic ascending aorta is a high-risk procedure. *Ann Thorac Surg* 1998;66:396–401.
177. Karanjia PN, Madden KP, Lobner S. Coexistence of abdominal aortic aneurysm in patients with carotid stenosis. *Stroke* 1994;25:627–630.
178. Besson G, Hommel M, Perret J. Historical aspects of the lacunar concept. *Cerebrovasc Dis* 1991;1:306–310.
179. Arboix A, Marti-Vilalta JL, Garcia JH. Clinical study of 227 patients with lacunar infarcts. *Stroke* 1990;21:842–847.
180. You R, McNeil JJ, O'Malley HM, Davis SM, Donnan GA. Risk factors for lacunar infarction syndromes. *Neurology* 1995;45:1483–1487.
181. Sacco SE, Whisnant JP, Broderick JP, Phillips SJ, O'Fallon WM. Epidemiological characteristics of lacunar infarcts in a population. *Stroke* 1991;22:1236–1241.
182. Brower MC, Rollins N, Roach ES. Basal ganglia and thalamic infarction in children. Cause and clinical features. *Arch Neurol* 1996;53: 1252–1256.
183. Fisher CM. A lacunar stroke. The dysarthria-clumsy hand syndrome. *Neurology* 1967;17: 614–617.
184. Fisher CM. Lacunar strokes and infarcts: a review. *Neurology* 1982;32:871–876.
185. Fisher CM. Ataxic hemiparesis. A pathologic study. *Arch Neurol* 1978;35:126–128.
186. Fisher CM, Caplan LR. Basilar artery branch occlusion: a cause of pontine infarction. *Neurology* 1971;21:900–905.
187. Fisher CM, Curry HB. Pure motor hemiplegia. *Trans Am Neurol Assoc* 1964;89:94–97.
188. Fisher CM, Cole M. Homolateral ataxia and rural paresis. A vascular syndrome. *J Neurol Neurosurg Psychiatry* 1965;28:48–55.
189. Fisher CM. Pure sensory stroke involving face, arm and leg. *Neurology* 1965;15:76–80.
190. Fisher CM. Lacunes: small, deep cerebral infarcts. *Neurology* 1965;50:841–852.
191. Bogousslavsky J, Martin R, Moulin T. Homolateral ataxia and crural paresis: a syndrome of anterior cerebral artery territory infarction. *J Neurol Neurosurg Psychiatry* 1992; 55:1146–1149.
192. Bogousslavsky J, Regli F. Capsular genu syndrome. *Neurology* 1990;40:1499–1502.
193. Chamorro A, Sacco RL, Mohr JP, et al. Clinical-computed tomographic correlations of lacunar infarction in the Stroke Data Bank. *Stroke* 1991; 22:175–181.
194. Terai S, Hori T, Miake S, Tamaki KSA. Mechanism in progressive lacunar infarction: A case report with magnetic resonance imaging. *Arch Neurol* 2000;57:225–232.
195. Landau WM. Clinical neuromythology VI. Au clair de lacune: holy, wholly, holey logic. *Neurology* 1989;39:725–730.
196. Gordon DL, Bendixen BH, Adams HP, Jr., et al. Interphysician agreement in the diagnosis of

subtypes of acute ischemic stroke: implications for clinical trials. The TOAST Investigators. *Neurology* 1993;43:1021–1027.
197. Toni D, Fiorelli M, De Michele M, et al. Clinical and prognostic correlates of stroke subtype misdiagnosis within 12 hours from onset. *Stroke* 1995;26:1837–1840.
198. Landi G, Anzalone N, Cella E, Boccardi E, Musicco M. Are sensorimotor strokes lacunar strokes? A case-control study of lacunar and non-lacunar infarcts. *J Neurol Neurosurg Psychiatry* 1991;54:1063–1068.
199. Hommel M, Besson G, Le Bas JF, et al. Prospective study of lacunar infarction using magnetic resonance imaging. *Stroke* 1990;21: 546–554.
200. Boiten J, Lodder J. Lacunar infarcts: pathogenesis and validity of the clinical syndromes. *Stroke* 1991;22:1374–1378.
201. Kappelle LJ, van Latum JC, Koudstaal PJ, van Gijn J. Transient ischaemic attacks and small-vessel disease. Dutch TIA Study Group. *Lancet* 1991;337:339–341.
202. Lodder J, Bamford J, Kappelle J, Boiten J. What causes false clinical prediction of small deep infarcts? *Stroke* 1994;25:86–91.
203. Bladin PF, Berkovic SF. Striatocapsular infarction. *Neurology* 1984;34:1423–1430.
204. Donnan GA, Bladin PF, Berkovic SF, Longley WA, Saling MM. The stroke syndrome of striatocapsular infarction. *Brain* 1991;114:51–70.
205. Ghika J, Bogousslavsky J, Regli F. Infarcts in the territory of lenticulostriate branches from the middle cerebral artery. Etiological factors and clinical features in 65 cases. *Schweiz Arch Neurol Psychiatr* 1991;142:5–18.
206. Mast H, Thompson JL, Voller H, Mohr JP, Marx P. Cardiac sources of embolism in patients with pial artery infarcts and lacunar lesions. *Stroke* 1994;25:776–781.
207. Kappelle LJ, Koudstaal PJ, van Gijn J, Ramos LM, Keunen JE. Carotid angiography in patients with lacunar infarction. A prospective study. *Stroke* 1988;19:1093–1096.
208. Luijckx G, Boiten J, Lodder J, Heuts-van Raak L, Kessels F. Cardiac and carotid embolism, and other rare definite disorders are unlikely causes of lacunar ischaemic stroke in young patients. *Cerebrovasc Dis* 1996;6:28–31.
209. Fisher CM. Lacunar Infarcts—a review. *Cerebrovasc Dis* 1991;1:311–320.
210. Mohr JP. Lacunes. *Stroke* 1982;13:3–11.
211. Vishteh AG, Marciano FF, David CA, Schievink WI, Zabramski JM, Spetzler RF. Long-term graft patency rates and clinical outcomes after revascularization for symptomatic traumatic internal carotid artery dissection. *Neurosurgery* 1998; 43:761–768.
212. Bamford J, Sandercock P, Dennis M, Burn J, Warlow C. Classification and natural history of clinically identifiable subtypes of cerebral infarction. *Lancet* 1991;337:1521–1526.
213. Anderson CS, Jamrozik KD, Broadhuest RJ, Stewart-Wynne EG. Predicting survival for one year among different subtypes of stroke. *Stroke* 1994;25:1935–1944.
214. Landi G, Cella E, Boccardi E, Musicco M. Lacunar versus non-lacunar infarcts: pathogenetic and prognostic differences. *J Neurol Neurosurg Psychiatry* 1992;55:441–445.
215. Boiten J, Lodder J. Prognosis for survival, handicap, and recurrence of stroke in lacunar and superficial infarction. *Cerebrovasc Dis* 1993;3: 221–226.
216. Kappelle LJ, van Latum JC, van Swieten JC, et al. Recurrent stroke after transient ischaemic attack or minor ischaemic stroke: does the distinction between small and large vessel disease remain true to type? Dutch TIA Trial Study Group. *J Neurol Neurosurg Psychiatry* 1995;59:127–131.
217. Benesch CG, Chimowitz MI, for the WASID Investigators. Best treatment of intracranial arterial stenosis? 50 years of uncertainty. *Neurology* 2000;55:465–466.
218. Thijs VN, Albers GW. Symptomatic intracranial atherosclerosis. Outcome of patients who fail antithrombotic therapy. *Neurology* 2000;55: 490–497.

Chapter 6

CARDIAC SOURCES OF EMBOLISM

Heart disease is a leading potential cause of ischemic neurological symptoms. In addition to causing ischemic stroke secondary to cardioembolism, heart disease also produces recurrent neurological complaints that are included in the differential diagnosis of transient ischemic attack (TIA). Symptoms including wooziness, dizziness, or syncope often are secondary to heart diseases that lead to transient declines in cardiac output. Intermittent cardiac arrhythmias, most commonly *intermittent complete heart block* or *the bradycardia–tachycardia* (*sick sinus syndrome*), are frequent cardiac causes of recurrent syncope in the elderly. Although these cardiac rhythm disturbances are important markers of severe heart disease that lead to transient episodes of loss of consciousness, they generally do not lead to embolism to the brain. Despite the relatively low risk of stroke directly related to these cardiac arrhythmias, they are associated with high risk of cardiac death.[1]

Cardioembolism accounts for approximately 20%–25% of ischemic strokes and is a leading cause of stroke in persons of all

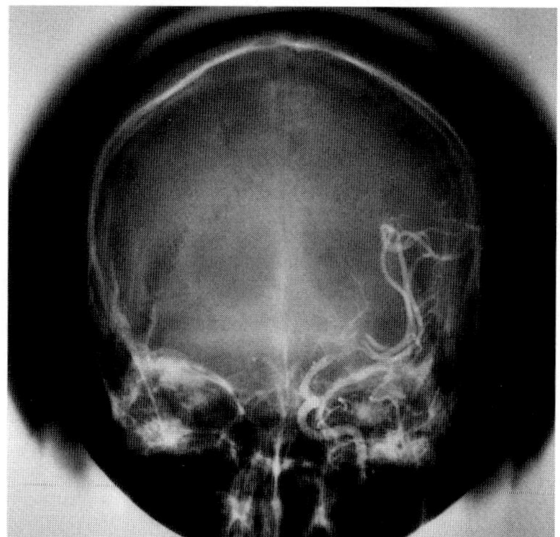

Figure 6–1. Middle cerebral artery occlusion secondary to cardioembolism.

ages (Fig. 6–1). Emboli from the heart can go to any intracranial artery. Both proximal and distal intracranial arterial occlusions can develop. As a result, cardioembolism should be considered in the differential diagnosis for cause of symptoms in any patient with a TIA or an ischemic stroke in either the carotid or the vertebrobasilar circulation.[2,3] Because of the widespread prevalence and age-related effects of atherosclerosis in persons older than 65, the relative importance of cardioembolism is less in this group. In contrast, because atherosclerosis is less common in children and young adults, the relative incidence of cardioembolism is greater in children and young adults, and heart diseases account for a sizeable proportion of strokes in these age groups. The types of heart disease leading to stroke also varies by age; coronary artery disease and atrial fibrillation are leading etiologies in persons older than 45, whereas valvular diseases are more prominent in younger persons. Cardioembolic stroke affects men and women of all ethnic groups. No data report a particular relationship between race and the frequency of cardioembolism. Because symptomatic coronary artery disease appears at earlier ages in men, it is a leading substrate for cardioembolic stroke in middle-age men. Conversely, atrial fibrillation is a leading cause of stroke in women, especially in those older than 75.

Most patients with cardioembolic stroke have a prior history of heart disease. Still, stroke can be a first presentation of otherwise occult heart disease. In general, patients have cardiac symptoms, including chest pain, fatigue, or dyspnea, and clinical evidence of heart disease, such as a murmur, cardiomegaly, cyanosis, or peripheral edema. Patients also may have been treated with cardiovascular medications or cardiac procedures. A past history of an abnormal chest x-ray or electrocardiogram also might suggest structural heart disease.

CATEGORIES OF HEART DISEASE THAT LEAD TO EMBOLISM

The cardiac lesions that lead to embolism can be divided into several categories, including arrhythmias, structural abnormalities of the cardiac valves (particularly mitral and aortic), structural abnormalities of the left ventricle or the atrium, and structural abnormalities that permit an intracardiac left-to-right flow of blood (Fig. 6–2). A combination of conditions may be detected in many patients. In particular, arrhythmias are likely to complicate structural lesions. Cardioembolic stroke is a potential complication of a number of cardiovascular procedures, including coronary artery bypass grafting, valve replacement, and cardiac transplantation (Table 6–1). Although stroke less commonly complicates other cardiac procedures, such as cardiac catheterization, neurological sequelae also are possible in this setting.

Table 6–1. **Cardiovascular Procedures Associated with Embolism to the Brain**

Cardiac catheterization
Electrophysiological studies of the heart
Placement of pacemaker
Cardioversion
Cardiac assist devices
Coronary artery bypass grafting
Valvular replacement
Valvuloplasty
Cardiac transplantation

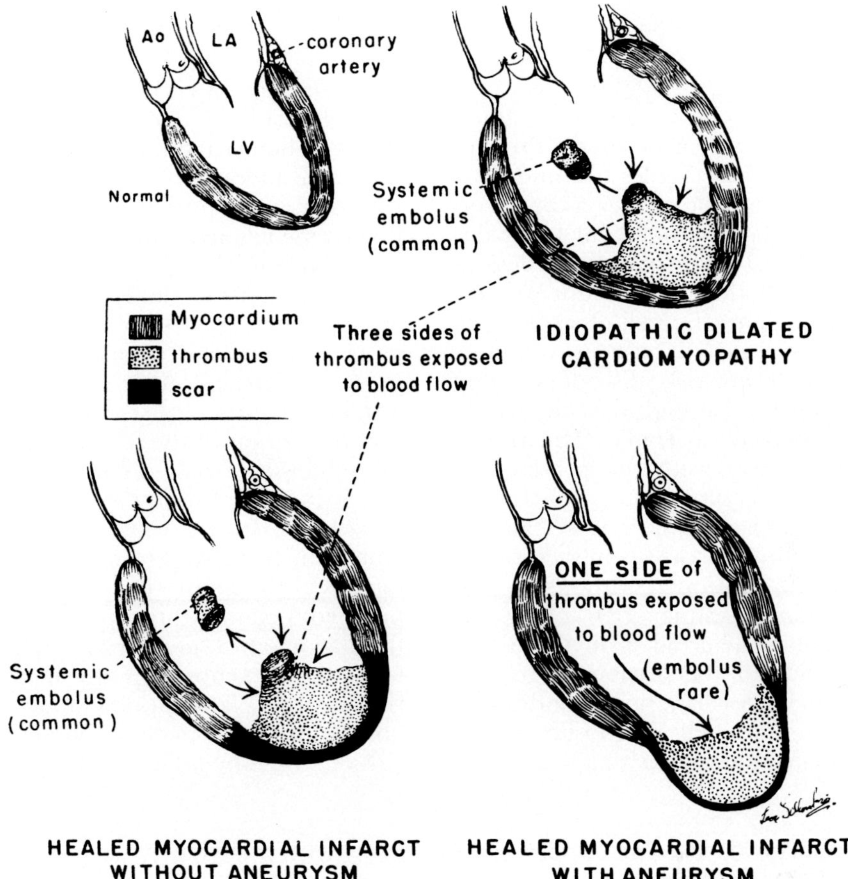

Figure 6–2. Features predisposing to embolization from a mural thrombus arising within the left ventricle. (Reprinted from Cabin HS, Roberts WC. Left ventricular aneurysm, intra-aneurysmal thrombus, and systemic embolus in coronary heart disease. *Chest* 1980;77:586, with permission.)

Besides acute procedure-related neurological events, embolism to the brain is a long-term risk following cardiovascular interventions, such as placement of a mechanical valve or heart transplantation.

The advent of new imaging studies to assess the heart, in particularly transesophageal echocardiography (TEE) has led to the detection of a number of structural abnormalities that foster embolism to the brain. Among the cardiac findings that have received considerable recent attention are patent foramen ovale, atrial septal aneurysm, left atrial turbulence, fibrous strands on the mitral valve, and Lambl excrescences. Several of these cardiac findings are prevalent in the general population and can be detected in healthy persons. Thus, their significance is unclear when they are detected by TEE performed as part of the evaluation of a patient with a stroke. Because these abnormalities have received attention only during the last few years, epidemiological and natural history data about these changes are not yet available. More research on the importance of several cardiac abnormalities is needed to provide solid information about the risks of embolism to the brain. Once this information is available, the usefulness of interventions to lower these risks can be tested in clinical trials.[4] In the meantime, caution should be exercised in ascribing stroke to cardioembolism when one of these newly described findings is the only cardiac abnormality identified.

Higher- and Lower-Risk Cardiac Diseases

Cardiac lesions can be divided into higher- and lower-risk categories based on currently available data (Tables 6–2 and 6–3). A high risk for embolic stroke has been correlated with a large number of heart diseases.[5] The list of lower-risk cardiac lesions involves some degree of uncertainty. Because data about the risk of stroke with some of these heart diseases are limited, some of the lower-risk disorders might need to be denoted as high risk when additional data become available. The risk of embolism increases with the presence of cardiovascular complications, including arrhythmias and congestive heart failure. As a rule of thumb, cardioembolic stroke usually can be diagnosed without a great deal of additional testing when a high-risk cardiac lesion is detected. Conversely, the stroke should not be attributed to cardioembolism if a low-risk heart condition is found until additional diagnostic studies have eliminated alternative diagnoses.

ATRIAL FIBRILLATION

Atrial fibrillation is the most common cardiac abnormality correlated with embolic stroke. The arrhythmia appears to predispose thromboembolism by reducing the contraction of the left atrium, decreasing flow in the left atrial appendage, increasing turbulence in the left atrium, and leading to enlargement of the left atrium and left atrial appendage.[6] All of these factors promote stasis and the formation of clots within the left atrium.[7] It is not clear whether atrial fibrillation is the cause or a complication of dilation of the left atrium. The risk of embolism in patients with the arrhythmia is increased by the presence of structural heart disease. Conversely, the risk of embolism from structural heart disease is increased by the presence of atrial fibrillation. For example, the presence of atrial fibrillation after myocardial infarction or with mitral stenosis greatly increases the risk of stroke. The finding of atrial fibrillation is associated with an increase in the risk of stroke by a factor of 5–7 times that

Table 6–2. **Cardiac Conditions Associated with a Higher Risk for Embolism**

Atrial fibrillation with structural heart disease	Acute myocardial infarction
Left intraventricular thrombus	Dilated cardiomyopathy
Rheumatic mitral stenosis	Infective endocarditis
Non-bacterial thrombotic endocarditis	Libman-Sacks endocarditis
Mechanical prosthetic mitral valve	Atrial myxoma
Left atrial appendage thrombus	Left atrial thrombus

Table 6–3. **Cardiac Conditions Associated with an Uncertain or Lower Risk for Embolism**

Lone atrial fibrillation	Sick sinus syndrome
Ventricular akinetic or hypokinetic segment	Ventricular aneurysm
Rheumatic aortic stenosis	Bicuspid aortic valve
Mitral annulus calcification	Calcific aortic stenosis
Mitral valve prolapse	Atrial septal aneurysm
Bioprosthetic mitral valve	Patent foramen ovale
Mechanial prosthetic aortic valve	Atrial septal defect
Lambl excresence	Mitral valve strands
Aneurysm of the sinus of Valsalva	Idiopathic hypertrophic subaortic stenosis

found in persons with sinus rhythm.[8] In persons who have heart disease not complicated by atrial fibrillation, the risk of stroke is approximately 6% per year. The presence of arrhythmia increases this risk to approximately 15% per year.[8,9]

Approximately 10% of patients with ischemic stroke will have atrial fibrillation diagnosed.[10] Clinically silent strokes that are found on brain imaging studies also are more common in persons with atrial fibrillation. European investigators found a prevalence of 14% among asymptomatic patients with atrial fibrillation.[11] Asymptomatic embolization can be detected by transcranial Doppler ultrasonography in a sizeable proportion of patients with non-valvular atrial fibrillation.[12] The assumption is that some of these emboli are producing the small infarctions detected by brain imaging.

Although the presence of atrial fibrillation is not associated with an increased risk of early recurrent stroke, the overall mortality is high in persons with the arrhythmia.[13] The 30-day fatality rate after stroke in persons in the Oxfordshire Community Stroke Project was 23% when atrial fibrillation was present and 8% if sinus rhythm was found.[10] Some of the increased early mortality is secondary to the more severe strokes associated with cardioembolism and the presence of serious heart disease. Mortality within 1 year after stroke also is high in persons with cardiac arrhythmia.[13] Deaths are largely due to the underlying heart disease. Recovery after stroke also is poor in patients with atrial fibrillation.[14]

The impact of atrial fibrillation on overall mortality, stroke, and health care costs is huge; for example, the presence of the arrhythmia increases medical spending in both men and women by a factor of 8–22 times.[9] Many of these associations with atrial fibrillation may not be directly related to the arrhythmia. Rather, they correspond to the propensity for embolic occlusions of large cerebral arteries leading to multilobar infarctions.

Atrial fibrillation is a risk factor for stroke in all age groups.[15] Still, the arrhythmia is relatively uncommon in children and young adults. The prevalence of atrial fibrillation significantly increases with advancing age.[16,17] Kannel et al[18] reported that the prevalence increased from a rate of 0.5% in persons ages 50–59 to a frequency of 9% in persons 80–89 years old. Furberg et al[19] report that the prevalence of atrial fibrillation in the elderly ranges from 7% to 14%. Atrial fibrillation appears to be an important predictor of stroke, especially in women older than 70. The major effect of atrial fibrillation on the chances of stroke has been shown in a number of studies. An autopsy study of persons older than 70 found brain infarctions in 82 of 136 patients with non-rheumatic atrial fibrillation and in 55 of 231 persons with no arrhythmia history.[20] In persons older than 80, atrial fibrillation is the primary cardiac condition that increases the risk of stroke.[21] In most age groups, the likelihood of atrial fibrillation in men is approximately 1.5 times that in women.[16] Still, because of the longer life expectancy of women and the strong age correlation between stroke and atrial fibrillation, atrial fibrillation is a leading risk factor for stroke in women. In one series, clinically silent strokes were found in 76 of 516 patients with atrial fibrillation.[22]

Atrial fibrillation is more common in persons who have a history of hypertension, diabetes mellitus, and smoking, even if they do not have symptoms of heart disease.[18] Atrial fibrillation is also more common in persons with a history of congestive heart failure.[16] Atrial fibrillation complicates several heart diseases, and a majority of patients with atrial fibrillation have an underlying cardiac abnormality (Table 6–4). With the decline in the prevalence of rheumatic heart disease secondary to improved antibiotic treatment, coronary artery disease and hypertension are the most common heart diseases associated with atrial fibrillation. Nevertheless, the frequency of atrial fibrillation is very high in persons with rheumatic mitral stenosis. Some of the relatively uncommon causes of atrial fibrillation (eg, thyrotoxicosis) also are associated with a relatively high risk for embolic stroke.[23] The presence of congestive heart failure as a complication of structural heart disease

Table 6–4. **Factors Predisposing to Atrial Fibrillation**

Risk factors
- Increasing age
- Hypertension
- Diabetes mellitus—particularly for women
- Smoking
- Chronic lung disease
- Congestive heart failure
- Left ventricular hypertrophy

Conditions associated with increased risk of atrial fibrillation
- Coronary artery disease
- Recent myocardial infarction
- Cardiovascular operations
- Valvular heart disease
- Congenital heart disease
- Hypertrophic or dilated cardiomyopathy
- Thyrotoxicosis

Table 6–5. **Risk of Embolism: Subgroups of Patients with Atrial Fibrillation**

Clinical Findings

Highest-risk patients
- Acute atrial fibrillation
  - Acute myocardial infarction
  - Cardiovascular procedures
  - Cardioversion
- Sustained atrial fibrillation
  - Prior neurological events—embolism
  - Rheumatic mitral stenosis

Higher-risk patients with sustained atrial fibrillation
- History of diabetes mellitus
- History of hypertension
- Known coronary artery disease
- Past history of congestive heart failure
- Women older than 75 years

Moderate-risk patients
- Men or women 65 or older with no high-risk features

Lower-risk patients
- Persons younger than 65 with no high-risk features

Echocardiographic Findings

Highest-risk patients
- Intra-atrial or intra-ventricular thrombus
- Spontaneous echocardiographic contrast in left atrium

Higher-risk patients
- Left ventricular enlargement
- Left atrial enlargement

Lower-risk patients
- Normal

increases the risk of atrial fibrillation by a factor of 4.5–5.9 times.[18] The presence of valvular heart disease of any cause increases the likelihood of atrial fibrillation by a factor of 1.8 in men and 3.4 in women.[18] Post-operative atrial fibrillation is relatively common after coronary artery bypass surgery. One study noted that the arrhythmia was detected in 27% of 2417 patients; the complication was more common in older patients, men, and those with a history of atrial fibrillation or congestive heart failure.[24] The likelihood of atrial fibrillation also increases with a past history of atrial fibrillation, previous heart surgery, pericarditis, or prior myocardial infarction.[25] An increased risk of stroke and length of stay in an intensive care unit are associated with the presence of post-operative atrial fibrillation.

Higher- and Lower-Risk Situations

The risk of embolism is highest in the elderly and persons with diabetes mellitus, hypertension, and a history of stroke. The likelihood of embolism is very low in persons younger than 65 who have no evidence of structural heart disease (lone atrial fibrillation).[26,27] (See Table 6–5). Lone atrial fibrillation should not be diagnosed if other evidence of heart or vascular disease, such as a cardiac murmur, is present. The echocardiogram must be normal; the presence of cardiac abnormalities on the test is not compatible with the diagnosis of lone atrial fibrillation. The risk of stroke is so low in persons with lone atrial fibrillation that no anti-embolic treatment has been advocated.

A patient's age appears to be an important predictor of risk for embolism. It appears to be approximately 3 times higher in persons older than 75 than in younger persons.[28,29] The Stroke Prevention in Atrial Fibrillation (SPAF) investigators calculated that stroke risk increases by a factor of 1.8 per decade.[26,30] The presence of non-valvular atrial fibrillation increases the likelihood of stroke in elderly persons by a factor of 2.5.[31] In persons older than 65, the annual risk of stroke is approximately 3%, but this risk increases to approximately 6% if hypertension, diabetes, coronary artery disease, congestive heart failure, or left ventricular dysfunction is present.[26] The risk of stroke also is higher in women, persons with a history of hypertension or ischemic heart disease, and in those with a systolic blood pressure greater than 160 mm Hg.[29,30] The presence of left ventricular hypertrophy, an abnormal left ventricular ejection fraction, or rheumatic mitral stenosis also increases the risk of thromboembolic stroke in persons older than 62 who have chronic atrial fibrillation.[32] Conversely, mitral regurgitation appears to reduce the risk of stroke in patients with nonrheumatic atrial fibrillation.[33] The single most important clinical forecaster of embolic stroke is history of a prior TIA, stroke, or another embolic event.[29] In the patients enrolled in the SPAF trial, a history of previous neurological symptoms was associated with an estimated risk of 2.9 when compared with persons without a prior stroke.[30] The annual risk of stroke in patients with atrial fibrillation who have a history of previous neurological symptoms is estimated to be 12%.[26]

Echocardiographic Findings

Echocardiography can help define a high risk for embolism in persons whose clinical features portend a low risk.[28,34] (See Table 6–5.) Either transthoracic or transesophageal echocardiographic (TTE or TEE, respectively) studies are used; however, the yield of transesophageal echocardiography is higher because most detected clots in persons with atrial fibrillation will be in the left atrium (see Chapter 4). Several findings are associated with an increased rate of embolism in patients with atrial fibrillation, including moderate-to-severe dysfunction of the left ventricle or a complex plaque of the aorta.[28,35–38] Other echocardiographic abnormalities associated with an increased risk of stroke are an increased left ventricular mass, left atrial appendage thrombus, left atrial spontaneous contrast, left atrial enlargement, and decreased left atrial appendage flow.[35,37–45] For example, Benjamin et al[45] reported that the risk of stroke increased for each 10 mm. in left atrial size by a factor of 2.4 in men and 1.4 in women. In patients with a history of TIA or ischemic stroke, the use of TEE can be guided by clinical findings. Because neurological symptoms are the most important forecaster of future embolism and, in most instances, mandate anticoagulation, the results of the TEE likely will not increase the indication for the medication. In such a circumstance, the TEE may not be needed.

Sustained or Intermittent Atrial Fibrillation

Embolism can complicate either sustained or intermittent atrial fibrillation. The presence of arrhythmia for more than 1 year predicts a higher risk of embolism.[29] The duration also appears critical for the risk of embolism in persons with new-onset or intermittent atrial fibrillation. The arrhythmia needs to be present for a period of at least 48 hours to promote stagnation and thrombosis. Thus, the determination of the duration of the atrial fibrillation becomes critical. The usual symptoms of atrial fibrillation are the sudden onset of palpitations, dyspnea, or fatigue. Unfortunately, many patients have no symptoms and the time of onset, therefore, is unknown. In such circumstances, the assumption is that the arrhythmia has been sustained. Detection of new-onset atrial fibrillation should prompt evaluation for an acute cardiac disease, in particular acute myocardial infarction. Atrial fibrillation also may be a direct complication of the acute intracranial event or may be secondary to acute cardiac ischemia that complicates the stroke.[46] Ambulatory monitoring may allow detection of paroxysmal atrial fibrillation.[47]

Management of Atrial Fibrillation

Treating the arrhythmia (electrical or chemical cardioversion) and any underlying heart disease is a critical component of stroke prevention.[48] Detection of an arrhythmia within 2 days of onset allows for rapid treatment that prevents intra-atrial thrombi from having the opportunity to develop. Cardioversion can be performed without a high risk for embolism even without anticoagulation if the procedure is done within days of onset.[49] The highest risk of embolization appears to be after conversion to sinus rhythm. A sudden increase in atrial contractility may promote release of a thrombus that had developed in the left atrium or left atrial appendage during the arrhythmic period. One recent study found that the risk of embolism was 1.32% among 454 patients treated with direct current electrical cardioversion.[50]

If electrical or pharmacological cardioversion is planned for a patient with sustained atrial fibrillation, then anticoagulation usually is prescribed before and after the procedure. The usual regimen is for at least 3 weeks before cardioversion and at least 4 weeks after the procedure.[51] The anticoagulation is continued after electrical cardioversion because "stunning" of the atrium may lead to formation of new thrombi.[52] Persons at greatest risk for embolism after cardioversion are those older than 55 or with either hypertension or a cardiomyopathy.[53] In one study, 7% of patients having cardioversion without anticoagulant coverage had a stroke.[53] Manning et al[54] recommended TEE to assess the left atrium before cardioversion. Other investigators also have recommended using TEE to guide the timing of cardioversion and the pariprocedural use of anticoagulants.[55] If a thrombus is present, then cardioversion can be delayed and the patient should receive anticoagulants.[56]

Prevention of Embolism

Because of the high prevalence of atrial fibrillation associated with heart diseases other than mitral stenosis, considerable research has focused on strategies to prevent embolic stroke in patients with non-valvular atrial fibrillation. Much of the current information about prevention of cardioembolic stroke in general was derived from studies of interventions tested on persons with atrial fibrillation. Specific measures to forestall the formation of clots are the key to prevention of stroke in persons with atrial fibrillation. Several clinical trials have tested the usefulness of chronic treatment with oral anticoagulants or antiplatelet aggregating agents in preventing embolism in persons with non-valvular atrial fibrillation. (See Chapter 10.) These studies confirm the usefulness of an adjusted dose regimen of oral anticoagulants in prevention of stroke in persons judged to be at high risk for stroke, including those with recent neurological symptoms.[57–62] Oral anticoagulants can lessen the risk of stroke by approximately 80% in persons with atrial fibrillation. In most situations, the desired level of anticoagulation is an International Normalized Ratio (INR) of 2–3; in persons with prosthetic heart valves, the preferred INR is 2.5–4.0.[63,64] The role of treatment with oral anticoagulants in prevention of stroke is discussed in more detail in Chapter 10. Anticoagulation appears to be an underused therapy. Many high-risk patients with atrial fibrillation are not being treated, and many others have inadequate dosages prescribed.[65–69]

Major bleeding complications and the risk of hemorrhage increases with advancing age.[57,70] In persons with atrial fibrillation, another factor that predicts bleeding complications is an excessive level of anticoagulation.[60,69] Antiplatelet aggregating agents, in particular aspirin, are effective in lowering the risk of stroke in persons with atrial fibrillation who cannot be treated with oral anticoagulants. (See Chapter 10.) Aspirin should be prescribed if warfarin cannot be used safely. The role of ticlopidine or clopidogrel is not known. Dipyridamole is another potential antiplatelet aggregating agent that probably has a role as an adjunct to treatment with warfarin. The combination of warfarin and aspirin or dipyridamole can be administered if a patient has ischemic symptoms when being treated with warfarin alone.

CORONARY ARTERY DISEASE

Acute Myocardial Infarction

Ischemic stroke is a leading non-cardiac complication of acute myocardial infarction. Some patients, especially diabetics, have relatively little pain at the time of myocardial infarction, and the acute cardiac event is not recognized. Thus, embolic stroke may be a presenting symptom. The risk of stroke following myocardial infarction probably has been reduced by the widespread administration of thrombolytic, antithrombotic, and antiplatelet aggregating medications to treat acute myocardial ischemia.[71,72] The risk of stroke in persons with acute myocardial infarction appears to range from 1% to 6%. In a survey of 4808 patients with myocardial infarction, 48 strokes were recorded.[73] Although a complicating stroke is relatively uncommon, it has a major affect on prognosis following myocardial infarction. The occurrence of a neurological event is associated with an increased risk of death.[73,74] In part, the increased mortality is secondary to the brain injury. It also reflects the serious ventricular injury that leads to thromboembolism.

A strong time relationship for embolic complications is present (Fig. 6–3). The first days and weeks after myocardial infarction are the period of highest risk for embolism.[75] Moore et al[76] calculated that the daily risk for stroke was approximately 9/10,000 during the first 28 days after myocardial infarction. This interaction

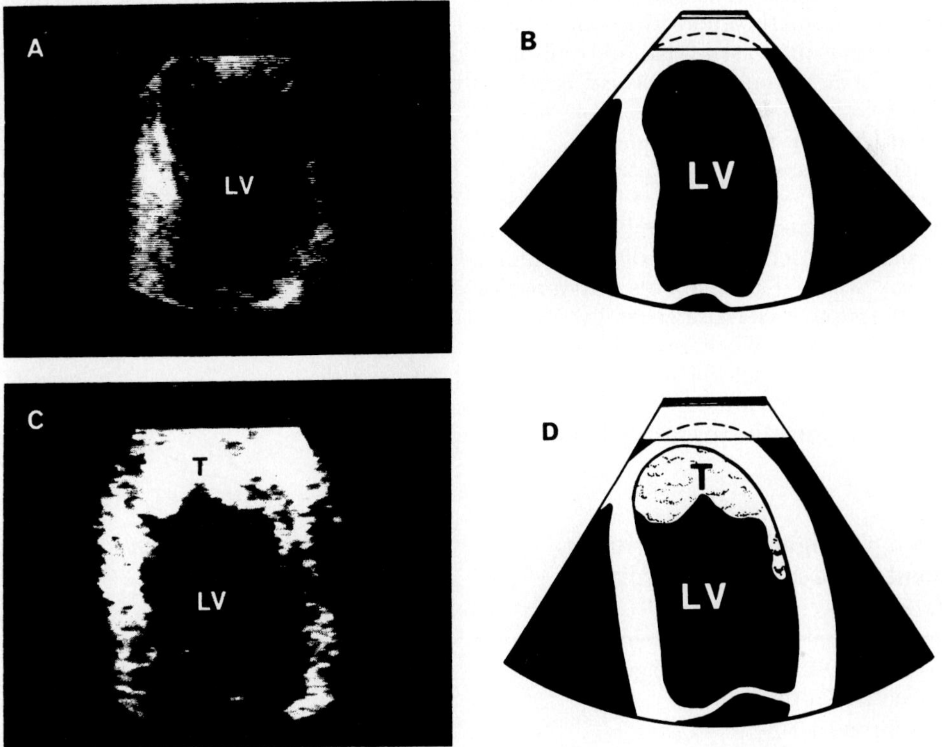

Figure 6–3. Apical views of transthoracic echocardiograms done 7 and 11 days after myocardial infarction show the development of a thrombus (T) in the left ventricle (LV). (Reprinted from Asinger RW et al. Incidences of left-ventricular thromboses after acute transmural myocardial infarction. *N Engl J Med* 1981;305:297, with permission.)

should not be surprising because the first few days after the acute heart injury are when cardiac instability, fresh myocardial injury, and changes in coagulation are most likely. By 6 months after the cardiac event, the likelihood of a complicating stroke is relatively low. This time interval is important when making recommendations about anticoagulant treatment to prevent cardioembolic stroke after myocardial infarction.

The risk of stroke after myocardial infarction is increased with an *anterior myocardial infarction,* a history of previous myocardial infarction, hypertension, atrial fibrillation, or age greater than 70.[73,75] (See Table 6–6.) The risk in persons with non-anterior myocardial infarction is less than 1%, whereas anterior injuries are associated with a risk of approximately 2%–6%. Although most reports describe a strong relationship between embolization and an anterior location of the myocardial infarction, Bodenheimer et al[77] could not find a relationship between stroke and the location. Echocardiographic detection of an intraventricular or mural thrombus is associated with a markedly increased risk of embolization.[78,79] The thrombus usually is adjacent to a *hypokinetic* or *akinetic segment of the left ventricle.* Martin and Bogousslavsky[80] noted that all patients with stroke after myocardial infarction had evidence of an akinetic segment. Left ventricular thrombi are rare in patients with inferior myocardial infarctions, whereas up to 40% of patients with anterior infarctions have clots detected by imaging tests.[81] Embolism also is more likely in persons who have atrial fibrillation, congestive heart failure, or poor left ventricular function complicating the myocardial injury.[82]

Table 6–6. **Highest Risk of Stroke: Patients with Acute Myocardial Infarction**

Anterior wall myocardial infarction
Intraventricular thrombus
Mural thrombus
Congestive heart failure
Atrial fibrillation
Lysis with thrombolytic agents
Hypokinetic or akinetic segment

Thrombolytic therapy after myocardial infarction also is complicated by a modest but real risk for *hemorrhagic stroke.*[83–86] Systemic embolization secondary to lysis of a complicating intraventricular thrombus can follow thrombolytic therapy for treatment of acute myocardial infarction.[87–90]

Anticoagulation is a key component of the regimen to prevent cardioembolic stroke after myocardial infarction.[91] Turpie et al[92] reported that heparin therapy lowered the frequency of mural thrombi from 32% to 11% in a group of high-risk patients, reducing the risk by a ratio of 0.46–0.60 (0.30–0.90).[93,94] Most patients are treated with anticoagulants, antiplatelet aggregating agents, and thrombolytic agents during the first hours after myocardial infarction. Both anticoagulants and thrombolytic agents appear to prevent formation of a mural thrombosis, but evidence that antiplatelet aggregating agents are effective is lacking.[78,95] The key to stroke prevention is to identify the highest-risk patients and continue anticoagulation for at least 6 months. (See Chapter 10.) The desired level of anticoagulation is an INR of 2–3.

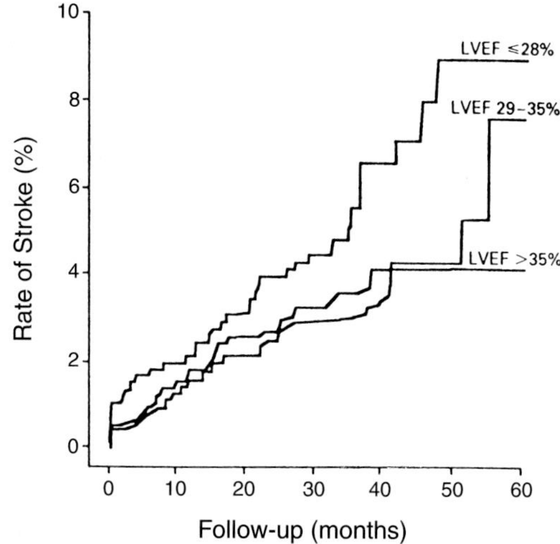

Figure 6–4. Cumulative rate of stroke within 60 months of myocardial infarction as influenced by the severity of reduction in the left ventricular ejection fraction. Patients with a left ventricular ejection fraction of 28% or less than normal had the highest risk of stroke. (Reprinted from Loh E et al. Ventricular dysfunction and the risk of stroke after myocardial infarction. *N Engl J Med* 1997;336:251–257, with permission of publisher)

Ventricular Aneurysm or Ischemic Cardiomyopathy

A long-term risk for embolization complicates a *ventricular aneurysm* or a *dilated ischemic cardiomyopathy* as delayed sequelae of a myocardial infarction.[82] (See Figs. 6–4 and 6–5.) In general, the risk of embolism is fairly low in persons with a chronic left ventricular aneurysm or reduced left ventricular ejection fraction.[82,96] Anticoagulation may not be needed in this

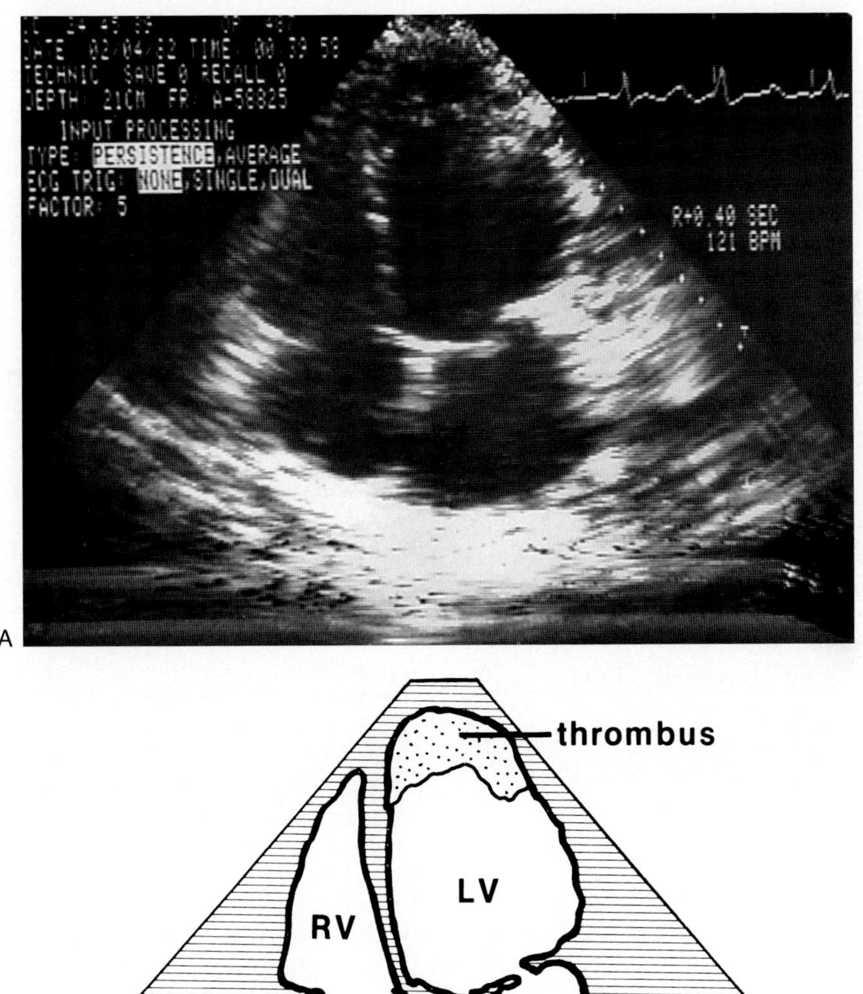

Figure 6–5. Two-dimensional transthoracic echocardiogram (*A*) and diagram (*B*) of a patient with cardiomyopathy and a left ventricular apical thrombus, apical four-chamber view. (Courtesy of DR Boughner, MD, University of Western Ontario.)

setting unless the patient has complications, such as atrial fibrillation or congestive heart failure. In addition, some of these patients are treated with cardiac assist devices that lead to embolization. The risk of stroke secondary to cardiac assist devices is described subsequently in this chapter.

CONGENITAL HEART DISEASE

Cyanotic Congenital Heart Disease

Cyanotic congenital heart disease is an important cause of cardioembolic stroke in childhood. A key factor in these cases is a right-to-left shunt that predisposes to embolization of clots or septic material that bypasses the lungs and goes directly to the brain. For example, stroke can occur in children with a ventricular septal aneurysm.[97] Because the material often is infected, these children are also at high risk for development of a *brain abscess*. Anaerobic organisms are the most likely pathogens. Progressive hemiparesis in a cyanotic child should prompt consideration of a brain abscess developing as the result of a septic embolus. Congenital heart disease is associated with cardiac conduction abnormalities that can cause stroke in childhood.[98]

Patent Foramen Ovale

Approximately 10%–20% of healthy adults have a right-to-left intracardiac shunt, which is detected by contrast or color Doppler echocardiography.[99,100] These abnormalities can be detected by either TTE or TEE. The congenital anomaly usually affects the inter-atrial septum. The most common form is a *patent foramen ovale (PFO)*. In this circumstance, the foramen ovale does not regress completely shortly after birth. The resulting hole permits a clinically occult transgress of blood from the right atrium into the left. The minor shunting does not produce cyanosis. It can be transient and become augmented by increased pressure on the right side of the heart. Thus, a sudden increase in pulmonary artery pressure secondary to pulmonary embolism may lead to an increase in flow through a PFO.[101] A *Valsalva maneuver* also can lead to increased right-to-left flow through a PFO. *Paradoxical embolism* results when a clot of peripheral venous origin bypasses the lung via an intracardiac shunt to reach the brain.[102] In the past, the diagnosis of paradoxical embolism required demonstration of a *venous thrombus* in addition to the right-to-left shunt; however, in most patients with a PFO and a stroke, a venous clot is not detected.[103] Rarely, a paradoxical embolism can occur in conjunction with a clinically overt pulmonary embolus.

In general, a PFO is clinically occult; the patient will have no signs or symptoms that point to a cardiac abnormality. A PFO can be suspected by the presence of an *"M"- shape notch in the "R" wave on electrocardiographic leads II, III, and AVF.*[104] It usually is detected by contrast-enhanced transesophageal echocardiography during the evaluation of patients with ischemic stroke.[105] The high prevalence of PFO in the general population is reflected among groups of patients with stroke. The likelihood of finding a PFO increases in persons with cryptogenic stroke and younger persons.[105–108] The relative size of the PFO may be important, and a greater risk of embolization may be associated with a larger shunt. Size can be predicted by the volume of bubbles moving from the right to the left side of the heart during contrast echocardiography (Fig. 6–6). A large volume of bubbles appearing soon after injection of agitated saline is correlated with a large PFO and *may be associated with an increased* risk for embolism.[108–111]

The overall risk of stroke in persons with a PFO is relatively low, and the chance for recurrent stroke is relatively low; the annual risk is approximately 1.9%.[112,113] The optimal treatment to prevent cerebral embolism is uncertain, as the relatively low risk for embolic events means that any treatment must be very safe.[4] Choices include anticoagulants,

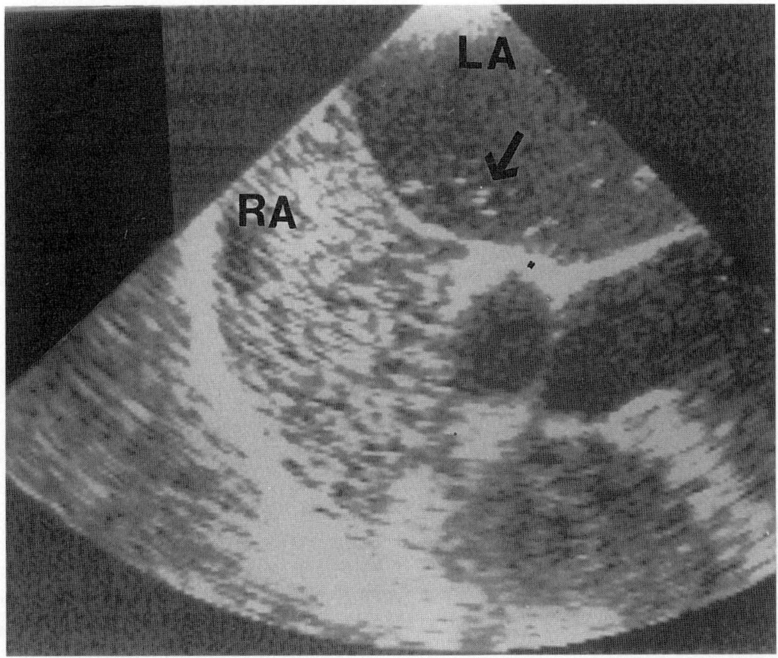

Figure 6–6. Transesophageal echocardiographic view of the base of the heart in a patient with a patent foramen ovale. Microbubbles from intravenous agitated saline injection fill the right atrium, and a few microbubbles are traversing the inter-atrial septum through a patent foramen ovale and appearing in the left atrium (arrow). (LA = left atrium; RA = right atrium.) Courtesy of Richard E. Kerber, MD, Department of Medicine, University of Iowa, Iowa City.)

antiplatelet aggregating agents, percutaneously placed devices, and surgical closure.[113–115] Although anticoagulants are often prescribed, their long-term necessity is not established. Trials are comparing the safety and efficacy of antiplatelet and anticoagulant agents. In addition, the superiority of any therapy is not known.[274] (See Chapters 10 and 11.)

Atrial Septal Aneurysm

An atrial septal aneurysm can be an isolated defect or can be associated with a PFO.[116–118] It also appears to be associated with an intra-cardiac right-to-left shunt. The risk of stroke appears to be low in persons with an isolated atrial septal aneurysm. Still, Agmon et al[118] reported that atrial septal aneurysms were found in 7.9% of patients with stroke and in 2.2% of controls. The relationship between atrial septal aneurysm and stroke risk needs additional study; especially when a PFO is absent.

VALVULAR HEART DISEASE

Rheumatic Valvular Disease

Rheumatic heart disease remains an important cause of stroke in young adults in many developing countries. Since the advent of antibiotic treatment for rheumatic fever and other acute infectious diseases, the prevalence of rheumatic heart disease has dropped greatly. Still, some adults who had rheumatic fever in childhood will present with stroke secondary to *rheumatic mitral stenosis* or *aortic stenosis*. These persons are at high risk for embolism. The combination of *mitral stenosis* and *atrial fibrillation* is particularly dangerous; one epidemiological study calculated a relative risk of approximately 13. Coulshed et al[119] reported that embolization occurred in 8%

of patients with mitral stenosis and 32% of patients with the combination of mitral stenosis and atrial fibrillation. The presence of rheumatic mitral stenosis doubles the risk of embolization in patients with atrial fibrillation.[32] The risk of stroke also increases with advancing age, decreased mitral valve area, aortic insufficiency, and the presence of poor cardiac output.[120,121] In addition to stroke, patients with severe mitral stenosis often have cardiac murmurs and signs of cardiomegaly and congestive heart failure. They also are prone to infective endocarditis that, in turn, also leads to embolization to the brain. Anticoagulation is the key medication for prevention of stroke in patients with rheumatic mitral stenosis.[122] (See Chapter 10.) Surgical replacement of a valve or valvuloplasty may be needed if the mitral stenosis is very severe. (See Chapter 11.)

Mitral Valve Prolapse

The clinical findings of *mitral valve prolapse (MVP)* include a cardiac murmur and a click most commonly auscultated during examination of thin, young women (Fig. 6–7). A recent report from the Framingham Study shows that the prevalence of MVP is not as common as previously thought.[123] The investigators found a rate of approximately 2.5%. During the 1970s and 1980s, MVP was speculated to be a leading cause of stroke in young adults.[124,125] This conclusion was based primarily on studies using echocardiography and probably reflects selection bias in the patients who were assessed. This idea has since been refuted, and the risk of stroke in persons with MVP probably is very small.[123,126,127] Gilon et al[128] recently found that MVP was not more common in young adults with stroke or TIA than in age-matched controls. Mitral valve prolapse also was not more common in persons with cryptogenic stroke than other young persons. Most young patients will have strokes ascribed to causes other than MVP. Many patients also have a PFO detected during evaluation of the heart.[129] The youth-relationship of MVP and stroke also has changed. Orencia et al[130] found that MVP was as common in older persons as in young adults. They also found that MVP did not predict a high risk for stroke and concluded that persons with uncomplicated MVP do not have an increased risk of stroke.[131]

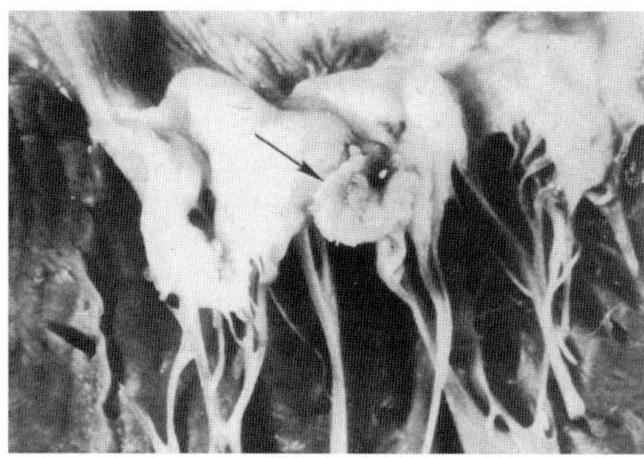

Figure 6–7. Posterior mitral valve leaflet with a large vegetation, a potential site for thrombus formation and cerebral embolism. Bramlet et al. South Med J, 1982; 75:1134, with permission. (Courtesy of Dr. H.J.M. Barnett.)

In most patients, stroke should not be ascribed to MVP. Clinical or echocardiographic evidence of MVP should not cause a clinician to make a diagnosis of cardioembolic stroke or to stop further investigation. Because the risk of stroke appears to be low in persons with MVP, oral anticoagulants usually are not needed. Conversely, MVP can be an underlying cardiac lesion that predisposes to *infective endocarditis,* which can then lead to stroke. Patients with a redundant valve with MVP have an increased risk for endocarditis, and they should receive *prophylactic antibiotics* when undergoing dental or surgical procedures.[132] Patients with MVP and stroke should have blood cultures obtained to screen for infection.

Mitral Annulus Calcification

Mitral annulus calcification is relatively common in older persons. In one series, the mean age of persons with calcification of the mitral annulus was 73 years.[133] The condition is more common in women. It is associated with an increased risk of stroke.[134,135] Its presence is associated with an increased frequency of atrial fibrillation. Mitral annulus calcification can lead to stroke by the embolization of clots and pieces of calcified spicules.[134] Still, the risk for cardioembolic stroke in persons with mitral annulus calcification is low. Rather than being a cause of stroke, mitral annulus calcification appears to be a marker for atherosclerosis of the internal carotid artery.[136] A finding of mitral annulus calcification should not automatically lead to a diagnosis of cardioembolism as the cause of stroke, nor should it prompt anticoagulant treatment unless other cardiac risk factors are identified. Calcific embolism to the brain secondary to mitral annular calcification can occur in association with chronic renal disease secondary to hyperparathyroidism.[137]

Aortic Valve Calcification and Aortic Stenosis

Calcification of the aortic valve with or without *aortic stenosis* appears not to be a major risk factor for stroke.[138] Still, a calcified aortic valve can be a source of microthrombi or turbulent flow that leads to embolization.[139,140] The risk of stroke with a *bicuspid aortic valve* also appears to be low.[141] An *aneurysm of the sinus of Valsalva* (the portion of the aorta immediately behind the cusps of the aortic valve) can be the source of clots that embolize to the brain.[142]

Prosthetic Heart Valves

Ischemic stroke is a well-known complication of a *mechanical prosthetic valve*. The risk of embolization is greater with *mitral valve prostheses* than with *aortic valve prostheses*. The risk for clot formation is extraordinarily high with mitral valve prostheses. In the absence of anticoagulant treatment, the risk for embolization with a mechanical mitral valve is approximately 25% per year.[143] The risk in a patient with mechanical aortic valves who is not treated with anticoagulants is approximately 12% per year. With both mitral and aortic valve prostheses, the annual risk approaches 90%.[143] The presence of a hypercoagulable state can increase the risk of thrombosis in patients with mechanical valves.[144]

The risk for embolization varies among types of prostheses. Using transcranial doppler ultrasonography (TCD) monitoring, investigators found the highest number of embolic signals in patients with *Bjork-Shiley valves*.[145,146] *Medtronic* and *Carpentier* valves have lower rates of embolization.[147] Geiser et al[148] found that microemboli in patients with prosthetic valves is related to platelet microparticles and increased levels of prothrombotic factors. The presence of complicating atrial fibrillation further increases the risk of cardioembolic stroke. Mechanical valves are vulnerable to *infective endocarditis*. A *bioprosthetic mitral* or *aortic valve* does not have the high risk of embolization associated with mechanical valves, especially while anticoagulants are administered.[149]

Cardioembolism should be the working diagnosis for cause of stroke in most patients with either a mechanical or a bioprosthetic valve. Additional evaluation will depend on the patient's presentation. Long-term anticoagulation is the treatment of choice for patients with mechanical valves in the mitral position. Patients with a tilting disk type of valve should be treated with doses of warfarin to achieve an INR valve of 3.5.[150,151] (See Chapter 10.) Anticoagulation of most other patients with mechanical valves should have an INR of at least 2.5–4.0.[150,152,153] Pregnant women usually are treated with heparin or a low molecular weight heparin.[154] Aspirin or dipyridamole can be added to warfarin in treating high-risk patients.[150,155] Patients with bioprosthetic aortic valves can be treated with antiplatelet aggregating agents with or without a short course of anticoagulation immediately after surgery.[150,156] (See Chapter 10.)

OTHER CARDIAC CONDITIONS

Infective Endocarditis

Stroke is a leading complication of infective endocarditis. In addition to embolism, infective endocarditis can lead to *meningitis*, *encephalitis*, a *brain abscess*, or an *intracranial*

Table 6–7. **Neurological Complications and Clinical Features of Infective Endocarditis**

Clinical features
Fever
Changing cardiac murmur
Congestive heart failure
Systemic embolism
Splenic infarction
Visceral infarction
Roth spots
Janeway lesions
Osler nodes
Neurological complications
Embolic stroke
Infective aneurysm
Subarachnoid hemorrhage
Encephalitis
Brain abscess

(infective) aneurysm.[157,158] (See Table 6–7.) Both the mitral and aortic valves are involved. The most common infectious organisms are *Staphylococcus aureus, enterococci,* and *streptococcal* species. A *fulminant infectious endocarditis* leading to cardiac failure and stroke can occur in persons who are using intravenously administered illegal drugs. These patients have a very high mortality risk, largely as the result of acute and severe cardiac failure.

Most patients have an underlying cardiac valvular abnormality or a prosthesis, which predisposes to infection. Both *native valves* and *prostheses* are vulnerable.[159] Transient bacteremia following a procedure or trauma may incite an infectious illness. Patients with infective endocarditis usually have a subacute course (*subacute bacterial endocarditis*) consisting of low-grade fever and constitutional symptoms.[158] In addition to stroke, patients with infective endocarditis also can present with headache or seizures. Most patients also have findings of embolization to other organs, including the skin. Abdominal pain secondary to splenic or visceral infarction, hematuria secondary to renal involvement, and skin or eye

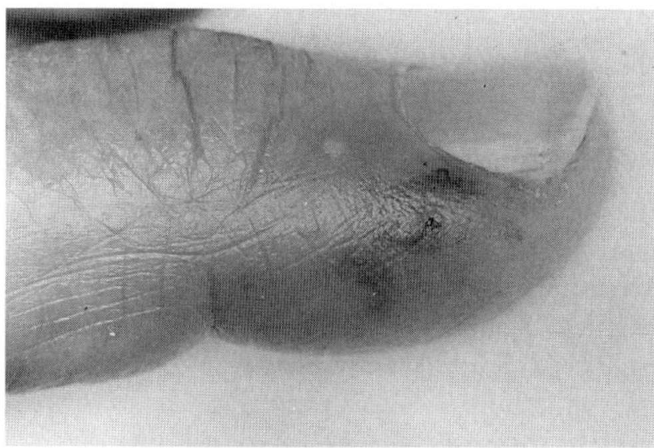

A

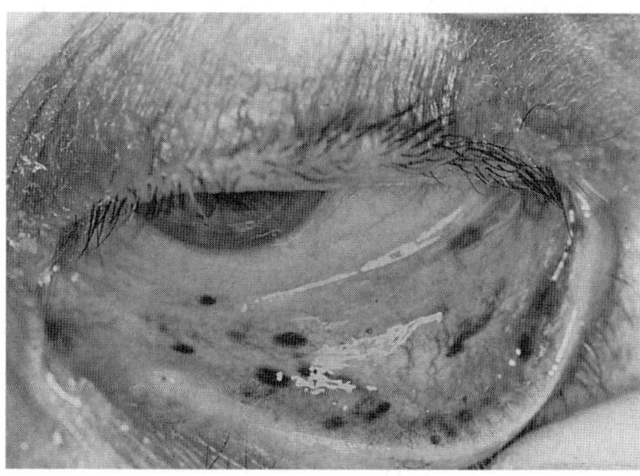

B

Figure 6–8. Cutaneous (*A*) and mucosal (*B*) petechiae noted in a patient with infective endocarditis.

lesions often are present. The latter abnormalities include Roth spots, Janeway lesions, and Osler nodes (Fig. 6–8). An evolving cardiac murmur usually is detected. An elevated erythrocyte sedimentation rate and leucocytosis are markers of the infectious disease. Cerebrospinal fluid also will often demonstrate signs of infection.[158] Although echocardiography can show vegetations of the mitral and aortic valves, the diagnostic procedure of choice is obtaining aerobic and anaerobic blood cultures.

A prolonged course of antibiotics is the treatment of choice for managing a patient with infective endocarditis. Patients with an infected prosthetic valve might need to have the valve replaced. A native valve that is severely damaged by infection likely will need replacement. Anticoagulants are not given to patients with embolic stroke secondary to infective endocarditis due to the high risk of bleeding as a result of the *infective aneurysm.*[160] Although intracranial aneurysm is a potential complication of infective endocarditis, most patients do not have arteriography to screen for this finding.[161] Still, the risk of an infective aneurysm is relatively low, and cerebral arteriography is not routinely indicated for evaluation of patients with infective endocarditis.[162] Treatment can include surgical resection of the aneurysm.

Non-bacterial Thrombotic Endocarditis

Non-bacterial thrombotic endocarditis (*marantic endocarditis/NBTE*) is a relatively uncommon disorder that can complicate a *mucin-producing adenocarcinoma* of the pancreas, ovary, lung, or bowel. Autopsy evidence of NBTE can be found in approximately 1% of patients with adenocarcinoma.[163–165] (See Table 6–8.) Non-bacterial thrombotic endocarditis also can complicate diabetes mellitus, pregnancy, surgery, AIDS, or dehydration.[166] Although the condition is relatively uncommon, the risk of stroke with NBTE is quite high. Approximately one-third of patients with NBTE have a history of cerebral embolism.[167] In addition to ischemic stroke, the patients often have mental status changes or multifocal hemorrhages.[168,169] Adding to the neurological symptoms, patients exhibit abdominal or flank pain secondary to ischemia in the kidneys, spleen, or intestines. An acute abdomen or hematuria can be found.

The pathogenesis of NBTE involves abnormal coagulation factors leading to a *disseminated intravascular coagulation.* Thrombocytopenia, decreased fibrinogen concentration, abnormal D-dimer, and increased fibrinogen degradation products can be detected.[167] Coagulation disturbance leads to the formation of *vegetations* on the surface and thickening of the cardiac valves.[170,171] The mitral and aortic valves are most commonly implicated.[163,165,167] The vegetations usually are small and may not be detected by cardiac imaging.[170]

Embolization of pieces of a vegetation leads to stroke, which can be the first symptom of NBTE. Multiple neurological events can mimic cerebral vasculitis.[172] Treatment involves anticoagulation to halt the disseminated intravascular coagulation and management of the underlying tumor. Because of its relationship to advanced malignancies and the presence of coagulopathy, the prognosis of patients with NBTE is very poor.

Table 6–8. **Non-bacterial Thrombotic Endocarditis**

- Complication of the following conditions
  - Malignancy, especially adenocarcinomas
    - Pancreas
    - Ovary
    - Lung
    - Bowel
  - Diabetes mellitus
  - Pregnancy
  - Surgery
  - Acquired immune deficiency syndrome
  - Dehydration
- Clinical findings
  - Embolic stroke
  - Venous thrombosis
  - Abdominal pain
  - Subtle cardiac changes
- Diagnostic tests
  - Disseminated intravascular coagulopathy
  - Subtle vegetations on cardiac valves

Libman-Sacks Endocarditis

Libman-Sacks endocarditis is a potential complication of *systemic lupus erythematosus,* which is correlated with the presence of *lupus anticoagulants* or the *antiphospholipid antibody syndrome.* Patients with *Sneddon's syndrome* (stroke, livedo reticularis, and digital ischemia) have a high rate of changes on the mitral valve that are secondary to deposits of antibody-antigen complexes.[173,174] These abnormalities can be detected by echocardiography. Mitral valve disease with antiphospholipid antibodies can lead to recurrent cerebral infarctions in patients with polyarteritis nodosa.[175] Microembolism to the brain can be detected by TCD.[176] Treatment involves long-term anticoagulation.

Atrial Myxoma

A *left atrial myxoma* can cause obstructive symptoms, constitutional symptoms, or embolic events, including stroke.[177,178] The tumor can arise in men and women of all age groups; a slight predominance is noted in women.[179] Obstruction of the mitral orifice can lead to a sudden decrease in cardiac output or sudden death. Constitutional symptoms include a subacute fever, fleeting neurological symptoms, skin eruption, and arthralgias. An elevated erythrocyte sedimentation rate and abnormal serum proteins may lead to a misdiagnosis of systemic lupus erythematosus. The usual cardiac finding is a change in a murmur that accompanies a change in posture. The electrocardiogram usually shows non-specific changes.[179] Neurological symptoms usually are secondary to the embolization of tumor cells that occlude an intracranial artery. Pieces of a superimposed thrombus also can go to the brain. Approximately one-third of patients with atrial myxoma will have neurological symptoms. Stroke can be an initial symptom of the cardiac tumor.[179] The tumor embolus can serve as the nidus for the formation of an intracranial aneurysm.[180–182] Occasionally, a *fibroelastoma* or *malignant tumor of the heart* also can lead to embolization to the brain.[183] In general, anticoagulants are not effective in preventing stroke in patients with cardiac tumors, including atrial myxoma. Surgical resection of the cardiac tumor is the recommended treatment.

Dilated Cardiomyopathy

A *dilated cardiomyopathy* is associated with intracavitary thrombus and can be secondary to *ischemic heart disease, pregnancy,* or *chronic alcohol use;* or it can follow a *viral infection.*[82,184–187] (See Table 6–9.) The risk of systemic embolization in patients with dilated cardiomyopathies who have not received anticoagulants approaches 20%.[186] Trials are planned to test the usefulness of anticoagulants or antiplatelet agents in preventing stroke among patients with heart failure and dilated cardiomyopathy.[82]

Table 6–9. **Causes of Dilated Cardiomyopathy**

Ischemic heart disease
Pregnancy—post-partum
Chronic alcohol abuse
Viral illnesses
Neuromuscular diseases
Mitochondrial diseases

Cardiomyopathy also is a complication of inherited mitochondrial disorders, including *mitochondrial encephalopathy, lactic acidosis,* and *stroke* (*MELAS*); *Kearns-Sayre syndrome*; and *myoclonus epilepsy with ragged red fibers.*[188] Successful management of the cardiac arrhythmias with these neuromuscular disorders leading to conduction abnormalities in the heart may leave the patient at risk for embolization from the developing cardiomyopathy.[189] Conduction defects and cardiomyopathy also can complicate scapuloperoneal, limb-girdle, and myotonic dystrophy.[190] Primary oxalosis is a rare cause of nephrolithiasis that can be complicated by intracardiac calcification and secondary embolism.[191]

Idiopathic Hypertrophic Subaortic Stenosis

Stroke is a potential complication of *idiopathic hypertrophic subaortic stenosis* (*IHSS*). Furlan et al[192] reported that ischemic strokes had occurred in 7% of 150 patients followed over a period of 5 years. Russell et al[193] noted that stroke can be the presenting feature of IHSS. The risk of cardioembolic stroke in persons with IHSS has been associated with the presence of concomitant atrial fibrillation, mitral annulus calcification, or left atrial enlargement.[128,193] Still, the chances of cardioembolism are low in patients with IHSS, and another cause for the neurological symptoms should be sought.

CARDIAC ABNORMALITIES DETECTED DURING EVALUATION

Discovery of cardiac abnormalities during diagnostic evaluation, especially by TEE, helps to define a population of patients with other heart diseases that are at high risk for embolism. The importance of ancillary cardiac findings is highlighted by data from the studies of patients with atrial fibrillation. Still, detection of some of these abnormalities also can lead to uncertainty because the significance of the findings remains unclear. Some of these changes, alone, may not predict a high risk for embolism. Considerable epidemiological research is needed to determine the long-term risk of embolism in persons who have these findings. Because risks of stroke are not obvious, the best treatment to lower the risks has not been determined.

Spontaneous Echocardiographic Contrast

Spontaneous echocardiographic contrast (*smoke*) can be seen in the left atrium. Presumably, this change reflects turbulence with the chamber. Chimowitz et al[194] found that spontaneous echocardiographic contrast in the left atrium is associated with an increased risk of stroke in patients with mitral stenosis or atrial fibrillation. A combination of mitral regurgitation and mitral stenosis is associated with a higher rate of spontaneous echocardiographic contrast than mitral stenosis alone.[195,196]

Valvular Strands

Detection of *valvular stands,* more commonly found on the mitral valve than on the aortic valve, is associated with an increased risk of stroke.[197] The strands are thin pieces of material attached to the surface of the valves. These lesions are more common in younger persons.[198] Freedberg et al[199] found strands in 63 of 597 (10.6%) patients with signs of embolism and in 23 of 962 (2.3%) patients without emboli. Roberts[198] concluded that the observed risk for stroke in patients with valvular stands is increased by a factor of approximately 4.4 (2.0–9.6). Cohen et al[200] concluded that the risk of stroke was increased by a factor of 2.2 when strands were present. They showed that strands were more common with *mitral valve dystrophy* but not with MVP, mitral annulus calcification, or spontaneous echocardiographic contrast in the left atrium. These lesions also can be found among patients with *prosthetic valves,* particularly mechanical mitral valves.[197]

Lambl Excrescence

Lambl excrescence, which is a filiform outgrowth on the free border of the mitral valve, can be detected during echocardiographic evaluation of persons with stroke.[201] Its significance as a risk factor for embolic stroke is not known.

CARDIOVASCULAR PROCEDURES

Embolism to the brain is the leading noncardiac complication of most cardiovascular procedures. Most of the events occur within a few hours or days of the cardiac intervention. In general, the risks of embolism are greater in patients having operations or major cardiovascular procedures than they are in persons having angiography. The presence of stroke following cardiac operations is associated with increased health care costs, length of stay, and mortality.[202,203]

Cardiac Catheterization and Coronary Arteriography

The chances of neurological sequelae are very low following *cardiac catheterization* and *coronary arteriography*; the risks are estimated to be from <0.1% to 1%.[204–206] Patients can have a migrainous event secondary to *transient neurotoxicity* of the contrast agent leading to visual loss and confusion.[205,207] Embolism of clots that develop on the catheter or local arterial trauma also may cause stroke.[204,205,207,208] Air embolism also can complicate cardiac catheterization.[209]

Stroke is a potential complication of other invasive cardiological techniques, including *coronary artery angioplasty*, placement of a *pacemaker, ablation procedures*, and *electrophysiological studies*.[210–212] Ischemic stroke may complicate right ventricular *endomyocardial biopsy* and *transmyocardial laser revascularization* procedures.[213,214] Embolism also is a complication of *percutaneous balloon valvuloplasty*.[215] These events are uncommon, and a relationship usually is entertained by the timing of the neurological event and the cardiac procedure.

Left Ventricular Assist Devices

Thromboembolism has been reported in approximately 20% of patients who have *left* or *right ventricular assist devices*.[216–218] These pumps are associated with altered blood flow patterns, increased blood viscosity, increased fibrinogen, infections, and increased blood-arterial surface interactions that lead to a pro-thrombotic state.[219] Strokes can occur at any time during the use of the device. The risk persists as long as the device is used. Heparin-bonded devices may lower the risk of thromboembolism.[220]

Coronary Artery Bypass Graft Surgery and Other Cardiac Operations

The frequency of neurological complications following *cardiopulmonary operations* depends on the intensity of observation. Neuropsychological impairments, encephalopathy, psychiatric disturbances, and visual loss are very common.[221–229] Intellectual decline is relatively common after major cardiovascular operations.[202] Visual impairments include retinal infarction, visual field defects, and decreased visual acuity.[230,231] A major stroke can be detected in approximately 6% of patients who have coronary bypass surgery, and the likelihood of stroke is higher in persons who have valvular surgery.[202,203,224,232–235] Borger et al[236] reported that the incidence of stroke following valvular surgery decreased from 3.8% in operations done between 1982 and 1986 to 2.6% in procedures performed from 1992 to 1996. Approximately 60% of these strokes are recognized within 2 days of the operation.[237]

The causes of stroke include *shock, septic embolization, atherosclerotic embolization*, and the *embolization of air, fat, or thrombotic material*.[238–242] Fracturing of a plaque during clamping of the aorta in persons with advanced aortic atherosclerosis can lead to massive embolization of debris.[202,243,244] *Endocarditis* also can occur.[202] *Microemboli* arising in the *extracorporeal device* can occur as well, and an increased time on this device alone also predicts stroke.[237,245] The periods during the filling of the empty beating heart and during the redistribution of blood from the heart–lung machine appear to be those with greatest risk for embolization.[246]

Borger et al[236] found that neurological complications after valve operations were more common if the patient had endocarditis, needed surgery urgently, was older than 74, or had concomitant coronary artery bypass grafting surgery (Fig. 6–9). The risk of stroke is high in patients who have atrial fibrillation following coronary artery bypass grafting operations.[24] Increased cross clamp time or increased ventricular resistance also predicts a high risk of stroke.[233] Persons older than 70 and those with a history of diabetes, congestive heart failure, peripheral vascular disease, or neurological symptoms are at higher risk.[203,245] However, Beall et al[247] did not find that a past history of stroke was an important marker for stroke following heart operations. Patients having a second operation or advanced stenosis of the internal carotid artery may be at increased risk.[203] Although the data are mixed, the risk of stroke appears to be increased in persons who have severe carotid artery atherosclerosis.[248–251] Still, the relationship between carotid stenosis and stroke following cardiac surgery has not been established.[252,253] The presence of aortic atherosclerosis also is associated with an increased risk of stroke following coronary artery surgery.[254]

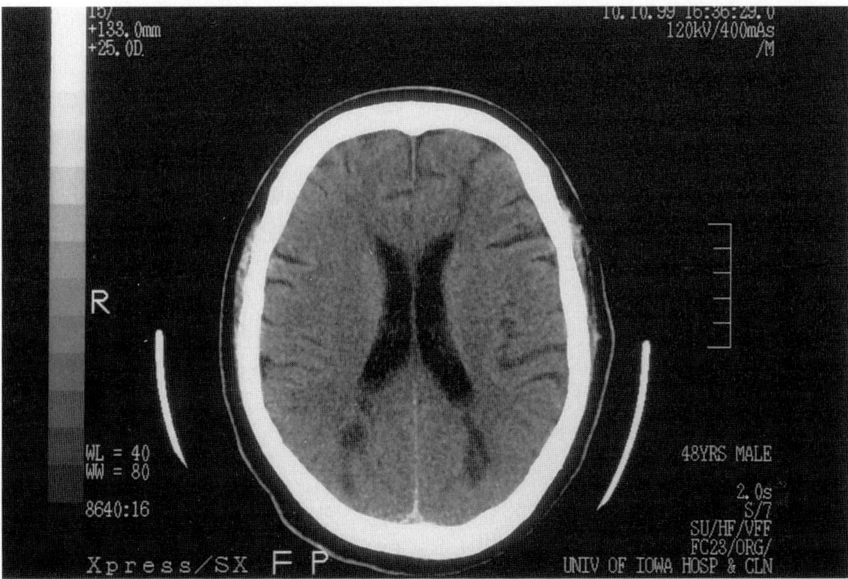

Figure 6–9. A computed tomographic scan obtained from a patient with hypotension demonstrates bilateral watershed infarctions in the border between the middle and the posterior cerebral arteries. This pattern of stroke could be found following a cardiovascular operation.

Stroke can complicate *pediatric cardiac operations.*[255] Approximately 30% of children and infants having pediatric cardiopulmonary bypass have some neurological morbidity.[256] Causes of stroke in children differ from those found in adults having operations for atherosclerotic cardiac diseases. The leading etiologies include arterial dissection and pro-thrombotic states.[255] Stroke also can complicate a *fenestrated fontan procedure.*[257]

Cardiac Transplantation

Stroke also is a recognized complication of *cardiac transplantation.* It occurs in approximately 15%–20% of patients.[258,259] The strokes can be secondary to the procedure itself or secondary to infectious or thrombotic complications.[260] One autopsy series found evidence of stroke in approximately 75% of patients who had cardiac transplantation.[261] Embolic events, including thrombi, fat, or air can occur with the operation.[262] Other neurological complications include anoxia and laminar necrosis, metabolic encephalopathies, seizures, central nervous system infections, and peripheral nerve palsies. An *angiodestructive infection* with *aspergillus* can lead to hemorrhagic infarction.[258]

NON-CARDIAC OR NON-THROMBOTIC CAUSES OF EMBOLISM

A number of unusual, non-thrombotic conditions can lead to embolism to the brain. Many of these embolic events are related to medical procedures. Materials that can reach the brain include air, fat, amniotic fluid, tumor, or foreign bodies.

Air Embolism

Air embolism to the brain can occur during *cardiovascular procedures, hemodialysis, esophageal operations,* or *neurosurgical interventions.*[209,263] It also can occur in placing an *arterial line* or during an *abortion.* Air emboli also can reach the brain during decompression (*Caisson disease*). Air embolism should be suspected when a neurological event occurs immediately after a procedure. Neurological impairments usually reflect diffuse or multifocal brain injury. Brain imaging (CT of the brain) can be diagnostic—bubbles of air will be found in the cerebral arteries.[264] Hyperbaric oxygen has been used to treat air embolism with neurological symptoms.[265]

Fat Embolism

Fat embolism to the brain most commonly occurs in the setting of a *long bone fracture* (usually the shaft of the femur) as part of severe multisystem trauma resulting from a motor vehicle accident.[266] The usual scenario is the sudden onset of acute respiratory distress and neurological impairments following trauma. The patient is hypoxic or cyanotic. A chest radiograph shows multiple areas of infiltration in both lungs. Fat emboli in the retina can be seen by direct ophthalmoscopic examination. Neurological impairments usually reflect bilateral or multifocal brain dysfunction. Brain imaging can detect fat embolization.[267]

Intravenous lipid infusions have caused encephalopathy, seizures, and focal neurological signs.[268] Inadvertent infusion of lipid-containing fluids into the internal carotid artery also can cause neurological impairments. Fat embolism also has followed injection of a melted suppository.[269]

Amniotic Fluid Embolism

Embolism of *amniotic fluid* is a rare complication of delivery.[270] It should be considered when a young woman develops neurological impairments reflecting bilateral or multifocal brain injuries that occur immediately after labor and delivery.

Other Types of Embolism

Foreign bodies, including talc or pieces of lint or gauze, can reach the brain as a complication of surgical procedures, including cardiovascular operations. Persons taking drugs of abuse through an intravenous route can inject adulterants into the body that can embolize to the brain. Tumor embolism has accompanied thoracic surgery.[271,272]

Pulmonary Arteriovenous Malformation

A pulmonary arteriovenous malformation can be the source of paradoxical embolism leading to ischemic stroke or brain abscess.[273] An intra-pulmonary right-to-left shunt will permit venous emboli to bypass the lung to reach the brain. Often a pulmonary arteriovenous malformation is a manifestation of *hereditary hemorrhagic telangiectasia* (*Rendu-Osler-Weber disease*). Patients can have cyanosis, dyspnea, or hemoptysis. This condition should be suspected by the presence of a bruit over the lateral wall of the chest. A chest x-ray or CT usually will detect the vascular lesion in the lung.

SUMMARY

Heart disease accounts for one quarter of strokes, with valvular disease predominating in the young, coronary disease in those of middle age, and atrial fibrillation in the elderly. Abnormal valves breed emboli and are prone to infection. Coronary heart disease can lead to myocardial infarction, hypokinetic segments, and cerebral embolism. Atrial fibrillation predisposes to left atrial thrombosis and embolization. The role of a patent foramen ovale in the causation of stroke remains uncertain, but it plausibly accounts for a minority of cases in the young.

Cardiovascular investigations (eg, cardiac catheterization), pacemaker implantations, and procedures such as Cardiolversion, cardiac transplantation, and coronary artery bypass grafting carry their own risk for stroke. Recognition of risk is an important first step in prevention. When a definite source of emboli can be identified (eg, a diseased or mechanical heart valve, a clot in an akinetic segment of the heart, atrial fibrillation), anticoagulation has a proven role.

REFERENCES

1. Koudstaal PJ, Algra A, Pop GA, Kappelle LJ, van Latum JC, van Gijn J. Risk of cardiac events in atypical transient ischaemic attack or minor stroke. The Dutch TIA Study Group. *Lancet* 1992;340:630–633.
2. Caplan LR. Brain embolism, revisited. *Neurology* 1993;43:1281–1287.
3. Oder W, Siostrzonek P, Lang W, et al. Distribution of ischemic cerebrovascular events in cardiac embolism. *Klin Wochenschr* 1991;69: 757–762.
4. Devuyst G, Bogousslavsky J. Status of patent foramen ovale, atrial septal aneurysm, atrial septal defect and aortic arch atheroma as risk factors for stroke. *Neuroepidemiology* 1997;16: 217–223.
5. Kistler JP. The risk of embolic stroke. Another piece of the puzzle. *N Engl J Med* 1994;331: 1517–1519.
6. Panagiotopoulos K, Toumanidis S, Saridakis N, Vemmos K, Moulopoulos S. Left atrial and left atrial appendage functional abnormalities in patients with cardioembolic stroke in sinus rhythm and idiopathic atrial fibrillation. *J Am Soc Echocardiogr* 1998;11:711–719.
7. Shively BK, Gelgand EA, Crawford MH. Regional left atrial stasis during atrial fibrillation and flutter: determinants and relation to stroke. *J Am Coll Cardiol* 1996;27:1722–1729.
8. Petersen P. Thromboembolic complications in atrial fibrillation. *Stroke* 1990;21:4–13.
9. Wolf PA, Mitchell JB, Baker CS, Kannel WB, D'Agostino RB. Impact of atrial fibrillation on mortality, stroke, and medical costs. *Arch Intern Med* 1998;158:229–234.
10. Sandercock P, Bamford J, Dennis M, et al. Atrial fibrillation and stroke: prevalence in different types of stroke and influence on early and long term prognosis (Oxfordshire Community Stroke Project). *BMJ* 1992;305:1460–1465.
11. EAFT Study Group. Silent brain infarction in nonrheumatic atrial fibrillation. European Atrial Fibrillation Trial. *Neurology* 1996;46:159–165.
12. Cullinane M, Wainwright R, Brown A, Monaghan M, Markus HS. Asymptomatic embolization in subjects with atrial fibrillation not taking anticoagulants: a prospective study. *Stroke* 1998;29:1810–1815.
13. Kaarisalo MM, Immonen-Raiha P, Marttila RJ, et al. Atrial fibrillation and stroke. Mortality and causes of death after the first acute ischemic stroke. *Stroke* 1997;28:311–315.
14. Lin HJ, Wolf PA, Kelly-Hayes M, et al. Stroke severity in atrial fibrillation. The Framingham Study. *Stroke* 1996;27:1760–1764.
15. You RX, McNeil JJ, Farish SJ, O'Malley HM, Donnan GA. The influence of age on atrial fibrillation as a risk factor for stroke. *Clin Exp Neurol* 1991;28:37–42.
16. Benjamin EJ, Levy D, Vaziri SM, D'Agostino RB, Belanger AJ, Wolf PA. Independent risk factors for atrial fibrillation in a population-based cohort. *JAMA* 1994;271:840–844.
17. Gold AE, Marshall SM. Cortical blindness and cerebral infarction associated with severe hypoglycemia. *Diabetes Care* 1996;19:1001–1003.
18. Kannel WB, Wolf PA, Benjamin EJ, Levy D. Prevalence, incidence, prognosis, and predisposing conditions for atrial fibrillation: population-based estimates. *Am J Cardiol* 1998;82:2N–9N.
19. Furberg CD, Psaty BM, Manolio TA, Gardin JM, Smith VE, Rautaharju PM. Prevalence of atrial fibrillation in elderly subjects (the Cardiovascular Health Study). *Am J Cardiol* 1994;74:236–241.
20. Yamanouchi H, Nagura H, Mizutani T, Matsushita S, Esaki Y. Embolic brain infarction in nonrheumatic atrial fibrillation: a clinicopathologic study in the elderly. *Neurology* 1997;48:1593–1597.
21. Wolf PA, Abbott RD, Kannel WB. Atrial fibrillation as an independent risk factor for stroke: the Framingham Study. *Stroke* 1991;22:983–988.
22. Ezekowitz MD, James KE, Nazarian SM, et al. Silent cerebral infarction in patients with nonrheumatic atrial fibrillation. The Veterans Affairs Stroke Prevention in Nonrheumatic Atrial Fibrillation Investigators. *Circulation* 1995;92: 2178–2182.
23. Presti CF, Hart RG. Thyrotoxicosis, atrial fibrillation, and embolism, revisited. *Am Heart J* 1989; 117:976–977.
24. Mathew JP, Parks R, Savino JS, et al. Atrial fibrillation following coronary artery bypass graft surgery: predictors, outcomes, and resource utilization. MultiCenter Study of Perioperative Ischemia Research Group. *JAMA* 1996;276:300–306.
25. Crosby LH, Pifalo WB, Woll KR, Burkholder JA. Risk factors for atrial fibrillation after coronary artery bypass grafting. *Am J Cardiol* 1990;66: 1520–1522.
26. Hart RG, Sherman DG, Easton JD, Cairns JA. Prevention of stroke in patients with nonvalvular atrial fibrillation. *Neurology* 1998;51:674–681.
27. Scardi S, Mazzone C, Pandullo C, Goldstein D, Poletti A, Humar F. Lone atrial fibrillation: prognostic differences between paroxysmal and chronic forms after 10 years of follow-up. *Am Heart J* 1999;137:686–691.
28. Atrial Fibrillation Investigators. Echocardiographic predictors of stroke in patients with atrial fibrillation: a prospective study of 1066 patients from 3 clinical trials. *Arch Intern Med* 1998;158:1316–1320.
29. van Latum JC, Koudstaal PJ, Venables GS, van Gijn J, Kappelle LJ, Algra A. Predictors of major vascular events in patients with a transient ischemic attack or minor ischemic stroke and with nonrheumatic atrial fibrillation. European Atrial Fibrillation Trial (EAFT) Study Group. *Stroke* 1995;26:801–806.
30. Hart RG, Pearce LA, McBride R, Rothbart RM, Asinger RW. Factors associated with ischemic stroke during aspirin therapy in atrial fibrillation: analysis of 2012 participants in the SPAF I–III clinical trials. *Stroke* 1999;30:1223–1229.
31. Yamanouchi H, Nagura H, Mizutani T, Matsushita S, Esaki Y. Embolic brain infarction in nonrheumatic atrial fibrillation: a

clinicopathologic study in the elderly. *Neurology* 1997;48:1593–1597.
32. Aronow WS, Ahn C, Kronzon I, Gutstein H. Risk factors for new thromboembolic stroke in patients > or = 62 years of age with chronic atrial fibrillation. *Am J Cardiol* 1998;82:119–121.
33. Nakagami H, Yamamoto K, Ikeda U, Mitsuhashi T, Goto T, Shimada K. Mitral regurgitation reduces the risk of stroke in patients with nonrheumatic atrial fibrillation. *Am Heart J* 1998; 136:528–532.
34. Manning WJ, Douglas PS. Transesophageal echocardiography and atrial fibrillation: added value or expensive toy? *Ann Intern Med* 1998; 128:685–687.
35. The Stroke Prevention in Atrial Fibrillation Investigators Committee on Echocardiography. Transesophageal echocardiographic correlates of thromboembolism in high-risk patients with nonvalvular atrial fibrillation. *Ann Intern Med* 1998;128:639–647.
36. Blackshear JL, Pearce LA, Hart RG, et al. Aortic plaque in atrial fibrillation: prevalence, predictors, and thromboembolic implications. *Stroke* 1999;30:834–840.
37. Zabalgoitia M, Halperin JL, Pearce LA, Blackshear JL, Asinger RW, Hart RG. Transesophageal echocardiographic correlates of clinical risk of thromboembolism in nonvalvular atrial fibrillation. Stroke Prevention in Atrial Fibrillation III Investigators. *J Am Coll Cardiol* 1998;31:1622–1626.
38. Igarashi Y, Yamaura M, Ito M, Inuzuka H, Ojima K, Aizawa Y. Elevated serum lipoprotein(a) is a risk factor for left atrial thrombus in patients with chronic atrial fibrillation: a transesophageal echocardiographic study. *Am Heart J* 1998;136:965–971.
39. Stollberger C, Chnupa P, Kronik G, et al. Transesophageal echocardiographic to assess embolic risk in patients with atrial fibrillation. ELAT Study Group. Embolism in Left Atrial Thrombi. *Ann Intern Med* 1998;128:630–638.
40. Mugge A, Kuhn H, Nikutta P, Grote J, Lopez JA, Daniel WG. Assessment of left atrial appendage function by biplane transesophageal echocardiographic in patients with nonrheumatic atrial fibrillation: identification of a subgroup of patients at increased embolic risk. *J Am Coll Cardiol* 1994; 23:599–607.
41. Jones EF, Calafiore P, McNeil JJ, Tonkin AM, Donnan GA. Atrial fibrillation with left atrial spontaneous contrast detected by transesophageal echocardiographic is a potent risk factor for stroke. *Am J Cardiol* 1996;78:425–429.
42. Di Pasquale G, Urbinati S, Pinelli G. New echocardiographic markers of embolic rsik in atrial fibrillation. *Cerebrovasc Dis* 1995;5: 315–322.
43. Di Tullio MR, Sacco RL, Sciacca RR, Homma S. Left atrial size and the risk of ischemic stroke in an ethnically mixed population. *Stroke* 1999;30:2019–2024.
44. Stoddard MF, Dawkins PR, Prince CR, Ammash NM. Left atrial appendage thrombus is not uncommon in patients with acute atrial fibrillation and a recent embolic event: a transesophageal echocardiographic study. *J Am Coll Cardiol* 1995;25:452–459.
45. Benjamin EJ, D'Agostino RB, Belanger AJ, Wolf PA, Levy D. Left atrial size and the risk of stroke and death. *Circulation* 1995;92:835–841.
46. Lin HJ, Wolf PA, Benjamin EJ, Belanger AJ, D'Agostino RB. Newly diagnosed atrial fibrillation and acute stroke. The Framingham Study. *Stroke* 1995;26:1527–1530.
47. Bell C, Kapral M. Use of ambulatory electrocardiography for the detection of paroxysmal atrial fibrillation in patients with stroke. *Can J Neurol Sci* 2000;27:25–31.
48. Giardina EG. Atrial fibrillation and stroke: elucidating a newly discovered risk factor. *Am J Cardiol* 1997;80:11D–18D.
49. Weigner MJ, Caulfield TA, Danias PG, Silverman DI, Manning WJ. Risk for clinical thromboembolism associated with conversion to sinus rhythm in patients with atrial fibrillation lasting less than 48 hours. *Ann Intern Med* 1997;126:615–620.
50. Zeiler AA, Mick MJ, Mazurer RP, Loop FD, Trohman RG. Role of prophylactic anticoagulation for direct current cardioversion in patients with atrial fibrillation or atrial flutter. *J Am Coll Cardiol* 1992;19:851–855.
51. Kinch JW, Davidoff R. Prevention of embolic events after cardioversion of atrial fibrillation. Current and evolving strategies. *Arch Intern Med* 1995;155:1353–1360.
52. Fatkin D, Kuchar DL, Thorburn CW, Feneley MP. Transesophageal echocardiographic before and during direct current cardioversion of atrial fibrillation: evidence for "atrial stunning" as a mechanism of thromboembolic complications. *J Am Coll Cardiol* 1994;23:307–316.
53. Weinberg DM, Mancini J. Anticoagulation for cardioversion of atrial fibrillation. *Am J Cardiol* 1989;63:745–746.
54. Manning WJ, Silverman DI, Gordon SP, Krumholz HM, Douglas PS. cardioversion from atrial fibrillation without prolonged anticoagulation with use of transesophageal echocardiographic to exclude the presence of atrial thrombi. *N Engl J Med* 1993;328:750–755.
55. Klein AL, Grimm RA, Black IW, et al. cardioversion guided by transesophageal echocardiographic: the ACUTE Pilot Study. A randomized, controlled trial. Assessment of Cardioversion Using Transesophageal Echocardiographic. *Ann Intern Med* 1997;126:200–209.
56. Ewy GA. Optimal technique for electrical cardioversion of atrial fibrillation. *Circulation* 1992; 86:1645–1647.
57. Stroke Prevention in Atrial Fibrillation Investigators. Warfarin versus aspirin for prevention of thromboembolism in atrial fibrillation: Stroke Prevention in Atrial Fibrillation II Study. *Lancet* 1994;343:687–691.
58. EAFT (European Atrial Fibrillation Trial) Study Group. Secondary prevention in non-rheumatic atrial fibrillation after transient ischaemic attack or minor stroke. *Lancet* 1993;342:1255–1262.
59. Stroke Prevention in Atrial Fibrillation Investigators, . Adjusted-dose warfarin versus

low-intensity, fixed-dose warfarin plus aspirin for high-risk patients with atrial fibrillation: Stroke Prevention in Atrial Fibrillation III randomised clinical trial. *Lancet* 1996;348:633–638.
60. Pengo V, Zasso A, Barbero F, et al. Effectiveness of fixed minidose warfarin in the prevention of thromboembolism and vascular death in nonrheumatic atrial fibrillation. *Am J Cardiol* 1998;82:433–437.
61. Stroke Prevention in Atrial Fibrillation Investigators. Stroke prevention in atrial fibrillation study. Final results. *Circulation* 1991;84: 527–539.
62. Connolly SJ, Laupacis A, Gent M, Roberts RS, Cairns JA, Joyner C. Canadian Atrial Fibrillation Anticoagulation (CAFA) Study. *J Am Coll Cardiol* 1991;18:349–355.
63. Albers GW. Choice of antithrombotic therapy for stroke prevention in atrial fibrillation. *Arch Intern Med* 1998;158:1487–1491.
64. Atrial Fibrillation Investigators. Risk factors for stroke and efficacy of antithrombotic therapy in atrial fibrillation. Analysis of pooled data from five randomized controlled trials. *Arch Intern Med* 1994;154:1449–1457.
65. Albers GW, Yim JM, Belew KM, et al. Status of antithrombotic therapy for patients with atrial fibrillation in university hospitals. *Arch Intern Med* 1996;156:2311–2316.
66. Albers GW, Bittar N, Young L, et al. Clinical characteristics and management of acute stroke in patients with atrial fibrillation admitted to US university hospitals. *Neurology* 1997;48:1598–1604.
67. Sudlow M, Thomson R, Thwaites B, Rodgers H, Kenny RA. Prevalence of atrial fibrillation and eligibility for anticoagulants in the community. *Lancet* 1998;352:1167–1171.
68. Brass LM, Krumholz HM, Scinto JD, Mathur D, Radford M. Warfarin use following ischemic stroke among Medicare patients with atrial fibrillation. *Arch Intern Med* 1998;158:2093–2100.
69. Brass LM, Krumholz HM, Scinto JM, Radford M. Warfarin use among patients with atrial fibrillation. *Stroke* 1997;28:2382–2389.
70. The Stroke Prevention in Atrial Fibrillation Investigators. Bleeding during antithrombotic therapy in patients with atrial fibrillation. *Arch Intern Med* 1996;156:409–416.
71. Maggioni AP, Franzosi MG, Santoro E, White H, Van de Werf F, Tognoni. The risk of stroke in patients with acute myocardial infarction after thrombolytic and antithrombotic treatment. Gruppo Italiano per lo Studio della Sopravvivenza nell'Infarto Miocardico II (GISSI–2), and The International Study Group. *N Engl J Med* 1992;327:1–6.
72. Sloan MA, Price TR, Terrin ML, et al. Ischemic cerebral infarction after rt-PA and heparin therapy for acute myocardial infarction. The TIMI-II pilot and randomized clinical trial combined experience. *Stroke* 1997;28:1107–1114.
73. Tanne D, Goldbourt U, Zion M, Reicher-Reiss H, Kaplinsky E, Behar S. Frequency and prognosis of stroke/TIA among 4808 survivors of acute myocardial infarction. The SPRINT Study Group. *Stroke* 1993;24:1490–1495.
74. Maggioni AP, Franzosi MG, Farina ML, et al. Cerebrovascular events after myocardial infarction: analysis of the GISSI trial. Gruppo Italiano per lo Studio della Streptochinasi nell'Infarto Miocardico (GISSI). *BMJ* 1991; 302:1428–1431.
75. Moore T, Eriksson P, Stegmayr B. Ischemic stroke after acute myocardial infarction. A population–based study. *Stroke* 1997;28:762–767.
76. Moore T, Olofsson B-O, Stegmayr B, Eriksson P. Ischemic stroke. Impact of a recent myocardial infarction. *Stroke* 1999;30:997–1001.
77. Bodenheimer MM, Sauer D, Shareef B, Brown MW, Fleiss JL, Moss AL. Relation between myocardial infarct location and stroke. *J Am Coll Cardiol* 1994;24:61–66.
78. Vaitkus PT, Barnathan ES. Embolic potential, prevention and management of mural thrombus complicating anterior myocardial infarction: a meta-analysis. *J Am Coll Cardiol* 1993;22: 1004–1009.
79. Johannessen KA, Nordrehaug JE, von der L. Left ventricular thrombosis and cerebrovascular accident in acute myocardial infarction. *Br Heart J* 1984;51:553–556.
80. Martin R, Bogousslavsky J. Mechanism of late stroke after myocardial infarct: the Lausanne Stroke Registry. *J Neurol Neurosurg Psychiatry* 1993;56:760–764.
81. Asinger RW, Mikell FL, Elsperger J, Hodges M. Incidence of left-ventricular thrombosis after acute transmural myocardial infarction. Serial evaluation by two-dimensional echocardiographic. *N Engl J Med* 1981;305:297–302.
82. Pullicino PM, Halperin JL, Thompson JLP. Stroke in patients with heart failure and reduced left ventricular ejection fraction. *Neurology* 2000;54:288–294.
83. Longstreth WT, Jr., Litwin PE, Weaver WD. Myocardial infarction, thrombolytic therapy, and stroke. A community-based study. The MITI Project Group. *Stroke* 1993;24:587–590.
84. Gore JM, Sloan M, Price TR, et al. Intracerebral hemorrhage, cerebral infarction, and subdural hematoma after acute myocardial infarction and thrombolytic therapy in the Thrombolysis in Myocardial Infarction Study. Thrombolysis in Myocardial Infarction, Phase II, pilot and clinical trial. *Circulation* 1991;83:448–459.
85. Uglietta JP, O'Connor CM, Boyko OB, Aldrich H, Massey EW, Heinz ER. CT patterns of intracranial hemorrhage complicating thrombolytic therapy for acute myocardial infarction. *Radiology* 1991;181:555–559.
86. Bellone P, Domenicucci S, Chiarella F, Bellotti P, Lupi G, Vecchio C. Chronic aneurysmatic dilatation: a possible source of lethal embolization in patients with acute myocardial infarction undergoing thrombolysis. *Internat J Cardiol* 1996;56: 201–204.
87. Zahger D, Weiss AT, Anner H, Waksman R. Systemic embolization following thrombolytic therapy for acute myocardial infarction. *Chest* 1990;97:754–756.
88. Bautista RE. Embolic stroke following thrombolytic therapy for myocardial infarction in a

patient with preexisting ventricular thrombi. *Stroke* 1995;26:324–325.
89. Gordon MF, Coyle PK, Golub B. Eales' disease presenting as stroke in the young adult. *Ann Neurol* 1988;24:264–266.
90. Stafford PJ, Strachan CJ, Vincent R, Chamberlain DA. Multiple microemboli after disintegration of clot during thrombolysis for acute myocardial infarction. *BMJ* 1989;299:1310–1312.
91. Smith P. Oral anticoagulants are effective long-term after acute myocardial infarction. *J Intern Med* 1999;245:383–387.
92. Turpie AG, Robinson JG, Doyle DJ, et al. Comparison of high-dose with low-dose subcutaneous heparin to prevent left ventricular mural thrombosis in patients with acute transmural anterior myocardial infarction. *N Engl J Med* 1989;320:352–357.
93. Vaitkus PT, Berlin JA, Schwartz JS, Barnathan ES. Stroke complicating acute myocardial infarction. A meta-analysis of risk modification by anticoagulation and thrombolytic therapy. *Arch Intern Med* 1992;152:2020–2024.
94. Azar AJ, Koudstaal PJ, Wintzen AR, et al. Risk of stroke during long-term anticoagulant therapy in patients after myocardial infarction. *Ann Neurol* 1996;39:301–307.
95. Anand SS, Yusuf S. Oral anticoagulant therapy in patients with coronary artery disease: A meta-analysis. *JAMA* 1999;282:2058–2067.
96. Lapeyre AC, Steele PM, Kazmier FJ, Chesebro JH, Vlietstra RE, Fuster V. Systemic embolism in chronic left ventricular aneurysm: incidence and the role of anticoagulation. *J Am Coll Cardiol* 1985;6:534–538.
97. Kowalski M, Hoffman P, Rozanski J, Rydlewska-Sadowska W. Ischemic neurologic event in a child as a result of ventricular septal aneurysm. *J Am Soc Echocardiogr* 1998;11:1161–1162.
98. Hayabuchi Y, Matsuoka S, Nii M, Suzuya H, Kuroda Y. Cerebral infarction in a patient with congenital complete heart block. *Clin Cardiol* 1998;21:302–303.
99. Schneider B, Zienkiewicz T, Jansen V, Hofmann T, Noltenius H, Meinertz T. Diagnosis of patent foramen ovale by transesophageal echocardiographic and correlation with autopsy findings. *Am J Cardiol* 1996;77:1202–1209.
100. Fisher DC, Fisher EA, Budd JH, Rosen SE, Goldman ME. The incidence of patent foramen ovale in 1,000 consecutive patients. A contrast transesophageal echocardiographic study. *Chest* 1995;107:1504–1509.
101. Konstantinides S, Geibel A, Kasper W, Olschewski M, Blumel L, Just H. Patent foramen ovale is an important predictor of adverse outcome in patients with major pulmonary embolism. *Circulation* 1998;97:1946–1951.
102. Ward R, Jones D, Haponik EF. Paradoxical embolism. An underrecognized problem. *Chest* 1995;108:549–558.
103. Lethen H, Flachskampf FA, Schneider R, et al. Frequency of deep vein thrombosis in patients with patent foramen ovale and ischemic stroke or transient ischemic attack. *Am J Cardiol* 1997; 80:1066–1069.
104. Ay H, Buonanno FS, Abraham SA, Kistler JP, Koroshetz WJ. An electrocardiographic criterion for diagnosis of patent foramen ovale associated with ischemic stroke. *Stroke* 1998;29:1393–1397.
105. Serena J, Segura T, Perez-Ayuso MJ, Bassaganyas J, Molins A, Davalos. The need to quantify right-to-left shunt in acute ischemic stroke: a case-control study. *Stroke* 1998;29: 1322–1328.
106. Petty GW, Khandheria BK, Chu CP, Sicks JD, Whisnant JP. Patent foramen ovale in patients with cerebral infarction. A transesophageal echocardiographic study. *Arch Neurol* 1997;54: 819–822.
107. Jones EF, Calafiore P, Donnan GA, Tonkin AM. Evidence that patent foramen ovale is not a risk factor for cerebral ischemia in the elderly. *Am J Cardiol* 1994;74:596–599.
108. Steiner MM, Di Tullio MR, Rundek T, et al. Patent foramen ovale size and embolic brain imaging findings among patients with ischemic stroke. *Stroke* 1998;29:944–948.
109. Stone DA, Godard J, Corretti MC, et al. Patent foramen ovale: association between the degree of shunt by contrast transesophageal echocardiographic and the risk of future ischemic neurologic events. *Am Heart J* 1996;131:158–161.
110. Van Camp G, Schulze D, Cosyns B, Vandenbossche JL. Relation between patent foramen ovale and unexplained stroke. *Am J Cardiol* 1993;71:596–598.
111. Homma S, Di Tullio MR, Sacco RL, Mihalatos D, Li MG, Mohr JP. Characteristics of patent foramen ovale associated with cryptogenic stroke. A biplane transesophageal echocardiographic study. *Stroke* 1994;25:582–586.
112. Bogousslavsky J, Garazi S, Jeanrenaud X, Aebischer N, Van Melle G. Stroke recurrence in patients with patent foramen ovale: the Lausanne Study. Lausanne Stroke with Paradoxal Embolism Study Group. *Neurology* 1996;46:1301–1305.
113. Nendaz MR, Sarasin FP, Junod AF, Bogousslavsky J. Preventing stroke recurrence in patients with patent foramen ovale: antithrombotic therapy, foramen closure, or therapeutic abstention? A decision analytic perspective. *Am Heart J* 1998;135:532–541.
114. Homma S, Di Tullio MR, Sacco RL, Sciacca RR, Smith C, Mohr JP. Surgical closure of patent foramen ovale in cryptogenic stroke patients. *Stroke* 1997;28:2376–2381.
115. Hanna JP, Sun JP, Furlan AJ, Stewart WJ, Sila CA, Tan M. Patent foramen ovale and brain infarct. Echocardiographic predictors, recurrence, and prevention. *Stroke* 1994;25:782–786.
116. Nater B, Bogousslavsky J, Regli J, Stauffer JC. Stroke patterns with atrial septal aneurysm. *Cerebrovasc Dis* 1992;2:342–346.
117. Mugge A, Daniel WG, Angermann C, et al. Atrial septal aneurysm in adult patients. A multicenter study using transthoracic and transesophageal echocardiographic. *Circulation* 1995;91: 2785–2792.
118. Agmon Y, Khandheria BK, Meissner I, et al. Frequency of atrial septal aneurysms in patients

with cerebral ischemic events. *Circulation* 1999; 99:1942–1944.

119. Coulshed N, Epstein EJ, McKendrick CS, Galloway RW, Walker E. Systemic embolism in mitral valve disease. *Br Heart J* 1970;32:26–34.
120. Dewar HA, Weightman D. A study of embolism in mitral valve disease and atrial fibrillation. *Br Heart J* 1983;49:133–140.
121. Chiang CW, Lo SK, Ko YS, Cheng NJ, Lin PJ, Chang CH. Predictors of systemic embolism in patients with mitral stenosis. A prospective study. *Ann Intern Med* 1998;128:885–889.
122. Adams GF, Merrett JD, Hutchinson WM, Pollock AM. Cerebral embolism and mitral stenosis. Survival with and without anticoagulants. *J Neurol Neurosurg Psychiatry* 1974;37: 378–383.
123. Freed LA, Levy D, Levine RA, et al. Prevalence and clinical outcome of mitral-valve prolapse. *N Engl J Med* 1999;341:1–7.
124. Jackson AC, Boughner DR, Barnett HJM. Mitral valve prolapse and cerebral ischemic events in young patients. *Neurology* 1984;34:784–787.
125. Barnett HJM, Boughner DR, Taylor DW, Cooper PE, Kostuk WJ, Nichol PM. Further evidence relating mitral-valve prolapse to cerebral ischemic events. *N Engl J Med* 1980;302: 139–144.
126. Hart RG, Easton JD. Mitral valve prolapse and cerebral infarction. *Stroke* 1982;13:429–430.
127. Petty GW, Orencia AJ, Khandheria BK, Whisnant JP. A population-based study of stroke in the setting of mitral valve prolapse: risk factors and infarct subtype classification. *Mayo Clin Proc* 1994;69:632–634.
128. Gilon D, Buonanno F, Joffe MM, et al. Lack of evidence of an association between mitralvalve prolapse and stroke in young adults. *N Engl J Med* 1999;341:8–13.
129. Besson G, Bogousslavsky J, Hommel M, Stauffer JC, Siche JP. Patent foramen ovale in young stroke patients with mitral valve prolapse. *Acta Neurol Scand* 1994;89:23–26.
130. Orencia AJ, Petty GW, Khandheria BK, O'Fallon WM, Whisnant JP. Mitral valve prolapse and the risk of stroke after initial cerebral ischemia. *Neurology* 1995;45:1083–1086.
131. Orencia AJ, Petty GW, Khandheria BK, et al. Risk of stroke with mitral valve prolapse in population-based cohort study. *Stroke* 1995;26:7–13.
132. Nishimura RA, McGoon MD, Shub C, Miller FAJ, Ilstrup DM, Tajik AJ. Echocardiographically documented mitral-valve prolapse. Long-term follow-up of 237 patients. *N Engl J Med* 1985;313:1305–1309.
133. Fulkerson PK, Beaver BM, Auseon JC, Graber HL. Calcification of the mitral annulus: etiology, clinical associations, complications and therapy. *Am J Med* 1979;66:967–977.
134. Benjamin EJ, Plehn JF, D'Agostino RB, et al. Mitral annular calcification and the risk of stroke in an elderly cohort. *N Engl J Med* 1992;327: 374–379.
135. Savage DD, Garrison RJ, Castelli WP, et al. Prevalence of submitral (annular) calcium and its correlates in a general population-based sample (the Framingham Study). *Am J Cardiol* 1983; 51:1375–1378.
136. Adler Y, Koren A, Fink N, et al. Association between mitral annulus calcification and carotid atherosclerotic disease. *Stroke* 1998;29: 1833–1837.
137. Katsamakis G, Lukovits TG, Gorelick PB. Calcific cerebral embolism in systemic calciphylaxis. *Neurology* 1998;51:295–297.
138. Boon A, Lodder J, Cheriex E, Kessels F. Risk of stroke in a cohort of 815 patients with calcification of the aortic valve with or without stenosis. *Stroke* 1996;27:847–851.
139. Stein PD, Sabbah HN, Pitha JV. Continuing disease process of calcific aortic stenosis. Role of microthrombi and turbulent flow. *Am J Cardiol* 1977;39:159–163.
140. Shanmugam V, Chhablani R, Gorelick PB. Spontaneous calcific cerebral embolus. *Neurology* 1997;48:538–539.
141. Pleet AB, Massey EW, Vengrow ME. TIA, stroke, and the bicuspid aortic valve. *Neurology* 1981;31:1540–1542.
142. Stollberger C, Seitelberger R, Fenninger C, Prainer C, Slany J. Aneurysm of the left sinus of Valsalva. An unusual source of cerebral embolism. *Stroke* 1996;27:1424–1426.
143. Deklunder G, Roussel M, Lecroart JL, Prat A, Gautier C. Microemboli in cerebral circulation and alteration of cognitive abilities in patients with mechanical prosthetic heart valves. *Stroke* 1998;29:1821–1826.
144. Gencbay M, Turan F, Degertekin M, Eksi N, Mutlu B, Unalp A. High prevalence of hypercoagulable states in patients with recurrent thrombosis of mechanical heart valves. *J Heart Valve Dise* 1998;7:601–609.
145. Georgiadis D, Grosset DG, Kelman A, Faichney A, Lees KR. Prevalence and characteristics of intracranial microemboli signals in patients with different types of prosthetic cardiac valves. *Stroke* 1994;25:587–592.
146. Baudet EM, Oca CC, Roques XF, et al. A 5 1/2 year experience with the St. Jude Medical cardiac valve prosthesis. Early and late results of 737 valve replacements in 671 patients. *J Thorac Cardiovasc Surg* 1985;90:137–144.
147. Hutchinson K, Hafeez F, Woods TD, et al. Recurrent ischemic strokes in a patient with Medtronic-Hall prosthetic aortic valve and valve strands. *J Am Soc Echocardiogr* 1998;11:755–757.
148. Geiser T, Sturzenegger M, Genewein U, Haeberli A, Beer JH. Mechanisms of cerebrovascular events as assessed by procoagulant activity, cerebral microemboli, and platelet microparticles in patients with prosthetic heart valves. *Stroke* 1998;29:1770–1777.
149. Cohn LH, Collins JJJ, Rizzo RJ, Adams DH, Couper GS, Aranki SF. Twenty-year followup of the Hancock modified orifice porcine aortic valve. *Ann Thorac Surg* 1998;66:S30–S34.
150. Tiede DJ, Nishimura RA, Gastineau DA, et al. Modern management of prosthetic valve anticoagulation. *Mayo Clin Proc* 1998;73:665–680.
151. Stein PD, Alpert JS, Dalen JE, Horstkotte D, Turpie AG. Antithrombotic therapy in patients

with mechanical and biological prosthetic heart valves. *Chest* 1998;114:602S–610S.

152. Cannegieter SC, Rosendal FR, Wintzen AR, van der Meer FJM, Vandenbroucke JP, Briet E. Optimal oral anticoagulant therapy in patients with mechanical heart valves. *N Engl J Med* 1995;333:11–17.

153. Altman R, Rouvier J, Gurfinkel E, et al. Comparison of two levels of anticoagulant therapy in patients with substitute heart valves. *J Thorac Cardiovasc Surg* 1991;101:427–431.

154. Ginsberg JS, Barron WM. Pregnancy and prosthetic heart valves. *Lancet* 1994;344:1170–1172.

155. Sullivan JM, Harken DE, Gorlin R. Pharmacologic control of thromboembolic complications of cardiac-valve replacement. *N Engl J Med* 1971;284:1391–1394.

156. Moinuddeen K, Quin J, Shaw R, et al. Anticoagulation is unnecessary after biological aortic valve replacement. *Circulation* 1998;98: II95–II98.

157. Tunkel AR, Kaye D. Neurologic complications of infective endocarditis. *Neurol Clin* 1993;11: 419–440.

158. Bitsch A, Nau R, Hilgers RA, Verheggen R, Werner G, Prange HW. Focal neurologic deficits in infective endocarditis and other septic diseases. *Acta Neurol Scand* 1996;94:279–286.

159. Delahaye JP, Poncet P, Malquarti V, Beaune J, Gare JP, Mann JM. Cerebrovascular accidents in infective endocarditis: role of anticoagulation. *Eur Heart J* 1990;11:1074–1078.

160. Shetty PC, Krasicky GA, Sharma RP, Vemuri BR, Burke MM. Mycotic aneurysms in intravenous drug abusers: the utility of intravenous digital subtraction angiography. *Radiology* 1985;155: 319–321.

161. Keyser DL, Biller J, Coffman TT, Adams HP, Jr. Neurologic complications of late prosthetic valve endocarditis. *Stroke* 1990;21:472–475.

162. van der Meulen JH, Weststrate W, van Gijn J, Habbema JD. Is cerebral angiography indicated in infective endocarditis? *Stroke* 1992;23: 1662–1667.

163. Lopez JA, Ross RS, Fishbein MC, Siegel RJ. Nonbacterial thrombotic endocarditis: a review. *Am Heart J* 1987;113:773–784.

164. Kooiker JC, MacLean JM, Sumi SM. Cerebral embolism, marantic endocarditis, and cancer. *Arch Neurol* 1976;33:260–264.

165. Edoute Y, Haim N, Rinkevich D, Brenner B, Reisner SA. Cardiac valvular vegetations in cancer patients: a prospective echocardiographic study of 200 patients. *Am J Med* 1997;102: 252–258.

166. Pinto AN. AIDS and cerebrovascular disease. *Stroke* 1996;27:538–543.

167. Biller J, Challa VR, Toole JF, Howard VJ. Nonbacterial thrombotic endocarditis. *Arch Neurol* 1982;39:95–98.

168. Schwartzman RJ, Hill JB. Neurologic complications of disseminated intravascular coagulation. *Neurology* 1982;32:791–797.

169. Rogers LR, Cho ES, Kempin S, Posner JB. Cerebral infarction from non-bacterial thrombotic endocarditis. Clinical and pathological study including the effects of anticoagulation. *Am J Med* 1987;83:746–756.

170. Lopez JA, Fishbein MC, Siegel RJ. Echocardiographic features of nonbacterial thrombotic endocarditis. *Am J Cardiol* 1987;59: 478–480.

171. Blanchard DG, Ross RS, Dittrich HC. Nonbacterial thrombotic endocarditis. Assessment by transesophageal echocardiographic. *Chest* 1992;102:954–956.

172. Vassallo R, Remstein ED, Parisi JE, Huston J, Brown RD. Multiple cerebral infarctions from nonbacterial thrombotic endocarditis mimicking cerebral vasculitis. *Mayo Clin Proc* 1999;74: 798–802.

173. Galve E, Ordi J, Barquinero J, Evangelista A, Vilardell M, Soler-Soler J. Valvular heart disease in the primary antiphospholipid syndrome. *Ann Intern Med* 1992;116:293–298.

174. Antoine JC, Michel D, Garnier P, Genin C. Rheumatic heart disease and Sneddon's syndrome. *Stroke* 1994;25:689–691.

175. Morelli S, Perrone C, Paroli M. Recurrent cerebral infarctions in polyarteritis nodosa with circulating antiphospholipid antibodies and mitral valve disease. *Lupus* 1998;7:51–52.

176. Sitzer M, Sohngen D, Siebler M, et al. Cerebral microembolism in patients with Sneddon's syndrome. *Arch Neurol* 1995;52:271–275.

177. Markel ML, Waller BF, Armstrong WF. Cardiac myxoma. A review. *Medicine* 1987;66:114–125.

178. Sandok BA, von E, I, Giuliani ER. CNS embolism due to atrial myxoma: clinical features and diagnosis. *Arch Neurol* 1980;37:485–488.

179. Knepper LE, Biller J, Adams HP, Jr., Bruno A. Neurologic manifestations of atrial myxoma. A 12-year experience and review. *Stroke* 1988;19:1435–1440.

180. Damasio H, Seabra-Gomes R, da Silva JP, Damasio AR, Antunes JL. Multiple cerebral aneurysms and cardiac myxoma. *Arch Neurol* 1975;32:269–270.

181. Furuya K, Sasaki T, Yoshimoto Y, Okada Y, Fujimaki T, Kirino T. Histologically verified cerebral aneurysm formation secondary to embolism from cardiac myxoma. Case report. *J Neurosurg* 1995;83:170–173.

182. Suzuki T, Nagai R, Yamazaki T, et al. Rapid growth of intracranial aneurysms secondary to cardiac myxoma. *Neurology* 1994;44:570–571.

183. Brown RD, Jr., Khandheria BK, Edwards WD. Cardiac papillary fibroelastoma: a treatable cause of transient ischemic attack and ischemic stroke detected by transesophageal echocardiographic. *Mayo Clin Proc* 1995;70:863–868.

184. Sauer CM. Recurrent embolic stroke and cocaine-related cardiomyopathy. *Stroke* 1991;22:1203–1205.

185. Hodgman MT, Pessin MS, Homans DC, et al. Cerebral embolism as the initial manifestation of peripartum cardiomyopathy. *Neurology* 1982;32:668–671.

186. Fuster V, Gersh BJ, Giuliani ER, Tajik AJ, Brandenburg RO, Frye RL. The natural history of idiopathic dilated cardiomyopathy. *Am J Cardiol* 1981;47:525–531.

187. Karande SC, Kulthe SG, Lahiri KR, Jain MK. Embolic stroke in a child with idiopathic dilated cardiomyopathy. *J Postgrad Med* 1996;42:84–86.
188. Kosinski C, Mull M, Lethen H, Topper R. Evidence for cardioembolic stroke in a case of Kearns-Sayre syndrome. *Stroke* 1995;26: 1950–1952.
189. Provenzale JM, VanLandingham K. Cerebral infarction associated with Kearns-Sayre syndrome-related cardiomyopathy. *Neurology* 1996; 46:826–828.
190. Lambert CD, Fairfax AJ. Neurological associations of chronic heart block. *J Neurol Neurosurg Psychiatry* 1976;39:571–575.
191. Di Pasquale G, Ribani M, Andreoli A, Zampa GA, Pinelli G. Cardioembolic stroke in primary oxalosis with cardiac involvement. *Stroke* 1989; 20:1403–1406.
192. Furlan AJ, Craciun AR, Raju NR, Hart N. Cerebrovascular complications associated with idiopathic hypertrophic subaortic stenosis. *Stroke* 1984;15:282–284.
193. Russell JW, Biller J, Hajduczok ZD, Jones MP, Kerber RE, Adams HP, Jr. Ischemic cerebrovascular complications and risk factors in idiopathic hypertrophic subaortic stenosis. *Stroke* 1991;22:1143–1147.
194. Chimowitz MI, DeGeorgia MA, Poole RM, Hepner A, Armstrong WM. Left atrial spontaneous echo contrast is highly associated with previous stroke in patients with atrial fibrillation or mitral stenosis. *Stroke* 1993;24:1015–1019.
195. Karatasakis GT, Gotsis AC, Cokkinos DV. Influence of mitral regurgitation on left atrial thrombus and spontaneous echocardiographic contrast in patients with rheumatic mitral valve disease. *Am J Cardiol* 1995;76:279–281.
196. Uzui H, Lee JD, Shimizu H, et al. Echocardiographic and hematological variables as a risk factor for stroke in chronic nonvalvular atrial fibrillation. *J Cardiol* 1998;32:15–20.
197. Orsinelli DA, Pearson AC. Detection of prosthetic valve strands by transesophageal echocardiographic: clinical significance in patients with suspected cardiac source of embolism. *J Am Coll Cardiol* 1995;26:1713–1718.
198. Roberts JK, Omarali I, Di Tullio MR, Sciacca RR, Sacco RL, Homma S. Valvular strands and cerebral ischemia. Effect of demographics and strand characteristics. *Stroke* 1997;28:2185–2188.
199. Freedberg RS, Goodkin GM, Perez JL, Tunick PA, Kronzon I. Valve strands are strongly associated with systemic embolization: a transesophageal echocardiographic study. *J Am Coll Cardiol* 1995;26:1709–1712.
200. Cohen A, Tzourio C, Chauvel C, et al. Mitral valve strands and the risk of ischemic stroke in elderly patients. The French Study of Aortic Plaques in Stroke (FAPS) Investigators. *Stroke* 1997;28:1574–1578.
201. Nighoghossian N, Derex L, Loire R, et al. Giant Lambl excrescences. An unusual source of cerebral embolism. *Arch Neurol* 1997;54:41–44.
202. Wolman R, Nussmeier N, Aggarwal A, et al. Cerebral injury after cardiac surgery. *Stroke* 1999;30:514–522.
203. Ricotta JJ, Faggioli GL, Castilone A, Hassett JM. Risk factors for stroke after cardiac surgery: Buffalo Cardiac-Cerebral Study Group. *J Vasc Surg* 1995;21:359–363.
204. Dawson DM, Fischer EG. Neurologic complications of cardiac catheterization. *Neurology* 1977; 27:496–497.
205. Kosmorsky G, Hanson MR, Tomsak RL. Neuro-ophthalmologic complications of cardiac catheterization. *Neurology* 1988;38:483–485.
206. Vik-Mo H, Todnem K, Folling M, Rosland GA. Transient visual disturbance during cardiac catheterization with angiography. *Cathet Cardiovasc Diagn* 1986;12:1–4.
207. Kinn RM, Breisblatt WM. Cortical blindness after coronary angiography: a rare but reversible complication. *Cathet Cardiovasc Diagn* 1991;22:177–179.
208. Fischer A, Ozbek C, Bay W, Hamann GF. Cerebral microemboli during left heart catheterization. *Am Heart J* 1999;137:162–168.
209. Wijman CA, Kase CS, Jacobs AK, Whitehead RE. Cerebral air embolism as a cause of stroke during cardiac catheterization. *Neurology* 1998;51:318–319.
210. Dimarco JP, Garan H, Ruskin JN. Complications in patients undergoing cardiac electrophysiologic procedures. *Ann Intern Med* 1982;97:490–493.
211. Bladin CF, Bingham L, Grigg L, Yapanis AG, Gerraty R, Davis SM. Transcranial Doppler detection of microemboli during percutaneous transluminal coronary angioplasty. *Stroke* 1998;29:2367–2370.
212. Galbreath C, Salgado ED, Furlan AJ, Hollman J. Central nervous system complications of percutaneous transluminal coronary angioplasty. *Stroke* 1986;17:616–619.
213. Adair JC, Call GK, O'Connell JB. A complication of right ventricular endomyocardial biopsy. *Cathet Cardiovasc Diagn* 1991;23:32–33.
214. Grocott HP, Amory DW, Lowry E, Newman MF, Lowe JE, Clements FM. Cerebral embolization during transmyocardial laser revascularization. *J Thorac Cardiovasc Surg* 1997;114:856–858.
215. Davidson CJ, Skelton TN, Kisslo KB, et al. The risk for systemic embolization associated with percutaneous balloon valvuloplasty in adults. A prospective comprehensive evaluation. *Ann Intern Med* 1988;108:557–560.
216. Goldstein DJ, Oz MC, Rose EA. Implantable left ventricular assist devices. *N Engl J Med* 1998; 339:1522–1533.
217. Schmid C, Weyand M, Nabavi DG, et al. Cerebral and systemic embolization during left ventricular support with the Novacor N100 device. *Ann Thorac Surg* 1998;65:1703–1710.
218. Moazami N, Roberts K, Argenziano M, et al. Asymptomatic microembolism in patients with long-term ventricular assist support. *ASAIO Journal* 1997;43:177–180.
219. Eidelman BH, Obrist WD, Wagner WR, Kormos R, Griffith B. Cerebrovascular complications associated with the use of artificial circulatory support services. *Neurol Clin* 1993;11:463–474.
220. Lazar HL, Bao Y, Rivers S, Treanor PR, Shemin RJ. Decreased incidence of arterial thrombosis

using heparin-bonded intraaortic balloons. *Ann Thorac Surg* 1999;67:446–449.
221. Brillman J. Central nervous system complications in coronary artery bypass graft surgery. *Neurol Clin* 1993;11:475–495.
222. Savageau JA, Stanton BA, Jenkins CD, Frater RW. Neuropsychological dysfunction following elective cardiac operation. II. A six-month reassessment. *J Thorac Cardiovasc Surg* 1982;84: 595–600.
223. Savageau JA, Stanton BA, Jenkins CD, Klein MD. Neuropsychological dysfunction following elective cardiac operation. I. Early assessment. *J Thorac Cardiovasc Surg* 1982;84:585–594.
224. Barbut D, Caplan LR. Brain complications of cardiac surgery. *Current Problems in Cardiol* 1997; 22:449–480.
225. Barbut D, Grassineau D, Lis E, Heier L, Hartman GS, Isom OW. Posterior distribution of infarcts in strokes related to cardiac operations. *Ann Thorac Surg* 1998;65:1656–1659.
226. Aberg T, Ronquist G, Tyden H, et al. Adverse effects on the brain in cardiac operations as assessed by biochemical, psychometric, and radiologic methods. *J Thorac Cardiovasc Surg* 1984; 87:99–105.
227. Hogue CWJ, Murphy SF, Schechtman KB, Davila-Roman VG. Risk factors for early or delayed stroke after cardiac surgery. *Circulation* 1999;100:642–647.
228. Sweeney PJ, Breuer AC, Selhorst JB, et al. Ischemic optic neuropathy: a complication of cardiopulmonary bypass surgery. *Neurology* 1982;32:560–562.
229. Taylor KM. Central nervous system effects of cardiopulmonary bypass. *Ann Thorac Surg* 1998; 66:S20–S24.
230. Shaw PJ, Bates D, Cartlidge NE, et al. Neuro-ophthalmological complications of coronary artery bypass graft surgery. *Acta Neurol Scand* 1987;76:1–7.
231. Taugher PJ. Visual loss after cardiopulmonary bypass. *Am J Ophthalmol* 1976;81:280–288.
232. Lynn GM, Stefanko K, Reed JF, Gee W, Nicholas G. Risk factors for stroke after coronary artery bypass. *J Thorac Cardiovasc Surg* 1992;104: 1518–1523.
233. Braekken SK, Russell D, Brucher R, Abdelnoor M, Svennevig JL. Cerebral microembolic signals during cardiopulmonary bypass surgery. Frequency, time of occurrence, and association with patient and surgical characteristics. *Stroke* 1997;28:1988–1992.
234. Roach GW, Kanchuger M, Mangano CM, et al. Adverse cerebral outcomes after coronary bypass surgery. Multicenter Study of Perioperative Ischemia Research Group and the Ischemia Research and Education Foundation Investigators. *N Engl J Med* 1996;335:1857–1863.
235. Carrascal Y, Guerrero AL, Maroto LC, et al. Neurological complications after cardiopulmonary bypass: an update. *Eur Neurol* 1999; 41:128–134.
236. Borger MA, Ivanov J, Weisel RD, et al. Decreasing incidence of stroke during valvular surgery. *Circulation* 1998;98:II137–II143
237. Libman RB, Wirkowski E, Neystat M, Barr W, Gelb S, Graver M. Stroke associated with cardiac surgery. Determinants, timing, and stroke subtypes. *Arch Neurol* 1997;54:83–87.
238. Mills NL, Ochsner JL. Massive air embolism during cardiopulmonary bypass. Causes, prevention, and management. *J Thorac Cardiovasc Surg* 1980;80:708–717.
239. Tettenborn B, Caplan LR, Sloan MA, et al. Postoperative brainstem and cerebellar infarcts. *Neurology* 1993;43:471–477.
240. Brown WR, Moody DM, Challa VR. Cerebral fat embolism from cardiopulmonary bypass. *J Neuropathol Exp Neurol* 1999;58:109–119.
241. Brooker RF, Brown WR, Moody DM, et al. Cardiotomy suction: a major source of brain lipid emboli during cardiopulmonary bypass. *Ann Thorac Surg* 1998;65:1651–1655.
242. Pugsley W, Klinger L, Paschalis C, Treasure T, Harrison M, Newman S. The impact of microemboli during cardiopulmonary bypass on neuropsychological functioning. *Stroke* 1994; 25:1393–1399.
243. Masuda J, Yutani C, Ogata J, Kuriyama Y, Yamaguchi T. Atheromatous embolism in the brain: a clinicopathologic analysis of 15 autopsy cases. *Neurology* 1994;44:1231–1237.
244. Choudhary SK, Bhan A, Sharma R, et al. Aortic atherosclerosis and perioperative stroke in patients undergoing coronary artery bypass: role of intra-operative transesophageal echocardiographic. *Internat J Cardiol* 1997;61:31–38.
245. Reed GL, Singer DE, Picard EH, DeSanctis RW. Stroke following coronary-artery bypass surgery. A case-control estimate of the risk from carotid bruits. *N Engl J Med* 1988;319:1246–1250.
246. van der Linden J, Casimir-Ahn H. When do cerebral emboli appear during open heart operations? A transcranial Doppler study. *Ann Thorac Surg* 1991;51:237–241.
247. Beall AC, Jr., Jones JW, Guinn GA, Svensson LG, Nahas C. Cardiopulmonary bypass in patients with previously completed stroke. *Ann Thorac Surg* 1993;55:1383–1385.
248. Brener BJ, Brief DK, Alpert J, et al. A four-year experience with preoperative noninvasive carotid evaluation of two thousand twenty-six patients undergoing cardiac surgery. *J Vasc Surg* 1984;1:326–328.
249. Brener BJ, Brief DK, Alpert J, Goldenkranz RJ, Parsonnet V. The risk of stroke in patients with asymptomatic carotid stenosis undergoing cardiac surgery. A followup study. *J Vasc Surg* 1987;5:269–279.
250. Dashe JF, Pessin MS, Murphy RE, Payne DD. Carotid occlusive disease and stroke risk in coronary artery bypass graft surgery. *Neurology* 1997;49:678–686.
251. Gerraty RP, Gates PC, Doyle JC. Carotid stenosis and perioperative stroke risk in symptomatic and asymptomatic patients undergoing vascular or coronary surgery. *Stroke* 1993;24:1115–1118.
252. Furlan AJ, Craciun AR. Risk of stroke during coronary artery bypass graft surgery in patients with internal carotid artery disease documented by angiography. *Stroke* 1985;16:797–799.

253. Safa TK, Friedman S, Mehta M, et al. Management of coexisting coronary artery and asymptomatic carotid artery disease: report of a series of patients treated with coronary bypass alone. *Eur J Vasc Endovasc Surg* 1999;17:249–252.
254. Barbut D, Lo YW, Hartman GS, et al. Aortic atheroma is related to outcome but not numbers of emboli during coronary bypass. *Ann Thorac Surg* 1997;64:454–459.
255. Kirkham FJ. Recognition and prevention of neurological complications in pediatric cardiac surgery. *Ped Cardiol* 1998;19:331–345.
256. Pua HL, Bissonnette B. Cerebral physiology in paediatric cardiopulmonary bypass. *Can J Anaesth* 1998;45:960–978.
257. Quinones JA, Deleon SY, Bell TJ, et al. Fenestrated fontan procedure: evolution of technique and occurrence of paradoxical embolism. *Ped Cardiol* 1997;18:218–221.
258. Sila CA. Spectrum of neurologic events following cardiac transplantation. *Stroke* 1989;20: 1586–1589.
259. Patchell RA. Neurological complications of organ transplantation. *Ann Neurol* 1994;36:688–703.
260. Adair JC, Call GK, O'Connell JB, Baringer JR. Cerebrovascular syndromes following cardiac transplantation. *Neurology* 1992;42:819–823.
261. Ang LC, Gillett JM, Kaufmann JCE. Neuropathology of heart transplantation. *Can J Neurol Sci* 1989;16:291–298.
262. Andrews BT, Hershon JJ, Calanchini P, Avery GJ, II, Hill JD. Neurologic ecomplications of cardiac transplantation. *West J Med* 1991;153: 146–148.
263. Yu AS, Levy E. Paradoxical cerebral air embolism from a hemodialysis catheter. *Am J Kidney Dise* 1997;29:453–455.
264. Jensen ME, Lipper MH. CT in atrogenic cerebral air embolism. *Am J Neuroradiol* 1986;7: 823–827.
265. Bitterman H, Melamed Y. Delayed hyperbaric treatment of cerebral air embolism. *Isr J Med Sci* 1993;29:22–26.
266. Thomas JE, Ayyar DR. Systemic fat embolism. A diagnostic profile in 24 patients. *Arch Neurol* 1972;26:517–523.
267. Saito A, Meguro K, Matsumura A, Komatsu Y, Oohashi N. Magnetic resonance imaging of a fat embolism of the brain: case report. *Neurosurgery* 1990;26:882–884.
268. Schulz PE, Weiner SP, Haber LM, Armstrong DD, Fishman MA. Neurological complications from fat emulsion therapy. *Ann Neurol* 1994; 35:628–630.
269. Bitar S, Gomez CR. Stroke following injection of a melted suppository. *Stroke* 1993;24: 741–743.
270. Mainprize TC, Maltby JR. Amniotic fluid embolism: a report of four probable cases. *Can Anaesth Soc J* 1986;33:382–387.
271. Lefkovitz NW, Roessmann U, Kori SH. Major cerebral infarction from tumor embolus. *Stroke* 1986;17:555–557.
272. Ben-Hur T, Siegal T. Brainstem infarction due to a tumor embolus. *Cerebrovasc Dis* 1996;6: 52–53.
273. Swanson KL, Prakash UBS, Stanson AW. Pulmonary arteriovenous fistulas: Mayo Clinic experience, 1982–1997. *Mayo Clin Proc* 1999; 74:671–680.
274. Albers GW, Easton JD, Sacco RL, Teal P. Antithrombotic and thrombolytic therapy for ischemic stroke. *Chest* 1998;114:683S–698S.

Chapter 7

NON-ATHEROSCLEROTIC VASCULOPATHIES

Several non-atherosclerotic vascular diseases can cause ischemic stroke. When compared with atherosclerosis and cardioembolism, the number of persons with stroke secondary to non-atherosclerotic vasculopathies is relatively small. In one clinical trial, stroke attributed to non-atherosclerotic vasculopathies accounted for less than 5% of cases.[1] Although these disorders can occur in any age group, the impact of non-atherosclerotic vasculopathies is most prominent in young adults and children because atherosclerosis is relatively uncommon in this population. Non-atherosclerotic vasculopathies can be categorized as non-inflammatory, infectious, and inflammatory but non-infectious (Table 7–1). Most patients do not have non-atherosclerotic vascular diseases, but these conditions should be considered in cases of atypical stroke. Each of these disorders has relatively distinct clinical findings that point to the likely cause for stroke. In addition, brain and vascular imaging studies, examination of the cerebrospinal fluid (CSF), and results of serological blood tests often are pivotal in diagnosis.

Table 7–1. **Non-atherosclerotic Vasculopathies**

Non-inflammatory
Arterial dissection
Arterial trauma
Radiation-induced vasculopathy
Fibromuscular dysplasia
Buerger disease
Saccular aneurysm
Moyamoya disease and syndrome
Infectious
Syphilis
Acquired immune deficiency syndrome
Herpes zoster and varicella
Cysticercosis
Bacterial meningitis
Aspergillosis
Mucormycosis
Cat scratch disease
Malaria
Whipple disease
Behçet disease
Inflammatory, non-infectious
Isolated central nervous system vasculitis (granulomatous angiitis)
Multisystem vasculitis
Cogan syndrome
Eale disease
Necrotizing vasculitis
Periarteritis nodosa
Wegener disease
Churg-Strauss angiitis
Giant cell arteritis
Giant cell arteritis (temporal arteritis)
Takayasu disease
Other vasculitis
Systemic lupus erythematosus
Scleroderma
Rheumatoid arthritis
Mixed connective tissue disease
Inflammatory bowel disease
Ulcerative colitis
Regional enteritis (Crohn disease)
Sarcoidosis

NON-INFLAMMATORY VASCULOPATHIES

Arterial Dissection

Dissection of intracranial or extracranial arteries was not widely detected as a cause of stroke until approximately 1975. As findings of the disease have begun to be increasingly recognized, the number of individuals diagnosed as having an arterial dissection has grown considerably. Now, it probably is second only to atherosclerosis as an arterial cause of stroke. Based on the number of events reported from the Rochester, Minnesota, community, Schievink et al[2] estimated that incidence for symptomatic arterial dissections was 2.6 (0.9–4.2)/100,000. The same group reported that the peak occurrence of spontaneous cervical dissections was in autumn.[3] The reason for this seasonal association is not clear. Arterial dissection can occur in any age group, but it is most commonly diagnosed in young adults and children.[4] The strong age relationship may be attributed partially to a heightened index of suspicion of dissection when a stroke occurs in a child or a young adult. The predominance of young people with dissections also may be related to underlying conditions that predispose to stroke and the higher risk for trauma secondary to sports and other vigorous activity among children and young adults. The following scenario often summarizes it: an acute ischemic stroke accompanied by intense neck or head pain occurring in a young person who has no obvious reason for the vascular event.

PATHOPHYSIOLOGY

Arterial dissection can occur spontaneously or can follow cranial or cervical trauma. The severity of the trauma does not need to be extreme, and arterial dissection can complicate even a brief, intense neck movement such as that which occurs with sneezing or coughing. The trauma usually involves rotation and torsion of the neck, with stretching of the artery over a bony prominence while the artery is tethered by structures such as a foramen at the base of the skull, the dura

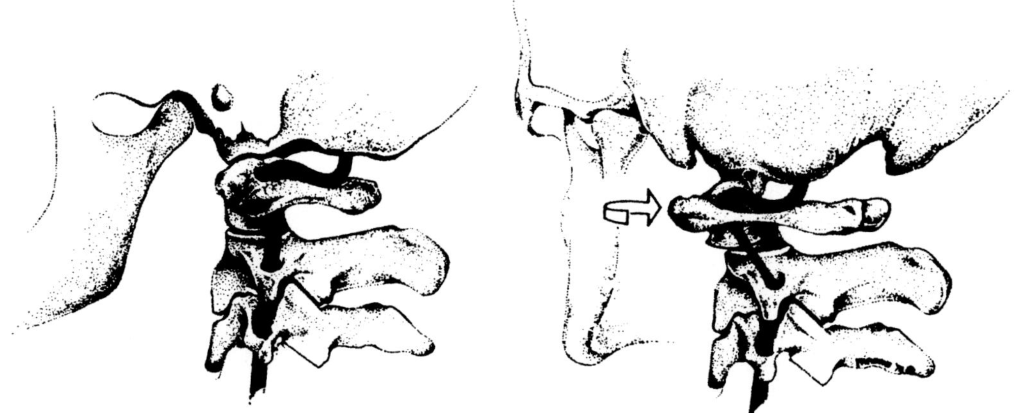

Figure 7–1. Vulnerability of the vertebral artery at the cranio-cervical junction that occurs with rotation of the head. (Reprinted from Barnett HJM. Progress towards stroke prevention. Robert Wartenberg lecture. *Neurology* 1980;30:1212, with permission.)

mater, soft tissues in the neck, and the vertebra (Fig. 7–1). The movement places stress on the artery, which leads to tearing of the intima. A tear in the endothelial surface permits an egress of blood from the normal lumen into the arterial wall itself. The resulting tearing (dissection) of tissue in the medial layer leads to severe stenosis or collapse of the normal lumen, leading to an arterial occlusion. The normal lumen usually has a tapered narrowing or occlusion just distal from the proximal site of the endothelial tear. The dissection can lead to occlusion of the orifices of small branches of the injured artery. A large intramural hematoma can promote formation of a false aneurysm that can be sufficiently large to produce compression on adjacent structures. Occasionally, the stream of blood will return into the normal lumen and produce a double lumen in the artery. Dissections of intracranial arteries can be transmural and lead to a subarachnoid hemorrhage. The ischemic complications of arterial dissection can be secondary to hypoperfusion or emboli that arise from the arterial flap.

LOCATIONS

A segment of the internal carotid artery approximately 1.5–2 cm. above the bifurcation is the most common location for extracranial dissection (Table 7–2). The artery is tethered adjacent to the body of the second cervical vertebra. From this site, the dissection can span up the length of the artery to the base of the skull (Fig. 7–2). The lumen usually tapers to a very constricted section or to an occlusion. Intracranial extension can occur, although differentiating the dissection from a secondary collapse of the arterial lumen from slow flow distal to the high-grade stenosis is difficult.

The most common location for vertebral artery dissection is adjacent to the body of the first cervical vertebra.[5] At this point, the artery is injured as it penetrates the

Table 7–2. **Most Common Locations for Arterial Dissection**

Internal carotid artery
1.5–2 cm. above bifurcation (body of C-2 vertebra)
Base of skull
Distal penetration of dura
Vertebral artery
Distal segment—penetrates dura at C-1 vertebra
Proximal artery
Middle cerebral artery
Proximal portion—adjacent to skull base
Basilar artery
Middle segment

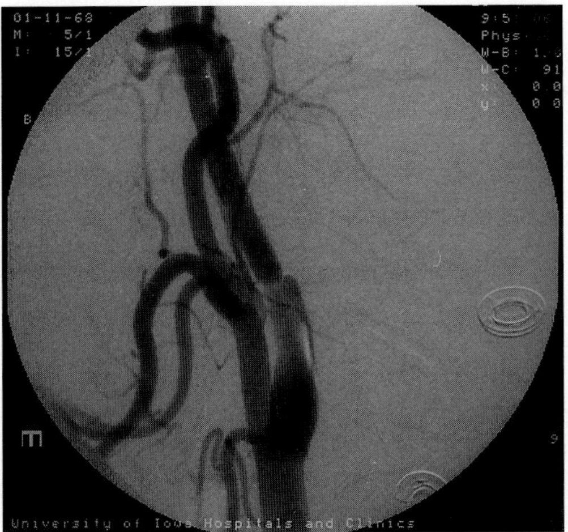

Figure 7–2. A lateral view of a carotid arteriogram using subtraction techniques demonstrates a dissection of the internal carotid artery. A second channel (double lumen) is found.

dura to enter the foramen magnum. The origin of the posterior inferior cerebellar artery and small penetrating vessels that arise from the vertebral artery usually are affected secondarily. In this situation, dissection frequently extends into the intracranial portion of the vertebral artery. It also can arise at proximal portions of the vertebral artery at the base of the neck. The dissection can occur near the origin of the vertebral artery from the subclavian artery. Although primary dissections of the intracranial arteries are much less common than those in cervical locations, they can arise in the distal segment of the internal carotid artery adjacent to the sella turcica, in the proximal segment of the middle cerebral artery, or in the mid-portion of the basilar artery. Presumably these dissections involve an element of traction against bony prominences at the base of the skull.

TRAUMATIC DISSECTION

Arterial dissection of cervical arteries causing stroke has been described as a complication of major cranio-cervical trauma including *motor vehicle accidents* or *falls*.[6] It also can be a complication of a number of *sports* that are popular among children and young adults.[7–9] (See Table 7–3.) All of these sports have common features, including sudden, brief, and often violent rotational or torsional movements of the neck. The sports also can be associated with falls that could lead to little or no overt neck injury. The injury, which most commonly affects the distal vertebral artery and extracranial portion of the internal carotid artery, might not become symptomatic for several hours or days after the trauma.

Table 7–3. **Sports Associated with Traumatic Dissections of the Cervical Arteries**

Skiing	Cycling
Wrestling	Golf
Basketball	Football
Volleyball	Archery
Horseback riding	Baseball
Softball	

In addition to sports, arterial dissection has been described as a complication of *yoga* and *self-manipulation of the neck*. In particular, dissection of the vertebral artery with secondary lateral medullary infarction is reported as a complication of *chiropractic treatment* of the cervical spine.[10–12] Hyperextension of the neck during *endotracheal intubation, anesthesia, labor* and *delivery*, or *surgical procedures* also can cause arterial dissection and stroke.[13] Malek et al[239] reported three patients with carotid dissections secondary to manual compression of the artery (attempted strangulation) as the result of domestic violence. Increased intrathoracic and intrapharyngeal pressure occuring while playing a wind sinstrument also has been associated with carotid artery dissection.[240] It also has occurred secondary to violent *sneezing* or *coughing*.

Although dissections in these cases are induced by trauma, many persons will have similar trauma and not have arterial complications. The relatively low frequency of arterial dissections in active children and young adults raises the possibility of some underlying process that makes the artery more vulnerable to the trauma.

Table 7–4. **Conditions Predisposing Spontaneous Arterial Dissections**

Fibromuscular dysplasia	Marfan syndrome
Cystic medial necrosis	Migraine
Osteogenesis imperfecta	Ehlers-Danlos III collagen deficiency
Alpha anti-trypsin deficiency	Dilated aortic root
Congenital heart disease	

SPONTANEOUS DISSECTION

Many patients with dissection do not have a history of trauma or activity that could have induced the arterial pathology. Such spontaneous cases are secondary to a number of arterial diseases and, in some instances, familial cases are described.[14–20] (See Table 7–4.) Dissection can complicate *infection* in the neck.[21,22] The relatively large number of associated conditions suggests that arterial dissection is a relatively non-specific complication of a number of diseases that weaken the structure of the arterial wall.

Still, familial clustering of cases raises the possibility of a genetic cause or predisposition for developing the arterial pathology. In one series of 200 patients with dissections, 10 reported other family members with similar arterial problems.[23] *Ehlers-Danlos type III collagen deficiency* is the inherited disorder most frequently correlated with arterial dissection.[17,24–26] Dissections also have described in patients with *dilation of the aortic root, mitral dystrophy, mitral valve prolapse,* and *aortic valve dystrophy.* Ultrastructural abnormalities resembling Ehlers-Danlos syndrome can be found in arteries with dissections.[27] These findings point to a generalized defect of the extracellular matrix.[28] Gap defects in the internal elastic lamina are speculated to be the pathological substrate for a dissection of the intracranial arteries.[29] A similar abnormality might play a role in extracranial dissections.

CLINICAL FEATURES

The lag from the time of dissection until the appearance of symptoms is variable. Biousse et al[30] noted that this interval ranged from a few minutes to 1 month. Most patients had ischemic symptoms within 1 week of the dissection. Clinical presentations include ischemic stroke, transient ischemic attack (TIA), ocular complaints, cranial nerve palsies, headache, or subarachnoid hemorrhage.[31–33] Ischemic stroke or TIA is the most common scenario (Table 7–5).

With dissections of the internal carotid artery, hemispheric or retinal ischemic symptoms predominate. Orbital ischemia can lead to amaurosis fugax, acute visual

Table 7–5. **Clinical Features of Arterial Dissections**

- Dissection of the internal carotid artery
  - Ocular ischemia
    - Amaurosis fugax
    - Anterior or posterior ischemic optic neuropathy
    - Optic disk edema
  - Hemispheric ischemia
    - Transient ischemic attack
    - Infarction—territory of middle cerebral artery
      - Lenticulostriate infarction
      - Watershed infarction
  - Neck, eye, ear, or face pain
  - Carotidynia
  - Horner syndrome
  - Isolated or multiple cranial nerve palsies
- Dissection of the vertebral artery
  - Brain stem—cerebellar ischemia
    - Dorsolateral medullary infarction
    - Inferior cerebellar infarction
  - Occipital or nuchal pain
  - Subarachnoid hemorrhage
  - Cranial nerve palsies secondary to aneurysmal mass

loss, proptosis, ophthalmoparesis, chemosis, and optic disk edema.[33–35] Ocular features include anterior or posterior ischemic optic neuropathy.[36] The ocular symptoms can precede other ischemic events, and the visual disturbances can be provoked by bright light—a finding that reflects borderline perfusion to the eye.[35] Hemispheric infarctions usually are in the territory of the middle cerebral artery and often include large lenticulostriate or subcortical watershed lesions.[37] Hemiparesis, hemisensory loss, dysarthria, and language impairments are the most common signs.

Vertebral artery dissection most commonly leads to an infarction in the dorsolateral medulla and the inferior cerebellum, causing Wallenberg syndrome.[32,38–40] Other signs of brain stem ischemia result from propagation of the arterial lesion or superimposed thrombus into the basilar artery. Distal embolism may lead to bilateral visual loss or the top-of-the-basilar syndrome.

Pain is a prominent symptom in most patients. In one series, headache or neck pain was noted in 20 of 21 patients with carotid dissections.[41] Severe ipsilateral headache, facial pain, eye pain, or neck pain accompanies dissections of the internal carotid artery.[41,42] The pain can be sufficiently severe to be the chief complaint. Neck pain usually is localized along the sternocleidomastoid muscle and the angle of the jaw. Dissection is a leading cause of carotidynia. The pain is usually described as steady or continuous. It can precede ischemic symptoms by hours to days.[43] Dissections of the vertebral artery produce ipsilateral nuchal and occipital pain.[43] The pain can lead to stiffness of the neck that can mimic the findings of meningeal irritation. An intense occipital-holocranial headache occurs when subarachnoid hemorrhage complicates a vertebral artery dissection. Pulsatile tinnitus and a cervical bruit can be heard in patients with dissection of the internal carotid artery.[32]

Horner syndrome is detected in approximately 50%–75% of cases.[44] Biousse et al[35] noted Horner syndrome and ipsilateral neck pain in 65 of 146 patients with internal carotid artery dissections; in 32, it was an isolated or primary finding. A brief, transient Horner syndrome may be the only finding of a dissection of the internal carotid artery.[45]

Dissections of the internal carotid artery can lead to either isolated or multiple cranial nerve palsies. Cranial neuropathy may be secondary to compression by the arterial lesion or from ischemia secondary to involvement of small penetrating arterioles that perfuse the nerves. Cranial nerves III, IV, VI, VII, IX, X, XI, and XII may be implicated.[44,46,47] A unilateral dilated pupil has been described with dissections presumably as a result of III nerve ischemia.[48] Facial weakness or sensory loss and oculomotor palsies are reported. Lower cranial nerve palsies can cause dysphonia, dysarthria, dysphagia, and numbness of the throat.[46]

False aneurysms can develop in approximately 5%–40% of patients with cervical dissections of the internal carotid artery.[49] (See Fig. 7–3.) The aneurysms are called *false* because the enlargement does not involve all three layers of the arterial wall. Because the dissection is below the intimal layer, the aneurysmal sac does not have an intimal lining. The lower cranial nerve palsies seen in patients with dissection of the internal carotid artery may be secondary

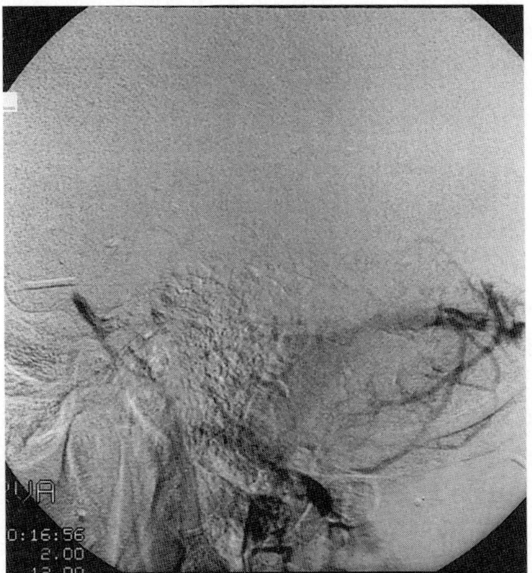

Figure 7–3. A lateral view of a vertebral arteriogram using subtraction techniques. The study was obtained in a patient with a vertebral artery dissection. A false aneurysm is seen opposite to the first cervical vertebral body.

to their compression from a false aneurysm. Approximately one-half will have resolution or reduction in the size of the aneurysm during a period of follow up. Symptoms of rupture or embolization are rare.[49] A chronic vertebral artery dissection may lead to an aneurysm that compresses the brain stem and the lower cranial nerves.[38]

A dissection aneurysm of the posterior circulation also can produce subarachnoid hemorrhage. The lesion may be confused with a fusiform or a dolichoectatic aneurysm. Subarachnoid hemorrhage can result from dissection of the distal vertebral artery or the basilar artery.[38,40,50] The bleeding reflects a transmural extravasation of blood from the lumen to the subarachnoid space.[51] The presence of only one elastic membrane in the intracranial arteries may contribute to this complication of dissection because extravascular hemorrhage is unusual with extracranial dissections. The clinical features of subarachnoid hemorrhage secondary to an arterial dissection mimic those of intracranial bleeding from other causes. Intracranial bleeding also can complicate dissections of the basilar, distal internal carotid artery or proximal middle cerebral artery.[52]

Bilateral vertebral artery dissections can develop.[53] Signs usually reflect medullary or rostral spinal cord involvement. Patients with intracranial dissections in the anterior circulation usually have headache, focal neurological impairments, seizures, syncope, or decreased consciousness.[54] The focal neurological impairments can be secondary to ischemic stroke.

EVALUATION

The evaluation of a patient with a presumed dissection focuses on the affected artery. Arteriography or intra-arterial digital subtraction angiography is the usual way to detect arterial dissection (Table 7–6). The usual finding is a tapered narrowing that can progress to an occlusion or a long segment of minimal flow (*string sign*).[50](See Figs. 7–4, 7–5, and 7–6.) The pattern of occlusion includes a distal point or tape and differs from the more horizontal cut-off pattern seen with athero-

Table 7–6. **Evaluation of the Patient with Arterial Dissection**

Brain imaging
- Computed tomography—semilunar hyperdensity with eccentric lumen
- Magnetic resonance imaging—semilunar hyperintensity with eccentric lumen
  - Patterns
    - Curvilinear
    - Crescentic
    - Band-like
    - Bamboo-cut

Vascular imaging
- Carotid duplex—decreased flow distal to bifurcation
- Transcranial Doppler ultrasonography—decreased flow
- Arteriography
  - String sign
    - Marked narrowing of artery
    - Not at usual site for atherosclerosis
    - Internal carotid—2.5 cm. above bifurcation
    - Vertebral—distal segment
  - Aneurysm
  - Double lumen

sclerotic lesions. An important clue in differentiating a dissection from severe atherosclerotic stenosis of the internal carotid artery is the site of the lesion. The usual location for a dissection is approximately 1.5–2 cm. above the carotid bifurcation. Other arteriographic findings of dissection include a *flap, pearl reaction, false aneurysm,* or *double lumen.*[50] The latter is the most specific finding for dissection, but it is relatively uncommon. Aneurysms secondary to a dissection usually do not arise at arterial bifurcations. They often are *fusiform* or *globular* in appearance and adjacent to the narrowed segment of the artery. Occlusion of cortical branches secondary to distal embolism can be detected by arteriography (See Fig. 7–5).

Computed tomography (CT) and magnetic resonance imaging (MRI) can be used to assess the extent and location of an infarction. In addition, MRI can assess the artery, which is an important attribute for

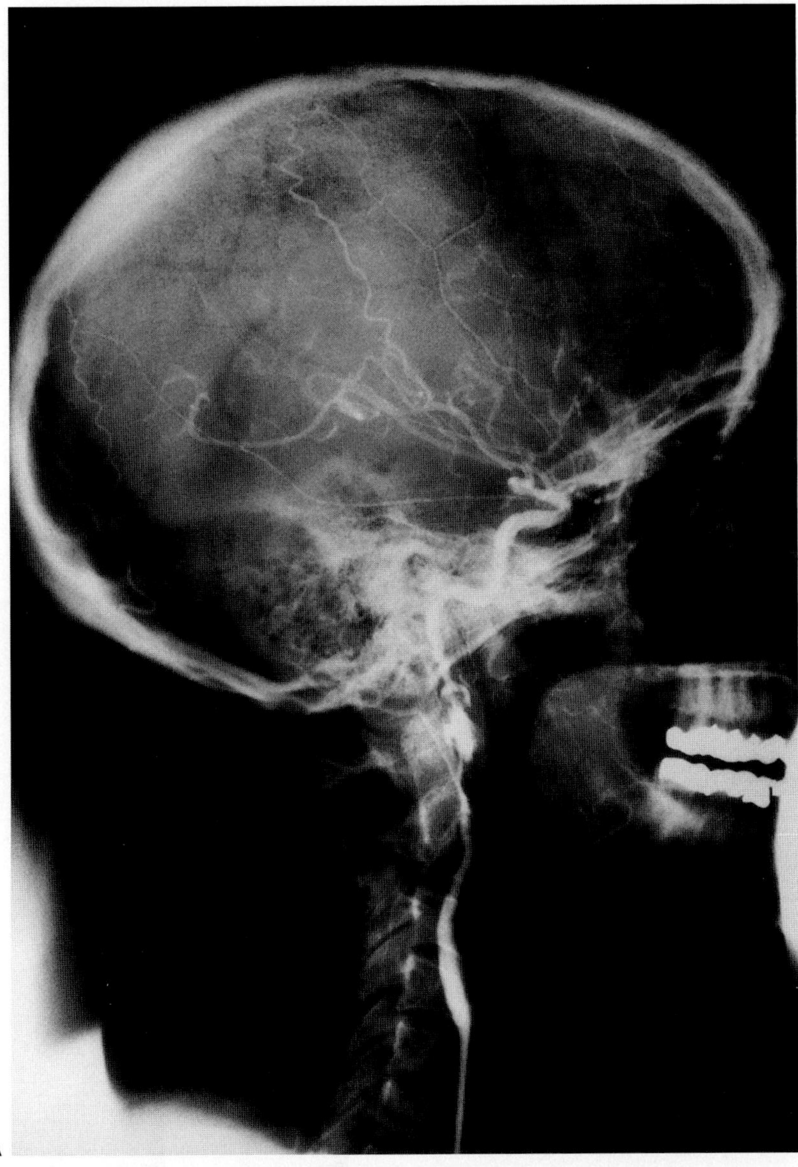

Figure 7–4. A left carotid arteriogram *(A)* and diagram *(B)* demonstrates an arterial dissection in a 33-year-old woman with neck pain, aphasia, and a right hemiparesis. *(continued)*

the evaluation of patients with dissection (See Table 7–6). The MRI hallmark of arterial dissection is an *eccentric flow void* of decreased caliber in the artery adjacent to a *semilunar hyperintensity.*[40,55–59] The hyperintensity is due to the intramural hematoma, and the lesion is described as curvilinear, crescentic, band-like, or bamboo-cut in shape.[60] The flow void may be lost if the artery is occluded, in which case the MRI may give non-specific data. The hyperintensity usually clears over 1–2 months as the arterial injury heals. The sensitivity and specificity of MRI in detecting dissections in the internal carotid artery are approximately 84% and 99%, respectively; in persons with vertebral dissections, the sensitivity and specificity are 60% and 95%, respectively.[61] The lower yield with posterior circulation dissections may reflect the

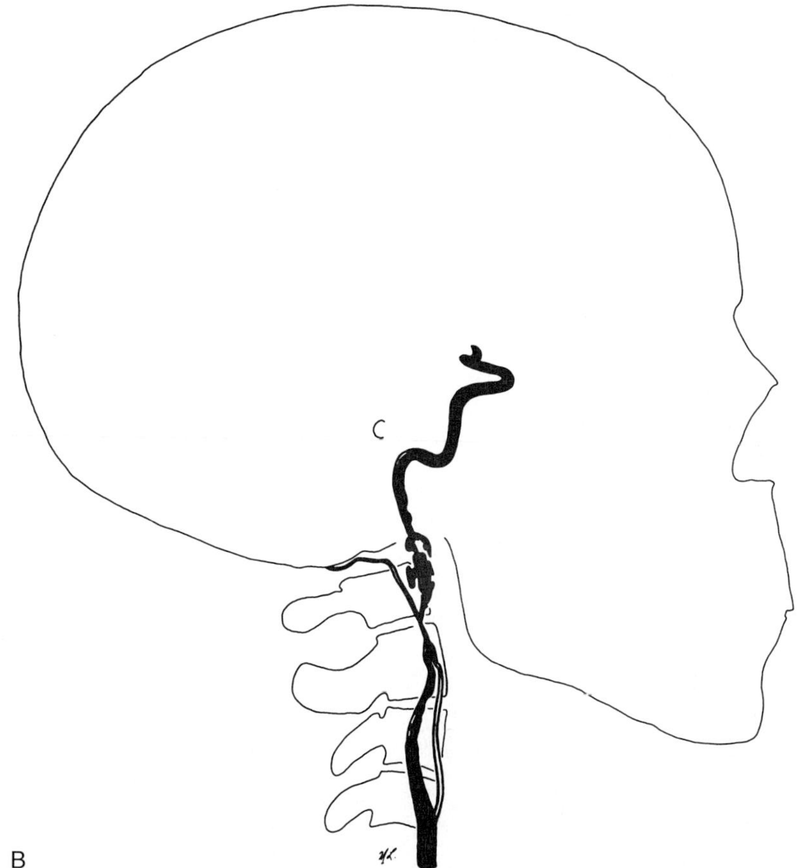

Figure 7–4. (*continued*)

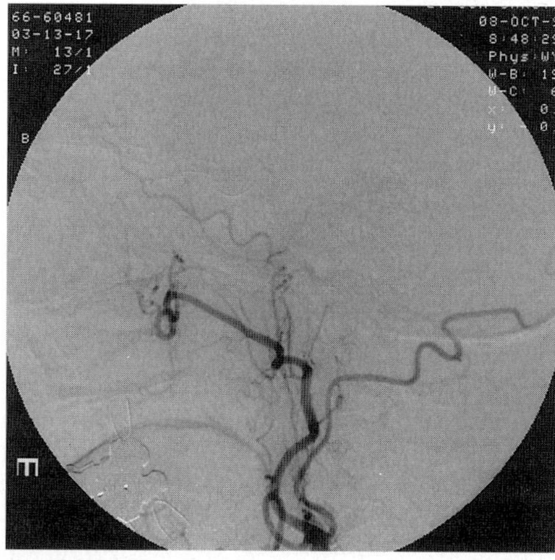

Figure 7–5. Left carotid arteriogram using subtraction techniques demonstrates a dissection of the left internal carotid arteriogram. A narrow lumen (string sign) is noted at the base of the skull.

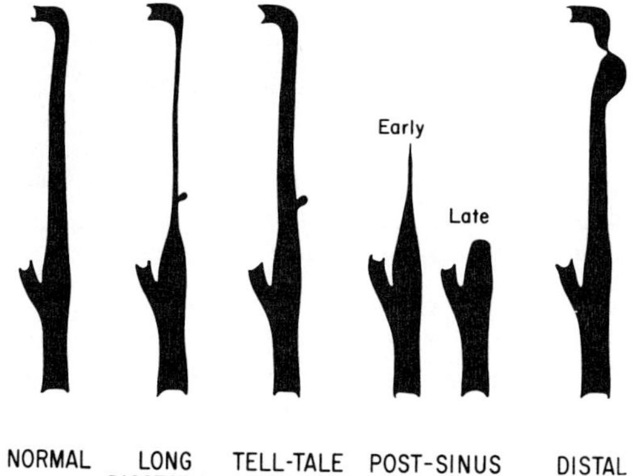

Figure 7–6. Diagrams of angiographic profiles of dissection of the internal carotid artery. (Reprinted from Fisher CM, Ojemann RG, Robertson GH. Spontaneous dissection of cervico-cerebral arteries. *Can J Neurol Sci* 1978;5:9, with permission.)

smaller caliber of the artery and its anatomic course. Dissections often occur at a location where the angle of the artery is changing. Magnetic resonance angiography (MRA) also provides data that are useful in defining the presence and extent of arterial pathology. It is very sensitive and specific in detecting a dissection of the internal carotid artery.[61] It also can detect vertebral or basilar artery lesions. A combination of MRI and MRA often can substitute for conventional arteriography.[31] If MRI and MRA are consistent with dissection, then arteriography can be avoided.

Ultrasound arterial studies provide some helpful information.[59,62,63] Although the carotid duplex does not visualize the distal extracranial portion of the internal carotid artery, which is the usual site for dissection, a finding of decreased flow in the vessel without an atheroma at the bifurcation suggests that a dissection may be present.[64,65] Patterns of decreased flow in the internal carotid artery include an *absent signal*, a *biphasic flow*, and a *high-resistance pattern*.[66] Sturzenegger[66] reported that the carotid duplex has a sensitivity of approximately 80% in predicting a dissection of the internal carotid artery. The carotid duplex could be combined with MRI and MRA to increase its sensitivity and specificity. (See Chapter 4.) Non-invasive findings of dissections of the vertebral artery are a high-resistance signal or no flow.[5,63,67] Transcranial Doppler ultrasonography (TCD) also might demonstrate decreased flow in the distal vertebral artery or the basilar artery.

PROGNOSIS

Acute prognosis after arterial dissection largely reflects the nature and severity of neurological injury. Patients with subarachnoid hemorrhage have a poor prognosis; in one series, deaths occurred in three-fourths of patients with intracranial bleeding.[52] This mortality figure exceeds that associated with ruptured saccular aneurysms and probably reflects the amount of intracranial hemorrhage. Unfavorable outcomes (death or severe disability) are reported in 15% of patients with hemispheric infarctions secondary to dissection of the internal carotid artery.[31] Deaths usually result from multilobar injuries that cause brain edema and herniation. Large subcortical or brain stem infarctions often can produce severe disability. Patients with ischemic ocular symptoms can have permanent visual sequelae. Patients with minor stroke, TIA, or local signs generally do very well.[31]

The long-term prognosis of patients with arterial dissections is generally very good, probably reflecting the young age of these patients and their lack of serious comorbid diseases. Gradual recanalization of the affected artery during the first 2 months occurs in a majority of patients.[68–70] Recurrent TIA or stroke appears to be relatively uncommon in this setting, and the risk of a second stroke seems lower than with atherosclerosis. Recurrent arterial dissection also occurs infrequently. Leys et al[69] followed 105 patients for an average of 3 years; 92 did very well. Five patients died, and 21 had residual headaches. Five patients had either a recurrent TIA or stroke in the distribution of the previously affected artery. Three patients had recurrent dissections. Bassetti et al[71] reported recurrent dissections in 3 of 74 patients; in some cases, the injury recurred at the level of the original dissection. The risk of recurrent dissection may be increased in patients with a family history of dissection.[23]

TREATMENT

Because the prognosis of patients with arterial dissection appears to be better than those with symptomatic atherosclerosis, caution should be used when prescribing interventions to prevent recurrent ischemic stroke. Although emergent anticoagulation (heparin) often is prescribed, no data exist on its effectiveness. The anticoagulants might forestall an intraluminal thrombosis and distal embolism; however, its presence could aggravate the intramural hemorrhage that denotes dissection. Additional bleeding within the arterial wall could promote collapse of the normal lumen. Emergent anticoagulation of a patient with an acute vertebral or intracranial dissection may be particularly dangerous because of the potential for subarachnoid hemorrhage. The safety and efficacy of thrombolytic therapy in patients with arterial dissections is unknown. Concerns about the effects of anticoagulants might be magnified with the thrombolytic agents.

Long-term oral anticoagulant therapy often is advised, but the relative usefulness of these agents is unknown when compared with antiplatelet aggregating agents. (See Chapter 10.) Many affected patients are active young adults who are prone to trauma that could increase morbidity with anticoagulation. Compliance with the anticoagulant regimen also is an issue. For this reason, antiplatelet aggregating agents appear to be the treatment of choice to prevent recurrent TIA or ischemic stroke. Surgical revascularization, including intracranial-to-extracranial bypass operations, can be used to lessen the risk of ischemic stroke in patients with dissection of the internal carotid artery.[72,73] Surgical treatment of aneurysms secondary to dissection of the internal carotid artery includes ligation, resection of the involved segment, or reconstruction of the artery.[73] Although arterial dissection is a potential complication of arteriography, endovascular placement of a stent could preserve the normal lumen and help compress the intramural lesion. (See Chapter 11.)

Arterial Injuries

Blunt or penetrating injuries to extracranial arteries can cause brain ischemia. These injuries can complicate motor vehicle accidents, falls, sports-related trauma, or other neck injuries.[6,74–76]

INTERNAL CAROTID ARTERY TRAUMA

A carotid artery occlusion, secondary to dissection or blunt intramural thrombosis, can occur immediately or shortly after a motor vehicle crash.[6,77] It should be suspected when a patient has signs of a major hemispheric injury that are seen within hours of the trauma but whose brain imaging study does not demonstrate intracerebral hemorrhage. Duplex imaging or TCD may be critical in detecting an occluded artery during the first hours of treatment. Less commonly, occlusion of the middle cerebral artery can complicate a blunt head injury.[78] In most patients with traumatic occlusion, treatment is influenced by the nature of the other injuries. Anticoagulant or thrombolytic agents probably cannot be given.

Compression of the internal carotid artery can lead to stroke as a complication of attempted strangulation.[79–81] External signs of soft tissue injury usually point to this etiology. Compression of the carotid artery during a sustained posture also could lead to arterial occlusion.[82] In an older person, blunt trauma to the carotid artery could fracture an atherosclerotic plaque that leads to thrombosis. Blunt trauma to the internal carotid artery can complicate a penetrating or compressive injury in the tonsillar fossa. A child could fall forward while running with a stick in his or her mouth, and the stick could traumatize the internal carotid artery at the back of the mouth.[83] This stroke sometimes is called *lollypop palsy*. The internal carotid artery also can be injured during tonsillectomy. With severe bleeding in the operative site, ill-advised deep ligature could cause a carotid occlusion.

Blunt trauma at the base of the skull can lead to injury of the internal carotid artery and the development of pseudoaneurysms or a carotid cavernous fistula.[77] These lesions cause mass symptoms, ocular symptoms, headaches, and facial edema. Symptoms of brain ischemia are uncommon. Treatment of these lesions often involves endovascular embolization. Preservation of the integrity of the lumen of the internal carotid artery is a critical part of the planning. Penetrating carotid arterial trauma can lead to ischemic stroke. The most common causes of the injury are gunshot wounds and stabbing with sharp objects.[84] Less commonly, the vertebral artery can be involved with a penetrating neck wound. Because life-threatening hemorrhage usually is prominent, surgical treatment of the injured artery, including ligation, usually is needed. Ischemia can complicate treatment of the arterial injury.

VERTEBRAL ARTERY TRAUMA

Cervical spine trauma can injure the vertebral artery and cause secondary infarction of the spinal cord, cerebellum, or brain stem.[76,85–87] Stroke may be the underlying cause of spinal cord dysfunction in a sizeable proportion of patients with cervical spine trauma. The frequency of vertebral artery injury secondary to blunt trauma to the neck probably is more common than is believed. Among the injuries is vertebral arterial dissection that occurs with a fracture of the cervical spine. Willis et al[88] reported vertebral artery changes in 12 of 26 patients with unstable cervical spine injuries. Ischemic symptoms can be delayed for days after the trauma. Tulyapronchote et al[89] found that neurological symptoms secondary to arterial injury could occur more than 1 week after a motor vehicle crash. A patient should be evaluated for vertebral artery injury if a posterior circulation infarction follows a neck injury. Evaluation of the vertebral artery should be performed if a patient develops ischemic symptoms of either the spinal cord or the brain stem following trauma to the neck.

Mechanical occlusion or stenosis of the vertebral artery also can occur with head rotation.[90] The obstruction can be independent of dissection. An arthritic spur also can compress the vertebral artery. Patients with severe osteoarthritis or rheumatoid arthritis appear to be at greatest risk. Patients with laxity of the ligaments of the odontoid secondary to rheumatoid arthritis may develop ischemic symptoms secondary to vertebral artery compression in addition to the signs of spinal cord dysfunction. External compression of the vertebral artery should be suspected if a patient describes a strong relationship between ischemic symptoms and head turning.

VASOSPASM

Patients with craniocerebral trauma often have subarachnoid bleeding associated with the development of vasospasm approximately 5–10 days after head injury. This complication usually occurs in patients who do not have traumatic intracerebral hemorrhage but have blood restricted to the subarachnoid space. The appearance of cerebral ischemic symptoms approximately 1 week after head injury should prompt consideration of post-traumatic vasospasm. Markedly increased flow velocities detected by TCD points to the diagnosis of post-traumatic vasospasm. Ischemia secondary to vasospasm can be treated by volume expansion, hemodilution, and drug-induced hypertension in an effort to improve flow beyond the vasospastic segment. This complication is sufficiently unusual that prophylactic administration of nimodipine usually is not prescribed.

Radiation-Induced Vasculopathy

Large doses of cranial or cervical therapeutic radiation used to treat malignancies of the head and the neck can induce arterial changes. Radiation is toxic to the metabolically active endothelial cells. Occlusion of the vasa vasorum of the larger intracranial or extracranial arteries can lead to a proliferation of cellular and fibrous elements, which, in turn, lead to narrowing of the arterial lumen. Stenosis or occlusion of the larger arteries can develop up to 20 years after radiation exposure.[91] Radiation-injured arterial necrosis can cause arterial rupture in patients who have had radical neck dissections. Intracranial arterial occlusions and moyamoya syndrome may follow radiation therapy for a brain tumor, craniopharyngioma, pituitary adenoma, medulloblastoma, retinoblastoma, facial hemangioma, and optic glioma.[92–96]

Diagnosis of radiation-induced vasculopathy usually is influenced by a history of exposure to therapeutic radiation in the area of the affected artery. Magnetic resonance imaging is helpful in diagnosing the radiation angiopathy.[97] Treatment usually involves antiplatelet aggregating agents or anticoagulants. Surgical treatment of post-irradiation stenosis of the internal carotid artery can be difficult because post-operative healing can be poor. Kashyap et al[98] reported that carotid endarterectomy can be done safely in this condition. They noted no major complications among 20 patients who had the surgery. Endovascular treatment of the stenosis appears to be a promising therapy for a symptomatic stenosis of the internal carotid artery. (See Chapter 11.) Bleeding secondary to rupture of an injured artery may mandate emergent ligation. In such a situation, stroke is a likely complication of the treatment.

Fibromuscular Dysplasia

While fibromuscular dysplasia (FMD) most commonly affects the renal artery, the internal carotid artery also is involved frequently. The internal carotid artery is, in fact, the second most commonly affected vessel after the renal artery. The usual site of FMD is the extracranial portion of the internal carotid artery approximately 1.5–2 cm. above the bifurcation.[99] Fibromuscular dysplasia seems to be less common than arterial dissection and is found in less than 1% of patients who have arteriography for evaluation of ischemic symptoms.[100] Very rarely, the vertebral arteries or the basilar artery may be affected.[101–103] The other intracranial arteries appear not to be affected. Fibromuscular dysplasia is found more commonly in women than in men. The peak frequency appears to be in young adults.[102] Corrin et al[100] reported that 74 of 82 patients with FMD were women. The cause of FMD is unknown, although one report associated the condition with *Ollier disease*.[104]

Fibromuscular dysplasia usually is first diagnosed by arteriography. It often is found as an incidental finding during arteriographic evaluation for another illness. Radiologic findings include a *string of beads*, a *long tapered segment*, or a *false aneurysm*. The first is the most common and specific finding for FMD. The usual location for FMD of the internal carotid artery is approximately 1.5 cm. above the bifurcation. Many of the abnormalities mimic those seen with arterial dissection. Dissection is a potential complication of FMD, and some of the cases that were ascribed to FMD in the past likely were due to dissection. The differential diagnosis also includes vasospasm secondary to the arteriographic procedure itself.

Stroke is a common presentation of FMD. In one series of 44 patients with cervical FMD, 22 had ischemic symptoms.[105] So et al[102] reported that 18 of 32 patients with FMD had either TIA or ischemic stroke. In a series of 30 patients, Wessen and Elliott[106] reported that 23 had ischemia, including TIA, amaurosis fugax, stroke, or global neurological symptoms. Besides causing symptoms of TIA or ischemic stroke, a patient with FMD may have pulsatile tinnitus or an asymptomatic carotid bruit. Fibromuscular dysplasia also has been associated with an increased frequency of *intracranial saccular aneurysms*. The relationship of between FMD and aneurysm is uncertain because changes in the internal carotid artery often are detected during an evaluation for the aneurysm. Thus, an element of selection bias may be present. Fibromuscular dysplasia also may be an asymptomatic finding detected by arteriography performed for another indication.[100]

The prognosis of patients with FMD appears to be relatively benign. Most patients do well. The rate of recurrent stroke appears to be much lower than that associated with atherosclerotic disease. Treatment with antiplatelet aggregating agents usually is prescribed. Surgical resection or dilation of the arterial segment with the FMD can be performed. (See Chapter 11.)

Buerger Disease

Digital ischemia leading to ulceration, *Raynaud phenomenon, claudication* of the upper or lower limbs, and superficial *thrombophlebitis* are the hallmarks of *Buerger disease*.[107,108] Virtually all patients with Buerger disease have a long-term history of heavy tobacco use. Approximately three-fourths of the patients are men, and most are young or middle-age.[108] Neurological symptoms are uncommon, but TIA or ischemic stroke has been reported in exceptional cases.[109] The risk of recurrent ischemic symptoms is uncertain. In addition to smoking cessation, treatment generally follows that prescribed to persons with atherosclerosis.

Intracranial Saccular Aneurysms

Laminar formation of a thrombus may occur with a large (10–25 mm. diameter) or giant (> 25 mm. diameter) *intracranial saccular aneurysm.* (Figs. 7–7 and 7–8). Flow usually is slow within the aneurysmal sac, and clotting factors are activated. Turbulence of flow within the aneurysm can promote fragmentation of the thrombus, leading to distal embolism.[110] Recurrent TIA or ischemic stroke is a potential but rare presentation of patients with these aneurysms.[111–113] These large aneurysms also may compress adjacent vascular and neural structures and produce signs of an intracranial mass. The basilar bifurcation is the most common site for aneurysms that cause vertebrobasilar ischemic symptoms. The intracavernous or intracranial portions of the internal carotid artery are the most common sites for those that cause hemispheric ischemia.

Because aneurysms that are the source for emboli usually are larger than 1 cm. in size, CT or MRI of the brain usually detects them. Magnetic resonance angiography or CT angiography can define the size and location of the aneurysm as well as the location of adjacent vessels. These aneurysms usually have not ruptured at the time of clinical presentation. Treatment options include endovascular embolization to the

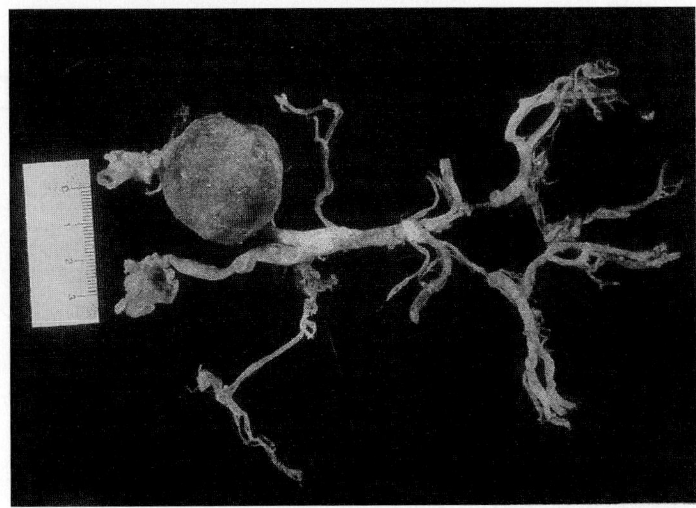

Figure 7–7. Giant saccular aneurysm of the vertebral artery. (Courtesy of Dr. Robert Hammond, University of Western Ontario, London Ontario.)

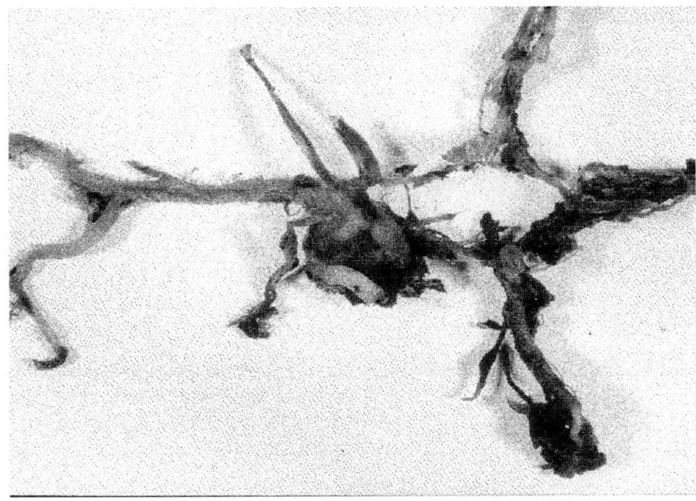

Figure 7–8. Giant saccular aneurysm of the posterior cerebral artery. (Courtesy of Dr. Robert Hammond, University of Western Ontario, London Ontario.)

aneurysm or surgical ligation of the aneurysm. Their large size means that surgical procedures to clip the aneurysm can be difficult.

Pseudoxanthoma Elasticum

Pseudoxanthoma elasticum is a rare inherited condition that leads to laxity of the skin, redundant skin, and abnormalities in the ocular fundus. It appears to be associated with mitral valve prolapse and cardiac abnormalities. Ischemic stroke, intracranial hemorrhage, seizures, and dementia are among its neurological complications.[114] The mechanism of stroke has not been determined, but it might involve changes in elastic tissue elements in the arteries. This very uncommon illness rarely will arise in the differential diagnosis of causes of stroke.

Table 7–7. **Radiological Features of Moyamoya Disease or Syndrome**

Usually bilateral involvement
  Can start unilaterally
  Asymmetrical
Occlusion or severe stenosis
  Proximal middle cerebral artery
  Proximal anterior cerebral artery
  Distal internal carotid artery
  Posterior cerebral artery affected late
Prominent basal network of small-caliber vessels (moyamoya)
Prominent collateral channels
  Leptomeningeal vessels
  Ethmoidal arteries
  Branches of posterior cerebral artery
Saccular aneurysms—especially of posterior circulation

Moyamoya Disease and Moyamoya Syndrome

Moyamoya disease is a progressive, largely intracranial, vasculopathy that causes ischemic or hemorrhagic stroke in children and young adults. Moyamoya disease was first described in Japan but, subsequently, cases have been described around the world. The hallmark of moyamoya is occlusion of the distal portions of both internal carotid arteries and obliteration of the proximal portions of both the anterior and the middle cerebral arteries (Table 7–7). These vessels are replaced by a bilateral basal meshwork of small-caliber vessels that look like a puff of smoke, an appearance that is the source of the name (Fig. 7–9). Collateral channels from the posterior circulation and the ethmoidal and other basal vessels are prominent so that adequate perfusion is maintained.[115] As the disease progresses, the small collateral channels also become obliterated. Rather than growth of new arterioles, the disease appears to promote dilation of existing vessels.[116,117] Occasionally, the changes of moyamoya may be unilateral when first detected.[118] Some asymmetry in the vascular changes between the hemispheres often is noted early in the disease. As it progresses, arterial changes usually become symmetrical. If they are strictly unilateral, then the findings should be considered atypical from moyamoya and alternative diagnoses, including embolic occlusions, should be sought.

Moyamoya disease occurs primarily in northeastern Asia and is not associated with other conditions. A sizeable proportion of patients in Japan report that other family members also have the disease, a feature that suggests a genetic cause or predisposition. Yamauchi et al[241] located the responsible gene to chromosome 17 q 25. Moyamoya syndrome is more commonly described elsewhere in the world. In this situation, patients have arteriographic findings consistent with moyamoya but with an identified underlying condition that promotes the vasculopathy.[96,119–121] (See Table 7–8.) A large number of predisposing conditions have been described, a finding that supports the contention that moyamoya syndrome may be a nonspecific radiologic finding. A relationship between moyamoya and radiation therapy to the base of the brain is reported.[122] An association may exist in young women between moyamoya syndrome and smoking and oral contraceptives use. In contrast, pregnancy does not seem to aggravate the effects of moyamoya.[123]

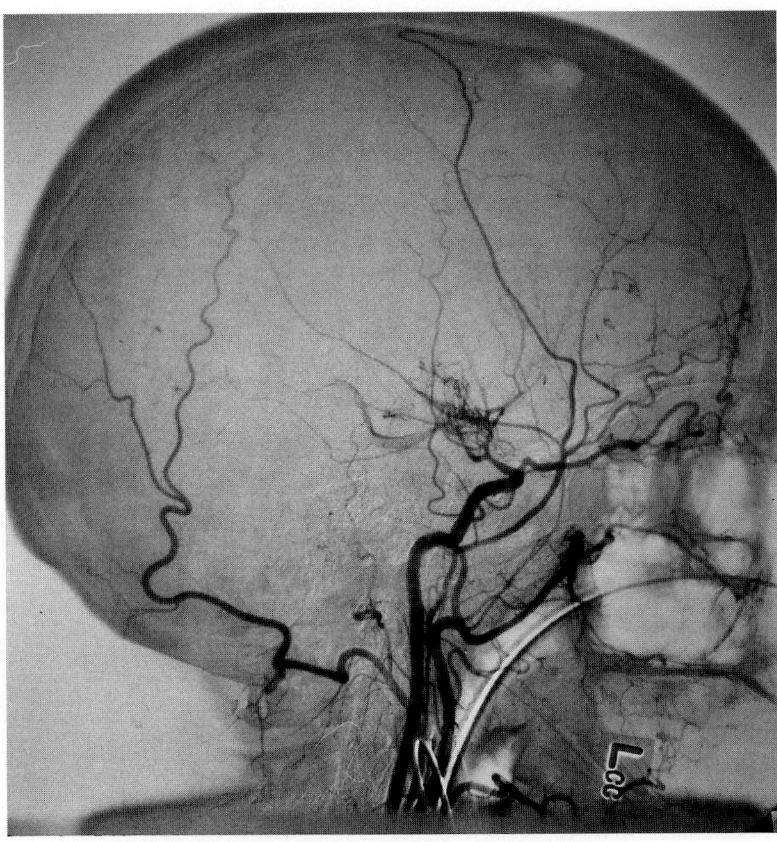

Figure 7–9. Right carotid arteriogram with subtraction technique obtained in a patient with moyamoya disease. Occlusions are noted in the proximal portion of the anterior and middle cerebral arteries. Small vessels are present at the base of the brain.

Table 7–8. **Conditions Associated with Moyamoya Syndrome**

Neurofibromatosis
Turner syndrome
Down syndrome
Glycogen storage disease type I
Thalassemia
Eosinophilic granuloma
Type II plasminogen deficiency
Leptospirosis
Ebstein-Barr virus
Tonsillitis
Proprionibacterium acnes
Systemic lupus erythematosus
Periarteritis nodosa
Kawasaki disease
Oral contraceptive use
Tobacco use
Atherosclerosis
Renal artery stenosis
Arteriovenous malformation
Tuberous sclerosis
Retinitis pigmentosa
Pseudoxanthoma elasticum
Sickle cell disease
Polycystic kidney disease
Protein C deficiency
Protein S deficiency
Anaerobic meningitis
Tuberculous meningitis
Pharyngitis
Vasculitis
Sjögren syndrome
Parasellar neoplasms
Craniocerebral trauma
Alcohol use
Cranial/basal irradiation
Fibromuscular dysplasia
Dissecting aneurysm
Saccular aneurysm

CLINICAL FEATURES

Clinical features of moyamoya include recurrent TIA or ischemic stroke, progressive neurological and cognitive decline, and intracranial hemorrhage.[124,125] (See Table 7–9.) The course appears to be more fulminant in children. The ischemic symptoms are secondary to effects of hypoperfusion and thrombosis, whereas the bleeding events are due to rupture of one of the small basal collaterals or associated intracranial saccular aneurysms.[126] The latter are located primarily in the vertebrobasilar circulation.

EVALUATION

Brain imaging shows multiple small bilateral subcortical lesions and brain atrophy.[127] (See Fig. 7–10.) Magnetic resonance imaging may demonstrate a lack of flow voids in the basal arteries at the circle of Willis and the pial collaterals.[127,128] Magnetic resonance angiography and CT angiography also demonstrate vascular changes.[129–131] Arteriography is the most definitive way to discern the presence and extent of the characteristic pattern of vessels (Fig. 7–11). Cerebral blood flow and metabolism studies show changes consistent with hypoperfusion and hypometabolism that are in excess of the vascular changes. Flow changes in the middle and anterior cerebral arteries are found by TCD.[132]

Table 7–9. **Clinical Features of Moyamoya Disease or Syndrome**

Children
Recurrent ischemic stroke
Recurrent transient ischemic attack
Epilepsy
Cognitive decline
Mental retardation
Adults
Recurrent ischemic stroke
Recurrent transient ischemic attack
Intracerebral hemorrhage
Subarachnoid hemorrhage
Cognitive decline

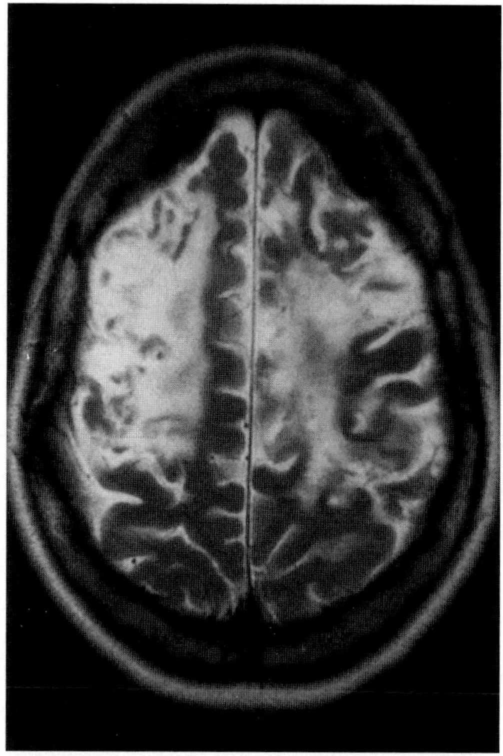

Figure 7–10. A T_2-weighted magnetic resonance imaging of the brain obtained in a patient with moyamoya syndrome. Bilateral cortical and subcortical ischemic lesions are found.

PROGNOSIS AND TREATMENT

Patients with moyamoya are at high risk for recurrent events. Children may have a higher risk for recurrent strokes than do young adults. Recurrent events lead to a progressive neurological decline that often causes severe cognitive impairments or the need for long-term institutional care. Because of the poor prognosis of patients with moyamoya disease, measures to prevent recurrent cerebrovascular events are critical. Most medical and surgical therapies are aimed at preventing the ischemic events. Treatment of the underlying condition that predisposes to moyamoya syndrome is fundamental. In particular, young women should be advised not to smoke and to stop use of oral contraceptives. Because of the small number of patients with moyamoya and the limited experience of most physicians, clinical trials have not been done to test

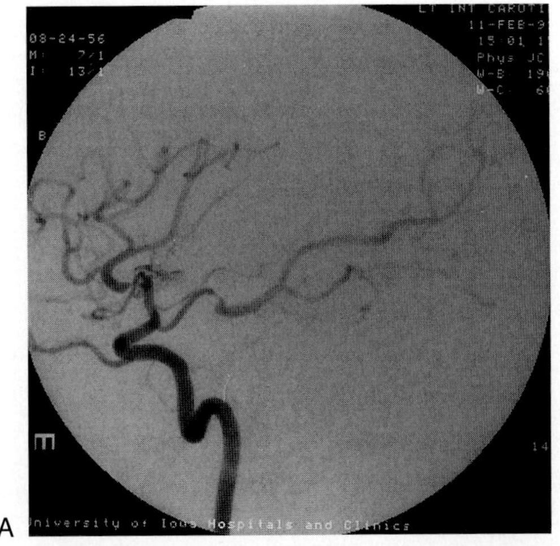

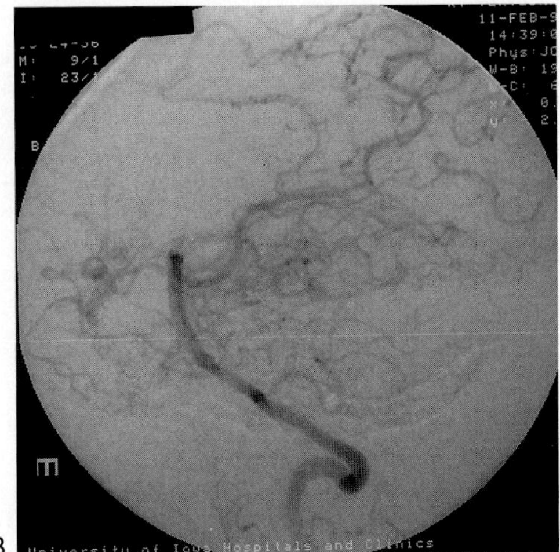

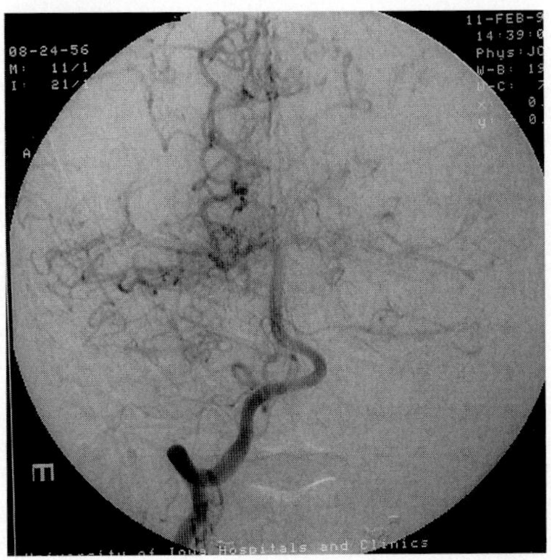

the usefulness of these interventions. The high risk of intracranial hemorrhage inhibits the use of oral anticoagulants. Antiplatelet aggregating agents often are prescribed. Direct or indirect cerebral revascularization procedures also are recommended.[133–135] An extracranial-to-intracranial anastomosis involves surgical creation of a collateral channel from the branch of the superior temporal artery to a distal branch of the anterior or middle cerebral artery.[136] Indirect revascularization operations involve the placement of tissue and blood supply onto the surface of the hemisphere.[137,138] (See Chapter 11.) These operations have been successful in patients who have not responded well to medical treatment.

INFECTIOUS VASCULOPATHIES

Ischemic stroke is a potential complication of infectious diseases that usually affect the intracranial arteries. Infections can cause an angiitis that leads to thromboembolism or a perivascular inflammatory process that causes an arterial occlusion.[139] Local suppurative processes in the head and neck can lead to occlusion of an adjacent artery. Inflammation also can lead to formation of intracranial aneurysms.[140] The clinical presentations of infectious vasculopathies usually differ greatly from other causes of stroke. A key component of diagnosis is examination of the CSF; findings of patients with an infectious intracranial vasculopathy include leucocytosis, an elevated protein, and a depressed glucose. Serological studies often are needed to confirm a diagnosis. Treatment of the underlying infection is the key to prevention of ischemic

Figure 7–11. Arteriography using subtraction techniques performed in a patient with moyamoya syndrome. The lateral view of the left carotid angiogram (*A*) shows occlusion of the middle cerebral artery and a mesh of fine vessels at the base of the brain. The lateral (*B*) and anterior posterior (*C*) views of a right vertebral angiogram show prominent collateral vessels arising from the posterior circulation to the anterior and the middle artery territories. Particularly prominent are the collateral channels along the corpus callosum.

cerebrovascular complications. In most instances, antimicrobial agents are the mainstays of treatment.

Syphilis

Stroke is a well-recognized complication of neurosyphilis. Since the advent of antibiotic treatment for syphilis, the frequency of tabes dorsalis or dementia has declined considerably, and the relative importance of *meningovascular syphilis* has grown. In this situation, stroke occurs in conjunction with clinical findings of an acute or subacute meningitis and encephalitis. Patients have a low-grade fever, headache, and nuchal rigidity. The stroke usually is a cortical infarction secondary to an occlusion of a branch of the middle cerebral artery.[141] The CSF will show leucocytosis, increased protein and immune globulins, and decreased glucose. Serological tests in the blood and CSF will be positive. Arteriographic findings of meningovascular syphilis include an arteritis and an atheromatous stenosis.[142] Treatment involves antibiotics and antiplatelet aggregating agents.

Acquired Immune Deficiency Syndrome

The problem of stroke in persons with *acquired immune deficiency syndrome* (*AIDS*) has received scant attention. Still, an autopsy study of 83 patients dying of AIDS reported brain infarctions in 24.[143] Qureshi et al[144] estimated that AIDS increases the risk of ischemic stroke among young adults who are ages 19–44 by a factor of 3.4. In many instances, individual infarctions are clinically silent, but their cumulative effects may lead to cognitive impairments. Vascular events may be secondary to central nervous system infection by the human immunodeficiency virus (HIV) itself or due to other complicating infectious illnesses, such as syphilis, or non-bacterial thrombotic endocarditis.[145] Reduced immunity increases the risk of central nervous system opportunistic infections, such as herpes zoster or fungal meningitis, that lead to arterial occlusion. Because of many common factors, including sexual promiscuity and intravenous drug abuse, persons with AIDS also have a high risk for syphilis. Meningovascular syphilis can lead to stroke, which, in turn, may represent the presentation of AIDS.[146] Patients with AIDS and neurosyphilis often do not respond well to the usual antibiotic treatment for syphilis.[147] Screening for AIDS should be performed if a stroke happens in a patient who has identified high-risk behaviors that could lead to the illness.

Herpes Zoster

Herpes zoster infection of the ophthalmic division of the trigeminal nerve can cause an intense arteritis of the intracranial portion of the internal carotid artery.[148,149] The virus appears to spread to the artery via nerve fibers and leads to intense perivascular inflammation and secondary thrombosis. The usual site of arteritis is the proximal intracranial or intracavernous portion. Both secondary retinal and hemispheric ischemic symptoms can occur.[150] In general, strokes do not occur at the time of acute cutaneous infection; rather, ischemic symptoms usually occur several weeks later.[151] Diagnosis is suspected when an ischemic stroke in the territory of the internal carotid artery occurs in a patient with a recent history of ipsilateral herpes zoster. Residuals from the cutaneous vesicles also provide a clue. Arteriography usually shows a segmental narrowing of the artery. Because of the limited number of cases, choices for treatment are based on anecdotal experiences. Anti-inflammatory agents (corticosteroids) appear to be critical in successfully treating herpes zoster arteritis. Antithrombotic agents may lessen the likelihood of thrombosis. One case of delayed hemiparesis secondary to cerebral angiitis has been described in a patient with chickenpox.[152]

Cysticercosis

Cysticercosis usually results from parasitic contamination of food, and it is most likely to occur in developing countries that have limited sanitation facilities. Neurocysticercosis that invades the meninges can lead to an intense inflammatory reaction at the base of the brain. This form of basilar meningitis leads to occlusion of major arteries in the anterior or the posterior circulation.[153–155] The usual presentation of neurocysticercosis is seizures, headaches, or an enlarging intracranial mass. Levy et al[156] reported that stroke occurs in 2%–12% of patients with neurocysticercosis and most of these strokes are lacunes. Besides stroke, progressive dementia may be a presenting sign. Brain imaging studies usually will show multiple intracranial lesions that are calcified. Many are adjacent to the arteries.[154] Besides leucocytosis, examination of the CSF permits assay for the antibody to the parasite. Treatment usually involves administration of albendazole or praziquantel. Corticosteroids can be given to reduce the meningeal inflammatory reaction. Surgical removal of a large, mass-producing cyst also can be performed.

Bacterial or Fungal Meningitis

Stroke secondary to intracranial arterial (pial) or cortical venous thrombosis can complicate either bacterial or fungal meningitis.[157,158] Stroke is a relatively uncommon complication and usually appears after the other signs of the illness are present. Patients with these ischemic complications and usually are critically ill. Thus, a vascular event should be considered if new focal neurological impairments and seizures occur in the clinical situation of acute or subacute meningitis. The signs of ischemia usually reflect cortical dysfunction. Brain imaging may show ischemic or hemorrhagic lesions in the cortex and adjacent structures. Ries et al[158] and Muller[157] found that changes in flow as detected by TCD are associated with ischemic complications of meningitis. Vasculitis occlusion of major intracranial arteries can complicate brain infections with *Candida albicans*.[159] The primary focus of management is the use of antibiotics or anti-fungal agents to treat the meningitis.

Aspergillosis

Aspergillosis is an opportunistic infection that can invade the intracranial blood vessels of persons with compromised immune responses.[160] Cerebrovascular aspergillosis most commonly affects persons who have malignancies or AIDS or who have had a transplant.[161] The fungus causes progressive vascular occlusion. Clinical manifestations include ischemic stroke, hemorrhagic infarction, and a progressively expanding intracranial mass. Patients usually have signs of increased intracranial pressure secondary to the mass. Sequential brain imaging studies usually show a progressively enlarging mass with hypodensity. Treatment, including surgical resection, can be done, but the prognosis of these patients is very poor.

Mucormycosis

Mucormycosis usually affects the paranasal or cavernous sinuses in diabetic or immunocompromised patients. A secondary *cavernous sinus thrombosis* can lead to occlusion of the internal carotid artery and stroke.[162,163] The patient has signs of cavernous sinus thrombosis, including bilateral exophthalmos, proptosis, chemosis, ocular movement impairments, and visual loss. In general, the signs of the stroke are overshadowed by the findings of the sinusitis and cavernous sinus occlusion. The treatment involves administration of amphotericin B and surgical debridement.

Cat-Scratch Disease

Cat-scratch disease is secondary to infection with *Bartonella henselae* and possibly other bacteria in the same family. The usual clinical findings include fever, malaise, and lymphadenopathy. Patients can have a retinitis or encephalopathy. A cerebral arteritis secondary to cat-scratch disease can lead to ischemic stroke.[164]

Malaria

The disseminated vasculopathy of cerebral malaria can cause occlusion of multiple intracranial arteries leading to an acute encephalopathy or stroke.[165] However, evidence is lacking for hypoperfusion secondary to obstruction or hemodynamic problems.[166] The neurological signs typically reflect a multifocal process. The usual organism leading to stroke is *Plasmodium falciparum.* A history of travel to an endemic area and the presence of high fevers usually point toward malaria. Microscopic examination of the blood can detect the organism. Treatment of malaria is the main component of treatment.

Whipple Disease

Whipple disease is an intestinal infectious process caused by *Tropheyma whippellii* that can be complicated by a multifocal neurological syndrome included in the differential diagnosis of cerebral vasculitis. Patients usually have prominent gastrointestinal symptoms, including malabsorption, diarrhea, and abdominal pain. Arthralgias are prominent. Neurological presentations include dementia, supranuclear ophthalmoplegia, and ocular and facial tics.[167] The test usually required for the diagnosis of whipple disease is an endoscopic intestinal biopsy to look for characteristic changes.

Behçet Disease

Behçet disease presents with migratory arthralgia, mucosal ulcerations, and meningitis.[168] The most common locations for the ulcers are the mouth and genital areas. There is uncertainty if it the disease an infectious or primary autoimmune disorder. Neurological symptoms, including stroke, cerebral vasculitis, encephalopathy, and cerebral venous thrombosis, are uncommon complications.[169] Behçet disease usually is diagnosed if the patient has the characteristic clinical findings. Brain imaging studies can show findings of meningeal irritation and small lesions consistent with a microangiopathy. Treatment usually involves the administration of immunosuppressive agents.

INFLAMMATORY, NON-INFECTIOUS VASCULOPATHIES

Symptoms and signs of peripheral or central nervous system dysfunction are prominent in patients with multisystem vasculitides. These autoimmune inflammatory diseases present with myriad neurological problems, including ischemic stroke. Although the mechanism of central neurological dysfunction in these patients often is vasculitis-induced ischemia, the course of illness usually does not mimic stroke. Most patients with involvement of the brain do not present with a single or recurrent stroke; rather, there is a more indolent, subacute course of gradual neurological decline marked by impairments in cognition. (Tables 7–10 and 7–11).[170–172] Seizures, meningitis, headaches, cranial nerve palsies, peripheral neuropathy, or a myopathy also develop.[173,174]

Brain imaging studies can show cortical atrophy, ventricular dilation, or multiple small grey and white matter lesions, or the tests may be normal (Figs. 7–12 and 7–13).

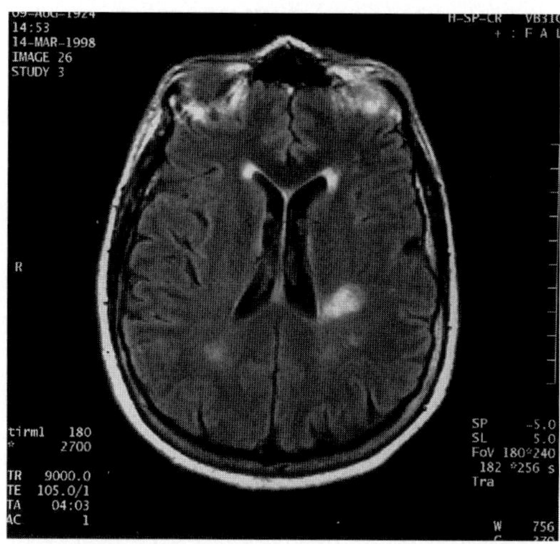

Figure 7–12. A magnetic resonance imaging study of the brain demonstrates an area of hyperintensity in the periventricular area of the left hemisphere. This lesion does not fit the usual vascular pattern of most infarctions and was noted in a patient with vasculitis.

Table 7–10. **Clinical and Diagnostic Features of Cerebral Vasculitis**

Neurological signs	Electroencephalogram
Recurrent ischemic stroke	Diffuse slow activity
Personality change and cognitive decline	Cerebrospinal fluid
Decrease in consciousness	Normal
Seizures	Elevated white blood cell count
Headaches	Elevated protein
Cranial nerve palsies	Serological studies
Peripheral neuropathy	Arteriography
Meningitis	Can be normal
Myopathy	Multiple vessels involved
Brain imaging	Segmental, sausage-like areas of dilations and narrowing
Normal	Medium-caliber (pial–branch cortical) arteries
Cortical atrophy	
Enlarged ventricles	
Multiple grey and white matter lesions	

Table 7–11. **Common Non-neurological Clinical Findings of the Leading Multisystem Vasculitides**

Condition	Symptoms
Cogan syndrome	Uveitis, blindness
	Hearing loss
Periarteritis nodosa	Pulmonary symptoms
	Renal dysfunction
	Skin abnormalities
Wegener disease	Pulmonary symptoms
	Sinus abnormalities
Giant cell arteritis	Visual loss
	Headache
	Jaw claudication
	Polymyalgia rheumatica
Sjögren syndrome	Dry eyes and mouth
Systemic lupus erythematosus	Fever and malaise
	Arthralgias
	Renal dysfunction
	Skin abnormalities
	Pulmonary symptoms
Scleroderma	Calcinosis
	Raynaud phenomenon
	Esophageal dysmotility
	Sclerodactyly
Rheumatoid arthritis	Arthritis

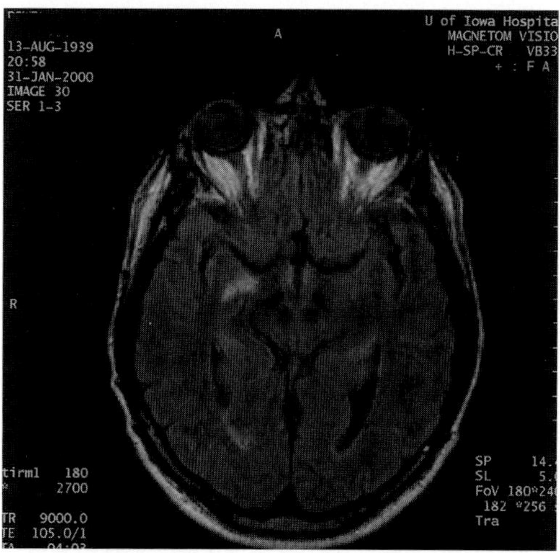

Figure 7–13. A small area of infarction in the anterior–medial aspect of the right temporal lobe was noted in a patient with vasculitis.

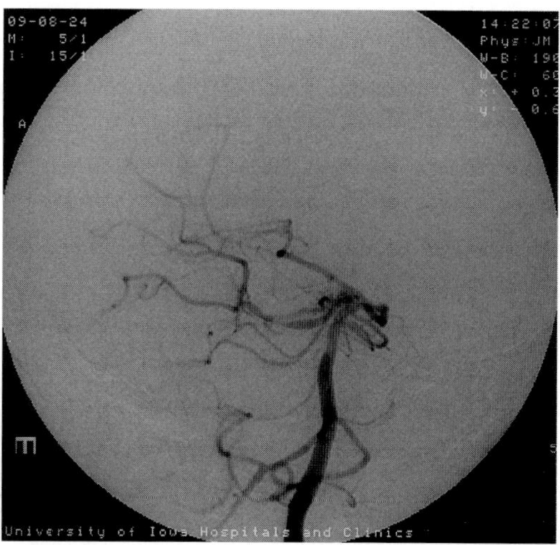

Figure 7–14. A lateral view of a vertebral arteriogram reveals segmental narrowing in the posterior cerebral artery in a patient with vasculitis.

Cerebrospinal fluid usually shows signs of inflammation. In particular, lymphocytosis is observed; however, it, too, can be normal. The electroencephalogram can reveal diffuse slow activity. Serological studies can help define a multisystem vasculitis with brain involvement, but results may be normal if the patient has an isolated central nervous system vasculitis.[170] Because most vasculitides involve moderate-or small-size vessels, non-invasive studies of the extracranial or intracranial arteries do not provide assistance in diagnosis (Fig. 7–14). Many vasculitides involve a necrotizing arteritis of moderate-size vessels and, in these instances, arteriography can point to a diagnosis.[173] The study will be inconclusive in approximately 50% of patients; the usual signs, if visible, are multiple areas of segmental, sausage-like narrowing involving multiple arteries of the brain. Brain and meningeal biopsy may be the only way to establish a diagnosis, but even this invasive procedure may be falsely negative.

Treatment of the inflammatory vasculitides that lead to brain ischemia is markedly different from that prescribed to persons with stroke of other causes. Immunosuppressive agents (corticosteroids, azathioprine, or cyclophosphamide) are mainstays of treatment. Angioplasty to dilate the vasculitic stenoses has been performed, but the results have not been promising.[175]

Isolated Central Nervous System Vasculitis

Isolated central nervous system vasculitis can occur in persons of any age. It more commonly affects men than women. Persons with isolated central nervous system vasculitis usually do not have symptoms of involvement of other organs or systemic serological changes. Fever, malaise, and uveitis can be present. Patients present with headache, seizures, cognitive impairments, and multifocal neurological impairments that develop insidiously and subacutely.[171,172,176–179] An encephalopathy, delirium, decreased consciousness, and coma can develop. Although stroke is an uncommon presentation, focal motor, sensory, or visual impairments can be found.[180]

Serological studies of the blood usually are negative. Brain imaging and electroencephalographic findings usually are nonspecific.[181] The CSF usually exhibits lymphocytosis and modest elevations of immune globulins. Arteriography usually is done to define the presence of the vasculitis.[181,182] Changes include segmental narrowing and dilation, prolongation of the circulation time, and vascular occlusions.[182] The arteriographic changes often progress despite treatment with immunosuppressive therapy.[181,182] Leptomeningeal and brain biopsy may be needed to establish the diagnosis.[181] Most patients are treated with cyclophosphamide and corticosteroids. If diagnosed and treated early, some patients can have a satisfactory outcome.

Although most patients have a progressive course, a subset of patients can have a more benign course.[183] The benign form of primary central nervous system vasculitis is more common in young women.[183]

Cogan Syndrome

Cogan syndrome is due a vasculitis that appears to be similar to periarteritis nodosa. It causes deafness, uveitis, and blindness.[184] The hearing loss, which usually is secondary to ischemia, usually is sudden and bilateral. The visual loss is secondary to retinal ischemia. Patients also present with fever, chills, weight loss, headache, psychiatric symptoms, aortic insufficiency, thrombocytopenia, and an abnormal CSF.[172,185] The neurological symptoms, including stroke, presumably are due to ischemia secondary to the vasculitis.[185] The prognosis of these patients generally is poor. Treatment involves immunosuppressive agents.[186]

Eale Disease

Retinal perivasculitis and recurrent vitreous hemorrhages are the hallmarks of *Eale disease,* which largely strikes young men. Ischemic stroke is a potential complication of Eale disease.[172,187]

Periarteritis Nodosa

Periarteritis nodosa occurs in persons of all ages.[171,172] It more commonly affects men than women. It produces a multisystem necrotizing vasculitis that leads to pulmonary, cutaneous, and renal dysfunction. Fever and malaise are prominent symptoms. Retinal vasculitis, hemorrhages, or ischemia may develop. Neurological symptoms include mononeuropathy multiplex, headache, encephalopathy seizures, and stroke. Reichart[81] reported lacunar strokes secondary to a microangiopathy of small, penetrating arterioles. Although ischemic stroke, including lacunar infarctions, is a potential complication, the necrotizing nature of this vasculopathy also produces intracerebral hemorrhage.[81] Intracranial bleeding may be more common than ischemic stroke. The patient usually has an abnormal urinalysis, elevated erythrocyte sedimentation rate, eosinophilia, and abnormal serological test. The chest x-ray usually is normal. The presence of antiphospholipid antibodies can lead to stroke complicating periarteritis nodosa.[188] Treatment focuses on the use of immunosuppressive medications.

Wegener Disease

Wegener granulomatosis is a necrotizing vasculitis that usually presents with pulmonary and nasal sinus symptoms. Ocular findings include uveitis and retinal vasculitis, ischemia, or hemorrhage. Neurological complications include a mononeuropathy, cranial neuropathy, myelopathy, meningitis, and cerebritis.[172,189,190] The most commonly involved cranial nerves are the optic, abducens, and facial.[191] Involvement of the central nervous system is less common than the cranial or peripheral neuropathies. Still, 13 patients in a series of 324 patients with Wegener disease had strokes.[191] These strokes probably were the result of vasculitis. Arteritis of the basilar artery leading to ischemic stroke has been described.[192] Treatment largely involves the use of immunosuppressives.

Churg-Strauss Angiitis

Churg-Strauss angiitis is a multisystem allergic vasculitis that leads to rhinitis, sinusitis, and asthma. Prominent eosinophilia is a hallmark of the disease. In addition to a mild neuropathy, neurological complications include an anterior ischemic optic neuropathy.[171,193,194]

Takayasu Disease

Takayasu arteritis is an inflammatory giant cell vasculitis that most commonly affects women younger than 40. It primarily affects the major branches of the arch of the aorta. Involvement of the subclavian arteries can lead to the loss of pulses in the upper limbs and posterior circulation ischemia.[171,172,195,196] A subclavian steal syndrome can lead to vertebrobasilar ischemia.[197] Hemispheric or ocular ischemia can complicate involvement of the common carotid artery. Ocular findings include hypertensive retinopathy, retinal ischemia, and retinal hemorrhage. In addition to ischemic symptoms, patients often present with fever, malaise, weight loss, arm claudication, myalgia, weight loss, headache, and carotidynia. Arterial hypertension and cervical bruits can be prominent.[198] The erythrocyte sedimentation rate and serological studies often are abnormal. Ultrasonography can detect a homogenous increase in the thickness of the wall of the common carotid artery, a finding that is relatively specific for Takayasu disease.[199] The usual treatment is with steroids and cyclophosphamide.[200]

Giant Cell Arteritis

Giant cell arteritis usually occurs in persons older than 60 and more commonly affects women than men. It causes an intense segmental inflammation of medium-caliber arteries of the head, and the pathological hallmark is an aggregation of giant cells within the wall. Patients usually present with fever, malaise, weight loss, and pain and stiffness of the proximal muscles of the upper and lower limbs (*polymyalgia rheumatica*).[172,201–203] Jaw pain (*jaw claudication*) also can occur with chewing. A unilateral temporal headache is the most common neurological symptom. The superficial temporal artery usually is tender and palpably enlarged. It may be tortuous. Carotid artery involvement can lead to a cervical bruit or a diminished pulse.[204] Ocular ischemia secondary to occlusion of the ciliary artery may cause blindness, which is the most common serious complication. Stroke, most commonly in the posterior circulation, has been reported.[205] Caselli et al[204] reported that a TIA or a stroke occurred in 12 of 166 patients with giant cell arteritis. The erythrocyte sedimentation rate and the level of C-reactive protein usually are markedly prolonged. Because it is a segmental arteritis, temporal artery biopsy can be negative. Bilateral resection of large segments of the temporal artery may be needed to establish the diagnosis. Large doses of corticosteroids are the mainstay of treatment.

Sjögren Syndrome

Ischemic stroke has been the presentation of Sjögren syndrome.[171,206,207] The primary features of Sjögren syndrome involve ocular symptoms and dryness of the mouth. The most common neurological findings involve trigeminal neuropathy and other cranial nerve palsies. Patients with Sjögren syndrome often have other evidence of a multisystem vasculitis.

Systemic Lupus Erythematosus

Systemic lupus erythematosus (*SLE*) is most common in young women. Fever, malaise, arthralgias, renal dysfunction, pulmonary symptoms, and dermatological changes are prominent. Mental status changes or cognitive impairments are the most common central nervous system complications of SLE.[172] Many patients present with psychiatric disturbances, seizures, headaches, or coma.[208] Stroke is a relatively uncommon complication. Kitagawa et al[209] reported stroke in only 13 of 326 patients (5.6%). Most events are not due to vasculitis.[208,210] Rather, strokes often are attributed to *circulating anticoagulants* (lupus anticoagulant/antiphospholipid antibody syndrome) and *Libman-Sacks endocarditis*.[209,211–218] Intramural platelet deposition has been found in patients with cerebral vasculopathy secondary to systemic lupus erythematosus.[219] In addition, patients with systemic lupus erythematosus may have a risk for *thrombotic thrombocytopenia purpura* and the hemolytic-uremia syndrome secondary to a multiorgan thrombotic disorder.[218]

Patients with SLE may have elevated antibodies or changes in the activated partial thromboplastin time alone or in combination.[211] A variation of the antiphospholipid/lupus anticoagulant syndrome is the *Sneddon syndrome.*[220] It presents with ischemic stroke, digital ischemia, and prominent livedo reticularis. Pathologic evaluation of a skin biopsy will show inflammation and subendothelial proliferation and fibrosis of small to medium arteries.[221] Serological tests, especially antinuclear antibodies, erythrocyte sedimentation rate, and cryoglobulins are abnormal. The urinalysis usually is abnormal. Treatment involves the administration of immunosuppressive agents.

Scleroderma

Scleroderma and the *CREST* (*Calcinosis, Raynaud's phenomenon, esophageal dysfunction, sclerodactyly and telangiectasias*) *syndrome* can be complicated by central nervous system dysfunction. Scleroderma is most common in middle-age women. The primary findings include calcinosis, Raynaud's phenomenon, disturbed esophageal motility, sclerodactyly and telangiectasias. Vasculitis of the central nervous system has been described.[222,223]

Rheumatoid Arthritis

Rheumatoid arthritis affects both young men and young women. The most prominent symptoms are arthralgias. Spine involvement can be especially prominent in young men. Mononeuropathy multiplex is the most common neurological complication. Signs of central nervous system dysfunction are less common, and stroke is unusual. Rheumatoid arthritis can be accompanied by a necrotizing vasculitis of the central nervous system.[172,224] Laxity of the longitudinal ligament of the cervical spine can lead to subluxation at the atlanto-occipital junction.[225] Displacement the spine at the rostral portion of the cervical spine can lead to compression of the vertebral artery with different head positions.[225,226] Serological studies (See Chapter 4) usually will help confirm the diagnosis.

Inflammatory Bowel Disease

Stroke has been reported as a complication of *ulcerative colitis* and *regional enteritis.*[227,228] In one series of 638 patients with inflammatory bowel disease, 4 patients had stroke.[229] Talbot et al[230] found that strokes occurred in approximately 1% of 7199 patients with inflammatory bowel disease. Most cases presumably are secondary to a coagulopathy attributed to elevated fibrinogen levels, increased clotting factors, or decreased levels of protein S.[227,230–234] However, Nelson et al[235] have reported a case of cerebral vasculitis secondary to ulcerative colitis that was successfully treated with immunosuppressives. Ischemic optic neuropathy and uveitis also has been described.[236] Penix[237] reported two cases of stroke among patients with Crohn's disease and attributed the vascular events to increased concentrations of homocysteine that were a result of malabsorption of vitamin B12. A difference in the rate of neurological complications may occur between those with ulcerative colitis and those with regional enteritis.[229]

Sarcoidosis

Sarcoidosis is a relatively uncommon infectious, inflammatory disease that has neurological complications, including subacute meningitis. Ischemic stroke and TIA are rare complications of sarcoidosis.[238] A vasculitis is the presumed cause of the ischemic symptoms. Diagnosis of sarcoidosis is supported by the presence of hilar lymphadenopathy, hypocalcemia, and anergy. Elevations in angiotensin converting enzyme levels can help confirm the diagnosis. Cerebrospinal fluid findings typically are consistent with a subacute inflammatory process. Treatment usually involves administration of immunosuppressive agents.

SUMMARY

Non-atherosclerotic vasculopathies account for a broad and bewildering range of entities. Non-inflammatory vasculopathies include arterial dissection, a leading cause of stroke in the young. Infectious vasculopathies encompass AIDS and syphilis, important causes of stroke in developing countries and a growing menace in Western subpopulations.

Inflammatory, non-infectious vasculopathies pose a particular challenge. The many types of vasculitis have neither satisfactory explanation nor treatment, with the possible exception of temporal arteritis, which responds empirically to corticosteroids. A distressing aspect of the non-atherosclerotic vasculopathies is that they tend to affect people who are young or in the prime of their lives. The solutions lie not only in the better understanding of genetics, autoimmunity, and infections but also in the prevention of risky behaviors that lead to some of the avoidable non-atherosclerotic vasculopathies.

REFERENCES

1. The Publications Committee for the Trial of ORG 10172 in Acute Stroke Treatment (TOAST) Investigators. Low molecular weight heparinoid, ORG 10172 (danaparoid), and outcome after acute ischemic stroke: a randomized controlled trial. *JAMA* 1998;279:1265–1272.
2. Schievink WI, Mokri B, Whisnant JP. Internal carotid artery dissection in a community. Rochester, Minnesota, 1987–1992. *Stroke* 1993;24:1678–1680.
3. Schievink WI, Wijdicks EF, Kuiper JD. Seasonal pattern of spontaneous cervical artery dissection. *J Neurosurg* 1998;89:101–103.
4. Schievink WI, Mokri B, Piepgras DG. Spontaneous dissections of cervicocephalic arteries in childhood and adolescence. *Neurology* 1994;44:1607–1612.
5. Bartels E, Flugel KA. Evaluation of extracranial vertebral artery dissection with duplex colorflow imaging. *Stroke* 1996;27:290–295.
6. Thie A, Hellner D, Lachenmayer L, Janzen RWC, Kunze K. Bilateral blunt traumatic dissections of the extracranial internal carotid artery: report of eleven cases and review literature. *Cerebrovasc Dis* 1993;3:295–303.
7. Noelle B, Clavier I, Besson G, Hommel M. Cervicocephalic arterial dissections related to skiing. *Stroke* 1994;25:526–527.
8. Zimmerman AW, Kumar AJ, Gadoth N, Hodges FJ. Traumatic vertebrobasilar occlusive disease in childhood. *Neurology* 1978;28:185–188.
9. Schievink WI, Atkinson JL, Bartleson JD, Whisnant JP. Traumatic internal carotid artery dissections caused by blunt softball injuries. *Am J Emerg Med* 1998;16:179–182.
10. Peters M, Bohl J, Thomke F, et al. Dissection of the internal carotid artery after chiropractic manipulation of the neck. *Neurology* 1995; 45:2284–2286.
11. Lee KP, Carlini WG, McCormick GF, Albers GW. Neurologic complications following chiropractic manipulation: a survey of California neurologists. *Neurology* 1995;45:1213–1215.
12. Frumkin LR, Baloh RW. Wallenberg's syndrome following neck manipulation. *Neurology* 1990; 40:611–615.
13. Van de Kelft E, Kunnen J, Truyen L, Heytens L. Postpartum dissecting aneurysm of the basilar artery. *Stroke* 1992;23:114–116.
14. Neau JP, Masson C, Vandermarcq P, et al. Familial occurence of dissection of the cervical arteries. *Cerebrovasc Dis* 1995;5:310–312.
15. Schievink WI, Mokri B, OFFpgras DG, Gittenberger-de Groot AC. Intracranial aneurysms and cervicocephalic arterial dissections associated with congenital heart disease. *Neurosurgery* 1996;39:685–689.
16. Skljarevski V, Turek M, Hakim AM. Cervical artery dissection is associated with wedined aortic root diameter. *Can J Neurol Sci* 1998; 25:315–319.
17. Youl BD, Coutellier A, Dubois B, Leger JM, Bousser MG. Three cases of spontaneous extracranial vertebral artery dissection. *Stroke* 1990;21:618–625.
18. Schievink WI, Prakash UB, Piepgras DG, Mokri B. Alpha 1-antitrypsin deficiency in intracranial aneurysms and cervical artery dissection. *Lancet* 1994;343:452–453.
19. Schievink WI, Bjornsson J, Piepgras DG. Coexistence of fibromuscular dysplasia and cystic medial necrosis in a patient with Marfan's syndrome and bilateral carotid artery dissections. *Stroke* 1994;25:2492–2496.
20. Schievink WI, Limburg M, Oorthuys JW, Fleury P, Pope FM. Cerebrovascular disease in Ehlers-Danlos syndrome type IV. *Stroke* 1990;21: 626–632.
21. Grau AJ, Brandt T, Forsting M, Winter R, Hacke W. Infection-associated cervical artery dissection. Three cases. *Stroke* 1997;28:453–455.
22. Grau AJ, Brandt T, Buggle F, et al. Association of cervical artery dissection with recent infection. *Arch Neurol* 1999;56:851–856.
23. Schievink WI, Mokri B, Piepgras DG, Kuiper JD. Recurrent spontaneous arterial dissections:

risk in familial versus nonfamilial disease. *Stroke* 1996;27:622–624.
24. van den Berg JS, Limburg M, Kappelle LJ, Pals G, Arwert F, Westerveld. The role of type III collagen in spontaneous cervical arterial dissections. *Ann Neurol* 1998;43:494–498.
25. Schievink WI, Michels VV, Piepgras DG. Neurovascular manifestations of heritable connective tissue disorders. A review. *Stroke* 1994;25:889–903.
26. Grond-Ginsbach C, Weber R, Haas J, et al. Mutations in the COL5A1 coding sequence are not common in patients with spontaneous cervical artery dissections. *Stroke* 1999;30: 1887–1890.
27. Brandt T, Hausser I, Orberk E, et al. Ultrastructural connective tissue abnormalities in patients with spontaneous cervicocerebral artery dissections. *Ann Neurol* 1998;44:281–285.
28. Tzourio C, Cohen A, Lamisse N, Biousse V, Bousser MG. Aortic root dilatation in patients with spontaneous cervical artery dissection. *Circulation* 1997;95:2351–2353.
29. Deck JH. Pathology of spontaneous dissection of intracranial arteries. *Can J Neurol Sci* 1987;14: 88–91.
30. Biousse V, d'Anglejan-Chatillon J, Touboul PJ, Amarenco P, Bousser MG. Time course of symptoms in extracranial carotid artery dissections. A series of 80 patients. *Stroke* 1995;26:235–239.
31. Guillon B, Levy C, Bousser MG. Internal carotid artery dissection: an update. *J Neurol Sci* 1998; 153:146–158.
32. Hart RG, Easton JD. Dissections. *Stroke* 1985;16:925–927.
33. Fisher CM, Ojemann RG, Roberson GH. Spontaneous dissection of cervico-cerebral arteries. *Can J Neurol Sci* 1978;5:9–19.
34. Galetta SL, Leahey A, Nichols CW, Raps EC. Orbital ischemia, ophthalmoparesis, and carotid dissection. *J Clin Neuro-Ophthalmol* 1991;11: 284–287.
35. Biousse V, Touboul PJ, d'Anglejan-Chatillon J, Levy C, Schaison M, Bousser MG. Ophthalmologic manifestations of internal carotid artery dissection. *Am J Ophthalmol* 1998;126:565–577.
36. Biousse V, Schaison M, Touboul PJ, d'Anglejan-Chatillon J, Bousser MG. Ischemic optic neuropathy associated with internal carotid artery dissection. *Arch Neurol* 1998;55:715–719.
37. Steinke W, Schwartz A, Hennerici M. Topography of cerebral infarction associated with carotid artery dissection. *J Neurol* 1996; 243:323–328.
38. Caplan LR, Baquis GD, Pessin MS, et al. Dissection of the intracranial vertebral artery. *Neurology* 1988;38:868–877.
39. Greselle JF, Zenteno M, Kien P, Castel JP, Caille JM. Spontaneous dissection of the vertebro-basilar system. A study of 18 cases (15 patients). *J Neuroradiol* 1987; 14:115–123.
40. Hosoya T, Adachi M, Yamaguchi K, Haku T, Kayama T, Kato T. Clinical and neuroradiological features of intracranial vertebrobasilar artery dissection. *Stroke* 1999;30:1083–1090.
41. Fisher CM. The headache and pain of spontaneous carotid dissection. *Headache* 1982;22: 60–65.
42. Cox LK, Bertorini T, Laster RE, Jr. Headaches due to spontaneous internal carotid artery dissection magnetic resonance imaging evaluation and follow up. *Headache* 1991;31:12–16.
43. Silbert PL, Mokri B, Schievink WI. Headache and neck pain in spontaneous internal carotid and vertebral artery dissections. *Neurology* 1995;45:1517–1522.
44. Schievink WI, Mokri B, Garrity JA, Nichols DA, Piepgras DG. Ocular motor nerve palsies in spontaneous dissections of the cervical internal carotid artery. *Neurology* 1993;43: 1938–1941.
45. Leira EC, Bendixen BH, Kardon RH, Adams HP, Jr. Brief, transient Horner's syndrome can be the hallmark of a carotid artery dissection. *Neurology* 1998;50:289–290.
46. Mokri B, Schievink WI, Olsen KD, Piepgras DG. Spontaneous dissection of the cervical internal carotid artery. Presentation with lower cranial nerve palsies. *Arch Otolaryngol Head Neck Surg* 1992;118:431–435.
47. Gout O, Bonnaud I, Weill A, et al. Facial diplegia complicating a bilateral internal carotid artery dissection. *Stroke* 1999;30:681–686.
48. Koennecke H, Seyfert S. Mydriatic pupil as the presenting sign of common carotid artery dissection. *Stroke* 1998;29:2653–2655.
49. Guillon B, Brunereau L, Biousse V, Djouhri H, Levy C, Bousser MG. Long-term follow-up of aneurysms developed during extracranial internal carotid artery dissection. *Neurology* 1999; 53:117–122.
50. Pozzati E, Andreoli A, Padovani R, Nuzzo G. Dissecting aneurysms of the basilar artery. *Neurosurgery* 1995;36:254–258.
51. Redekop G, TerBrugge K, Willinsky R. Subarachnoid hemorrhage from vertebrobasilar dissecting aneurysm treated with staged bilateral vertebral artery occlusion: The importance of early follow-up angiography: technical case report. *Neurosurgery* 1999;45:1258–1263.
52. Bassetti C, Bogousslavsky J, Eskenasy-Cottier AC, Janzen RWC, Regli F. Spontaneous intracranial dissection in the anterior circulation. *Cerebrovasc Dis* 1994;4:170–174.
53. Chang AJ, Mylonakis E, Karanasias P, De Orchis DF, Gold R. Spontaneous bilateral vertebral artery dissections: case report and literature review. *Mayo Clin Proc* 1999;74:893–896.
54. Sharif AA, Remley KB, Clark HB. Middle cerebral artery dissection: a clinicopathologic study. *Neurology* 1995;45:1929–1931.
55. Gelbert F, Assouline E, Hodes JE, et al. MRI in spontaneous dissection of vertebral and carotid arteries. 15 cases studied at 0.5 tesla. *Neuroradiology* 1991;33:111–113.
56. Sue DE, Brant-Zawadzki MN, Chance J. Dissection of cranial arteries in the neck: correlation of MRI and arteriography. *Neuroradiology* 1992;34:273–278.
57. van Putten MJ, Bloem BR, Smit VT, Aarts NJ, Lammers GJ. An uncommon cause of

stroke in young adults. *Arch Neurol* 1999;56: 1018–1020.
58. Iwama T, Andoh T, Sakai N, Iwata T, Hirata T, Yamada H. Dissecting and fusiform aneurysms of vertebro-basilar systems. MR imaging. *Neuroradiology* 1990;32:272–279.
59. Auer A, Felber S, Schmidauer C, Waldenberger P, Aichner F. Magnetic resonance angiographic and clinical features of extracranial vertebral artery dissection. *J Neurol Neurosurg Psychiatry* 1998;64:474–481.
60. Kitanaka C, Tanaka J, Kuwahara M, Teraoka A. Magnetic resonance imaging study of intracranial vertebrobasilar artery dissections. *Stroke* 1994;25:571–575.
61. Levy C, Laissy JP, Raveau V, et al. Carotid and vertebral artery dissections: three-dimensional time-of-flight MR angiography and MR imaging versus conventional angiography. *Radiology* 1994;190:97–103.
62. Mullges W, Ringelstein EB, Leibold M. Non-invasive diagnosis of internal carotid artery dissections. *J Neurol Neurosurg Psychiatry* 1992; 55:98–104.
63. Rother J, Schwartz A, Rautenberg W, Hennerici M. Magnetic resonance angiography of spontaneous vertebral artery dissection suspected on Doppler ultrasonography. *J Neurol* 1995; 242:430–436.
64. Eljamel MS, Humphrey PR, Shaw MD. Dissection of the cervical internal carotid artery. The role of Doppler/duplex studies and conservative management. *J Neurol Neurosurg Psychiatry* 1990;53:379–383.
65. Sidhu PS, Jonker ND, Khaw KT, et al. Spontaneous dissections of the internal carotid artery: appearances on colour Doppler ultrasound. *Br J Radiol* 1997;70:50–57.
66. Sturzenegger M, Mattle HP, Rivoir A, Baumgartner RW. Ultrasound findings in carotid artery dissection: analysis of 43 patients. *Neurology* 1995;45:691–698.
67. Hoffmann M, Sacco RL, Chan S, Mohr JP. Noninvasive detection of vertebral artery dissection. *Stroke* 1993;24:815–819.
68. Steinke W, Rautenberg W, Schwartz A, Hennerici M. Noninvasive monitoring of internal carotid artery dissection. *Stroke* 1994;25: 998–1005.
69. Leys D, Moulin T, Stojkovic T, Begey S, Chavot D. Follow-up of patients with history of cervical artery dissection. *Cerebrovasc Dis* 1995;5: 43–49.
70. Kasner SE, Hankins LL, Bratina P, Morgenstern LB. Magnetic resonance angiography demonstrates vascular healing of carotid and vertebral artery dissections. *Stroke* 1997;28:1993–1997.
71. Bassetti C, Carruzzo A, Sturzenegger M, Tuncdogan E. Recurrence of cervical artery dissection. A prospective study of 81 patients. *Stroke* 1996;27:1804–1807.
72. Vishteh AG, Marciano FF, David CA, Schievink WI, Zabramski JM, Spetzler RF. Long-term graft patency rates and clinical outcomes after revascularization for symptomatic traumatic internal carotid artery dissection. *Neurosurgery* 1998; 43:761–768.
73. Schievink WI, Piepgras DG, McCaffrey TV, Mokri B. Surgical treatment of extracranial internal carotid artery dissecting aneurysms. *Neurosurgery* 1994;35:809–815.
74. Prall JA, Brega KE, Coldwell DM, Breeze RE. Incidence of unsuspected blunt carotid artery injury. *Neurosurgery* 1998;42:495–498.
75. Krauss JK, Jankovic J. Hemidystonia secondary to carotid artery gunshot injury. *Childs Nervous System* 1997;13:285–288.
76. Rommel O, Niedeggen A, Tegenthoff M, Kiwitt P, Botel U, Malin J. Carotid and vertebral artery injury following severe head or cervical spine trauma. *Cerebrovasc Dis* 1999;9:202–209.
77. Welling RE, Saul TG, Tew JMJ, Tomsick TA, Kremchek TE, Bellamy MJ. Management of blunt injury to the internal carotid artery. *J Trauma* 1987;27:1221–1226.
78. De Caro R, Munari PF, Parenti A. Middle cerebral artery thrombosis following blunt head trauma. *Clin Neuropathol* 1998;17:1–5.
79. Hilton-Jones D, Warlow CP. Non-penetrating arterial trauma and cerebral infarction in the young. *Lancet* 1985;1:1435–1438.
80. Milligan N, Anderson M. Conjugal disharmony: a hitherto unrecognised cause of strokes. *BMJ* 1980;281:421–422.
81. Reichhart MD, Bogousslavsky J, Janzer RC. Early lacunar strokes complicating polyarteritis nodosa. Thrombotic microangiopathy. *Neurology* 2000;54:883–889.
82. Amarenco P, Biousse V, Bousser MG. The archer's eye. *Cerebrovasc Dis* 1993;3:180.
83. Moriarty KP, Harris BH, Benitez-Marchand K. Carotid artery thrombosis and stroke after blunt pharyngeal injury. *J Trauma* 1997;42: 541–543.
84. Padberg FT, Jr., Hobson RW, Yeager RA, Lynch TG. Penetrating carotid arterial trauma. *Am Surg* 1984;50:277–282.
85. Bogousslavsky J, Cachin C, Regli F, Despland PA, Van Melle G, Kappenberger L. Cardiac sources of embolism and cerebral infarction—clinical consequences and vascular concomitants. *Neurology* 1991;41:855–859.
86. Garg BP, Ottinger CJ, Smith RR, Fishman MA. Strokes in children due to vertebral artery trauma. *Neurology* 1993;43:2555–2558.
87. Pryse-Phillips W. Infarction of the medulla and cervical cord after fitness exercises. *Stroke* 1989;20:292–294.
88. Willis BK, Greiner F, Orrison WW, Benzel EC. The incidence of vertebral artery injury after midcervical spine fracture or subluxation. *Neurosurgery* 1994;34:435–441.
89. Tulyapronchote R, Selhorst JB, Malkoff MD, Gomez CR. Delayed sequelae of vertebral artery dissection and occult cervical fractures. *Neurology* 1994;44:1397–1399.
90. Matsuyama T, Morimoto T, Sakaki T. Bow Hunter's stroke caused by a nondominant vertebral artery occlusion: case report. *Neurosurgery* 1997;41:1393–1395.

91. Murros KE, Toole JF. The effect of radiation on carotid arteries. *Arch Neurol* 1989;46: 449–455.
92. Zuber M, Khoubesserian P, Meder JF, Mas JL. A 34-year delayed and focal postirradiation intracranial vasculopathy. *Cerebrovasc Dis* 1993; 3:181–182.
93. Bowen J, Paulsen CA. Stroke after pituitary irradiation. *Stroke* 1992;23:908–911.
94. Bitzer M, Topka H. Progressive cerebral occlusive disease after radiation therapy. *Stroke* 1995; 26:131–136.
95. Grenier Y, Tomita T, Marymont MH, Byrd S, Burrowes DM. Late postirradiation occlusive vasculopathy in childhood medulloblastoma. Report of two cases. *J Neurosurg* 1998; 89:460–464.
96. Grill J, Couanet D, Cappelli C, et al. Radiation-induced cerebral vasculopathy in children with neurofibromatosis and optic pathway glioma. *Ann Neurol* 1999;45:393–396.
97. Chung TS, Yousem DM, Lexa FJ, Markiewicz DA. MRI of carotid angiopathy after therapeutic radiation. *J Comput Assist Tomogr* 1994;18:533–538.
98. Kashyap VS, Moore WS, Quinones-Baldrich WJ. Carotid artery repair for radiation-associated atherosclerosis is a safe and durable procedure. *J Vasc Surg* 1999;29:90–96.
99. Balaji MR, DeWeese JA. Fibromuscular dysplasia of the internal carotid artery: its occurrence with acute stroke and its surgical reversal. *Arch Surg* 1980;115:984–986.
100. Corrin LS, Sandok BA, Houser OW. Cerebral ischemic events in patients with carotid artery fibromuscular dysplasia. *Arch Neurol* 1981; 38:616–618.
101. Hegedus K, Nemeth G. Fibromuscular dysplasia of the basilar artery. Case report with autopsy verification. *Arch Neurol* 1984;41:440–442.
102. So EL, Toole JF, Dalal P, Moody DM. Cephalic fibromuscular dysplasia in 32 patients: clinical findings and radiologic features. *Arch Neurol* 1981;38:619–622.
103. Arunodaya GR, Vani S, Shankar SK, Taly AB, Swamy HS, Sarala D. Fibromuscular dysplasia with dissection of basilar artery presenting as "locked-in-syndrome." *Neurology* 1997; 48:1605–1608.
104. Slagsvold JE, Bergsholm P, Larsen JL. Fibromuscular dysplasia of intracranial arteries in a patient with multiple enchondromas (Ollier disease). *Neurology* 1977;27:1168–1171.
105. Sandok BA, Houser OW, Baker WLJ, Holley KE. Fibromuscular dysplasia. Neurologic disorders associated with disease involving the great vessels in the neck. *Arch Neurol* 1971;24: 462–466.
106. Wesen CA, Elliott BM. Fibromuscular dysplasia of the carotid arteries. *Am J Surg* 1986; 151:448–451.
107. Joyce JW. Buerger's disease (thromboangiitis obliterans). *Rheum Dis Clin N Am* 1990;16: 463–470.
108. Olin JW, Young JR, Graor RA, Ruschhaupt WF, Bartholomew JR. The changing clinical spectrum of thromboangiitis obliterans (Buerger's disease). *Circulation* 1990;82:IV3–IV8.
109. Inzelberg R, Bornstein NM, Korczyn AD. Cerebrovascular symptoms in thromboangiitis obliterans. *Acta Neurol Scand* 1989;80:347–350.
110. Brownlee RD, Tranmer BI, Sevick RJ, Karmy G, Curry BJ. Spontaneous thrombosis of an unruptured anterior communicating artery aneurysm. An unusual cause of ischemic stroke. *Stroke* 1995;26:1945–1949.
111. Antunes JL, Correll JW. Cerebral emboli from intracranial aneurysms. *Surg Neurol* 1976; 6:7–10.
112. Sakaki T, Kinugawa K, Tanigake T, Miyamoto S, Kyoi K, Utsumi S. Embolism from intracranial aneurysms. *J Neurosurg* 1980;53:300–304.
113. Steinberger A, Ganti SR, McMurtry JG, Hilal SK. Transient neurological deficits secondary to saccular vertebrobasilar aneurysms. Report of two cases. *J Neurosurg* 1984;60:410–413.
114. Iqbal A, Alter M, Lee SH. Pseudoxanthoma elasticum: a review of neurological complications. *Ann Neurol* 1978;4:18–20.
115. Miyamoto S, Kikuchi H, Karasawa J, Nagata I, Ikota T, Takeuchi S. Study of the posterior circulation in moyamoya disease. Clinical and neuroradiological evaluation. *J Neurosurg* 1984; 61:1032–1037.
116. Hojo M, Hoshimaru M, Miyamoto S, et al. Role of transforming growth factor-beta1 in the pathogenesis of moyamoya disease. *J Neurosurg* 1998;89:623–629.
117. Masuda J, Ogata J, Yutani C. Smooth muscle cell proliferation and localization of macrophages and T cells in the occlusive intracranial major arteries in moyamoya disease. *Stroke* 1993; 24:1960–1967.
118. Kawada N, Sakuma H, Yamakado T, et al. Hypertrophic cardiomyopathy: MR measurement of coronary blood flow and vasodilator flow reserve in patients and healthy subjects. *Radiology* 1999;211(1):129–135.
119. Berg JM, Armstrong D. On the association of moyamoya disease with Down's syndrome. *J Ment Defic Res* 1991;35:398–403.
120. Cramer SC, Robertson RL, Dooling EC, Scott RM. Moyamoya and Down syndrome. Clinical and radiological features. *Stroke* 1996; 27:2131–2135.
121. Bruno A, Adams HP, Jr., Biller J, Rezai K, Cornell S, Aschenbrener CA. Cerebral infarction due to moyamoya disease in young adults. *Stroke* 1988;19:826–833.
122. Servo A, Puranen M. Moyamoya syndrome as a complication of radiation therapy. Case report. *J Neurosurg* 1978;48:1026–1029.
123. Komiyama M, Yasui T, Kitano S, Sakamoto H, Fujitani K, Matsuo S. Moyamoya disease and pregnancy: case report and review of the literature. *Neurosurgery* 1998;43:360–368.
124. Chiu D, Shedden P, Bratina P, Grotta JC. Clinical features of moyamoya disease in the United States. *Stroke* 1998;29:1347–1351.
125. Sun JCL, Yakimov M, Al-Badawi I, Honey CR. Hemorrhagic moyamoya disease during pregnancy. *Can J Neurol Sci* 2000;27:73–76.

126. Kawaguchi S, Sakaki T, Morimoto T, Kakizaki T, Kamada K. Characteristics of intracranial aneurysms associated with moyamoya disease. *Acta Neurochir* 1996;138:1287–1294.
127. Bruno A, Yuh WT, Biller J, Adams HP, Jr., Cornell SH. Magnetic resonance imaging in young adults with cerebral infarction due to moyamoya. *Arch Neurol* 1988;45:303–306.
128. Fujisawa I, Asato R, Nishimura K, et al. Moyamoya disease: MR imaging. *Radiology* 1987;164:103–105.
129. Houkin K, Aoki T, Takahashi A, Abe H. Diagnosis of moyamoya disease with magnetic resonance angiography. *Stroke* 1994;25: 2159–2164.
130. Yamada I, Matsushima Y, Suzuki S. Moyamoya disease: diagnosis with three-dimensional time-of-flight MR angiography. *Radiology* 1992; 184:773–778.
131. Barboriak DP, Provenzale JM. MR arteriography of intracranial circulation. *Am J Roentgenol* 1998;171:1469–1478.
132. Laborde G, Harders A, Klimek L, Hardenack M. Correlation between clinical, angiographic and transcranial Doppler sonographic findings in patients with moyamoya disease. *Neurol Res* 1993;15:87–92.
133. Ueki K, Meyer FB, Mellinger JF. Moyamoya disease: the disorder and surgical treatment. *Mayo Clin Proc* 1994;69:749–757.
134. Golby AJ, Marks MP, Thompson RC, Steinberg GK. Direct and combined revascularization in pediatric moyamoya disease. *Neurosurgery* 1999;45:50–60.
135. Karasawa J, Touho H, Ohnishi H, Miyamoto S, Kikuchi H. Long-term follow-up study after extracranial-intracranial bypass surgery for anterior circulation ischemia in childhood moyamoya disease. *J Neurosurg* 1992;77:84–89.
136. Iwama T, Hashimoto N, Miyake H, Yonekawa Y. Direct revascularization to the anterior cerebral artery territory in patients with moyamoya disease: report of five cases. *Neurosurgery* 1998; 42:1157–1161.
137. Kinugasa K, Mandai S, Kamata I, Sugiu K, Ohmoto T. Surgical treatment of moyamoya disease: operative technique for encephalo-duro-arterio-myo-synangiosis, its follow-up, clinical results, and angiograms. *Neurosurgery* 1993; 32:527–531.
138. Kinugasa K, Mandai S, Tokunaga K, et al. Ribbon enchephalo-duro-arterio-myo-synangiosis for moyamoya disease. *Surg Neurol* 1994; 41:455–461.
139. Bollen AE, Krikke AP, de Jager AEJ. Painful Horner syndrome due to arteritis of the internal carotid artery. *Neurology* 1998;51:1471–1472.
140. Chyatte D, Bruno G, Desai S, Todor R. Inflammation and intracranial aneurysms. *Neurosurgery* 1999;45:1137–1147.
141. Holmes MD, Brant-Zawadzki MM, Simon RP. Clinical features of meningovascular syphilis. *Neurology* 1984;34:553–556.
142. Landi G, Villani F, Anzalone N. Variable angiographic findings in patients with stroke and neurosyphilis. *Stroke* 1990;21:333–338.
143. Mizusawa H, Hirano A, Llena JF, Shintaku M. Cerebrovascular lesions in acquired immune deficiency syndrome (AIDS). *Acta Neuropathol* 1988;76:451–457.
144. Qureshi AI, Janssen RS, Karon JM, et al. Human immunodeficiency virus infection and stroke in young patients. *Arch Neurol* 1997; 54:1150–1153.
145. Pinto AN. AIDS and cerebrovascular disease. *Stroke* 1996;27:538–543.
146. Tyler KL, Sandberg E, Baum KF. Medical medullary syndrome and meningovascular syphilis: a case report in an HIV-infected man and a review of the literature. *Neurology* 1994; 44:2231–2235.
147. Gordon SM, Eaton ME, George R, et al. The response of symptomatic neurosyphilis to high-dose intravenous penicillin G in patients with human immunodeficiency virus infection. *N Engl J Med* 1994;331:1469–1473.
148. Eidelberg D, Sotrel A, Horoupian DS, Neumann PE, Pumarola-Sune T, Price RW. Thrombotic cerebral vasculopathy associated with herpes zoster. *Ann Neurol* 1986;19:7–14.
149. Hilt DC, Buchholz D, Krumholz A, Weiss H, Wolinsky JS. Herpes zoster ophthalmicus and delayed contralateral hemiparesis caused by cerebral angiitis: diagnosis and management approaches. *Ann Neurol* 1983;14: 543–553.
150. Amlie-Lefond C, Kleinschmidt-DeMasters BK, Mahalingam R, Davis LE, Gilden DH. The vasculopathy of varicella-zoster virus encephalitis. *Ann Neurol* 1995;37:784–790.
151. Bourdette DN, Rosenberg NL, Yatsu FM. Herpes zoster ophthalmicus and delayed ipsilateral cerebral infarction. *Neurology* 1983; 33:1428–1432.
152. Kamholz J, Tremblay G. Chickenpox with delayed contralateral hemiparesis caused by cerebral angiitis. *Ann Neurol* 1985;18: 358–360.
153. McCormick GF, Giannotta S, Zee C, Fisher M. Carotid occlusion in cysticercosis. *Neurology* 1983;33:1078–1080.
154. Monteiro L, Almeida-Pinto J, Leite I, Xavier J, Correia M. Cerebral cysticercus arteritis: five angiographic cases. *Cerebrovasc Dis* 1994; 4:125–133.
155. Cantu C, Barinagarrementeria F. Cerebrovascular complications of neurocysticercosis. Clinical and neuroimaging spectrum. *Arch Neurol* 1996; 53:233–239.
156. Levy AS, Lillehei KO, Rubinstein D, Stears JC. Subarachnoid neurocysticercosis with occlusion of the major intracranial arteries: case report. *Neurosurgery* 1995;36:183–188.
157. Muller M, Merkelbach S, Huss GP, Schimrigk K. Clinical relevance and frequency of transient stenoses of the middle and anterior cerebral arteries in bacterial meningitis. *Stroke* 1995; 26:1399–1403.
158. Ries S, Schminke U, Fassbender K, Daffertshofer M, Steinke W, Hennerici M. Cerebrovascular involvement in the acute phase of bacterial meningitis. *J Neurol* 1997;244:51–55.

159. Grimes DA, Lach B, Bourque PR. Vasculitic basilar artery thrombosis in chronic *Candida albicans* meningitis. *Can J Neurol Sci* 1998;25:76–78.
160. Walsh TJ, Hier DB, Caplan LR. Aspergillosis of the central nervous system: clinicopathological analysis of 17 patients. *Ann Neurol* 1985; 18:574–582.
161. Sila CA, Spectrum of neurologic events following cardiac transplantation. *Stroke* 1989;20: 1586–1589.
162. Galetta SL, Wulc AE, Goldberg HI, Nichols CW, Glaser JS. Rhinocerebral mucormycosis: management and survival after carotid occlusion. *Ann Neurol* 1990;28:103–107.
163. Wilson WB, Grotta JC, Schold C, Fisher LE. Cerebral mucormycosis: an unusual case. *Arch Neurol* 1979;36:725–726.
164. Selby G, Walker GL. Cerebral arteritis in cat-scratch disease. *Neurology* 1979;29:1413–1418.
165. Toro G, Roman G. Cerebral malaria. A disseminated vasculomyelinopathy. *Arch Neurol* 1978; 35:271–275.
166. Clavier N, Rahimy C, Falanga P, Ayivi B, Payen D. No evidence for cerebral hypoperfusion during cerebral malaria. *Crit Care Med* 1999;27:628–632.
167. Knox DL, Green WR, Troncoso JC, Yardley JH, Hsu J, Zee DS. Cerebral ocular Whipple's disease: a 62-year odyssey from death to diagnosis. *Neurology* 1995;45:617–625.
168. Devlin T, Gray L, Allen NB, Friedman AH, Tien R, Morgenlander JC. Neuro-Behcet's disease: factors hampering proper diagnosis. *Neurology* 1995;45:1754–1757.
169. Shakir RA, Sulaiman K, Kahn RA, Rudwan M. Neurological presentation of neuro-Behcet's syndrome: clinical categories. *Eur Neurol* 1990; 30:249–253.
170. Moore PM, Richardson B. Neurology of the vasculitides and connective tissue diseases. *J Neurol Neurosurg Psychiatry* 1998;65:10–22.
171. Ferro JM. Vasculitis of the central nervous system. *J Neurol* 1998;245:766–776.
172. Sigal LH. The neurologic presentation of vasculitic and rheumatologic syndromes. A review. *Medicine* 1987;66:157–180.
173. Moore PM, Cupps TR. Neurological complications of vasculitis. *Ann Neurol* 1983;14:155–167.
174. Berlit P, Moore PM, Bluestein HG. Vasculitis, rheumatic disease and the neurologist: the pathophysiology and diagnosis of neurologic problems in systemic disease. *Cerebrovasc Dis* 1993;3:139–145.
175. McKenzie JD, Wallace RC, Dean BL, Flom RA, Khayata MH. Preliminary results of intracranial angioplasty for vascular stenosis caused by atherosclerosis and vasculitis. *Am J Neuroradiol* 1996;17:263–268.
176. Moore PM. Diagnosis and management of isolated angiitis of the central nervous system. *Neurology* 1989;39:167–173.
177. Woolfenden AR, Tong DC, Marks MP, Ali AO, Albers GW. Angiographically defined primary angiitis of the CNS: is it really benign? *Neurology* 1998;51:183–188.
178. Calabrese LH, Furlan AJ, Gragg LA, Ropos TJ. Primary angiitis of the central nervous system: diagnostic criteria and clinical approach. *Cleve Clin J Med* 1992;59:293–306.
179. Hankey GJ. Isolated angiitis/angiopathy of the central nervous system. *Cerebrovasc Dis* 1991; 1:2–15.
180. Vollmer TL, Guarnaccia J, Harrington W, Pacia SV, Petroff OA. Idiopathic granulomatous angiitis of the central nervous system. Diagnostic challenges. *Arch Neurol* 1993;50:925–930.
181. Chu CT, Gray L, Goldstein LB, Hulette CM. Diagnosis of intracranial vasculitis: a multi-disciplinary approach. *J Neuropathol Exp Neurol* 1998;57:30–38.
182. Alhalabi M, Moore PM. Serial angiography in isolated angiitis of the central nervous system. *Neurology* 1994;44:1221–1226.
183. Calabrese LH, Gragg LA, Furlan AJ. Benign angiopathy: a distinct subset of angiographically defined primary angiitis of the central nervous system. *J Rheumatol* 1993;20:2046–2050.
184. Vollertsen RS, McDonald TJ, Younge BR, et al. Cogan's syndrome: 18 cases and a review of the literature. *Mayo Clin Proc* 1986;61:344–361.
185. Bicknell JM, Holland JV. Neurologic manifestations of Cogan syndrome. *Neurology* 1978; 28:278–281.
186. Allen NB, Cox CC, Cobo M, et al. Use of immunosuppressive agents in the treatment of severe ocular and vascular manifestations of Cogan's syndrome. *Am J Med* 1990;88: 296–301.
187. Gordon MF, Coyle PK, Golub B. Eales' disease presenting as stroke in the young adult. *Ann Neurol* 1988;24:264–266.
188. Morelli S, Perrone C, Paroli M. Recurrent cerebral infarctions in polyarteritis nodosa with circulating antiphospholipid antibodies and mitral valve disease. *Lupus* 1998;7:51–52.
189. Nishino H, Rubino FA, Parisi JE. The spectrum of neurologic involvement in Wegener's granulomatosis. *Neurology* 1993;43:1334–1337.
190. Fauci AS, Haynes BF, Katz P, Wolff SM. Wegener's granulomatosis: prospective clinical and therapeutic experience with 85 patients for 21 years. *Ann Intern Med* 1983;98:76–85.
191. Nishino H, Rubino FA, DeRemee RA, Swanson JW, Parisi JE. Neurological involvement in Wegener's granulomatosis: an analysis of 324 consecutive patients at the Mayo Clinic. *Ann Neurol* 1993;33:4–9.
192. Savitz JM, Young MA, Ratan RR. Basilar artery occlusion in a young patient with Wegener's granulomatosis. *Stroke* 1994;25:214–216.
193. Kattah JC, Chrousos GA, Katz PA, McCasland B, Kolsky MP. Anterior ischemic optic neuropathy in Churg-Strauss syndrome. *Neurology* 1994; 44:2200–2202.
194. Sehgal M, Swanson JW, DeRemee RA, Colby TV. Neurologic manifestations of Churg-Strauss syndrome. *Mayo Clin Proc* 1995;70:337–341.
195. Kerr GS, Hallahan CW, Giordano J, et al. Takayasu arteritis. *Ann Intern Med* 1994; 120:919–929.
196. Ishikawa K, Uyama M, Asayama K. Occlusive thromboaortopathy (Takayasu's disease): cervical arterial stenoses, retinal arterial pressure,

retinal microaneurysms and prognosis. *Stroke* 1983;14:730–735.
197. Takano K, Sadoshima S, Ibayashi S, Ichiya Y, Fujishima M. Altered cerebral hemodynamics and metabolism in Takayasu's arteritis with neurological deficits. *Stroke* 1993;24:1501–1506.
198. Hall S, Barr W, Lie JT, Stanson AW, Kazmier FJ, Hunder GG. Takayasu arteritis. A study of 32 North American patients. *Medicine* 1985; 64:89–99.
199. Sun Y, Yip PK, Jeng JS, Hwang BS, Lin WH. Ultrasonographic study and long-term follow-up of Takayasu's arteritis. *Stroke* 1996;27:2178–2182.
200. Shelhamer JH, Volkman DJ, Parrillo JE, et al. Takayasu's arteritis and its therapy. *Ann Intern Med* 1985;103:121–126.
201. Turnbull J. Temporal arteritis and polymyalgia rheumatica: nosographic and nosologic considerations. *Neurology* 1996;46:901–906.
202. Berlit P. Clinical and laboratory findings with giant cell arteritis. *J Neurol Sci* 1992;111:1–12.
203. Brack A, Martinez-Taboada V, Stanson A, Goronzy JJ, Weyand CM. Disease pattern in cranial and large-vessel giant cell arteritis. *Arthritis & Rheumatism* 1999;42:311–317.
204. Caselli RJ, Hunder GG, Whisnant JP. Neurologic disease in biopsy-proven giant cell (temporal) arteritis. *Neurology* 1988;38:352–359.
205. Reich KA, Giansiracusa DF, Strongwater SL. Neurologic manifestations of giant cell arteritis. *Am J Med* 1990;89:67–72.
206. Bragoni M, Di P, V, Priori R, Valesini G, Lenzi GL. Sjogren's syndrome presenting as ischemic stroke. *Stroke* 1994;25:2276–2279.
207. Alexander E. Central nervous system disease in Sjogren's syndrome. New insights into immunopathogenesis. *Rheum Dis Clin N Am* 1992;18:637–672.
208. Wong KL, Woo EK, Yu YL, Wong RW. Neurological manifestations of systemic lupus erythematosus: a prospective study. *Q J Med* 1991;81:857–870.
209. Kitigawa Y, Gotoh F, Koto A, Okayasu H. Stroke in systemic lupus erythematosus. *Stroke* 1990; 21:1533–1539.
210. D'Cruz D. Vasculitis in systemic lupus erythematosus. *Lupus* 1998;7:270–274.
211. Trimble M, Bell DA, Brien W, et al. The antiphospholipid syndrome: prevalence among patients with stroke and transient ischemic attacks. *Am J Med* 1990;88:593–597.
212. Verro P, Levine SR, Tietjen GE. Cerebrovascular ischemic events with high positive anticardiolipin antibodies. *Stroke* 1998;29:2245–2253.
213. Ware AE, Mongey AB. Lupus and cerebrovascular accidents. *Lupus* 1997;6:420–424.
214. Lie JT, Kobayashi S, Tokano Y, Hashimoto H. Systemic and cerebral vasculitis coexisting with disseminated coagulopathy in systemic lupus erythematosus associated with antiphospholipid syndrome. *J Rheumatol* 1995;22:2173–2176.
215. Postiglione A, De Chiara S, Soricelli A, et al. Alterations of cerebral blood flow and antiphospholipid antibodies in patients with systemic lupus erythematosus. *Internati J Clin Lab Res* 1998;28:34–38.
216. Asherson RA, Khamashta MA, Gil A, et al. Cerebrovascular disease and antiphospholipid antibodies in systemic lupus erythematosus, lupus-like disease, and the primary antiphospholipid syndrome. *Am J Med* 1989;86:391–399.
217. Donders RC, Kappelle LJ, Derksen RH, et al. Transient monocular blindness and antiphospholipid antibodies in systemic lupus erythematosus. *Neurology* 1998;51:535–540.
218. Asherson RA, Cervera R, Font J. Multiorgan thrombotic disorders in systemic lupus erythematosus: a common link?. *Lupus* 1992; 1:199–203.
219. Ellison D, Gatter K, Heryet A, Esiri M. Intramural platelet deposition in cerebral vasculopathy of systemic lupus erythematosus. *J Clin Pathol* 1993;46:37–40.
220. Tourbah A, Piette JC, Iba-Zizen MT, Lyon-Caen O, Godeau P, Frances C. The natural course of cerebral lesions in Sneddon syndrome. *Arch Neurol* 1997;54:53–60.
221. Stockhammer G, Felber SR, Zelger B, et al. Sneddon's syndrome: diagnosis by skin biopsy and MRI in 17 patients. *Stroke* 1993;24:685–690.
222. Pathak R, Gabor AJ. Scleroderma and central nervous system vasculitis. *Stroke* 1991;22: 410–413.
223. Estey E, Lieberman A, Pinto R, Meltzer M, Ransohoff J. Cerebral arteritis in scleroderma. *Stroke* 1979;10:595–597.
224. Ramos M, Mandybur TI. Cerebral vasculitis in rheumatoid arthritis. *Arch Neurol* 1975;32: 271–275.
225. Shim SC, Yoo DH, Lee JK, et al. Multiple cerebellar infarction due to vertebral artery obstruction and bulbar symptoms associated with vertical subluxation and atlanto-occipital subluxation in ankylosing spondylitis. *J Rheumatol* 1998; 25:2464–2468.
226. Robinson BP, Seeger JF, Zak SM. Rheumatoid arthritis and positional vertebrobasilar insufficiency. Case report. *J Neurosurg* 1986;65: 111–114.
227. Mevorach D, Goldberg Y, Gomori JM, Rachmilewitz D. Antiphospholipid syndrome manifested by ischemic stroke in a patient with Crohn's disease. *J Clin Gastroenterol* 1996; 22:141–143.
228. Ryan FP, Timperley WR, Preston FE, Holdsworth CD. Cerebral involvement with disseminated intravascular coagulation in intestinal disease. *J Clin Pathol* 1977;30:551–555.
229. Lossos A, River Y, Eliakim A, Steiner I. Neurologic aspects of inflammatory bowel disease. *Neurology* 1995;45:416–421.
230. Talbot RW, Heppell J, Dozois RR, Beart RW, Jr. Vascular complications of inflammatory bowel disease. *Mayo Clin Proc* 1986;61:140–145.
231. Mayeux R, Fahn S. Strokes and ulcerative colitis. *Neurology* 1978;28:571–574.
232. Calderon R, Cruz-Correa MR, Torres EA. Cerebral thrombosis associated with active Crohn's disease. *Puerto Rico Health Sciences Journal* 1998;17:293–295.
233. Vaezi MF, Rustagi PK, Elson CO. Transient protein S deficiency associated with cerebral venous

thrombosis in active ulcerative colitis. *Am J Gastroenterol* 1995;90:313–315.

234. Weber P, Husemann S, Vielhaber H, Zimmer KP, Nowak-Gottl U. Coagulation and fibrinolysis in children, adolescents, and young adults with inflammatory bowel disease. *J Ped Gastroenterol Nutr* 1999;28:418–422.
235. Nelson J, Barron MM, Riggs JE, Gutmann L, Schochet SS, Jr. Cerebral vasculitis and ulcerative colitis. *Neurology* 1986;36:719–721.
236. Heuer DK, Gager WE, Reeser FH. Ischemic optic neuropathy associated with Crohn's disease. *J Clin Neuro-Ophthalmol* 1982;2:175–181.
237. Penix LP. Ischemic strokes secondary to vitamin B12 deficiency-induced hyperhomocystinemia. *Neurology* 1998;51:622–624.
238. Brown MM, Thompson AJ, Wedzicha JA, Swash M. Sarcoidosis presenting with stroke. *Stroke* 1989;20:400–405.
239. Malek AM, Higashida RT, Halbach VV, et al. Patient presentation, angiographic features, and treatment of strangulation-induced bilateral dissection of the cervical internal carotid artery. Report of three cases. *J Neurosurg* 2009; 92:481–487.
240. Evers S. Altenmuller E, Ringelstein EB. Cerebrovascular ischemic events in wind instrument players. *Neurology* 2000;55:865–867.
241. Yamauchi T, Tada M, Houkin K, et al. Linkage of familial moyamoya disease (spontaneous occlusion of the Circle of Willis) to chromosome17q25. *Stoke* 2000;31:930–935.

Chapter 8

PRO-THROMBOTIC STATES

Regardless of the underlying vascular disease, activation of hemostatic mechanisms plays a critical role in the development of arterial or venous thromboembolism. Hemostasis involves a very complex set of interactions between cellular elements and circulating plasma proteins to maintain blood in a fluid state within the body's arteries, capillaries, and veins. These factors can respond with thrombosis formation at the time of a vascular injury. Disturbances in the homeostasis between factors that either promote or limit thrombosis are critical in clinical complications of vascular disease. An acquired or inherited lack of a procoagulant factor can lead to major hemorrhage. For example, intracranial bleeding can occur in patients with hemophilia or thrombocytopenia. Conversely, both acquired and inherited changes that tip the balance in favor of

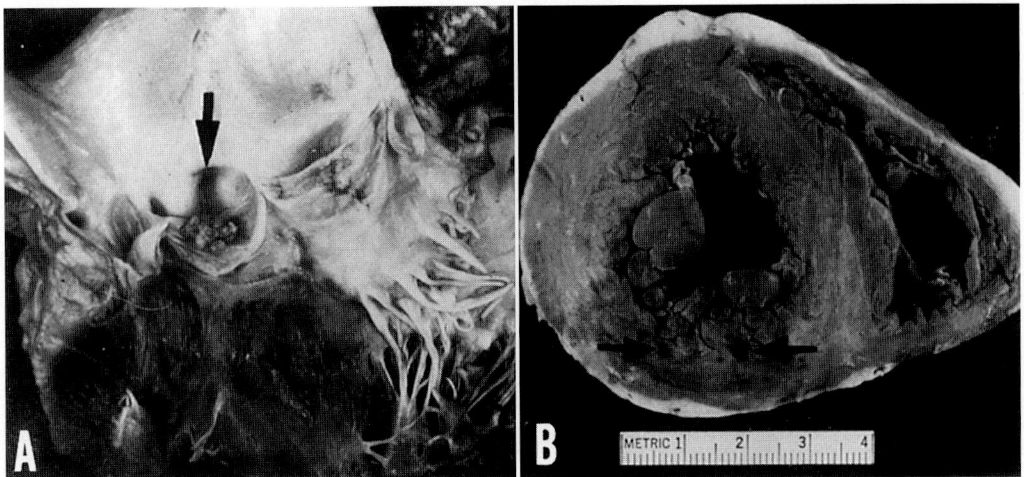

Figure 8–1. Cardiac vegetations (*A* and *B*) focussed in on Pathological examinations in a patient with Marantic endocarditis. The arrow in (A) denotes vegetations on a cardiac value. (Reprinted from Olney BA et al. The consequences of the nonsequential Marantic [nonbacterial thrombotic] endocarditis. *Am Heart J* 1979;98:513, with permission.)

thrombosis can lead to ischemic stroke secondary to either arterial or venous occlusion. Because of the key role of hemostasis in the development of ischemic vascular disease, many interventions prescribed to prevent or treat ischemic stroke aim at inhibiting factors that encourage thrombosis. Unfortunately, because these agents also limit coagulation, bleeding, including intracranial hemorrhage, is an important complication of their use.

A detailed description of the physiology of coagulation that maintains normal hemostasis is beyond the purview of this book. The endothelium is increasingly recognized as a critical player in the maintenance of hemostasis and in the development of thrombosis.[1] Expression of tissue factors from ruptured atherosclerotic plaques or denuded subendothelial cells prompts activation of platelets and procoagulant proteins. Knowledge about the interactions between the endothelium and circulating procoagulant and anticoagulant factors and platelets is changing rapidly.[2–8] Platelets continue to be critical in initiating arterial thrombosis, and both red blood cells and white cells contribute to the formation of clots.[9] A number of plasma proteins, including plasminogen, protein C, protein S, and antithrombin III, limit or reverse the formation of thrombi. Adequate concentrations of these proteins and their prompt activation are crucial in halting the development of large intraluminal thrombi and arterial occlusions. Concentrations of both procoagulant and anticoagulant elements in the blood change in response to a number of factors. For example, with advancing age and after menopause in women, concentrations of the natural anticoagulants (protein C, protein S, and antithrombin III) rise in response to an age-related increase in procoagulant factors.[10]

GENERAL FEATURES OF PRO-THROMBOTIC DISEASES

This chapter discusses acquired and inherited disorders of hemostasis that promote the development of thromboembolism, affecting either cellular elements (erythrocytes, leucocytes, or platelets) or circulating proteins in the blood (Table 8–1). These hemorheological alterations can lead to hypercoagulable states and both venous and arterial thrombosis.[11–13] As such, they may cause life-threatening ischemic events, including pulmonary embolism, myocardial infarction, or ischemic stroke. An acquired pro-thrombotic (hypercoagulable) disorder is presumed to

Table 8–1. **Inherited or Acquired Pro-thrombotic Disorders**

Cellular
Polycythemia
Severe anemia
Sickle cell disease
Thrombocytosis
Thrombotic thrombocytopenia purpura
Heparin-associated thrombocytopenia—white clot syndrome
Leukemia
Plasma proteins
Decreased protein C activity
Decreased protein S activity
Antithrombin III deficiency
Factor V-Leiden
Prothrombin G20210A mutation
Deficiency of heparin cofactor II
Deficiency of plasminogen
Increased fibrinogen
Thalassemia
Carbohydrate-deficient glycoprotein syndrome
Waldenstrom macroglobulinemia
Antiphospholipid antibody syndrome—lupus anticoagulant
Warfarin-induced skin necrosis
Disseminated intravascular coagulation

play an important role in vascular thrombosis in persons with a number of serious medical illnesses. (Table 8–2). Although a discrete disorder of a hemostatic factor has not been described in some of these conditions, combinations of changes in cellular elements or plasma proteins likely play a role.

General Clinical Features

Most patients with a transient ischemic attack (TIA) or an ischemic stroke do not have a primary acquired or inherited pro-thrombotic disorder.[14,15] Still, disorders of hemostasis can lead to stroke. In some instances, a pro-thrombotic state can compound the effects of an arterial lesion. Nighoghossian et al[16] estimated that

Table 8–2. **Diseases Presumably Associated with a Pro-thrombotic State**

Pregnancy and puerperium
Oral contraceptives
Cancer and chemotherapy
Dehydration
Inflammatory bowel disease
Nephrotic syndrome
Hemolytic-uremic syndrome
Sepsis and inflammation
Trauma
Surgery

approximately 4% of all ischemic strokes are secondary to a pro-thrombotic disturbance. The risks of stroke secondary to disordered coagulation are not uniform. A hypercoagulable state may be more likely to cause ischemic stroke in persons younger than 45, especially children.[17] Some of the age relationship may be secondary to more detailed screening for abnormalities in coagulation in this population.

Some clinical features point to pro-thrombotic disease as a cause of ischemic stroke. A past history of recurrent or recent *arterial* or *venous thrombosis* might point to a hypercoagulable state. An inherited hypercoagulable state should be suspected if one or more relatives have a history of arterial or venous thrombosis, particularly, if thrombotic events occurred before the age of 45. Patients should be asked about a personal or family history of *myocardial infarction, venous thrombosis,* or *pulmonary embolism.* An acquired or inherited pro-thrombotic state also should be considered if a female patient or female relatives have a history of recurrent spontaneous abortion. *Fetal demise* leading to abortion may be ascribed to pro-thrombotic–induced placental thrombosis, such as in patients with antiphospholipid syndrome.

SCREENING

Screening for a hypercoagulable disorder is described in Chapter 4. The timing of these tests is important. A *complete blood count, platelet count, pro-thrombin time/international normalized ratio (INR),* and *activated partial thromboplastin time (aPTT)* can be obtained at any time. They should be ordered on an emergent basis when a patient is seen with an acute ischemic stroke or a recent TIA.

However, the results of several other tests can be influenced by the neurological event. Coagulation and fibrinolytic pathways are activated during the acute phase of ischemic stroke secondary to atherosclerosis, small artery disease, or cardioembolism.[14,18,19] Elevations in hemostatic markers, such as *fibrinopeptide A, D-dimer,* or *beta-thromboglobulin* have been correlated with the severity of acute ischemic stroke.[20,21] Levels of circulating anticoagulant proteins may drop during the first few weeks after a neurological event and a false-positive test might suggest a pro-thrombotic disorder. Franke et al[22] reported increases in levels of *fibrin monomers, thrombin-antithrombin III complex,* D-dimer, and *tissue plasminogen* activity after a recent stroke. Fon et al[23] found evidence of both increased thrombogenesis and fibrinolysis after acute TIA; they noted increases in levels of both fibrinopeptide A and thrombin-antithrombin III complexes.

Because the results of testing for *protein C, protein S,* and *antithrombin III* can be spurious, these tests should not be performed within the first 6 weeks after stroke or TIA. Conversely, testing can be done immediately for other hematologic conditions that could promote thrombosis, such as *Factor V-Leiden, antiphospholipid antibody,* or *sickle cell* studies.

The presence of a coagulation abnormality that predisposes to deep vein thrombosis could be the substrate for paradoxical embolism among persons with a patent foramen ovale (PFO). Chaturvedi[24] noted that almost one-third of patients with a PFO and cryptogenic stroke had hematologic risk factors. The combination of a PFO and evidence of a pro-thrombotic state likely would lead to recommending long-term anticoagulant therapy for these patients. The presence of a pro-thrombotic state also may potentiate the risk of embolism in persons with structural diseases of the heart. This type of patient would likely be treated with long-term oral anticoagulants instead of antiplatelet aggregating medications. Elevations in *von Willebrand factor, factor VIII, fibrinogen,* D-dimer, and beta thromboglobulin may play a role in increasing the risk of stroke in persons with atrial fibrillation.[25] Hypercoagulable states appear to increase risk of recurrent thrombosis in patients with prosthetic heart valves.[26] Libman-Sacks endocarditis and non-bacterial thrombotic endocarditis also are manifestations of pro-thrombotic disorders that can lead to cardioembolic stroke.

Frequency of Hypercoagulable Causes of Ischemic Stroke

Approximately 1%–25% of young adults and children with ischemic stroke are identified with an abnormality in coagulation.[27–30] The broad range probably, in part, reflects the intensity of screening for a coagulation disorder. Several studies have focused on the frequency and types of pro-thrombotic diseases in young adults and children with ischemic stroke. Douay et al[31] assessed levels of protein C, protein S, and antithrombin III in 127 patients under the age of 45; 9 had abnormal levels. Still, 7 of these patients had other risk factors (pregnancy, inflammation, or oral contraceptive use) that helped to explain the low levels of these clotting factors. Munts et al[32] evaluated 120 patients under the age of 45 for evidence of a coagulation defect. The most common problems observed were elevated anticardiolipin antibodies, lupus-like anticoagulant, and decreased protein S activity. They could not find a relationship between an abnormality of coagulation and stroke subtype. Another series of 67 children with cerebral arterial thromboses were evaluated for pro-thrombotic states.[33] Eight had inherited disorders of coagulation. DeVeber et al[34] confirmed the high rate of pro-thrombotic disorders among children. They found abnormal tests in 35 of 92 children with stroke. In 21 of these children, multiple abnormalities were detected.

CELLULAR PRO-THROMBOTIC DISORDERS

Polycythemia

Red blood cells are active in both normal and pathologic aspects of hemostasis, and their role in clot formation is becoming clearer. The red blood cell now is recognized as having an active role in the formation of intravascular thrombi.[8] At present, no red blood cell–mediated coagulant state is known; however, increases in red blood cell concentrations (*polycythemia*) do have affects on viscosity and blood flow. An elevated hematocrit increases *blood viscosity* and slows cerebral blood flow.[35] Polycythemia is recognized as a potential cause of ischemic stroke.[36–39] In general, a *hematocrit value* greater than 50% identifies a high risk for stroke.

Polycythemia can occur as part of a *myeloproliferative disease* or secondary to a tumor that produces *erthyropoetin,* such as a cerebellar hemangioblastoma or renal cell carcinoma. The administration of epoetin alfa aslo can cause an elevated hematocrit.[301] A familial form also has been associated with ischemic stroke.[40] It also can complicate pulmonary disease or cyanotic congenital heart disease. Assessment of the complete blood count is the usual way to screen for polycythemia.

In general, lowering the blood hematocrit to a value of approximately 40% will increase cerebral blood flow by reducing viscosity. Patients with polycythemia can be treated with periodic removal of a volume of blood (500 mL) in an attempt to lower the hematocrit and blood viscosity. This approach should used with caution in elderly patients. Chemotherapy or administration or radioactive phosphorus may be prescribed to treat the myeloproliferative disease underlying polycythemia. Some patients with acute ischemic stroke have been treated with hemodilution in an effort to improve viscosity and cerebral blood flow. These acute trials have been unsuccessful.[41–44] (See Chapter 12.)

Anemia

Profound *anemia* could contribute to global cerebral ischemia by reducing the oxygen-carrying capacity of the blood. The level of hematocrit that is critical for causing global ischemic symptoms is uncertain, but it likely is a value less than 30%. Anemia can be secondary to blood loss, hemolysis, or one of a large number of conditions that suppress bone marrow function. The latter may be the most common reason for chronic anemia. Patients with severe anemia usually have symptoms of syncope or a multifocal neurological syndrome rather than focal symptoms of a TIA or an ischemic stroke. High flows needed to maintain adequate cerebral oxygenation may cause a cranial bruit.[45]

Sickle Cell Disease

The *hemoglobinopathies* are inherited diseases that increase the risk of ischemic stroke in both young adults and children.[17,36,37,40] *Hemoglobin S* (*HgbS*) results from a mutation that causes the substitution of valine for glutamic acid in the protein structure of the globin chain. Normal hemoglobin is labeled *hemoglobin A* (*Hgb A*). The abnormal hemoglobin structure causes abnormalities in the red blood cell plasticity that is aggravated by the presence of acidosis or hypoxia. The sickled cells lead to increased viscosity of the blood and a sludging of flow in the microcirculation.[46]

An ethnic association of hemoglobinopathy is strong. Approximately 8% of African Americans have a heterozygous *sickle cell trait* (*Hgb SA*), whereas less than 0.2% have homozygous *Hgb SS* (*sickle cell disease*). Sickle hemoglobinopathies also occur in persons of Middle Eastern or Eastern Mediterranean ancestry. Children with Hgb SS have very severe disease and are symptomatic at young ages. Children and young adults with Hg SA may be asymptomatic until they develop either acidosis or hypoxia. Approximately 4%–10% of patients with sickle cell disease have a history of clinical stroke. Another 10%–15% of patients have brain imaging findings of an asymptomatic stroke.[47,48] The incidence of stroke among persons with sickle cell disease is estimated to be 0.61/100 patient-years.[48] Sickle cell disease is recognized as a leading cause of stroke in children.[48–50] Children with a low hemoglobin concentration or leucocytosis have an increased risk of silent brain infarctions.[48,51] A hemoglobin S concentration greater than 30% also predicts an increased risk of ischemic stroke.[52]

Most children and young adults with sickle cell disease also have anemia. In young adults with sickle cell disease, chronic hypoxia and a decreased hematocrit can lead to a decreased intellect and changes consistent with multiple ischemic strokes detected by brain imaging.[53,54] Neuropsychological impairments can be prominent secondary to multiple areas of subcortical or cortical infarction.[55] The silent brain infarctions also are associated with an increased risk of seizures.[51] Children with sickle cell disease can have either hemorrhagic or ischemic stroke. Strokes can be compatible with occlusions of either large- or small-caliber vessels. The features of stroke secondary to sickle cell disease are described in more detail in Chapter 9.

Magnetic resonance angiography often demonstrates stenosis or occlusions of the intracranial arteries in patients with sickle cell disease, suggesting that it leads to a progressive arteriopathy as well as a pro-thrombotic state.[56–58] Positron emission tomography and magnetic resonance imaging also can detect areas of hypoperfusion.[59] Sequential transcranial Doppler ultrasound (TCD) examinations can be used to monitor vascular disease in children with sickle cell disease.[57,60,61] In particular, intracranial arterial stenoses can be detected by TCD.[58] Children with evidence of increased blood flow velocity on TCD are at an increased risk of ischemic stroke.[62] Changes in flow velocities can prompt early transfusion to lower the concentration of hemoglobin S and prevent ischemic stroke.[63]

Some patients have been reported to have sickle cell disease and decreased free and total levels of protein S or heparin cofactor II or increased thrombin–antithrombin complex or prothrombin F1 + 2.[47] Tam[64] noted that children with stroke complicating sickle cell disease also had low levels of protein C and protein S. An elevation of blood homocysteine is associated with stroke in children with sickle cell disease.[65] These comorbid pro-thrombotic factors may further increase the risk of ischemia in persons with sickle cell disease.

Thrombocytosis

Because platelets play a leading role in the initiation and propagation of intravascular thrombosis, an abnormality in platelet number or function can lead to arterial occlusion and ischemic stroke.[4,9,13,36,37,66,67] *Essential thrombocytosis* (*thrombocythemia*) usually is diagnosed when platelet count exceeds 600,000 per cubic mm. and when there is a marked proliferation of bone marrow megakaryocytes. Rarely, the platelet count can surpass 1 million. Essential thrombocytosis may result from an increase in megakaryocyte as in essential thrombocythemia or from the clonal expansion of erythroid precursors, such as in *polycythemia vera* or *chronic myelogenous leukemia*.[68] Stroke can be the first clinical manifestation of an elevated platelet count.[69,70]

In addition to an increase in platelet count, a change in platelet morphology or platelet activity can induce arterial occlusions. An increase in platelet volume has been reported during both the acute and the non-acute phases of ischemic stroke.[71] *Sticky platelet syndrome* is a rare but potential cause of ischemic stroke in young adults.[72,73] Increases in levels of *platelet factor 4* or *beta-thromboglobulin* have been noted in patients with ischemic stroke; these findings may represent ongoing platelet activation.[74] These platelet-specific proteins presumably mean that increased rates of platelet adhesion and aggregation underlie acute arterial thrombosis. Antiplatelet agents, in particular aspirin, are the usual treatment for patients with essential thrombocythemia.[75]

Thrombotic Thrombocytopenia Purpura/Hemolytic-Uremic Syndrome

Thrombotic thrombocytopenia purpura (*TTP*) is a thrombotic microangiopathy that produces purpura and skin ischemia, bleeding and hemolysis, neurological symptoms, fever, and renal failure.[36,37,76,77] The microangiopathy appears to be secondary to endothelial dysfunction, which leads to a direct interaction with circulating platelets.[78,79] Thrombotic thrombocytopenia purpura presumably is attributed to an autoimmune process, but evidence suggesting that TTP is a true autoimmune disorder is not definitive.[80] Recent data suggest that an inherited or acquired *antibody to the von Willebrand factor metalloprotenase* leads to the circulation of large von Willebrand factor proteins.[81] The presence of the large protein leads to increases in platelet aggregation. The same factors seem to be important in patients with TTP secondary to the use of ticlopidine.[302]

Hemolytic-uremic syndrome, which is described in this chapter, often is associated with TTP. Although fibrinogen levels usually are not affected in patients with both conditions, the platelet count usually drops and the von Willebrand factor is increased.[79,82] Familial cases of stroke secondary to TTP have been reported.[83] Thrombotic thrombocytopenia purpura also has been associated with *systemic lupus erythematosus, pregnancy, transplantation, AIDS, and infection.*[78,79,84–87] A potential association between TTP and the presence of *antiphospholipid antibodies* and systemic lupus erythematosus also is reported.[88,89]

Thrombotic thrombocytopenia purpura can occur in persons of any age, and it has been reported in children.[77,90] Approximately 70% of affected patients are women.[77] Ischemic stroke can complicate TTP and the hemolytic-uremic syndrome. The neurological symptoms can fluctuate and be the presenting feature.[91] The usually reflect global dysfunction or an encephalopathy. Focal signs may not be prominent. Progression to coma is a poor prognostic sign.[77] A polyneuropathy also can develop.[86] In addition to stroke, brain imaging findings among patients with TTP show reversible cerebral edema with a posterior predominance mimicking a posterior leucoencephalopathy syndrome.[92] Thrombotic thrombocytopenia purpura is a life-threatening disease. Treatment options for TTP include *plasma exchange,* steroids, aspirin, and vincristine.[79,93] Plasma exchange appears to be the best choice for treatment of acute TTP.[87]

Thrombotic thrombocytopenia purpura is a potential complication of treatment with ticlopidine. (See Chapter 10.) *Ticlopidine-associated TTP* appears to be an idiosyncratic reaction. The frequency of this complication is not clear, but it is approximately <0.5%. Based on a survey of patients receiving ticlopidine following stenting of the coronary arteries, Steinhubl et al[94] estimated that the rate of TTP was 0.02%. They did not note a relationship between the duration of use of ticlopidine and TTP; some patients with the complication had taken the medication for less than 2 weeks. Bennett et al[95] reported 60 cases of patients with TTP following the use of ticlopidine. Approximately 80% had the complication within 1 month of starting treatment. Cases of TTP developing several months after starting ticlopidine have not been reported. The risk of TTP is sufficiently high to mandate that all patients receiving ticlopidine should have their platelet count checked when their white blood cell count is monitored. Even this monitoring might not predict a sudden fulminant TTP reaction. The mortality of patients with ticlopidine-induced TTP is approximately 50% but, with plasma exchange, mortality can be reduced by approximately one-half.

Heparin-Associated Thrombocytopenia

Heparin is a glycosaminoglycan of bovine or porcine origin. Because it is a foreign protein, its use can be associated with an immune reaction. The most common consequence is thrombocytopenia. Abnormal *IgG* or *IgM antibodies* and platelet active antibodies can be found among a sizeable proportion of persons exposed to heparin.[96–99] The presence of platelet factor 4 is required for the immune binding of the platelets that occurs with *heparin-associated thrombocytope-*

nia.[100] No dosage of heparin or duration of exposure has been correlated with the risk of thrombocytopenia. Thrombocytopenia can occur even with the tiny amount of heparin given to maintain patency of intravenous catheters. A modest decline in platelet count develops in approximately 80% of patients treated with heparin for 3–7 days.[98,101] Although these declines are frequently found, they are of borderline significance. More severe declines in platelet counts (<100,000 or greater than 40% decline) can be associated with the so-called white clot syndrome and a high risk of arterial occlusion and ischemic stroke. This more severe type of thrombocytopenia is immune mediated and generally appears approximately 1 week after starting treatment with heparin.[102] Prior administration of heparin may sensitize a patient to a second exposure to the agent. Severe thrombocytopenia may occur within hours of restarting treatment.

The neurological complications of heparin-associated thrombocytopenia may mimic those of TTP.[103,104] Multiple cerebral infarctions can occur. In addition to stroke, white clot syndrome has been implicated as a cause of limb ischemia, myocardial infarction, and venous thromboembolism.[105,106] Perioperative use of heparin can affect cerebrovascular and peripheral vascular reconstruction procedures. Atkinson et al[107] reported 18 carotid occlusions among 2527 patients undergoing carotid endarterectomy; 6 of the 18 patients had heparin-associated coagulopathies. Calaitges et al[97] noted a 2.6-fold increase in perioperative thrombotic events among patients treated with heparin.

Patients receiving heparin should have their platelet count assessed every 2–3 days. A decline to less than 100,000 platelets/cubic mm. is a source of concern. Values less than 50,000 are particularly dangerous.[102] Diagnosis can be confirmed in the laboratory by demonstrating the presence of the antibody or by platelet aggregation studies in the presence of heparin. Treatment involves stopping heparin. Patients with a high risk for thrombosis may require another antithrombotic agent if the heparin is discontinued. Patients with heparin-associated thrombocytopenia should not receive *low molecular weight heparin* because of the high risk of cross-reactivity. *Low molecular weight heparinoid* or a thrombin inhibitor, such as *hirudin* or *argatroban,* might be prescribed if the patient requires antithrombotic treatment.[108–110]

Leukemia

Knowledge is expanding about the role of white blood cells in the maintenance of hemostasis. *Adhesion molecules* on circulating *leukocytes* appear to be important in local thrombus regulation.[111,112] Thus, information will grow about the role of abnormal white blood cells (either in number or functional activity) in the development of thromboembolism.

Stroke is a potential complication of leukemia in children.[28,36] The elevated white blood cell count presumably increases blood viscosity, slows cerebral blood flow, and promotes thrombosis in intracranial arteries and veins.[113] Leukemia is also a rare cause of stroke among adults. Thrombosis has been associated with *acute lymphoblastic leukemia* or, as a complication of its treatment, with *L-asparaginase.*[114] *Acute promyelocytic leukemia* can induce *disseminated intravascular coagulation.* Treating leukemia can affect levels of clotting factors and promote either hemorrhagic or ischemic stroke. Monitoring coagulation and replacing clotting factors during treatment have been recommended.[114] Stroke also is a complication of the *hypereosinophilia syndrome.*[115,116] This neoplastic proliferation of eosinophils can cause a microvasculopathy and multifocal ischemic encephalopathy.

PRO-THROMBOTIC DISORDERS OF PLASMA PROTEINS

Decreased Protein C Activity

Protein C is a natural anticoagulant that, in conjunction with protein S, inhibits the function of activated *factors V* and *VIII.*[10] *Thrombomodulin,* which is expressed by endothelial cells, activates protein C.

Protein C also may have an indirect thrombolytic effect by reducing thrombin generation. A deficiency in protein C can occur as part of an *inherited disease* or it can be acquired secondary to *disseminated intravascular coagulation, malignancies, liver disease, acute respiratory distress syndrome, sepsis,* or *L-asparaginase* therapy.[12,40] Inherited cases of protein C deficiency are caused by a genetic mutation resulting in changes in the polypeptide sequence of the natural anticoagulant protein.[117] Homozygous protein C deficiency can cause *neonatal purpura fulminans.*

Deficiency in protein C is most commonly associated with deep vein thrombosis.[2] Although venous thrombosis is the leading complication, cerebral infarction also has been described in a patient with an inherited disorder of protein C deficiency.[118] A deficiency of protein C is not a leading cause of stroke in middle-age adults or the elderly; however, a low level of protein C is associated with ischemic stroke in children and young adults.[27,30,34,36,118–121] Overall, the frequency of a protein C deficiency even among young persons with ischemic stroke seems to be low. Nighoghossian et al[16] could not find any cases of protein C deficiency among a population of young adults with stroke. Martinez et al[122] found low concentrations of protein C in only 3 of 60 young adults with ischemic stroke. Overall, protein C deficiency plays a minor role in the pathogenesis of ischemic stroke or arterial occlusions. Kiechl et al[123] reported that poor responses to activated protein C are a predictor of advanced atherosclerotic disease. This observation implies that changes in the protein C could be the result of arterial disease.

Determination of the protein C level probably is not required as part of the evaluation of patients with ischemic stroke. Only young adults with other history of thrombosis or patients with either a family history suggestive of a pro-thrombotic state or one of the previously described medical conditions that could lead to protein C deficiency should be screened. Low levels of protein C need verification in most patients because the changes may be an epiphenomenon. The test probably should not be performed until at least 6 weeks after the ischemic event.

Decreased Protein S Activity

Protein S is a cofactor for the activity of protein C, as described, and a deficiency is most commonly correlated with deep vein thrombosis.[2] The frequency of protein S deficiency is approximately 1:1000 to 1:5000 persons. The inherited form of protein S deficiency appears to be secondary to the development of abnormal polypeptide chains secondary to a change in the nucleotide sequence.[117]

Protein S deficiency is an unusual cause of ischemic stroke in children and young adults.[17,27,30,36,40,119] A low level of free protein S was detected in approximately 11% of 92 children with stroke.[34] Munts et al[32] reported that 20 of 120 young patients with ischemic stroke had decreased protein S activity, but only 2 had the abnormality confirmed by a second test. Another study tested free protein S levels 1 month after stroke among 26 young adults with stroke. Only 2 cases were identified; 1 had an acquired decline in protein S, and the other had an inherited disorder.[16] Another study of 60 young adults with ischemic stroke found protein S deficiency in 2 cases.[122] A deficiency of both protein C and protein S in a family with ischemic strokes in multiple young adults has been reported.[124] A transient decline in protein S concentration has been associated with cerebral venous thrombosis and stroke in a patient with active ulcerative colitis.[125]

Cautions about diagnosing stroke secondary to protein C deficiency also apply to protein S. Persons with protein S deficiency and thromboembolic events should be treated with oral anticoagulants on a long-term basis. Proteins C and S activity are reduced by warfarin and, thus, the diagnosis of these conditions is unreliable if the patient is receiving the anticoagulant.

Decreased Antithrombin III Activity

Antithrombin III plays a pivotal role in the prevention of thrombosis. It binds heparin to thrombin to halt coagulation and also neutralizes *activated factor X* and other pro-thrombotic proteases.[126] *Heparin sulfate* activates antithrombin III, a feature that is important in understanding the therapeutic actions of heparin. Heparin sulfate, a natural constituent of the vascular endothelium, is also a cofactor for antithrombin III, an important feature for the therapeutic effect of heparin and for physiological hemostasis. The antibody detected in heparin-associated thrombocytopenia exhibits a cross-reactivity with heparin sulfate—hence another mechanism for its pro-thrombotic propensity. Both inherited and acquired deficiency of antithrombin III can occur. The inherited form is due to a substitution, a deletion, or an insertion mutation leading to development of aberrant polypeptide chains.[117] A heterozygous deficiency in antithrombin III activity is correlated with an increased risk of venous thrombosis, whereas arterial or venous occlusions are complications of the homozygous recessive state.[2]

Antithrombin III deficiency can cause ischemic stroke in young adults and children.[27,30,36,127,128] Decreased antithrombin III activity was identified in 3 of 120 patients with acute ischemic stroke.[32] Martinez et al[122] reported that 5 of 60 young patients with ischemic stroke had low levels of antithrombin III. In a series of deVeber et al,[34] a low level of antithrombin III was detected in 12.5% of 92 children. Conversely, no cases of antithrombin III deficiency were noted among the young adults with stroke studies by Nighoghossian et al.[16] Co-existence of antithrombin III deficiency and Factor V Leiden has been reported in a family with recurrent thrombosis.[129] Levels of antithrombin III change with age, and these changes may lead to the increased risk of ischemia in the elderly.[130] Still, antithrombin III deficiency probably is not a major cause of ischemic stroke in persons older than 45. Because stroke can affect blood levels of antithrombin III, it should not be checked until several weeks after the ischemic event.

Factor V Leiden/Activated Protein C Resistance

The genetic disease that increases *resistance to protein C activation* (*Factor V-Leiden*) is due to a 1691 G A point mutation of nucleotides in the factor V gene (Arg506Glu).[131–134] The resultant factor V amino acid sequence is altered, making it resistant to inactivation by the actions of activated protein C.[135] Clinicians should differentiate the homozygous or heterozygous form deficiency of factor V; the former is much less common and causes a marked bleeding diathesis.[136] Most patients have a heterozygous condition. A homozygous state usually is associated with stroke and multiple arterial thromboses at a very early age.[133,137]

The interactions between Factor V-Leiden and protein C need additional clarification. Van der Bom et al[138] concluded that only part of the reduced response to activated protein C is independent on the presence of Factor V-Leiden. Some resistance to activated protein C may also be acquired, and this can occur without Factor V-Leiden.[139] This finding suggests that other factors influence the interaction between factor V and activated protein C. For example, Aznar et al[140] noted that antiphospholipid antibodies affect activation of protein C. A genetic link between migraine with aura and abnormalities leading to protein C resistance has been speculated as a cause of migrainous stroke.[141] Resistance to activated protein C may be worsened by the use of oral contraceptives.[142,143] A poor response to activated protein C also has been associated with advanced atherosclerosis and arterial disease.[123]

Price and Ridker[143] and Eskandari et al[144] estimated that 4%–6% of the American population has Factor V-Leiden. This high prevalence means that Factor V-Leiden probably is the leading inherited hypercoagulable cause of arterial or venous occlusions in children or adults.[2,34,36,128,135,144–147] Its presence increases the risk of venous thromboembolism by a factor of 3–6.[143] One study demonstrated that a decreased response to activated protein C increases the risk of stroke by a factor of 1.43 (1.12–1.81).[138] Factor V-Leiden also is a potential cause of otherwise unexplained recurrent pregnancy loss.[148,149]

Eskandari et al[144] reported that Factor V-Leiden is a potential cause of either myocardial infarction or ischemic stroke in persons younger than 50. Although Factor V-Leiden is implicated commonly as a cause of ischemic stroke, the associated risk may persist among persons older than 50. Factor V-Leiden appears to be the most common inherited pro-thrombotic cause of brain ischemia. Factor V-Leiden can cause stroke or myocardial infarction in persons of all ages.[146] The prevalence of Factor V-Leiden is not increased in elderly patients with ischemic stroke.[131]

The presence of Factor V-Leiden is recognized as a risk factor for cerebral venous thrombosis.[145] De Lucia et al[134] reported finding resistance to activated protein C in 9 of 14 young adults with ischemic stroke. These 9 patients were from three different families. In a study of young women, Longstreth et al[150] did not find that Factor V-Leiden was a risk factor for ischemic stroke. In a series of 67 children with stroke, 6 had Factor V-Leiden identified. One study evaluated 28 patients younger than 55 for the presence of activated protein C resistance; 9 patients had the hematologic abnormality.[72] Most of the 9 patients had other pro-thrombotic abnormalities, including anticardiolipin antibodies, protein S deficiency, sticky platelet syndrome, or lupus anticoagulant. Brain imaging tests will show multiple ischemic lesions among patients with factor V-Leiden.[151] The diagnosis of Factor V-Leiden can be established by either a coagulation assay evaluating the effect of activated protein C or by polymerase chain reaction.

Gruppo et al[152] described a syndrome of strokes, cutis marmorata, telangiectasia, and Factor V-Leiden. Factor V-Leiden also appears to increase the risk of ischemia among patients with thalassemia.[135] Elevated blood levels of homocysteine may increase the risk of thrombosis secondary to Factor V-Leiden.[143] Martinelli et al[153] found a high risk of venous thrombosis among persons who have Factor V-Leiden and who use oral contraceptives. A similar relationship with arterial thrombosis was not described. Lalouschek et al[154] recently reported a series of patients with Factor V-Leiden and a C 677 T mutation. These patients also had elevated levels of homocysteine. They concluded that the presence of this new mutation could increase the risk of stroke by a ratio of 2.75.

Oral anticoagulation has been advocated to lower the risk of recurrent arterial or venous thrombosis in persons with Factor V-Leiden. Baglin et al[155] recommended that long-term anticoagulation not be prescribed if a patient has had only one episode of thrombosis.

Prothrombin G20210A Mutation

A change in the gene leading to *prothrombin G20210A mutation* is associated with a prothrombotic state.[2] It leads to increased plasma concentrations of thrombin, prothrombin, thrombin-AT III complex, and prothrombin fragment 1 + 2.[156,157] The highest risk for thrombosis is among persons who are homozygous for the mutation.[158] The presence of G20210A mutation and factor V-Leiden are associated with a high risk of deep vein thrombosis.[159,160] Investigators of a large study of American men concluded that the genetic mutation also is associated with an increased risk of myocardial infarction or ischemic stroke but that the magnitude of the risk is less than with Factor V-Leiden.[161] Still, the prothrombin G20210A mutation now appears to be the second most important inherited prothrombotic risk factor. Its presence greatly increases the risk of thrombosis in conjunction with other risk factors.[157]

The genetic mutation has been associated with severe vascular occlusive events in children with sickle cell disease.[162] Arkel et al[163] described ischemic stroke in a young patient who had protein C deficiency and the prothrombin gene mutation G20210A. They recommended long-term oral anticoagulant therapy to prevent recurrent stroke in this situation. However, Longstreth et al[150] did not find that the G20210A gene mutation was a risk factor for stroke in young women. A Danish study concluded that the genetic mutation was not a risk factor for juvenile stroke.[164] Ferraresi et al[160] concluded that the heterozygous genotype was not associated with an increased risk of arterial occlusions. Further research on the importance of both the homozygous and the heterozygous genotypic mutations of prothrombin

G20210A will be needed to clarify the role of this inherited disorder in ischemic stroke.

A homozygous variant of the G20210A mutation leading to polymorphism at the gene 3′-untranslated region has been associated with massive thrombosis.[165]

Deficiency of Heparin Cofactor II

Deficiency of heparin cofactor II is a potential cause of thrombosis or hypercoagulability.[12] It is a very rare cause of ischemic stroke.[36,37]

Deficiency of Plasminogen

Low concentrations or abnormalities of *plasminogen* are associated with ischemic stroke in children and young adults.[27,32,34,37,166] Based on an evaluation of 23 patients with pro-thrombotic states and plasminogen deficiency and their family members, Demarmels et al[167] found that 2.2% had venous thrombosis and 1.4% had arterial events. The frequency of plasminogen deficiency in patients with ischemic stroke or in the general population is not known.

Increased Fibrinogen Concentration

High concentrations of *fibrinogen* are associated with an increased risk of ischemic stroke or myocardial infarction.[37,39,168–174] Resch et al[175] concluded that the presence of *hyperfibrinogenemia* increased risk of subsequent cardiovascular events by a ratio of approximately 3.67 in persons who have survived stroke. Qizilbash et al[176] estimated that the risk of stroke is increased by a factor of 1.78 if the fibrinogen concentration is >3.6 gm/L. Elevations in fibrinogen are more common in men and African Americans. Levels of fibrinogen also increase with advancing age, smoking, inactivity, or the use of oral contraceptives. Elevations of fibrinogen also can follow an acute ischemic process or be seen with an acute inflammatory or infectious illness.[177] Elevations of fibrin or D-dimer and increased blood viscosity are associated with an increased risk of stroke in persons with peripheral vascular disease.[178]

Hyperfibrinogenemia probably is not a primary factor causing stroke, but it may contribute to a pro-thrombotic state. The frequency of hyperfibrinogenemia is not known among persons with ischemic stroke or in the general population. Increases in fibrinogen and blood viscosity presumably lead to decreased cerebral blood flow and a high risk of ischemic stroke.[35,175,179–181] Reducing fibrinogen levels can help to lower blood viscosity and improve blood flow. Several strategies, including volume expansion, removal of one or more units of blood, or plasma exchange, can be employed. Walzl et al[172] described the success of extracorporeal precipitation in lowering fibrinogen concentrations and blood viscosity.

Thalassemia

Thromboembolic events and ischemic stroke are potential complications of *beta-thalassemia*. In one series of 495 patients with either *thalassemia major* or *intermedia*, the prevalence of thromboembolic events was 5.2%.[144,182] Borgna et al[183] reported that thromboembolism occurred in 16 of 32 affected patients.

Carbohydrate-Deficient Glycoprotein Syndrome

The *carbohydrate-deficient glycoprotein syndrome* is an autosomal recessive disorder that leads to a problem in the glycosylation of glycoproteins.[184] Affected patients have seizures, hypotonia, and stroke-like events. Bleeding or thrombosis can be due to defects in protein C, protein S, antithrombin III, or factor XI.

Waldenstrom Macroglobulinemia

The *paraproteinemias* increase blood viscosity by augmenting concentrations of immune globulins. The pentameric structure of IgM, the paraprotein elevated in most cases of *Waldenstrom macroglobulinemia,* makes it particularly prone to increases in plasma viscosity. Cerebral blood flow declines, and the risk of ischemic stroke grows with increases in blood protein.[179,180] Alpha-2 globulin and gamma globulin are the macroproteins that have the greatest effect on viscosity and blood flow.[180] The paraproteinemia most commonly associated with an elevated risk of ischemic stroke is Waldenstrom macroglobulinemia.[36,126]

Antiphospholipid Antibodies/Lupus Anticoagulant

An *elevated antiphospholipid antibody* is the most common acquired thrombophilia leading to ischemic stroke.[185] Although the presence of antiphospholipid antibodies is common among persons with stroke or in the general population, these antibodies may not be the cause of stroke in most persons with elevations. Increases in antiphosphoplipid antibodies are not a leading cause of stroke among large, unselected populations with ischemic stroke.[128,186,187] The mechanism for promoting thrombosis in the presence of elevated antiphospholipid antibodies has not been fully elucidated, but it appears to relate to interactions with cardiolipin found in endothelial cells or to beta-2-glycoprotein I.[188–194] The pro-thrombotic effects also might through interference with the activation of protein C or an increase in concentration of fibrinogen and factors VII and VIII.[140,195]

Antiphospholipid antibodies and *lupus anticoagulants* are recognized as a leading cause of ischemic stroke among subgroups of patients, especially among young adults and children.[32,34,66,196–200] Tuhrim et al[201] found that the impact of antiphospholipid antibodies was seen in all ethnic groups. A high rate of positive anticardiolipin antibodies is found in elderly patients who have an otherwise unexplained stroke.[202]

Advanced age, or the presence of atrial fibrillation, congestive heart failure, or valvular heart disease, is associated with elevations of *IgG anticardiolipin* antibodies.[203,204] Tuhrim et al[201] calculated that the risk of stroke increased by a factor of 3.9 with the presence of IgG anticardiolipin antibodies and by a factor of 3.4 with *IgM anticardiolipin* antibodies. The degree of increase of IgG antibodies appears to correlate with an increase in the number of risk factors for stroke.[203] This finding was not confirmed by another study.[201] Other investigators have not established a relationship between thrombosis and elevation of either IgG or IgM anticardiolipin antibodies.[192,200] An elevated IgG antiphospholipid antibody level appears to be critical for ischemic symptoms, although a relationship has not been established between the level of antibody titers and the occurrence of ischemic events. Elevated levels of these antibodies can be detected within the first hours after stroke.[205] Finazzi et al[206] found that the risk of stroke among patients with antiphosphoplipid antibodies was approximately 2.5% per year.

Anti–prothrombin antibodies also may have a relation to the lupus anticoagulant and thrombosis.[207,208] Toschi et al[209] noted that patients with cerebral ischemia of undetermined cause had a high prevalence of *antiphosphatidylinositol antibodies.* The most common are antibodies to cardiolipin and phosphatidaylinositol. Approximately one-third of patients with anticardiolipin antibodies had antibodies to other compounds.[209] The lupus anticoagulant syndrome is associated with thromboembolism, rather than bleeding. Prolongation of aPTT is a key finding for the lupus anticoagulant. Although the association is strong between an elevated antiphospholipid antibody and the lupus anticoagulant, the relationship is not uniform.[210]

Clinical features of the antiphospholipid antibody-lupus anticoagulant syndrome are fairly stereotyped. Patients have recurrent arterial and venous thromboses, including stroke, myocardial infarction, deep vein thrombosis, and pulmonary embolism.[211] A strong relationship between anticoardiolipin antibodies and cerebral venous thrombosis also has been found. Christopher et al[212] found abnormal IgG and IgM antibodies in 22% of 31 patients with cerebral venous thrombosis. Pregnant women with antiphospholipid antibodies have a very high risk for fetal demise and spontaneous abortion.[185,213,214] Approximately one-half of the patients have other evidence of systemic lupus erythematosus (SLE).[215,216] Interactions among SLE, ischemic stroke, and antiphospholipid antibodies are strong.[217–219] Elevated antiphospholipid antibodies are the primary cause of stroke among persons with SLE.[216,220] A multicenter study found that approximately 16% of patients with stroke and antiphospholipid antibodies had other evidence of systemic lupus erythematosus.[214]

Libman-Sacks endocarditis is a potential cause of stroke in patients with antiphospholipid syndrome.[221] Cardiac abnormalities suggestive of Libman-Sacks endocarditis were found in 16 of 72 patients studied by echocardiography in one multicenter series.[214] The vegetations can embolize and cause cardioembolic occlusion of a major intracranial vessel.

Sneddon syndrome, consisting of prominent trunk and limb livedo reticularis, digital ischemia, behavioral signs, and stroke, is a hallmark of the antiphospholipid antibody syndrome.[185,222–224] Sneddon syndrome also can be found among patients with rheumatic heart disease or SLE.[225,226] Familial cases of Sneddon syndrome and families with elevated antiphospholipid antibodies have been reported.[227,228] Still, the disease is considered to be an acquired, rather than an inherited, illness.

Elevated antiphospholipid antibodies may complicate cardiac or arterial diseases, causing stroke or ocular ischemia in young adults.[229,230] Stroke is the most common neurological complication among patients with elevated antiphospholipid antibodies.[185,216] Other neurological symptoms include seizures, chorea, cognitive impairments, depression, psychosis, and myelitis.[213] Antiphospholipid antibodies have been associated with cerebral atrophy and Binswanger's disease.[231,232] Many patients have non-specific abnormalities found in the cerebral hemispheres by brain imaging studies.[213] Migraine also has been associated with antiphospholipid antibodies.[233] The latter relationship has been debated. Brey and Escalante[213] have not found an increased frequency of migraine in persons with elevated antiphospholipid antibodies. Hinse et al[230] found elevated anticardiolipin antibodies in only 1 of 25 young adults with migraine.

Laboratory evaluation of a patient with suspected antiphospholipid antibody syndrome includes measurements of both the IgG and the IgM anticardiolipin antibodies.[199] A *falsely positive* serological test for *syphilis* can be detected in approximately one-fourth of cases.[216] The syphilis serology is another useful tool in screening for an autoimmune disorder. Elevated titers of *antinuclear antibodies* can be found in up to one-half of affected patients.[210] Either thrombocytosis or thrombocytopenia can be found. [210,213] Increased platelet activity (adhesion and aggregation) also has been described.[234] In the absence of heparin, a prolongation of the aPTT that does not reverse with the addition of normal plasma is the key finding for the presence of a lupus anticoagulant. The *dilute Russel viper time* and *kaolin clotting* also can add supportive evidence.[235] Echocardiography will be abnormal in approximately 30%–75% of patients.[210,214] Both thickening of the valves and vegetations may be detected. Microemboli can be detected by TCD.[236] One study using Single photon electron computed tomography evaluated 22 patients with antiphospholipid antibodies and SLE.[237] Abnormalities in blood flow were detected in 13. No difference in blood flow patterns was observed between the patients who had elevated antibody titers and those who had the lupus anticoagulant. Arteriography can demonstrate occlusions of small- to moderate-caliber intracranial arteries.[220,238] Skin biopsy in a patient with Sneddon syndrome can show inflammation, subendothelial proliferation, and fibrosis of small- to medium-caliber vessels at the border between the dermis and the subdermal tissues.[239]

The risk for recurrent thromboembolism is very high among persons with antiphospholipid antibody syndrome.[210,215] The rate of early recurrent stroke appears to be approximately 10% within the first year.[214] The likelihood of a second stroke is highest during the first 6 months after a thrombotic event.[215] Because of the high risk for thrombosis, patients with antiphospholipid antibody syndrome usually are treated with long-term oral anticoagulants. The desired level of International Normalized Ratio is greater than 3.[215] In general, no effect on the level of antibodies is found with the use of anticoagulants, steroids, or other immunosuppressives.[192]

Warfarin-Induced Skin Necrosis

The administration of warfarin slows hepatic production of functional *vitamin K–dependent factors* that affect hemostasis (factors II, VII, IX, and X; proteins C and S). The long-term effect of warfarin is suppression of procoagulant clotting factor activity leading to effective anticoagulation. However, the initial actions of warfarin reduce the synthesis of natural anticoagulant proteins (proteins C and S), and a transient hypercoagulable state can occur. Changes in thrombin–antithrombin III complex and D-dimer levels can be used to detect the presence of a hypercoagulable state in the presence of low levels of anticoagulation with warfarin.[240] The most common clinical consequence of *warfarin-induced hypercoagulation* is skin necrosis, but stroke also is a potential complication.[241,242] The incidence of warfarin-induced skin necrosis has been estimated to be 1:100 to 1:10,000 treated patients.[243] Skin changes usually occur within 3–10 days following the start of treatment and are most commonly associated with protein C deficiency.[243,244] Warfarin-induced skin necrosis in a patient with a mutation of the pro-thrombin gene has been reported.[245] Skin changes also have occurred after stopping the anticoagulant.[246]

Warfarin also can induce the *purple toe syndrome* or a vasculitis leading to skin necrosis.[242,247,248] *Heparin-induced skin necrosis* can mimic the findings ascribed to warfarin among patients treated with both agents.

Disseminated Intravascular Coagulation

Ischemic stroke can be a complication or presentation of *disseminated intravascular coagulation* (*DIC*), which most commonly occurs in critically ill patients, including persons with advanced malignancies, severe metabolic diseases, multiple trauma, sepsis, or severe brain illnesses. Both cortical and brain stem hemorrhage and infarction can result from large- or small-vessel occlusions.[249] Clinical findings include coma and obtundation, as well as focal neurological impairments. Typically, patients with DIC have reductions in platelet count and plasma fibrinogen, as well as prolongation of pro-thrombin, thrombin, and aPTT times. Elevations in D-dimer and fibrin split products usually are found. Disseminated intravascular coagulation is a feature of *non-bacterial thrombotic endocarditis* (*NBTE*/ *marantic endocarditis*) (see Fig. 8–1 on page 255). NBTE is a potential complication of malignancies. Approximately one-third of patients will have cerebral embolism.[250–252] This condition is described in more detail in Chapter 6. In the absence of major bleeding, treatment of DIC and NBTE may involve administration of anticoagulants, including heparin.

Other Disorders of Coagulation

Several other disorders of coagulation have been described in persons with ischemic vascular disease. These conditions appear to be relatively uncommon, and testing for their presence should be considered only in exceptional circumstances. A decline in *plasminogen activator inhibitor* has been seen in patients with atherosclerosis.[253] This decline may promote the development of atherosclerotic lesions or thrombosis. Conversely, increases in plasminogen activator inhibitor concentrations are associated with an increased risk of stroke.[37,168] An elevation of *tissue plasminogen activator antigen* also has been associated with an increased risk of stroke in young women ages 15–45.[168,254,255] Additional research is needed on this finding. An *inherited disorder of factor XII* activity may be associated with an increased risk of ischemic stroke.[40] An abnormality in the *dilute pro-thrombin assay* has been described in 28 of 120 young patients with ischemic stroke.[32] The significance of this finding is unclear. Changes in *fibrinopeptide A, von Willebrand factor, D-dimer, beta-thromboglobulin, factor VIII activity, factor*

V activity, factor XII, prekallikreins, or *prothrombin fragment 1.2* concentrations occur in persons with cardioembolic, lacunar, or cortical ischemic strokes.[19,37,168,256–259] Stroke also is a potential complication of cryoglobuinemia.[260]

HYPERCOAGULABLE STATES SECONDARY TO OTHER CONDITIONS

Pregnancy and Puerperium

Ischemic stroke occurring late in *pregnancy* and during the *puerperium* often is attributed to a hypercoagulable state.[37,126,171] *Venous thrombosis* is more common than arterial occlusion. Abnormalities in levels of protein C, protein S, and antithrombin III have been identified in young women who are pregnant.[31,261] Ischemic stroke complicating pregnancy and puerperium is described in more detail in Chapter 9.

Oral Contraceptives

Ischemic stroke developing in young women taking *oral contraceptives* has been attributed to a medication-induced pro-thrombotic state.[37,126,171] Oral contraceptives have been associated with a decline in tissue factor pathway inhibitors. Declines in protein C, protein S, or antithrombin III activity have been associated with oral contraceptive use.[12,31,262] A resistance to activated protein C also can be worsened by oral contraceptives.[142] Ischemic stroke related to the use of oral contraceptives is discussed in Chapter 9.

Cancer and Chemotherapy

Ischemic stroke is a potential complication of *malignancy* and *chemotherapy*.[171,263–266] In an autopsy-based study, Rogers[267] found evidence of stroke in approximately 15% of 4326 patients who had cancer. Strokes usually occur when a patient has advanced or disseminated disease.[268] Occasionally, a thrombotic event, including an ischemic stroke or unexplained and recurrent deep vein thrombosis, may be the initial presentation of an occult malignancy.[269] Immobility, surgery, chemotherapy, or the use of central venous lines can be associated with an increased risk of thrombosis among patients with cancer.[270]

Although stroke seems to be most common in patients with *mucin-producing adenocarcinomas,* it also can complicate lymphoreticular malignancies.[267,271,272] Stroke also can result from disseminated intravascular coagulation with or without evidence of non-bacterial thrombotic endocarditis.[267,273,274] Occlusions of large cerebral arteries and microvascular occlusions both can be seen.[273] In addition to focal neurological impairments such as hemiparesis, severe encephalopathy or delirium can present the cerebrovascular complications of a cancer-related pro-thrombotic state.[273] Other features of a malignancy-related pro-thrombotic state include clot formation at unusual sites and resistance to treatment with warfarin or heparin.[269]

This mechanism of stroke presumably is due to the production of proteins or antibodies that foster production or activity of coagulation factors.[275,276] Malignancy can be associated with a deficiency of protein C, a deficiency of von Willebrand factor, or an increase in the thrombin–antithrombin complex.[12,268,277] Disturbances in concentrations of fibrinogen and alpha-2-antiplasmin also have been described.[278] In addition, malignancy may promote thrombosis by altering the functioning of blood cells and the endothelium.[275] Still, many patients with malignancy and recurrent thromboembolism will not have a specific defect in coagulation identified.[269]

Changes in coagulation, fibrinolysis, endothelial function, platelet reactivity, and monocyte function that occur with cancer can be exacerbated by chemotherapy.[279,280] Administration of *L-asparaginase* for treatment of leukemia has been associated with an increased risk of thrombosis and ischemia.[114,281–283] L-asparaginase therapy also has been correlated with a decline in levels of protein C, plasminogen, or antithrombin III.[12,284] Ischemic stroke also is a potential complication of treatment with *5-fluorouracil, cisplatinum,* or *methotrexate.*[271,283,285,286] Administration of erythropoietic agents to a patient with a malignancy could lead to an elevated hematocrit and possibly thrombosis.[301] Stroke also has been diagnosed as a potential complication among patients having *bone marrow transplantation.*[287]

Dehydration

Dehydration causes hemoconcentration, an increase in the levels of blood clotting factors, and increased viscosity that may progress to a pro-thrombotic state leading to ischemic stroke in children and young adults.[17] Dehydration also can lead to stroke in older persons. Deyhdration can complicate infectious illnesses, malignancies, or multisystem inflammatory disease.

Inflammatory Bowel Disease

Ischemic stroke is a potential complication of inflammatory bowel disease. Approximately 10% of patients with hypercoagulable states secondary to inflammatory bowel disease have strokes.[288] Disorders of coagulation that have been reported among persons with ulcerative colitis or regional enteritis include a decreased level of protein S, increased fibrinogen concentration, thrombocytosis, increased prothrombin F1+2 level, increased level of plasminogen activator inhibitor, and increased thrombomodulin.[125,289] Elevated anticardiolipin antibodies also have been reported.[288] See Chapter 7 for additional information about the relationship of stroke and inflammatory bowel disease.

Paroxysmal Nocturnal Hemoglobinuria

Paroxysmal nocturnal hemoglobinuria is a rare pro-thombotic cause of ischemic stroke.[36] It can be related to genetic modifiers or associated with nutritional or infectious diseases.[182] A case of moyamoya syndrome complicating paroxysmal nocturnal hemoglobinuria has been described.[290]

Nephrotic Syndrome

Nephrotic syndrome is a potential cause of a hypercoagulable state.[12,126,171] The urinary loss of proteins, in particular proteins C and S, leads to hypercoagulablity that promotes thrombosis and ischemic stroke.[291,292] Chaturvedi[293] reported stroke as a complication of membranous nephropathy. Proteinuria appears to be an independent risk factor for stroke in persons with diabetes mellitus, presumably because of its effects on blood levels of proteins C and S.[294]

Sepsis and Inflammation

Reductions in the activity of the protein C pathway and fibrinolysis have been described in patients with infections. These reductions might explain the association of ischemic stroke with recent febrile or infectious illness.[295] Abnormalities of protein C, protein S, and antithrombin III have been associated with acute inflammation.[31] Brain ischemia can be secondary to a pro-thrombotic state and NBTE among patients *with acquired immune deficiency syndrome.*[296]

Other Diseases

An acquired thrombophilia has been associated with *acute respiratory distress syndrome* or *liver disease.*[12,171] Liver disease can be complicated by a decline in the production of vitamin K–dependent clotting factors, including proteins C and S. Prolonged *hyperglycemia* can enhance thrombin generation and thrombosis.[297] Lip and Gibbs[298] reported that *heart failure* might confer a hypercoagulable state. Thrombophilia leading to ischemic stroke has been reported as a complication of prolonged bed rest, surgery, burns, or trauma.[37,171]

A pro-thrombotic state has not been found to occur as a complication of use of *anabolic steroids.*[299] *Alcohol* consumption increases concentrations of plasminogen activator inhibitor and tissue-type plasminogen activator antigen.[300] These changes in coagulation may be a partial explanation for the high rates of stroke reported shortly after heavy alcohol consumption.

SUMMARY

Altered coagulation underlies the development of arterial and venous thromboembolism regardless of the initiating cause. Although the tendency to coagulate increases with advancing age, it is the young in whom coagulation disorders are an important cause of stroke, especially in children and young adults.

The dynamic equilibrium between fluid and clotted blood is maintained by a complex interaction of blood cells, plasma factors, and the vascular endothelium. Disturbances of this equilibrium, as occurs around the time of a stroke, renders measurement of certain plasma factors, such as protein C, protein S, and antithrombin III, unreliable until about 6 weeks after a stroke or a TIA. The coagulation balance can also be tilted by systemic diseases and by therapies, sometimes paradoxically, such as the development of thrombocytopenia with heparin.

Although genetic defects of coagulation affect a minority of patients and account for only a fraction of all strokes, their presence may prove important in interaction with other factors and at the time of urgent therapy, such as the infusion of tissue plasminogen activator factor. The time will come when high-risk, asymptomatic patients will have their coagulation profiles documented so that their treatments can be tailored appropriately.

REFERENCES

1. Maruyama I. Biology of endothelium. *Lupus* 1998;7(Suppl 2):S41–S43.
2. Rosenberg RD, Aird WC. Vascular-bed—specific hemostasis and hypercoagulable states. *N Engl J Med* 1999;340:1555–1564.
3. Beguin S, Kumar R, Keularts I, Seligsohn U, Coller BS, Hemker HC. Fibrin-dependent platelet procoagulant activity requires GPIb receptors and von Willebrand factor. *Blood* 1999;93:564–570.
4. Eisenberg PR, Ghigliotti G. Platelet-dependent and procoagulant mechanisms in arterial thrombosis. *Internat J Cardiol* 1999;68,(Suppl 1): S3–S10.
5. Bennett JS. Both sides of the hypercoagulable state. *Hospital Practice (Office Edition)* 1997; 32:105–108.
6. Harker LA. Therapeutic inhibition of thrombin activities, receptors, and production. *Hematol Oncol Clin North Am* 1998;12:1211–1230.
7. Nagamatsu Y, Tsujioka Y, Hashimoto M, Giddings JC, Yamamoto J. The differential effects of aspirin on platelets, leucocytes and vascular endothelium in an in vivo model of thrombus formation. *Clin Laborat Haematol* 1999;21:33–40.
8. Andrews DA, Low PS. Role of red blood cells in thrombosis. *Curr Opin Hematol* 1999;6:76–82.
9. del Zoppo GJ. The role of platelets in ischemic stroke. *Neurology* 1998;51:S9–S14.
10. Sagripanti A, Carpi A. Natural anticoagulants, aging, and thromboembolism. *Experimental Gerontology* 1998;33:891–896.
11. Mira Y, Vaya A, Martinez M, et al. Hemorheological alterations and hypercoagulable state in deep vein thrombosis. *Clin Hemorheol Microcirculation* 1998;19:265–270.
12. Bick RL. Hypercoagulability and thrombosis. *Med Clin N Am* 1994;78:635–665.
13. Greaves M. Coagulation abnormalities and cerebral infarction. *J Neurol Neurosurg Psychiatry* 1993;56:433–439.
14. Habel RL, Biniasch O, Ott M, Peinemann A, Wick M, Kempter B. Infrequency of stroke caused by specific coagulation disorders. *Cerebrovasc Dis* 1995;5:391–396.
15. Levine J, Swanson PD. Nonatherosclerotic causes of stroke. *Ann Intern Med* 1969;70:807–816.
16. Nighoghossian N, Berruyer M, Getenet JC, Trouillas P. Free protein S spectrum in young patients with stroke. *Cerebrovasc Dis* 1994; 4:304–308.
17. Mendoza PL, Conway EE, Jr. Cerebrovascular events in pediatric patients. *Pediatr Ann* 1998; 27:665–674.
18. Altes A, Abellan MT, Mateo J, Avila A, Marti-Vilalta JL, Fontcuberta J. Hemostatic disturbances in acute ischemic stroke: a study of 86 patients. *Acta Haematologica* 1995;94:10–15.
19. Giroud M, Dutrillaux F, Lemesle M, et al. Coagulation abnormalities in lacunar and cortical ischemic stroke are quite different. *Neurol Res* 1998;20:15–18.
20. Feinberg WM, Erickson LP, Bruck D, Kittelson J. Hemostatic markers in acute ischemic stroke. Association with stroke type, severity, and outcome. *Stroke* 1996;27:1296–1300.
21. Takano K, Yamaguchi T, Uchida K. Markers of a hypercoagulable state following acute ischemic stroke. *Stroke* 1992;23:194–198.
22. Franke CL, Buscher MJJ, van Wersch JWJ. Haemostasis and fibrinolysis after recent stroke. *Cerebrovasc Dis* 1992;2:365–368.
23. Fon EA, Mackey A, Cote R, et al. Hemostatic markers in acute transient ischemic attacks. *Stroke* 1994;25:282–286.
24. Chaturvedi S. Coagulation abnormalities in adults with cryptogenic stroke and patent foramen ovale. *J Neurol Sci* 1998;160:158–160.
25. Gustafsson C, Blomback M, Britton M, Hamsten A, Svensson J. Coagulation factors and the

increased risk of stroke in nonvalvular atrial fibrillation. *Stroke* 1990;21:47–51.
26. Gencbay M, Turan F, Degertekin M, Eksi N, Mutlu B, Unalp A. High prevalence of hypercoagulable states in patients with recurrent thrombosis of mechanical heart valves. *J Heart Valve Dis* 1998;7:601–609.
27. Barinagarrementeria F, Cantu-Brito C, De La Pena A, Izaguirre R. Prothrombotic states in young people with idiopathic stroke. A prospective study. *Stroke* 1994;25:287–290.
28. Gore RM, Weinberg PE, Anandappa E, Shkolnik A, White H. Intracranial complications of pediatric hematologic disorders: computed tomographic assessment. *Investigative Radiology* 1981; 16:175–180.
29. Gobel U. Inherited or acquired disorders of blood coagulation in children with neurovascular complications. *Neuropediatrics* 1994;25:4–7.
30. Bonduel M, Sciuccati G, Hepner M, Torres AF, Pieroni G, Frontroth JP. Prethrombotic disorders in children with arterial ischemic stroke and sinovenous thrombosis. *Arch Neurol* 1999; 56:967–971.
31. Douay X, Lucas C, Caron C, Goudemand J, Leys D. Antithrombin, protein C and protein S levels in 127 consecutive young adults with ischemic stroke. *Acta Neurol Scand* 1998; 98:124–127.
32. Munts AG, van Genderen PJ, Dippel DW, van Kooten F, Koudstaal PJ. Coagulation disorders in young adults with acute cerebral ischaemia. *J Neurol* 1998;245:21–25.
33. Ganesan V, McShane MA, Liesner R, Cookson J, Hann I, Kirkham FJ. Inherited prothrombotic states and ischaemic stroke in childhood. *J Neurol Neurosurg Psychiatry* 1998;65:508–511.
34. deVeber G, Monagle P, Chan A, et al. Prothrombotic disorders in infants and children with cerebral thromboembolism. *Arch Neurol* 1998;55:1539–1543.
35. Lowe GD, Lee AJ, Rumley A, Price JF, Fowkes FG. Blood viscosity and risk of cardiovascular events: the Edinburgh Artery Study. *Br J Haematol* 1997;96:168–173.
36. Tatlisumak T, Fisher M. Hematologic disorders associated with ischemic stroke. *J Neurol Sci* 1996;140:1–11.
37. Hart RG, Kanter MC. Hematologic disorders and ischemic stroke. A selective review. *Stroke* 1990;21:1111–1121.
38. Grotta JC, Manner C, Pettigrew LC, Yatsu FM. Red blood cell disorders and stroke. [Review]. *Stroke* 1986;17:811–817.
39. Forconi S, Turchetti V, Cappelli R, Guerrini M, Bicchi M. Haemorheological disturbances and possibility of their correction in cerebrovascular diseases. [Review]. *Journal des Maladies Vasculaires* 1999;24:110–116.
40. Natowicz M, Kelley RI. Mendelian etiologies of stroke. *Ann Neurol* 1987;22:175–192.
41. Italian Acute Stroke Study Group. Haemodilution in acute stroke. Results of the Italian haemodilution trial. *Lancet* 1988;1:318–321.
42. Asplund K. Hemodilution in acute stroke. *Cerebrovasc Dis* 1991;1(Suppl 1):129–138.
43. Scandinavian Stroke Study Group. Multicenter trial of hemodilution in acute ischemic stroke. Results of subgroup analyses. *Stroke* 1988; 19:464–471.
44. The Hemodilution in Stroke Study Group. Hypervolemic hemodilution treatment of acute stroke. Results of a randomized multicenter trial using pentastarch. *Stroke* 1989;20:317–323.
45. Gareeboo H. Severe anaemia as a cause of cranial bruit in adults. *Br Med J* 1968;1:294.
46. French JA, Kenny D, Scott JP, et al. Mechanisms of stroke in sickle cell disease: sickle erythrocytes decrease cerebral blood flow in rats after nitric oxide synthase inhibition. *Blood* 1997;89: 4591–4599.
47. Liesner R, Mackie I, Cookson J, et al. Prothrombotic changes in children with sickle cell disease: relationships to cerebrovascular disease and transfusion. *Br J Haematol* 1998;103: 1037–1044.
48. Ohene-Frempong K, Weiner SJ, Sleeper LA, et al. Cerebrovascular accidents in sickle cell disease: rates and risk factors. *Blood* 1998;91: 288–294.
49. Earley CJ, Kittner SJ, Feeser BR, et al. Stroke in children and sickle-cell disease: Baltimore-Washington Cooperative Young Stroke Study. *Neurology* 1998;51:169–176.
50. Dover GJ. A new look at neuropathology in sickle cell disease. *Ann Neurol* 1999;45:277–278.
51. Kinney TR, Sleeper LA, Wang WC, et al. Silent cerebral infarcts in sickle cell anemia: a risk factor analysis. The Cooperative Study of Sickle Cell Disease. *Pediatrics* 1999;103:640–645.
52. Pegelow CH, Adams RJ, McKie V, et al. Risk of recurrent stroke in patients with sickle cell disease treated with erythrocyte transfusions. *J Pediatr* 1995;126:896–899.
53. Steen RG, Xiong X, Mulhern RK, Langston JW, Wang WC. Subtle brain abnormalities in children with sickle cell disease. Relationship to blood hematocrit. *Ann Neurol* 1999;45:279–286.
54. DeBaun MR, Schatz J, Siegel MJ, et al. Cognitive screening examinations for silent cerebral infarcts in sickle cell disease. *Neurology* 1998; 50:1678–1682.
55. Cohen MJ, Branch WB, McKie VC, Adams RJ. Neuropsychological impairment in children with sickle cell anemia and cerebrovascular accidents. *Clin Pediatr* 1994;33:517–524.
56. Kandeel AY, Zimmerman RA, Ohene-Frempong K. Comparison of magnetic resonance angiography and conventional angiography in sickle cell disease: clinical significance and reliability. *Neuroradiology* 1996;38:409–416.
57. Seibert JJ, Glasier CM, Kirby RS, et al. Transcranial Doppler, MRA, and MRI as a screening examination for cerebrovascular disease in patients with sickle cell anemia: an 8-year study. *Pediatr Radiol* 1998;28:138–142.
58. Verlhac S, Bernaudin F, Tortrat D, et al. Detection of cerebrovascular disease in patients with sickle cell disease using transcranial Doppler sonography: correlation with MRI, MRA and conventional angiography. *Pediatr Radiol* 1995;25(Suppl 1):S14–S19.

59. Powars DR, Conti PS, Wong WY, et al. Cerebral vasculopathy in sickle cell anemia: diagnostic contribution of positron emission tomography. *Blood* 1999;93:71–79.
60. Seibert JJ, Miller SF, Kirby RS, et al. Cerebrovascular disease in symptomatic and asymptomatic patients with sickle cell anemia: screening with duplex transcranial Doppler US—correlation with MR imaging and MR angiography. *Radiology* 1993;189:457–466.
61. Adams RJ, McKie VC, Nichols FT, et al. The use of transcranial untrasonography to predict stroke in sickle cell disease. *N Engl J Med* 1992;326:605–610.
62. Adams RJ, McKie VC, Carl EM, et al. Long-term stroke risk in children with sickle cell disease screened with transcranial Doppler. *Ann Neurol* 1997;42:699–704.
63. Adams RJ, McKie VC, Hsu L, et al. Prevention of a first stroke by transfusions in children with sickle cell anemia and abnormal results on transcranial Doppler ultrasonography. *N Engl J Med* 1998;339:5–11.
64. Tam DA. Protein C and protein S activity in sickle cell disease and stroke. *J Child Neurol* 1997;12:19–21.
65. Houston PE, Rana S, Sekhsaria S, Perlin E, Kim KS, Castro OL. Homocysteine in sickle cell disease: relationship to stroke. *Am J Med* 1997; 103:192–196.
66. Weksler BB. Hematologic disorders and ischemic stroke. *Curr Opin Neurol* 1995;8:38–44.
67. Fisher M, Levine PH, Fullerton AL, et al. Marker proteins of platelet activation in patients with cerebrovascular disease. *Arch Neurol* 1982; 39:692–695.
68. Casto L, Camerlingo M, Finazzi G, Censori B, Barbui T, Mamoli A. Essential thrombocytemia and ischemic stroke: report of six cases. *Ital J Neurol Sci* 1994;15:359–362.
69. Arboix A, Besses C, Acin P, et al. Ischemic stroke as first manifestation of essential thrombocythemia. Report of six cases. *Stroke* 1995; 26:1463–1466.
70. Benassi G, Ricci P, Calbucci F, Cacciatore FM, D'Alessandro R. Slowly progressive ischemic stroke as first manifestation of essential thrombocythemia. *Stroke* 1989;20:1271–1272.
71. O'Malley T, Langhorne P, Elton RA, Stewart C. Platelet size in stroke patients. *Stroke* 1995; 26:995–999.
72. Chaturvedi S, Dzieczkowski J. Multiple hemostatic abnormalities in young adults with activated protein C resistance and cerebral ischemia. *J Neurol Sci* 1998;159:209–212.
73. Chaturvedi S, Dzieczkowski JS. Protein S deficiency, activated protein C resistance and sticky platelet syndrome in a young woman with bilateral strokes. *Cerebrovasc Dis* 1999;9:127–130.
74. Levine PH, Fisher M, Fullerton AL, Duffy CP, Hoogasian JJ. Human platelet factor 4: preparation from outdated platelet concentrates and application in cerebral vascular disease. *Am J Hematol* 1981;10:375–385.
75. Griesshammer M, Bangerter M, van Vliet HH, Michiels JJ. Aspirin in essential thrombocythemia: status quo and quo vadis. *Semin Thromb Hemost* 1997;23:371–377.
76. George JN, Gilcher RO, Smith JW, Chandler L, Duvall D, Ellis C. Thrombotic thrombocytopenic purpura-hemolytic uremic syndrome: diagnosis and management. *J Clin Apheresis* 1998; 13:120–125.
77. Sarode R, Gottschall JL, Aster RH, McFarland JG. Thrombotic thrombocytopenic purpura: early and late responders. *Am J Hematol* 1997; 54:102–107.
78. Ruggenenti P, Remuzzi G. Pathophysiology and management of thrombotic microangiopathies. *J Nephrol* 1998;11:300–310.
79. Eldor A. Thrombotic thrombocytopenic purpura: diagnosis, pathogenesis and modern therapy. *Baillieres Clin Haematol* 1998;11:475–495.
80. Porta C, Caporali R, Montecucco C. Thrombotic thrombocytopenic purpura and autoimmunity: a tale of shadows and suspects. *Haematologica* 1999;84:260–269.
81. Moake JL. Thrombotic thrombocytopenic purpura today. *Hospital Practice (Office Edition)* 1999;53–59.
82. Gordjani N, Sutor AH. Coagulation changes associated with the hemolytic uremic syndrome. *Semin Thromb Hemost* 1998;24:577–582.
83. Kelly PJ, McDonald CT, Neill GO, Thomas C, Niles J, Rordorf G. Middle cerebral artery main stem thrombosis in two siblings with familial thrombotic thrombocytopenic purpura. *Neurology* 1998;50:1157–1160.
84. Musio F, Bohen EM, Yuan CM, Welch PG. Review of thrombotic thrombocytopenic purpura in the setting of systemic lupus erythematosus. *Semin Arth Rheum* 1998;28:1–19.
85. Gordon LI, Kwaan HC. Cancer- and drug-associated thrombotic thrombocytopenic purpura and hemolytic uremic syndrome. *Semin Hematol* 1997;34:140–147.
86. Miller A, Ryan PF, Dowling JP. Vasculitis and thrombotic thrombocytopenic purpura in a patient with limited scleroderma. *J Rheumatol* 1997;24:598–600.
87. Nesher G, Hanna VE, Moore TL, Hersh M, Osborn TG. Thrombotic microangiographic hemolytic anemia in systemic lupus erythematosus. *Semin Arth Rheum* 1994;24:165–172.
88. Trent K, Neustater BR, Lottenberg R. Chronic relapsing thrombotic thrombocytopenic purpura and antiphospholipid antibodies: a report of two cases. *Am J Hematol* 1997;54:155–159.
89. Hess DC, Sethi K, Awad E. Thrombotic thrombocytopenic purpura in systemic lupus erythematosus and antiphospholipid antibodies: effective treatment with plasma exchange and immunosuppression. *J Rheumatol* 1992;19: 1474–1478.
90. Lawlor ER, Webb DW, Hill A, Wadsworth LD. Thrombotic thrombocytopenic purpura: a treatable cause of childhood encephalopathy. *J Pediatr* 1997;130:313–316.
91. Druschky A, Erbguth F, Strauss R, Helm G, Heckmann J, Neundorfer B. Central nervous system involvement in thrombotic thrombocytopenic purpura. *Eur Neurol* 1998;40:220–224.

92. Bakshi R, Shaikh ZA, Bates VE, Kinkel PR. Thrombotic thrombocytopenic purpura: brain CT and MRI findings in 12 patients. *Neurology* 1999;52:1285–1288.
93. Hirasawa H, Sugai T, Oda S, et al. Efficacy and limitation of apheresis therapy in critical care. *Therapeutic Apheresis* 1997;1:228–232.
94. Steinhubl SR, Tan WA, Foody JM, Topol EJ. Incidence and clinical course of thrombotic thrombocytopenic purpura due to ticlopidine following coronary stenting. EPISTENT Investigators. Evaluation of Platelet IIb/IIIa Inhibitor for Stenting. *JAMA* 1999;281:806–810.
95. Bennett CL, Weinberg PD, Rozenberg-Bendror K, Yarnold PR, Kwaan HC, Green D. Thrombotic thrombocytopenia purpura associated with ticlopidine. *Ann Intern Med* 1998; 128:541–544.
96. Kappers-Klunne MC, Boon DM, Hop WC, et al. Heparin-induced thrombocytopenia and thrombosis: a prospective analysis of the incidence in patients with heart and cerebrovascular diseases. *Br J Haematol* 1997;96:442–446.
97. Calaitges JG, Liem TK, Spadone D, Nichols WK, Silver D. The role of heparin-associated antiplatelet antibodies in the outcome of arterial reconstruction. *J Vasc Surg* 1999;29:779–785.
98. Becker PS, Miller VT. Heparin-induced thrombocytopenia. *Stroke* 1989;20:1449–1459.
99. Greinacher A, Potzsch B, Amiral J, Dummel V, Eichner A, Mueller-Eckhardt C. Heparin-associated thrombocytopenia: isolation of the antibody and characterization of a multimolecular PF4-heparin complex as the major antigen. *Thromb Haemost* 1994;71:247–251.
100. Horne MK, Alkins BR. Platelet binding of IgG from patients with heparin-induced thrombocytopenia. *J Lab Clin Med* 1996;127:435–442.
101. Ramirez-Lassepas M, Cipolle RJ, Rodvold KA, et al. Heparin induced thrombocytopenia in patients with cerebrovascular ischemic disease. *Neurology* 1986;34:736–740.
102. Gupta AK, Kovacs MJ, Sauder DN. Heparin-induced thrombocytopenia. *Ann Pharmacother* 1998;32:55–59.
103. Boon DM, Michiels JJ, Tanghe HL, Kappers-Klunne MC. Heparin-induced thrombocytopenia with multiple cerebral infarctions simulating thrombotic thrombocytopenic purpura. A case report. *Angiology* 1996;47:407–411.
104. Pohl C, Klockgether T, Greinacher A, Hanfland P, Harbrecht U. Neurological complications in heparin-induced thrombocytopenia. *Lancet* 1999;353:1678–1679.
105. Warkentin TE, Elavathil LJ, Hayward CP, Johnston MA, Russett JI, Kelton JG. The pathogenesis of venous limb gangrene associated with heparin-induced thrombocytopenia. *Ann Intern Med* 1997;127:804–812.
106. Warkentin TE, Levine MN, Hirsh J, et al. Heparin-induced thrombocytopenia in patients treated with low-molecular-weight heparin or unfractionated heparin. *N Engl J Med* 1995; 332:1330–1335.
107. Atkinson JL, Sundt TMJ, Kazmier FJ, Bowie EJ, Whisnant JP. Heparin-induced thrombocytopenia and thrombosis in ischemic stroke. *Mayo Clin Proc* 1988;63:353–361.
108. Magnani HN. Heparin-induced thrombocytopenia (HIT): an overview of 230 patients treated with orgaran (Org 10172). *Thromb Haemost* 1993;70:554–561.
109. Lewis BE, Walenga JM, Wallis DE. Anticoagulation with Novastan (argatroban) in patients with heparin-induced thrombocytopenia and heparin-induced thrombocytopenia and thrombosis syndrome. *Semin Thromb Hemost* 1997;23:197–202.
110. Kanagasabay RR, Unsworth-White MJ, Robinson G, et al. Cardiopulmonary bypass with danaparoid sodium and ancrod in heparin-induced thrombocytopenia. *Ann Thorac Surg* 1998;66:567–569.
111. Galante A, Silvestrini M, Stanzione P, et al. Leucocyte aggregation in acute cerebrovascular disease. *Acta Neurol Scand* 1992;86:446–449.
112. Hagberg IA, Roald HE, Lyberg T. Adhesion of leukocytes to growing arterial thrombi. *Thromb Haemost* 1998;80:852–858.
113. Hagner G, Iglesias-Rozas JR, Kolmel HW, Gerhartz H. Hemorrhagic infarction of the basal ganglia. An unusual complication of acute leukemia. *Oncology* 1983;40:387–391.
114. Alberts SR, Bretscher M, Wiltsie JC, O'Neill BP, Mokri B, Witzig TE. Thrombosis related to the use of L-asparaginase in adults with acute lymphoblastic leukemia: a need to consider coagulation monitoring and clotting factor replacement. *Leukemia & Lymphoma* 1999;32: 489–496.
115. Cogan E, Schandene L, Crusiaux A, Cochaux P, Velu T, Goldman M. Brief report: clonal proliferation of type 2 helper T cells in a man with the hypereosinophilic syndrome. *N Engl J Med* 1994;330:535–538.
116. Rothenberg ME. Eosinophilia. *N Engl J Med* 1998;338:1592–1600.
117. Aiach M, Gandrille S, Emmerich J. A review of mutations causing deficiencies of antithrombin, protein C, and protein S. *Thromb Haemost* 1995;74:81–89.
118. Kato H, Shirahama M, Ohmori K, Sunaga T. Cerebral infarction in a young adult associated with protein C deficiency. A case report. *Angiology* 1995;46:169–173.
119. Ferrera PC, Curran CB, Swanson H. Etiology of pediatric ischemic stroke. *Am J Emerg Med* 1997;15:671–679.
120. van Kuijck MA, Rotteveel JJ, van Oostrom CG, Novakova I. Neurological complications in children with protein C deficiency. *Neuropediatrics* 1994;25:16–19.
121. Camerlingo M, Finazzi G, Casto L, Laffranch C, Barbui T, Mamoli A. Inherited protein C deficiency and nonhemorrhagic arterial stroke in young adults. *Neurology* 1991;41:1371–1373.
122. Martinez HR, Rangel-Guerra RA, Marfil LJ. Ischemic stroke due to deficiency of coagulation inhibitors. Report of 10 young adults. *Stroke* 1993;24:19–25.
123. Kiechl S, Muigg A, Santer P, et al. Poor response to activated protein C as a prominent

risk predictor of advanced atherosclerosis and arterial disease. *Circulation* 1999;99:614–619.

124. Koller H, Stoll G, Sitzer M, Burk M, Schottler B, Freund HJ. Deficiency of both protein C and protein S in a family with ischemic strokes in young adults. *Neurology* 1994;44:1238–1240.
125. Vaezi MF, Rustagi PK, Elson CO. Transient protein S deficiency associated with cerebral venous thrombosis in active ulcerative colitis. *Am J Gastroenterol* 1995;90:313–315.
126. Nachman RL, Silverstein R. Hypercoagulable states. *Ann Intern Med* 1993;119:819–827.
127. Graham JA, Daly HM, Carson PJ. Antithrombin III deficiency and cerebrovascular accidents in young adults. *J Clin Pathol* 1992;45:921–922.
128. Mohanty S, Saxena R, Behari M. Risk factors for thrombosis in nonembolic cerebrovascular disease. *Am J Hematol* 1999;60:239–241.
129. Gemmati D, Serino ML, Moratelli S, Mari R, Ballerini G, Scapoli GL. Coexistence of antithrombin deficiency, factor V Leiden and hyperhomocysteinemia in a thrombotic family. *Blood Coagulation & Fibrinolysis* 1998;9:173–176.
130. Arai H, Miyakawa T, Ozaki K, Sakuragawa N. Changes of the levels of antithrombin III in patients with cerebrovascular diseases. *Thromb Res* 1983;31:197–202.
131. Press RD, Liu XY, Beamer N, Coull BM. Ischemic stroke in the elderly. Role of the common factor V mutation causing resistance to activated protein C. *Stroke* 1996;27:44–48.
132. Sanchez J, Roman J, de la Torre MJ, Velasco F, Torres A. Low prevalence of the factor V Leiden among patients with ischemic stroke. *Haemostasis* 1997;27:9–15.
133. Simioni P, de Ronde H, Prandoni P, Saladini M, Bertina RM, Girolami. Ischemic stroke in young patients with activated protein C resistance. A report of three cases belonging to three different kindreds. *Stroke* 1995;26:885–890.
134. De Lucia D, Nina P, Papa ML, et al. Activated protein C resistance due to a factor V mutation associated with familial ischemic stroke. *J Neurosurg Sci* 1997;41:373–378.
135. Giordano P, Sabato V, Schettini F, De Mattia D, Iolascon A. Resistance to activated protein C as a risk factor of stroke in a thalassemic patient. *Haematologica* 1997;82:698–700.
136. Girolami A, Simioni P, Scarano L, Girolami B, Marchiori A. Hemorrhagic and thrombotic disorders due to factor V deficiencies and abnormalities: an updated classification. *Blood Reviews* 1998;12:45–51.
137. Rosendaal FR, Koster T, Vandenbroucke JP, Reitsma PH. High risk of thrombosis in patients homozygous for factor V Leiden (activated protein C resistance). *Blood* 1995;85:1504–1508.
138. van der Bom JG, Bots ML, Haverkate F, et al. Reduced response to activated protein C is associated with increased risk for cerebrovascular disease. *Ann Intern Med* 1996;125:265–269.
139. Fisher M, Fernandez JA, Ameriso SF, et al. Activated protein C resistance in ischemic stroke not due to factor V arginine506 → glutamine mutation. *Stroke* 1996;27:1163–1166.
140. Aznar J, Villa P, Espana F, Estelles A, Grancha S, Falco C. Activated protein C resistance phenotype in patients with antiphospholipid antibodies. *J Lab Clin Med* 1997;130:202–208.
141. D'Amico D, Moschiano F, Leone M, et al. Genetic abnormalities of the protein C system: shared risk factors in young adults with migraine with aura and with ischemic stroke? *Cephalalgia* 1998;18:618–621.
142. James RH, O'Dell MW. Resistance to activated protein C as an etiology for stroke in a young adult: a case report. *Arch Phys Med Rehabil* 1999;80:343–345.
143. Price DT, Ridker PM. Factor V Leiden mutation and the risks for thromboembolic disease: a clinical perspective. *Ann Intern Med* 1997;127:895–903.
144. Eskandari MK, Bontempo FA, Hassett AC, Faruki H, Makaroun MS. Arterial thromboembolic events in patients with the factor V Leiden mutation. *Am J Surg* 1998;176:122–125.
145. Ludemann P, Nabavi DG, Junker R, et al. Factor V Leiden mutation is a risk factor for cerebral venous thrombosis: a case-control study of 55 patients. *Stroke* 1998;29:2507–2510.
146. Ridker PM, Hennekens CH, Lindpaintner K, Stampfer MJ, Eisenberg PR, Miletich JP. Mutation in the gene coding for coagulation factor V and the risk of myocardial infarction, stroke, and venous thrombosis in apparently healthy men. *N Engl J Med* 1995;332:912–917.
147. Marinella MA, Greene K. Bilateral thalamic infarction in a patient with factor V leiden mutation. *Mayo Clin Proc* 999;74:795–797.
148. Ridker PM, Miletich JP, Buring JE, et al. Factor V Leiden mutation as a risk factor for recurrent pregnancy loss. *Ann Intern Med* 1998;128:1000–1003.
149. Espana F, Villa P, Mira Y, et al. Factor V Leiden and antibodies against phospholipids and protein S in a young woman with recurrent thromboses and abortion. *Haematologica* 1999;84:80–84.
150. Longstreth WT, Jr., Rosendaal FR, Siscovick DS, et al. Risk of stroke in young women and two prothrombotic mutations: factor V Leiden and prothrombin gene variant (G20210A). *Stroke* 1998;29:577–580.
151. Provenzale JM, Barboriak DP, Davey IC, Ortel TL. Cerebrovascular disease risk factors: neuroradiologic findings in patients with activated protein C resistance. *Radiology* 1998;207:85–89.
152. Gruppo RA, DeGrauw TJ, Palasis S, Kalinyak KA, Bofinger MK. Strokes, cutis marmorata telangiectatica congenita, and factor V Leiden. *Ped Neurol* 1998;18:342–345.
153. Martinelli I, Sacchi E, Landi G, Taioli E, Duca F, Mannucci PM. High risk of cerebral-vein thrombosis in carriers of a prothrombin-gene mutation and in users of oral contraceptives. *N Engl J Med* 1998;338:1793–1797.
154. Lalouschek W, Aull S, Serles W, et al. C677T MTHFR mutation and factor V Leiden mutation in patients with TIA/minor stroke: a case-control study. *Thromb Res* 1999;93:61–69.

155. Baglin C, Brown K, Luddington R, Baglin T. Risk of recurrent venous thromboembolism in patients with the factor V Leiden (FVR506Q) mutation: effect of warfarin and prediction by precipitating factors. East Anglian Thrombophilia Study Group. *Br J Haematol* 1998;100:764–768.
156. Franco RF, Trip MD, ten Cate H, et al. The 20210 G → A mutation in the 3'-untranslated region of the prothrombin gene and the risk for arterial thrombotic disease. *Br J Haematol* 1999; 104:50–54.
157. Vicente V, Gonzalez-Conejero R, Rivera J, Corral J. The prothrombin gene variant 20210A in venous and arterial thromboembolism. *Haematologica* 1999;84:356–362.
158. Eikelboom JW, Ivey L, Ivey J, Baker RI. Familial thrombophilia and the prothrombin 20210A mutation: association with increased thrombin generation and unusual thrombosis. *Blood Coagulation & Fibrinolysis* 1999;10:1–5.
159. De Stefano V, Martinelli I, Mannucci PM, et al. The risk of recurrent deep venous thrombosis among heterozygous carriers of both factor V leiden and the G20210A prothrombin mutation. *N Engl J Med* 1999;341:801–806.
160. Ferraresi P, Marchetti G, Legnani C, et al. The heterozygous 20210 G/A prothrombin genotype is associated with early venous thrombosis in inherited thrombophilias and is not increased in frequency in artery disease. *Arterioscler Thromb Vasc Biol* 1997;17:2418–2422.
161. Ridker PM, Hennekens CH, Miletich JP. G20210A mutation in prothrombin gene and risk of myocardial infarction, stroke, and venous thrombosis in a large cohort of US men. *Circulation* 1999;99:999–1004.
162. Favier R, Neonato MG, Maillet F, Feingold J, Cayre Y, Girot R. Incidence of G20210A mutation in severe vaso-occlusive events complicating sickle cell anemia. *Blood Coagulation & Fibrinolysis* 1999;10:111–112.
163. Arkel YS, Ku DH, Gibson D, Lam X. Ischemic stroke in a young patient with protein C deficiency and prothrombin gene mutation G20210A. *Blood Coagulation & Fibrinolysis* 1998; 9:757–760.
164. Gaustadnes M, Rudiger N, Ingerslev J. The 20210 A allele of the prothrombin gene is not a risk factor for juvenile stroke in the Danish population [letter; comment]. *Blood Coagulation & Fibrinolysis* 1998;9:663–664.
165. Howard TE, Marusa M, Channell C, Duncan A. A patient homozygous for a mutation in the prothrombin gene 3′-untranslated region associated with massive thrombosis. *Blood Coagulation & Fibrinolysis* 1997;8:316–319.
166. Furlan AJ, Lucas FV, Craciun R, Wohl RC. Stroke in a young adult with familial plasminogen disorder. *Stroke* 1991;22:1598–1602.
167. Demarmels BF, Sulzer I, Stucki B, Wuillemin WA, Furlan M, Lammle B. Is plasminogen deficiency a thrombotic risk factor? A study on 23 thrombophilic patients and their family members. *Thromb Haemost* 1998;80:167–170.
168. Kienast J. Coagulation and fibrinolysis. *Cerebrovasc Dis* 1995;5:89–92.
169. Fisher M, Meiselman HJ. Hemorheological factors in cerebral ischemia. *Stroke* 1991;22: 1164–1169.
170. Ernst E, Resch KL. Fibrinogen as a cardiovascular risk factor: a meta-analysis and review of the literature. *Ann Intern Med* 1993;118:956–963.
171. Eby CS. A review of the hypercoagulable state. *Hematol Oncol Clin North Am* 1993;7:1121–1142.
172. Walzl M, Schied G, Walzl B. Effects of ameliorated haemorheology on clinical symptoms in cerebrovascular disease. *Atherosclerosis* 1998;139: 385–389.
173. Meade TW. Fibrinogen and cardiovascular disease. *J Clin Pathol* 1997;50:13–15.
174. Kowal P. Quantitative study of fibrinogen molecules' contribution to the inter-red cells connections in selected clinical groups of stroke patients. *Clin Hemorheol Microcirculation* 1998;18:37–41.
175. Resch KL, Ernst E, Matrai A, Paulsen HF. Fibrinogen and viscosity as risk factors for subsequent cardiovascular events in stroke survivors. *Ann Intern Med* 1992;117:371–375.
176. Qizilbash N, Jones L, Warlow C, Mann J. Fibrinogen and lipid concentrations as risk factors for transient ischaemic attacks and minor ischaemic strokes. *BMJ* 1991;303:605–609.
177. Ernst E. Fibrinogen as a cardiovascular risk factor–interrelationship with infections and inflammation. *Eur Heart J* 1993;14 (Suppl K):82–87.
178. Smith FB, Rumley A, Lee AJ, Leng GC, Fowkes FG, Lowe GD. Haemostatic factors and prediction of ischaemic heart disease and stroke in claudicants. *Br J Haematol* 1998;100:758–763.
179. Di Perri T, Guerrini M, Pasini FL, et al. Hemorheological factors in the pathophysiology of acute and chronic cerebrovascular disease. *Cephalalgia* 1985;5 (Suppl 2):71–77.
180. Elwan O, al-Ashmawy S, el-Karaksy S, Hassan AA. Hemorheology, stroke and the elderly. *J Neurol Sci* 1991;101:157–162.
181. Tsuda Y, Satoh K, Kitadai M, Takahashi T. Hemorheologic profiles of plasma fibrinogen and blood viscosity from silent to acute and chronic cerebral infarctions. *J Neurol Sci* 1997; 147:49–54.
182. Barker JE, Wandersee NJ. Thrombosis in heritable hemolytic disorders. *Curr Opin Hematol* 1999;6:71–75.
183. Borgna PC, Carnelli V, Caruso V, et al. Thromboembolic events in beta thalassemia major: an Italian multicenter study. *Acta Haematologica* 1998;99:76–79.
184. Young G, Driscoll MC. Coagulation abnormalities in the carbohydrate-deficient glycoprotein syndrome: case report and review of the literature. *Am J Hematol* 1999;60:66–69.
185. Triplett DA. Many faces of lupus anticoagulants. *Lupus* 1998;7 (Suppl) 2:S18–S22
186. Metz LM, Edworthy S, Mydlarski R, Fritzler MJ. The frequency of phospholipid antibodies in an unselected stroke population. *Can J Neurol Sci* 1998;25:64–69.
187. Muir KW, Squire IB, Alwan W, Lees KR. Anticardiolipin antibodies in an unselected stroke population. *Lancet* 1994;344:452–456.

188. Feldmann E, Levine SR. Cerebrovascular disease with antiphospholipid antibodies: immune mechanisms, significance, and therapeutic options. *Ann Neurol* 1995;37(Suppl) 1:S114–S130.
189. Arnout J. The pathogenesis of the antiphospholipid syndrome: a hypothesis based on parallelisms with heparin-induced thrombocytopenia. *Thromb Haemost* 1996;75:536–541.
190. The Antiphospholipid Antibodies and Stroke Study Group (APASS). Anticardiolipin antibodies and the risk of recurrent thrombo-occlusive events and death. *Neurology* 1997;48:91–94.
191. Tanne D, Triplett DA, Levine SR. Antiphospholipid-protein antibodies and ischemic stroke: not just cardiolipin any more. *Stroke* 1998;29:1755–1758.
192. Gomez-Pacheco L, Villa AR, Drenkard C, Cabiedes J, Cabral AR, Alarcon-Segovia D. Serum anti-beta2-glycoprotein-I and anticardiolipin antibodies during thrombosis in systemic lupus erythematosus patients. *Am J Med* 1999; 106:417–423.
193. Inanc M, Donohoe S, Ravirajan CT, et al. Anti-beta2-glycoprotein I, anti-prothrombin and anticardiolipin antibodies in a longitudinal study of patients with systemic lupus erythematosus and the antiphospholipid syndrome. *Br J Rheumatol* 1998;37:1089–1094.
194. McCrae KR, DeMichele A, Samuels P, et al. Detection of endothelial cell-reactive immunoglobulin in patients with anti-phospholipid antibodies. *Br J Haematol* 1991; 79:595–605.
195. Coull BM, Goodnight SH. Antiphospholipid antibodies, prethrombotic states, and stroke. *Stroke* 1990;21:1370–1374.
196. Baca V, Garcia-Ramirez R, Ramirez-Lacayo M, Marquez-Enriquez L, Martinez I, Lavalle C. Cerebral infarction and antiphospholipid syndrome in children. *J Rheumatol* 1996;23: 1428–1431.
197. Schoning M, Klein R, Krageloh-Mann I, et al. Antiphospholipid antibodies in cerebrovascular ischemia and stroke in childhood. *Neuropediatrics* 1994;25:8–14.
198. Levine SR, Welch KM. Antiphospholipid antibodies. *Ann Neurol* 1989;26:386–389.
199. Nagaraja D, Christopher R, Manjari T. Anticardiolipin antibodies in ischemic stroke in the young: Indian experience. *J Neurol Sci* 1997;150:137–142.
200. Greaves M. Antiphospholipid antibodies and thrombosis. *Lancet* 1999;353:1348–1353.
201. Tuhrim S, Rand JH, Weinberger J, Horowitz DR, Goldman ME, Godbold JH. Elevated anticardiolipin antibody titer is a stroke risk factor in a multiethnic population independent of isotype or degree of positivity. *Stroke* 1999;30: 1561–1565.
202. Tohgi H, Takahashi H, Kashiwaya M, Watanabe K, Hayama K. The anticardiolipin antibody in elderly stroke patients: its effects on stroke types, recurrence, and the coagulation-fibrinolysis system. *Acta Neurol Scand* 1994;90:86–90.
203. Tanne D, D'Olhaberriague L, Schultz LR, Salowich-Palm L, Sawaya L, Levine SR. Anticardiolipin antibodies and their associations with cerebrovascular risk factors. *Neurology* 1999;52:1368–1373.
204. D'Olhaberriague L, Levine SR, Salowich-Palm L, et al. Specificity, isotype, and titer distribution of anticardiolipin antibodies in CNS diseases. *Neurology* 1998;51:1376–1380.
205. Camerlingo M, Casto L, Censori B, et al. Anticardiolipin antibodies in acute non-hemorrhagic stroke seen within six hours after onset. *Acta Neurol Scand* 1995;92:69–71.
206. Finazzi G, Brancaccio V, Moia M, et al. Natural history and risk factors for thrombosis in 360 patients with antiphospholipid antibodies: a four-year prospective study from the Italian Registry. *Am J Med* 1996;100:530–536.
207. de Groot PG, Horbach DA, Simmelink MJ, van Oort E, Derksen RH. Anti-prothrombin antibodies and their relation with thrombosis and lupus anticoagulant. *Lupus* 1998;7(Suppl 2): S32–S36.
208. Kalashnikova LA, Korczyn AD, Shavit S, Rebrova O, Reshetnyak T, Chapman J. Antibodies to prothrombin in patients with Sneddon's syndrome. *Neurology* 1999;53: 223–225.
209. Toschi V, Motta A, Castelli C, Paracchini ML, Zerbi D, Gibelli A. High prevalence of antiphosphatidylinositol antibodies in young patients with cerebral ischemia of undetermined cause. *Stroke* 1998;29:1759–1764.
210. Verro P, Levine SR, Tietjen GE. Cerebrovascular ischemic events with high positive anticardiolipin antibodies. *Stroke* 1998;29:2245–2253.
211. Vaarala O, Manttari M, Manninen V, et al. Anticardiolipin antibodies and risk of myocardial infarction in a prospective cohort of middle-aged men. *Circulation* 1995;91:23–27.
212. Christopher R, Nagaraja D, Dixit NS, Narayanan CP. Anticardiolipin antibodies: a study in cerebral venous thrombosis. *Acta Neurol Scand* 1999;99:121–124.
213. Brey RL, Escalante A. Neurological manifestations of antiphospholipid antibody syndrome. *Lupus* 1998;7(Suppl 2):S67–S74.
214. The Antiphospholipid Antibodies in Stroke Study Group. Clinical and laboratory findings in patients with antiphospholipid antibodies and cerebral ischemia. *Stroke* 1990;21: 1268–1273.
215. Khamashta MA, Cuadrado MJ, Mujic F, Taub NA, Hunt BJ, Hughes GR. The management of thrombosis in the antiphospholipid-antibody syndrome. *N Engl J Med* 1995;332:993–997.
216. Asherson RA, Khamashta MA, Gil A, et al. Cerebrovascular disease and antiphospholipid antibodies in systemic lupus erythematosus, lupus-like disease, and the primary antiphospholipid syndrome. *Am J Med* 1989; 86:391–399.
217. Trimble M, Bell DA, Brien W, et al. The antiphospholipid syndrome: prevalence among patients with stroke and transient ischemic attacks. *Am J Med* 1990;88:593–597.
218. Kitagawa Y, Gotoh F, Koto A, Okayasu H. Stroke in systemic lupus erythematosus. *Stroke* 1990; 21:1533–1539.

219. Lie JT, Kobayashi S, Tokano Y, Hashimoto H. Systemic and cerebral vasculitis coexisting with disseminated coagulopathy in systemic lupus erythematosus associated with antiphospholipid syndrome. *J Rheumatol* 1995;22:2173–2176.
220. Ellison D, Gatter K, Heryet A, Esiri M. Intramural platelet deposition in cerebral vasculopathy of systemic lupus erythematosus. *J Clin Pathol* 1993;46:37–40.
221. Galve E, Ordi J, Barquinero J, Evangelista A, Vilardell M, Soler-Soler J. Valvular heart disease in the primary antiphospholipid syndrome. *Ann Intern Med* 1992;116:293–298.
222. Sohngen D, Wehmeier A, Specker C, Schneider W. Antiphospholipid antibodies in systemic lupus erythematosus and Sneddon's syndrome. *Semin Thromb Hemost* 1994;20:55–63.
223. Tourbah A, Piette JC, Iba-Zizen MT, Lyon-Caen O, Godeau P, Frances C. The natural course of cerebral lesions in Sneddon syndrome. *Arch Neurol* 1997;54:53–60.
224. Weissenborn K, Ruckert N, Ehrenheim C, Schellong S, Goetz C, Lubach. Neuropsychological deficits in patients with Sneddon's syndrome. *J Neurol* 1996;243:357–363.
225. Antoine JC, Michel D, Garnier P, Genin C. Rheumatic heart disease and Sneddon's syndrome. *Stroke* 1994;25:689–691.
226. Asherson RA, Cervera R. 'Primary,' 'secondary' and other variants of the antiphospholipid syndrome. *Lupus* 1994;3:293–298.
227. Pettee AD, Wasserman BA, Adams NL, et al. Familial Sneddon's syndrome: clinical, hematologic, and radiographic findings in two brothers. *Neurology* 1994;44:399–405.
228. Ford PM, Brunet D, Lillicrap DP, Ford SE. Premature stroke in a family with lupus anticoagulant and antiphospholipid antibodies. *Stroke* 1990;21:66–71.
229. Brey RL, Hart RG, Sherman DG, Tegeler CH. Antiphospholipid antibodies and cerebral ischemia in young people. *Neurology* 1990; 40:1190–1196.
230. Hinse P, Schulz A, Haag F, Carvajal-Lizano M, Thie A. Anticardiolipin antibodies in oculocerebral ishaemia and migraine: prevalence and prognostic value. *Cerebrovasc Dis* 1993;3:168–173.
231. Amoroso A, Del Porto F, Garzia P, Mariotti A, Addessi MA, Afeltra A. Primary antiphospholipid syndrome and cerebral atrophy: a rare association?. *Am J Med Sci* 1999;317:425–428.
232. Akiguchi I, Tomimoto H, Kinoshita M, et al. Effects of antithrombin on Binswanger's disease with antiphospholipid antibody syndrome. *Neurology* 1999;52:398–401.
233. Silvestrini M, Cupini LM, Matteis M, De Simone R, Bernardi G. Migraine in patients with stroke and antiphospholipid antibodies. *Headache* 1993;33:421–426.
234. Joseph JE, Harrison P, Mackie IJ, Machin SJ. Platelet activation markers and the primary antiphospholipid syndrome (PAPS). *Lupus* 1998;7 (Suppl 2):S48–S51.
235. Exner T, Triplett DA, Taberner D, Machin SJ. Guidelines for testing and revised criteria for lupus anticoagulants. SSC Subcommittee for the Standardization of Lupus Anticoagulants. *Thromb Haemost* 1991;65:320–322.
236. Sitzer M, Sohngen D, Siebler M, et al. Cerebral microembolism in patients with Sneddon's syndrome. *Arch Neurol* 1995;52:271–275.
237. Postiglione A, De Chiara S, Soricelli A, et al. Alterations of cerebral blood flow and antiphospholipid antibodies in patients with systemic lupus erythematosus. *Internat J Clin Lab Res* 1998;28:34–38.
238. Provenzale JM, Barboriak DP, Allen NB, Ortel TL. Antiphospholipid antibodies: findings at arteriography. *Am J Neuroradiol* 1998;19:611–616.
239. Stockhammer G, Felber SR, Zelger B, et al. Sneddon's syndrome: diagnosis by skin biopsy and MRI in 17 patients. *Stroke* 1993;24:685–690.
240. Takano K, Iino K, Ibayashi S, Tagawa K, Sadoshima S, Fujishima M. Hypercoagulable state under low-intensity warfarin anticoagulation assessed with hemostatic markers in cardiac disorders. *Am J Cardiol* 1994;74:935–939.
241. Gelwix TJ, Beeson MS. Warfarin-induced skin necrosis. *Am J Emerg Med* 1998;16:541–543.
242. Sallah S, Thomas DP, Roberts HR. Warfarin and heparin-induced skin necrosis and the purple toe syndrome: infrequent complications of anticoagulant treatment. *Thromb Haemost* 1997; 78:785–790.
243. Sallah S, Abdallah JM, Gagnon GA. Recurrent warfarin-induced skin necrosis in kindreds with protein S deficiency. *Haemostasis* 1998;28:25–30.
244. Essex DW, Wynn SS, Jin DK. Late-onset warfarin-induced skin necrosis: case report and review of the literature. *Am J Hematol* 1998;57:233–237.
245. Yang Y, Algazy KM. Warfarin-induced skin necrosis in a patient with a mutation of the prothrombin gene [letter]. *N Engl J Med* 1999; 340:735.
246. Wynn SS, Jin DK, Essex DW. Warfarin-induced skin necrosis occurring four days after discontinuation of warfarin. *Haemostasis* 1997;27: 246–250.
247. Krahn MJ, Pettigrew NM, Cuddy TE. Unusual side effects due to warfarin. *Can J Cardiol* 1998;14:90–93.
248. Hyman BT, Landas SK, Ashman RF, Schelper RL, Robinson RA. Warfarin-related purple toes syndrome and cholesterol microembolization. *Am J Med* 1987;82:1233–1237.
249. Schwartzman RJ, Hill JB. Neurologic complications of disseminated intravascular coagulation. *Neurology* 1982;32:791–797.
250. Biller J, Challa VR, Toole JF, Howard VJ. Nonbacterial thrombotic endocarditis. *Arch Neurol* 1982;39:95–98.
251. Kooiker JC, MacLean JM, Sumi SM. Cerebral embolism, marantic endocarditis, and cancer. *Arch Neurol* 1976;33:260–264.
252. Blanchard DG, Ross RS, Dittrich HC. Nonbacterial thrombotic endocarditis. Assessment by transesophageal echocardiography. *Chest* 1992; 102:954–956.
253. Salomaa V, Stinson V, Kark JD, Folsom AR, Davis CE, Wu KK. Association of fibrinolytic parameters with early atherosclerosis. The ARIC

Study. Atherosclerosis Risk in Communities Study. *Circulation* 1995;91:284–290.
254. Macko RF, Kittner SJ, Epstein A, et al. Elevated tissue plasminogen activator antigen and stroke risk: The Stroke Prevention in Young Women Study. *Stroke* 1999;30:7–11.
255. Lindgren A, Lindoff C, Norrving B, Astedt B, Johansson BB. Tissue plasminogen activator and plasminogen activator inhibitor-1 in stroke patients. *Stroke* 1996;27:1066–1071.
256. Quattrone A, Colucci M, Donati MB, et al. Stroke in two young siblings with congenital dysfibrinogenemia. *Ital J Neurolog Sci* 1983;4:229–232.
257. Landi G, D'Angelo A, Boccardi E, et al. Hypercoagulability in acute stroke: prognostic significance. *Neurology* 1987;37:1667–1671.
258. Feinberg WM, Cornell ES, Nightingale SD, et al. Relationship between prothrombin activation fragment F1.2 and international normalized ratio in patients with atrial fibrillation. Stroke Prevention in Atrial Fibrillation Investigators. *Stroke* 1997;28:1101–1106.
259. Qizilbash N, Duffy S, Prentice CR, Boothby M, Warlow C. Von Willebrand factor and risk of ischemic stroke. *Neurology* 1997;49:1552–1556.
260. Abramsky O, Slavin S. Neurologic manifestations in patients with mixed cryoglobulinemia. *Neurology* 1974;24:245–249.
261. Ballem P. Acquired thrombophilia in pregnancy. *Semin Thromb Hemost* 1998;24(Suppl 1):41–47.
262. Harris GM, Stendt CL, Vollenhoven BJ, Gan TE, Tipping PG. Decreased plasma tissue factor pathway inhibitor in women taking combined oral contraceptives. *Am J Hematol* 1999;60:175–180.
263. Chaturvedi S, Ansell J, Recht L. Should cerebral ischemic events in cancer patients be considered a manifestation of hypercoagulability? *Stroke* 1994;25:1215–1218.
264. Collins RC, Al-Mondhiry H, Chernik NL, Posner JB. Neurologic manifestations of intravascular coagulation in patients with cancer. A clinicopathologic analysis of 12 cases. *Neurology* 1975;25:795–806.
265. Graus F, Rogers LR, Posner JB. Cerebrovascular complications in patients with cancer. *Medicine* 1985;64:16–35.
266. Packer RJ, Rorke LB, Lange BJ, Siegel KR, Evans AE. Cerebrovascular accidents in children with cancer. *Pediatrics* 1985;76:194–201.
267. Rogers LR. Cerebrovascular complications in cancer patients. *Neurol Clin* 1991;9:889–899.
268. Oleksowicz L, Bhagwati N, DeLeon-Fernandez M. Deficient activity of von Willebrand's factor-cleaving protease in patients with disseminated malignancies. *Cancer Res* 1999;59:2244–2250.
269. Frenkel EP, Bick R. Issues of thrombosis and hemorrhagic events in patients with cancer. *In Vivo* 1998;12:625–628.
270. Kakkar AK, Williamson RC. Thromboprophylaxis in the cancer patient. *Haemostasis* 1998;28(Suppl 3):61–65.
271. Grotta J. Cerebrovascular disease in young patients. *Thromb Haemost* 1997;78:13–23.
272. Amico L, Caplan LR, Thomas C. Cerebrovascular complications of mucinous cancers. *Neurology* 1989;39:522–526.
273. Reagan TJ, Okazaki H. The thrombotic syndrome associated with carcinoma. A clinical and neuropathologic study. *Arch Neurol* 1974;31: 390–395.
274. Edoute Y, Haim N, Rinkevich D, Brenner B, Reisner SA. Cardiac valvular vegetations in cancer patients: a prospective echocardiographic study of 200 patients. *Am J Med* 1997;102:252–258.
275. Schwartz JD, Simantov R. Thrombosis and malignancy: pathogenesis and prevention. *In Vivo* 1998;12:619–624.
276. Edwards RL, Silver J, Rickles FR. Human tumor procoagulants: registry of the Subcommittee on Haemostasis and Malignancy of the Scientific and Standardization Committee, International Society on Thrombosis and Haemostasis. *Thromb Haemost* 1993;69:205–213.
277. Seitz R, Heidtmann HH, Wolf M, Immel A, Egbring R. Prognostic impact of an activation of coagulation in lung cancer. *Ann Oncol* 1997;8: 781–784.
278. Meijer K, Smid WM, Geerards S, van der Meer J. Hyperfibrinogenolysis in disseminated adenocarcinoma. *Blood Coagulation & Fibrinolysis* 1998;9:279–283.
279. Falanga A. Mechanisms of hypercoagulation in malignancy and during chemotherapy. *Haemostasis* 1998;28(Suppl 3):50–60.
280. Doll DC, Ringenberg QS, Yarbro JW. Vascular toxicity associated with antineoplastic agents. *J Clin Oncol* 1986;4:1405–1417.
281. Priest JR, Ramsay NK, Latchaw RE, et al. Thrombotic and hemorrhagic strokes complicating early therapy for childhood acute lymphoblastic leukemia. *Cancer* 1980;46:1548–1554.
282. Feinberg WM, Swenson MR. Cerebrovascular complications of L-asparaginase therapy. *Neurology* 1988;38:127–133.
283. Kelly MA, Gorelick PB, Mirza D. The role of drugs in the etiology of stroke. *Clin Neuropharmacol* 1992;15:249–275.
284. Kucuk O, Kwaan HC, Gunnar W, Vazquez RM. Thromboembolic complications associated with L-asparaginase therapy. Etiologic role of low antithrombin III and plasminogen levels and therapeutic correction by fresh frozen plasma. *Cancer* 1985;55:702–706.
285. Doll DC, List AF, Greco FA, Hainsworth JD, Hande KR, Johnson DH. Acute vascular ischemic events after cisplatin-based combination chemotherapy for germ-cell tumors of the testis. *Ann Intern Med* 1986;105:48–51.
286. El Amrani M, Heinzlef O, Debroucker T, Roullet E, Bousser MG, Amarenco P. Brain infarction following 5-fluorouracil and cisplatin therapy. *Neurology* 1998;51:899–901.
287. Graus F, Saiz A, Sierra J, et al. Neurologic complications of autologous and allogeneic bone marrow transplantation in patients with leukemia: a comparative study. *Neurology* 1996;46:1004–1009.
288. Mevorach D, Goldberg Y, Gomori JM, Rachmilewitz D. Antiphospholipid syndrome manifested by ischemic stroke in a patient with Crohn's disease. *J. Clin Gastroenterol* 1996;22: 141–143.

289. Weber P, Husemann S, Vielhaber H, Zimmer KP, Nowak-Gottl U. Coagulation and fibrinolysis in children, adolescents, and young adults with inflammatory bowel disease. *J Pediatr Gastroenterol Nutr* 1999;28:418–422.
290. Lin HC, Chen RL, Wang PJ. Paroxysmal nocturnal hemoglobinuria presenting as moyamoya syndrome. *Brain & Development* 1996;18:157–159.
291. Fuh JL, Teng MM, Yang WC, Liu HC. Cerebral infarction in young men with nephrotic syndrome. *Stroke* 1992;23:295–297.
292. Marsh EE, Biller J, Adams HP, Jr., Kaplan JM. Cerebral infarction in patients with nephrotic syndrome. *Stroke* 1991;22:90–93.
293. Chaturvedi S. Fulminant cerebral infarctions with membranous nephropathy. *Stroke* 1993;24:473–475.
294. Guerrero-Romero F, Rodriguez-Moran M. Proteinuria is an independent risk factor for ischemic stroke in non-insulin-dependent diabetes mellitus. *Stroke* 1999;30:1787–1791.
295. Macko RF, Ameriso SF, Gruber A, et al. Impairments of the protein C system and fibrinolysis in infection-associated stroke. *Stroke* 1996;27:2005–2011.
296. Pinto AN. AIDS and cerebrovascular disease. *Stroke* 1996;27:538–543.
297. Rao AK, Chouhan V, Chen X, Sun L, Boden G. Activation of the tissue factor pathway of blood coagulation during prolonged hyperglycemia in young healthy men. *Diabetes* 1999;48:1156–1161.
298. Lip GY, Gibbs CR. Does heart failure confer a hypercoagulable state? Virchow's triad revisited. *J Am Coll Cardiol* 1999;33:1424–1426.
299. Ansell JE, Tiarks C, Fairchild VK. Coagulation abnormalities associated with the use of anabolic steriods. *Am Heart J* 1993;125:367–371.
300. Hendriks HF, Veenstra J, Velthuis-te WE, Schaafsma G, Kluft C. Effect of moderate dose of alcohol with evening meal on fibrinolytic factors. *BMJ* 1994;308:1003–1006.
301. Finelli PF, Carley MD. Cerebral venous thrombosis associated with epoetin alfa therapy. *Arch Neurol* 2000;57:260–262.
302. Tsai HM, Rice L, Sarode R, Chow TW, Moake JL. Antibody inhibitors to von willebrand factor metalloproteinase and increased binding of von willebrand factor to platelets in ticlopidine-associated thrombotic thrombocytopenic purpura. *Ann Intern Med* 2000;132:794–799.

Chapter 9

STROKE IN CHILDREN AND YOUNG ADULTS AND GENETIC CAUSES OF STROKE

Although most ischemic strokes occur in persons older than 65, approximately 3% of events occur in those under 45. The number of young persons having stroke may be increasing. This increase may be a true increase in incidence, or it may be secondary to a greater awareness that stroke does occur in this patient population. Because children and young adults have a long life expectancy, a stroke that leads to death or prolonged disability has a huge economic impact. The economic and societal effects of stroke are exacerbated by the absence of other serious medical illnesses in this population. Although congenital hemiparesis and other focal impairments often are due to an in utero vascular event or a neonatal stroke, these events usually are not included when defining the population of children with stroke. For the purposes of this chapter, stroke in childhood includes events in persons ages 1–15 year. Because the causes of stroke among adolescents ages 15–18 generally are the same as those among slightly older persons, they are included in the population of young adults, ages 15–45. By the age of 45, ischemic stroke begins to mimic that which occurs in older age groups.

Stroke is among the leading causes of death in children and young adults, but a majority of fatal strokes in these groups are hemorrhages. Approximately two-thirds of strokes in children and young adults are due to intracerebral or subarachnoid hemorrhage. The relative importance of intracranial hemorrhage as an alternative diagnosis for ischemic stroke in a young adult is highlighted by the results of epidemiological studies. Still, ischemic stroke does occur at a frequency sufficient to be considered in the differential diagnosis of any sudden focal neurological impairment in these populations.[1] In general, the clinical and brain imaging features of stroke in children and young adults are similar to those in older persons. Headache and seizures are, however, relatively more common in young persons, whereas lacunar syndromes are relatively less frequent.[2] Most young people do not have transient ischemic attack (TIA) as a warning of ischemic stroke and, in particular, transient vertebrobasilar events are uncommon.[3] The relationship between TIA and ischemic stroke is not as clear in young adults as in older persons. The lack of a strong association between TIA and stroke in young adults reflects the relatively high rate of cardioembolism and acute non-atherosclerotic vasculopathies in this group and the relatively low rate of extracranial atherosclerosis.

The causes of ischemic stroke in children and young adults are multiple (Tables 9–1 and 9–2). Hospital-based registries report up to approximately 60 different etiologies for ischemic stroke in young persons.[4,5] The diversity of causes and subsequent potential for differences in management mean that an extensive evaluation often is needed to screen for the cause of stroke. The leading causes of stroke in older persons—atherosclerosis, structural heart disease, and secondary atrial fibrillation—are not common etiologies of stroke in children and young adults. Because of the relatively low frequency of atherosclerosis in young adults, *non-atherosclerotic vasculopathies, cardioembolism,* and *hypercoagulable states* have increased importance as etiologies of stroke in both children and young adults. *Migraine, pregnancy* and the *post-partum state, oral contraceptive use,* and *alcohol and drug abuse* also are included in the differential diagnosis of causes of stroke in young adults. In addition, an increasing number of *inherited diseases* and *metabolic disorders* are being identified as causes of stroke.

Table 9–1. **Leading Causes of Ischemic Stroke in Children**

Non-inflammatory vasculopathies
Arterial dissection
Trauma
Moyamoya disease and moyamoya syndrome
Fibromuscular dysplasia
Migraine
Vasculitis
Systemic lupus erythematosus
Kawasaki disease
Takayasu disease
Infectious vasculopathies or complications of infections
Lyme disease
Mycoplasma pneumonia
Coxsackie disease
Acquired immune deficiency syndrome
Meningitis
Pro-thrombotic states
Sickle cell disease
Deficiency of protein C, protein S, or antithrombin III
Factor V-Leiden deficiency
Leukemia
Chemotherapy
Cardioembolism
Cyanotic congenital heart disease
Pulmonary atresia
Tetrology of Fallot
Transposition
Patent foramen ovale
Patent ductus arteriosus
Atrial or ventricular septal defect
Cardiovascular operations
Dilated cardiomyopathy—neuromuscular diseases

Tests that might not be ordered for an elderly patient might be obtained in an effort to establish stroke subtype in a younger person. For example, younger patients often need arteriography, cardiac imaging studies, and a broad battery of hematologic studies because of the very extensive differential diagnosis for the cause of stroke. The yield of both transesophageal echocardiography and

Table 9–2. **Leading Causes of Ischemic Stroke in Young Adults**

- Large artery atherosclerosis
- Small artery occlusion (lacunar infarction)
- Non-atherosclerotic vasculopathies
  - Susac syndrome
  - Arterial dissection
  - Trauma
  - Fibromuscular dysplasia
  - Moyamoya disease and moyamoya syndrome
  - Infectious diseases
  - Non-infectious vasculopathies
  - Migraine
- Cardioembolism
  - Myocardial infarction
  - Rheumatic heart disease (mitral stenosis)
  - Mechanical prosthetic valve
  - Patent foramen ovale
  - Mital valve prolapse
- Disorders of coagulation
  - Deficiencies of protein C, protein S, or antithrombin III
  - Antiphospholipid antibodies
  - Factor V-Leiden deficiency
- Pregnancy and puerperium
- Oral contraceptives
- Alcohol abuse
- Drug abuse
- Genetic causes
  - Homocystinuria
  - Fabry-Anderson disease
  - Cerebral autosomal dominant arteriopathy and subcortical ischemic leukoencephalopathy
  - Mitochondrial encephalopathy, lactic acidosis, and stroke-like episodes
  - Kearns-Sayre syndrome
  - Myoclonus epilepsy with ragged red fibers
  - Ehlers-Danlos disease type III
  - Marfan disease
  - Osteogenesis imperfecta

transthoracic echocardiography in detecting important cardiac abnormalities associated with an increased risk of embolism is higher in young adults than in older persons.[6–8] (See Chapter 4.) As a result, cardiac imaging is done in a young adult who has no cardiological findings detected on examination; the same test is not conducted in a similar situation if the patient is older than 45. An arteriogram may be needed to define the presence of an intracranial, non-atherosclerotic vasculopathy, such as moyamoya disease or a vasculitis, in a child or a young adult.

ISCHEMIC STROKE IN CHILDHOOD

The risk of stroke, of all types, among white children of ages 1–14 in the United States appears to be approximately 2.6/100,000, and the rate among African American children is slightly higher at 3.1/100,000.[9] The above rates include both hemorrhagic and ischemic stroke. The rate of ischemic stroke is lower; Earley et al[10] estimated that this incidence was 0.58/100,000. The higher rate of stroke in African American children probably reflects the high risk for stroke in persons affected with *sickle cell disease.* In the series by Earley et al,[10] which included a large African American population, sickle cell disease was the leading cause of stroke in childhood. Homocystinuria can predispose children to stroke. Hyperhomocysteinemia is also a potential risk factor for ischemic stroke in children; a Dutch study calculated that moderate increases in homocysteine increased the risk of stroke among children under the age of 18 by a factor of 4.4.[11] The differential diagnosis of ischemic stroke in children ages 1–14 is broad and includes hypercoagulable states, congential heart diseases, and infections.[12] (See Table 9–1.) In addition, multiple risk factors can be found in children with stroke.[284] Still, despite an extensive evaluation, the cause of stroke likely will not be determined in a sizeable proportion of children with ischemic stroke.[10]

Arterial Diseases

Atherosclerosis is not included in the differential diagnosis of stroke in childhood, even among children with inherited disorders of lipid metabolism. Several non-atherosclerotic vasculopathies, however, can lead to stroke in this population.[13] The clinical features of several of these arteriopathies are described in Chapter 7. Arteriography is a critical component of the evaluation of children with ischemic stroke. The test will accurately detect intracranial arterial lesions, including occlusion, stenosis, and moyamoya syndrome.[14] An *arterial dissection* can follow blunt or penetrating trauma to the neck or the pharynx.[12] A fall experienced while a child has a foreign body, such as a stick, in his or her mouth can lead to occlusion of the internal carotid artery in the *tonsillar fossa.* Falls or extreme movements of the neck during sports, playing, or other vigorous activities can lead to dissection of the internal carotid or vertebral artery in a child.[15] Spontaneous dissections do occur, particularly in children with inherited disorders, such as Ehlers-Danlos syndrome.[10,16] (See Chapter 7.) In one series of 263 patients with dissection, 18 persons were under the age of 18 and, as in young adults, both cervical and intracranial dissections were found.[17] Still, Schievink et al[17] noted a relatively high frequency of spontaneous intracranial dissections in this group (7 of 18 cases), and all of the intracranial lesions were in the anterior circulation. The prognosis of arterial dissections in childhood and adolescence generally is similar to that noted for young adults.[17]

In Japan, childhood is a peak period for stroke secondary to *moyamoya disease.* A similar peak for childhood moyamoya disease is reported in other countries.[16,18] A relationship between moyamoya syndrome in childhood and Down syndrome or sickle cell disease also has been reported.[19,20] (See Chapter 7.) Congenital arterial anomalies also can predispose to stroke in childhood.[21] The inherited mitochondrial diseases described subsequently in this chapter also induce stroke in childhood.[21] A study by Chabrier et al[22] described a type of transient arteriopathy characterized by multifocal lesions of the basal arteries and subcortical infarctions. The mean age of affected children was 6 years. The relationship of this arteriopathy with other illnesses, including moyamoya disease, is not clear, and additional research is needed. Pediatric stroke also can complicate *migraine.*[23] A dolichoectatic abnormality of the vertebrobasilar circulation leading to migraine headaches and stroke in childhood also has been described.[24] Occlusive vasculopathy can lead to stroke occurring up to 20 years following irradiation for a medulloblastoma.[25] These *radiation-induced changes* typically occur in medium-size arteries. (See Chapter 7.)

Infectious diseases that directly cause a vasculitis or secondarily affect the cerebral vasculature are leading causes of stroke in childhood.[12,26] (See Table 9–1.) Among the implicated infections are *varicella, Lyme disease, Mycoplasma pneumonia, bacterial meningitis,* and *tonsillitis.*[10,16] Severe multisystem infectious illnesses also can lead to arterial or venous thrombosis. Dehydration and a hematologic derangement that prompts thrombosis can follow severe diarrhea and vomiting. Infectious endocarditis is a potential complication of several congenital heart conditions, and stroke can be a consequence. Non-infectious, inflammatory vasculitides, including multisystem vasculitis, can lead to stroke in children. Although autoimmune diseases are relatively uncommon in children, *Kawasaki disease, Takayasu disease,* and *systemic lupus erythematosus* are among the inflammatory vasculitides that lead to stroke in childhood.

Pro-thrombotic Conditions

Williams et al[2] concluded that an acquired or inherited pro-thrombotic state was the leading cause of ischemic stroke in childhood (see Table 9–1). This experience is similar to that reported by other investigators.[10,21,27,28] Increased viscosity of the blood can lead to stasis and thrombotic stroke among children with *leukemia.*[27,29] Stroke is also a relatively common neurological complication in children with *solid cancers.*[30] Stroke also is seen as a complication of *hemolytic-uremic syndrome,* shock, or dehydration.[31,32] Primary disorders of platelets or polycythemia are uncommon. An elevated hematocrit or hemoglobin can be detected among children with severe cyanotic congenital heart disease.

Sickle cell disease is a leading cause of brain ischemia in children.[33–39] Approximately 4%–10% of children with sickle cell disease have clinically overt stroke, and another 14% of patients have brain imaging evidence of asymptomatic infarction.[40,41] Children with sickle cell disease appear to be at high risk for recurrent ischemic or hemorrhagic stroke. An ischemic stroke occurring in a child of African or Middle Eastern ancestry should prompt an assessment for sickle cell disease using hemoglobin electrophoresis. (See Chapter 8.) Screening of asymptomatic children with sickle cell disease using transcranial Doppler ultrasonography can identify patients at greatest risk for brain ischemia.[42–44] Transcranial Doppler detection of changes in blood flow could prompt the use of transfusions in an effort to prevent stroke.[45] Disorders of protein C, protein S, heparin cofactor II, and thrombin–antithrombin complex have been described in children with sickle cell disease.[40,46] These abnormalities complicate management of these patients.

In one series, inherited pro-thrombotic disorders were noted in 8 of 67 children with arterial strokes; the most common was resistance to activated protein C (Factor V–Leiden).[47] (See Chapter 8.) DeVeber et al[48] reported abnormal coagulation tests in approximately one-third of children with thromboembolism; in many cases, multiple abnormalities were found. Among the disorders are activated protein C resistance; decreased levels of protein C, protein S, or antithrombin III; decreased concentrations of plasminogen; elevated anticardiolipin antibodies; and lupus anticoagulant.[16] Baca et al[49] found a high rate of elevated anticardiolipin antibodies in children with stroke. Kenet et al[285] found a relationship of elevated antibodies and Factor V Leiden with stroke in children. Bonduel et al[50] evaluated 40 children with either arterial or venous thrombosis of the brain. Nine had an identified acquired or inherited pro-thrombotic disorder. Conversely, Tosetto et al[51] did not find a higher frequency of inherited abnormalities of blood coagulation among children with stroke when compared with age-matched controls. They concluded that most children do not need to be screened for disorders of protein C, protein S, or antithrombin III. Despite these results, screening for a hypercoagulable state probably remains a key component of the evaluation of young patients with ischemic stroke. A strategy would be to limit testing for the inherited disorders of coagulation to circumstances when another cause of stroke has not been detected or when a family history of premature thrombosis is reported.

Cardioembolism

Cardioembolism should be a primary diagnostic consideration whenever a stroke occurs in a child.[16] (See Chapter 6.) In most instances, heart disease is clinically obvious. Still, a less apparent cardiac lesion can be found during a more detailed evaluation. In one series of stroke in childhood, approximately 15% of the events were ascribed to cardioembolism.[2] Cerebral ischemia is a complication of congenital heart disease, including *pulmonary artery atresia, tetralogy of Fallot, transposition of the great vessels, patent foramen ovale, patent ductus arteriosus, atrial* or *ventricular septal defects,* and surgical repair of cardiac abnormalities.[12,21,52–54] Dilated cardiomyopathy also can lead to cerebral embolism.[55] The causes of brain ischemia following cardiovascular procedures in childhood are similar to those reported in adults, except for the absence of embolism of atherosclerotic debris. Pua and Bissonnette[56] estimated that neurological sequelae could be detected in up to 30% of children having major cardiovascular operations. The Fontan procedure appears to have the highest risk for embolism.[57] Cyanotic congenital heart diseases that have a right-to-left shunt can lead to paradoxical embolism. Ischemic stroke and brain abscesses are potential complications.

Prognosis

Most children recover remarkably well after a stroke. Focal neurological impairments, such as hemiparesis or ataxia, often resolve. *Dystonia* and seizures are potential long-term sequelae.[12,58] Development of a dystonia after a subcortical hemispheric stroke seems to be restricted to children, as this complication does not occur in young adults. Less commonly, cognitive impairments and mental retardation are residual effects from recurrent stroke. Children with sickle cell disease have a risk for cognitive impairments secondary to recurrent brain ischemia.[39,59] Children with moyamoya disease have a high risk for recurrent stroke, progressively worsening neurological impairments, mental retardation, and seizures. As a result, revascularization procedures are often prescribed to prevent recurrent stroke and cognitive decline, although the value of these procedures has not been established.[60] (See Chapter 11.) In general, medical therapies to prevent recurrences in children parallel those prescribed to adults.[61] (See Chapter 10.)

ISCHEMIC STROKE IN YOUNG ADULTS

The differential diagnosis for etiologies of ischemic stroke in young adults are listed in Table 9–2. Despite an extensive evaluation, a specific etiology will not be determined in sizeable proportion of young patients. Depending on the strictness of the criteria used for making a subtype diagnosis, the cause of stroke cannot be established in 25%–40% of these patients.[4,5,62,63,286] The difficulty in making an accurate subtype diagnosis is considerable. Presentations of stroke in young adults can be atypical. In addition, many young patients might not have a thorough evaluation.[286] The number of illnesses causing stroke continues to expand and now includes *mitochondrial cytopathies* and *cerebral autosomal dominant arteriopathy and subcortical ischemic leucoencephalopathy* (*CADASIL*).[64] The number of patients at risk for stroke secondary to drug abuse is growing as *illicit drug use* becomes more widespread.[64] Stroke is recognized as a potential complication of *acquired immune deficiency syndrome* (*AIDS*).[65] In addition, strokes continue to be attributed to pregnancy, use of oral contraceptives, and migraine.[66] As information accrues, the contributions of several of these conditions to the problem of stroke in young adults likely will become clearer.

The differential diagnosis of stroke differs between young men and women. Atherosclerosis is uncommon in women younger than 45, whereas cardioembolism, non-atherosclerotic vasculopathies and hematologic disorders are the leading etiologies.[67] Strokes related to pregnancy or the use of oral contraceptives also are considerations.[68]

Atherosclerosis

After the age of 35, atherosclerosis becomes an important diagnostic consideration among men, especially those who have traditional risk factors for accelerated atherosclerotic disease, including smoking, hypertension, diabetes mellitus, and hyperlipidemia (Table 9–3). Atherosclerosis is uncommon in men and women younger than 35. A number of life-style–associated risk factors have been identified that are associated with a high risk of ischemic stroke among young persons of both sexes. Some of these might be modifiable. Among young men, heavy alcohol use, smoking,

Table 9–3. **Premature Atherosclerosis in Young Adults**

Uncommon among men <35 years, women <45 years

Can lead to large artery disease or small artery occlusion

Higher-risk patients
- Familial hypercholesterolemia
- Tobacco use
- Hypertension
- Diabetes mellitus
- Homocystinuria—hyperhomocysteinemia
- Fabry-Anderson disease

hypertension, diabetes mellitus, and heart disease are stroke risk factors.[69] Among young women, pregnancy and the use of oral contraceptives, smoking, and heavy alcohol consumption predispose to stroke.[68,69] You et al[70] estimated that diabetes mellitus increased the risk of stroke in young adults by a factor of approximately 11, and hypertension was associated with a risk ratio of approximately 7. Most young adults who have stroke secondary to large artery atherosclerosis have a history of heavy tobacco use. Although Love et al[71] found a strong relationship between cigarette smoking and stroke, they could not find an association with a specific stroke subtype. They found a strong interaction between stroke and both the duration of smoking and the average daily consumption. Efforts to stop smoking can lower the risk of stroke in persons younger than 45.

In large, hospital-based studies, approximately 10%–25% of cases of stroke in young adults are due to cerebrovascular atherosclerosis or small vessel occlusive disease.[2,4,72,73] (See Chapter 5.) Atherosclerosis can be identified in young men, usually older than 35, and rarely young women who have risk factors for premature atherosclerosis, including diabetes mellitus, hypertension, or heavy tobacco use.[73–75] Lacunar infarctions also can be detected in the same population of patients, especially among those with hypertension.[74] Because of a high prevalence of hypertension in young African American patients, lacunar infarctions are seen with an increased frequency in this group.[76]

Non-atherosclerotic Vascular Diseases

Non-atherosclerotic vasculopathies account for approximately 25% of ischemic strokes in persons ages 15–45.[63] (See Table 9–2.) This proportion is much higher than that noted in persons older than 45. *Arterial dissection* is the most common non-atherosclerotic arterial disease leading to stroke in young men and women.[72] Instances of familial cases with arterial dissection have been reported.[77] The classic scenario of stroke secondary to arterial dissection is a young adult who does not have any identified risk factors for the vascular event and who has prominent head or neck pain. Often the stroke follows sports or other activities during which arterial trauma can occur. *Direct blunt or penetrating trauma* also lead to intracranial or extracranial arterial occlusions.[78–81] *Dissection of the aorta* leading to stroke in a young adult also may be secondary to *Erdheim-Gsell cystic medial necrosis*.[82] *Fibromuscular dysplasia* of the internal carotid artery is most commonly found among young women.[83] A second peak of incidence of moyamoya disease and moyamoya syndrome is seen among young adults.[84] Ischemic stroke secondary to *moyamoya syndrome* is most commonly found among young women who smoke and use oral contraceptive agents.[85,86] Infectious diseases, such as *acquired immune deficiency syndrome* or meningovascular *syphilis,* and non-infectious inflammatory vasculopathies, such as *Takayasu disease* or systemic lupus erythematosus, should be included in the differential diagnosis of the cause of ischemic stroke among young adults.[87] The non-atherosclerotic vasculopathies are discussed in more detail in Chapter 7.

Cardioembolism

Emboli arising from cardiac abnormalities account for approximately 12%–30% of ischemic strokes in young adults.[63,72] (See Table 9–3.) Atrial fibrillation is relatively rare in this population. When present, it usually complicates severe structural heart diseases. Despite the low frequency of atrial fibrillation, its presence in a young adult with ischemic stroke should prompt investigation of the heart for a source of emboli. *Myocardial infarction* is a potential cause of cardioembolic stroke in a young adult with risk factors for accelerated atherosclerosis. This scenario usually is noted in a young diabetic or hypertensive man who smokes and is older than 35. *Rheumatic heart disease* (*mitral stenosis*) with or without atrial fibrillation is recognized as a cardiac cause of embolism. Previously, this condition was a leading cause of cardioembolism in young adults but, with improved treatment of rheumatic fever, it has largely disappeared in industrialized societies. Young patients with severe rheumatic valvular disease may require a mechanical prosthetic valve. These patients have an unusually high risk of embolic stroke. Most serious congenital heart diseases become symptomatic in childhood and, in the modern era, probably will be corrected surgically if the abnormality is severe. Thus, the number of *congenital abnormalities of the heart* that might cause cardioembolic stroke in young adults is relatively small. The most common congenital cardiac abnormality in young adults is a patent foramen ovale, which often is detected in patients with cryptogenic stroke.[88] Although *mitral valve prolapse* was speculated to be a leading cardiac cause of stroke in young adults, recent data show that embolism to the brain is not related to this cardiac condition.[89–92] The cardiac lesions predisposing to stroke are discussed in Chapter 6.

Pro-thrombotic Conditions

Disorders of coagulation account for approximately 4%–20% of ischemic strokes in young adults.[4,63,72,73,93] (See Table 9–2.) The most common abnormalities are deficiencies of protein C, protein S, antithrombin III, and plasminogen.[93–95] Increased anticardiolipin antibodies also are cause stroke in young adults.[96] The pro-thrombotic disorders are described in Chapter 8.

Prognosis

The acute prognosis for ischemic stroke among young adults generally reflects the severity of the neurological injury. Young adults may be particularly prone to development of malignant brain edema complicating a multilobar infarction. Biller et al[97] reported that the 1-month mortality was 6.6% among 213 young adults with ischemic stroke. Marini et al[98] also found a high mortality among young adults with recent stroke. In one series, acute mortality was highest in patients with stroke secondary to large artery atherosclerosis.[99] However, most young adults do not have serious co-morbid diseases, and acute care usually can focus on the neurological injury, thereby making the long-term prognosis better than among older persons. During follow up that spanned several years, Kappelle et al[99] reported that recurrent strokes developed in approximately 10% of young patients. The long-term prognosis for recurrent stroke depends on the cause. For example, patients with arterial dissections have a relatively low risk for recurrent events. Adunsky et al[100] reported that 81% of 30 young people were able to return to work. In a study of a larger cohort of patients, Kappelle et al[99] found that only 42% were able to return to prestroke activities and that most survivors had residual emotional, physical, or social impairments.

CAUSES OF STROKE LARGELY RESTRICTED TO YOUNG ADULTS

Some causes of ischemic stroke rarely are diagnosed among children or persons older than 45. For example, the likelihood of atherosclerotic disease is relatively low. In addition, coronary artery disease and atrial fibrillation peak at later ages. Some of the differences in causes of stroke reflect the prevalence of risk factors among people ages 15–45. However, the causes of stroke described in Chapters 5–8 can develop in young adults. Conversely, some of the other causes of stroke appear to be largely restricted to young persons.

Susac Syndrome

Susac syndrome is a rare disease usually diagnosed in young women who present with a microangiopathy that affects the retina, ear, and brain (*RED-M syndrome/Susac syndrome*).[101] (See Table 9–4.) Changes in small-caliber arteries lead to infarctions in the uvea, retina, cochlea, and brain.[102] Multiple subcortical lesions are found deep in the cerebral hemispheres.[102] The clinical findings include visual symptoms, deafness, and an encephalopathy.[101,103] Confusion and cognitive impairments accompany decreased visual acuity or visual field loss

Table 9–4. **Susac Syndrome**

Most commonly affects women <40 years
Microangiopathy
Retina
Ear
Brain
Findings
Visual loss, visual field defects
Unilateral or bilateral deafness
Encephalopathy
Stepwise progression
Waxing and waning

and unilateral or bilateral declines in hearing. Focal motor or sensory impairments are uncommon. The course of Susac syndrome is subacute and is associated with recurrent symptoms and waxing and waning or a stepwise progression. The cause of the microangiopathy has not been determined, but a vasculitis, a disturbance in coagulation, or recurrent embolization have been proposed as causes.[104,105] Potential therapies include antiplatelet aggregating agents, anticoagulants, calcium channel blockers, corticosteroids, cyclophosphamide, and plasma exchange.[104–107]

Migraine

Approximately 10% of men and 20% of women in the United States have a history of *migraine with* or *without aura*.[108] Because migraine is very prevalent among young adults and because stroke often occurs in this population of patients, a possible relationship between migraine and stroke has been proposed (Table 9–5). An interrelationship also is assumed because migraine involves changes in both brain metabolism and cerebral blood flow.[109] The sequence of events that causes migraine is not established, but headache usually is accompanied by dilation of intracranial and scalp arteries, whereas focal neurological symptoms (aura) are presumably associated with vasoconstriction. Still, in many patients, a cause-and-effect relationship has not been established

Table 9–5. **Migraine and Ischemic Stroke**

Both migraine and ischemic stroke are common
Cause-and-effect relationship is uncertain
Migraine does cause stroke
Migraine is not a common cause of stroke
Migraine may account for 5% of strokes
Risk of stroke may be greater among young women
Risk of stroke may be greater with migraine with aura
Hemiplegic migraine—CADASIL
Visual loss secondary to occipital infarction
Ocular migraine can lead to unilateral visual loss
Stroke can complicate use of migraine medications
Ergots
Triptans

between migraine and ischemic stroke. The mechanism for a migrainous stroke might involve a prolongation of the migrainous process beyond usual time limits that leads to ischemic stroke and permanent neurological sequelae.[110] Protein C resistance also may play a role in migrainous stroke.[111]

A young adult will have a vascular event ascribed to migraine if it is accompanied by headache. Undoubtedly, this sequence leads to over-diagnosis of migraine-induced stroke. The presence of headache should not automatically lead to a diagnosis of migraine because a number of other arterial diseases cause head pain.[112,113] For example, headache or neck pain is prominent among persons with cervical or intracranial *arterial dissection*. The presence of this arteriopathy should be eliminated before a diagnosis of migrainous stroke is made. Other vascular diseases, including atherosclerosis, can masquerade as migraine-related stroke.[114] Regardless of the cause, headache is more common with stroke among younger persons, women, those with posterior circulation events, and those with a past history of migraine.[115]

The frequency of stroke attributed to migraine is not clear; hospital-based studies report that approximately 5% of cases in young adults are of migrainous origin.[4,5] In a large Italian study, Carolei et al[116] noted that approximately 14% of young adults with ischemic stroke had a history of migraine. Even if migraine does not directly induce stroke, it does appear to be associated with a higher risk of stroke among young people.[117] Migraine increased the risk of ischemic stroke by a factor of 2 among men in the Physicians' Health Study.[118] An Australian study of older men found that migraine increased the risk of stroke by a factor of 2.2.[119] Carolei et al[116] concluded that the relative risk of stroke increased by a factor of 3.5 among women with a history of migraine and, if the migraine was accompanied by aura, then relative risk was even higher.[116] In two studies, Tzourio et al[120,121] found an increased risk of stroke among women with migraine. Women with migraine without aura had a relative risk of 3.0 (1.5–5.8), and those with migraine with aura had a risk of 6.2 (2.1–18). The authors also found that the use of oral contraceptives or smoking greatly increased the risk of stroke among women who had migraine. An epidemiological study in the United States found that the risk of stroke among persons with migraine also was influenced by an individual's age; relative risk was increased by a ratio of 2.81 among persons under age 40 but, thereafter, the relative risk declined.[122] An international collaborative study evaluated the role of migraine as a cause of stroke in young women.[123] Classic migraine (migraine with visual aura) was associated with an increase in relative risk of 3.81, whereas migraine without aura had a relative risk of 2.97. The risk of stroke among young women with migraine was increased if the patient smoked, used oral contraceptives, or had hypertension.[123] Silvestrini et al[124] found an increased risk of stroke among migrainous persons who also had elevated antiphospholipid antibodies. These studies, taken as a group, provide supportive evidence that migraine is a contributing factor to ischemic stroke among young adults.[125,126] Persons with ischemic stroke, especially those under the age of 40, should be quizzed about a past history of migraine headaches.

Patients with *ocular migraine* may have episodes of transient monocular visual disturbance, including visual loss that mimics an attack of amaurosis fugax. A vasospastic form of amaurosis fugax presumably due to migraine has been described.[127] Migraine is a leading alternative diagnosis when a young patient complains of recurrent episodes of transient monocular visual loss. If positive visual phenomena or headache are noted, then the likelihood of migraine increases considerably. Rarely, a severe episode of ocular migraine may lead to a permanent loss of part of vision in the eye secondary to an ischemic optic neuropathy.[128]

Most auras accompanying migraine involve visual phenomena, including positive visual disturbances, scintillating scotoma, or visual field loss in one or both visual fields (Table 9–6). Transient episodes of visual obscuration, visual loss, or positive visual phenomena without headache can occur in persons of all ages. The events appear to be more frequent with increasing age.[129] These events often are included in the differential diagnosis of vertebrobasilar TIA. Differentiating relatively benign *migraine equivalents* from true TIA is critical because the former usually begin after the age of 50.[130] They are not associated with a high risk of ischemic stroke or the traditional risk factors for stroke.[130,131] Migraine accompaniments usually involve visual disturbances without other neurological

Table 9–6. **Diagnosis of Stroke Secondary to Migraine**

- The presence of headache with stroke is not sufficient for diagnosis
- Most strokes among persons with migraine are secondary to other diseases
- The diagnosis of stroke secondary to migraine should be made with caution
- Most common scenario
  - Prior attacks of migraine with transient focal neurological symptoms
  - Focal neurological symptoms persist after event
  - Positive visual phenomena or a march of symptoms at onset

symptoms. These events are stereotyped and usually last 15–60 minutes.[130] The management of persons with migraine equivalents generally involves preventive therapies, such as beta-blockers or calcium channel blockers. Abortive therapies usually have a limited role because most patients with migraine equivalents do not have headache and autonomic nervous system symptoms.

Most strokes attributed to migraine occur in the posterior circulation and usually involve infarction in the territory of the posterior cerebral artery.[132,133] Most infarctions are located in the occipital or medial temporal lobes.[134] In general, the symptoms of *migrainous stroke* mimic those of a migraine, but neurological findings persist.[110,132,134] A homonymous hemianopia is the most common neurological residual. Patients with complex neurological symptoms (hemiparesis, aphasia, cranial nerve palsies) may have a higher risk of permanent sequelae (stroke) than do persons who have only visual symptoms. A risk of stroke appears to be particularly high among persons with *familial hemiplegic migraine;* some of these patients may subsequently be diagnosed with CADASIL.[135–137]

Stroke can precede the development of migraine headaches in some patients.[133] Diagnosis in this situation is difficult because the patient does not have a prior history of migraine with or without aura. Stroke may be a trigger for migraines or a component of a "first" migraine. Ferbert et al[138] found patchy subcortical lesions suggestive of small stroke on magnetic resonance imaging (MRI) studies performed among persons with classic migraine.[138]

Stroke also is a potential complication of both abortive and prophylactic agents used to treat migraine.[139] Concerns about permanent neurological residuals are greatest when vasoconstrictors are given. In general, *ergots* or the *triptans* are not prescribed to patients with complex migraine because of the risk of stroke. Stroke also might be a complication when propranolol therapy is prescribed for migraine.[140] Still, prophylactic therapies are a key strategy in preventing stroke among persons with migraine. Aspirin also appears to be effective in lessening the risk of stroke and migraine. Dipyridamole may be associated with an increased frequency of migraine headaches. Physicians have worried that arteriography may be dangerous in the setting of migraine; however, Shuaib and Hachinski[141] concluded that arteriography is not associated with an increased risk of stroke.

In general, diagnosis of migrainous stroke should not be made until other causes of stroke are excluded.[4,142] It should be made with considerable caution if a patient has not had prior migraine headaches. The presence of headache, nausea, vomiting, and positive visual phenomena may not be sufficient for a diagnosis of migraine-induced stroke unless the patient has had prior similar events that are consistent with migraines.[142]

Recently, Ojaimi et al[143] screened a series of patients with cryptogenic stroke or migraine with aura for disorders of mitochondrial DNA. Abnormalities detected at two sites were likened to Leber's hereditary optic neuropathy. These findings support the concept that some young persons with ischemic stroke and migraine may have an underlying genetic abnormality. Further research on this promising finding is needed.

Pregnancy and Puerperium

Stroke is a leading complication of *pregnancy* and *puerperium* (Table 9–7). Both hemorrhagic and ischemic strokes and arterial and venous occlusions are recognized as potentially life-threatening complications. The decline in fatal obstetrical complications of pregnancy during the past century means that non-obstetrical complications, including neurological events, have increased in importance as a cause of maternal mortality or morbidity.[144] In a survey of more than 50 million deliveries in the United States, Lanska and Kryscio[145] calculated that the risks of stroke and venous thrombosis are 17.7 and 11.4 per 100,000 pregnancies respectively. A French study reported that the frequencies of hemorrhagic and ischemic stroke were approximately equal.[146] Leys et al[147] reported that arterial ischemic strokes occur at a rate of

Table 9–7. **Pregnancy and Puerperium in Stroke**

Stroke is a leading non-obstetrical cause of maternal mortality or disability
Pregnancy-related events are a leading cause of stroke among young women
The highest risk of arterial occlusions is in the third trimester and <6 weeks of delivery
Multiple pregnancies
History of eclampsia or pre-eclampsia
Pregnancy-related conditions
Pro-thrombotic states
Post-partum cerebral angiopathy
Paradoxical embolism
Peripartum cardiomyopathy
Air embolism
Amniotic fluid embolism
Metastatic choriocarcinoma

3.8–5/100,000 pregnancies. Venous thrombosis is a potential complication of pregnancy.[148] In general, the risk of arterial occlusions is highest during the second and third trimesters and within 6 weeks of delivery.[149] Kittner et al[66,150] demonstrated that the relative risk of cerebral infarction is higher during the puerperium than during pregnancy. They suggested that the greatest risk of ischemic stroke is during the first 6 weeks after delivery. The number of pregnancies also appears to be important. Risk of stroke in women who have had six or more pregnancies is approximately 1.6 times that of women with fewer pregnancies.[151] Stroke also appears to be more common in women who have evidence of *eclampsia* or *pre-eclampsia*.[147,152,153] Besides pregnancy-related hypertension, Cesarean delivery also has been associated with an increased risk of stroke.[287] However, the latter relationship might be a reflection of the women's health.

Ischemic stroke during pregnancy and the puerperium is attributed to a broad group of conditions.[154] In addition to many of the other diseases that cause ischemic stroke in young women, several pregnancy-related conditions lead to stroke. Changes in concentrations of clotting factors can lead to a pro-thrombotic state.[146,149,155,156] Arterial diseases, including fibromuscular dysplasia, dissection, and moyamoya disease, can lead to ischemic stroke in a pregnant woman.[87] Overall, pregnancy does not seem to increase the risk of stroke among women with moyamoya disease.[157] Pregnant women with moyamoya disease have been treated successfully. Still, additional care is needed. Efforts to control blood pressure and to avoid toxemia of pregnancy may lower the risk of cerebrovascular complications of moyamoya disease. Komiyama et al[157] recommended that delivery be done either vaginally or by caesarean section. The latter recommendation is aimed primarily at reducing the risk of intracranial bleeding. Dissection of an extracranial artery also can induce stroke following delivery.[158] Presumably straining and hyperextension of the neck during the delivery can lead to trauma of the artery.

Post-partum cerebral angiopathy has been reported. Symptoms included headache, seizures, and focal signs.[87] A patient can have stroke with multifocal signs or an encephalopathy. Brain imaging tests show abnormalities consistent with multiple infarctions. Arteriographic findings include multiple areas of vascular narrowing that mimic the appearance of a vasculitis. Post-partum angiopathy may be related to migraine, eclampsia, or the administration of *bromocriptine* or *ergots* following delivery.[87,159–161] The angiopathy usually resolves spontaneously.

Pregnant women can have embolism from a structural heart disease, including rheumatic mitral stenosis, prosthetic cardiac valves, or congenital lesions. Infective endocarditis or paradoxical embolism via a patent foramen ovale can be potential cardiac causes of embolic stroke during pregnancy. Paradoxical embolism may be secondary to clots from deep vein thrombosis in the lower limbs or the pelvis. In addition, a pregnancy-specific heart condition that leads to embolism is *peripartum cardiomyopathy*.[146,162] Peripartum cardiomyopathy is more common in women of African American background, multiparous women, and those with multiple pregnancies. It produces dilation and intraventricular thrombosis, usually leading to an embolic stroke within the first 2–3 months after delivery.

Air or amniotic fluid emboli are potential causes of stroke during pregnancy, delivery, and the puerperium.[149] *Air embolism* can complicate a criminal abortion or a dilatation and curettage of the uterus. *Amniotic fluid embolism* can complicate delivery and usually develops within the first few hours of childbirth.[147,163] Women with amniotic fluid embolism have blood studies compatible with disseminated intravascular coagulation. Amniotic fluid embolism also can complicate dilatation and curettage performed during the second trimester.[163] *Metastatic choriocarcinoma* more commonly presents with an intracranial hemorrhage, but a tumor embolus could cause an infarction.[147] Choriocarcinoma most commonly causes symptoms within 6 months of delivery and usually is associated with pulmonary metastases. Elevated levels of beta human chorionic gonodotropin are a hallmark of the disease.

In general, evaluating a pregnant patient with acute ischemic stroke is similar to the process for a non-pregnant woman. If appropriate, radiologic studies, including arteriography, can be done with efforts to protect the fetus during the procedures. Magnetic resonance imaging and echocardiography are relatively safe for both the mother and the child. Other tests, such as examination of the blood or the cerebrospinal fluid do not require special protection of the fetus. The pregnancy can affect blood levels of procoagulation and anticoagulation factors.

Careful prenatal care and the prompt prescription of interventions to prevent eclampsia are important components of managing pregnant women. Transcranial Doppler ultrasonography can detect changes in flow velocities in the middle cerebral artery among patients with eclampsia.[153] Changes in flow may predict the ischemic complications of eclampsia and prompt increased efforts to maintain adequate cerebral perfusion. These efforts are critical to prevent both hemorrhagic and ischemic cerebrovascular complications.

Pregnancy also influences choices of medications to prevent stroke.[164,165] Because of high risks of teratogenicity, oral anticoagulants are contraindicated. Administering oral anticoagulants in the third trimester is further complicated by fetal deficiency of vitamin K. Neonatal bleeding secondary to vitamin K deficiency can occur even if the mother has not taken an oral anticoagulant.[166] Women at high risk for stroke, such as those with prosthetic heart valves, can be treated with unfractionated heparin, low molecular weight heparin, or low molecular weight heparinoid.[167] Aspirin has been prescribed to prevent eclampsia and can be given to pregnant women to prevent stroke. Data are not available about the safety of ticlopidine, clopidogrel, or dipyridamole during pregnancy.

Oral Contraceptives

The potential of an increased risk of ischemic stroke among young women taking *oral contraceptives* has been a concern since the introduction of these medications in the 1960s (Table 9–8). Oral contraceptives were thought to promote arterial occlusion by causing a pro-thrombotic state. Studies give conflicting evidence about the effects of these medications on coagulation factors.[168,169,288] The medications have changed drastically over time. Dosages of estrogen and progesterone have

Table 9–8. **Relationships Between Ischemic Stroke and Oral Contraceptives**

Oral contraceptives modestly increase the risk of stroke
Lower-dose estrogen preparations lower the risk
May be associated with increased risk of moyamoya syndrome
Women at higher risk of stroke
Age >30, especially >35
Smoking
Hypertension
Obesity
Migraine
Diabetes mellitus
Probably a contributing factor, not a cause of stroke
Contraceptive-related stroke is a diagnosis of exclusion

been reduced. The risk of stroke seems to be lowest among women using the most recent formulations.[170] Heinemann et al[171] noted that the likelihood of ischemic stroke was increased by a factor of 4.4 (2.0–9.9) among women taking the first generation of oral contraceptives. The relative risk was lowered modestly to a factor of 3.9 (2.3–6.6) among users of the third generation (current) of medications. Based on these results, Schwartz et al[172] recently concluded that the use of low-dose formulations of oral contraceptives is not associated with an increased risk of stroke among young women. Reducing the dosage of these medications and restricting their use among some groups of young women with other risk factors for stroke have resulted in a decline in the number of ischemic strokes that can be ascribed to the use of oral contraceptives.[172]

Recent epidemiological and clinical studies give mixed data about the risk of stroke associated with the use of oral contraceptives, but, in general, the risk appears to be low.[173] Hannaford et al[174] reported that a history of oral contraceptive use (current or past) increased the chances of stroke by an odds ratio of 1.5 (1.1–2.0.) A very large international study in Europe and third-world countries sponsored by the World Health Organization concluded that the use of oral contraceptives increased the risk of stroke by a factor of 2.99 and 2.93 in Europe and developing countries, respectively.[175] In a study that compared the likelihood of stroke among women using oral contraceptives to that noted among either former users or non-users, Petitti et al[176] found a marginal increase in risk; the odds ratio was 1.18 (0.54–2.59.) In two studies, Schwartz et al[172,177] compared the chances of ischemic stroke among women who were current users, non-users, or former users of low-dose preparations of oral contraceptives. No significant differences in rates were noted among the three groups.

These large studies identified several groups of women who might have a higher risk of ischemic stroke when using oral contraceptives. The most important factor is advancing age. No increase in risk is seen among women under the age of 30; however, the chances of stroke escalate rapidly among older women. By the age of 35, a risk of stroke appears to be considerable. One study showed it increases by a factor of 16.2 (13.4–19.4) among women older than 40 years.[178] Other factors identifying a patient at higher risk for stroke include smoking, hypertension, obesity, or migraine.[172,174,175,179,180] Diabetic women probably also have an elevated risk of ischemic stroke. Oral contraceptives should be prescribed only with caution to women with any one of the previously identified risk factors. In particular, women who are older than 35 or who have more than one of the previously identified risk factors probably should not use oral contraceptives. Other forms of birth control should be recommended.

Some ischemic strokes do occur in young women using oral contraceptives and probably are related to their use of these medications.[66,117] However, oral contraceptives should not be considered as a primary cause of stroke; rather, the medication should be considered to be a contributing factor. In most instances, another cause of stroke, such as arterial dissection or cardioembolism, will be discovered.[4] An ischemic stroke should not be attributed to the use of oral contraceptives alone until other causes of stroke have been excluded. Oral contraceptives should be discontinued if a woman has a stroke. Another birth control method should be recommended.

Ovarian hyperstimulation syndrome also has been described as a cause of stroke.[181] Presumably the relationship is mediated via a change in coagulation factors. The frequency of stroke as a complication of this uncommon illness has not been determined.

Alcohol Abuse

The interactions between alcohol consumption and the frequency of stroke are complex. Epidemiological and clinical studies demonstrate that light-to-moderate consumption of alcohol lessens the progression of atherosclerosis and lowers the risk of myocardial infarction and stroke.[182–186] Light consumption of alcohol (approximately 1 glass of wine or beer or a comparable amount of distilled spirits per day) is associated with a slowing of the progression of intimal-medial thickness (IMT) of the internal carotid arteries.[187] Consumption of alcohol also has beneficial effects on atherosclerosis by lowering low-density lipoprotein cholesterol and increasing high-density lipoprotein cholesterol concentrations.[183,185] Although modest alcohol consumption appears to have protective effects, either *heavy daily consumption* or *binge drinking* appears to be dangerous and is associated with a markedly increased risk of stroke.[188] This increase seems to occur in both men and women of any age and of any race.[182] Rodgers et al[186] reported that daily heavy consumption of alcohol (>180 gm./week) increased the risk of stroke by a ratio of approximately 2.9. Other studies found that intermittent heavy bouts of alcohol consumption increased the risk of stroke by a factor of 1.8–2.1.[189–191] Heavy alcohol consumption can help to explain the increased risk of ischemic strokes on weekends and holidays.[190,192]

Multiple factors explain why persons who abuse alcohol have an increased risk of stroke (Table 9–9). Chronic heavy alcohol consumption may promote progression of atherosclerosis. This relationship is supported by observations by Kiechl et al,[187] who found that heavy alcohol consumption (>100 gm./day) was associated with an accelerated progression of IMT. It also increased blood pressure, heart rate, and cardiac output.[193,194] Cardioembolism can arise from an alcohol-induced dilated cardiomyopathy.[191,194] Alcohol also can have a diuretic effect, leading to hemoconcentration and a disturbance in levels of clotting factors. In addition, ingestion of relatively low doses of alcohol transiently enhance thromboxane-medicated platelet activation.[289]

Table 9–9. **Relationships Between Alcohol and Ischemic Stroke**

Light-to-moderate alcohol use lowers stroke risk
- Slows progression of atherosclerosis
- Lowers low-density lipoprotein cholesterol and increases high-density lipoprotein cholesterol
- Reduces risk of myocardial infarction—cardioembolism

Heavy daily consumption increases stroke risk
- Progression of atherosclerosis
- Increase blood pressure
- Disturbances in clotting factors
- Diuretic effect—hemoconcentration
- Alcohol-induced dilated cardiomyopathy

Binges may explain risk of stroke on weekends and holidays, especially in young adults

When evaluating for ischemic stroke in a young adult, the patient and the family should be asked about heavy alcohol consumption in the past and during the previous 24 hours. A blood sample for alcohol concentration should be obtained if clinical findings suggest that the patient has been consuming large amounts of alcohol in the previous 24 hours. Still, even if heavy alcohol consumption is documented, other causes of stroke should be sought. For example, a patient could have symptomatic atherosclerosis, a recent myocardial infarction, or traumatic arterial injury from a fall. In addition to measures to treat the ischemic brain injury, management to prevent signs of alcohol withdrawal should be included in treating alcoholic patients who have had a stroke. Because many alcoholic patients have poor diets, supplemental administration of thiamine should be given. These patients also have poor compliance with complex treatment regimens and are at a high risk for falls, so oral anticoagulants usually cannot be prescribed for the long-term prevention of recurrent stroke. Antiplatelet aggregating agents probably are safe.

Illicit Drug Abuse

Information on the role of the use of *illicit drugs* in the pathogenesis of ischemic stroke continues to accumulate (Table 9–10). Drug abuse now is recognized as a cause or a contributing factor for ischemic stroke in a sizeable proportion of young adults.[188,195,196] In one series of 214 young adults with stroke, 73 patients had a history of drug abuse.[197] In another series, approximately 10% of cases of stroke were associated with recent drug abuse.[198] The most commonly implicated drugs are

Table 9–10. **Relationships Between Ischemic Stroke and Drug Abuse**

Contributing factor for ischemic stroke, especially young adults
Heroin, cocaine, and amphetamines most commonly implicated
Most persons who abuse drugs also abuse alcohol and tobacco
Causes of stroke secondary to drug abuse
Drug-induced cardiomyopathy
Drug-induced myocardial infarction
Drug-induced arterial hypertension
Infective endocarditis
Vasculitis

heroin, cocaine, and *amphetamines.*[199] In addition to these, stroke has been reported in persons who were abusing *phencyclidine* or *marijuana.*[198,200,201] Because persons who abuse drugs also may abuse alcohol and tobacco, these latter habits may play a contributing role in the increased risk of ischemic stroke.[202]

Among persons abusing drugs, stroke can be secondary to *infective endocarditis, drug-induced vasoconstriction* of the cerebral vessels, a *vasculitis,* or *markedly elevated blood pressure.* Persons who abuse drugs also have a high risk for traumatic arterial occlusions. Embolic stroke also has been described as a complication of drug-induced cardiomyopathy or myocardial infarction.[203–205] Effects of the drugs also may potentiate cerebrovascular complications of primary arterial diseases, including atherosclerosis, aneurysms, or vascular malformations. This latter effect is particularly important in understanding drug-induced intracranial hemorrhage. Arterial hypertension secondary to cocaine or methamphetamine abuse may provoke rupture of an intracranial aneurysm or a vascular malformation.

Ischemic stroke is most commonly described with the abuse of cocaine and amphetamines. Petitti et al[206] found that the use of these drugs increases the risk of stroke among young adults by a ratio of approximately 7–8.5. Cocaine and amphetamines are both potent vasoconstrictors that lead to increased blood pressure, increased cardiac output, and coronary artery vasospasm; myocardial infarction or a cardiac arrhythmia can result.[203] Cocaine also affects platelet function.[207] Narrowing (vasoconstriction) of the intracranial arteries has been found in persons with ischemic stroke following abuse of cocaine or methamphetamines.[202] In one experimental model, Wang et al[208] found that a combination of the two drugs reliably induced cerebral vasospasm. Arterial narrowing also has been ascribed to a drug-induced vasculitis.[202,209] (See Fig. 9–1.) The presence of an amphetamine- or cocaine-induced cerebral vasculitis has not been established. Pathologic confirmation of a vasculitic process is not available and radiologic changes of vasculitis often are not seen in patients with stroke following cocaine abuse.[210] The arterial narrowing attributed to vasculitis may be drug-induced vasoconstriction rather than a true inflammatory reaction.

Although stroke is a potential complication of a single exposure to cocaine or amphetamines, chronic or repeated use seems to be associated with a higher likelihood of neurological complications. A case of recurrent ischemic stroke associated with repeated use of cocaine has been reported.[211] The risk of ischemic stroke may be even greater with the alkaloidal form of cocaine (crack) than the hydrochloride form.[210,212] Other investigators have not confirmed this observation.[213]

Ischemic stroke also has been reported among patients abusing heroin.[214] Rather than leading to hypertension or vasoconstriction, heroin probably causes hypotension and bilateral borderzone infarctions.[215] Because heroin often causes a profound depression in consciousness, stroke also may result from hypoxia secondary to compromise of the airway or direct compression of the carotid artery.[216] The fact that heroin abusers usually inject the agent intravenously also puts them at high risk for infective endocarditis. The cardiac infection can be fulminant, and secondary acute heart failure usually is life threatening. Cardiac infection tends to be severe, and patients often do not survive long enough for embolic complications, although such a situation could occur.

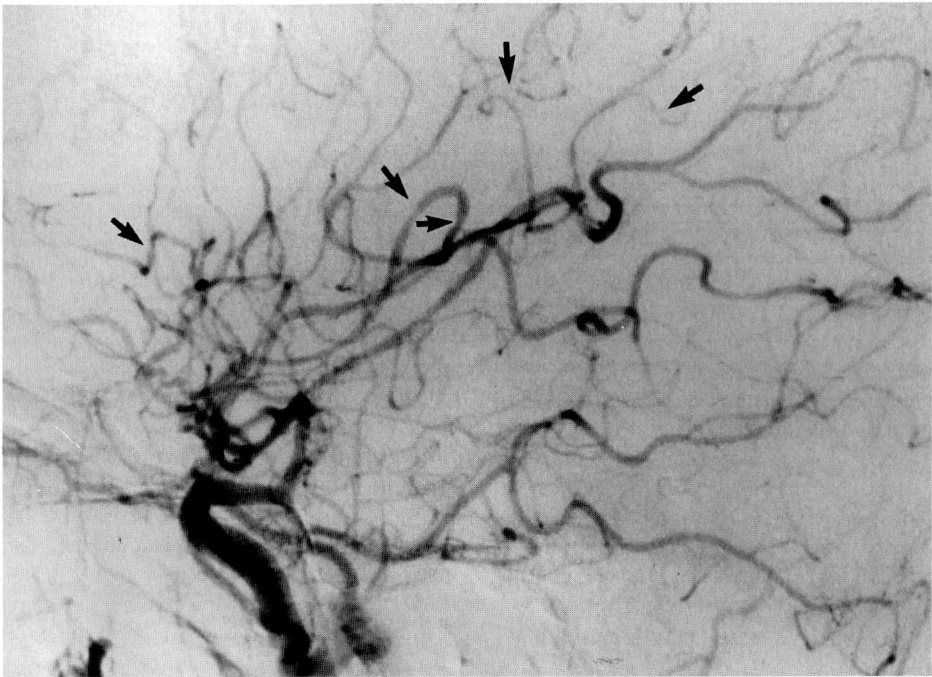

Figure 9–1. Arteriogram obtained from a 25-year-old man who had a stroke following injection of amphetamines. Several areas of segmental narrowing (beading) are noted with arrows in the intracranial vasculature.

Heroin users also may inadvertently inject the drug into an artery, and brain ischemia could result from the direct neurotoxic effects of the heroin. Stroke also may be due to adulterants that are added to the heroin, such as talc, that lead to embolism to the brain.

The most prudent approach for the physician is to be aware of drug abuse as a potential cause of stroke in young adults. In particular, drug abuse should be suspected in cases of cryptogenic or "atypical" stroke. Because the body often clears drugs quickly, urine or blood samples to screen for drug abuse should be obtained as quickly as possible after the patient arrives in the emergency room or hospital. Abstinence from the drugs is fundamental for prevention of recurrent stroke.

Stroke Complicating Use of Medications

Stroke is a potential complication of other medications that have vasoconstrictive properties. Among the medications that have been implicated are *phenylpropanolamine* and *ephedrine*.[198,202,217–219] The former agent is a component of medications that are used to suppress appetite or to rhinitis (decongestant), whereas ephedrine is available as a prescribed stimulant. Young patients with cryptogenic stroke should be asked about recent use of these medications. A cerebral arteritis leading to stroke has been associated with use of *ginseng*.[220] Stroke also has complicated the use of *anabolic steroids* in young men.[199,202,221] Stroke also is a potential complication of chemotherapy with *5-fluorouracil, cisplatin, methotrexate,* or *L-asparaginase*.[53,199,222–224] These agents probably cause stroke by the induction of a prothrombotic state. The issues that are related to stroke complicating cancer and chemotherapy also are described in Chapter 8. Screening for the use of these medications should be included when an ischemic stroke occurs in a patient who is receiving chemotherapy for a malignancy.

GENETIC CAUSES OF ISCHEMIC STROKE

Several inherited diseases lead to ischemic stroke by inducing changes in coagulation, leading to structural diseases of the heart, or producing arterial pathology.[225–228,240] The *inherited disorders of coagulation,* including sickle cell disease, are reviewed in Chapter 8. *Inherited diseases that predispose to atherosclerosis,* such as familial hypercholesterolemia, are discussed in Chapters 2 and 5.[229] The NOS 3 gene polymorphism has not been found to be a risk factor for stroke.[230]

Homocystinuria

Homocystinuria results from a genetic deficiency of cystathionine beta-synthase, leading to increased concentrations of methionine and homocysteine in the cells and body fluids (Table 9–11). This accumulation of homocysteine affects the vascular walls, leading to arterial and venous thrombosis. Homocysteine appears to be toxic to the vessels because it causes endothelial dysfunction, smooth muscle proliferation, changes in the extracellular matrix, and lipoprotein oxidation.[231] (See Chapter 2.) Homocystinuria also may cause changes in coagulation that promote thrombosis.[232] Affected patients typically have mental retardation, dislocated optic lenses, and osteoporosis. Most patients have recurrent ischemic events, including stroke, myocardial infarction, retinal infarction, or renal infarction, before the age of 30.[233,234] Young adults with homocystinuria can have an increase in the IMT detected by sonography of the internal carotid artery.[235] Supplementing the diet with additional pyridoxine, folate, and vitamin B12 appears to lessen the risk of stroke or vascular death among this population.[236] See Chapter 2 for a review of hyperhomocysteinemia as a risk factor for stroke.

Fabry-Anderson Disease

Fabry-Anderson disease is caused by a genetic mutation of the long arm of the X chromosome (Table 9–12). The mutation reduces the production of alpha-galactosidase and, secondarily, deposition of ceramide trihexosides in the arterial walls, myocardium, renal epithelium, dorsal root ganglia, and autonomic nerves.[237] Affected men usually have symptoms of painful neuropathy, renal dysfunction, Maltese cross crystals in the urine, corneal opacities, and red punctate lesions (angiokeratoma diffusum) on the scrotum and the perineum. The intramural deposits of lipid cause arterial occlusions leading to myocardial infarction or recurrent stroke. Mitsias and Levine[238] described 53 patients with stroke complicating Fabry-Anderson disease; the average age of onset of stroke was approximately 35. Two-thirds of the patients had symptoms in the vertebrobasilar circulation, and they found elongated and ectatic basilar arteries

Table 9–11. **Homocystinuria**

Genetic deficiency of cystathionine beta-synthase
Increased levels of methionine and homocysteine
Endothelial dysfunction and smooth muscle proliferation
Changes in extracellular matix
Pro-thrombotic
Clinical features
  Mental retardation
  Dislocated lens
  Osteoporosis
  Recurrent stroke or myocardial infarction

Table 9–12. **Fabry-Anderson Disease**

X-linked genetic deficiency of alpha-galactosidase
Ceramide trihexosidase deposited in arteries, myocardium, kidneys, and nerves
Clinical features in young men
  Recurrent stroke or myocardial infarction
  Painful neuropathy
  Renal dysfunction
  Corneal opacities
  Maltese cross crystals in the urine
  Angiokeratoma diffusum of the scrotum and groin

in many cases. This latter finding confirms the observation of Maisey and Cosh,[239] who reported the relationship between a dolichoectatic basilar artery and Fabry-Anderson disease. Recurrent stroke and progressive neurological impairments can occur. In an MRI-based study, Crutchfield et al[237] noted that a progressive increase in the number of brain lesions was associated with the age of the patient. Treatment to prevent recurrent stroke generally involves antiplatelet aggregating agents.

Mitochondrial Encephalopathy, Lactic Acidosis, and Stroke-Like Episodes

Mitochondrial encephalopathy, lactic acidosis, and stroke-like episodes (*MELAS*) is a relatively uncommon inherited disease that is included in the differential diagnosis of strokes in children and young adults.[240,241] It is caused by a translational mutation of segment 3243 of mitochondrial transfer RNA.[242,243] The mutation leads to a mitchondrial myopathy that promotes changes in the capillaries, epithelial cells, and smooth muscle cells in arteries.[244] (See Table 9–13.) However, Molnar et al[291] concluded that MELAS does not appear to be due to arteriolar disturbances leading to ischemia. The authors concluded that the primary mitochondrial problem may be located in the neurons and glia instead of the blood vessels. Patients also can have headaches, seizures, cognitive decline, vomiting, decreased hearing, and ileus. The presence of lactic acidosis in the blood and cerebrospinal fluid is characteristic of MELAS. Managing a pregnant patient with MELAS appears to be particularly problematic.[245,246]

Table 9–13. **Mitochondrial Encephalopathy, Lactic Acidosis, and Stroke-Like Episodes (MELAS)**

Translational mutation of mitochondrial transfer RNA
Mitochondrial myopathy
Capillaries
Epithelial cells
Smooth muscle cells
Lactic acidosis in blood and cerebrospinal fluid
Clinical findings
Recurrent stroke
Headaches
Seizures
Cognitive decline
Vomiting
Hearing loss
Ileus

Kearns-Sayre Syndrome and Other Mitochondrial Diseases

Kearns-Sayre syndrome is an inherited mitochondrial disease that leads to progressive external ophthalmoplegia, retinitis pigmentosa, a characteristic myopathy, and cardiac disturbances.[247] Maternal transmission appears to be particularly critical for this genetic disease. The higher the amount of maternal mutant mitochondrial DNA, the greater the risk that children will be affected.[248] Cardioembolic stroke is a potential complication of the cardiomyopathy or cardiac conduction defect.[249] In the past, the cardiac conduction problems usually were fatal. Now, placement of pacemakers to control these problems can prolong survival but leave the patient at risk for ischemic stroke.[247] Because heart disease is a complication of *myoclonus epilepsy with ragged red fibers* (*MERRF*), embolic stroke also may be possible. Stroke-like episodes have been described in children with *Saguenay Lac St. Jean syndrome*.[250] This autosomal recessive disease causes a deficiency of cytochrome oxidase and lactic acidosis. It can evolve into an illness that resembles Leigh disease.

Cerebral Autosomal Dominant Arteriopathy and Subcortical Ischemic Leukoencephalopathy

Cerebral autosomal dominant arteriopathy and subcortical ischemic leukoencephalopathy was first described in France in the early 1990s, but, since then, cases have been reported from around the world. The condition is due to an autosomal dominant notch 3 mutation on chromosome 19.[135,251–253] An accumulation of granular osmiophilic material leads to degeneration of vascular smooth muscle.[254,255] The changes in the endothelium of affected blood vessels cause a decrease in the number of cells, increased density of the endothelial cytoplasm, and impaired permeability.[256] In addition to the cerebral vessels, changes can be detected in the peripheral nerve, skin, or muscle.[257,258]

The clinical hallmark of CADASIL is recurrent subcortical ischemic strokes occurring in multiple young adults from one family.[251,253] (See Table 9–14.) Approximately one-half of the patients have associated cognitive impairments, progressive dementia, depression, or psychiatric disturbances.[251,253–255] Because of preferential involvement of both frontal lobes, patients with dementia also have evidence of gait disturbances, incontinence, and pseudobulbar palsy.[259,260] Prominent neuropsychological impairments include decreased attention, processing speed, abstract thinking, short-term memory, and learning as well as poor constructional praxis.[261] Dementia can develop in the absence of distinct vascular events.[260] Its course can mimic the findings of a neurodegenerative process.[262] Approximately 10% of patients have a history of seizures.[259] Most patients are symptomatic before the age of 45 and are bedridden by the age of 55.[137,259] Affected patients usually die in their 60s.[259] Other patients may have migraine with or without aura.[135] Symptoms of migraine usually begin before the age of 30.[137] In particular, hemiplegic migraine is associated with CADASIL. A genetic link between the two conditions is proposed because a gene for familial hemiplegic migraine also maps to chromosome 19.[136,263] However, Dichgans et al[264] argue against a common allele for CADASIL and familial hemiplegic migraine.

Multiple white matter and subcortical hyperintense abnormalities in the cerebral hemispheres are characteristic findings on MRI.[265] The changes on MRI are worse in symptomatic patients.[266] The combination of diffuse bilateral MRI findings and clinical features are highly characteristic of CADASIL. Early involvement of the basal ganglia, thalamus, and deep white matter can be seen in demented patients with CADASIL.[262] Chabriat et al[266] found that MRI shows periventricular white matter lesions in 96% of cases, basal ganglia lesions in 60%, brain stem lesions in 45%, and supraventricular white matter lesions in 25%. Brain stem lesions often can be found.[267] The severity and extent of MRI abnormalities are correlated with declines in cognitive performance and advancing age.[268] Abnormalities in perfusion can be detected in the basal ganglia, and the severity of the changes correlates with the patients' clinical status.[292] Genetic testing can detect the abnormality on chromosome 19 and confirm a diagnosis.[269] At autopsy, abnormalities of the medial layer of the arteries of the brain can be found.[253] In addition, skin biopsy can detect distinctive changes in the arterioles, including the presence of a granular osmiophilic material within the basement membrane of vascular smooth muscle cells.[251,256,270] Treatment usually involves antiplatelet aggregating agents or anticoagulants.

Table 9–14. **Cerebral Autosomal Dominant Arteriopathy and Subcortical Leucoencephalopathy (CADASIL)**

- Genetic notch 3 mutation on chromosome 19
- Granular osmiophilic material accumulates in vascular smooth muscle
- Clinical features
  - Premature stroke and mental decline in young adults
  - Progressive dementia and psychiatric disturbances
  - Gait disturbance, incontinence, and pseudobulbar palsy
  - Seizures
  - Possibly related to hemiplegic migraine
- Imaging
  - Multiple deep white matter and subcortical infarctions
  - Early involvement in basal ganglia and thalamus
  - Bilateral periventricular white matter lesions

Despite treatment, patients usually deteriorate and have a high risk of recurrent stroke and dementia.

Other Genetic Diseases

New genetic diseases that cause stroke are being described. Fukutake and Hirayama[271] described a *familial illness of alopecia, lumbago,* and *atherosclerotic leucoencephalopathy* that produces symptoms in young adults and appears to be distinct from CADASIL. A rare hereditary disorder can produce a *cerebroretinal vasculopathy* that can mimic a brain tumor.[272] This newly described disorder presents with changes in the retina and progressive development of an intracerebral mass.

Inherited Connective Tissue Disorders

Several inherited connective tissue disorders are associated with cerebrovascular complications. These diseases are relatively rare, and many of them lead to changes in the arterial wall that promote the development of dissection. *Ehlers-Danlos disease type III* is most commonly associated with the development of intracranial aneurysms, dissection, and a carotid-cavernous fistula.[273–275] *Marfan syndrome* is caused by a mutation of chromosome 15q21.1, which leads to a build-up of fibrillin that affects the function of the arterial wall.[276] *Dissections of the aorta* and the formation of aneurysms complicate it.[273] Patients with Marfan syndrome also can have *cervical artery dissections.*[277] Clinically, patients with Marfan syndrome usually have a tall, thin habitus with long digits. A cardiac murmur and dislocation of the lens also can be found. Surgical treatment of persons with severe aortic disease including dissection of the aorta can be performed successfully.[278,279] Vertebral arterial dissection and a carotid-cavernous fistula are complications of *osteogenensis imperfecta.*[273] Mitral valve prolapse is a potential cause of embolic stroke among persons with osteogenesis imperfecta. Premature arterial changes similar to atherosclerosis and stroke have been described in patients with *pseudoxanthoma elasticum.*[273,280] Schievink et al[281] found a deficiency of alpha-1 antitrypsin among four patients with cervical artery dissection.

Stroke as a Complication of Other Inherited Diseases

Stroke has been described as a complication of *neurofibromatosis* (von Recklinghausen disease) or *tuberous sclerosis.*[32] Moyamoya disease is the vascular condition leading to stroke that is most commonly associated with neurofibromatosis. Stroke may be caused by radiation therapy for an optic nerve glioma.[282,283] Moyamoya syndrome also has been described as a complication of sickle cell disease and Down syndrome. Moyamoya disease likely is an inherited illness, although further research is needed to define its genetic basis.

SUMMARY

Although persons under the age of 45 years present a small minority of strokes, the greatest number of causes of stroke occur in this population. In children, hemorrhagic strokes predominate over ischemic ones, and coagulation disorders are important factors in both. Moyamoya disease afflicts children of predominantly Eastern Asian origin, and sickle cell disease affects those of African or Middle Eastern origin.

Atherosclerosis is a relatively uncommon cause of stroke in young adults. Cardioembolism, pro-thrombotic states, and non-atheroslcerotic vasculopathies account for a majority of cases; however, up to one-third of patients will not have a definitive cause found even after an extensive investigation.

In women, pregnancy and puerperium mark times of increased risk for stroke. Young men are more likely to have stroke secondary to illegal drug use, binge drinking, or trauma. Although migraine is very prevalent in young adults, its relationship to stroke remains obscure. Opinions waver between declaring migraine as a cause of stroke or considering it a marker for increased risk.

Strokes in young adults and children are seldom heralded by TIA and, when strokes occur, they often are associated with headache and seizures. Brain edema following stroke may be more severe among young adults than older persons. Still, because the young often do not have severe co-morbid conditions and their brains have remarkable potential for recovery, their prognosis can be surprisingly good. Because of the potential for recovery and because the large number of possible causes, extensive investigations usually are warranted.

Genetic causes of stroke are becoming recognized increasingly. The list of genetic causes of stroke likely will grow. Some genetic defects, such as those leading to homocystinemia, can cause stroke in children in their homozygous form and pose a stroke risk in adults in their more attenuated heterozygous form.

The brains of children have great plasticity in the healthiest systemic milieu. Thus, they offer the most promising population to study the brain's recovery from stroke and to test the utility of agents to speed restoration. Once proven, these treatments could be used across populations of patients that span a wide chronological range. Thus, discovering causes of, and devising treatment for, stroke in the young could benefit not only them but also persons of all ages.

REFERENCES

1. Yamamoto LG, Yim GK, Bart RD, Jr. Emergency department presentations of cerebrovascular disease in children. *Am J Emerg Med* 1999;17: 163–171.
2. Williams LS, Garg BP, Cohen M, Fleck JD, Biller J. Subtypes of ischemic stroke in children and young adults. *Neurology* 1997;49:1541–1545.
3. Giovannoni G, Fritz VU. Transient ischemic attacks in younger and older patients. A comparative study of 798 patients in South Africa. *Stroke* 1993;24:947–953.
4. Adams HP, Jr., Kappelle LJ, Biller J, Gordon DL, Love BB. Ischemic stroke in young adults. *Arch Neurol* 1995;52:491–495.
5. Adams HP, Jr., Butler MJ, Biller J, Toffol GJ. Nonhemorrhagic cerebral infarction in young adults. *Arch Neurol* 1986;43:793–796.
6. Biller J, Johnson MR, Adams HP, Jr., Kerber RE, Toffol GJ, Butler MJ. Echocardiographic evaluation of young adults with nonhemorrhagic cerebral infarction. *Stroke* 1986;17:608–612.
7. Vandenberg B, Biller J. Cardiac evaulation of the patient with stroke. *Cerebrovasc Dis* 1991; 1(Suppl 1):73–82.
8. Urbinati S, Di Pasquale G, Andreoli A, et al. Role and indication of two-dimensional echocardiography in young adults with cerebral ishcemia: a prospective study in 125 patients. *Cerebrovasc Dis* 1992;2:14–21.
9. Broderick J, Talbot GT, Prenger E, Leach A, Brott T. Stroke in children within a major metropolitan area: the surprising importance of intracerebral hemorrhage. *J Child Neurol* 1993; 8:250–255.
10. Earley CJ, Kittner SJ, Feeser BR, et al. Stroke in children and sickle-cell disease: Baltimore-Washington Cooperative Young Stroke Study. *Neurology* 1998;51:169–176.
11. van Beynum I, Smeitink JA, den Heijer M, te Poele Pothoff MT, Blom HJ. Hyperhomocysteinemia: a risk factor for ischemic stroke in children. *Circulation* 1999;99:2070–2072.
12. Giroud M, Lemesle M, Madinier G, Manceau E, Osseby GV, Dumas R. Stroke in children under 16 years of age. Clinical and etiological difference with adults. *Acta Neurol Scand* 1997;96: 401–406.
13. Brower MC, Rollins N, Roach ES. Basal ganglia and thalamic infarction in children. Cause and clinical features. *Arch Neurol* 1996;53:1252–1256.
14. Ganesan V, Savvy L, Chong WK, Kirkham FJ. Conventional cerebral angiography in children with ischemic stroke. *Pediatr Neurol* 1999;20: 38–42.
15. Zimmerman AW, Kumar AJ, Gadoth N, Hodges FJ. Traumatic vertebrobasilar occlusive disease in childhood. *Neurology* 1978;28:185–188.
16. Ferrera PC, Curran CB, Swanson H, . Etiology of pediatric ischemic stroke. *Am J Emerg Med* 1997;15:671–679.
17. Schievink WI, Mokri B, Piepgras DG. Spontaneous dissections of cervicocephalic arteries in childhood and adolescence. *Neurology* 1994;44:1607–1612.
18. Chiu D, Shedden P, Bratina P, Grotta JC. Clinical features of moyamoya disease in the United States. *Stroke* 1998;29:1347–1351.
19. Cramer SC, Robertson RL, Dooling EC, Scott RM. Moyamoya and Down syndrome. Clinical and radiological features. *Stroke* 1996;27: 2131–2135.
20. Berg JM, Armstrong D. On the association of moyamoya disease with Down's syndrome. *J Ment Defic Res* 1991;35:398–403.
21. Garcia JH, Pantoni L. Strokes in childhood. *Semin Pediatr Neurol* 1995;2:180–191.
22. Chabrier S, Rodesch G, Lasjaunias P, Tardieu M, Landrieu P, Sebire G. Transient cerebral arteriopathy: a disorder recognized by serial angiograms in children with stroke. *J Child Neurol* 1998;13:27–32.
23. Wober-Bingol C, Wober C, Karwautz A, Feucht M, Brandtner S, Scheidinger H. Migraine and stroke in childhood and adolescence. *Cephalalgia* 1995;15:26–30.

24. Zambrino CA, Berardinelli A, Martelli A, Vercelli P, Termine C, Lanzi. Dolicho-vertebrobasilar abnormality and migraine-like attacks. *Eur Neurol* 1999;41:10–14.
25. Grenier Y, Tomita T, Marymont MH, Byrd S, Burrowes DM. Late postirradiation occlusive vasculopathy in childhood medulloblastoma. Report of two cases. *J Neurosurg* 1998;89:460–464.
26. Kerr LM, Anderson DM, Thompson JA, Lyver SM, Call GK. Ischemic stroke in the young: evaluation and age comparison of patients six months to thirty-nine years. *J Child Neurol* 1993; 8:266–270.
27. Gore RM, Weinberg PE, Anandappa E, Shkolnik A, White H. Intracranial complications of pediatric hematologic disorders: computed tomographic assessment. *Investigative Radiology* 1981; 16:175–180.
28. Gobel U. Inherited or acquired disorders of blood coagulation in children with neurovascular complications. *Neuropediatrics* 1994;25:4–7.
29. Priest JR, Ramsay NK, Latchaw RE, et al. Thrombotic and hemorrhagic strokes complicating early therapy for childhood acute lymphoblastic leukemia. *Cancer* 1980;46: 1548–1554.
30. Packer RJ, Rorke LB, Lange BJ, Siegel KR, Evans AE. Cerebrovascular accidents in children with cancer. *Pediatrics* 1985;76:194–201.
31. Gordjani N, Sutor AH. Coagulation changes associated with the hemolytic uremic syndrome. *Semin Thromb Hemost* 1998;24:577–582.
32. Mendoza PL, Conway EE, Jr. Cerebrovascular events in pediatric patients. *Pediatr Ann* 1998; 27:665–674.
33. Adams RJ, McKie VC, Carl EM, et al. Long-term stroke risk in children with sickle cell disease screened with transcranial Doppler. *Ann Neurol* 1997;42:699–704.
34. Steen RG, Xiong X, Mulhern RK, Langston JW, Wang WC. Subtle brain abnormalities in children with sickle cell disease. Relationship to blood hematocrit. *Ann Neurol* 1999;45:279–286.
35. Dover GJ. A new look at neuropathology in sickle cell disease. *Ann Neurol* 1999;45:277–278.
36. Kinney TR, Sleeper LA, Wang WC, et al. Silent cerebral infarcts in sickle cell anemia: a risk factor analysis. The Cooperative Study of Sickle Cell Disease. *Pediatrics* 1999;103:640–645.
37. Powars DR, Conti PS, Wong WY, et al. Cerebral vasculopathy in sickle cell anemia: diagnostic contribution of positron emission tomography. *Blood* 1999;93:71–79.
38. Wood DH. Cerebrovascular complications of sickle cell anemia. *Stroke* 1978;9:73–75.
39. DeBaun MR, Schatz J, Siegel MJ, et al. Cognitive screening examinations for silent cerebral infarcts in sickle cell disease. *Neurology* 1998; 50:1678–1682.
40. Liesner R, Mackie I, Cookson J, et al. Prothrombotic changes in children with sickle cell disease: relationships to cerebrovascular disease and transfusion. *Br J Haematol* 1998;103: 1037–1044.
41. Ohene-Frempong K, Weiner SJ, Sleeper LA, et al. Cerebrovascular accidents in sickle cell disease: rates and risk factors. *Blood* 1998;91: 288–294.
42. Seibert JJ, Miller SF, Kirby RS, et al. Cerebrovascular disease in symptomatic and asymptomatic patients with sickle cell anemia: screening with duplex transcranial Doppler US—correlation with MR imaging and MR angiography. *Radiology* 1993;189:457–466.
43. Adams RJ, McKie VC, Nichols FT, et al. The use of transcranial ultrasonography to predict stroke in sickle cell disease. *N Engl J Med* 1992;326: 605–610.
44. Verlhac S, Bernaudin F, Tortrat D, et al. Detection of cerebrovascular disease in patients with sickle cell disease using transcranial Doppler sonography: correlation with MRI, MRA and conventional angiography. *Pediatr Radiol* 1995;25(Suppl 1):S14–S19.
45. Adams RJ, McKie VC, Hsu L, et al. Prevention of a first stroke by transfusions in children with sickle cell anemia and abnormal results on transcranial Doppler ultrasonography. *N Engl J Med* 1998;339:5–11.
46. Tam DA. Protein C and protein S activity in sickle cell disease and stroke. *J Child Neurol* 1997; 12:19–21.
47. Ganesan V, McShane MA, Liesner R, Cookson J, Hann I, Kirkham FJ. Inherited prothrombotic states and ischaemic stroke in childhood. *J Neurol Neurosurg Psychiatry* 1998;65:508–511.
48. deVeber G, Monagle P, Chan A, et al. Prothrombotic disorders in infants and children with cerebral thromboembolism. *Arch Neurol* 1998;55:1539–1543.
49. Baca V, Garcia-Ramirez R, Ramirez-Lacayo M, Marquez-Enriquez L, Martinez I, Lavalle C. Cerebral infarction and antiphospholipid syndrome in children. *J Rheumatol* 1996;23: 1428–1431.
50. Bonduel M, Sciuccati G, Hepner M, Torres AF, Pieroni G, Frontroth JP. Prethrombotic disorders in children with arterial ischemic stroke and sinovenous thrombosis. *Arch Neurol* 1999;56: 967–971.
51. Tosetto A, Ruggeri M, Castaman G, Rodeghiero F. Inherited abnormalities of blood coagulation in juvenile stroke. A case-control study. *Blood Coagulation & Fibrinolysis* 1997;8:397–402.
52. Kirkham FJ. Recognition and prevention of neurological complications in pediatric cardiac surgery. *Pediatr Cardiol* 1998;19:331–345.
53. Grotta J. Cerebrovascular disease in young patients. *Thromb Haemost* 1997;78:13–23.
54. Kowalski M, Hoffman P, Rozanski J, Rydlewska-Sadowska W. Ischemic neurologic event in a child as a result of ventricular septal aneurysm. *J Am Soc Echocardiogr* 1998;11:1161–1162.
55. Karande SC, Kulthe SG, Lahiri KR, Jain MK. Embolic stroke in a child with idiopathic dilated cardiomyopathy. *J Postgrad Med* 1996;42: 84–86.
56. Pua HL, Bissonnette B. Cerebral physiology in pediatric cardiopulmonary bypass. *Can J Anaesth* 1998;45:960–978.
57. Quinones JA, Deleon SY, Bell TJ, et al. Fenestrated fontan procedure: evolution of

technique and occurrence of paradoxical embolism. *Pediatr Cardiol* 1997;18:218–221.
58. Krauss JK, Jankovic J. Hemidystonia secondary to carotid artery gunshot injury. *Childs Nervous System* 1997;13:285–288.
59. Cohen MJ, Branch WB, McKie VC, Adams RJ. Neuropsychological impairment in children with sickle cell anemia and cerebrovascular accidents. *Clin Pediatr* 1994;33:517–524.
60. Karasawa J, Touho H, Ohnishi H, Miyamoto S, Kikuchi H. Long-term follow-up study after extracranial-intracranial bypass surgery for anterior circulation ischemia in childhood moyamoya disease. *J Neurosurg* 1992;77:84–89.
61. Streif W, Mitchell LG, Andrew M. Antithrombotic therapy in children. *Curr Opin Pediatr* 1999;11:56–64.
62. van den Berg JS, Limburg M. Ischemic stroke in the young: influence of diagnostic criteria. *Cerebrovasc Dis* 1993;3:227–230.
63. Kittner SJ, Stern BJ, Wozniak M, et al. Cerebral infarction in young adults: the Baltimore-Washington Cooperative Young Stroke Study. *Neurology* 1998;50:890–894.
64. Martin PJ, Enevoldson TP, Humphrey PR. Causes of ischaemic stroke in the young. *Postgrad Med J* 1997;73:8–16.
65. Qureshi AI, Janssen RS, Karon JM, et al. Human immunodeficiency virus infection and stroke in young patients. *Arch Neurol* 1997;54: 1150–1153.
66. Kittner SJ. Stroke in young adults: progress and opportunities. *Neuroepidemiology* 1998;17: 174–178.
67. Barinagarrementeria F, Gonzalez-Duarte A, Miranda L, Cantu C. Cerebral infarction in young women: analysis of 130 cases. *Eur Neurol* 1998;40:228–233.
68. Knepper LE, Giuliani MJ. Cerebrovascular disease in women. *Cardiology* 1995;86:339–348.
69. Haapaniemi H, Hillbom M, Juvela S. Lifestyle-associated risk factors for acute brain infarction among persons of working age. *Stroke* 1997; 28:26–30.
70. You RX, McNeil JJ, O'Malley HM, Davis SM, Thrift AG, Donnan GA. Risk factors for stroke due to cerebral infarction in young adults. *Stroke* 1997;28:1913–1918.
71. Love BB, Biller J, Jones MP, Adams HP, Jr., Bruno A. Cigarette smoking. A risk factor for cerebral infarction in young adults. *Arch Neurol* 1990;47:693–698.
72. Lisovoski F, Rousseaux P. Cerebral infarction in young people. A study of 148 patients with early cerebral angiography. *J Neurol Neurosurg Psychiatry* 1991;54:576–579.
73. Carolei A, Marini C, Nencini P, et al. Prevalence and outcome of symptomatic carotid lesions in young adults. National Research Council Study Group. *BMJ* 1995;310:1363–1366.
74. Ferro JM, Crespo M, Ferro H. Role of vascular risk factors in lacunar and unexplained stokes in young adults: a case-control study. *Cerebrovasc Dis* 1995;5:188–193.
75. Caplan LR. Brain embolism, revisited. *Neurology* 1993;43:1281–1287.
76. Qureshi AI, Safdar K, Patel M, Janssen RS, Frankel MR. Stroke in young black patients. Risk factors, subtypes, and prognosis. *Stroke* 1995; 26:1995–1998.
77. Neau JP, Masson C, Vandermarcq P, et al. Familial occurence of dissection of the cervical arteries. *Cerebrovasc Dis* 1995;5:310–312.
78. Hilton-Jones D, Warlow CP. Non-penetrating arterial trauma and cerebral infarction in the young. *Lancet* 1985;1:1435–1438.
79. Thie A, Hellner D, Lachenmayer L, Janzen RWC, Kunze K. Bilateral blunt traumatic dissections of the extracranial internal carotid artery; report of eleven cases and review literature. *Cerebrovasc Dis* 1993;3:295–303.
80. Welling RE, Saul TG, Tew JMJ, Tomsick TA, Kremchek TE, Bellamy MJ. Management of blunt injury to the internal carotid artery. *J Trauma* 1987;27:1221–1226.
81. Schievink WI, Atkinson JL, Bartleson JD, Whisnant JP. Traumatic internal carotid artery dissections caused by blunt softball injuries. *Am J Emerg Med* 1998;16:179–182.
82. van Putten MJ, Bloem BR, Smit VT, Aarts NJ, Lammers GJ. An uncommon cause of stroke in young adults. *Arch Neurol* 1999;56:1018–1020.
83. Wesen CA, Elliott BM. Fibromuscular dysplasia of the carotid arteries. *Am J Surg* 1986;151:448–451.
84. Bruno A, Yuh WT, Biller J, Adams HP, Jr., Cornell SH. Magnetic resonance imaging in young adults with cerebral infarction due to moyamoya. *Arch Neurol* 1988;45:303–306.
85. Levine SR, Fagan SC, Pessin MS, et al. Accelerated intracranial occlusive disease, oral contraceptives, and cigarette use. *Neurology* 1991;41:1893–1901.
86. Bruno A, Adams HP, Jr., Biller J, Rezai K, Cornell S, Aschenbrener CA. Cerebral infarction due to moyamoya disease in young adults. *Stroke* 1988;19:826–833.
87. Bousser MG. Stroke in women: the 1997 Paul Dudley White International Lecture. *Circulation* 1999;99:463–467.
88. Van Camp G, Schulze D, Cosyns B, Vandenbossche JL. Relation between patent foramen ovale and unexplained stroke. *Am J Cardiol* 1993;71:596–598.
89. Barnett HJM, Boughner DR, Taylor DW, Cooper PE, Kostuk WJ, Nichol PM. Further evidence relating mitral-valve prolapse to cerebral ischemic events. *N Engl J Med* 1980;302: 139–144.
90. Jackson AC, Boughner DR, Barnett HJM. Mitral valve prolapse and cerebral ischemic events in young patients. *Neurology* 1984;34:784–787.
91. Gilon D, Buonanno F, Joffe MM, et al. Lack of evidence of an association between mitral-valve prolapse and stroke in young adults. *N Engl J Med* 1999;341:8–13.
92. Freed LA, Levy D, Levine RA, et al. Prevalence and clinical outcome of mitral-valve prolapse. *N Engl J Med* 1999;341:1–7.
93. Barinagarrementeria F, Cantu-Brito C, De La Pena A, Izaguirre R. Prothrombotic states in young people with idiopathic stroke. A prospective study. *Stroke* 1994;25:287–290.

94. Douay X, Lucas C, Caron C, Goudemand J, Leys D. Antithrombin, protein C and protein S levels in 127 consecutive young adults with ischemic stroke. *Acta Neurol Scand* 1998;98:124–127.
95. Munts AG, van Genderen PJ, Dippel DW, van Kooten F, Koudstaal PJ. Coagulation disorders in young adults with acute cerebral ischaemia. *J Neurol* 1998;245:21–25.
96. Nagaraja D, Christopher R, Manjari T. Anticardiolipin antibodies in ischemic stroke in the young: Indian experience. *J Neurol Sci* 1997; 150:137–142.
97. Biller J, Adams HP, Jr., Bruno A, Love BB, Marsh EE. Mortality in acute cerebral infarction in young adults—a ten-year experience. *Angiology* 1991;42:224–230.
98. Marini C, Totaro R, Carolei A, for the National Research Council Study Group on Stroke in the Young. Long-term prognosis of cerebral ischemia in young adults. *Stroke* 1999;30: 2320–2325.
99. Kappelle LJ, Adams HP, Jr., Heffner ML, Torner JC, Gomez F, Biller J. Prognosis of young adults with ischemic stroke. A long-term follow-up study assessing recurrent vascular events and functional outcome in the Iowa Registry of Stroke in Young Adults. *Stroke* 1994;25: 1360–1365.
100. Adunsky A, Hershkowitz M, Rabbi R, Asher-Sivron L, Ohry A. Functional recovery in young stroke patients. *Arch Phys Med Rehabil* 1992;73: 859–862.
101. Susac JO, Hardman JM, Selhorst JB. Microangiopathy of the brain and retina. *Neurology* 1979;29:313–316.
102. Papo T, Biousse V, Lehoang P, et al. Susac syndrome. *Medicine* 1998;77:3–11.
103. Bogousslavsky J, Gaio JM, Caplan LR, et al. Encephalopathy, deafness and blindness in young women: a distinct retinocochleocerebral arteriolopathy? *J Neurol Neurosurg Psychiatry* 1989;52:43–46.
104. Gordon DL, Hayreh SS, Adams HP, Jr. Microangiopathy of the brain, retina, and ear: improvement without immunosuppressive therapy. *Stroke* 1991;22:933–937.
105. Vila N, Graus F, Blesa R, Santamaria J, Ribalta T, Tolosa E. Microangiopathy of the brain and retina (Susac's syndrome): two patients with atypical features. *Neurology* 1995;45:1225–1226.
106. Wildemann B, Schulin C, Storch-Hagenlocher B, et al. Susac's syndrome: improvement with combined antiplatelet and calcium antagonist therapy. *Stroke* 1996;27:149–151.
107. Notis CM, Kitei RA, Cafferty MS, Odel JG, Mitchell JP. Microangiopathy of brain, retina, and inner ear. *Journal of Neuro-Ophthalmology* 1995;15:1–8.
108. Launer LJ, Terwindt GM, Ferrari MD. The prevalence and characteristics of migraine in a population-based cohort. *Neurology* 1999;53: 537–542.
109. Lance JW. The pathophysiology of migraine: a tentative synthesis. *Pathologie Biologie* 1992;40: 355–360.
110. Bogousslavsky J, Regli F, Van Melle G, Payot M, Uske A. Migraine stroke. *Neurology* 1988;38: 223–227.
111. D'Amico D, Moschiano F, Leone M, et al. Genetic abnormalities of the protein C system: shared risk factors in young adults with migraine with aura and with ischemic stroke? *Cephalalgia* 1998;18:618–621.
112. Ferro JM, Melo TP, Oliveira V, et al. A multivariate study of headache associated with ischemic stroke. *Headache* 1995;35:315–319.
113. Gorelick PB, Hier DB, Caplan LR, Langenberg P. Headache in acute cerebrovascular disease. *Neurology* 1986;36:1445–1450.
114. Shuaib A. Stroke from other etiologies masquerading as migraine-stroke. *Stroke* 1991;22: 1068–1074.
115. Jorgensen HS, Jespersen HF, Nakayama H, Raaschou HO, Olsen TS. Headache in stroke: the Copenhagen Stroke Study. *Neurology* 1994; 44:1793–1797.
116. Carolei A, Marini C, De Matteis G. History of migraine and risk of cerebral ischaemia in young adults. The Italian National Research Council Study Group on Stroke in the Young. *Lancet* 1996;347:1503–1506.
117. Weinberger J, Azhar S, Danisi F, Hayes R, Goldman M. A new noninvasive technique for imaging atherosclerotic plaque in the aortic arch of stroke patients by transcutaneous real-time B-mode ultrasonography: an initial report. *Stroke* 1998;29:673–676.
118. Buring JE, Hebert P, Romero J, et al. Migraine and subsequent risk of stroke in the Physicians' Health Study. *Arch Neurol* 1995;52:129–134.
119. Mitchell P, Wang JJ, Currie J, Cumming RG, Smith W. Prevalence and vascular associations with migraine in older Australians. *Aust N Z J Med* 1998;28:627–632.
120. Tzourio C, Tehindrazanarivelo A, Iglesias S, et al. Case-control study of migraine and risk of ischaemic stroke in young women. *BMJ* 1995; 310:830–833.
121. Tzourio C, Iglesias S, Hubert JB, et al. Migraine and risk of ischaemic stroke: a case-control study. *BMJ* 1993;307:289–292.
122. Merikangas KR, Fenton BT, Cheng SH, Stolar MJ, Risch N. Association between migraine and stroke in a large-scale epidemiological study of the United States. *Arch Neurol* 1997;54:362–368.
123. Chang CL, Donaghy M, Poulter N. Migraine and stroke in young women: case-control study. The World Health Organisation Collaborative Study of Cardiovascular Disease and Steroid Hormone Contraception. *BMJ* 1999;318:13–18.
124. Silvestrini M, Cupini LM, Matteis M, De Simone R, Bernardi G. Migraine in patients with stroke and antiphospholipid antibodies. *Headache* 1993; 33:421–426.
125. Narbone MC, Leggiadro N, La Spina P, Rao R, Grugno R, Musolino R. Migraine stroke: a possible complication of both migraine with and without aura. *Headache* 1996;36:481–483.
126. Rothrock J, North J, Madden K, Lyden P, Fleck P, Dittrich H. Migraine and migrainous stroke: risk factors and prognosis. *Neurology* 1993;43: 2473–2476.
127. Winterkorn JM, Kupersmith MJ, Wirtschafter JD, Forman S. Brief report: treatment of

vasospastic amaurosis fugax with calcium-channel blockers. *N Engl J Med* 1993;329:396–398.
128. Katz B, Bamford CR. Migrainous ischemic optic neuropathy. *Neurology* 1985;35:112–114.
129. Meyer JS, Terayama Y, Konno S, et al. Age-related cerebrovascular disease alters the symptomatic course of migraine. *Cephalalgia* 1998; 18:202–208.
130. Wijman CA, Wolf PA, Kase CS, Kelly-Hayes M, Beiser AS. Migrainous visual accompaniments are not rare in late life: the Framingham Study. *Stroke* 1998;29:1539–1543.
131. Dennis M, Warlow C. Migraine aura without headache: transient ischaemic attack or not? *J Neurol Neurosurg Psychiatry* 1992;55:437–440.
132. Broderick JP, Swanson JW. Migraine-related strokes. Clinical profile and prognosis in 20 patients. *Arch Neurol* 1987;44:868–871.
133. Caplan LR. Migraine and vertebrobasilar ischemia. *Neurology* 1991;41:55–61.
134. Hoekstra-van Dalen RA, Cillessen JP, Kappelle LJ, van Gijn J. Cerebral infarcts associated with migraine: clinical features, risk factors and follow-up. *J Neurol* 1996;243:511–515.
135. Chabriat H, Tournier-Lasserve E, Vahedi K, et al. Autosomal dominant migraine with MRI white-matter abnormalities mapping to the CADASIL locus. *Neurology* 1995;45:1086–1091.
136. Hutchinson M, O'Riordan J, Javed M, et al. Familial hemiplegic migraine and autosomal dominant arteriopathy with leukoencephalopathy (CADASIL). *Ann Neurol* 1995;38:817–824.
137. Desmond DW, Moroney JT, Lynch T, Chan S, Chin SS, Mohr JP. The natural history of CADASIL: a pooled analysis of previously published cases. *Stroke* 1999;30:1230–1233.
138. Ferbert A, Busse D, Thron A. Microinfarction in classic migraine? A study with magnetic resonance imaging findings. *Stroke* 1991;22: 1010–1014.
139. Meschia JF, Malkoff MD, Biller J. Reversible segmental cerebral arterial vasospasm and cerebral infarction: possible association with excessive use of sumatriptan and Midrin. *Arch Neurol* 1998;55:712–714.
140. Bardwell A, Trott JA. Stroke in migraine as a consequence of propranolol. *Headache* 1987;27: 381–383.
141. Shuaib A, Hachinski VC. Migraine and the risks from angiography. *Arch Neurol* 1988;45:911–912.
142. Welch KM. Relationship of stroke and migraine. *Neurology* 1994;44:S33–S36.
143. Ojaimi J, Katsabanis S, Bower S, Quigley A, Byrne E. Mitochondrial DNA in stroke and migraine with aura. *Cerebrovasc Dis* 1998;8:102–106.
144. Grosset DG, Ebrahim S, Bone I, Warlow C. Stroke in pregnancy and the puerperium: what magnitude of risk? *J Neurol Neurosurg Psychiatry* 1995;58:129–131.
145. Lanska DJ, Kryscio RJ. Stroke and intracranial venous thrombosis during pregnancy and puerperium. *Neurology* 1998;51:1622–1628.
146. Sharshar T, Lamy C, Mas JL. Incidence and causes of strokes associated with pregnancy and puerperium. A study in public hospitals of Ile de France. Stroke in Pregnancy Study Group. *Stroke* 1995;26:930–936.
147. Leys D, Lamy C, Lucas C, et al. Arterial ischemic strokes associated with pregnancy and puerperium. *Acta Neurologica Belgica* 1997;97:5–16.
148. Cantu C, Barinagarrementeria F. Cerebral venous thrombosis associated with pregnancy and puerperium. *Stroke* 1993;24:1880–1884.
149. Wiebers DO. Ischemic cerebrovascular complications of pregnancy. *Arch Neurol* 1985;42: 1106–1113.
150. Kittner SJ, Stern BJ, Feeser BR, et al. Pregnancy and the risk of stroke. *N Engl J Med* 1996;335: 768–774.
151. Qureshi AI, Giles WH, Croft JB, Stern BJ. Number of pregnancies and risk for stroke and stroke subtypes. *Arch Neurol* 1997;54:203–206.
152. Kaplan PW. Neurologic issues in eclampsia. *Rev Neurol* 1999;155:335–341.
153. Qureshi AI, Frankel MR, Ottenlips JR, Stern BJ. Cerebral hemodynamics in preeclampsia and eclampsia. *Arch Neurol* 1996;53:1226–1231.
154. Donaldson JO, Lee NS. Arterial and venous stroke associated with pregnancy. *Neurol Clin* 1994;12:583–599.
155. Ballem P. Acquired thrombophilia in pregnancy. *Semin Thromb Hemost* 1998;24(Suppl 1):41–47.
156. Mas JL, Lamy C. Stroke in pregnancy and the puerperium. *J Neurol* 1998;245:305–313.
157. Komiyama M, Yasui T, Kitano S, Sakamoto H, Fujitani K, Matsuo S. Moyamoya disease and pregnancy: case report and review of the literature. *Neurosurgery* 1998;43:360–368.
158. Van de Kelft E, Kunnen J, Truyen L, Heytens L. Postpartum dissecting aneurysm of the basilar artery. *Stroke* 1992;23:114–116.
159. Raroque HGJ, Tesfa G, Purdy P. Postpartum cerebral angiopathy. Is there a role for sympathomimetic drugs? *Stroke* 1993;24:2108–2110.
160. Janssens E, Hommel M, Mounier-Vehier F, Leclerc X, Guerin dM, Leys D. Postpartum cerebral angiopathy possibly due to bromocriptine therapy. *Stroke* 1995;26:128–130.
161. Barinagarrementeria F, Cantu C, Balderrama J. Postpartum cerebral angiopathy with cerebral infarction due to ergonovine use. *Stroke* 1992;23: 1364–1366.
162. Hodgman MT, Pessin MS, Homans DC, et al. Cerebral embolism as the initial manifestation of peripartum cardiomyopathy. *Neurology* 1982;32: 668–671.
163. Mainprize TC, Maltby JR. Amniotic fluid embolism: a report of four probable cases. *Can Anaesth Soc J* 1986;33:382–387.
164. Gilmore J, Pennell PB, Stern BJ. Medication use during pregnancy for neurologic conditions. *Neurol Clin* 1998;16:189–206.
165. Ginsberg JS, Hirsh J. Use of antithrombotic agents during pregnancy. *Chest* 1998;114: 524S–530S.
166. Zipursky A. Prevention of vitamin K deficiency bleeding in newborns. *Br J Haematol* 1999;104: 430–437.
167. Ginsberg JS, Barron WM. Pregnancy and prosthetic heart valves. *Lancet* 1994;344:1170–1172.
168. Samsioe G. Coagulation and anticoagulation effects of contraceptive steroids. *Am J Obstet Gynecol* 1994;170:1523–1527.

169. Harris GM, Stendt CL, Vollenhoven BJ, Gan TE, Tipping PG. Decreased plasma tissue factor pathway inhibitor in women taking combined oral contraceptives. *Am J Hematol* 1999;60: 175–180.
170. Lidegaard O, Kreiner S. Cerebral thrombosis and oral contraceptives. A case-control study. *Contraception* 1998;57:303–314.
171. Heinemann LA, Lewis MA, Thorogood M, Spitzer WO, Guggenmoos H, Bruppacher R. Case-control study of oral contraceptives and risk of thromboembolic stroke: results from International Study on Oral Contraceptives and Health of Young Women. *BMJ* 1997;315: 1502–1504.
172. Schwartz SM, Petitti DB, Siscovick DS, et al. Stroke and use of low-dose oral contraceptives in young women: a pooled analysis of two US studies. *Stroke* 1998;29:2277–2284.
173. Archie JP, Jr. The outcome of external carotid endarterectomy during routine carotid endarterectomy. *J Vasc Surg* 1998;28:585–590.
174. Hannaford PC, Croft PR, Kay CR. Oral contraception and stroke. Evidence from the Royal College of General Practitioners' Oral Contraception Study. *Stroke* 1994;25:935–942.
175. WHO Collaborative Study of Cardiovascular Disease and Steroid Hormone Contraception. Ischaemic stroke and combined oral contraceptives: results of an international, multicentre, case-control study. *Lancet* 1996;348:498–505.
176. Petitti DB, Sidney S, Bernstein A, Wolf S, Quesenberry C, Ziel HK. Stroke in users of low-dose oral contraceptives. *N Engl J Med* 1996; 335:8–15.
177. Schwartz SM, Siscovick DS, Longstreth WT, Jr., et al. Use of low-dose oral contraceptives and stroke in young women. *Ann Intern Med* 1997; 127:596–603.
178. Thorogood M. Stroke and steroid hormonal contraception. *Contraception* 1998;57:157–167.
179. Chasan-Taber L, Stampfer MJ. Epidemiology of oral contraceptives and cardiovascular disease. *Ann Intern Med* 1998;128:467–477.
180. Becker WJ. Migraine and oral contraceptives. *Can J Neurol Sci* 1997;24:16–21.
181. Yoshii F, Ooki N, Shinohara Y, Uehara K, Mochimaru F. Multiple cerebral infarctions associated with ovarian hyperstimulation syndrome. *Neurology* 1999;53:225–227.
182. Sacco RL, Eikind M, Boden-Albala B, et al. The potential effect of moderate alcohol consumption on ischemic stroke. *JAMA* 1999;281:53–60.
183. Kiechl S, Willeit J, Rungger G, Egger G, Oberhollenzer F, Bonora E. Alcohol consumption and atherosclerosis: what is the relation? Prospective results from the Bruneck Study. *Stroke* 1998;29:900–907.
184. Shinton R, Sagar G, Beevers G. The relation of alcohol consumption to cardiovascular risk factors and stroke. The West Birmingham Stroke Project. *J Neurol Neurosurg Psychiatry* 1993;56: 458–462.
185. Steinberg D, Pearson TA, Kuller LH. Alcohol and atherosclerosis. *Ann Intern Med* 1991;114: 967–976.
186. Rodgers H, Aitken PD, French JM, Curless RH, Bates D, James OF. Alcohol and stroke. A case-control study of drinking habits past and present. *Stroke* 1993;24:1473–1477.
187. Kiechl S, Willeit J, Egger G, Oberhollenzer M, Aichner F. Alcohol consumption and carotid atherosclerosis: evidence of dose-dependent atherogenic and antiatherogenic effects. Results from the Bruneck Study. *Stroke* 1994;25:1593–1598.
188. Gorelick PB. Stroke from alcohol and drug abuse. A current social peril. *Postgrad Med* 1917; 88:171–174.
189. Hansagi H, Romelsjo A, Gerhardsson d, V, Andreasson S, Leifman BA. Alcohol consumption and stroke mortality. 20-year follow-up of 15,077 men and women. *Stroke* 1995;26: 1768–1773.
190. Haapaniemi H, Hillbom M, Juvela S. Weekend and holiday increase in the onset of ischemic stroke in young women. *Stroke* 1996;27: 1023–1027.
191. Hillbom M, Numminen H, Juvela S. Recent heavy drinking of alcohol and embolic stroke. *Stroke* 1999;30:2307–2312.
192. Hillbom M, Haapaniemi H, Juvela S, Palomaki H, Numminen H, Kaste M. Recent alcohol consumption, cigarette smoking, and cerebral infarction in young adults. *Stroke* 1995;26:40–45.
193. Wannamethee SG, Shaper AG. Patterns of alcohol intake and risk of stroke in middle-aged British men. *Stroke* 1996;27:1033–1039.
194. Friedman HS. Cardiovascular effects of alcohol. *Recent Developments in Alcoholism* 1998;14: 135–166.
195. Caplan LR, Hier DB, Banks G. Current concepts of cerebrovascular disease—stroke: stroke and drug abuse. *Stroke* 1982;13:869–872.
196. Daras M, Tuchman AJ, Marks S. Central nervous system infarction related to cocaine abuse. *Stroke* 1991;22:1320–1325.
197. Kaku DA, Lowenstein DH. Emergence of recreational drug abuse as a major risk factor for stroke in young adults. *Ann Intern Med* 1990; 113:821–827.
198. Sloan MA, Kittner SJ, Rigamonti D, Price TR. Occurrence of stroke associated with use/abuse of drugs. *Neurology* 1991;41:1358–1364.
199. Kelly MA, Gorelick PB, Mirza D. The role of drugs in the etiology of stroke. *Clin Neuropharmacol* 1992;15:249–275.
200. Zachariah SB. Stroke after heavy marijuana smoking. *Stroke* 1991;22:406–409.
201. Lawson TM, Rees A. Stroke and transient ischaemic attacks in association with substance abuse in a young man. *Postgrad Med* 1996;72: 692–693.
202. Kokkinos J, Levine SR. Stroke. *Neurol Clin* 1993;11:577–590.
203. Sloan MA, Mattioni TA. Concurrent myocardial and cerebral infarctions after intranasal cocaine use. *Stroke* 1992;23:427–430.
204. Petty GW, Brust JC, Tatemichi TK, Barr ML. Embolic stroke after smoking "crack" cocaine. *Stroke* 1990;21:1632–1635.
205. Sauer CM. Recurrent embolic stroke and cocaine-related cardiomyopathy. *Stroke* 1991;22: 1203–1205.

206. Petitti DB, Sidney S, Quesenberry C, Bernstein A. Stroke and cocaine or amphetamine use. *Epidemiology* 1998;9:596–600.
207. Jennings LK, White MM, Sauer CM, Mauer AM, Robertson JT. Cocaine-induced platelet defects. *Stroke* 1993;24:1352–1359.
208. Wang AM, Suojanen JN, Colucci VM, Rumbaugh CL, Hollenberg NK. Cocaine- and methamphetamine-induced acute cerebral vasospasm: an angiographic study in rabbits. *Am J Neuroradiol* 1990;11:1141–1146.
209. Talbot RW, Heppell J, Dozois RR, Beart RW, Jr. Vascular complications of inflammatory bowel disease. *Mayo Clin Proc* 1986;61:140–145.
210. Levine SR, Brust JC, Futrell N, et al. Cerebrovascular complications of the use of the "crack" form of alkaloidal cocaine. *N Engl J Med* 1990;323:699–704.
211. Tuchman AJ, Marks S, Daras M. Recurring strokes with repeated cocaine use. *Cerebrovasc Dis* 1992;2:369–371.
212. Levine SR, Brust JC, Futrell N, et al. A comparative study of the cerebrovascular complications of cocaine: alkaloidal versus hydrochloride—a review. *Neurology* 1991;41:1173–1177.
213. Qureshi AI, Akbar MS, Czander E, Safdar K, Janssen RS, Frankel MR. Crack cocaine use and stroke in young patients. *Neurology* 1997;48: 341–345.
214. Brust JCM, Richter RW. Stroke associated with addiction to heroin. *J Neurol Neurosurg Psychiatry* 1976;39:194–199.
215. Niehaus L, Meyer BU. Bilateral borderzone brain infarctions in association with heroin abuse. *J Neurol Sci* 1998;160:180–182.
216. Jensen R, Olsen TS, Winther BB. Severe non-occlusive ischemic stroke in young heroin addicts. *Acta Neurol Scand* 1990;81:354–357.
217. Edwards M, Russo L, Harwood-Nuss A. Cerebral infarction with a single oral dose of phenylpropanolamine. *Am J Emerg Med* 1987;5: 163–164.
218. Bruno A, Nolte KB, Chapin J. Stroke associated with ephedrine use. *Neurology* 1993;43: 1313–1316.
219. Kaye BR, Fainstat M. Cerebral vasculitis associated with cocaine abuse. *JAMA* 1987;258: 2104–2106.
220. Ryu SJ, Chien YY. Ginseng-associated cerebral arteritis. *Neurology* 1995;45:829–830.
221. Akhter J, Hyder S, Ahmed M. Cerebrovascular accident associated with anabolic steroid use in a young man. *Neurology* 1994;44:2405–2406.
222. El Amrani M, Heinzlef O, Debroucker T, Roullet E, Bousser MG, Amarenco P. Brain infarction following 5-fluorouracil and cisplatin therapy. *Neurology* 1998;51:899–901.
223. Alberts SR, Bretscher M, Wiltsie JC, O'Neill BP, Mokri B, Witzig TE. Thrombosis related to the use of L-asparaginase in adults with acute lymphoblastic leukemia: a need to consider coagulation monitoring and clotting factor replacement. *Leukemia & Lymphoma* 1999;32:489–496.
224. Kucuk O, Kwaan HC, Gunnar W, Vazquez RM. Thromboembolic complications associated with L-asparaginase therapy. Etiologic role of low antithrombin III and plasminogen levels and therapeutic correction by fresh frozen plasma. *Cancer* 1985;55:702–706.
225. Natowicz M, Kelley RI. Mendelian etiologies of stroke. *Ann Neurol* 1987;22:175–192.
226. Rastenyte D, Tuomilehto J, Sarti C. Genetics of stroke—a review. *J Neurol Sci* 1998;153:132–145.
227. Martin JB. Molecular genetics in neurology. *Ann Neurol* 1993;34:757–773.
228. Auburger G. New genetic concepts and stroke prevention. *Cerebrovasc Dis* 1998;8 (Suppl 5): 28–32.
229. Goldbourt U, Neufeld HN. Genetic aspects of arteriosclerosis. *Arteriosclerosis* 1986;6:357–377.
230. MacLeod MJ, Dahiyat MT, Cumming A, Meiklejohn D, Shaw D, St.Clair D. No association between Glu/Asp polymorphism of NOS3 gene and ischemic stroke. *Neurology* 1999;53:418–420.
231. Bellamy MF, McDowell IF. Putative mechanisms for vascular damage by homocysteine. *Journal of Inherited Metabolic Disease* 1997;20:307–315.
232. Lobo CA, Millward SF. Homocystinuria: a cause of hypercoagulability that may be unrecognized. *J Vasc Interv Radiol* 1998;9:971–975.
233. Paoli D, Pierro L. Bilateral occlusion of the central retinal artery in a homocystinuric patient: the role of echography. *Ophthalmologica* 1998; 212(Suppl 1):95–98.
234. Cardo E, Campistol J, Caritg J, et al. Fatal haemorrhagic infarct in an infant with homocystinuria. *Developmental Medicine & Child Neurology* 1999;41:132–135.
235. Megnien JL, Gariepy J, Saudubray JM, et al. Evidence of carotid artery wall hypertrophy in homozygous homocystinuria. *Circulation* 1998; 98:2276–2281.
236. Wilcken DE, Wilcken B. The natural history of vascular disease in homocystinuria and the effects of treatment. *Journal of Inherited Metabolic Disease* 1997;20:295–300.
237. Crutchfield KE, Patronas NJ, Dambrosia JM, et al. Quantitative analysis of cerebral vasculopathy in patients with Fabry disease. *Neurology* 1998; 50:1746–1749.
238. Mitsias P, Levine SR. Cerebrovascular complications of Fabry's disease. *Ann Neurol* 1996; 40:8–17.
239. Maisey DN, Cosh JA. Basilar artery aneurysm and Anderson-Fabry disease. *J Neurol Neurosurg Psychiatry* 1980;43:85–87.
240. Liou CW, Huang CC, Chee EC, et al. MELAS syndrome: correlation between clinical features and molecular genetic analysis. *Acta Neurol Scand* 1994;90:354–359.
241. Ohno K, Isotani E, Hirakawa K. MELAS presenting as migraine complicated by stroke: case report. *Neuroradiology* 1997;39:781–784.
242. Gilchrist JM, Sikirica M, Stopa E, Shanske S. Adult-onset MELAS. Evidence for involvement of neurons as well as cerebral vasculature in strokelike episodes. *Stroke* 1996;27:1420–1423.
243. Driscoll PF, Larsen PD, Gruber AB. MELAS syndrome involving a mother and two children. *Arch Neurol* 1987;44:971–973.
244. Sakuta R, Nonaka I. Vascular involvement in mitochondrial myopathy. *Ann Neurol* 1989; 25:594–601.

245. Kokawa N, Ishii Y, Yamoto M, Nakano R. Pregnancy and delivery complicated by mitochondrial myopathy, encephalopathy, lactic acidosis, and stroke-like episodes. *Obstetrics & Gynecology* 1998;91:865.
246. Yanagawa T, Sakaguchi H, Nakao T, et al. Mitochondrial myopathy, encephalopathy, lactic acidosis, and stroke-like episodes with deterioration during pregnancy. *Intern Med* 1998;37: 780–783.
247. Provenzale JM, VanLandingham K. Cerebral infarction associated with Kearns-Sayre syndrome-related cardiomyopathy. *Neurology* 1996; 46:826–828.
248. Chinnery PF, Howell N, Lightowlers RN, Turnbull DM. MELAS and MERRF. The relationship between maternal mutation load and the frequency of clinically affected offspring. *Brain* 1998;121:1889–1894.
249. Kosinski C, Mull M, Lethen H, Topper R. Evidence for cardioembolic stroke in a case of Kearns-Sayre syndrome. *Stroke* 1995;26: 1950–1952.
250. Morin C, Dube J, Robinson BH, et al. Stroke-like episodes in autosomal recessive cytochrome oxidase deficiency. *Ann Neurol* 1999;45:389–392.
251. Desmond DW, Moroney JT, Lynch T, et al. CADASIL in a North American family: clinical, pathologic, and radiologic findings. *Neurology* 1998;51:844–849.
252. Joutel A, Corpechot C, Ducros A, et al. Notch3 mutations in CADASIL, a hereditary adult-onset condition causing stroke and dementia. *Nature* 1996;383:707–710.
253. Sabbadini G, Francia A, Calandriello L, et al. Cerebral autosomal dominant arteriopathy with subcortical infarcts and leucoencephalopathy (CADASIL). Clinical, neuroimaging, pathological and genetic study of a large Italian family. *Brain* 1995;118:207–215.
254. Bergmann M, Ebke M, Yuan Y, Bruck W, Mugler M, Schwendemann G. Cerebral autosomal dominant arteriopathy with subcortical infarcts and leukoencephalopathy (CADASIL): a morphological study of a German family. *Acta Neuropathol* 1996;92:341–350.
255. Adair JC, Hart BL, Kornfeld M, et al. Autosomal dominant cerebral arteriopathy: neuropsychiatric syndrome in a family. *Neuropsychiatry, Neuropsychology, & Behavioral Neurology* 1998;11: 31–39.
256. Ruchoux MM, Maurage CA. Endothelial changes in muscle and skin biopsies in patients with CADASIL. *Neuropathology & Applied Neurobiology* 1998;24:60–65.
257. Rubio A, Rifkin D, Powers JM, et al. Phenotypic variability of CADASIL and novel morphologic findings. *Acta Neuropathol* 1997;94:247–254.
258. Ebke M, Dichgans M, Bergmann M, et al. CADASIL: skin biopsy allows diagnosis in early stages. *Acta Neurol Scand* 1997;95:351–357.
259. Dichgans M, Mayer M, Uttner I, et al. The phenotypic spectrum of CADSIL: clinical findings in 102 cases. *Ann Neurol* 1998;44:731–739.
260. Taillia H, Chabriat H, Kurtz A, et al. Cognitive alterations in non-demented CADASIL patients. *Cerebrovasc Dis* 1998;8:97–101.
261. Trojano L, Ragno M, Manca A, Caruso G. A kindred affected by cerebral autosomal dominant arteriopathy with subcortical infarcts and leukoencephalopathy (CADASIL). A 2-year neuropsychological follow-up. *J Neurol* 1998;245: 217–222.
262. Hedera P, Friedland RP. Cerebral autosomal dominant arteriopathy with subcortical infarcts and leukoencephalopathy: study of two American families with predominant dementia. *J Neurol Sci* 1997;146:27–33.
263. Joutel A, Bousser MG, Biousse V, et al. A gene for familial hemiplegic migraine maps to chromosome 19. *Nature Genetics* 1993;5:40–45.
264. Dichgans M, Mayer M, Muller-Myhsok B, Straube A, Gasser T. Identification of a key recombinant narrows the CADASIL gene region to 8 cM and argues against allelism of CADASIL and familial hemiplegic migraine. *Genomics* 1996;32:151–154.
265. Hu WY, Hudon M. Neuroimaging highlight. Cerebral autosomal dominant arteriopathy withsubcortical infarcts and leukoencephalopathy (CADASIL). *Can J Neurol Sci* 1999;26:311–312.
266. Chabriat H, Levy C, Taillia H, et al. Patterns of MRI lesions in CADASIL. *Neurology* 1998;51: 452–457.
267. Chabriat H, Mrissa R, Levy C, et al. Brain stem MRI signal abnormalities in CADASIL. *Stroke* 1999;30:457–459.
268. Dichgans M, Filippi M, Bruning R, et al. Quantitative MRI in CADASIL. *Neurology* 1999;52:1361–1367.
269. Wielaard R, Bornebroek M, Ophoff RA, et al. A four-generation Dutch family with cerebral autosomal dominant arteriopathy with subcortical infarcts and leukoencephalopathy (CADASIL), linked to chromosome 19p13. *Clin Neurol Neurosurg* 1995;97:307–313.
270. Ruchoux MM, Chabriat H, Bousser MG, Baudrimont M, Tournier-Lasserve E. Presence of ultrastructural arterial lesions in muscle and skin vessels of patients with CADASIL. *Stroke* 1994;25:2291–2292.
271. Fukutake T, Hirayama K. Familial young-adult-onset arteriosclerotic leukoencephalopathy with alopecia and lumbago without arterial hypertension. *Eur Neurol* 1995;35:69–79.
272. Weil S, Reifenberger G, Dudel C, Yousry TA, Schriever S. Cerebroretinal vasculopathy mimicking a brain tumor: A case of a rare hereditary syndrome. *Neurology* 1999;53:629–631.
273. Schievink WI, Michels VV, Piepgras DG. Neurovascular manifestations of heritable connective tissue disorders. A review. *Stroke* 1994; 25:889–903.
274. Schievink WI, Limburg M, Oorthuys JW, Fleury P, Pope FM. Cerebrovascular disease in Ehlers-Danlos syndrome type IV. *Stroke* 1990;21: 626–632.
275. van den Berg JS, Limburg M, Kappelle LJ, Pals G, Arwert F, Westerveld. The role of type III collagen in spontaneous cervical arterial dissections. *Ann Neurol* 1998;43:494–498.
276. Hayward C, Brock DJ. Fibrillin-1 mutations in Marfan syndrome and other type-1

fibrillinopathies. *Human Mutation* 1997;10: 415–423.
277. Schievink WI, Bjornsson J, Piepgras DG. Coexistence of fibromuscular dysplasia and cystic medial necrosis in a patient with Marfan's syndrome and bilateral carotid artery dissections. *Stroke* 1994;25:2492–2496.
278. Mingke D, Dresler C, Pethig K, Heinemann M, Borst HG. Surgical treatment of Marfan patients with aneurysms and dissection of the proximal aorta. *J Cardiovasc Surg* 1998;39:65–74.
279. Gott VL, Greene PS, Alejo DE, et al. Replacement of the aortic root in patients with Marfan's syndrome. *N Engl J Med* 1999;340: 1307–1313.
280. Iqbal A, Alter M, Lee SH. Pseudoxanthoma elasticum: a review of neurological complications. *Ann Neurol* 1978;4:18–20.
281. Schievink WI, Prakash UB, Piepgras DG, Mokri B. Alpha 1-antitrypsin deficiency in intracranial aneurysms and cervical artery dissection. *Lancet* 1994;343:452–453.
282. Sobata E, Ohkuma H, Suzuki S. Cerebrovascular disorders associated with von Recklinghausen's neurofibromatosis: a case report. *Neurosurgery* 1988;22:544–549.
283. Grill J, Couanet D, Cappelli C, et al. Radiation-induced cerebral vasculopathy in children with neurofibromatosis and optic pathway glioma. *Ann Neurol* 1999;45:393–396.
284. Lanthier S, Carmant L, David M, Larbrisseau A, de Veber G. Stroke in children. The coexistence of multiple risk factors predicts poor outcome. *Neurology* 2000; 54:371–378.
285. Kenet G, Sadetzki S, Murad H, et al. Factor V Leiden and antiphospholipid antibodies are significant risk factors for ischemic stroke in children. *Stroke* 2000;31:1283–1288.
286. Chan MT, Nadareishvili ZG, Norris JW. Diagnostic strategies in young patients with ischemic stroke in Canada. *Can J Neurol Sci* 2000; 27:120–124.
287. Lanska DJ, Kryscio RJ. Risk factors for peripartum and postpartum stroke and intracranialvenous thrombosis. *Stroke* 2000;31:1274–1282.
288. Rosing J, Middeldorp S, Curvers J, et al. Low-dose oral contraceptives and acquired resistance to activated protein C: a randomised cross-over study. *Lancet* 2000;354:2036–2040.
289. Numminen H, Syrjala M, Benthin G, Kaste M, Hillbom M. The effect of acute ingestion of a large dose of alcohol on the hemostatic system and its circadian variation. *Stroke* 2000;31: 1269–1273.
290. Yamauchi T, Tada M, Houkin K, et al. Linkage of familial moyamoya disease (spontaneous occlusion of the Circle of Willis) to chromosome 17q25. *Stroke* 2000;31:930–935.
291. Molnar MJ, Valikovics A, Molnar S, et al. Cerebral blood flow and glucose metabolism in mitochondrial disorders. *Neurology* 2000;55: 544–548.
292. Chabriat H, Pappata S, Ostergaard L, et al. Cerebral hemodynamics in CADASIL before and after acetazolamide challenge assessed with MRI bolus tracking. *Stroke* 2000;31: 1904–1912.

Chapter 10

MEDICAL THERAPY FOR PREVENTION OF ISCHEMIC STROKE

GENERAL PRINCIPLES IN PREVENTION OF ISCHEMIC STROKE

Prevention of ischemic stroke is the most cost-effective strategy for treatment of patients with cerebrovascular disease[1,367] Economically, prevention of stroke eliminates the costs of acute hospital care and rehabilitation. Prevention is key in lowering mortality and morbidity from ischemic stroke. Effective therapies to forestall stroke also improve quality of life for both the persons who otherwise would have had a vascular event and their families. Since the 1970s, detection of risk factors that promote premature and advanced atherosclerosis has permitted the development of therapies to slow the progression of this leading vascular disease.[367] Guidelines for treatment are available.[368] Future advances in development of interventions that affect the course of atherosclerosis are likely. Also since the 1970s, medical and surgical therapies of proven usefulness have become available for treatment of high-risk patients. Additional improvements in medical or surgical care should be anticipated.

Identification of High-Risk Patients

Although stroke can potentially affect any person, several conditions identify a person as being at increased risk. The details about the leading risk factors for accelerated atherosclerosis, heart disease, and stroke are discussed in Chapter 2. Effective management of these factors has a major impact on lessening the likelihood of stroke. The most important components in risk-factor reduction are controlling hypertension, stopping smoking, avoiding heavy alcohol consumption, losing weight, and treating hypercholesteroleima.[2] Because atherosclerosis evolves over many years, treatment to halt its progression should span an individual's lifetime. Early treatment may be the most effective strategy because halting development of the initial stages of atherosclerosis might be more successful than trying to alter the composition or extent of a complex, symptomatic plaque. Still, evidence demonstrating the long-term efficacy of this approach is not available from clinical trials. One must remember that a healthy patient might be treated at a young age with the goal of forestalling a potential event that might not occur until as much as 50 years later. The cost-effectiveness and public acceptance of some of the more expensive and potentially dangerous interventions likely will be low; however, public health measures aimed toward changing life-style and avoiding risky behaviors make considerable sense.

Public health efforts to control weight should begin in childhood or adolescence and continue throughout life. Most people find weight loss a difficult goal to achieve. A sustained program of reducing caloric intake and maintaining an active life-style likely will be more effective than fad diets or weight-loss medications. Ways to maintain a high level of physical activity should start at the same time. Exercise can result in weight loss and improve cardiovascular fitness. Exercise also is a good tonic to control stress. Efforts to teach avoidance of tobacco and alcohol abuse should focus on adolescents and young adults, the most vulnerable groups in the population. The best plan is never to start smoking or abusing alcohol, and education is the core of this effort. Young people should be warned that tobacco or alcohol abuse causes several adverse consequences on health, including increasing the risk of stroke. Unfortunately, peer and societal pressures run counter to these activities. As a result, even coordinated educational programs by governmental and public health groups are making a very small impact. Despite failures, the most reasonable course seems to be to continue these efforts. Treatment of hypercholesterolemia also should focus on younger persons. This program can be extended to older patients. The initial emphasis should be on dietary modifications, rather than the use of medications. Treatment of hypertension also is a lifetime process. Although most patients eventually need medications, weight loss, exercise, and life-style modifications may be effective for some persons.

Some asymptomatic persons have a much higher risk for stroke than the general population. In these circumstances, additional surgical or medical therapies may be indicated even though the patient has no neurological complaints. Persons with atrial fibrillation have a much higher risk for cardioembolic stroke than do persons with normal sinus rhythm.[3,4] (See

Chapter 6.) Patients with atrial fibrillation often do not have either neurological or cardiac symptoms. Because atrial fibrillation is very prevalent among persons older than 60 years and because it is such a potent risk factor for stroke, measures to lower the likelihood of secondary cardioembolism can have a major impact on stroke rates.[5] Patients older than 75 and with ischemic heart disease, cardiomegaly, hypertension, or sustained atrial fibrillation benefit most from treatment.[3,6] Treatment of the atrial fibrillation itself (with medical or electrical cardioversion) also is an important way to prevent embolism to the brain.[7,8] Hart et al[9] recently concluded that post-menopausal use of estrogen and moderate alcohol consumption might be additional ways to lower the risk of stroke in patients with atrial fibrillation. Other high-risk cardiac lesions include mitral stenosis or an intracardiac thrombus; patients with these cardiac conditions need medical treatment and, on occasion, surgical therapy.[10] Thus, measures that directly treat high-risk heart diseases can effectively lower the chances of complicating stroke.

Patients with symptomatic atherosclerotic disease in the coronary or peripheral arteries have a high risk for ischemic stroke. Therefore, management of patients with these illnesses should incorporate stroke-prevention strategies. In general, the most commonly prescribed medications to prevent limb or cardiac ischemia, antiplatelet aggregating agents, also are useful in lowering the risk of ischemic stroke. Patients with an asymptomatic bruit or stenosis of the internal carotid artery also have a high risk for myocardial infarction, ischemic stroke, or vascular death.[11–13] (See Chapter 5.) The risks of stroke are greatest among persons younger than 75.

Management of Risk Factors

Management of risk factors for accelerated atherosclerosis is a fundamental component of treatment to prevent ischemic stroke or recurrent stroke (Table 10–1).

Table 10–1. **General Measures to Control Risk Factors for Prevention of Ischemic Stroke**

- Life-style
  - Control weight
  - Increase exercise
  - No smoking
  - Alcohol consumption in moderation
  - No use of drugs of abuse
- Specific interventions
  - Treat hypertension
  - Treat diabetes
  - Treat hyperlipidemia—hypercholesterolemia
  - Treat hyperhomocystinemia

Public education about the importance of these risk factors is critical. Unfortunately, knowledge about the conditions that increase the chance of stroke is low.[14] The presence of multiple risk factors greatly increases the risk of stroke, and each should be addressed.[15] Treatment of arterial hypertension is the single most effective strategy in primary prevention of ischemic stroke.[2,5,16–20] Patients with untreated and treated but uncontrolled hypertension have a high risk for stroke.[20] Both diastolic and isolated systolic hypertension increase the risk of stroke, and an elevation of a diastolic blood pressure >90 mm Hg or systolic blood pressure >140 mm Hg should prompt treatment.[21,22] The goal for blood pressure values should be 80–85 mm Hg diastolic and 130–140 mm Hg systolic.[19,23] Blood pressure can be lowered through dietary changes, exercise, weight loss, or medications.[5,24–26] The choices for anti-hypertensive medications are listed in Table 2–5. A clinical trial tested the combination of aspirin and atenolol in prevention of stroke among high-risk patients, but the addition of the beta-blocking agent did not prove to be effective.[27] Thus, the administration of an antihypertensive agent should not be considered as a direct stroke-prevention therapy. Rather, these agents indirectly lower the risk of stroke by slowing the progression of extracranial or intracranial arterial disease or preventing heart disease.

Vigorous treatment of hyperglycemia is not established as a useful way to prevent stroke in diabetic patients. Still, lowering of blood sugars to normoglycemic values is recommended, and this strategy may lessen the risk of stroke.[17,28] A goal is a concentration of <126 mg/dL (<6.99 mmol/L), although the desired level of blood glucose also is unknown.[19] Patients with either type I or type II diabetes could be treated with diet alone or in combination with an oral agent or insulin. Weight loss can lessen the risk of hypertension and diabetes mellitus.[17] Exercise can lower weight, blood pressure, serum glucose, and serum cholesterol. Although patients should be encouraged to participate in exercise on a regular basis, the activities must be tailored to the individual needs of patients with a prior stroke or other motor impairments. Stopping smoking is a very cost-effective strategy. The patient does not incur the expense of the tobacco. Abstinence for 5 years results in risk lowered, to that of a non-smoker.[17,29,30] Medications can be used to help a patient stop smoking.[31] Elevated plasma homocysteine levels are increasingly recognized as an important risk factor for ischemic vascular disease, including stroke.[32,33] Vitamin supplementation with folate, 0.5–5 mg/day; pyridoxine, 20 mg/day; and vitamin B12, 0.5 mg/day, can lower homocysteine levels and might be helpful in preventing stroke.[33] Still undetermined is the effectiveness of hormone replacement therapy in lowering the risk of stroke among post-menopausal women.[34]

Unfortunately, Joseph et al[35] reported that a stroke-prevention program that emphasizes modification of risk factors for treatment of patients with stroke results in little improvement in controlling weight, smoking, hyperglycemia, hypercholesterolemia, or smoking. Most patients do not stop smoking, do not lose weight, and do not change their diets. Although these results are discouraging, this component of management to prevent stroke cannot be abandoned. Additional tactics are needed to improve the control of risk factors of persons at high risk for ischemic stroke. Education and emotional support likely will be key. Continued reinforcement of the importance of risk-factor management should occur at the time of each clinic visit. Monitoring of blood pressure, serum glucose, and blood lipids should be repeated at regular intervals and at the time of follow-up clinic visits. The results of the assessments should be discussed and new ways (diet, medications, etc.) explored to address these risk factors. Medications to control risk factors, including stopping smoking, could be prescribed in conjunction with dietary and life-style modifications. Still, the prescription of medical therapies to control risk factors likely will be futile unless the patient's behavior changes.

Treatment of co-developing ischemic heart disease is an important component of management. Persons with ischemic neurological symptoms, especially those with atherosclerosis, are at very high risk for cardiac ischemia.[36] Myocardial infarction is a leading long-term cause of death among persons who have survived a stroke or who have had a transient ischemic attack (TIA).[37] In addition to prevention of premature death or disability, secondary artery disease treatment of the coronary artery disease can also lower the risk of cardioembolic stroke from a myocardial infarction complicated by atrial fibrillation or an intraventricular thrombus (see Chapter 6). Thus, effective management of coronary artery disease is a prudent stroke-prevention strategy in its own right. The coronary artery disease may be asymptomatic at the time of the neurological event.[38] Thus, an effort to screen for coronary artery disease should be included in the evaluation of patients identified as being at high risk for ischemic stroke. The proposed evaluation is included in Chapter 4.

Prevention of Stroke with the HMG Co A Reductase Inhibitor Medications

Treatment of hypercholesterolemia is a leading component of management to lessen the risk of ischemic events among patients with atherosclerosis.[39–41,369] In the past, the primary aim of therapies to lower cholesterol levels was to prevent coronary artery disease and myocardial infarction. Now the benefit of reducing cholesterol levels for prevention of ischemic stroke, especially among persons younger than 75 years, is becoming increasingly obvious. Treatment of hypercholesterolemia is as critical for prevention of cerebral infarction as it is for prevention of myocardial infarction. Lowering serum cholesterol values can be effective in slowing the progression of the early changes of atherosclerotic lesions. Furberg et al[42] showed that agents slow development of intimal-medial thickness of the internal carotid artery, a finding on carotid duplex that is a surrogate for the earliest changes of atherosclerosis. Early treatment of the evolving atherosclerotic plaque could focus on reducing inflammation, smooth muscle proliferation, and lipid deposition in the arterial wall. At this point, the changes might be reversible. At present, no medical therapies, including cholesterol-lowering medications, are likely to reverse the abnormalities found in a mature, complex atherosclerotic plaque.

In 1993, Atkins et al[43] reported that the use of cholesterol-lowering medications did not reduce the risk of stroke. They also concluded that clofibrate actually might increase the risk of a cerebrovascular event. An overview performed in 1995 found a modest or no effect in the reduction of risk of stroke by treatment of hypercholesterolemia.[44] Since then, several clinical trials have tested the usefulness of HMG Co A reductase inhibitors and found that these medications were very effective in preventing both ischemic cerebrovascular and cardiovascular events.[41,45–47] A Scandinavian study noted that strokes occurred in 4.3% of patients treated with placebo and 2.7% of patients given simvastatin; although the overall risk of stroke was relatively low, the relative reduction in risk with treatment with significant.[48] (See Table 10–2.) Plehn et al[49] found that prescribing pravastatin after a myocardial infarction reduced the risk of stroke by approximately 32%. Lewis et al[50] reported that pravastatin lowered the risk of ischemic stroke among older patients who had a history of a myocardial infarction but average blood levels of cholesterol. The risk of stroke was 7.3% among the placebo-treated patients and 4.5% among those receiving pravastatin (2.9% absolute risk reduction/40% relative risk reduction). Several meta-analyses demonstrate that the HMG Co A reductase inhibitors reduce the risk of stroke by approximately 30%–60%.[51–54] These studies provide compelling

Table 10–2. **Clinical Trials of HMG Co A Reductase Inhibitors and Prevention of Stroke**

Study	Medication	Patients Treatment Strokes Strokes	Patients Control
WOSCOPS	Pravastatin	46/3302	51/3292
4 S	Simvastatin	75/2221	102/2223
CARE	Pravastatin	54/2081	78/2078
LIPID	Pravastatin	171/4512	198/4502
ACAPS	Lovastatin	0/460	2/459
KAPS	Pravastatin	2/224	4/223
Totals		348/12,800	435/12,777

WOSCOPS = West of Scotland Coronary Prevention Study[353]; 4 S = Scandinavian Simvastatin Survival Study[48]; CARE = Cholesterol and Recurrent Events[49,354]; LIPID = Long-term Intervention with Pravastatin in Ischaemic Disease[355]; ACAPS = Asymptomatic Carotid Artery Progression Study[42]; KAPS = Kuopio Atherosclerosis Prevention Study.[41]

evidence that prescription of a HMG Co A reductase inhibitor can dramatically reduce the risk of stroke among patients with hypercholesterolemia, including those with a history of myocardial ischemia.[40] By implication, the same benefit should accrue with treatment of patients with ischemic neurological symptoms and hypercholesterolemia, including older patients.[369,370,371]

The reduction in risk with the HMG Co A reductase inhibitors is approximately the same as that obtained with the prescription of antiplatelet aggregating agents.[40] These reductions truly are impressive. Although most of the available data involve patients with a history of symptomatic coronary artery disease, ongoing trials are testing the usefulness of the HMG Co A reductase inhibitors in prevention of recurrent stroke among patients with symptomatic cerebrovascular disease. The mechanism for the lowering of ischemic events is not clear, but it may be independent of the cholesterol-lowering effects of the HMG Co A reductase inhibitors.[40] This scenario is proposed because the declines in the number of vascular events seem far greater than the documented effects on reducing cholesterol values. In addition, the responses appear relatively soon after starting treatment, and it seems improbable that declines in cholesterol will rapidly alter or shrink atherosclerotic plaques resulting in fewer events. Corsini et al[55] reported that the statins interfered with smooth muscle proliferation in the arterial wall. The changes in cholesterol concentrations might change endothelial function, but data to support this hypothesis are not available. These changes may modify arterial wall contractility or the fracturing of atherosclerotic plaques. The medications themselves may affect platelets or influence the production of natural anticoagulant proteins. Further research about the affects of these medications on hemostasis is needed.

These medications already are indicated for the management of patients with hypercholesterolemia whether or not the patient has had ischemic symptoms. The role of these medications as an adjunctive therapy among persons with normal or modestly elevated cholesterol levels needs exploration. Experimental studies have shown that the HMG Co A reductase inhibitors may reduce the volume of ischemic strokes by affecting production of nitric oxide.[56] Recently, Vaughan and Delanty[57] speculated that the HMG Co A reductase inhibitors might offer neural protection by altering production of endothelial nitric oxide synthase, by reducing inflammatory cytokines, and through antioxidant properties. Additional research likely will clarify the role of these agents in the protection of the brain among patients at high risk for ischemic stroke. An increasingly important role in the prophylaxis of stroke can be anticipated.

PREVENTION OF ISCHEMIC STROKE AMONG HIGH-RISK PATIENTS

In addition to controlling risk factors that promote vascular disease, the prevention of ischemic stroke among high-risk patients usually involves the prescription of medications that prevent thromboembolism. Regardless of the underlying vascular pathology, a thromboembolic process incites the actual occurrence of acute ischemia. Thus, prevention of thrombosis is the cornerstone in ischemic stroke prophylaxis. The medical therapies often are complemented by surgical procedures to restore or improve blood flow to the brain or to correct an underlying cardiac or vascular process that promotes the formation of thrombi. As such, surgical interventions should be considered as adjunctive therapies to the basic medical regimen. The decision is not surgical versus medical therapy to prevent stroke. Rather, the key aspect of management is a decision about surgical and medical therapy versus medical treatment alone.

Patients with amaurosis fugax, TIA, or ischemic stroke are at the greatest risk for ischemic stroke. Of these groups, the likelihood is highest among patients with a prior ischemic stroke.[13] (See Table 10–3.) The outcomes of patients who have recurrent stroke are poorer than among those patients who have only one event.[58]

Table 10–3. **Persons at Highest Risk for Ischemic Stroke or Recurrent Ischemic Stroke**

Clinical
- Ischemic stroke
- Transient ischemic attack
  - Crescendo events
  - Prolonged or severe event
- Amaurosis fugax
- Atrial fibrillation with structural heart disease
- Recent anterior myocardial infarction
- Asymptomatic carotid bruit or stenosis
- Atrial fibrillation without structural heart disease

Vascular imaging
- Intraluminal thrombus in artery
- Severe stenosis of the internal carotid artery
- Ulcerated plaque of the internal carotid artery
- Extensive atherosclerotic disease

Cardiac imaging
- Intraventricular or intra-atrial thrombus
- Valvular vegetations or dysfunction
- Dilated left atrium or ventricle

Patients do not recover as well or as fast after a second stroke as after the first. The risk of recurrent neurological symptoms is time linked and is at a peak in the first days and weeks after the ischemic event. Thus, the evaluation and treatment of patients with recent ischemic symptoms should be started to forestall another event.

Still, separating acute and long-term stroke-prevention therapy is clinically important. The emphasis of treatment for a patient who is seriously ill or medically unstable likely will be aimed at saving the patient's life, ameliorating the neurological consequences of the stroke, or controlling complications. Differentiating the first days after stroke seems arbitrary, but some of the therapies to prevent recurrent stroke might be dangerous if they were administered within the first few days after an acute ischemic event. For example, carotid endarterectomy may be complicated by increased brain edema if the operation is done soon after stroke. Intracranial hemorrhage is a potential complication of the administration of anticoagulants within the first days after ischemic stroke. Differentiating acute and long-term care also is important when reviewing data from clinical trials. Information about both safety and efficacy is affected by the interval from stroke. For example, the benefits and risks of treatment with long-term anticoagulation to prevent recurrent cardioembolism should not be confused with the benefits and risks of emergent anticoagulation. With careful patient selection and treatment, long-term anticoagulation is effective and relatively safe. In contrast, acute anticoagulation has not been shown to be either safe or effective. Conversely, a patient with a mild stroke probably has a low risk for complications from the disease or the therapies to prevent recurrences. In this situation, the best approach is to emulate the strategy for treatment of patients with recent TIA. The timing of starting therapies to prevent recurrent stroke should be made on a case-by-case basis.

Because patients with previous neurological symptoms have the highest risk, the benefit for medical or surgical therapies to prevent stroke will be highest among this population. Treatments of proven value include anticoagulants, antiplatelet aggregating agents, and carotid endarterectomy (Table 10–4). Extracranial–intracranial

Table 10–4. **Antithrombotic Agents That Could Be Used to Prevent Ischemic Stroke**

- Heparin
- Low molecular weight heparins
- Danaparoid
- Oral anticoagulants (vitamin K antagonists) (warfarin)
- Hirudin and hirulog
- Thrombin inhibitors (argatroban, napsagatran, inogatran, melagatran)
- Factor Xa inhibitors (tick anticoagulant peptide, antistatin)
- Activated protein C
- Thrombomodulin
- Tissue factor inhibitors
- Factor VII inhibitors

bypass procedures, angioplasty and stenting, and other vascular operations can be prescribed to treat exceptional cases. Cardiovascular operations also can be used to prevent ischemic stroke.

Most therapies have a risk for potentially serious or life-threatening complications. In most circumstances, the likelihood for significantly lowering the chances of stroke justifies the potential side effects. Still, the decision for treatment should be based on a careful calculation of the likely risks and benefits of treatment. The risks and benefits of alternative forms of management, including no specific intervention, should be included in these calculations. The choice of therapies is influenced by several variables, including the patient's age, overall health, and presence of co-morbid diseases. Specific contraindications, such as an allergy, previous adverse experiences, or a medical illness such as peptic ulcer disease, also can affect decisions about treatment. The occurrence of neurological symptoms during treatment with a specific therapy or major complications from the agent also affect decisions about future management. The preferences of the patient, the availability of follow-up care, and patient compliance also are critical.

The presumed vascular territory reflecting the patient's neurological symptoms greatly affects decisions about surgical procedures. Carotid endarterectomy and other revascularization operations are prescribed more frequently for patients with symptoms of carotid circulation ischemia than among those with vertebrobasilar events. In the future, angioplasty might find a role in local treatment of vertebrobasilar atherosclerosis. If angioplasty proves to be helpful, then it would greatly influence plans for evaluation and treatment of most patients with symptoms of ischemia in the posterior circulation.

Most patients with atherosclerotic cerebrovascular disease are treated with antiplatelet aggregating agents regardless of a decision about surgical management. Antiplatelet aggregating agents usually are prescribed to patients with non-atherosclerotic vasculopathies, although anticoagulants are given on occasion to persons with severely stenotic arterial diseases. Etiology-specific treatments are the mainstay of management of patients with some of the uncommon non-atherosclerotic vasculopathies. For example, antibiotics are prescribed to patients with meningovascular syphilis, and immunosuppressive agents are key to management of patients with autoimmune vasculitis. Anticoagulants are the usual treatment to prevent stroke among patients with high-risk cardiac lesions, including persons with neurological symptoms. Although antiplatelet aggregating agents do lessen the risk of embolism among patients with "low-risk" heart diseases, the occurrence of a TIA or an ischemic stroke automatically denotes the cardiac lesion as being high risk. Combinations of antiplatelet aggregating agents or antiplatelet aggregating agents with anticoagulants also can be prescribed. The usual scenario is when a patient has had recurrent symptoms despite treatment with one medical agent alone.

ANTICOAGULANTS

Anticoagulants are a fundamental component of medical management to prevent ischemic stroke. The rationale for these therapies is that most ischemic strokes are secondary to thromboembolism that leads to an occlusion of an extracranial or intracranial artery. The anticoagulants inhibit the action of several native procoagulant proteins, including thrombin. This inhibition would limit formation of a large intraluminal thrombus, which leads to arterial occlusion or can be a source of emboli to the brain. Intravenously or orally administered anticoagulants can be prescribed to patients with a TIA or an ischemic stroke. Despite the widespread use of these therapies to prevent stroke, they have been controversial because of the limited data about either their safety or efficacy. Recently, several clinical studies evaluated the usefulness of anticoagulants in the management of patients with ischemic cerebrovascular disease. The results of these studies, described subsequently in this chapter, are mixed. Delineating the data from trials testing chronic anticoagulation from the information from trials evaluating acute treatment is critical to understand the role of anticoagulation in prevention of stroke. The role of long-term anticoagulation for prevention of cardioembolic stroke has been strengthened; these agents now are the treatment of choice for this indication. The results of recent trials have highlighted the limited utility of emergent anticoagulant treatment. The usefulness of anticoagulants in acute treatment of patients with recent neurological symptoms probably is far from established. Data do not demonstrate that anticoagulants effectively reduce the early risk of recurrent stroke. The role of long-term oral anticoagulant therapy for treatment of patients with ischemic symptoms secondary to arterial diseases remains uncertain. Data are limited about the use of anticoagulants in conjunction with other medical or surgical therapies to prevent stroke.

The most commonly prescribed agents are warfarin, heparin, the low molecular weight heparins, and danaparoid. These agents are discussed in this chapter. Additional agents that affect coagulation are under development or are being tested (see Table 10–4). Although these agents are listed in this chapter for updating purposes, they are not discussed in detail because of marginal information about their clinical utility. Some of these agents have attributes that might make them useful, but their potential role in ischemic stroke prevention is unclear.

HEPARIN

Pharmacology

Heparin is a complex and heterogeneous glycosaminoglycan that has been used for more than 40 years for the prevention of arterial or venous thromboembolism.[59] It is a biological product derived from bovine or porcine sources. Heparin has a wide range of pharmacologic and pharmacokinetic properties. Heparin is not one compound; rather, it is a mixture of pieces of glycosaminoglycans. The molecular weight of heparin ranges from 5000 to 30,000 Daltons, with the usual weight being approximately 15,000 Daltons. Only approximately one-third of the heparin molecules actually produce an anticoagulant effect.[60] The clearance of heparin by the body is influenced by the size of the compound; the higher molecular weight components are cleared from the circulation more quickly than are the lower molecular weight compounds.[60] Heparin cannot be given orally; the preferred routes of administration are subcutaneous or intravenous injections. Intramuscular injection is avoided because of the high risk for local hematoma. Adequate levels of anticoagulation can be achieved with either intravenous or subcutaneous injections, but a several hour lag in achieving responses occurs with subcutaneous administration. Patients receiving subcutaneous heparin may not have therapeutic levels of anticoagulation until 24 hours after starting treatment. If an immediate anticoagulant effect is needed, then the preferred route of administration is an intravenous bolus dose followed by a continuous intravenous infusion.[60] Because heparin is negatively charged, it binds to a number of plasma proteins, platelet derived proteins, and proteins released by endothelial cells.[60] Variations in concentrations of these proteins among patients partially explain the marked inter-individual differences in clinical response to heparin.

The anticoagulant properties of heparin are due to its structure, which permits high-affinity binding to antithrombin III.[60] Heparin alters the conformation of antithrombin III and results in a marked increase in the ability of antithrombin III to inactivate thrombin, activated factor X, and activated factor IX. The inactivation of thrombin is the primary mechanism of the anticoagulant actions of heparin. Heparin does not affect either thrombin or activated factor X already bound to a formed clot.[61] Heparin also affects the inactivation of thrombin via heparin cofactor II. This effect is separated from its actions on antithrombin III function and occurs only with high concentrations of the agent.[60] In addition, the larger molecular weight components of heparin appear to perturb endothelial modulation of clotting factors and platelet factor IV.[61] In particular, the interaction with platelet factor IV may explain some of the anti-thrombotic properties of heparin.

Unfortunately, heparin has a narrow therapeutic window; the difference between a safe but effective dose and a dangerous one is relatively small.[61] A clear association is present between the risk of serious bleeding and escalating doses of heparin. The optimal dose for heparin for effective treatment of patients with recent TIA or ischemic stroke still is not known. The relationships between the dose of heparin and either its safety or its efficacy are complex. The dosage of heparin usually is modified in reaction to biological responses. Thus, marked differences in response to a dose are found among patients. In addition, an individual patient's responses can change for no clinically obvious reason.

The activated partial thromboplastin time (aPTT) is the most widely used test to monitor responses to heparin. This test reacts to heparin's inhibition of thrombin, activated factor X, and activated factor IX. Despite its widespread use, the test has limitations. For example, patients with the lupus anticoagulant syndrome will have falsely elevated aPTT concentrations, and monitoring heparin therapy with aPTT levels in this situation is precarious. Because of the marked variability of heparin, its binding to proteins, and its biological activity, the correlations between heparin concentrations and aPTT levels are relatively poor.[60] The optimal level of aPTT remains unknown for the patient receiving heparin. The usual therapeutic aPTT level for heparin is assumed to be approximately 1.5 times control levels. Still, data to support this level of anticoagulation come largely from trials of treatment to prevent deep vein thrombosis, and information about the level of anticoagulation for prevention of arterial thrombosis is unknown.

As alternatives to the aPTT, blood concentrations of heparin or level of inhibition of activated factor X also can use used to monitor dosages and administration. However, these tests are not widely available and they are more cumbersome than the aPTT. The usual desired level of inhibition of activated factor X is 0.3—0.7 U/mL.[60] Measurements of levels of inhibition of activated factor X are needed to assess responses to treatment with heparin in persons with lupus anticoagulants.

Most patients receive approximately 24,000–30,000 units of heparin daily to maintain a therapeutic level of anticoagulation. Still, a broad range of doses can be expected. For the prevention of deep vein thrombosis, most patients receive 5000 units subcutaneously one or twice a day. A different regimen has been used to treat patients with acute thromboembolic disease. A dose of heparin (often 5000 or 10,000 units) has been given intravenously to initiate treatment. This dose was followed by an intravenous infusion—usually in the range of 1000 units/hour. Because the anticoagulant effects of an intravenous bolus of heparin are immediate, the aPTT level will be markedly prolonged if it is measured immediately after the administration of the medication. Thereafter, the aPTT will decline toward desired levels as the follow-up maintenance infusion is continued. Traditionally, at approximately 6 hours, the aPTT was measured and dosages adjusted upward or downward in increments of 100 units. Unfortunately, this time-honored approach does not take into consideration the marked variances in responses among patients. As a result, some patients were receiving excessive levels of anticoagulation, and others were inadequately treated. Both bleeding and ischemic complications could occur. This traditional strategy has been abandoned for both safety and lack of efficacy concerns. The patient's size is an important variable that affects responses to heparin. As a result, weight-based nomograms have been developed to ease the initial administration of heparin.[62,63] These nomograms are effective in safely achieving desired levels of anticoagulation within a reasonable length of time. The nomograms continue to include an initial intravenous

Table 10–5. **Weight-Based Nomogram for Initial Intravenous Administration of Treatment with Heparin**

- Initial dose: Give 80 U/kg bolus followed by infusion at 18 U/kg/hr
- Check aPTT at 6 hours, and adjust infusion in response to levels

aPTT <35 seconds (<1.2 × control)
  Give another 80 U/kg bolus followed by infusion at 22 U/kg/hr
  Net increase of 4 U/kg/hr
aPTT 35–45 seconds (1.2–1.5 × control)
  Give another 40 U/kg bolus followed by infusion at 20 U/kg/hr
  Net increase of 2 U/kg/hr
aPTT 46–70 seconds (1.5–2.3 × control)
  Do not change rate of infusion
aPTT 71–90 seconds (2.3–3 × control)
  Decrease infusion to 16 U/kg/hr
  Net decrease of 2 U/kg/hr
aPTT >91 seconds (>3 × control)
  Interrupt infusion for 1 hour; then start infusion at 15 U/kg/hr
  Net decrease of 3 U/kg/hr
Recheck the aPTT 6 hours after adjustment
Re-adjust treatment regimen in response to aPTT and most recent dosage

Adapted from Hirsh et al,[60] Raschke et al,[63] and Becker and Ansell.[62]

bolus dose to achieve anticoagulation immediately and, thereafter, is followed by a continuous infusion (Table 10–5). Subsequently, the infusion has a weight-based adjustment in response to the aPTT levels. This regimen is superior to the traditional approach of starting a relatively uniform dose.[63] This method of starting heparin treatment should be used when the agent is being given to patients with recent TIA. Adjustments to the treatment regimen can be made in response to the aPTT levels (see Table 10–5). The level of anticoagulation declines rapidly after a bolus if a follow-up intravenous infusion is not administered. Thus, intermittent intravenous boluses of heparin should be avoided. Not only will the intermittent dose regimen lead to long periods when the patient is not receiving adequate levels of anticoagulation, but the intermittent spikes in available drug following the boluses may increase the likelihood of bleeding complications. There is no indication for the subcutaneous administration of heparin to prevent stroke among patients who are neurologically unstable.

Safety

Bleeding is the most common major complication of treatment with heparin (Table 10–6). Petty et al[64] calculated that the risk of bleeding with heparin is 0.3/100 person-days. This risk is higher than with either

Table 10–6. **Complications of Heparin in Patients with Ischemic Cerebrovascular Disease**

Hemorrhagic transformation of an infarction
Other intracranial bleeding
Systemic bleeding
  Retroperitoneal hemorrhage
  Gastrointestinal hemorrhage
  Genitourinary hemorrhage
  Soft tissue hematoma
Thrombocytopenia—white clot syndrome
  Ischemic stroke
  Myocardial infarction
Digital ischemia—purple toe syndrome
Osteoporosis

aspirin or warfarin. The risk of bleeding generally is associated with the dose of heparin and level of aPTT.[65] There are no data about the risk of bleeding with different administration techniques. For example, subcutaneous administration of heparin may not be safer than intravenous treatment. Data also do not exist indicating that a bolus dose to rapidly achieve anticoagulation is particularly dangerous. A continuous intravenous infusion appears to be safer than intermittent bolus doses. Systemic or intracranial hemorrhage can occur in persons receiving heparin for treatment of either arterial or venous occlusive disease. Intracranial hemorrhage, including hemorrhagic transformation of the infarction, is the leading life-threatening complication of heparin treatment given to patients with a recent ischemic stroke. In general, the risk of central nervous system bleeding is associated with the severity of the patient's neurological impairments. Thus, the likelihood of major brain bleeding is not great among patients receiving heparin for treatment of a TIA unless the level of anticoagulation is markedly excessive. The risk of bleeding also appears to be increased among women, persons with renal failure, and patients older than 70.[65]

Minor hemorrhages (microscopic hematuria, epistaxis, bleeding hemorrhoids) may not necessitate stopping heparin; a dosage adjustment alone may be needed. More serious bleeding usually prompts discontinuance of the heparin. Protamine sulfate can be administered to patients with serious or life-threatening hemorrhagic complications secondary to heparin. Approximately 1 mg. of protamine sulfate neutralizes the anticoagulant effects of 100 units of heparin. The dose of protamine is calculated on an assumption of a 60-minute half-life for heparin and would correspond to the amount of heparin given during the immediately preceding hour and one-half of the dosage given during the previous hour.[60] Intravenous protamine should be given slowly (over at least 10 minutes) because it can cause hypotension, and rare cases of anaphylaxis secondary to protamine have been reported.[60]

A decline in platelet count commonly follows treatment with heparin. In one series of 137 patients with ischemic cerebrovascular disease, a >40% decline in platelet count was observed in 21.[66] In most cases, the drop in platelet count was asymptomatic. However, the administration of heparin is associated with an autoimmune-mediated thrombocytopenia that can lead to white clot syndrome and stroke.[67–69] In addition, digital ischemia and purple toe syndrome can complicate heparin treatment.[70] (See Table 10–6.) These prothrombotic conditions and their treatment are described in Chapter 8. In addition, long-term administration of heparin can lead to osteoporosis.

Potential Indications

Anticoagulation, initially with heparin and subsequently with warfarin, is a potential alternative to carotid endarterectomy for treatment of patients with a recent TIA or a minor stroke and an intraluminal thrombus in the ipsilateral internal carotid artery.[71] (See Table 10–7.) Carotid endarterectomy can be associated with a high risk of ischemic cerebrovascular complications when the operation is done in the presence of an intraluminal clot. A course of anticoagulants might foster resolution of the thrombus and permit scheduling of the carotid endarterectomy to remove the underlying plaque at a later date. Small studies have shown that this course of treatment can be successful with

Table 10–7. **Potential Indications for Heparin: Treatment of Patients with Transient Ischemic Attack or Stroke**

Presence of an intraluminal thrombus
High-grade arterial stenosis with or without thrombus
Perioperative management of patients undergoing vascular surgery
Intracardiac thrombus
Crescendo or recent transient ischemic attacks
Recent cardioembolic event
Initiation of treatment with oral anticoagulants

patients remaining symptom-free.[72,73] Although these studies support the use of heparin as an interim, pre-operative measure, the data are not definitive. A brief course of heparin is administered for treatment of patients with high-grade stenosis of the internal carotid artery and who are scheduled for carotid endarterectomy. Although this situation is a potential indication for anticoagulant therapy, clinical studies do not establish the efficacy of heparin for these high-risk patients. Heparin is used regularly as a perioperative treatment to lessen the risks of embolization during carotid endarterectomy and other reconstructive vascular procedures.[74,75] Still, the problem of heparin-associated thrombocytopenia persists, and the risk of post-operative arterial thrombosis increases by a ratio of 2.6 among patients who have this complication.[76] Heparin also has been given to prevent mural thrombi from developing after an anterior myocardial infarction.[77,78]

Intravenous heparin often is prescribed to patients considered to have an extraordinarily high risk for stroke, including those with recent or crescendo TIA. The anticoagulant would be given to stabilize the patient while the evaluation is under way. It also could be administered as a prelude to surgical or long-term medical treatment. Despite the frequent use of heparin for this reason, very few data are available to provide guidance. An uncontrolled study looked at the value of an intravenous heparin infusion given to 74 patients with recent TIA.[79] Despite treatment, 12 patients (16.4%) had recurrent TIA and 5 patients (6.8%) had strokes. One patient died of a complication attributed to treatment, heparin-associated thrombocytopenia. A small, randomized trial compared the efficacy of a short course of heparin or aspirin among patients with recent TIA.[80] No significant difference in the risk of stroke was noted between the two treatment groups. No other studies of emergent intravenous anticoagulant therapy for treatment of patients with recent TIA are available. Thus, the value of a short course of heparin to stabilize a patient remains undetermined. A course of intravenously administered heparin should not be considered as the standard treatment for patients with recent or crescendo TIA. An alternative treatment would be immediate treatment with aspirin. If heparin is administered, a subsequent medical therapy should be started before the heparin is stopped. Slivka et al[81] noted that clinical worsening occurred in 10 of 143 patients who did not receive either warfarin or aspirin before discontinuing the heparin, whereas only 3 of 215 patients who were taking a long-term medication had events. This information suggests that a possible rebound hypercoagulable state could follow the interim use of heparin.

Persons with acute ischemic stroke are considered to have a particularly high risk for another vascular event. In particular, patients with cardioembolic stroke are predicted to have a very high risk for a second embolic event.[82,83] One of the rationales for early administration of anticoagulants after cardioembolic stroke is to prevent another event within the next few days. For example, a study in Spain prescribed heparin to 231 patients within 48 hours of stroke with the goal of preventing recurrent stroke.[84] All of the patients had atrial fibrillation, and approximately one-third of the patients were treated within 6 hours of stroke. Despite anticoagulation, 5 patients had recurrent stroke during hospitalization, and 8 had symptomatic brain hemorrhages. Six of the hemorrhages were fatal. Unfortunately, this was an uncontrolled trial, and the data cannot be compared to other interventions or the natural history. Still, these data can be examined in light of the results of recent clinical trials and epidemiological studies. Several studies show that the rate of recurrent embolization during the first days after stroke, even among patients with atrial fibrillation or other cardiac causes of stroke, is relatively low. The approximate rates are 1%–2% within 1 week and 2%–3% within 2 weeks.[85,86] These rates are approximately the same as those reported with treatment with heparin in the study by Chamorro et al.[84] With these low rates of early recurrent embolism, demonstration of any benefit from a short course of any treatment will be difficult. In addition, because the risk of stroke is very low, any therapy to lower the risk of embolism must be extraordinarily safe.

Unfortunately, heparin cannot be given with impunity. An earlier report by Chamorro et al[87] associated the risk of bleeding following the administration of heparin with the severity of the patients' neurological impairments and the level of anticoagulation. The International Stroke Trial recently evaluated the usefulness of subcutaneously administered heparin given within 48 hours of stroke to a very large cohort of patients.[85] A modest reduction (<1%) in early recurrent ischemic stroke was noted with heparin, including among patients who had atrial fibrillation. However, this reduction was negated by an increase in the rate of intracranial bleeding. As a result, no net benefit was seen from treatment. Another trial tested a low molecular heparinoid (danaparoid) given intravenously.[86] The trial found that the rate of early recurrent stroke was quite low (approximately 2%) among persons with all subtypes of stroke, including cardioembolism. Recurrent events occurred at equal rates among patients treated with danaparoid or placebo. No benefit in lowering this risk was seen with the antithrombotic agent, and an increased risk of bleeding was seen with treatment. Another trial tested the usefulness of either aspirin or low molecular weight heparin in prevention of recurrent cardioembolic stroke among persons with atrial fibrillation.[88] Anticoagulation was not more effective than aspirin in preventing recurrent embolism within 2 weeks of stroke. These data suggest that the role of emergent anticoagulation for prevention of early recurrent stroke is minimal. Caplan[89] concluded that heparin still might be useful in treating a subset of patients with recent stroke and atrial fibrillation. Decisions about early anticoagulation would be based on the relative risks of early recurrent stroke in comparison to the risks of bleeding. This advice seems sage. Factors such as a history of several previous neurological events or the presence cardiac abnormalities (left atrial size, atrial thrombus, ventricular abnormalities, etc.) might support early administration of heparin. Unfortunately, information about the prognostic importance of these changes is not available. Data also do not exist to identify patients who have such a high risk for stroke to justify the potential risks from treatment with anticoagulants. Pending more definitive data, one should conclude that heparin is of unproven value in preventing early recurrent embolism. This conclusion should not be confused with the established efficacy of long-term oral anticoagulant therapy in preventing cardioembolic stroke.

Heparin also has been given to "protect" patients from a transient hypercoagulable state during the initiation of treatment with oral anticoagulants. Warfarin-associated skin necrosis could occur with the initiation of treatment. The pharmacology of warfarin is reviewed subsequently in this chapter. Although a transient warfarin-induced pro-thrombotic state is a theoretical concern, the incidence of this complication is relatively low. The use of small doses of warfarin (2–5 mg./day) also may lessen the likelihood of this complication. In addition, the combination of heparin and warfarin has been associated with ischemic skin necrosis, and some of these events have been attributed to heparin. As a result, this indication for interim treatment with heparin probably is relatively uncommon.

Summary

The role of heparin in prevention of ischemic stroke appears to be limited. The use of heparin is complicated by a high risk of serious bleeding, particularly in patients who have had a recent ischemic stroke. Because the risk of early recurrent embolism is relatively low even among persons with a cardioembolic stroke, the agent must be very safe to demonstrate a net benefit from treatment. Unfortunately, heparin does not meet this criterion. As a result, the efficacy of emergent heparin therapy to prevent ischemic stroke will be difficult to establish. Although heparin is administered for several potential indications in stroke prophylaxis, it has not been established as efficacious in any of these situations. Its position likely will be as an adjunct to other therapies or as a treatment for patients who need anticoagulation but who cannot use oral agents.

LOW MOLECULAR WEIGHT HEPARINS AND DANAPAROID

Pharmacology

Because of the many major limitations of conventional heparin, other intravenously administered, rapidly acting medications are needed.[90] The leading alternatives are the low molecular weight (LMW) heparins and danaparoid (Table 10–8). These medications were created by chemical or enzymatic depolarization of conventional heparin and, thus, also are of biological origin.[60] These LMW fragments are approximately one-third the size of traditional heparin and most weigh 1000–10,000 Daltons. Danaparoid is slightly different from the other LMW compounds in that it consists primarily of heparan sulfate. Still, its actions are similar to the other LMW agents.[91] The fractionation into lower weight compounds leads to a reduced binding of the agents to platelets and platelet factor 4, endothelial cells, macrophages, and plasma proteins. These reductions result in longer periods of antithrombotic effects and a more predictable dose-antithrombotic response relationship than with conventional heparin.[92] The LMW heparins and danaparoid have a half-life that is at least 2–4 times that of conventional heparin. Because the LMW heparins and danaparoid are cleared renally, patients with renal failure should be given a lower dose of the medications.

The LMW heparins and danaparoid have a lessened ability to inhibit thrombin than does conventional heparin, but they retain their ability to inhibit activation of factor X.[60] Because activated factor X is at the key site of the merger of the intrinsic and extrinsic cascades for coagulation, its inhibition appears to be the major antithrombotic function of the LMW heparins.[92] As these medications do not affect thrombin activity except in very high concentrations, the anticoagulant responses of the LMW heparins cannot be monitored using aPTT. Instead, the anticoagulant actions are assessed by the determination of levels of anti-factor Xa activity.[60,93] Several different LMW heparins have been developed. As a result, the weights and the pharmacologic effects of the LMW heparins vary considerably. These agents should not be judged uniformly. Differences may affect both their therapeutic effects and the propensity for hemorrhagic complications. In particular, the ratio between inhibition of thrombin (factor II) and factor X varies markedly between the agents. As a result, one should use caution in assuming that the data about effectiveness and safety of one LMW heparin can be ascribed to another agent.

Table 10–8. **Potential Advantages of Low Molecular Weight Heparins or Danaproid over Unfractionated Heparin**

Longer periods of antithrombotic effects
Predictable dose–antithrombotic responses
Lessened ability to inhibit thrombin
Restricted antithrombotic effects—factor X activation
Lowered risk of bleeding and thrombocytopenia

Safety

As with conventional heparin, bleeding is the major potential complication of treatment with either the LMW heparins or danaparoid. Presumably the risk of bleeding is less than with heparin because of the more predictable dose–response relationships. Clinical studies comparing heparin and the LMW heparins or danaparoid report lower rates of bleeding with the latter medications.[60,94] Most of these studies have been in the setting of prophylaxis against venous thrombus. No studies have compared heparin and the LMW compounds for prevention of arterial thromboembolism. Intracranial or systemic bleeding has been an important problem in clinical trials testing the use of these agents in the treatment of patients with acute ischemic stroke. Protamine sulfate primarily counteracts heparin's effects on thrombin, but the antidote does not greatly influence the inhibition of activated factor X. Because the LMW heparins and danaparoid act primarily on factor X, protamine sulfate is not effective if hemorrhage develops secondary to the administration of an, LMW compound. If bleeding occurs, the long half-life of the medications also is a potential problem. Clotting factors can be given, but the usefulness of this tactic is uncertain.

The incidence of thrombocytopenia is less with the LMW heparins and danaparoid than with heparin.[69,95,96] However, patients with heparin-associated thrombocytopenia can have cross-reactivity with the LMW heparins.[60] The risk of thrombocytopenia secondary to danaparoid is much less, and it is even used as an anticoagulant to treat patients who have a high risk for thrombosis and a history of heparin-associated thrombocytopenia.[91] Patients receiving the LMW agents also appear to have a lower risk of osteoporosis than do patients given heparin.[60,95]

Potential Indications

A trial of danaparoid did not find the agent to be effective in preventing early recurrent stroke.[86] Another study tested the LMW heparin nadroparin; it did not describe any potential benefit in the number of early recurrent events that resulted from treatment.[97] Occasionally, a patient may need long-term anticoagulant therapy but cannot take oral medications. The LMW heparins and danaparoid can be given subcutaneously. An advantage of these medications is that they can be given less frequently than traditional heparin. Because of the high risk of teratogenicity of warfarin administration during pregnancy, women who have a high risk for stroke may need long-term administration of heparin, an LMW heparin, or danaparoid.[98,99] Both LMW heparins and danaparoid have been tested in treatment of patients with acute ischemic stroke.[86,97,88] No reduction in the risk of recurrent stroke was seen in these studies.[88] The usefulness of these agents in preventing embolism has not been tested among patient with TIA.

Summary

None of the currently available LMW heparins or danaparoid has demonstrated efficacy in prevention of ischemic stroke among high-risk patients. These agents appear to be associated with a considerable risk for serious bleeding, including intracranial hemorrhage. Their primary advantage over conventional heparin is their longer duration of action. Thus, they could be given as an alternative to an oral anticoagulant in long-term prophylaxis against stroke. The most obvious situation is prevention of thromboembolism in a pregnant woman with a high-risk cardiac lesion.

ORAL ANTICOAGULANTS

Pharmacology

Oral anticoagulants produce their antithrombotic action by hampering the cyclic interconversion of vitamin K and its 2,3 epoxide (vitamin K epoxide) through the blockade of vitamin K reductases in the liver.[100] As a result, vitamin K levels are depleted, and the vitamin K–dependent procoagulant factors, prothrombin, factor VII, factor IX, and factor X are lowered. In addition, the oral anticoagulants impair the carboxylation of the natural regulatory anticoagulant proteins (protein C and protein S) (Table 10–9). Warfarin is the most widely used oral and tested anticoagulant in patient care.[100] Warfarin has several advantages over the other vitamin K antagonists. It has a relatively predictable onset and duration of action. It is the standard oral agent against which other long-term

Table 10–9. **Actions of Oral Anticoagulants**

Decline in factor II (thrombin) levels
Decline in factor VII levels
Decline in factor IX levels
Decline in factor X levels
Decline in protein C levels
Decline in protein S levels

oral anticoagulants are compared. Warfarin is available in several dosage preparations to ease patient use. Although a parenteral form of warfarin is available, it usually is given in an oral preparation. Parental warfarin could be prescribed to patients who have severe gastrointestinal problems and cannot take the medication orally. It also might be prescribed to treat patients with recent cardiac operations. However, no major advantage is achieved. Parenteral administration does not produce therapeutic levels of anticoagulation more rapidly than oral administration. Warfarin is absorbed rapidly from the gastrointestinal tract and reaches maximal blood concentrations within 90 minutes.[100] The half-life of the medication is approximately 36–48 hours.

Although warfarin lowers levels of prothrombin, factor X, factor VII, and factor IX, the reductions in the two former proteins are the most important therapeutic actions.[100] Warfarin's primary actions in preventing thromboembolism relate best to its lowering of prothrombin concentrations. The reduction in prothrombin leads to a decline in concentrations of thrombin that can be subsequently bound to fibrin. In addition, fibrin-bound thrombin can amplify the generation of thrombosis. Thrombin mediates acute intravascular thrombosis, influences the activation of factor VII, binds with tissue factors, and simultaneously activates platelets, white blood cells, and endothelial cells.[101] Thus, inhibition of thrombin activity is key in preventing thrombosis and propagation of clots. Clinical research shows that the administration of warfarin lowers the blood levels of prothrombin activity among high-risk patients, such as those with atrial fibrillation.[102]

Still, the antithrombotic effects of warfarin are delayed for several days. The delay in therapeutic response means that warfarin cannot be used as an acute treatment to prevent recurrent ischemic events. This lag reflects the half-life of prothrombin, which is approximately 72 hours. The prolonged half-life of pro-thrombin means that warfarin's anticoagulant effects do not appear until several days after starting treatment, and they then persist for several days after stopping the medication. Conversely, the half-life of the anticoagulant proteins protein S and protein C are approximately 6–24 hours. Thus, these vitamin K–dependent factors inhibiting anticoagulation are affected by warfarin before prothrombin activity is reduced. As a result, the early administration of warfarin has the potential to cause an early transient hypercoagulable state. This prothrombotic state most commonly leads to skin necrosis. This complication of warfarin is relatively rare. Most patients do not have problems with hypercoagulability when starting treatment with warfarin. The complication is most common among patients who have an acquired or inherited deficiency of protein C or protein S.[70,103–106] A brief course of treatment with heparin has been used to protect against the prothrombotic effects of warfarin during the initiation of treatment with the oral anticoagulant.[107] However, the usefulness of this strategy is not clear. The heparin also might be associated with the skin necrosis and purple toe syndrome.[70] Most patients do not need "coverage" with heparin while starting treatment with warfarin. Starting with low doses of warfarin that gradually inhibit the vitamin K–dependent prothrombotic and antithrombotic factors also has been used.[108,109] The use of a relatively low maintenance dose probably is the best way to start oral anticoagulant treatment while avoiding any possible procoagulant complications.

The antithrombotic effects of warfarin were measured by assessing changes in the pro-thrombin time. The prothrombin time responds to depressions in concentrations of thrombin, factor VII and factor X.[100] For many years, the usual measure of therapeutic effects was the ratio of the prothrombin time from the treated patient compared with a control level. Unfortunately, laboratories around the world used different thromboplastin reagents in performing the test. The thromboplastins differ in their response to the anticoagulant actions of warfarin, depending on their tissue of origin, the concentration of phospholipids, and the method of their preparation.[100] As a result, the prothrombin times and ratios varied considerably among institutions.

Patients could be either under-treated and still be at high risk for stroke or over-treated and be at high risk for bleeding complications despite having the "same" prothrombin times. Adjusting doses of medication in response to the prothrombin time results from different laboratories created chaos in long-term care. In addition, the pro-thrombin time ratios reported to be effective and safe in a clinical trial might not be replicated by studies performed in laboratories in other parts of the world. The most important scenario is the underestimation of the significance of prothrombin values that leads the use of incorrect doses of warfarin in patients. In particular, levels of the prothrombin time that were "low" would lead to increased doses of warfarin and a high risk for serious bleeding complications. This problem probably was important as a cause for the high frequency of bleeding complications with warfarin. A whole generation of patients may have been inadvertently over-dosed.

Fortunately, the international normalized ratio (INR) was developed to help clarify issues about the level of anticoagulation among patients receiving warfarin.[110] The INR involves a mathematical conversion of the ratio of the patient's prothrombin time and the control prothrombin time as adjusted by the thromboplastin reagent. Thus, the level of anticoagulation should be the same regardless of the thromboplastin reagent used to do the test. This method should allow for assessment of a prothrombin time value from a patient at a clinical laboratory anywhere in the world. For most indications, the usual desired INR is approximately 2–3 (Table 10–10) and (Fig. 10–1). The INR now is the standard way to monitor responses to warfarin.

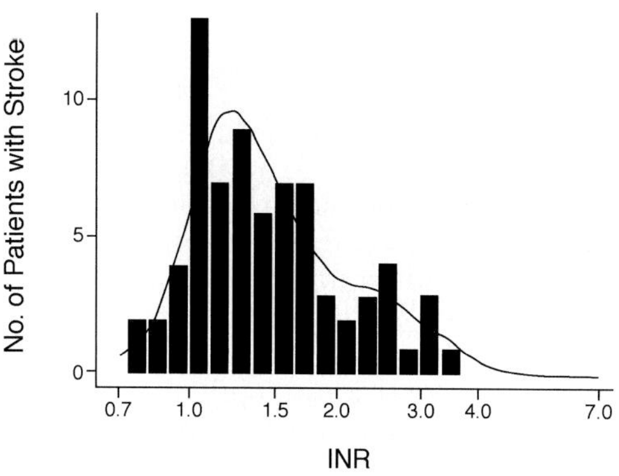

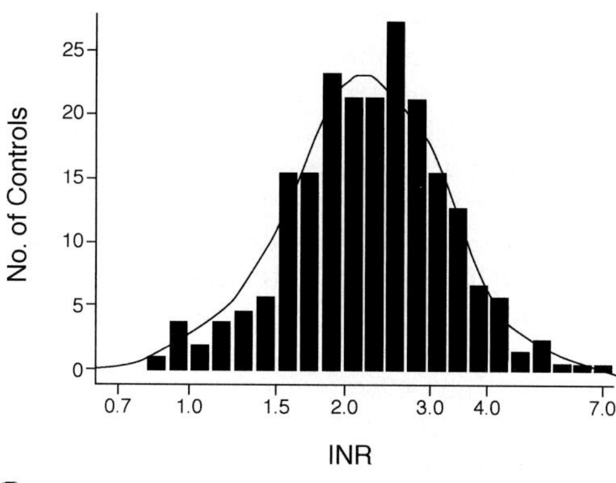

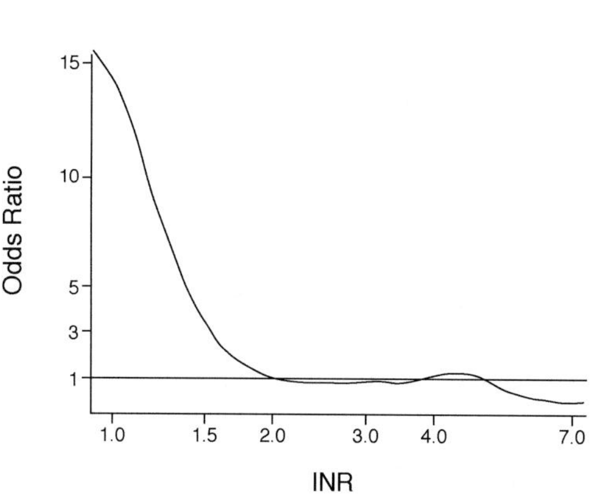

Figure 10–1. Odds ratio of stroke among persons with atrial fibrillation as influenced by the level of anticoagulation as measured by the international normalized ratio (INR). The odds ratios for stroke are estimated for a given INR value in comparison to an INR of 2. This calculation shows that the odds for a stroke are not reduced among persons with atrial fibrillation even if the level of anticoagulation is extended to above an INR of 3. (Reprinted from Hylek et al. An analysis of the lowest effective intensity of prophylactic anticoagulation for patients with non-rheumatic atrial fibrillation. *N Engl J Med* 1996;335: 540–546, with permission of publisher.)

Table 10–10. **Recommended Levels of Anticoagulation in Patients with Heart Disease**

Indication	Desired International Normalized Ratio Level
Recent (<6 months) myocardial infarction	2–3
Dilated cardiomyopathy	2–3
Rheumatic mitral stenosis with atrial fibrillation	2–3
Non-valvular atrial fibrillation	2–3
Prosthetic heart valves	
Aortic	
New bileaflet	2.5 +/–aspirin 81 mg/day
All other valves	3.0 +/–aspirin 81 mg/day
Bioprosthetic valves	2.5 in first 3 months; then aspirin 325 mg/day
Bioprosthetic valves + risk factors	2.5
Mitral	
Tilting disk	3.5 +/–aspirin 81 mg/day
All other valves	3.0 +/–aspirin 81 mg/day
Bioprosthetic valves	2.5 +/–aspirin 81 mg/day
Mitral valve repair	2.5 in first 3 months; then aspirin 325 mg/day

Pro-thrombin times and INR levels can be affected by the presence of antiphospholipid antibodies; in this situation, follow-up assessments of thrombin levels may be needed to assess anticoagulation of a patient treated with warfarin.

Administration

Oral anticoagulants have been used to treat patients at high risk for venous or arterial thromboembolism since the 1950s.[111] The use of these agents has changed dramatically in the intervening decades, partially due to improved monitoring with the use of the INR. In addition, clinical trials have defined the usefulness of oral anticoagulants in prevention of stroke among high-risk candidates. The strategy for starting treatment with oral anticoagulants also is changing. The method of starting with daily doses of approximately 10 mg. for 2 or 3 days to achieve rapid changes in the INR is being abandoned. The former tactic usually required in-patient treatment and daily adjustments of medications in response to INR values. Now a slower rate for initiation of anticoagulation can be done as an out-patient. This new approach is as effective as the old strategy and probably is safer. It also is more convenient for the patient and is less expensive than a prolonged hospitalization during which the doses of warfarin are being adjusted daily in response to INR levels. Crowther et al[108] found that a 10 mg loading dose was not more efficient than starting with 5 mg doses; most patients achieved therapeutic INR levels by 4–5 days with the latter regimen. This is the usual time for stability in INR levels in patients receiving the larger loading-dose regimen. The strategy for a slow initiation of anticoagulation is endorsed by the experience of Harrison et al,[109] who found that the 5 mg/day loading dose regimen caused less excessive levels of anticoagulation and also is less likely to cause a transient hypercoagulable state by a sudden decline in protein C concentrations. Oates et al[112] proposed starting warfarin at 2 mg/day and then making the first dosage adjustment at approximately 2 weeks. The dosage would be changed only if the INR was <1.5 or >4. Starting with low doses of warfarin is especially important among older patients and those with liver disease.

Responses to warfarin vary considerably among patients. Some patients require daily doses of up to 10 mg to maintain a therapeutic level of anticoagulation, whereas others may need doses as low as 1 mg. No reliable way is available to predict individual patients' responses to warfarin. In general, patients older than 75 often are more sensitive to warfarin than are younger persons.[113] A nomogram for warfarin dosage adjustments has been developed.[114] Hepatic or bowel disease can alter the affects of warfarin by changing absorption or metabolism of vitamin K (Table 10–11). For example, diarrhea can lead to an elevation of INR secondary to malabsorption of vitamin K.[115] A stable diet is important for maintaining a stable anticoagulant response to warfarin. Patients should be advised about foods that are high in vitamin K, including green leafy vegetables, peas and beans, tofu, soybean oil, and canola oil. Japanese green tea, herbal teas, ginseng, or garlic also can affect the INR level. Although these foods should not be forbidden, patients should eat them regularly so that the dose of warfarin can be adjusted accordingly. The oils of some fish may potentiate the anticoagulant effects of warfarin. Although consumption of fish should not be discouraged, patients should be advised to eat fish on a regular basis so that the warfarin regimen can be modified in response to any changes in the INR. Alcohol consumption can alter the anticoagulant affects of warfarin. If a patient has been previously advised not to drink alcoholic beverages, then that recommendation should be continued if warfarin is prescribed. Otherwise, a patient can be allowed to drink modest amounts of alcohol—a maximum of 1 or 2 drinks/day. Binges of alcohol consumption can raise the INR, whereas chronic alcohol ise may lower the INR. Patients need careful instruction about dietary issues and compliance with the treatment regimen to avoid complications of treatment. Differences between generic and proprietary formulations of warfarin also can lead to problems. A patient should not switch the "brand" of warfarin without monitoring for changes in the INR levels.

As a rule of thumb, a physician should assume that almost any medication could affect the actions of warfarin and either prolong or lessen the INR.[116] Several medications will prolong the INR, and others will lessen the level of anticoagulation (Tables 10–12 and 10–13). The medications listed are not comprehensive. The initiation of any new medication should prompt reconsideration of the warfarin dose and screening for the levels of INR. In particular, patients should be monitored when antibiotics are prescribed, as they can affect the absorption or metabolism of vitamin K or warfarin. Patients should be informed about the use of over-the-counter medications. In particular, they should be advised about the large number of medications that contain aspirin and non-steroidal anti-inflammatory agents. Patients also should be informed about which multiple vitamins do not contain vitamin K. Patients should take a multiple vitamin that includes vitamin K so they can maintain their normal level of anticoagulation. Patients taking warfarin should be told to contact their physician whenever they start taking a new medication. Follow-up measurements of the INR and subsequent

Table 10–11. **Conditions that Can Potentiate or Lessen the Effects of Oral Anticoagulants**

Potentiate
- Malignancy
- Autoimmune diseases
- Diarrhea
- Malabsorption
- Bowel disease
- Hepatic disease
- Hyperthyroidism
- Malnutrition
- Vitamin K deficiency

Lessen
- Inherited resistance to warfarin
- Hyperlipidemia
- Hypothyroidism
- Nephrotic syndrome

Table 10–12. **Medications that Potentiate the Effect of Oral Anticoagulants**

Major Effect	
Amiodarone	Anabolic steroids
Cimetidine	Clofibrate
Disulfiram	Erythromycin
Fluconazole	Methronidazole
Phenylbutazone	Sulfonamides
Moderate Effect	
Acetaminophen	Cisapride
Fluoxetine	Fluorouracil
Isoniazid	Omperazole
Propafenone	Propoxyphene
Quinidine	Tamoixifen
Tetracycline	Thyroid medications
Minimal Effect	
Allopurinol	Chloral hydrate
HMG Co A reductase inhibitors	Metrolazone
Nalidixic acid	Propranolol
Theophylline	Tricyclic antidepressants

adjustments of the dose of warfarin may be needed.

Treatment with warfarin might need to be suspended for an elective surgical procedure, such as a major dental operation, ocular surgery, or a hip replacement. Serious bleeding could complicate these operations if they are done in the presence of a therapeutic level of anticoagulation.

Table 10–13. **Medications that May Lessen the Effect of Warfarin**

Major Effect	
Barbiturates	Carbamezepine
Cholestyramine	Griseofulvin
Nafcillin	Rifampin
Moderate Effect	
Azathioprine	Cyclosporine
Dicloxacillin	Phenytoin
Propylthiouracil	
Minimal Effect	
Benzodiazepine	Sucralfate

Depending on the patient's neurological status and recent history, the operation might need to be postponed because of the continued need for anticoagulation. However, when the patient is stable or the operation needs to be done expeditiously, then the warfarin should be discontinued approximately 3–4 days before the procedure.[117] If the patient has a very high risk for thromboembolism—for example, a prosthetic heart valve—then, an interim course of treatment with heparin may be needed. The heparin could be stopped 4–6 hours before the surgery. The anticoagulation should be restarted as soon as possible after the operation. The surgeon should be asked beforehand about the timing of instituting the anticoagulants.

The suspension of anticoagulant treatment may be needed for urgent interventions, such as a laparotomy for an acute abdominal illness. In these situations, vitamin K or fresh frozen plasma are given to rapidly reverse the effects of warfarin. The goal would be to lower the INR <1.4 before the operation. As soon as the patient's condition permits, the anticoagulation should be re-instituted either with warfarin alone or with heparin followed by warfarin. If vitamin K was administered, then the achievement of therapeutic levels of the INR might be delayed.

Safety

The associated risk of hemorrhage remains the major safety issue with the use of oral anticoagulants.[65] (See Table 10–14.) A Danish study recently reported that the 3-year risk of bleeding was 41.1% among patients prescribed adjusted-dose warfarin.[118] A fixed, low-dose regimen of warfarin has lower risk of bleeding.[118] Petty et al[64] calculated that the bleeding complication rate with warfarin is 7.9/100 person-years. Major hemorrhages have been reported within 1 month of starting treatment in approximately 1.6% of patients.[119] Subsequently, the chances of bleeding are approximately 3.3% in 3 months, 5.3% in 12 months, and 10.6% at 2 years.[119] The risk of bleeding is reduced with the administration of a relatively low, fixed-dose regimen of warfarin. In this situation, the INR is relatively low and, not surprisingly, the risk of major hemorrhage also is low. Pengo et al[120] reported that major bleeding occurred in 1.0% of patients treated with a low-dose protocol and 2.6% among patients with adjusted doses of medication. They also found that the risk of hemorrhage increased when the INR exceeded 3.0. Another study estimated that warfarin-related mortality would be 1% at 6 months, 5% at 1 year, and 7% by 2–3 years.[121] Most of these deaths are secondary to major bleeding events, in particular intracranial hemorrhages. Van der Meer et al[122] evaluated 16,814 patients who received oral anticoagulant therapy; 1003 complications (162 major) were reported. The rate of major complications was estimated to be 2.7 per 100 patient-years. The risk of all hemorrhages and major bleeds increased by approximately 30%–40% for every decade in age. Green et al[123] concluded that warfarin given in the doses used in the recent clinical trials did not increase the risk of fatal bleeding but did increase the risk of major hemorrhage. Most major, non-fatal hemorrhages involve the urinary and gastrointestinal systems. As a result, patients should be warned about excessive nosebleeds or bruising, hematuria, gingival bleeding, rectal bleeding, dark stools, or coffee grounds emesis. Patients should also be advised to seek medical attention if new neurological symptoms or headaches appear. Although the new neurological symptoms might be secondary to a TIA or ischemic stroke, their occurrence in a patient who is taking warfarin should prompt screening for a symptomatic intracranial hemorrhage or a subdural hematoma. The latter is a particularly important potential complication that can present with increasing headaches and evolving personality changes. Subdural bleeding can occur with relatively trivial cranial trauma, and the patient may not remember the injury. Intracranial bleeding is the hemorrhagic complication most likely to threaten a patient's life. The risk of hemorrhage is increased among elderly patients and those with systolic hypertension, past myocardial infarction, or prior bleeding.[65,118,124,125] A large randomized trial testing anticoagulation among patients with atrial fibrillation

Table 10–14. **Complications of Oral Anticoagulants in Patients with Ischemic Cerebrovascular Disease**

Intracranial hemorrhage
Intracerebral hemorrhage
Subdural hematoma
Systemic bleeding
Retroperitoneal hemorrhage
Gastrointestinal hemorrhage
Genitourinary hemorrhage
Soft tissue hematoma
Epistaxis
Transient prothrombotic state
Purple toe syndrome
Osteopenia and compression fractures
Teratogenicity

Table 10–15. **Intracranial Bleeding Events During Treatment in Patients with Atrial Fibrillation**

Trial	Bleeding Events with Warfarin (%)	Control	Bleeding Events with Control (%)
AFASAK—1[135]	0.3	Placebo	0.0
		Aspirin	0.0
SPAF—I[146]	0.8	Placebo	0.8
BAATAF[136]	0.2	Placebo	0.0
CAFA[147]	0.4	Placebo	0.0
SPINAF[137]	0.0	Placebo	0.0
EAFT[257]	0.0	Placebo	0.2
SPAF—II[254]			
Age < 76	0.5	Aspirin	0.2
Age 76 +	1.8	Aspirin	0.8
SPAF—III[174]	0.5	Aspirin and Low-dose warfarin	0.9
AFASAK—2[173]	0.6	Aspirin	0.3
		Aspirin and Low-dose warfarin	0.0
SIFA[356]	0.0	Indobufen	0.0

AFASAK = Atrial Fibrillation
SPAF = Stroke Prevention in Atrial Fibrillation
BAATAF = Boston Area Anticoagulation Trial for Atrial Fibrillation
CAFA = Canadian Atrial Fibrillation Anticoagulation
SPINAF = Stroke Prevention in Non-rheumatic Atrial Fibrillation
EAFT = European Atrial Fibrillation Trial
SIFA = Studio Italiano Fibrillaizione Atriale (Italian Atrial Fibrillation Trial)

found that the risk of major hemorrhage with warfarin was 1.7% among patients <75 and 4.2% among older patients.[126] (See Table 10–15.) The risk of intracerebral hemorrhage was 0.6% in the younger patients and 1.8% among persons age >75. Although the risk of bleeding is increased among elderly patients, advanced age alone should not be a contraindication for treatment.[119] Patients older than 75 who have atrial fibrillation can tolerate adjusted doses of warfarin.[127] Elderly patients who are not at a high risk for falls and who can follow the treatment regimen should receive anticoagulants when indicated.

Patients with a history of stroke are identified as having a heightened risk of complications of anticoagulant therapy (Table 10–16) Some of the increased risk

Table 10–16. **Factors Associated with a High Risk for Bleeding—Treatment with Oral Anticoagulants**

- Past history of stroke, in particular brain hemorrhage
- Advancing age (increases with each decade)
- Poor balance or incoordination—at high risk for falls
- Dementia
- History of poor compliance with medical treatments
- Non-availability of laboratory monitoring
- Alcohol or drug abuse
- Prior adverse experience to an anticoagulant
- Serious medical diseases—cancer, peptic ulcer disease, hepatic failure, renal failure, terminal illnesses

may be secondary to a high risk for falls or cognitive impairments that could weaken compliance with the treatment regimen. Patients with liver dysfunction, gastrointestinal disease, or nephrotic syndrome also can have difficulty in maintaining a therapeutic but safe level of anticoagulation. Still, neither stroke nor these medical conditions by themselves should be considered as contraindications for treatment. Patients with a history of recent or recurrent serious bleeding, including those with intracranial bleeding, should be treated with caution. A potential scenario is long-term anticoagulation to prevent recurrent infarction in a patient who has a prosthetic valve and a hemorrhagic transformation of a cardioembolic stroke. In such a situation, the long-term risks of recurrent stroke greatly outweigh the risks of bleeding, and the question of timing of initiation of the anticoagulant therapy becomes the major issue. In general, the anticoagulants should be started once the patient's neurological condition has stabilized. In a small series of patients, Pessin et al[128] continued the oral anticoagulants despite a hemorrhagic transformation, and no untoward effects were noted. Still, the prudent course is probably to wait a few days after the hemorrhage to start or re-institute treatment with warfarin.

Patients who might have problems with compliance with the treatment regimen probably should not be treated because of the issue of safety. Included in this group would be patients who abuse alcohol, prescription medications, or illegal drugs. The potential for interactions with the warfarin and an inability to conform to the treatment regimen are great. In addition, these patients have a chance of falling and having bleeding complications. If a patient and family do not understand the nuances of the treatment regimen, including taking medication and having laboratory follow up, then anticoagulation should be avoided. Patients at high risk for falls, including those with poor balance, probably should not be treated with oral anticoagulants.

The occurrence of systemic bleeding should prompt a search for an underlying structural pathology, particularly if the hemorrhage develops when a patient does not have an excessively high INR. The warfarin may unmask a source of minor bleeding that was otherwise asymptomatic; for example, a tumor of the urinary or gastrointestinal system may be uncovered. The warfarin can be interrupted if the patient has mild bleeding.[129] For example, suspending treatment may be appropriate if the patient has developed multiple bruises. For cases of serious bleeding and prolonged INR level, the patient should receive vitamin K—the antidote to the anticoagulant. If serious bleeding is occurring, then the recommended treatment is an intravenous infusion of 1–10 mg.[110,129,130] The infusion should administered slowly. Intravenous administration of vitamin K can be complicated by anaphylaxis. Subcutaneously administered vitamin K is not well absorbed and should not be given.[100] Vitamin K should be prescribed only after some deliberation over the consequences of giving the agent. Administration of a large dose of vitamin K can lead to a state of warfarin resistance that could last up to 1 week once the oral anticoagulant is restarted. This resistance could greatly complicate the re-institution of warfarin in treatment of a patient who has a high risk for stroke, such as a patient with a prosthetic heart valve. In critical circumstances, fresh frozen plasma can be given to immediately reverse the effects of the warfarin.[107] An intravenous infusion of these clotting factors is most commonly prescribed when a patient has an intracranial hemorrhage complicating warfarin therapy.

Vitamin K is needed for the formation of bone matrix proteins, and low levels of vitamin K can cause a decrease in bone density, osteopenia, and possibly compression fractures. Bone mineral density can be reduced among patients with stroke who are taking warfarin.[131] Patients should be advised about this potential complication of prolonged use of oral anticoagulants. The oral anticoagulants are associated with a high risk of teratogenicity.[99] These agents should not be prescribed to women who are pregnant, and counseling about the risks of stroke and fetal complications from treatment should be performed if a young woman needs oral anticoagulants but wants to become pregnant. Administration of heparin or an LMW heparin is recommended for treatment to prevent recurrent stroke among pregnant women who have a very high risk for embolism to the brain.[98,99]

The therapeutic level of anticoagulation for most patients is an INR of 2–3.[132,133] Higher levels of anticoagulation are recommended for patients with pro-thrombotic states or mechanical prosthetic heart valves. Occasionally, a patient will have a marked prolongation of the INR even though no evidence of bleeding is present. Over-anticoagulation (INR >6) is more common among older patients.[113] If the INR is <5–6, then the usual response is to interrupt the warfarin treatment.[110,130] After missing one or two doses, the patient usually can restart the warfarin at a slightly lower maintenance dose. If the INR is 6–10, then a small 0.5- to 1-mg dose of vitamin K can be given intravenously in addition to stopping the warfarin. The level of anticoagulation usually will decline within 24 hours.[110] Alternatively, 1–2.5 mg of vitamin K can be given orally. For INR levels >10, a larger dose of vitamin K (3–5 mg) usually is needed. Fresh frozen plasma should be reserved for situations in which a very prolonged INR is associated with serious bleeding.

If one or two doses of medication are missed, then the patient should be advised not to double up on doses of medication because an inadvertently high level of anticoagulation can result.

Potential Indications

Oral anticoagulants are the mainstay of medical management to prevent embolization to the brain among persons with severe structural heart diseases. A number of high-risk cardiac diseases have been identified. Anticoagulants are used in both primary and secondary prevention of embolism. Recent research has focused on the usefulness of warfarin in the primary prevention of stroke and other embolic events among patients with atrial fibrillation. Some groups of patients with atrial fibrillation are identified as having a high risk for embolic stroke.[134] The likelihood of stroke increases by a factor of 1.8 per decade of age, in women by a factor of 1.6, with a history of hypertension—2.0, with systolic blood pressure >160 mm Hg, and with a history of stroke—2.9.[4,9] (See Table 10–17.) The results of several clinical trials support the use of oral anticoagulants (Table 10–18). A Danish study found that warfarin was superior to either placebo or aspirin in preventing thromboembolism among patients with atrial fibrillation.[135] The Boston Area Anticoagulation Trial for Atrial Fibrillation found that warfarin reduced the risk of stroke by approximately 86%.[136] A reduction in mortality and no increase in intracranial bleeding were noted with treatment. A randomized, double-blind clinical trial performed in Veterans Affairs Hospitals in the United States found that warfarin reduced the risk of stroke by a factor of 0.79.[137] Warfarin also is effective in preventing silent cerebral infarctions or asymptomatic embolic signals detected by transcranial Doppler ultrasonography among patients with atrial fibrillation.[138–140] The use of oral anticoagulants has been associated with a resolution of left atrial appendage clots among patients with atrial fibrillation.[141]

Table 10–17. **Risk of Embolic Stroke Among Persons with Atrial Fibrillation**

Highest-risk patients—oral anticoagulants are the preferred medication
Advancing age (>75 years)
Women (especially >75 years)
History of hypertension
Systolic arterial blood pressure >160 mm Hg
Diabetes mellitus
History of coronary artery disease
History of congestive heart failure
Left ventricular dysfunction
Spontaneous contrast visualized
Left atrial appendage thrombus visualized
Intermediate risk patients—either oral anticoagulants or aspirin
Age >65 years but no other risk factors
Lowest-risk patients—aspirin or no special anti-embolic medication
Age <65 years but no other features

Table 10–18. **Trials of Prevention of Embolism with Atrial Fibrillation**

Trial	Warfarin INR Value	Events Annual Rate (%)	Events Other	Annual Rate (%)	RRR* (%)	p-value
AFASAK—1[135]	2.8–4.2	2.7	Placebo	6.2	56	<0.05
			Aspirin	5.2	48	<0.05
SPAF—I[146]	2.0–4.5	2.3	Placebo	7.4	67	0.01
BAATAF[136]	1.5–2.7	0.4	Placebo	3.0	86	0.002
CAFA[147]	2.0–3.0	3.4	Placebo	4.6	26	0.25
SPINAF[137]	1.4–2.8	0.9	Placebo	4.3	79	0.001
EAFT[257]	2.5–4.0	8.5	Placebo	16.5	47	0.001
SPAF—II[254]	2.0–4.5					
Age <76		1.3	Aspirin	1.9	33	0.24
Age 76+		3.6	Aspirin	4.8	27	0.39
SPAF—III[174]	2.0–3.0	1.9	Aspirin and low-dose warfarin	7.9	74	<0.0001
AFASAK—2[173]	2.0–3.0	3.4	Aspirin and low-dose warfarin	3.2	–6	NS*
			Aspirin alone	2.7	–21	NS*
SIFA[356]	2.0–3.0	9.0	Indobufen	10.6	15	NS*

*NS = Not significant; RRR = Relative Risk Reduction.

Anticoagulation reduces the risk of recurrent stroke among patients with ischemic stroke and atrial fibrillation.[142] A trial performed in Europe demonstrated that anticoagulants lessen the risk of embolism by approximately two-thirds.

Based on a meta-analysis of data from clinical trials in primary prevention of stroke, several groups concluded that anticoagulants reduce the annual risk of events from 12% to 4%.[143–147] Feinberg[134] calculated that the risk of stroke among all patients with atrial fibrillation could be reduced from approximately 4.5% per year to 1.5% per year with anticoagulant therapy. Anderson[148] concluded that warfarin reduced the risk of stroke by approximately 70% among patients with atrial fibrillation. Although anticoagulation lowers the risk of major strokes among patients with nonvalvular atrial fibrillation, it does not lessen the risk of fatal cerebral infarctions.[123] Koefoed et al[149] concluded that warfarin reduced the risk of embolism by approximately 68%. Oral anticoagulants are used for treatment of most patients with atrial fibrillation.[3,148,150–154] Patients who have a pacemaker and atrial fibrillation should be treated with anticoagulants.[155]

Anticoagulants should be given before chemical or electrical cardioversion of patients with sustained atrial fibrillation.[151,156–158] The medications might not be needed for treatment of new-onset atrial fibrillation or if echocardiography demonstrates no thrombus in the left atrium.[156, 59] Weinberg et al[151] found that anticoagulation was very effective in preventing embolism during cardioversion for atrial fibrillation. Among a series of high-risk patients, 7% of those who did not receive procedural anticoagulation had embolic events,whereas none of the patients who had medical treatment had events. Another series reported that embolic events occurred in 1.32% of 454 patients treated with electrical cardioversion; all of the events happened among patients who did not receive anticoagulants.[160] They were not able to identify any risk factors to predict a higher risk of embolic events among some patients with atrial fibrillation. In particular, the duration of atrial fibrillation was less than 1 week among 5 of the 6 patients who had embolic events. Because clots can develop after electrical cardioversion, the anticoagulant should be continued after the treatment.[161] A recommended regimen would be 3 weeks of anticoagulant therapy before cardioversion followed by another 4 weeks of treatment after the procedure.[159]

Anticoagulants are also recommended for patients with a large number of other heart diseases. Among the potential indications are sick sinus syndrome, a recent myocardial infarction, a patent foramen ovale, atrial septal aneurysm, left ventricular dysfunction, dilated cardiomyopathy, and rheumatic mitral stenosis with atrial fibrillation.[124,134,162,163] The levels of evidence to support the administration of anticoagulants vary considerably among these indications. For example, the severity and location of the cardiac injury influence the role of oral anticoagulant therapy in prevention of stroke following myocardial infarction. Anticoagulation is prescribed to patients with large anterior myocardial infarctions in an attempt to prevent development of a mural thrombus that can be the source of emboli to the brain.[77] Azar et al[164] evaluated the risk of stroke during long-term oral anticoagulant therapy among patients with recent myocardial infarction. The medication reduced the incidence of stroke from 1.2/100 patient-years to 0.7/100 patient-years. Seventeen patients receiving anticoagulants had hemorrhages, but 14 had had an INR >3 at the time of the bleeding event. Smith[165] found that oral anticoagulation after myocardial infarction can prevent recurrent myocardial infarction or stroke with a relatively low risk for bleeding. Patients with a large right-to-left shunt secondary to a patent foramen ovale appear to have the highest risk for embolism, and these patients might benefit from anticoagulation.[166] This situation has not been examined in a clinical trial setting.

Anticoagulants are the preferred medical regimen for treatment of patients with valvular heart diseases, including those with rheumatic heart disease, especially if atrial fibrillation is present.[167] Oral anticoagulants are the primary treatment for most patients with both mechanical and bioprosthetic cardiac valves.[125,168–170] (See Table 10–10.) The factors that predict a very high risk of embolism include the presence of two prostheses, atrial fibrillation, severe left ventricular dysfunction, a prior neurological event, or a hypercoagulable state.[125] The efficacy of oral anticoagulants in preventing stroke among patients with mechanical valves, especially mitral valve prostheses, is compelling. The usual desired level of anticoagulation is an INR of approximately 2.5 to approximately 4. Among patients with mechanical valves, the risk of ischemic stroke rises quickly when the INR is <2, and the likelihood of hemorrhagic stroke increases rapidly when the INR >5.[169] Patients receiving an oral anticoagulant that leads to an INR of 2–3 also can receive antiplatelet aggregating agents with an acceptable margin of safety.[170] Oral anticoagulants are recommended for treatment of patients with bioprosthetic valves during the first 3 months following surgery and if the patient has a history of embolism.[125,168]

The optimal level of anticoagulation for prevention of cardioembolic events appears to be relatively clear. For most indications, the desired level is an INR of 2–3. (See Table 10–10.) Brass et al[171] analyzed the risk of embolic stroke among patients with atrial fibrillation as influenced by the INR. When compared to an INR of 2–3, the risk of stroke was 4 times greater if the INR was <1.5 and approximately 2.5–3 times greater if the INF was 1.5–1.9. Modest additional protection was seen with INR greater than 3, but this benefit was negated by an increased risk of hemorrhage.[170,171] The usefulness of low-intensity warfarin therapy is uncertain.[172] A clinical trial in patients with atrial fibrillation found that the risk of ischemic stroke was 3.7% among patients receiving a fixed low dose of warfarin and 0% among patients having the conventional, adjusted-dose regimen.[120] Another trial found that the 1-year rate of stroke among patients with atrial fibrillation was 2.8% in persons taking adjusted doses of warfarin and 5.8% in patients using a mini-dose warfarin regimen.[173] The Stroke Prevention in Atrial Fibrillation Investigators[174] reported that the incidence of stroke was 7.9% among patients treated with aspirin and a low-intensity, fixed dose of aspirin and 1.9% among patients receiving the conventional, adjusted-dose regimen with an INR of 2–3. Not only was the fixed-dose regimen less effective in preventing stroke, but it also did not lessen the risk of hemorrhages. Among a group of high-risk patients, those with spontaneous contrast in the left atrium visualized by transesophageal echocardiography had a risk of stroke at 4.5% per year with adjusted-dose warfarin, and the risk was 18.2% per year among patients receiving a fixed, low dose of warfarin and aspirin.[175]

Anticoagulants have been the mainstay of prevention of recurrent thromboembolism among patients with prothrombotic states.[124] (See Chapter 8.) Warfarin is prescribed for treatment of patients with prothrombotic states, including those with antiphospholipid antibodies. The risk of recurrent thrombosis is high among this group of patients, and warfarin with a desired INR >3 is often recommended.[176]

Patients with atherosclerotic disease of the aorta with protruding or mobile plaques often are treated with anticoagulants (Table 10–19). Dressler et al[177] reported that warfarin appears to be helpful in preventing stroke among patients with mobile atherosclerotic plaques. Events occurred in 27% of patients who did not receive anticoagulants, whereas none of the treated patients had strokes. Another study showed that adjusted-dose warfarin (INR 2–3) was associated with a 5.9% annual risk of embolism among persons with thoracic aortic plaques and atrial fibrillation.[178] The risk of embolism was 17.3% per year among patients who received the combination of low-dose warfarin and aspirin. The investigators did not differentiate embolism from the heart from embolism arising from the aorta. No randomized clinical trials have demonstrated the efficacy of anticoagulation in this situation or its superiority over treatment with antiplatelet aggregating agents. Antiplatelet aggregating agents remain an alternative choice for treatment.

Oral anticoagulants often are used to avert stroke among patients with intracranial or extracranial arterial disease:[372] Potential indications include treatment of persons with intracranial lesions, high-grade arterial stenoses, or arterial dissection. Despite the widespread administration of warfarin for these reasons, limited data are available about its efficacy and safety in these situations. Patients with symptomatic intracranial atherosclerosis, who have symptoms despite treatment with anticoagulants, might have a poor prognosis.[373] One of the rationales for anticoagulation is that warfarin will prevent thrombosis in the environment of a slow-flow state, such as distal- to high-grade arterial stenosis. Unfortunately, no data are available to support this presumed pathogenetic mechanism for embolism distal to segments of arterial narrowing. If a slow-flow state is the primary reason to prescribe warfarin, then the uncommon nature of this condition portends that warfarin might not be shown to be effective. Patients with radiation-induced arteriopathy or dissection of an intracranial or extracranial artery often receive warfarin for prevention of stroke. A retrospective study concluded that warfarin might be superior to aspirin in prevention of vascular events in patients with symptomatic intracranial atherosclerosis.[179] Patients receiving warfarin had a stroke rate of 3.6/100 patient-years, whereas patients taking aspirin had a stroke rate of 10.4/100 patient-years. A subsequent report

Table 10–19. **Long-Term Oral Anticoagulants: Potential Indications**

- Established indications
  - Cardioembolism—high-risk heart diseases
  - Pro-thrombotic disorders
- Uncertain indications
  - Cardioembolism—low-risk heart diseases
  - Atherosclerotic disease of the aorta
  - Arterial dissections
  - Intracranial or extracranial atherosclerotic disease
    - High-grade stenosis
    - Intraluminal thrombus
    - Vertebrobasilar disease
  - Recurrent events despite treatment with antiplatelet aggregating agents

from a multi-center study reported that the risk of stroke was 10.7/100 patient-years among persons with basilar artery stenosis, 7.8/100 patient-years among patients with vertebral artery stenosis, and 6.0/100 patient-years among patients with stenosis of the posterior cerebral artery.[180] Unfortunately, a clinical trial tested warfarin or aspirin treatment in prevention of stroke among a series of patients with atherosclerosis and a prior neurological event.[181] The desired level of anticoagulation was higher than that generally recommended, and the trial was halted prematurely because of a high rate of intracranial hemorrhage. Ongoing trials should expand the information about the usefulness of anticoagulant therapy in prevention of stroke among patients with symptomatic intracranial or extracranial disease.

Summary

The previously described data provide robust evidence that oral anticoagulants are instrumental in lessening the chances of stroke among persons with heart diseases that cause embolization. (See Table 10–18.) Oral anticoagulants are under-used in persons younger than 75 and in older persons.[182,183] Among the proven indications is the prevention of embolization in patients with anterior wall myocardial infarction, mechanical prosthetic cardiac valves, rheumatic mitral stenosis complicated by atrial fibrillation, and atrial fibrillation complicating structural heart disease. Patients with a dilated cardiomyopathy likely will benefit from treatment with anticoagulants. Patients with other heart diseases, including a patent foramen ovale, might be treated with warfarin. However, definitive data are not available, and the results of clinical trials will be needed to guide decisions about treatment.

Although several epidemiological variables, such as age, and the results of cardiac imaging studies forecast which patients are at highest risk for embolization, these factors are most useful in guiding decisions about the use of warfarin as a primary stroke prevention strategy. The occurrence of a TIA or an ischemic stroke in a patient with one of the previously described underlying heart diseases automatically designates the situation as very high risk. In these circumstances, anticoagulants should be prescribed unless a specific contraindication for their use is present.

Oral anticoagulants should not be considered as a panacea. The risk of major hemorrhagic complications, including intracranial hemorrhage, is considerable. Even with advances in monitoring with the INR and efforts to develop the safest levels of anticoagulation, the chances for bleeding remain high. The use of a low, fixed dose of warfarin that slightly perturbs the INR generally is not as effective as the adjusted-dose regimen. This strategy should not substitute for the conventional, adjusted-dose regimen. Thus, the decisions for long-term oral anticoagulant care must continue to be made on a case-by-case basis that balances the risks versus the benefits from treatment.

The indications for long-term oral anticoagulant therapy among persons with stroke secondary to pro-thrombotic conditions also seem to be fairly clear. Warfarin is the preferred treatment for most patients with inherited or acquired conditions that lead to repeated venous or arterial occlusions, including those with the antiphospholipid antibody syndrome. Ongoing studies should provide guidance for the potential value of either anticoagulants or antiplatelet aggregating agents in prevention of stroke among patients with these antibodies.

The value of anticoagulation in preventing ischemic events among patients with arterial causes of stroke remains uncertain. Limited data from clinical trials are available, and the results from these studies are mixed. Still, the likelihood is high that warfarin may not be as effective in preventing stroke among patients with atherosclerotic cerebrovascular disease as it is in averting cardioembolic stroke. It is hoped that the results of ongoing studies will clarify the role of anticoagulation in prevention of stroke.[374] Pending the results of these trials, warfarin should not be considered to be the primary medical therapy for patients with symptomatic atherosclerosis. The exception might be patients who have advanced aortic plaque formation with superimposed thrombi. Even this situation has not been tested sufficiently to define the treatment role for anticoagulation. No data are available to define the status of anticoagulant treatment for patients who have recurrent ischemic symptoms despite management with antiplatelet aggregating agents.

Table 10–20. **Antiplatelet Aggregating Agents in Prevention of Ischemic Stroke**

Medication	Daily Dose
Aspirin	30–1300 mg
Ticlopidine	500 mg
Clopidogrel	75 mg
Dipyridamole	400 mg

OTHER ANTITHROMBOTIC AGENTS

The potential contribution of the direct inhibitors of thrombin function in preventing ischemia is being assessed in patients with a number of vascular diseases.[184] Most agents have been tested for the treatment of patients with unstable cardiac diseases, but these medications' efficacy to prevent ischemic stroke has not been examined (see Table 10–4). Argatroban inhibits platelet activation of the fibrin clot–associated thrombin, and it might be better than heparin for treatment of acute thromboembolic disease.[185] Argatroban also is used to treat patients with heparin-associated thrombocytopenia and thrombosis.[186] It might be effective in preventing recurrent emboli in a setting where heparin usually is prescribed. Recombinant hirudin has been used to treat patients with unstable angina and acute coronary artery syndromes.[187,188] Clinical trials of hirudin therapy for patients with unstable heart disease have been stopped because of high rates of intracranial hemorrhages. Hirudin has not been shown to be safer than heparin. Because of the high rate of intracranial bleeding following the use of hirudin for patients with ischemic heart disease, caution should be exercised with regard to the administration of this agent to patients with stroke. The bleeding risk seems to be considerable.

ANTIPLATELET AGGREGATING AGENTS

Antiplatelet aggregating agents are the standard medical therapy for prevention of stroke among high-risk patients with arterial disease.[189–193] (See Table 10–20.) These agents are widely used alone or in combination with oral anticoagulants or surgical procedures. Since the 1970s, clinical trials have demonstrated the benefit of aspirin, ticlopidine, clopidogrel, and the combination of aspirin and dipyridamole in prevention of stroke, myocardial infarction, or vascular death among high-risk patients, including those with a recent TIA or ischemic stroke. Based on data collected from more than 100,000 patients enrolled in multiple clinical trials for prevention of ischemic vascular disease, the Antiplatelet Trialists' Collaboration[194] show that antiplatelet aggregating agents lessen the risk of stroke by approximately 25%. Although antiplatelet aggregating agents are of proven usefulness in secondary prevention of stroke among persons who have had symptoms of ischemia, their value in the primary prevention of stroke is not established. A collaborative study found that antiplatelet aggregating agents were effective in both men and women, persons older or younger than 65, persons who did or did not have hypertension, and persons with or without diabetes mellitus.[194] Puranen et al[195] concluded that the risk reduction in stroke was greatest among persons with elevated diastolic blood pressure. Antiplatelet aggregating agents appear to be effective regardless of the number of risk factors for stroke, and all subgroups of patients seem to benefit.[196] However, despite their efficacy, considerable room exists for additional medical therapies that might be superior in their ability to prevent stroke.

In addition to being effective, the antiplatelet aggregating agents are easy to administer. The antiplatelet aggregating agents generally are safe, and the risk of major bleeding seems to be less than with oral anticoagulants. Still, surgeons report that perioperative bleeding can be brisk among patients who have been taking antiplatelet aggregating agents in the days before surgery. As a result, most surgeons favor stopping these medications approximately 7–10 days before an elective operation.

Unfortunately, population-based studies show that the antiplatelet aggregating agents are under-used among person at high risk for stroke or myocardial infarction.[197] Aspirin or other antiplatelet aggregating agents are not a substitute for management of risk factors; rather, they should be considered as adjuncts to efforts to control conditions that lead to atherosclerosis and stroke.[198]

Aspirin

Aspirin is the most widely used antiplatelet aggregating agent. It is the most extensively studied medication and was the first medical or surgical therapy to be established as useful in prevention of stroke among patients with TIA or stroke. It also effectively lowers the risk of myocardial infarction or vascular death. As such, aspirin usually is the control agent against which other medical or surgical therapies are compared. Aspirin has several advantages. It is inexpensive and easy to administer. It is relatively safe, and the side effects from treatment are well known. Still, aspirin is a potent drug and should be considered as such despite its status as an over-the-counter medication. Physicians and patients need to remain alert to the powerful actions of this common, almost prosaic, medication.

PHARMACOLOGY

Aspirin inhibits prostaglandin function and irreversibly blocks cyclooxygenase activity in both platelets and endothelial cells.[199–201] Aspirin's inhibition of thromboxane A2 synthetase is the primary mechanism for blocking platelet aggregation.[199,202] Secondary epinephrine and collagen-induced aggregation is effectively blocked by aspirin.[203] Aspirin also blocks the production of prostacyclin by endothelial cells via the same mechanism.[201] Additional antithrombotic effects of aspirin involve its actions on leucocytes and vascular endothelium.[204]

Aspirin is rapidly absorbed from the stomach and proximal portion of the small intestine. Platelet function usually is inhibited within 1 hour of taking the medication.[201] Absorption and secondary antiplatelet aggregating effects can be slower if an enteric-coated preparation is used. Aspirin given as rapid-release preparation seems to be more potent in blocking platelet aggregation than a slow- or delayed-release formulation.[205] Although the blood levels of aspirin rapidly decline, its effects persist for several days. In addition to arresting aggregation of circulating platelets, aspirin also acetylates the prostaglandin synthase in megakaryocytes. Thus, the aggregating functions of new platelets also are blocked. Aspirin's inhibitory affects on platelet function persist for the life of the platelet—approximately 10 days. Because approximately 10% of platelets are replaced daily, it takes approximately 1 week for the blood's platelet aggregating function to normalize.

Aspirin's actions on platelet function occur over a broad range of doses. Most research has focused on daily doses of 30–1300 mg of aspirin. A single 325 mg dose of aspirin has immediate effects on cyclooxygenase activity and platelet function.[206] Although low doses of aspirin (approximately 30 mg/day) lessen platelet aggregation and prolong bleeding times, these effects do not appear until after several doses (3–7 days).[206,207] Following a single, 325 mg dose of aspirin, subsequent daily doses of approximately 40–75 mg will maintain the inhibition of platelet aggregation.[208] Aspirin in daily doses of 40–160 mg cause a greater than 80% inhibition of platelet cyclooxygenase activity, which can be maintained.[209] Data suggest that low doses (approximately 30 mg) of aspirin affect platelet aggregation to the same extent as larger doses.[207] Gomes[210] recently reported that very high daily doses (4–6 gm) of aspirin could over a neuroprotective effect by inhibiting the actions of glutamate toxicity. These doses are far higher than those prescribed on a long-term basis to patients with ischemic cerebrovascular disease. The clinical utility of this observation has not been tested, but there has been a debate about the possibility that pre-treatment with aspirin can lessen the consequences of ischemic stroke.

Aspirin does prevent platelet aggregation among all persons with a history of ischemic stroke.[211] Helgason et al[212] noted that the dose of aspirin that blocks platelet aggregation may vary considerably among individual patients. A subsequent report suggested that some patients develop resistance to the antiplatelet aggregating actions of aspirin.[213] Approximately one-third of patients who initially have a complete inhibition of platelet function subsequently lose these effects. Although clinical correlates to the changes in platelet function subsequently lost these effects. Although clinical correlates to the changes in platelet function were not described, Helgason et al[213] proposed that an increase in the dose of aspirin might be needed to maintain antithrombtic effects. Grotemeyer et al[214] found that some patients do not maintain inhibition of platelet activity with the use of aspirin. This group of patients, called *secondary aspirin non-responders,* is at a high risk for ischemic stroke. Still, no data have demonstrated that a dose of aspirin will help if a patient has another stroke despite a low dose of aspirin. These experiences suggest that additional research is needed about individual responses to aspirin.

SAFETY

The leading side effects of aspirin are gastric irritation, peptic ulcer disease, and gastrointestinal bleeding (Table 10–21). Gastric distress and pain are the most common complaints. Sze et al[215] estimated that the use of aspirin increases the risk of gastrointestinal bleeding or peptic ulcer disease by approximately 350%. Gastrointestinal bleeding secondary to aspirin can be severe.[216] A dosage relationship is found for these complications. Many patients do not tolerate doses greater than 325 mg/day and will need a reduction in dose. For example, Hobson et al[217] noted that a majority of men in a large clinical trial could not tolerate a dose of 1300 mg/day. In a British trial, the risk of gastrointestinal symptoms was less among patients with a 300 mg daily dose than with a 1200 mg daily dose of aspirin.[218] The use of enteric-coated medication can lessen these complaints, but the formulation does not eliminate the risk of the more serious gastrointestinal complications. Although a low daily dose of aspirin (30–160 mg) does not eliminate the risk of bleeding or other gastrointestinal side effects, the likelihood of a major complication seems to be less than with larger doses.[219,220] Still, most patients tolerate the lower doses of aspirin much better than a daily dose of 1300 mg.[221]

The risk of bleeding complications with aspirin is estimated to be 3.5/100 person-years.[64] In general, aspirin does not cause a generalized bleeding disorder unless the patient has another factor (concomitant anticoagulant treatment or a hemostatic

Table 10–21. **Most Common Complications of Antiplatelet Aggregating Agents**

Aspirin
Allergic reactions
Gastritis and gastric ulcer
Gastrointestinal bleeding
Ticlopidine
Diarrhea and gastrointestinal distress
Skin eruptions
Neutropenia and agranulocytosis
Thrombotic thrombocytopenic purpura
Clopidogrel
Diarrhea and gastrointestinal distress
Skin eruptions
Thrombotic thrombocytopenic purpura
Dipyridamole
Headache

defect) to promote hemorrhage.[201] Still, potentially fatal bleeding complications can occur with aspirin.[198] Non-gastrointestinal hemorrhage can occur, and intracranial bleeding is a possibility. The use of aspirin has been associated with an increased risk of intracerebral hemorrhage among low-risk elderly men and women.[222] A study of aspirin in the primary prevention of myocardial infarction reported that a regimen of a 325 mg tablet taken every other day was associated with an increased risk of intracranial bleeding.[223] He et al[224] recently calculated that risk of hemorrhagic stroke among persons taking aspirin was 12/10,000. The risk of intracranial bleeding or other non-gastrointestinal bleeding has not been associated with the dosage of aspirin.[219] Recently, Thrift et al[225] concluded that a low or moderate dose of aspirin was not associated with intracranial hemorrhage. However, the odds of intracerebral hemorrhage were increased by a factor of 3.05 (1.02–9.14) when patients took more than 1225 mg/week in at least three divided doses. The lack of a strong dose relationship with the occurrence of intracranial bleeding supports the contention that aspirin's effects on platelet function occur over a wide range of doses.

POTENTIAL INDICATIONS

Aspirin is effective in both the primary and secondary prevention of myocardial infarction and vascular death.[201,223] Aspirin reduces the risk of stroke by approximately 30%, stroke and death by approximately 22%, or vascular death by 15% among patients with symptomatic atherosclerosis, especially among patients with ischemic neurological symptoms.[226] Although aspirin is an effective therapy for primary prevention of vascular events among men, its value is less obvious as a primary treatment for women. [227] Data are not available to support the assertion that aspirin is effective in primary prevention of stroke among asymptomatic patients. Aspirin was not effective in prevention of stroke among patients with asymptomatic carotid artery bruits.[228,229] In a primary prevention study of aspirin use among men and women older than 65, Kronmal et al[222] surprisingly showed that use of the medication was associated with an increased risk of ischemic stroke in women. In contrast, Iso et al[230] reported that women who take 1–6 aspirin tablets (325 mg) week have a markedly reduced risk of stroke secondary to large artery occlusion. The benefit was greatest in older women and among those who had hypertension or who smoked. Part of the lack of efficacy may be attributed to a lower risk of stroke than ischemic heart disease among asymptomatic patients. The average age at the time of onset of neurological symptoms is older than for the first cardiac symptoms. Thus, the impact of aspirin in the primary prevention strategy will be greater for heart disease than for stroke. The conflicting results of these studies do not settle the issue about the role of aspirin in primary prevention of stroke. Additional data about the role of aspirin in primary prevention of stroke is needed.

The best daily dose of aspirin for prevention of myocardial infarction is 75–325 mg.[194,201,231] (See Table 10–22.) Several studies strongly suggest that the mechanisms of action and dose requirements for the antithrombotic actions in prevention of ischemic stroke are similar to those for patients with coronary artery disease.[232] Despite agreement about the best dose of aspirin for treatment of patients with coronary artery disease, considerable controversy remains about the best dose for prevention of stroke.[201,233] Comparisons of data collected in the early 1970s with those reported from trials performed 20 years later should be done with caution because of the dramatic changes in health care during that time; for example, the treatment of hypertension has evolved considerably. The first clinical trials tested daily doses in excess of 1000 mg.[234–236] These large doses were selected without any particular knowledge about any dosage relationship on limiting platelet aggregation. A Canadian trial found that aspirin reduced the risk of stroke or death by approximately 31%, but the benefit was seen only in men.[234] In men, the benefit was a 48% reduction in ischemic events, but no effect from treatment with aspirin 1300 mg/day was found in women.[237] There was no

Table 10–22. **Trials of Aspirin in Prevention of Stroke or Death Among High-Risk Patients**

Trial	Daily Dose of Aspirin	Aspirin Events/Patients	Control Events/Patients
Aspirin vs Placebo/Control			
Heidelberg[357]	1/30	4/30	
Fields[236]	1300 mg	13/88	19/90
Canadian[234]	1300 mg	26/144	30/139
Bousser et al[360]	1000 mg	27/198	38/204
Danish[238]	1000 mg	21/101	17/102
Swedish[362]	1500 mg	57/253	55/252
Boysen[363]	50–100 mg	21/150	17/151
UK TIA[218]	1200 mg	168/815	195/814
300 mg	173/806	195/814	
SALT[240]	75 mg	138/676	171/685
Lindblad[241]	75 mg	13/117	23/115
ESPS–2[307]	50 mg	330/1649	378/1649
Aspirin and Diyprydamole vs Placebo/control			
Bousser et al[360]	1000mg	26/202	38/204
ESPS—1[364]	975 mg	190/1250	283/1250
ESPS—2[307]	50 mg	286/1650	378/1649

UKTIA = United Kingdom Transient Ischemic Attack
SALT = Swedish Aspirin Low dose Trial
ESPS = European Stroke Prevention Study

statistically significant difference in the numbers of adverse outcomes among persons taking aspirin alone in comparison to those prescribed placebo. Small trials in the United States found that aspirin was effective among patients who either did or did not have carotid endarterectomy but, because of the size of the studies, the results were not conclusive.[235,236] A Danish trial could not find that treatment with aspirin (1000 mg/day) was effective in reducing the chances of stroke or death, although the chances of myocardial infarction was lessened.[238] Subsequent clinical trials during the next 20 years tested progressively lower doses of aspirin. A British trial determined that 300 mg of aspirin was equal in effect to 1200 mg.[218] Still, when the two doses were examined independently, neither was superior to placebo, although the lower dose had fewer side effects. The Dutch TIA Trial found that aspirin in a dose of 30 mg/day was equal in effect to approximately a daily dose of 300 mg.[239] (See Fig. 10–2.) A Swedish study tested a daily dose of 75 mg and found aspirin to be effective.[240] The low dose of aspirin reduced the risk of both stroke and death. Lindblad et al[241] showed that aspirin (75 mg/day) is safe and effective in preventing disabling strokes following carotid endarterectomy. The lack of efficacy for aspirin among women that was reported in the first studies has been resolved.[237] The initial observation probably was secondary to the relatively low risk of stroke among women with TIA and the small number of women enrolled in the early trials. Aspirin is equally effective in preventing stroke among women and men with TIA or ischemic stroke.[227] Aspirin appears to be effective regardless of the patient's age or the presence or absence of diabetes mellitus or hypertension.[194] The trials have enrolled primarily persons of European ancestry. Although aspirin might be equally

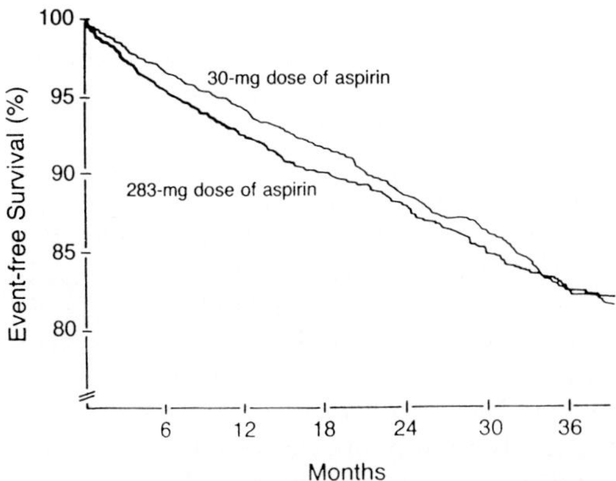

Figure 10–2. Kaplan-Meier curves for the combined outcome events from vascular death, non-fatal stroke, or non-fatal myocardial infarction among patients assigned treatment of daily doses of 30 mg or 283 mg of aspirin in the Dutch TIA Trial. (Reprinted from The Dutch TIA Trial Study Group. *N Engl J Med* 1991;325:1261–1266, with permission of publisher.)

effective in other ethnic groups, it has not been tested extensively.

Algra and van Gijn[242] evaluated the efficacy of aspirin in daily doses ranging from under 100 mg (low) to more than 900 mg (high), and they noted no major differences in responses (see Table 10–23). They calculated the risk reduction to be 13% with a low dose and 14% with a high dose. In a separate analysis, Tijssen[243] confirmed these results. These analyses are similar to the results of the analysis of Sze et al,[215] who estimated that aspirin reduced the risk of stroke by approximately 15%. Based on a meta-analysis, Johnson et al[244] found that aspirin reduced the risk of stroke by approximately 15% with administered doses that range from 50 mg to 1500 mg per day. Patrono and Roth[245] concluded that the preferred dose of aspirin for stroke prophylaxis is 75 mg/day. Conversely, Dyken[192] contended that circumstantial evidence supported the conclusion that larger doses of aspirin (>1000 mg/day) were more effective than lower doses. In a retrospective review of recurrent stroke, Bornstein et al[246] concluded that the likelihood for early recurrence was greater with low doses of aspirin and that a daily dose of 500 mg or greater should be prescribed for secondary stroke prophylaxis. Taylor et al[365] found that low doses of aspirin (81–325 mg/day) were superior to larger doses in preventing ischemic events following carotid endarterectomy. Although the equality of effectiveness of aspirin is over a broad range of doses, the frequency of side effects appears to have a strong dose relationship.[201,219] Thus, a risk–benefit analysis would favor the lower doses of aspirin.

The ischemic strokes occurring among patients taking aspirin have been attributed to a variety of causes, and the strokes among these patients often lead to moderate-to-severe disability.[247] Some of these events likely were of cardioembolic origin, and aspirin has limited usefulness to prevent these events. Aspirin might not be as effective among persons with high-grade stenoses of the internal carotid artery as other groups of patients.[247] This observation might be a reason to consider prescription of other antiplatelet aggregating agents or anticoagulants. Still, the potential superiority of other medical therapies has not been tested in this situation. The poor response to aspirin among patients with severe arterial stenoses also might partially explain the success of carotid endarterectomy. Grotta et al[248] concluded that aspirin might reduce the severity of ischemic

Table 10–23. **Comparisons of Doses of Aspirin**

	HIGHER DOSE OF ASPIRIN		LOWER DOSE OF ASPIRIN	
Trial	**Dose**	**Events/Patients**	**Dose**	**Events/Patients**
UK TIA[218]	1200 mg	168/815	300 mg	195/806
Dutch[239]	300 mg	216/1555	30 mg	195/1576
ACE[365]	650–1300 mg	118/1409	81–325 mg	87/1395

ACE = Aspirin Carotid Endarterectomy Trial.

strokes as well as the likelihood of a vascular event. However, recent studies could not provide evidence that low-dose aspirin reduced the severity of stroke or outcome after the event.[249–251]

Aspirin is not an effective agent in preventing the formation of mural thrombus in the left ventricle following a large anterior myocardial infarction.[77] It should not be considered as an effective way to reduce the risk of cardioembolic stroke among this group of high-risk patients. Aspirin alone is not effective in prevention of stroke among patients with mechanical prosthetic valves.[168] Still, aspirin has a place for prevention of embolism among patients with bioprosthetic aortic valves. Although warfarin usually is given during the first 3 months following surgery for patients with bioprosthetic valves, particularly aortic valve replacements, aspirin is administered subsequently.[168] Even this approach is being challenged. A recent report concluded that the 3-month course of anticoagulation might not be necessary after biological aortic valve replacement.[252] In a small, controlled study, no difference in the rate of embolism was noted in patients initially treated with anticoagulants versus those treated with antiplatelet aggregating agents. A low dose of aspirin can be added to oral anticoagulants for treatment of patients with mechanical prosthetic valves.[168] The usual scenario of combined treatment is the occurrence of embolism despite treatment with the anticoagulant.

Analyses show that the risk of stroke among persons with atrial fibrillation could be reduced by approximately 21% with treatment with aspirin, but no subgroups of patients appeared to be particularly benefited.[145,148,253] Another analysis concluded that aspirin's effects in reducing thromboembolism are in the range of an 18%–44% reduction in risk.[149] (See Table 10–18.) The only tested dose of aspirin for prevention of stroke among patients with atrial fibrillation is approximately 325 mg.[149] The Stroke Prevention Atrial Fibrillation Investigators evaluated the usefulness of either aspirin or warfarin in prevention of stroke among patients with non-valvular atrial fibrillation.[254] Among persons younger than 75, the risk of ischemic stroke was slightly higher in persons taking aspirin than those receiving warfarin (1.9% vs. 1.3%), but the risk of intracranial bleeding was higher in the patients taking the anticoagulant. As a result, aspirin and warfarin were approximately equal. Among persons older than 75, the risk of ischemic stroke was significantly higher among persons taking aspirin than among those using warfarin. But older patients also had a high chance of bleeding secondary to warfarin. Again, the net benefit from warfarin was marginal.

Other reports from the same group show that patients with atrial fibrillation considered to be at "low risk" for embolism could be treated with aspirin.[4,255] The risk of major bleeding events with aspirin was low—approximately 0.5% per year. Still, women and persons with advancing age, a history of hypertension, a systolic blood pressure >160 mm Hg, or a prior neurological event appear to have a high risk for cerebral embolism secondary to atrial fibrillation, despite treatment with aspirin.[9] A recent study of low-dose aspirin (125 mg/day or 125 mg every other day) for prevention of vascular events among patients with atrial fibrillation found benefit in preventing cardiac events but no efficacy in preventing strokes.[256] Patients with lone atrial fibrillation (those persons under the age of 60 and with no other risk factors) could be treated with aspirin, although the overall risk of embolism is low even without medical intervention.[4,149,154] A Norwegian trial showed that aspirin was at least equal to LMW heparin in preventing recurrent embolism among patients with atrial fibrillation and a recent ischemic stroke.[88]

A placebo-controlled trial performed in Europe compared the utility of aspirin or adjusted-dose anticoagulation in prevention of recurrent stroke among patients with atrial fibrillation.[257] Aspirin had a modest protective effect and was inferior to the anticoagulant. This finding is not surprising because the occurrence of neurological symptoms denotes the patient as having a very high risk for cardioembolism.

Patients are advised to take aspirin as part of the initial response to an acute myocardial infarction, but the value of this recommendation for lessening the consequences of ischemic stroke is less certain. Two clinical trials tested the value of aspirin in prevention of recurrent stroke or death following ischemic stroke.[85,258] In both trials, aspirin could be started up to 48 hours after the onset of the ischemic event. One trial prescribed approximately 300 mg/day, and the other used one-half that dose. Both trials found that aspirin was relatively safe and that the risk of intracranial hemorrhage was relatively low. They also found a modest benefit in prevention of recurrent ischemic events in the first months after stroke. In another trial of treatment for acute ischemic stroke, low-dose aspirin in combination with streptokinase was compared with aspiring alone, streptokinase alone, or placebo.[259] No particular benefit was seen with aspiring alone, and the combination of aspirin and streptokinase was extremely dangerous. The frequency of serious, often fatal intracranial hemorrhages was markedly increased with the combination of medications. This finding causes concerns about the administration of aspirin to prevent recurrent stroke within the first hours after treatment with a thrombolytic agent. Overall, the benefit of aspirin in treatment of acute stroke is minimal.[260] Although these trials do not prove that aspirin is an effective treatment for acute ischemic stroke itself, they do show that the medication can be safely started in the first days after the event. These trials' data suggest that aspirin can be started if thrombolytic therapy or another agent that acutely affects thrombosis is not being used to treat the stroke itself. Still, the initiation of aspirin should be considered as an urgent therapy because the risk of recurrent stroke seems to be relatively low during the first few days. The goal of early aspirin treatment should remain to prevent recurrent stroke, myocardial infarction, or vascular death.

SUMMARY

Aspirin's many attributes make it an attractive choice as a therapy that can be prescribed for either the primary or the secondary prevention of ischemic stroke. It also is the mainstay of medical treatments to avert myocardial infarction or vascular death. Still, aspirin is under-used among patients with a history of stroke.[197] Aspirin is the logical first therapy to avoid recurrent neurological symptoms among patients who have non-cardioembolic events and who have not been taking aspirin. Although aspirin's efficacy has been shown primarily among patients with non-atherosclerotic vasculopatheis, such as an arterial dissection. Aspirin is an important part of medical management following reconstructive cerebrovascular operations, including carotid endarterectomy. Low doses of aspirin (81–160 mg/day) are safer than and equal in efficacy to larger daily doses (>1000 mg). In contrast, aspirin's role in limiting the risks of cardioembolic stroke is limited. Aspirin should be reserved for cases that are judged to have a low risk for embolism or patients who have a contraindication for treatment with an oral anticoagulant.[152,261] An advantage of antiplatelet aggregating agents is the lower risk of major bleeding complications, including intracerebral hemorrhage. Aspirin is much safer than warfarin.[232] A large trial found that aspirin was associated with the approximately one-third the risk of major bleeding than was warfarin.[126] Aspirin can be added to warfarin for patients having recurrent neurological symptoms despite treatment with the anticoagulant. The major contraindications to treatment with aspirin are allergic reactions and active peptic ulcer disease.

Ticlopidine

PHARMACOLOGY

Ticlopidine is a thienopyridine that blocks platelet responses to adenosine diphosphate–induced aggregation and signal transduction.[199,201–203,262] It was the first medication specifically developed for its effects on platelet aggregation. Ticlopidine does not inhibit platelet function in in-vitro testing, a finding that suggests some in-vivo transformation of the medication is required for it to prevent thrombosis. Ticlopidine modifies platelet adelyate and thus effects the platelet IIb/IIIa receptor's interactions with fibrinogen.[62,199] The medication greatly prolongs the bleeding time. Ticlopidine suppresses platelet aggregation induced by either collagen or thrombin, but these actions can be overcome by increasing concentrations of agonists of thrombosis.[201,203] Droste et al[203] found that platelet counts were higher among patients taking ticlopidine than among those using aspirin. They concluded that the higher platelet counts probably reflects less platelet activation and degradation and a longer platelet survival time with ticlopidine than with aspirin. The importance of this observation is not clear.

Ticlopidine is rapidly absorbed after ingestion. It has a half-life of approximately 24–36 hours after a single dose.[201] Although it is rapidly absorbed, ticlopidine's antithrombotic effects may not reach therapeutic levels for up to 1–2 weeks after starting treatment. This feature means that ticlopidine is not a potential intervention for treatment of acute ischemic stroke. Aspirin has been prescribed in conjunction with ticlopidine for the first few days to protect the patient during the initiation of treatment. Yet, the necessity of this strategy has not been established because no period of high risk of thromboembolism has been reported during the first days after starting ticlopidine.

SAFETY

Gastrointestinal distress and diarrhea are the most common side effects from the use of ticlopidine.[263–265](See Table 10–21.) In addition, ticlopidine has been associated with rare cases of cholestatic hepatitis or jaundice.[266,267] A case of acute renal failure and interstitial nephritis also was ascribed to the medication.[268] Allergic reactions can lead to urticaria or other skin eruptions. Still, the most bothersome side effects of ticlopidine are neutropenia, thrombocytopenia, aplastic anemia, and thrombotic thrombocytopenia purpura.[265,269–272,375] Although many patients can have a mild decline in white blood cell count spontaneously after stroke or with the use of ticlopidine, the medication-related neutropenia can progress to agranulocytosis. Severe hematologic reactions usually develop within 3 months of starting treatment, but these complications peak approximately 1 month after starting treatment. Thus, patients need to have regular monitoring of the white blood cell and platelet counts during the first 3 months. The usual regimen is biweekly testing. If a decline in either the white blood cell or the platelet count is noted, then the medication should be discontinued. Most patients will be asymptomatic at the time of discovery of the hematologic changes. Still, a patient with severe neutropenia likely will be admitted to the hospital for observation and treatment of the severe neutropenia. The cause of the neutropenia is not established, but it may relate to an arrest in the maturation of white blood cell precursors in the bone marrow. The reaction appears to be idiosyncratic. The neutropenia has been complicated by serious infections that could be potentially life-threatening. In most cases, stopping the ticlopidine will permit recovery of the white blood cell count during the next few days. Granulocyte colony stimulating factor (GCSF) could be administered to stimulate recovery of the neutrophil count among patients with agranulocytosis and complicating infections. The complication of ticlopidine-associated thrombotic thrombocytopenia purpura is discussed in more detail in Chapter 8. Still this life-threatening complication makes a physician pause before treating with ticlopidine. The relatively high rate of serious adverse experiences is the major limitation for the use of ticlopidine.

POTENTIAL INDICATIONS

Ticlopidine has been found to be effective in treatment of patients with peripheral vascular disease and diabetic retinopathy[273,274] (see Fig. 10–3). Murray et al[275] concluded that ticlopidine was better than aspirin in treatment of unstable angina, intermittent claudication, or non-proliferative vascular retinopathies. In a clinical trial enrolling patients with peripheral vascular disease, ticlopidine reduced the risk of TIA, stroke, or myocardial infarction by 11.4% and mortality by 29.1%.[265] Ticlopidine has been tested for use as a perioperative procedure for patients having coronary artery angioplasty. [276–279] The combination

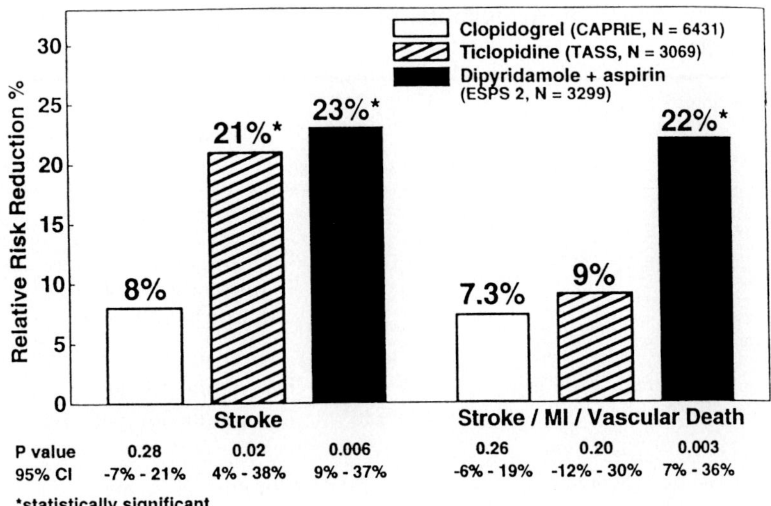

Figure 10–3. Comparisons of the efficacy of other antiplatelet agents (clopidogrel, ticlopidine, or dipyridamole and aspirin) against aspirin. Data are the major outcomes from three large trials—CAPRIE[296], TASS[263], and ESPS—2.[307] (Reprinted from Albers G et al. Antithrombotic and Thrombolytic Therapy for Ischemic Stroke *Chest*, 1998;114(Suppl)683, with permission of publisher.)

of aspirin and ticlopidine was superior to aspirin alone or warfarin in preventing thrombosis. A short (4-week) course of ticlopidine among patients having coronary angioplasty and stenting is prescribed commonly. Physicians doing cerebrovascular angioplasty and stenting have adopted this approach.

Ticlopidine was tested for its ability to prevent ischemic stroke in two large clinical trials. A placebo-controlled trial that enrolled patients with moderately severe stroke demonstrated the effectiveness of ticlopidine in prevention of recurrent ischemic stroke.[264] (See Table 10–24.) This trial found that ticlopidine was effective in both men and women; the relative risk reductions were 28.1% and 34.2%, respectively. Another trial compared aspirin (1300 mg/day) and ticlopidine (500 mg/day) in prevention of stroke among patients with warning ischemic symptoms.[263] During a period of follow up of approximately 3 years, ticlopidine achieved an approximately 12%–18% relative risk reduction in major events when compared to aspirin. This study found ticlopidine to be superior to aspirin.[192,260] Among patients with minor stroke followed for 1 year, stroke or death occurred in 6.2% of patients given ticlopidine and 10.8% of patients receiving aspirin.[280] In a series of post-hoc analyses based on the data collected for the Ticlopidine-Aspirin Stroke Study, ticlopidine was reported to be superior to aspirin in preventing stroke among women, African Americans, and persons with carotid stenosis, reversible ischemic neurological deficits, transient ischemic attacks, vertebrobasilar events.[281–285]

SUMMARY

Ticlopidine is effective in prevention of stroke. In a head-to-head comparison with aspirin, it was found to be superior. Easton[226] concluded that ticlopidine is superior to aspirin and that it provides an important reduction in the risk of thromboembolic events among patients with a history of stroke or warning symptoms of stroke. Despite the results of the clinical trials, the use of the medication has been controversial. Ticlopidine has been criticized for lack of efficacy and safety.[286] Notwithstanding these criticisms, it should be considered as an alternative to treatment with aspirin for

Table 10–24. **Comparisons of Medications in Prevention of Stroke or Death: High Risk Patients**

Medication/Trial	Group Medication Daily Dose	Events/Patients	Group Medication Daily Dose	Events/Patients
Sulfinpyrazone				
Canadian[234]	Aspirin 1300 mg	26/144	Sulfinpyrazone 800 mg	38/156
			Sulfinpyrazone 800 mg and aspirin 1300 mg	20/146
Ticlopidine				
TASS[263]	Aspirin 1300 mg	349/1540	Ticlopidine 500 mg	306/1529
CATS[264]	Placebo	134/528*	Ticlopidine 500 mg	106/525
Clopidogrel				
CAPRIE[296]	Aspirin 325 mg		Clopidogrel 75 mg	
All patients		1175/9586		1032/9599
TIA/stroke		424/3198†		400/3233
Dipyridamole				
Guiraud-Chaumeil[366]	Aspirin 900 mg	6/102	Aspirin 900 mg and dipyridamole 150 mg	7/105
Bousser el al[360]	Aspirin 1000 mg	27/198	Aspirin 1000 mg and dipyridamole 225 mg	26/202
Matias-Guiu[304]	Aspirin 100 mg Dipyridamole 300 mg	9/115	dipyridamole 400 mg	7/71
ACCSG[302]	Aspirin 325 mg	84/442	Aspirin 325 mg and dipyridamole 300 mg	85/448
ESPS—2[307]	Aspirin 50 mg	330/1649	Aspirin 50 mg and dipyridamole 400 mg	286/1650
			Dipyridamole 400 mg	321/1654

*Stroke, myocardial infarction, vascular death.
†Stroke or vascular death, including fatal myocardial infarction.
TASS = Ticlopidine Aspirin Stroke Study
CATS = Canadian American Ticlopidine Study
CAPRIE = Clopidogrel Aspirin Prevention Recurrent Ischemic Events
ACCSG = American-Canadian Cooperative Study Group
ESPS = European Stroke Prevention Study

patients with TIA or ischemic stroke.[287] Generally, it should be prescribed to patients who cannot tolerate aspirin or who have recurrent neurological symptoms despite treatment with aspirin.[287–289] The medication has serious limitations (see Table 10–15). It is more expensive than aspirin and requires hematologic monitoring for the first 3 months. Despite these expenses, ticlopidine appears to be cost-effective because of its added benefit in preventing disabling stroke.[290] The major limitation of treatment with ticlopidine is the risk of serious hematologic reactions. Although the potential for agranulocytosis or thrombotic thrombocytopenia purpura is low, these complications are potentially life-threatening. Patients and their families must be warned about these potential complications. The medication should not be prescribed if the necessary laboratory monitoring cannot be performed.[287,291] With the development of new medications to prevent stroke, the use of ticlopidine likely will diminish in the future.

Clopidogrel

PHARMACOLOGY

Clopidogrel also is a thenopyridine whose mechanism of action is similar to that of ticlopidine.[262] It also produces an irreversible, dose-dependent inhibition of thrombosis.[292] Clopidogrel is readily absorbed and some inhibition of platelet aggregation can be seen within hours of starting treatment.[201]

SAFETY

The new antiplatelet aggregating agent clopidogrel has been shown to be relatively safe.[293] (See Table 10–21.) It has not been accompanied by the frequent and potentially serious side effects that are described with use of ticlopidine. Apparently, it does not cause leucopenia, but it can cause gastrointestinal distress, diarrhea, and skin eruptions.[294] Recently, the use of clopidogrel has been associated with the developments of thrombotic thrombocytopenia purpura.[295,376] The comparative risk of ticlopidine or clopidogrel in causing this platelet disorder is not known. The risk of gastrointestinal bleeding is lower with clopidogrel than with aspirin.[294]

POTENTIAL INDICATIONS

The clinical information about the use of clopidogrel comes from one large trial (Table 10–24 and Fig. 10–3). This international study compared the usefulness of clopidogrel (75 mg/day) and aspirin (325 mg/day) in prevention of stroke, myocardial infarction, or vascular death among patients with symptomatic cerebrovascular disease, coronary artery disease, or peripheral vascular disease.[294,296] The overall results of the trial demonstrated that clopidogrel was superior to aspirin, but the benefit was confined largely to persons who presented with symptoms of peripheral artery disease. The trial showed only a modest reduction in vascular events among patients who had had either a TIA or an ischemic stroke. Unlike the results of the trial of ticlopidine, clopidogrel was not superior to aspirin among patients with neurological symptoms. No study has focused solely on the group of patients who have had TIA or ischemic stroke. No direct comparison between the efficacy of clopidogrel and ticlopidine has been performed. As a result, clopidogrel should be considered as possibly as effective as ticlopidine; its major advantage is its lower rate of complications.

SUMMARY

Creager[294] concluded that clopidogrel is more effective and safer than aspirin in preventing ischemic events in patients with atherosclerosis. This probably is an overstatement, especially when dealing with a population that presents with TIA or stroke. The basic premise of the large study of clopidogrel was that the medication would have equal efficacy in preventing vascular events regardless of the presentation of atherosclerosis. This assumption may not be totally correct. In particular, the diversity of causes of stroke, even in a population of patients with atherosclerosis, may limit application of the results from patients with peripheral artery disease. The fracturing of plaques that lead to acute coronary or cerebrovascular arterial thrombosis may not be the same problem among persons with peripheral atherosclerosis and intermittent claudication. Clopidiogrel might be effective in preventing ischemea in slow-flow situations, but it might not be at successful in preventing thrombosis secondary to a fractural plaque. Another analysis concluded that clopidogrel has a better safety profile than ticlopidine and has equal efficacy.[297] The safety of clopidogrel now is open to question.[295] Although experience shows that clopidogrel may have fewer side effects than ticlopidine, there are no data to state that the two drugs have equal efficacy. Only indirect evidence is available. Among patients with ischemic cerebrovascular disease, ticlopidine was shown to be superior to aspirin, but clopidogrel was not. A reasonable conclusion is that clopidogrel generally is equal to aspirin in efficacy and safety.[192,260,287,298] Some authors have concluded that clopidogrel should be the first treatment to prevent stroke among high-risk patients.[297] Still, the data about the efficacy of clopidogrel in prevention of stroke are not overwhelming, and there is room for doubt about its use.[299] The data do not show that clopidogrel is superior to aspirin in preventing ischemic events among patients with TIA or stroke.[232] There appears to be little reason to substitute clopidogrel for aspirin as the primary medical therapy to avoid stroke. The medication is more expensive than aspirin. Rather, its role likely will be as an alternative to aspirin if the patient has symptoms despite treatment with aspirin or if the patient has a contraindication for the use of aspirin.

Dipyridamole

PHARMACOLOGY

Dipyridamole is a pyrimidopyrimidine that is a potent vasodilator that increases coronary artery blood flow.[300] The agent also presumably inhibits cyclic nucleotide phosphodiesterase and blocks the uptake of adenosine in the platelet.[201] This results in decreased platelet aggregation, an effect that appears to be reversible. The medication also prolongs platelet survival.[300] Dipyridamole now is available in conventional and sustained-release formulations. The latter formulation may improve the bioavailability of the medication.[201] The half-life of dipyridamole is approximately 10 hours, which means that a minimum of a twice-per-day dosage regimen is needed to maintain pharmacologic effects even if the sustained- release formulation is prescribed.

SAFETY

Dipyridamole is relatively safe (see Table 10–21). Because it is a vasodilator, it does induce headaches. The risk of bleeding is relatively low. No other serious complication has been ascribed to dipyridamole, and no special laboratory monitoring is required.

POTENTIAL INDICATIONS

The role of dipyridamole in prevention of stroke remains controversial. For example, Gibbs and Lip[301] concluded that there are no data to support the use of dipyridamole alone in treatment of coronary artery disease or peripheral vascular disease. The studies of dipyridamole alone are few (see Table 10–24 and Fig. 10–3). The usefulness of the medication usually has been examined in combination with aspirin. Still, efficacy of the addition of dipyridamole to aspirin has been questioned. The extra cost of prescribing a second medication must be justified by an incremental increase in efficacy because the safety of dipyridamole is not an issue. French and North American clinical trials did not find any benefit in prevention of stroke among high-risk patients with the addition of dipyridamole.[302,303] Another trial found that the combination of aspirin, 50 mg/day, and dipyridamole, 300 mg/day, was not different in prevention of vascular events than the use of dipyridamole, 400 mg/day, alone.[304] A large European trial compared the combination of aspirin, 900 mg/day, and dipyridamole, 225 mg/day, against placebo and found a major reduction in the number of strokes.[305] The overall reduction in risk with the combination was approximately 30%. The results were better than those described in most studies of aspirin alone. Still, most of the benefit from treatment was ascribed to the aspirin.[226] A meta-analysis of antiplatelet therapies also was unable to detect a significant benefit from treatment with dipyridamole.[306] As a result, a second large trial tested the value of low-dose aspirin, dipyridamole, or the combination against placebo in prevention of vascular events.[307] This trial has been criticized on several grounds, but the results have not been refuted. Either aspirin or dipyridamole reduced the risk of vascular events by approximately 13%–15%, and the combination lowered the risk by approximately 24%.[306–308] Regardless of the patient's age, the antiplatelet aggregating agents (alone or combination) were effective.[309] Although the combination of aspirin and dipyridamole was effective in reducing the number of subsequent strokes, the agents were not useful in reducing the severity of the events that did occur.[251] Additional studies have examined dipyridamole in other situations. Sullivan et al[310] tested the comparison of dipyridamole, 400 mg/day, and warfarin to warfarin alone among patients with cardiac valve replacements. The combination reduced the risk of embolism from

14.3% to 1.3%. This study provides the rationale for dipyridamole in addition to warfarin to prevent cerebral embolism among high-risk patients. Dipyridamole might be an alternative to aspirin, but there are no data to show that dipyridamole is superior to aspirin.

SUMMARY

The status of dipyridamole as an agent to prevent stroke remains somewhat unclear. The combination of aspirin and dipyridamole appears to be effective.[192] Tijssen[243] and Easton[260] concluded that the addition of dipyridamole increased the efficacy of aspirin by approximately 15% regardless of the dose of aspirin. Another analysis concluded that there was substantial benefit with the combination of dipyridamole and aspirin; the relative risk reduction of stroke was estimated to be 23%.[311] Thus, its primary utility likely will be as an adjunct to aspirin, although the European study demonstrates that dipyridamole alone is approximately equal to aspirin in efficacy. Thus, monotherapy with dipyridamole likely will be restricted to patients who cannot tolerate aspirin, ticlopidine, or clopidogrel. Conversely the formulation of the combination of aspirin and dipyridamole is useful. It could be prescribed to patients who have symptoms despite treatment with aspirin. The status of the combination as a first-line treatment likely will evolve during the next few years.

Other Antiplatelet Aggregating Agents

Several compounds that block platelet aggregation and prevent ischemic vascular events are being developed.[312] The most promising are the glycoprotein IIb/IIIa receptor blocking agents. Because this receptor is the common site for platelet aggregation regardless of stimulus, its blockade should have marked affect on thrombosis. The agents that block the receptor might provide extra protection against ischemic stroke among high-risk patients. The new agents are platelet specific and affect platelet aggregation by interacting with the sites of the integrins, laminin and fibronectin.[313,314] The glycoprotein IIb/IIIa receptor inhibitors do not affect platelet adhesion. A bolus dose of 0.25 mg/Kg of one of these receptor inhibitors—abciximab—can block >80% of platelet receptors, and an infusion will maintain inhibition for several hours.[315] The antiplatelet affects are lost as new platelets enter the circulation.

The glycoprotein IIb/IIIa receptor blockers have been used successfully to treat patients with acute coronary artery disease.[316–320] Because *abciximab* is an intravenously administered antiplatelet aggregating agent, it will not be indicated for long-term care. It might be prescribed in a situation that is currently considered as an indication for heparin. Other glycoprotein IIb/IIIa blockers that are cyclic peptides or orally active blockers might be useful in chronic treatment.[321] These agents alone or in combination with other antiplatelet aggregating agents could be useful for prevention of stroke.[322] At present, little information is available about their clinical utility, and there is no current indication for their use in long-term care. Mahaffey et al[323] reviewed the frequency of stroke among patients who received a glycoprotein IIb/IIIa receptor blocker in treatment of acute coronary artery syndromes. No lessening in the risk of stroke was noted with treatment.

Several non-steroidal, anti-inflammatory agents besides aspirin can inhibit platelet cyclooxygenase activity.[201] *Sulfinpyrazone* is a uricosuric agent that weakly inhibits platelet cyclooxygenase activity.[324] A Canadian trial tested sulfinpyrazone alone and with aspirin in comparison to aspirin alone or placebo in a large clinical trial.[234] (See Table 10–24.) No benefit in lowering the risk of stroke or death was seen with sulfinpyrazone, although the patients who received the combination of aspirin and sulfinpyrazone appeared to do the best. Sze et al[215] concluded that the combination of aspirin and sulfinpyrazone reduced the risk of ischemic events by approximately 39%. Conversely, a review of the role of antiplatelet agents in prevention of stroke concluded that sulfinpyrazone was not effective.[226] At present, this agent should not be prescribed. *Indobufen* is another cyclooxygenase inhibitor that has been tested for its usefulness in prevention of stroke. This agent should not be confused with the over-the-counter analgesic ibuprofen. A clinical trial tested indobufen in comparison to ticlopidine in prevention of stroke among high-risk patients, but the medication was not as effective as the ticlopidine.[325] The frequencies of adverse reactions were similar in the two treatment groups, but gastrointestinal symptoms and bleeding were more common among the patients receiving indobufen. In addition to being an anti-inflammatory agent, *ibuprofen* also affects platelet aggregation. Ibuprofen has been proposed as an alternative to aspirin or warfarin for prevention of cardioembolic stroke, but no data are available about the usefulness of this medication.[142]

PENTOXIFYLLINE

Pentoxifylline reduces deformability of red blood cells and affects shear stress.[326] In addition, the agent can affect platelet aggregation, fibrinogen concentrations, and viscosity. These features may support the use of pentoxifylline to improve flow in the microcirculation of the brain.[327] Pentoxifylline is used to improve the symptoms of intermittent claudication among patients with peripheral vascular disease, but its value in preventing thromboembolism is not known. Because of its effects on blood flow, pentoxifylline might be helpful in preventing stroke among patients with critically severe stenotic disease of the intracranial or extracranial vasculature. No data have yet defined the role of pentoxifylline in the prevention of stroke among high-risk persons. The combination of ticlopidine and pentoxifylline has been tested in a small clinical trial.[328] The results of the trial showed that the combination might be useful, but additional research is needed to determine whether the conclusion was correct. Additional research is needed to determine the role of treatment with pentoxifylline in prevention of stroke. At present, it is a nonstandard intervention.

COMBINATIONS OF MEDICATIONS

Combinations of Antiplatelet Aggregating Agents

Because the pharmacologic effects of aspirin, ticlopidine (or clopidogrel), and dipyridamole differ, they could have complementary actions in lessening the risk of ischemic stroke.[260] The combination of dipyridamole and aspirin already has been tested extensively. The combination of dipyridamole and aspirin has a greater cumulative effect on platelet function than does aspirin alone.[207] A European trial showed that the combination was superior to either aspirin or dipyridamole alone in prevention of stroke.[306] The combination of aspirin and dipyridamole can reduce the chances of ischemic events by approximately 39%.[215] Presumably, the combination also is superior to ticlopidine or clopidogrel alone.[298] No comparison studies are available to judge that conclusion.

Because ticlopidine and clopidogrel act by mechanisms different from aspirin, their combination with aspirin could provide additional benefit in prevention of ischemic stroke.[322,329] Harker et al[292] concluded that the pharmacologic effects of clopidogrel are enhanced by the addition of aspirin. Already, ticlopidine or clopidogrel is combined with aspirin to prevent thrombosis following coronary artery angioplasty and stenting.[276–278] The combination has allure when a patient has symptoms despite treatment with single medications. Still, issues such as the potential for a marked increase in bleeding complications need additional attention. Further research is needed on the combination of clopidogrel or ticlopidine and aspirin. There is no reason to combine ticlopidine and clopidogrel.

Combinations of Anticoagulants and Antiplatelet Aggregating Agents

Antiplatelet aggregating agents and anticoagulants are used to treat patients with ischemic heart disease. For example, a large clinical trial in the United Kingdom showed that the combination of low-dose warfarin and aspirin was better than either medication alone in preventing death or non-fatal myocardial infarction.[330] The combination also has been tested in treatment of patients at high risk for stroke.[322] A large clinical trial compared the safety of warfarin (INR 2.5–4.2) or warfarin (INR 2.2–2.8) and aspirin, 150 mg/day.[331] No significant differences in major, fatal, or intracranial hemorrhages were noted between the two groups. The investigators concluded that the combination of warfarin and low-dose aspirin is safe. Another study found that the combination of aspirin and an anticoagulant is as safe as anticoagulation alone in treatment of patients with acute ischemic stroke.[332] In contrast, the addition of aspirin increases the risk of intracranial hemorrhage among patients taking an adjusted dose regimen of warfarin.[333] Although the combination of aspirin and low, fixed doses of warfarin generally is safe, clinical data about the efficacy among persons with atrial fibrillation are disappointing.[118] Clinical studies show that the combination is not as effective as an adjusted-dose regimen of warfarin.[173]

The addition of aspirin is recommended for treatment of patients with prosthetic heart valves who have neurological symptoms despite adequate levels of anticoagulation.[334] High-risk patients can benefit from treatment despite the increased chance of bleeding complications. The usual dose of aspirin is approximately 100 mg/day. Dipyridamole could be a substitute for aspirin in this situation.

NEUROPROTECTIVE AGENTS

Most recent research has focused on the ability of neuroprotective agents to lessen the neurological consequences of acute ischemic stroke. Presumably, the prophylactic administration of neuroprotective agents might help lessen the severity of ischemic neurological deficits.[335] Although these drugs would not prevent thromboembolism per se, they would be at therapeutic levels in areas of the brain that might be affected by the thromboembolic event. They would inhibit the acute cellular and metabolic consequences of the stroke. These medications could be given as a supplement to antiplatelet aggregating or anticoagulant agents to patients who have had recent TIA or those who are scheduled for cardiovascular or cerebrovascular operations. The assumption would be to treat during a time when risk for ischemia was high, such as the perioperative period. Although this strategy holds promise, to date, no neuroprotective therapy has been established as useful in acute treatment or an acute prevention mode.

SUMMARY AND ALGORITHM FOR MEDICAL MANAGEMENT

Summary

The use of antiplatelet aggregating agents and anticoagulants in prevention of ischemic stroke varies widely.[336] The physician's specialty and geographic location influence decisions for medical treatment. Even among stroke specialists, recommendations for surgical or medical therapies vary widely. For example, a survey noted that carotid endarterectomy would be recommended for treatment of a severe asymptomatic stenosis by 48% of specialists in North America and 28% in Europe.[337] These differences appear not to be secondary to the results of clinical trials and rather reflect physicians' personal preferences or experiences. Elderly patients with dementia, including those with multi-infarction dementia, often are not prescribed either antiplatelet aggregating agents or warfarin, despite the high risk of recurrent stroke in this group.[338,339] The reasons for these decisions are not clear. Despite extensive data about the usefulness of medical therapies in prevention of stroke, they remain under-prescribed. Aspirin remains the key medical intervention for prevention of stroke among most patients with vascular disease.[340] Unfortunately, aspirin also is under-used for secondary prevention of vascular disease.[341] Brass et al[342] noted that only 49 or 278 elderly patients with atrial fibrillation and recent stroke were treated with aspirin at the time of discharge while 81 reveived no medication. Thus, a sizeable group of high risk patients did not receive any stroke prophylaxis medication.

Clopidogrel may be useful in persons whose primary problem is peripheral vascular disease and for treatment of patients who have had either myocardial or brain ischemia and who have not responded to treatment with aspirin.[340,343] Ticlopidine also remains an option for treatment of patients who have had symptoms despite treatment with aspirin or who have a contraindication for treatment with aspirin. The combination of aspirin and dipyridamole also is an option for treating patients who have had ischemic symptoms despite the use of aspirin.[343]

The benefits of long-term oral anticoagulant therapy in preventing cardioembolic stroke are unequivocal.[150,261] Anticoagulants are the most effective medical therapy to prevent embolic stroke among patients with prosthetic heart valves.[169] Anticoagulants are clearly indicated for treatment of patients with atrial fibrillation and recent neurological symptoms.[143,150] Long-term anticoagulation to prevent stroke among asymptomatic patients with atrial fibrillation is safe, efficient, and cost-effective.[344–347] The benefits from anticoagulation begin immediately after starting treatment with warfarin, and managed care organizations and health care planners should support this therapy.[344] The use of oral anticoagulants among patients with atrial fibrillation increased during the early 1990s, but no increase in prescription has occurred more recently.[348] Warfarin is not contraindicated for the treatment of elderly patients with atrial fibrillation.[65] White et al[182] and Bath et al[349] found that many patients with atrial fibrillation who are at high risk for embolism are not receiving anticoagulation. Unfortunately, these agents are being under-used in treatment of patients at high risk for cardioembolic stroke, including those with atrial fibrillation.[342,350–352]

Algorithm

The selection of treatments to prevent stroke must continue to be made on an individual basis using the available data about efficacy and safety as guideposts. Any decision is influenced by the patient's presenting symptoms, the presumed cause of the ischemia, and the patient's overall health. The patient's personal preferences, the presence of any contraindications for a specific treatment, and prior use of therapies also influence management. The administration of medical or surgical interventions is built on the substrate of treatment of risk factors and co-developing heart disease.

Patients with unusual causes of stroke, such as inflammatory or infectious vasculitides, usually receive specific interventions, such as antibiotics or immunosuppressive agents. Most patients with pro-thrombotic conditions are treated with anticoagulants, and those with disorders of platelets often receive aspirin or other antiplatelet aggregating drugs. Clinical trials have not tested the usefulness of either medical or surgical therapies in stroke prevention among persons with non-atherosclerotic vasculopatheis. Thus, the results from trials of treatment of patients with atherosclerotic disease often are used as the foundation for decisions about management. Some special situations may alter these judgments. For example, anticoagulants often are prescribed to patients with arterial dissections because of the presumed high risk for recurrent embolism. Inversely, patients with moyamoya disease usually are not prescribed anticoagulants because of the high risk for bleeding.

Anticoagulants are the preferred treatment for the prevention of cardioembolic stroke (Figs. 10–4 and 10–5). The occcurrence of neurological symptoms automatically usually denotes the underlying cardiac cause as being a high-risk lesion. The only major exception to the recommendation for anticoagulation is the presence of infective endocarditis on a native valve. These patients are at a high risk for intracranial hemorrhage secondary to an infective aneurysm, and the presence of an anticoagulant may exacerbate the bleeding. Surgery is preferred over anticoagulant treatment among patients with atrial myxoma. In general, the aim of anticoagulant therapy is to achieve an INR level of 2–3. The desired INR level is 2.5–4 for persons with mechanical prosthetic valves. If symptoms occur

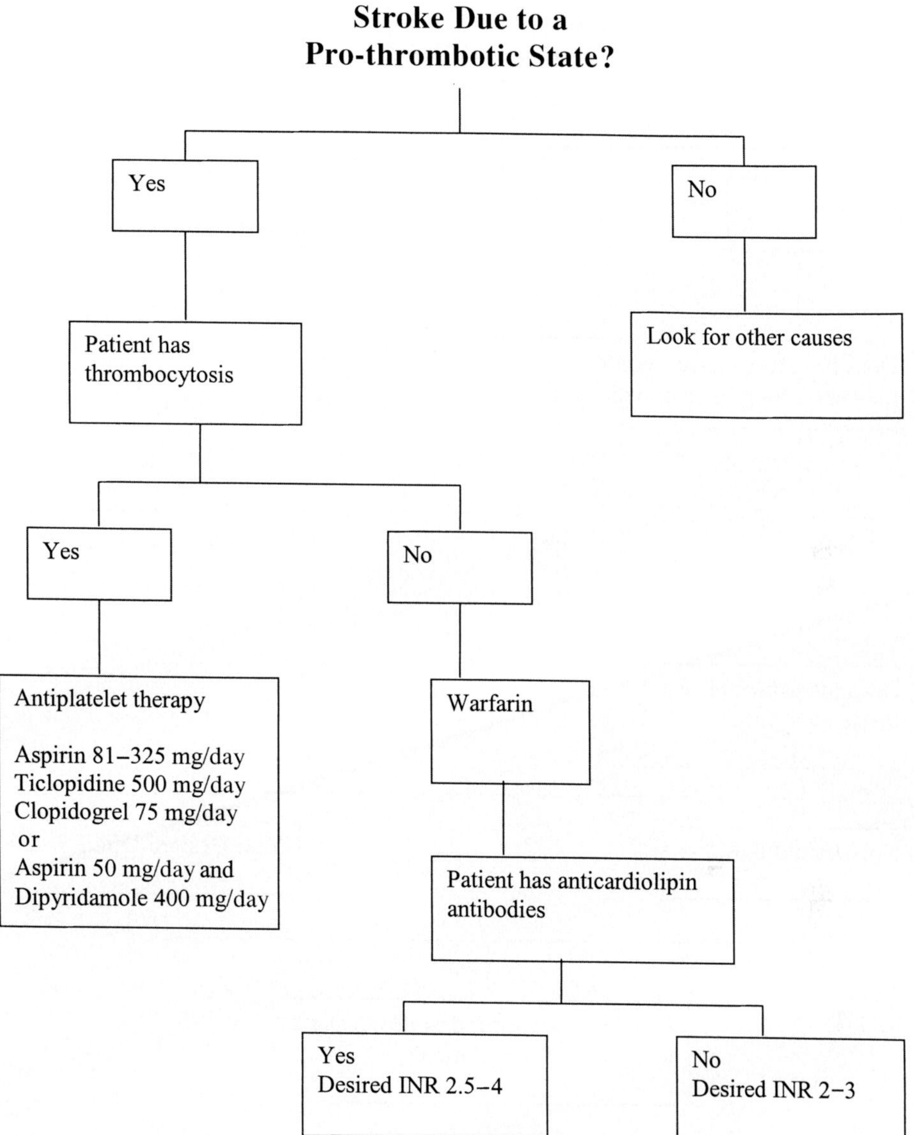

Figure 10–4. Algorithm for therapy to prevent stroke in a patient with a pro-thrombotic state.

when a patient's INR is subtherapeutic, then the best response is to increase the dose of the medication. If the INR level is at a low therapeutic range (ie, 2.1), then a modest increase in dose to achieve a higher therapeutic level is appropriate. Either low-dose aspirin, approximately 81 mg/day, or dipyridamole, approximately 400 mg/day, can be added to the warfarin if the patient has recurrent symptoms despite a therapeutic level of anticoagulation. Some patients who have a very high risk for embolism may warrant treatment with warfarin and an antiplatelet agent even if no neurological symptoms have occurred. Other medications should be prescribed to prevent embolism among patients who cannot receive warfarin. Pregnant patients and other persons who cannot tolerate warfarin can be treated with subcutaneously administered heparin or LMW heparin. Aspirin can be prescribed to patients who cannot receive warfarin for long-term stroke prophylaxis. The usual daily dose is 325 mg.

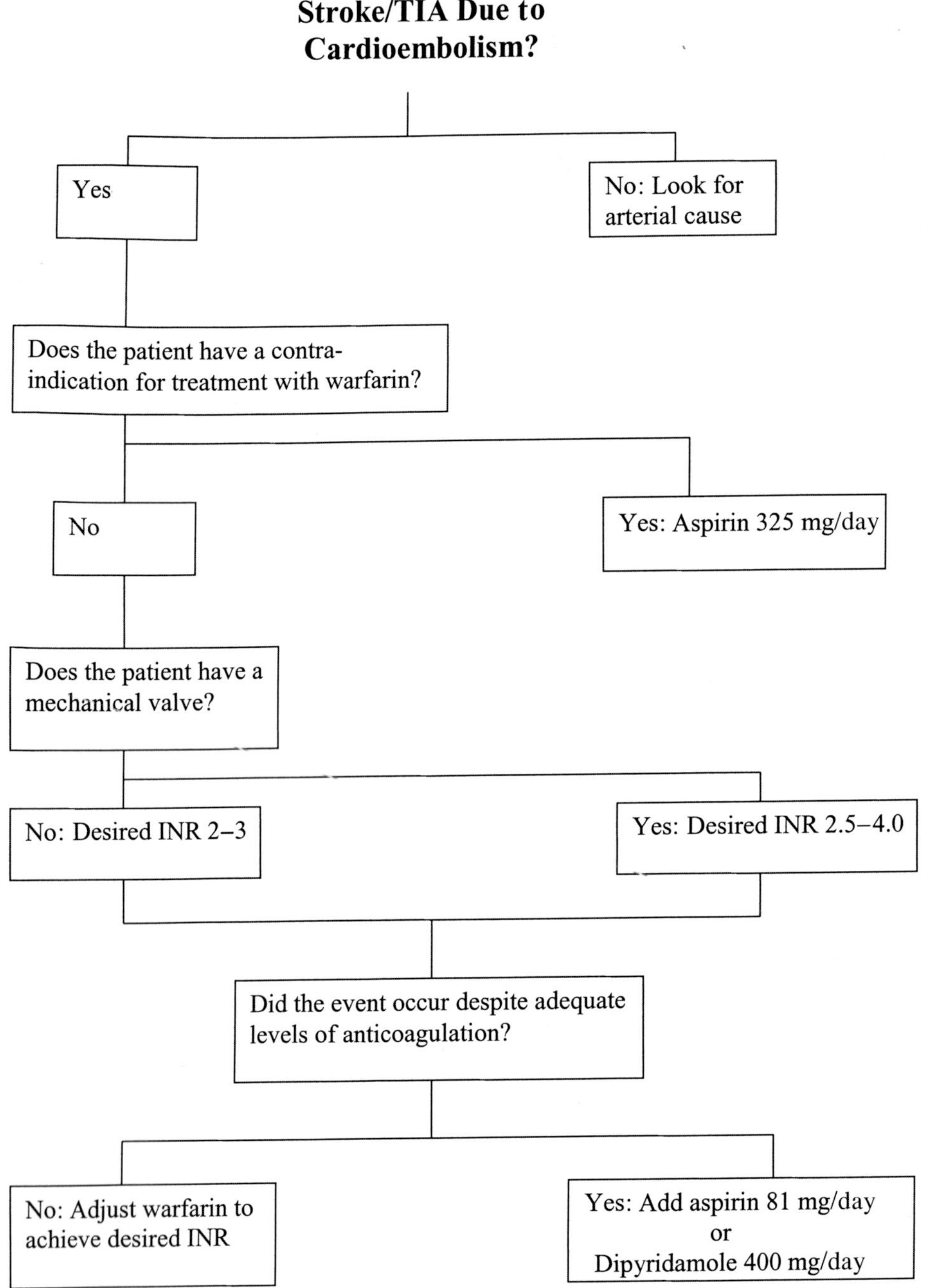

Figure 10–5. Algorithm for selection of therapy to prevent stroke or transient ischemic attack (TIA) secondary to cardioembolism.

The other antiplatelet aggregating agents are of unproven utility in prevention of cardioembolic stroke. They could be prescribed if a patient cannot take either aspirin or warfarin but the adequacy of the options is not clear.

Patients with stroke or TIA of undetermined cause should be prescribed the same medications as those prescribed to patients with large artery atherosclerosis (Figs. 10–6 and 10–7). In this situation, the patient has had an evaluation, and no likely explanation

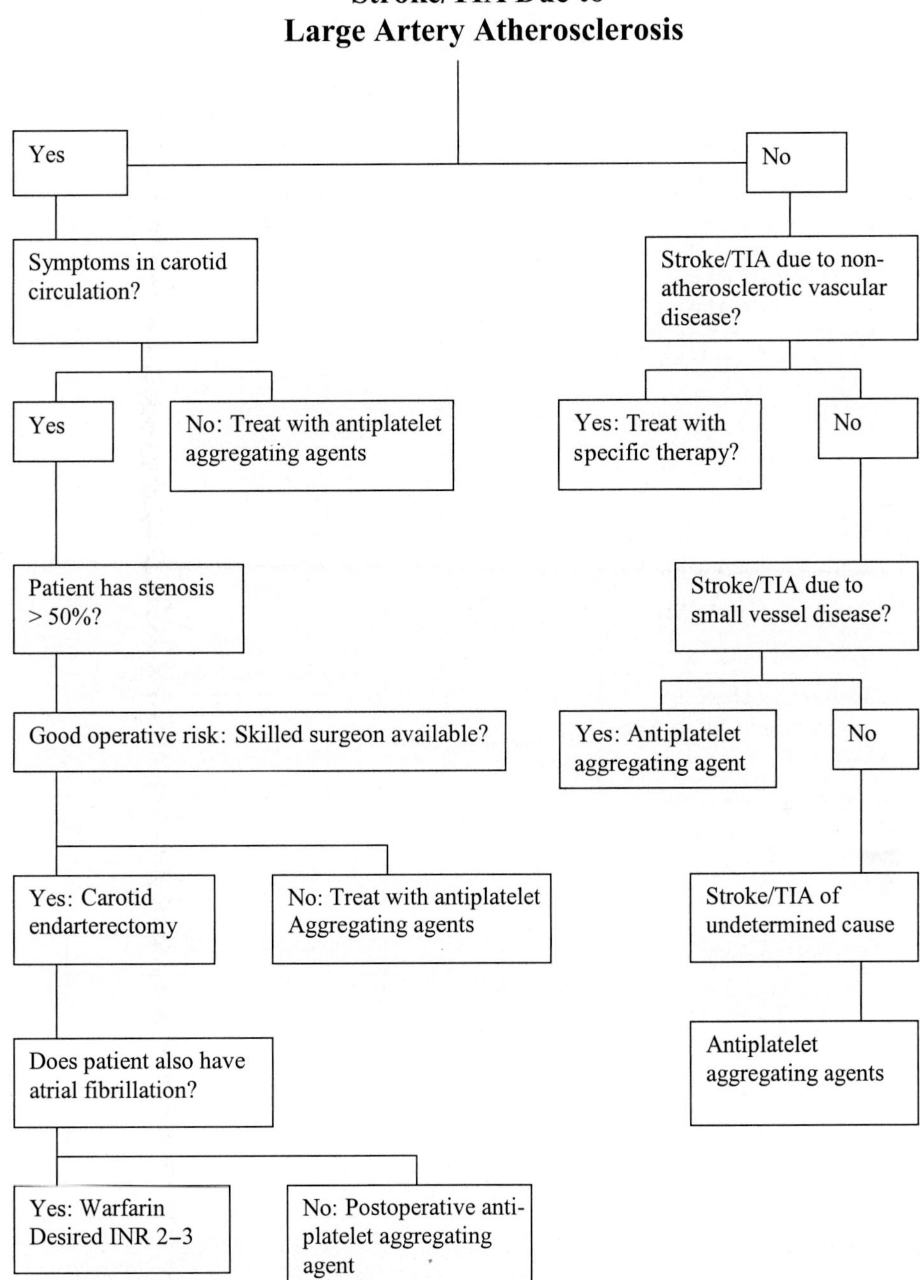

Figure 10–6. Algorithm for selection of therapies to prevent stroke or transient ischemic attack (TIA) among patients with large artery atherosclerosis.

is found. In particular, a cardiac cause has been excluded. Patients with lacunar infarctions have occlusions of small intracranial arteries. These patients usually have diabetes mellitus or hypertension. These patients often have some evidence of large artery atherosclerosis, and they are as likely to have a stroke secondary to occlusion of a major artery as from another lacunar infarction. Patients with lacunar strokes have been enrolled in clinical trials, and their responses have been combined with

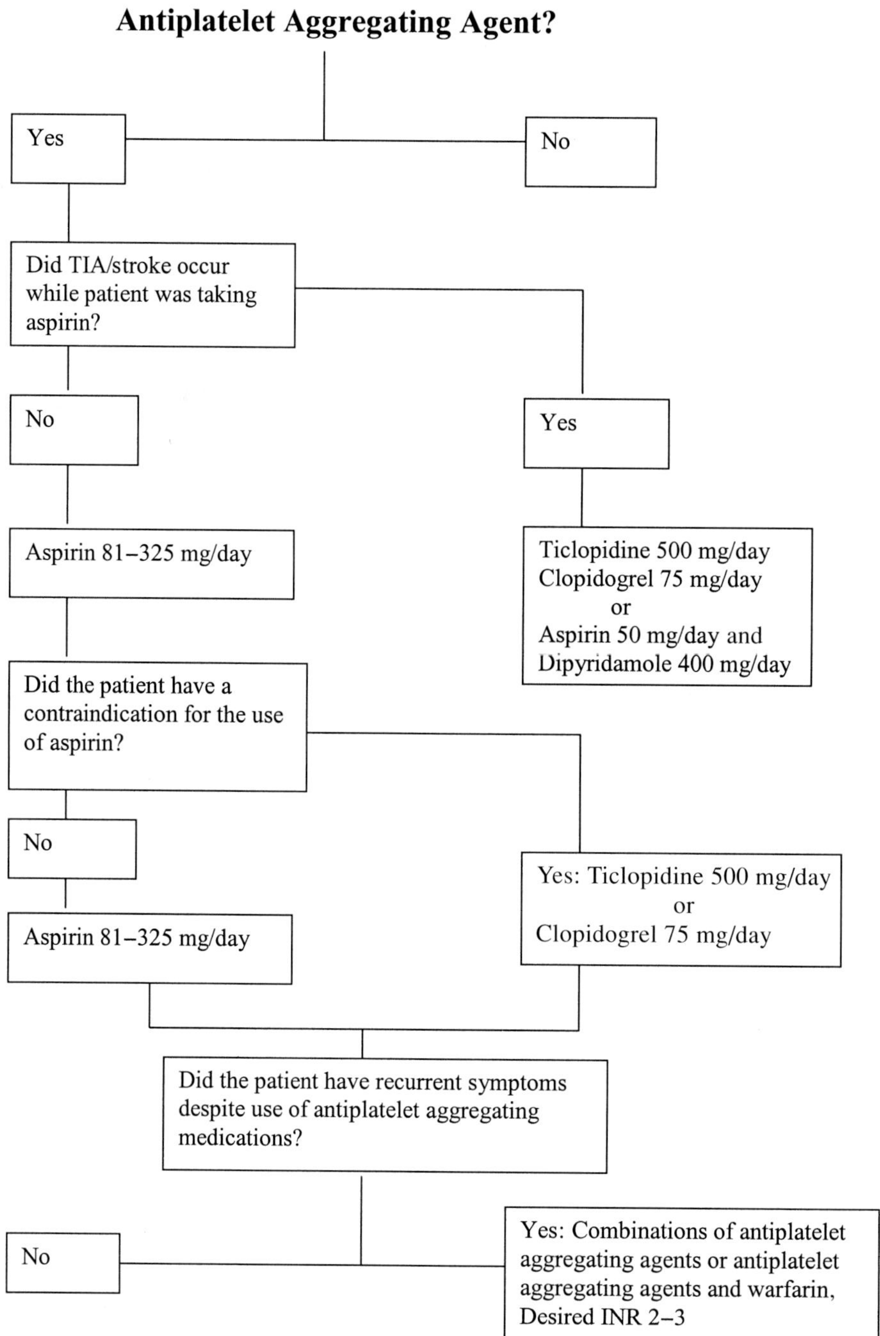

Figure 10–7. Algorithm for selection of antiplatelet aggregating agents to prevent stroke.

those reported by patients with documented large artery atherosclerosis. The differences in safety and efficacy of the medical therapies likely do not differ between persons with small or large artery disease. Until data show that responses are different among patients with lacunar strokes, the measures to prevent ischemic stroke should mimic those prescribed to patients with large artery atherosclerosis.

Aspirin, 81–325 mg/day, is the usual first choice for prevention of stroke among patients with arterial disease. A larger dose of aspirin is not superior to these doses, and increasing the dose of aspirin likely will not be helpful when a patient has recurrent symptoms. The combination of aspirin and dipyridamole, 50 mg and 400 mg/day, can be prescribed if a patient has recurrent symptoms despite treatment with aspirin alone. Ticlopidine, 500 mg/day, or clopidogrel, 75 mg, can be administered if the patient has a contraindication for aspirin or if the patient has recurrent ischemia despite treatment with aspirin. Although dipyridamole did demonstrate efficacy in one clinical trial, its role probably will be as an adjunct to aspirin. Aspirin can be combined with either ticlopidine or clopidogrel, but the safety and efficacy of aggregate treatment are undetermined. Oral anticoagulants should be considered as a second-line therapy for prevention of stroke among patients with arterial disease.

SUMMARY

Prevention is infinitely superior to the treatment of stroke. Luckily, a number of drugs are effective in the management of patients with the clinical manifestations of atherosclerosis, such as statins, and, most recently, the angiotensin converting enzyme inhibitor ramipril.

Heparin has a strong rationale and a poor record in the treatment of stroke. Despite decades of widespread use, the only proven indication is in the treatment of the attending physician's anxiety. Despite early promise, the same can be said for low molecular heparins and danaparoid.

Warfarin has a proven role in the prevention of cardiac embolism from atrial fibrillation and structural heart lesions and good bases for testing in the antiphospholipid/lupus anticoagulant syndrome. Warfarin often is prescribed to patients with pro-thrombotic disorders of coagulation.

Aspirin remains the mainstay of antiplatelet therapy and the second line drug in the prevention of atrial fibrillation. Ticlopidine, clopidogrel and dipyridamole offer alternatives for the aspirin intolerant or unresponsive. Most patients with neurological symptoms secondary to arterial diseases are treated with antiplatelet agents.

Combination therapy of different antiplatelet agents and of antiplatelet agents and anticoagulants offer a good rationale for clinical trials. Neuroprotectants and individual testing for drug responsiveness are likely to enhance and transform medical therapy for the prevention of stroke.

REFERENCES

1. Matchar DB. The value of stroke prevention and treatment. *Neurology* 1998;51:S31–S35.
2. Gorelick PB. Stroke prevention: windows of opportunity and failed expectations? A discussion of modifiable cardiovascular risk factors and a prevention proposal. *Neuroepidemiology* 1997; 16:163–173.
3. Petersen P. Thromboembolic complications in atrial fibrillation. *Stroke* 1990;21:4–13.
4. Hart RG, Sherman DG, Easton JD, Cairns JA. Prevention of stroke in patients with nonvalvular atrial fibrillation. *Neurology* 1998;51:674–681.
5. Gorelick PB, Sacco RL, Smith DB, et al. Prevention of a first stroke: a review of guidelines and a multidisciplinary consensus statement from the National Stroke Association. *JAMA* 1999;281:1112–1120.
6. van Latum JC, Koudstaal PJ, Venables GS, van Gijn J, Kappelle LJ, Algra A. Predictors of major vascular events in patients with a transient ischemic attack or minor ischemic stroke and with nonrheumatic atrial fibrillation. European Atrial Fibrillation Trial (EAFT) Study Group. *Stroke* 1995;26:801–806.
7. Hohnloser SH, Li YG. Drug treatment of atrial fibrillation: what have we learned?. *Curr Opin Cardiol* 1997;12:24–32.
8. Van Gelder I, Brugemann J, Crijns HJ. Pharmacological management of arrhythmias in the elderly. *Drugs Aging* 1997;11:96–110.
9. Hart RG, Pearce LA, McBride R, Rothbart RM, Asinger RW. Factors associated with ischemic stroke during aspirin therapy in atrial fibrillation: analysis of 2012 participants in the SPAF I-III clinical trials. *Stroke* 1999;30:1223–1229.
10. Kistler JP. The risk of embolic stroke. Another piece of the puzzle. *N Engl J Med* 1994;331: 1517–1519.
11. Norris JW, Zhu CZ, Bornstein NM, Chambers BR. Vascular risks of asymptomatic carotid stenosis. *Stroke* 1991;22:1485–1490.
12. Bock RW, Gray-Weale AC, Mock PA, Robinson DA, Irwig L, Lusby RJ. The natural history of asymptomatic carotid artery disease. *J Vasc Surg* 1993;17:160–171.

13. Norris JW. Risk of cerebral infarction, myocardial infarction and vascular death in patients with asymptomatic carotid disease, transient ischemic attack and stroke. *Cerebrovasc Dis* 1992; 2(Suppl):2–5.
14. Kattapong VJ, Longstreth WT, Jr., Kukull WA, et al. Stroke risk factor knowledge in Hispanic and non-Hispanic white women in New Mexico: implications for targeted prevention strategies. *Health Care for Women International* 1998;19: 313–325.
15. Wolf PA, D'Agostino RB, Belanger AJ, Kannel WB. Probability of stroke: a risk profile from the Framingham Study. *Stroke* 1991;22:312–318.
16. Phillips SJ, Whisnant JP. Hypertension and the brain. The National High Blood Pressure Education Program. *Arch Intern Med* 1992; 152:938–945.
17. Bronner LL, Kanter DS, Manson JE. Primary prevention of stroke. *N Engl J Med* 1995;333: 1392–1400.
18. Staessen JA, Thijs L, Gasowski J, Cells H, Fagard RH. Treatment of isolated systolic hypertension in the elderly: further evidence from the systolic hypertension in Europe (Syst-Eur) trial. *Am J Cardiol* 1998;82:20R–22R.
19. Wolf PA, Clagett P, Easton JD, et al. Preventing ischemic stroke in patients with prior stroke and transient ischemic attack. A statement for healt care professionals from the Stroke Council of the American Heart Association. *Stroke* 1999;30: 1991–1994.
20. Klungel OH, Stricker BHC, Paes AHP, et al. Excess stroke among hypertensive men and women attributable to undertreatment of hypertension. *Stroke* 1999;30:1312–1318.
21. Lindenstrom E, Boysen G, Nyboe J. Influence of systolic and diastolic blood pressure on stroke risk: a prospective observational study. *Am J Epidemiol* 1995;142:1279–1290.
22. Davis BR, Vogt T, Frost PH, et al. Risk factors for stroke and type of stroke in persons with isolated systolic hypertension. Systolic Hypertension in the Elderly Program Cooperative Research Group. *Stroke* 1998;29:1333–1340.
23. Hansson L. The Hypertension Optimal Treatment Study and the importance of lowering blood pressure. *J Hyperten* 1999;17 (Suppl): S9–513.
24. Kaplan NM, Gifford RW, Jr. Choice of initial therapy for hypertension. *JAMA* 1996;275: 1577–1580.
25. Pickering TG. Advances in the treatment of hypertension. *JAMA* 1999;281:114–116.
26. Kannel WB. Blood pressure as a cardiovascular risk factor: prevention and treatment. *JAMA* 1996;275:1571–1576.
27. The Dutch TIA Study Group. The Dutch TIA Trial: protective effects of low-dose aspirin and atenolol in patients with transient ischemic attacks or nondisabling stroke. *Stroke* 1988; 19:512–517.
28. Wolf PA. Prevention of stroke. *Lancet* 1998;352, (Suppl 3):SIII15–SIII18.
29. Tell GS, Polak JF, Ward BJ, Kittner SJ, Savage PJ, Robbins J. Relation of smoking with carotid artery wall thickness and stenosis in older adults. The Cardiovascular Health Study. The Cardiovascular Health Study (CHS) Collaborative Research Group. *Circulation* 1994; 90:2905–2908.
30. Wannamethee SG, Shaper AG, Whincup PH, Walker M. Smoking cessation and the risk of stroke in middle-aged men. *JAMA* 1995;274: 155–160.
31. Hughes JR, Goldstein MG, Hurt RD, Shiffman S. Recent advances in the pharmacotherapy of smoking. *JAMA* 1999;281:72–76.
32. Graham IM, Daly LE, Refsum HM, et al. Plasma homocysteine as a risk factor for vascular disease. The European Concerted Action Project. *JAMA* 1997;277:1775–1781.
33. Eikelboom JW, Lonn E, Genest J, Jr., Hankey G, Yusuf S. Homocyst(e)ine and cardiovascular disease: a critical review of the epidemiologic evidence. *Ann Intern Med* 1999;131:363–375.
34. Fung MM, Barrett-Connor E, Bettencourt RR. Hormone replacement therapy and stroke risk in older women. *J Womens Health* 1999;8:359–364.
35. Joseph LN, Babikian VL, Allen NC, Winter MR. Risk factor modification in stroke prevention: the experience of a stroke clinic. *Stroke* 1999; 30:16–20.
36. Estes JM, Guadagnoli E, Wolf R, LoGerfo FW, Whittemore AD. The impact of cardiac comorbidity after carotid endarterectomy. *J Vasc Surg* 1998;28:577–584.
37. Hankey GJ, Slattery JM, Warlow CP. The prognosis of hospital-referred transient ischaemic attacks. *J Neurol Neurosurg Psychiatry* 1991;54:793–802.
38. Chimowitz MI, Mancini GB. Asymptomatic coronary artery disease in patients with stroke. Prevalence, prognosis, diagnosis, and treatment. *Stroke* 1992;23:433–436.
39. Cleeman JI, Lenfant C. The National Cholesterol Education Program: progress and prospects. *JAMA* 1998;280:2099–2104.
40. Hess DC, Demchuk AM, Brass LM, Yatsu FM. HMG-CoA reductase inhibitors (statins). A promising approach to stroke prevention. *Neurology* 2000;54:790–796.
41. Salonen R, Nyyssonen K, Porkkala E, et al. Kuopio Atherosclerosis Prevention Study (KAPS). A population-based primary preventive trial of the effect of LDL lowering on atherosclerotic progression in carotid and femoral arteries. *Circulation* 1995;92:1758–1764.
42. Furberg CD, Adams HP, Jr., Applegate WB, et al. Effect of lovastatin on early carotid atherosclerosis and cardiovascular events. Asymptomatic Carotid Artery Progression Study (ACAPS) Research Group. *Circulation* 1994;90:1679–1687.
43. Atkins D, Psaty BM, Koepsell TD, Longstreth WT, Jr., Larson EB. Cholesterol reduction and the risk for stroke in men. *Ann Intern Med* 1993; 119:136–145.
44. Hebert PR, Gaziano JM, Hennekens CH. An overview of trials of cholesterol lowering and risk of stroke. *Arch Intern Med* 1995;155:50–55.
45. Adams RJ, McKie VC, Carl EM, et al. Long-term stroke risk in children with sickle cell disease screened with transcranial Doppler. *Ann Neurol* 1997;42:699–704.
46. Adams GF, Merrett JD, Hutchinson WM, Pollock AM. Cerebral embolism and mitral stenosis. Survival with and without anticoagulants. *J Neurol Neurosurg Psychiatry* 1974;37:378–383.

47. Adair JC, Call GK, O'Connell JB. A complication of right ventricular endomyocardial biopsy. *Cathet Cardiovasc Diagn* 1991;23:32–33.
48. The Scandinavian Simvastatin Survival Study Group. Randomised trial of cholesterol lowering in 4444 patients with coronary heart disease: the Scandinavian Simvastatin Survival Study (4S). *Lancet* 1994;344:1383–1389.
49. Plehn JF, Davis BR, Sacks FM, et al. Reduction of stroke incidence after myocardial infarction with pravastatin: the Cholesterol and Recurrent Events (CARE) study. The Care Investigators. *Circulation* 1999;99:216–223.
50. Lewis SJ, Moye LA, Sacks FM, et al. Effect of pravastatin on cardiovascular events in older patients with myocardial infarction and cholesterol levels in the average range. Results of the Cholesterol and Recurrent Events (CARE) trial. *Ann Intern Med* 1998;12:681–689.
51. Blauw GJ, Lagaay AM, Smelt AHM, Westendorp RGJ. Stroke, statins, and cholesterol. *Stroke* 1997;28:946–950.
52. Byington RP, Jukema JW, Salonen JT, et al. Reduction in cardiovascular events during pravastatin therapy. Pooled analysis of clinical events of the Pravastatin Atherosclerosis Intervention Program. *Circulation* 1995;922:2419–2425.
53. Hebert PR, Gaziano JM, Chan KS, Hennekens CH. Cholesterol lowering with statin drugs, risk of stroke, and total mortality. An overview of randomized trials. *JAMA* 1997;278:313–321.
54. Crouse JR, Byington RP, Furberg CD. HMG-CoA reductase inhibitor therapy and stroke risk reduction: an analysis of clinical trials data. *Atherosclerosis* 1998;138:11–24.
55. Corsini A, Pazzucconi F, Arnaboldi L, et al. Direct effects of statins on the vascular wall. *J Cardiovasc Pharmacol* 1998;31:773–778.
56. Endres M, Laufs U, Huang Z, et al. Stroke protection by 3-hydroxy-3-methylglutaryl (HMG)-CoA reductase inhibitors mediated by endothelial nitric oxide synthase. *Proceedings of the National Academy of Sciences of the United States of America* 1998;95:8880–8885.
57. Vaughan CJ, Delanty N. Neuroprotective properties of statins in cerebral ischemia and stroke. *Stroke* 1999;30:1969–1973.
58. Jorgensen HS, Nakayama H, Reith J, Raaschou HO, Olsen TS. Stroke recurrence: predictors, severity, and prognosis. The Copenhagen Stroke Study. *Neurology* 1997;48:891–895.
59. Hirsh J, Fuster V. Guide to anticoagulant therapy. Part 1: heparin. *Circulation* 1994;89:1449–1468.
60. Hirsh J, Warkentin TE, Raschke R, Granger C, Ohman EM, Dalen JE. Heparin and low-molecular-weight heparin: mechanisms of action, pharmacokinetics, dosing considerations, monitoring, efficacy, and safety. *Chest* 1998;114:489S–510S.
61. Fareed J, Callas D, Hoppensteadt DA, Walenga JM, Bick RL. Antithrombin agents as anticoagulants and antithrombotics. Implications in drug development. *Med Clin N Am* 1998;82:569–586.
62. Becker RC, Ansell J. Antithrombotic therapy. An abbreviated reference for clinicians. *Arch Intern Med* 1995;155:149–161.
63. Raschke RA, Reilly BM, Guidry JR, Fontana JR, Srinivas S. The weight-based heparin dosing nomogram compared with a "standard care" nomogram. A randomized controlled trial. *Ann Intern Med* 1993;119:874–881.
64. Petty GW, Brown RD, Jr., Whisnant JP, Sicks JD, O'Fallon WM, Wiebers DO. Frequency of major complications of aspirin, warfarin, and intravenous heparin for secondary stroke prevention. *Ann Intern Med* 1999;130:14–22.
65. Levine MN, Raskob G, Landefeld S, Kearon C. Hemorrhagic complications of anticoagulant treatment. *Chest* 1998;114:511S–523S.
66. Ramirez-Lassepas M, Cipolle RJ, Rodvold KA, et al. Heparin induced thrombocytopenia in patients with cerebrovascular ischemic disease. *Neurology* 1986;34:736–740.
67. Atkinson JL, Sundt TMJ, Kazmier FJ, Bowie EJ, Whisnant JP. Heparin-induced thrombocytopenia and thrombosis in ischemic stroke. *Mayo Clin Proc* 1988;63:353–361.
68. Becker PS, Miller VT. Heparin-induced thrombocytopenia. *Stroke* 1989;20:1449–1459.
69. Kappers-Klunne MC, Boon DM, Hop WC, et al. Heparin-induced thrombocytopenia and thrombosis: a prospective analysis of the incidence in patients with heart and cerebrovascular diseases. *Br J Haematol* 1997;96:442–446.
70. Sallah S, Thomas DP, Roberts HR. Warfarin and heparin-induced skin necrosis and the purple toe syndrome: infrequent complications of anticoagulant treatment. *Thromb Haemost* 1997; 78:785–790.
71. Biller J, Adams HP, Jr., Boarini D, Godersky JC, Smoker WRK, Kongable G. Intraluminal clot of the carotid artery. *Surg Neurol* 1986;25:467–477.
72. Pelz DM, Buchan A, Fox AJ, Barnett HJM, Vinuela F. Intraluminal thrombus of the internal carotid arteries: angiographic demonstration of resolution with anticoagulant therapy alone. *Radiology* 1986;160:369–373.
73. Caplan L, Stein R, Patel D, Amico L, Cashman N, Gewertz B. Intraluminal clot of the carotid artery detected radiographically. *Neurology* 1984;34:1175–1181.
74. Poisik A, Heyer EJ, Solomon RA, et al. Safety and efficacy of fixed-dose heparin in carotid endarterectomy. *Neurosurgery* 1999;45:434–442.
75. Groudine SB, Sakawi Y, Patel MK, et al. Low-dose heparin appears safe and can eliminate protamine use for carotid endarterectomy. *J Cardiothorac Vasc Anesth* 1998;12:295–298.
76. Calaitges JG, Liem TK, Spadone D, Nichols WK, Silver D. The role of heparin-associated antiplatelet antibodies in the outcome of arterial reconstruction. *J Vasc Surg* 1999;29:779–785.
77. Vaitkus PT, Barnathan ES. Embolic potential, prevention and management of mural thrombus complicating anterior myocardial infarction: a meta-analysis. *J Am Coll Cardiol* 1993;22: 1004–1009.
78. Turpie AG, Robinson JG, Doyle DJ, et al. Comparison of high-dose with low-dose subcutaneous heparin to prevent left ventricular mural thrombosis in patients with acute transmural anterior myocardial infarction. *N Engl J Med* 1989;320:352–357.
79. Putman SF, Adams HP, Jr. Usefulness of heparin in initial management of patients with recent

transient ischemic attacks. *Arch Neurol* 1985; 42:960–962.

80. Biller J, Bruno A, Adams HP, Jr., et al. A randomized trial of aspirin or heparin in hospitalized patients with recent transient ischemic attacks. A pilot study. *Stroke* 1989;20:441–447.
81. Slivka A, Levy DE, Lapinski RH. Risk associated with heparin withdrawal in ischaemic cerebrovascular disease. *J Neurol Neurosurg Psychiatry* 1989;52:1332–1336.
82. Cerebral Embolism Study Group. Immediate anticoagulation of embolic stroke: brain hemorrhage and management options. *Stroke* 1984; 15:779–789.
83. Cerebral Embolism Study Group. Cardioembolic stroke, early anticoagulation, and brain hemorrhage. *Arch Intern Med* 1987; 147:636–640.
84. Chamorro A, Vila N, Ascaso C, Blanc R. Heparin in acute stroke with atrial fibrillation. Clinical relevance of very early treatment. *Arch Neurol* 1999;56:1098–1102.
85. International Stroke Trial Collaborative Group. The International Stroke Trial (IST): a randomised trial of aspirin, subcutaneous heparin, both, or neither among 19435 patients with acute ischaemic stroke. *Lancet* 1997;1569–1581.
86. The Publications Committee for the Trial of ORG 10172 in Acute Stroke Treatment (TOAST) Investigators. Low molecular weight heparinoid, ORG 10172 (danaparoid), and outcome after acute ischemic stroke: a randomized controlled trial. *JAMA* 1998;279:1265–1272.
87. Chamorro A, Vila N, Saiz A, Alday M, Tolosa E. Early anticoagulation after large cerebral embolic infarction: a safety study. *Neurology* 1995; 45:861–865.
88. Berge E, Abdelnoor M, Nakstad PH, Sandset PM, on behalf of the HAEST Study Group. Low molecular-weight heparin versus aspirin in patients with acute ischaemic stroke and atrial fibrillation: a double-blind randomised study. *Lancet* 2000;355:1205–1210.
89. Caplan LR. When should heparin be given to patients with atrial fibrillation–related embolic brain infarcts? *Arch Neurol* 1999;56:1059–1060.
90. Hirsh J, Weitz JI. New antithrombotic agents. *Lancet* 1999;353:1431–1436.
91. Magnani HN. Heparin-induced thrombocytopenia (HIT): an overview of 230 patients treated with organ (Org 10172). *Thromb Haemost* 1993; 70:554–561.
92. Green D, Hirsh J, Heit J, Prins M, Davidson B, Lensing AW. Low molecular weight heparin: a critical analysis of clinical trials. *Pharmacol Rev* 1994;46:89–109.
93. Laposata M, Green D, Van Cott EM, Barrowcliffe TW, Goodnight SH, Sosolik RC. College of American Pathologists Conference XXXI on laboratory monitoring of anticoagulant therapy: the clinical use and laboratory monitoring of low-molecular-weight heparin, danaparoid, hirudin and related compounds, and argatroban. *Arch Pathol Lab Med* 1998;122: 799–807.
94. Turpie AG, Gent M, Cote R, et al. A low-molecular-weight heparinoid compared with unfractionated heparin in the prevention of deep vein thrombosis in patients with acute ischemic stroke. A randomized, double-blind study. *Ann Intern Med* 1992;117:353–357.
95. Bergqvist D. Low molecular weight heparins. *J Intern Med* 1996;240:63–72.
96. Warkentin TE, Levine MN, Hirsh J, et al. Heparin-induced thrombocytopenia in patients treated with low-molecular-weight heparin or unfractionated heparin. *N Engl J Med* 1995;332: 1330–1335.
97. Kay R, Wong KS, Yu YL, et al. Low-molecular-weight heparin for the treatment of acute ischemic stroke. *N Engl J Med* 1995;333: 1588–1593.
98. Wehrmacher WH, Karlman RL, Scanlon P, Messmore HL, Jr. Anticoagulant therapy of thromboembolic disease during pregnancy. *Compr Ther* 1998;24:289–294.
99. Ginsberg JS, Hirsh J. Use of antithrombotic agents during pregnancy. *Chest* 1998;114: 524S–530S.
100. Hirsh J, Dalen JE, Anderson DR, et al. Oral anticoagulants: mechanism of action, clinical effectiveness, and optimal therapeutic range. *Chest* 1998;114:445S–469S.
101. Harker LA. Therapeutic inhibition of thrombin activities, receptors, and production. *Hematol Oncol Clin North Am* 1998;12:1211–1230.
102. Kistler JP, Singer DE, Millenson MM, et al. Effect of low-intensity warfarin anticoagulation on level of activity of the hemostatic system in patients with atrial fibrillation. BAATAF Investigators. *Stroke* 1993;24:1360–1365.
103. Hyman BT, Landas SK, Ashman RF, Schelper RL, Robinson RA. Warfarin-related purple toes syndrome and cholesterol microembolization. *Am J Med* 1987;82:1233–1237.
104. Sallah S, Abdallah JM, Gagnon GA. Recurrent warfarin-induced skin necrosis in kindreds with protein S deficiency. *Haemostasis* 1998;28:25–30.
105. Essex DW, Wynn SS, Jin DK. Late-onset warfarin-induced skin necrosis: case report and review of the literature. *Am J Hematol* 1998;57: 233–237.
106. Krahn MJ, Pettigrew NM, Cuddy TE. Unusual side effects due to warfarin. *Can J Cardiol* 1998; 14:90–93.
107. Litin SC, Gastineau DA. Current concepts in anticoagulant therapy. *Mayo Clin Proc* 1995;70: 266–272.
108. Crowther MA, Ginsberg JB, Kearon C, et al. A randomized trial comparing 5-mg and 10-mg warfarin loading doses. *Arch Intern Med* 1999; 159:46–48.
109. Harrison L, Johnston M, Massicotte MP, Crowther M, Moffat K, Hirsh J. Comparison of 5-mg and 10-mg loading doses in initiation of warfarin therapy. *Ann Intern Med* 1997;126: 133–136.
110. Hirsh J, Poller L. The international normalized ratio. A guide to understanding and correcting its problems. *Arch Intern Med* 1994;154:282–288.
111. Ansell JE. Oral anticoagulant therapy—50 years later. *Arch Intern Med* 1993;153:586–596.
112. Oates A, Jackson PR, Austin CA, Channer KS. A new regimen for starting warfarin therapy in out-patients. *Br J Clin Pharmacol* 1998;46:157–161.

113. Gladman JR, Dolan G. Effect of age upon the induction and maintenance of anticoagulation with warfarin. *Postgrad Med* 1995;71:153–155.
114. Dalere GM, Coleman RW, Lum BL. A graphic nomogram for warfarin dosage adjustment. *Pharmacotherapy* 1999;19:461–467.
115. Smith JK, Aljazairi A, Fuller SH. INR elevation associated with diarrhea in a patient receiving warfarin. *Ann Pharmacother* 1999;33:301–304.
116. Weser JK, Sellers E. Drug interactions with coumarin anticoagulants. 2. *N Engl J Med* 1971; 285:547–558.
117. Kearon C, Hirsh J. Management of anticoagulation before and after elective surgery. *N Engl J Med* 1997;336:1506–1511.
118. Gullov AL, Koefoed BG, Petersen P. Bleeding during warfarin and aspirin therapy in patients with atrial fibrillation: the AFASAK 2 study. Atrial Fibrillation Aspirin and Anticoagulation. *Arch Intern Med* 1999;159:1322–1328.
119. Gitter MJ, Jaeger TM, Petterson TM, Gersh BJ, Silverstein MD. Bleeding and thromboembolism during anticoagulant therapy: a population-based study in Rochester, Minnesota. *Mayo Clin Proc* 1995;70:725–733.
120. Pengo V, Zasso A, Barbero F, et al. Effectiveness of fixed minidose warfarin in the prevention of thromboembolism and vascular death in no rheumatic atrial fibrillation. *Am J Cardiol* 1998; 82:433–437.
121. Petty GW, Lennihan L, Mohr JP, et al. Complications of long-term anticoagulation. *Ann Neurol* 1988;23:570–574.
122. van der Meer FJ, Rosendaal FR, Vandenbroucke JP, Briet E. Bleeding complications in oral anticoagulant therapy. An analysis of risk factors. *Arch Intern Med* 1993;153:1557–1562.
123. Green CJ, Hadorn DC, Bassett K, Kazanjian A. Anticoagulation in chronic nonvalvular atrial fibrillation: a critical appraisal and meta-analysis. Can *J Cardiol* 1997;13:811–815.
124. Hart RG. Oral anticoagulants for secondary prevention of stroke. *Cerebrovasc Dis* 1997;7(Suppl 6):24–29.
125. Tiede DJ, Nishimura RA, Gastineau DA, et al. Modern management of prosthetic valve anticoagulation. *Mayo Clin Proc* 1998;73:665–680.
126. The Stroke Prevention in Atrial Fibrillation Investigators. Bleeding during antithrombotic therapy in patients with atrial fibrillation. *Arch Intern Med* 1996;156:409–416.
127. Gullov AL, Koefoed BG, Petersen P. Bleeding during warfarin and aspirin therapy in patients with atrial fibrillation: the AFASAK 2 study. Atrial Fibrillation Aspirin and Anticoagulation. *Arch Intern Med* 1999;159:1322–1328.
128. Pessin MS, Estol CJ, Lafranchise F, Caplan LR. Safety of anticoagulation after hemorrhagic infarction. *Neurology* 1993;43:1298–1303.
129. Ortin M, Olalla J, Marco F, Velasco N. Low-dose vitamin K1 versus short-term with holding of acenocoumarol in the treatment of excessive anticoagulation episodes induced by acenocoumarol. A retrospective comparative study. *Haemostasis* 1998;28:57–61.
130. Weibert RT, Le DT, Kayser SR, Rapaport SI. Correction of excessive anticoagulation with low-dose oral vitamin K1. *Ann Intern Med* 1997; 126:959–962.
131. Sato Y, Honda Y, Kunoh H, Oizumi K. Long-term oral anticoagulation reduces bone mass in patients with previous hemispheric infarction and nonrheumatic atrial fibrillation. *Stroke* 1997; 28:2390–2394.
132. Aiach M, Gandrille S, Emmerich J. A review of mutations causing deficiencies of antithrombin, protein C, and protein S. *Thromb Haemost* 1995; 74:81–89.
133. Albers GW. Antithrombotic agents in cerebral ischemia. *Am J Cardiol* 1995;75:34B–38B.
134. Feinberg WM. Anticoagulation for prevention of stroke. *Neurology* 1998;51:S20–S22.
135. Petersen P, Boysen G, Godtfredsen J, Andersen ED, Andersen B. Placebo-controlled, randomised trial of warfarin and aspirin for prevention of thromboembolic complications in chronic atrial fibrillation. The Copenhagen AFASAK study. *Lancet* 1989;1:175–179.
136. The Boston Area Anticoagulation Trial for Atrial Fibrillation Investigators. The effect of low-dose warfarin on the risk of stroke in patients with nonrheumatic atrial fibrillation. *N Engl J Med* 1990;323:1505–1511.
137. Ezekowitz MD, Bridgers SL, James KE, et al. Warfarin in the prevention of stroke associated with nonrheumatic atrial fibrillation. Veterans Affairs Stroke Prevention in Nonrheumatic Atrial Fibrillation Investigators. *N Engl J Med* 1992;327:1406–1412.
138. Matsuo S, Nakamura Y, Kinoshita M. Warfarin reduces silent cerebral infarction in elderly patients with atrial fibrillation. *Coronary Artery Disease* 1998;9:223–226.
139. Ezekowitz MD, James KE, Nazarian SM, et al. Silent cerebral infarction in patients with nonrheumatic atrial fibrillation. The Veterans Affairs Stroke Prevention in Nonrheumatic Atrial Fibrillation Investigators. *Circulation* 1995;92: 2178–2182.
140. Cullinane M, Wainwright R, Brown A, Monaghan M, Markus HS. Asymptomatic embolization in subjects with atrial fibrillation not taking anticoagulants: a prospective study. *Stroke* 1998;29:1810–1815.
141. Corrado G, Tadeo G, Beretta S, et al. Atrial thrombi resolution after prolonged anticoagulation in patients with atrial fibrillation. *Chest* 1999;115:140–143.
142. Koudstaal PJ, Koudstaal A. Secondary stroke prevention in atrial fibrillation: indications, risks, and benefits. *J Thromb Thrombol* 1999;7:61–65.
143. Laupacis A. Anticoagulants for atrial fibrillation. *Lancet* 1993;342:1251–1252.
144. Blakely JA. Anticoagulation in chronic nonvalvular atrial fibrillation: appraisal of two meta-analyses. *Can J Cardiol* 1998;14:945–948.
145. Albers GW, Sherman DG, Gress DR, Paulseth JE, Petersen P. Stroke prevention in nonvalvular atrial fibrillation: a review of prospective randomized trials. *Ann Neurol* 1991;30:511–518.
146. Stroke Prevention in Atrial Fibrillation Investigators. Stroke prevention in atrial fibrillation study. Final results. *Circulation* 1991;84: 527–539.

147. Connolly SJ, Laupacis A, Gent M, Roberts RS, Cairns JA, Joyner C. Canadian Atrial Fibrillation Anticoagulation (CAFA) Study. *J Am Coll Cardiol* 1991;18:349–355.
148. Anderson DC. Primary and secondary stroke prevention in atrial fibrillation. *Semin Neurol* 1998;18:451–459.
149. Koefoed BG, Gullov AL, Petersen P. Prevention of thromboembolic events in atrial fibrillation. *Thromb Haemost* 1997;78:377–381.
150. Laupacis A, Albers G, Dalen J, Dunn MI, Jacobson AK, Singer DE. Antithrombotic therapy in atrial fibrillation. *Chest* 1998;114: 579S–589S.
151. Weinberg DM, Mancini J. Anticoagulation for cardioversion of atrial fibrillation. *Am J Cardiol* 1989;63:745–746.
152. Ezekowitz MD, Levine JA. Preventing stroke in patients with atrial fibrillation. *JAMA* 1999;281:1830–1835.
153. Atrial Fibrillation Investigators, . Risk factors for stroke and efficacy of antithrombotic therapy in atrial fibrillation. Analysis of pooled data from five randomized controlled trials. *Arch Intern Med* 1994;154:1449–1457.
154. Koefoed BG, Petersen P. Oral anticoagulation in nonvalvular atrial fibrillation. *J Intern Med* 1999;245:375–381.
155. Sparks PB, Mond HG, Kalman JM, Jayaprakash S, Lewis MA, Grigg LE. Atrial fibrillation and anticoagulation in patients with permanent pacemakers: implications for stroke prevention. *Pacing & Clinical Electrophysiology* 1998;21:1258–1267.
156. Manning WJ, Silverman DI, Gordon SP, Krumholz HM, Douglas PS. Cardioversion from atrial fibrillation without prolonged anticoagulation with use of transesophageal echocardiography to exclude the presence of atrial thrombi. *N Engl J Med* 1993;328:750–755.
157. Ewy GA. Optimal technique for electrical cardioversion of atrial fibrillation. *Circulation* 1992; 86:1645–1647.
158. Klein AL, Grimm RA, Black IW, et al. Cardioversion guided by transesophageal echocardiography: the ACUTE Pilot Study. A randomized, controlled trial. Assessment of Cardioversion Using Transesophageal Echocardiography. *Ann Intern Med* 1997;126: 200–209.
159. Kinch JW, Davidoff R. Prevention of embolic events after cardioversion of atrial fibrillation. Current and evolving strategies. *Arch Intern Med* 1995;155:1353–1360.
160. Zeiler AA, Mick MJ, Mazurer RP, Loop FD, Trohman RG. Role of prophylactic anticoagulation for direct current cardioversion in patients with atrial fibrillation or atrial flutter. *J Am Coll Cardiol* 1992;19:851–855.
161. Fatkin D, Kuchar DL, Thorburn CW, Feneley MP. Transesophageal echocardiography before and during direct current cardioversion of atrial fibrillation: evidence for "atrial stunning" as a mechanism of thromboembolic complications. *J Am Coll Cardiol* 1994;23:307–316.
162. Pullicino PM, Halperin JL, Thompson JLP. Stroke in patients with heart failure and reduced left ventricular ejection fraction. *Neurology* 2000;54:288–294.
163. Al-Khadra AS, Salem DN, Rand WM, Udelson JE, Smith JJ, Konstam MA. Warfarin anticoagulation and survival: a cohort analysis from the Studies of Left Ventricular Dysfunction. *J Am Coll Cardiol* 1998;31:749–753.
164. Azar AJ, Koudstaal PJ, Wintzen AR, et al. Risk of stroke during long-term anticoagulant therapy in patients after myocardial infarction. *Ann Neurol* 1996;39:301–307.
165. Smith P. Oral anticoagulants are effective long-term after acute myocardial infarction. *J Intern Med* 1999;245:383–387.
166. Serena J, Segura T, Perez-Ayuso MJ, Bassaganyas J, Molins A, Davalos. The need to quantify right-to-left shunt in acute ischemic stroke: a case-control study. *Stroke* 1998;29:1322–1328.
167. Salem DN, Levine HJ, Pauker SG, Eckman MH, Daudelin DH. Antithrombotic therapy in valvular heart disease. *Chest* 1998;114:590S–601S.
168. Stein PD, Alpert JS, Dalen JE, Horstkotte D, Turpie AG. Antithrombotic therapy in patients with mechanical and biological prosthetic heart valves. *Chest* 1998;114:602S–610S.
169. Cannegieter SC, Rosendal FR, Wintzen AR, van der Meer FJM, Vandenbroucke JP, Briet E. Optimal oral anticoagulant therapy in patients with mechanical heart valves. *N Engl J Med* 1995; 333:11–17.
170. Altman R, Rouvier J, Gurfinkel E, et al. Comparison of two levels of anticoagulant therapy in patients with substitute heart valves. *J Thorac Cardiovasc Surg* 1991;101:427–431.
171. Brass LM, Krumholz HM, Scinto JM, Radford M. Warfarin use among patients with atrial fibrillation. *Stroke* 1997;28:2382–2389.
172. Pengo V, Zasso A, Barbero F, Garelli E, Biasiolo A. Low intensity warfarin therapy. *Haematologica* 1997;82:710–712.
173. Gullov AL, Koefoed BG, Petersen P, et al. Fixed minidose warfarin and aspirin alone and in combination vs adjusted-dose warfarin for stroke prevention in atrial fibrillation: Second Copenhagen Atrial Fibrillation, Aspirin, and Anticoagulation Study. *Arch Intern Med* 1998;158:1513–1521.
174. Stroke Prevention in Atrial Fibrillation Investigators, . Adjusted-dose warfarin versus low-intensity, fixed-dose warfarin plus aspirin for high-risk patients with atrial fibrillation: Stroke Prevention in Atrial Fibrillation III randomised clinical trial. *Lancet* 1996;348: 633–638.
175. The Stroke Prevention in Atrial Fibrillation Investigators Committee on Echocardiography. Transesophageal echocardiographic correlates of thromboembolism in high-risk patients with nonvalvular atrial fibrillation. *Ann Intern Med* 1998;128:639–647.
176. Khamashta MA, Cuadrado MJ, Mujic F, Taub NA, Hunt BJ, Hughes GR. The management of thrombosis in the antiphospholipid-antibody syndrome. *N Engl J Med* 1995;332:993–997.
177. Dressler FA, Craig WR, Castello R, Labovitz AJ. Mobile aortic atheroma and systemic emboli: efficacy of anticoagulation and influence of plaque morphology on recurrent stroke. *J Am Coll Cardiol* 1998;31:134–138.

178. Blackshear JL, Zabalgoitia M, Pennock G, et al. Warfarin safety and efficacy in patients with thoracic aortic plaque and atrial fibrillation. SPAF TEE Investigators. Stroke Prevention and Atrial Fibrillation. Transesophageal echocardiography. *Am J Cardiol* 1999;83:453–455.
179. Chimowitz MI, Kokkinos J, Strong J, et al. The Warfarin-Aspirin Symptomatic Intracranial Disease Study. *Neurology* 1995;45:1488–1493.
180. The Warfarin-Aspirin Symptomatic Intracranial Disease (WASID) Study Group. Prognosis of patients with symptomatic vertebral or basilar artery stenosis. *Stroke* 1998;29:1389–1392.
181. The Stroke Prevention in Reversible Ischemia Trial (SPIRIT) Study Group. A randomized trial of anticoagulants versus aspirin after cerebral ischemia of presumed arterial origin. *Ann Neurol* 1997;42:857–865.
182. White RH, McBurnie MA, Manolio T, et al. Oral anticoagulation in patients with atrial fibrillation: adherence with guidelines in an elderly cohort. *Am J Med* 1999;106:165–171.
183. Kalra L, Perez I, Melbourn A. Risk assessment and anticoagulation for primary stroke prevention in atrial fibrillation. *Stroke* 1999;30:1218–1222.
184. Lefkovits J, Topol EJ. Direct thrombin inhibitors in cardiovascular medicine. *Circulation* 1994;90: 1522–1536.
185. Lunven C, Gauffeny C, Lecoffre C, O'Brien DP, Roome NO, Berry CN. Inhibition by argatroban, a specific thrombin inhibitor, of platelet activation by fibrin clot-associated thrombin. *Thromb Haemost* 1996;75:154–160.
186. Lewis BE, Walenga JM, Wallis DE. Anticoagulation with Novastan (argatroban) in patients with heparin-induced thrombocytopenia and heparin-induced thrombocytopenia and thrombosis syndrome. *Semin Thromb Hemost* 1997;23:197–202.
187. Topol EJ, Fuster V, Harrington RA, et al. Recombinant hirudin for unstable angina pectoris. A multicenter, randomized angiographic trial. *Circulation* 1994;89:1557–1566.
188. The Global Use of Strategies to Open Occluded Coronary Arteries (GUSTO) IIa Investigators. Randomized trial of intravenous heparin versus recombinant hirudin for acute coronary syndromes. *Circulation* 1994;90:1631–1637.
189. Albers GW, Easton JD, Sacco RL, Teal P. Antithrombotic and thrombolytic therapy for ischemic stroke. *Chest* 1998;114:683S–698S.
190. Adams HP, Jr., Davis PH. Management of transient ischemic attacks. *Compr Ther* 1995;21: 355–361.
191. Barnett HJM, Eliasziw M, Meldrum HE. Drugs and surgery in the prevention of ischemic stroke. *N Engl J Med* 1995;332:238–248.
192. Dyken ML. Antiplatelet agents and stroke prevention. *Semin Neurol* 1998;18:441–450.
193. Adams HP, Jr. Use of anticoagulants or antiplatelet aggregating drugs in the prevention of ischemic stroke. *Adv Intern Med* 1995;40:503–531.
194. Antiplatelet Trialists' Collaboration. Collaborative overview of randomised trials of antiplatelet therapy—I: prevention of death, myocardial infarction, and stroke by prolonged antiplatelet therapy in various categories of patients. *BMJ* 1994;308:81–106.
195. Puranen J, Laakso M, Riekkinen PJS, Sivenius J. Efficacy of antiplatelet treatment in hypertensive patients with TIA or stroke. *J Cardiovasc Pharmacol* 1998;32:291–294.
196. Puranen J, Laakso M, Riekkinen PS, Sivenius J. Risk factors and antiplatelet therapy in TIA and stroke patients. *J Neurol Sci* 1998;154:200–204.
197. Rojas-Fernandez CH, Kephart GC, Sketris IS, Kass K. Underuse of acetylsalicylic acid in individuals with myocardial infarction, ischemic heart disease or stroke: data from the 1995 population-based Nova Scotia Health Survey. *Can J Cardiol* 1999;15:291–296.
198. Lekstrom JA, Bell WR. Aspirin in the prevention of thrombosis. *Medicine* 1991;70:161–178.
199. Verstraete M, Zoldhelyi P. Novel antithrombotic drugs in development. *Drugs* 1995;49:856–884.
200. Roth GJ, Calverley DC. Aspirin, platelets, and thrombosis: theory and practice. *Blood* 1994; 83:885–898.
201. Patrono C, Coller B, Dalen JE, et al. Platelet-active drugs: the relationships among dose, effectiveness, and side effects. *Chest* 1998;114: 470S–488S.
202. Harker LA. Therapeutic inhibition of platelet function in stroke. *Cerebrovasc Dis* 1998;8(Suppl 5): 8–18.
203. Droste DW, Siemens HJ, Sonne M, Kaps M, Wagner T. Hemostaseologic and hematologic parameters with aspirin and ticlopidine treatment in patients with cerebrovascular disease: a cross-over study. *J Cardiovasc Pharmacol* 1996;28: 591–594.
204. Nagamatsu Y, Tsujioka Y, Hashimoto M, Giddings JC, Yamamoto J. The differential effects of aspirin on platelets, leucocytes and vascular endothelium in an in vivo model of thrombus formation. *Clin Lab Haematol* 1999;21:33–40.
205. Brandon RA, Eadie MJ. The basis for aspirin dosage in stroke prevention. *Clin Exp Neurol* 1987;23:47–54.
206. Burch JW, Stanford N, Majerus PW. Inhibition of platelet prostaglandin synthetase by oral aspirin. *J Clin Investig* 1978;61:314–319.
207. Weksler BB, Kent JL, Rudolph D, Scherer PB, Levy DE. Effects of low dose aspirin on platelet function in patients with recent cerebral ischemia. *Stroke* 1985;16:5–9.
208. Tohgi H, Tamura K, Kimura B, Kimura M, Suzuki H. Individual variation in platelet aggregability and serum thromboxane B2 concentrations after low-dose aspirin. *Stroke* 1988;19: 700–703.
209. Buchanan MR, Hirsh J. Effect of aspirin on hemostasis and thrombosis. *New England & Regional Allergy Proceedings* 1986;7:26–31.
210. Gomes I. Aspirin: a neuroprotective agent at high doses?. *National Medical Journal of India* 1998;11:14–17.
211. Grotemeyer KH. Effects of acetylsalicylic acid in stroke patients. Evidence of nonresponders in a subpopulation of treated patients. *Thromb Res* 1991;63:587–593.
212. Helgason CM, Tortorice KL, Winkler SR, et al. Aspirin response and failure in cerebral infarction. *Stroke* 1993;24:345–350.

213. Helgason CM, Bolin KM, Hoff JA, et al. Development of aspirin resistance in persons with previous ischemic stroke. *Stroke* 1994;25: 2331–2336.
214. Grotemeyer KH, Scharafinski HW, Husstedt IW. Two-year follow-up of aspirin responder and aspirin non responder. A pilot-study including 180 post-stroke patients. *Thromb Res* 1993;71: 397–403.
215. Sze PC, Reitman D, Pincus MM, Sacks HS, Chalmers TC. Antiplatelet agents in the secondary prevention of stroke: meta-analysis of the randomized control trials. *Stroke* 1988;19: 436–442.
216. Isles C, Norrie J, Paterson J, Ritchie L. Risk of major gastrointestinal bleeding with aspirin. *Lancet* 1999;353:148–150.
217. Hobson RW, Krupski WC, Weiss DG. Influence of aspirin in the management of asymptomatic carotid artery stenosis. VA Cooperative Study Group on Asymptomatic Carotid Stenosis. *J Vasc Surg* 1993;17:257–263.
218. UK-TIA Study Group. United Kingdom transient ischaemic attack (UK-TIA) aspirin trial: interim results. *Br Med J [Clin Res Ed]* 1988;. 296: 316–320.
219. Cappelleri JC, Lau J, Kupelnick B, Chalmers TC. Efficacy and safety of different aspirin dosages on vascular diseases in high-risk patients. A metaregression analysis. *Online Journal of Current Clinical Trials* 1995;174:6442.
220. Silagy CA, McNeil JJ, Donnan GA, Tonkin AM, Worsam B, Campion K. Adverse effects of low-dose aspirin in a healthy elderly population. *Clin Pharmacol Ther* 1993;54:84–89.
221. Adams HP, Jr., Bendixen BH. Low- versus high-dose aspirin in prevention of ischemic stroke. *Clin Neuropharmacol* 1993;16:485–500.
222. Kronmal RA, Hart RG, Manolio TA, Talbert RL, Beauchamp NJ, Newman A. Aspirin use and incident stroke in the cardiovascular health study. CHS Collaborative Research Group. *Stroke* 1998;29:887–894.
223. Steering Committee of the Physicians' Health Study Research Group. Final report on the aspirin component of the ongoing Physicians' Health Study. *N Engl J Med* 1989;321:129–135.
224. He J, Whelton PK, Vu B. Aspirin and risk of hemorrhagic stroke. *JAMA* 1998;280: 1930–1935.
225. Thrift AG, McNeil JJ, Forbes A, Donnan GA. Risk of primary intracerebral haemorrhage associated with aspirin and non-steroidal anti-inflammatory drugs: case-control study. *BMJ* 1999;318:759–764.
226. Easton JD. Antiplatelet therapy in the prevention of stroke. *Drugs* 1991;42, (Suppl 5): 39–50.
227. McAnally LE, Corn CR, Hamilton SF. Aspirin for the prevention of vascular death in women. *Ann Pharmacother* 1992;26:1530–1534.
228. Cote R, Battista RN, Abrahamowicz M, Langlois Y, Bourque F, Mackey A. Lack of effect of aspirin in asymptomatic patients with carotid bruits and substantial carotid narrowing. The Asymptomatic Cervical Bruit Study Group. *Ann Intern Med* 1995;123:649–655.
229. Cote R. Aspirin in asymptomatic carotid disease. *Health Reports* 1994;6:114–120.
230. Iso H, Hennekens CH, Stampfer MJ, et al. Prospective study of aspirin use and risk of stroke in women.*Stroke* 1999;30:1764–1771.
231. Cairns JA, Theroux P, Lewis HDJ, Ezekowitz M, Meade TW, Sutton GC. Antithrombotic agents in coronary artery disease. *Chest* 1998;114: 611S–633S.
232. Patrono C. Prevention of myocardial infarction and stroke by aspirin: different mechanisms? Different dosage? *Thromb Res* 1998;92:S7–S12.
233. Hart RG, Harrison MJ. Aspirin wars: the optimal dose of aspirin prevent stroke.*Stroke* 1996;27:585–587.
234. Canadian Cooperative Study Group. A randomized trial of aspirin and sulfinpyrazone in threatened stroke. *N Engl J Med* 1978;299:53–59.
235. Fields WS, Lemak NA, Frankowski RF, Hardy RJ. Controlled trial of aspirin in cerebral ischemia. Part II: surgical group. *Stroke* 1978;9:309–319.
236. Fields WS, Lemak NA, Frankowski RF, Hardy RJ, Bigelow RH. Controlled trial of aspirin in cerebral ischemia. *Circulation* 1980;62:V90–V96
237. Gent M, Barnett HJM, Sackett DL, Taylor DW. A randomized trial of aspirin and sulfinpyrazone in patients with threatened stroke. Results and methodologic issues. *Circulation* 1980;62: V97–V105.
238. Sorensen PS, Pedersen H, Marquardsen J, et al. Acetylsalicylic acid in the prevention of stroke in patients with reversible cerebral ischemic attacks. A Danish cooperative study. *Stroke* 1983; 14:15–22.
239. The Dutch TIA Trial Study Group. A comparison of two doses of aspirin (30 mg vs. 283 mg a day) in patients after a transient ischemic attack or minor ischemic stroke. *N Engl J Med* 1991; 325:1261–1266.
240. The SALT Collaborative Group. Swedish Aspirin Low-Dose Trial (SALT) of 75 mg aspirin as secondary prophylaxis after cerebrovascular ischaemic events. *Lancet* 1991;338:1345–1349.
241. Lindblad B, Persson NH, Takolander R, Bergqvist D. Does low-dose acetylsalicylic acid prevent stroke after carotid surgery? A double-blind, placebo-controlled randomized trial. *Stroke* 1993;24:1125–1128.
242. Algra A, van Gijn J. Aspirin at any dose above 30 mg offers only modest protection after cerebral ischaemia. *J Neurol Neurosurg Psychiatry* 1996;60: 197–199.
243. Tijssen JG. Low-dose and high-dose acetylsalicylic acid, with and without dipyridamole: a review of clinical trial results. *Neurology* 1998;51: S15–S16.
244. Johnson ES, Lanes SF, Wentworth CE, Satterfield MH, Abebe BL, Dicker LW. A metaregression analysis of the dose-response effect of aspirin on stroke. *Arch Intern Med* 1999;159: 1248–1253.
245. Patrono C, Roth GJ. Aspirin in ischemic cerebrovascular disease. How strong is the case for a different dosing regimen? *Stroke* 1996;27: 756–760.
246. Bornstein NM, Karepov VG, Aronovich BD, Gorbulev AY, Treves TA, Korczyn AD. Failure of aspirin treatment after stroke. *Stroke* 1994;25: 275–277.

247. Chimowitz MI, Furlan AJ, Nayak S, Sila CA. Mechanism of stroke in patients taking aspirin. *Neurology* 1990;40:1682–1685.
248. Grotta JC, Lemak NA, Gary H, Fields WS, Vital D. Does platelet antiaggregant therapy lessen the severity of stroke?. *Neurology* 1985;35: 632–636.
249. De Keyser J, Herroelen L, De Klippel N. Early outcome in acute ischemic stroke is not influenced by the prophylactic use of low-dose aspirin. *J Neurol Sci* 1997;145:93–96.
250. Karepov V, Bornstein NM, Hass Y, Korczyn AD. Does daily aspirin diminish severity of first-ever stroke? *Arch Neurol* 1997;54:1369–1371.
251. Sivenius J, Cunha L, Diener HC, et al. Antiplatelet treatment does not reduce the severity of subsequent stroke. *Neurology* 1999;53: 825–829.
252. Moinuddeen K, Quin J, Shaw R, et al. Anticoagulation is unnecessary after biological aortic valve replacement. *Circulation* 1998;98: II95–II98.
253. The Atrial Fibrillation Investigators. The efficacy of aspirin in patients with atrial fibrillation. Analysis of pooled data from 3 randomized trials. *Arch Intern Med* 1997;157: 1237–1240.
254. Stroke Prevention in Atrial Fibrillation Investigators. Warfarin versus aspirin for prevention of thromboembolism in atrial fibrillation: Stroke Prevention in Atrial Fibrillation II Study. *Lancet* 1994;343:687–691.
255. The SPAF III Writing Committee for the Stroke Prevention in Atrial Fibrillation. Patients with nonvalvular atrial fibrillation at low risk of stroke during treatment with aspirin: Stroke Prevention in Atrial Fibrillation III Study. *JAMA* 1998;279:1273–1277.
256. Posada IS, Barriales V. Alternate-day dosing of aspirin in atrial fibrillation. LASAF Pilot Study Group. *Am Heart J* 1999;138:137–143.
257. EAFT (European Atrial Fibrillation Trial) Study Group. Secondary prevention in nonrheumatic atrial fibrillation after transient ischaemic attack or minor stroke. *Lancet* 1993; 342:1255–1262.
258. CAST (Chinese Acute Stroke Trial) Collaborative Group. CAST: randomised placebo-controlled trial of early aspirin use in 20,000 patients with acute ischaemic stroke. *Lancet* 1997;349: 1641–1649.
259. Multicentre Acute Stroke Trial—Italy (MAST-I) Group. Randomised controlled trial of streptokinase, aspirin, and combination of both in treatment of acute ischaemic stroke. *Lancet* 1995;346: 1509–1514.
260. Easton JD. What have we learned from recent antiplatelet trials? *Neurology* 1998;51:S36–S38.
261. Nademanee K, Kosar EM. Long-term antithrombotic treatment for atrial fibrillation. *Am J Cardiol* 1998;82:N37–N42.
262. Sharis PJ, Cannon CP, Loscalzo J. The antiplatelet effects of ticlopidine and clopidogrel. *Ann Intern Med* 1998;129:394–405.
263. Hass WK, Easton JD, Adams HP, Jr., et al. A randomized trial comparing ticlopidine hydrochloride with aspirin for the prevention of stroke in high-risk patients. Ticlopidine Aspirin Stroke Study Group. *N Engl J Med* 1989;321:501–507.
264. Gent M, Blakely JA, Easton JD, et al. The Canadian American Ticlopidine Study (CATS) in thromboembolic stroke. *Lancet* 1989;1: 1215–1220.
265. Janzon L, Bergqvist D, Boberg J, et al. Prevention of myocardial infarction and stroke in patients with intermittent claudication; effects of ticlopidine. Results from STIMS, the Swedish Ticlopidine Multicentre Study. *J Intern Med* 1990;227:301–308.
266. Iqbal M, Goenka P, Young MF, Thomas E, Borthwick TR. Ticlopidine-induced cholestatic hepatitis: report of three cases and review of the literature. *Digestive Diseases & Sciences* 1998;43: 2223–2226.
267. Yim HB, Lieu PK, Choo PW. Ticlopidine induced cholestatic jaundice. *Singapore Med J* 1997;38:132–133.
268. Rosen H, el-Hennawy AS, Greenberg S, Chen CK, Nicastri AD. Acute interstitial nephritis associated with ticlopidine. *Am J Kid Dis* 1995;25:934–936.
269. Love BB, Biller J, Gent M. Adverse haematological effects of ticlopidine. Prevention, recognition and management. *Drug Saf* 1998;19:89–98.
270. Bennett CL, Weinberg PD, Rozenberg-Bendror K, Yarnold PR, Kwaan HC, Green D. Thrombotic thrombocytopenia purpura associated with ticlopidine. *Ann Intern Med* 1998;128:541–544.
271. Mallet L, Mallet J. Ticlopidine and fatal aplastic anemia in an elderly woman. *Ann Pharmacother* 1994;28:1169–1171.
272. Steinhubl SR, Tan WA, Foody JM, Topol EJ. Incidence and clinical course of thrombotic thrombocytopenic purpura due to ticlopidine following coronary stenting. EPISTENT Investigators. Evaluation of Platelet IIb/IIIa Inhibitor for Stenting. *JAMA* 1999;281:806–810.
273. Janzon L. The STIMS trial: the ticlopidine experience and its clinical applications. Swedish Ticlopidine Multicenter Study. *Vasc Med* 1996;1:141–143.
274. McTavish D, Faulds D, Goa KL. Ticlopidine. An updated review of its pharmacology and therapeutic use in platelet-dependent disorders. *Drugs* 1990;40:238–259.
275. Murray JC, Kelly MA, Gorelick PB. Ticlopidine: a new antiplatelet agent for the secondary prevention of stroke. *Clin Neuropharmacol* 1994; 17:23–31.
276. Madan M, Marquis JF, de May MR, et al. Coronary stenting in unstable angina: early and late clinical outcomes. *Can J Cardiol* 1998; 14:1109–1114.
277. Walter H, Neumann FJ, Hadamitzky M, Elezi S, Muller A, Schomig A. Coronary artery stent placement with postprocedural antiplatelet therapy in acute myocardial infarction. *Cor Art Dis* 1998;9:577–582.
278. van de Loo A, Nauck M, Noory E, Wollschlager H. Enhancement of platelet inhibition of ticlopidine plus aspirin vs aspirin alone given prior to elective PTCA. *Eur Heart J* 1998;19:96–102.
279. Goods CM, al-Shaibi KF, Liu MW, et al. Comparison of aspirin alone versus aspirin plus

ticlopidine after coronary artery stenting. *Am J Cardiol* 1996;78:1042–1044.
280. Harbison JW. Ticlopidine versus aspirin for the prevention of recurrent stroke. Analysis of patients with minor stroke from the Ticlopidine Aspirin Stroke Study. *Stroke* 1992;23:1723–1727.
281. Grotta JC, Norris JW, Kamm B. Prevention of stroke with ticlopidine: who benefits most? TASS Baseline and Angiographic Data Subgroup. *Neurology* 1992;42:111–115.
282. Bellavance A. Efficacy of ticlopidine and aspirin for prevention of reversible cerebrovascular ischemic events. The Ticlopidine Aspirin Stroke Study. *Stroke* 1993;24:1452–1457.
283. Hershey LA. Stroke prevention in women: role of aspirin versus ticlopidine. *Am J Med* 1991;91: 288–292.
284. Weisberg LA. The efficacy and safety of ticlopidine and aspirin in non-whites: analysis of a patient subgroup from the Ticlopidine Aspirin Stroke Study. *Neurology* 1993;43:27–31.
285. Pryse-Phillips W, for the Ticlopidine Aspirin Stroke Study Group. Ticlopidine Aspirin Stroke Study: Outcome by vascular distribution of the qualifying event. *J Stroke Cerebrovasc Dis* 1993; 3:49–56.
286. Warlow C. Ticlopidine, a new antithrombotic drug: but is it better than aspirin for longterm use? *J Neurol Neurosurg Psychiatry* 1990;53: 185–187.
287. Bendixen BH, Adams HP, Jr. Ticlopidine or clopidogrel as alternatives to aspirin in prevention of ischemic stroke. *Eur Neurol* 1996;36:256–257.
288. Haynes RB, Sandler RS, Larson EB, Pater JL, Yatsu FM. A critical appraisal of ticlopidine, a new antiplatelet agent. Effectiveness and clinical indications for prophylaxis of atherosclerotic events. *Arch Intern Med* 1992;152:1376–1380.
289. Noble S, Goa KL. Ticlopidine. A review of its pharmacology, clinical efficacy and tolerability in the prevention of cerebral ischaemia and stroke. *Drugs Aging* 1996;8:214–232.
290. Oster G, Huse DM, Lacey MJ, Epstein AM. Cost-effectiveness of ticlopidine in preventing stroke in high-risk patients. *Stroke* 1994;25:1149–1156.
291. Rothrock JF, Hart RG. Ticlopidine hydrochloride use and threatened stroke. *West J Med* 1994; 160:43–47.
292. Harker LA, Marzec UM, Kelly AB, et al. Clopidogrel inhibition of stent, graft, and vascular thrombogenesis with antithrombotic enhancement by aspirin in nonhuman primates. *Circulation* 1998;98:2461–2469.
293. Hankey GJ. Clopidogrel: a new safe and effective antiplatelet agent. But unanswered questions remain. *Med J Aust* 1997;167:120–121.
294. Creager MA. Results of the CAPRIE trial: efficacy and safety of clopidogrel. Clopidogrel versus aspirin in patients at risk of ischaemic events. *Vasc Med* 1998;3:257–260.
295. Bennett CL, Connors JM, Carwile MJ, et al. Thrombotic thrombocytopenic purpura associated with clopidogrel. *N Engl J Med* 2000;325: 1371–1372.
296. CAPRIE Steering Committee. A randomised, blinded, trial of clopidogrel versus aspirin in patients at risk of ischaemic events (CAPRIE). *Lancet* 1996;348:1329–1339.
297. Paciaroni M, Bogousslavsky J. Clopidogrel for cerebrovascular prevention. *Cerebrovasc Dis* 1999;9:253–260.
298. Harbison JW. Clinical considerations in selecting antiplatelet therapy in cerebrovascular disease. *Ame J Health-System Pharm* 1998;55:S17–S20.
299. Dippel DW. The results of CAPRIE, IST and CAST. Clopidogrel vs. Aspirin in Patients at Risk of Ischaemic Events. International Stroke Trial. Chinese Acute Stroke Trial. *Thromb Res* 1998; 92:S13–S16.
300. Rivey MP, Alexander MR, Taylor JW. Dipyridamole: a critical evaluation. *Drug Intelligence & Clinical Pharmacy* 1984;18:869–880.
301. Gibbs CR, Lip GY. Do we still need dipyridamole? *Br J Clin Pharmacol* 1998;45:323–328.
302. The American-Canadian Co-Operative Study Group. Persantine Aspirin Trial in cerebral ischemia. Part II: endpoint results. *Stroke* 1985; 16:406–415.
303. The Persantine-Aspirin Reinfarction Study (PARIS) Research Group. The Persantine-Aspirin Reinfarction Study. *Circulation* 1980;62: V85–V88.
304. Matias-Guiu J, Davalos A, Pico M, Monasterio J, Vilaseca J, Codina A. Low-dose acetylsalicylic acid (ASA) plus dipyridamole versus dipyridamole alone in the prevention of stroke in patients with reversible ischemic attacks. *Acta Neurol Scand* 1987;76:413–421.
305. Sivenius J, Riekkinen PJ, Laakso M, Smets P, Lowenthal A. European Stroke Prevention Study (ESPS): antithrombotic therapy is also effective in the elderly. *Acta Neurol Scand* 1993; 87:111–114.
306. Diener HC. Dipyridamole trials in stroke prevention. *Neurology* 1998;51:S17–S19.
307. Diener HC, Cunha L, Forbes C, Sivenius J, Smets P, Lowenthal A. European Stroke Prevention Study. 2. Dipyridamole and acetylsalicylic acid in the secondary prevention of stroke. *J Neurol Sci* 1996;143:1–13.
308. Forbes CD. Secondary stroke prevention with low-dose aspirin, sustained release dipyridamole alone and in combination. ESPS Investigators. European Stroke Prevention Study. *Thromb Res* 1998;92:S1–S6.
309. Sivenius J, Cunha L, Diener HC, et al. Second European Stroke Prevention Study: antiplatelet therapy is effective regardless of age. ESPS2 Working Group. Acta *Neurol Scand* 1999;99: 54–60.
310. Sullivan JM, Harken DE, Gorlin R. Pharmacologic control of thromboembolic complications of cardiac-valve replacement. *N Engl J Med* 1971;284:1391–1394.
311. Wilterkink JL, Easton JD. Dipyridamole plus aspirin in cerebrovascular disease. *Arch Neurol* 1999;56:1087–1092.
312. Califf RM. A perspective on the regulation of the evaluation of new antithrombotic drugs. *Am J Cardiol* 1998;82:P25–P35.
313. Coller BS, Anderson K, Weisman HF. New antiplatelet agents: platelet GPIIb/IIIa antagonists. *Thromb Haemost* 1995;74:302–308.

314. Theroux P. Oral inhibitors of platelet membrane receptor glycoprotein IIb/IIIa in clinical cardiology: issues and opportunities. *Am Heart J* 1998;135:S107–S112.
315. Tcheng JE, Ellis SG, George BS, et al. Pharmacodynamics of chimeric glycoprotein IIb/IIIa integrin antiplatelet antibody Fab 7E3 in high-risk coronary angioplasty. *Circulation* 1994;90:1757–1764.
316. Topol EJ. Prevention of cardiovascular ischemic complications with new platelet glycoprotein IIb/IIIa inhibitors. *Am Heart J* 1995;130: 666–672.
317. Topol EJ, Califf RM, Weisman HF, et al. Randomised trial of coronary intervention with antibody against platelet IIb/IIIa integrin for reduction of clinical restenosis: results at six months. The EPIC Investigators. *Lancet* 1994; 343:881–886.
318. Simoons ML, de Boer MJ, van den Brand MJ, et al. Randomized trial of a GPIIb/IIIa platelet receptor blocker in refractory unstable angina. European Cooperative Study Group. *Circulation* 1994;89:596–603.
319. Theroux P. Oral inhibitors of platelet membrane receptor glycoprotein IIb/IIIa in clinical cardiology: issues and opportunities. *Am Heart J* 1998; 135:S107–S112.
320. Cines DB. Glycoprotein IIb/IIIa antagonists: Potential induction and detection of drug-dependent antiplatelet antibodies. *Am Heart J* 1998;135:S152–S159.
321. Quinn M, Fitzgerald DJ. Long-term administration of glycoprotein IIb/IIIa antagonists. *Am Heart J* 1998;135:S113–S118.
322. Hankey GJ. One year after CAPRIE, IST and ESPS 2. Any changes in concepts?. *Cerebrovasc Dis* 1998;8(Suppl 5):1–7.
323. Mahaffey KW, Harrington RA, Simoons ML, et al. Stroke in patients with acute coronary syndromes: incidence and outcomes in the platelet glycoprotein IIb/IIIa in unstable angina. Receptor suppression using integrilin therapy (PURSUIT) trial. The PURSUIT Investigators. *Circulation* 1999;99:2371–2377.
324. Margulies EH, White AM, Sherry S. Sulfinpyrazone: a review of its pharmacological properties and therapeutic use. *Drugs* 1980;20: 179–197.
325. Bergamasco B, Benna P, Carolei A, Rasura M, Rudelli G, Fieschi C. A randomized trial comparing ticlopidine hydrochloride with indobufen for the prevention of stroke in high-risk patients (TISS Study). Ticlopidine Indobufen Stroke Study. *Funct Neurol* 1997;12:33–43.
326. Schneider R. Results of hemorheologically active treatment with pentoxifylline in patients with cerebrovascular disease. *Angiology* 1989;40: 987–993.
327. Frampton JE, Brogden RN. Pentoxifylline (oxpentifylline). A review of its therapeutic efficacy in the management of peripheral vascular and cerebrovascular disorders. *Drugs Aging* 1995;7:480–503.
328. Apollonio A, Castignani P, Magrini L, Angeletti R. Ticlopidine-pentoxifylline combination in the treatment of atherosclerosis and the prevention of cerebrovascular accidents. *Jo Internat Med Res* 1989;17:28–35.
329. Herbert JM, Bernat A, Samama M, Maffrand JP. The antiaggregating and antithrombotic activity of ticlopidine is potentiated by aspirin in the rat. *Thromb Haemost* 1996;76:94–98.
330. The Medical Research Council's General Practice Research Framework, . Thrombosis prevention trial: randomised trial of low-intensity oral anticoagulation with warfarin and low-dose aspirin in the primary prevention of ischaemic heart disease in men at increased risk. The Medical Research Council's General Practice Research Framework. *Lancet* 1998;351: 233–241.
331. Hurlen M, Erikssen J, Smith P, Arnesen H, Rollag A. Comparison of bleeding complications of warfarin and warfarin plus acetylsalicylic acid: a study in 3166 outpatients. *J Intern Med* 1994; 236:299–304.
332. Fagan SC, Kertland HR, Tietjen GE. Safety of combination aspirin and anticoagulation in acute ischemic stroke. *Ann Pharmacother* 1994;28: 441–443.
333. Golby AJ, Marks MP, Thompson RC, Steinberg GK. Direct and combined revascularization in pediatric moyamoya disease. *Neurosurgery* 1999; 45:50–60.
334. Loewen P, Sunderji R, Gin K. The efficacy and safety of combination warfarin and ASA therapy: a systematic review of the literature and update of guidelines. *Can J Cardiol* 1998;14:717–726.
335. Fisher M, Jonas S, Sacco RL, Jones S. Prophylactic neuroprotection for cerebral ischemia. *Stroke* 1994;25:1075–1080.
336. Goldstein LB, Bonito AJ, Matchar DB, Duncan PW, Samsa GP. US National Survey of Physician Practices for the Secondary and Tertiary Prevention of Ischemic Stroke. Medical therapy in patients with carotid artery stenosis. *Stroke* 1996;27:1473–1478.
337. Masuhr F, Busch M, Einhaupl KM. Differences in medical and surgical therapy for stroke prevention between leading experts in North America and Western Europe. *Stroke* 1998;29: 339–345.
338. Moroney JT, Tseng CL, Paik MC, Mohr JP, Desmond DW. Treatment for the secondary prevention of stroke in older patients: the influence of dementia status. *J Am Geriatr Soc* 1999;47: 824–829.
339. Gurwitz JH, Monette J, Rochon PA, Eckler MA, Avorn J. Atrial fibrillation and stroke prevention with warfarin in the long-term care setting. *Arch Intern Med* 1997;157:978–984.
340. Gorelick PB, Born GV, D'Agostino RB, Hanley DFJ, Moye L, Pepine CJ. Therapeutic benefit. Aspirin revisited in light of the introduction of clopidogrel. *Stroke* 1999;30:1716–1721.
341. Mollison LC, James-Wallace MJ, Kirke AB, Stein GR, Jamrozik KD. Underuse of aspirin for secondary prevention of vascular disease. *Med J Aust* 1934;170:339–341.
342. Brass LM, Krumholz HM, Scinto JD, Mathur D, Radford M. Warfarin use following ischemic stroke among Medicare patients with atrial fibrillation. *Arch Intern Med* 1998;158:2093–2100.

343. Davis SM, Donnan GA. Secondary prevention for stroke after CAPRIE and ESPS-2. Opinion 1. *Cerebrovasc Dis* 1977;8:73–75.
344. Singer DE. Anticoagulation to prevent stroke in atrial fibrillation and its implications for managed care. *Am J Cardiol* 1998;81:C35–C40.
345. Howard PA, Duncan PW. Primary stroke prevention in nonvalvular atrial fibrillation: implementing the clinical trial findings. *Ann Pharmacother* 1997;31:1187–1196.
346. Gage BF, Cardinalli AB, Owens DK. Cost-effectiveness of preference-based antithrombotic therapy for patients with nonvalvular atrial fibrillation. *Stroke* 1998;29:1083–1091.
347. Lightowlers S, McGuire A. Cost-effectiveness of anticoagulation in nonrheumatic atrial fibrillation in the primary prevention of ischemic stroke. *Stroke* 1998;29:1827–1832.
348. Stafford RS, Singer DE. Recent national patterns of warfarin use in atrial fibrillation. *Circulation* 1998;97:1231–1233.
349. Bath PM, Prasad A, Brown MM, MacGregor GA. Survey of use of anticoagulation in patients with atrial fibrillation. *BMJ* 1993;307:1045.
350. Sudlow M, Thomson R, Thwaites B, Rodgers H, Kenny RA. Prevalence of atrial fibrillation and eligibility for anticoagulants in the community. *Lancet* 1998;352:1167–1171.
351. Caplan LR. Migraine and vertebrobasilar ischemia. *Neurology* 1991;41:55–61.
352. Albers GW, Yim JM, Belew KM, et al. Status of antithrombotic therapy for patients with atrial fibrillation in university hospitals. *Arch Intern Med* 1996;156:2311–2316.
353. Shepherd J, Cobbe SM, Ford I, et al. Prevention of coronary heart disease with pravastatin in men with hypercholesterolemia. West of Scotland Coronary Prevention Study Group. *N Engl J Med* 1995;333:1301–1307.
354. Sacks FM, Pfeffer MA, Moye LA, et al. The effect of pravastatin on coronary events after myocardial infarction in patients with average cholesterol levels. Cholesterol and Recurrent Events Trial investigators. *N Engl J Medi* 1996;335:1001–1009.
355. The Long-Term Intervention with Pravastatin in Ischaemic Disease (LIPID) Study Group. Prevention of cardiovascular events and death with pravastatin in patients with coronary heart disease and a broad range of initial cholesterol levels. *N Engl J Med* 1998;339:1349–1357.
356. Morocutti C, Amabile G, Fattapposta F, et al. Indobufen versus warfarin in the secondary prevention of major vascular events in nonrheumatic atrial fibrillation. SIFA (Studio Italiano Fibrillazione Atriale) Investigators. *Stroke* 1997;28:1015–1021.
357. Reuther R, Domdorf W, Loew D. Behandlund transitorisch-ischamischer attacehn mit acetylsaliclsaure. *Munch Med Wochenschr* 1980;122: 795–798.
360. Bousser M-G, Eschwage E, Hauenau M. "A.I.C.L.A." controlled trial of aspirin and dipyridamole in the secondary prevention of atherothrombotic cerebral ischemia. *Stroke* 1983;14:5–14
362. A Swedish Cooperative Study. High-dose acetylsalicyclic acid after cerebral infarction. *Stroke* 1987;18:325–334.
363. Boysen G, Sorensen PS, Juhler M. Danish very-low-dose aspirin after carotid endarterectomy trial. *Stroke* 1988;19:1211–1215.
364. The ESPS Group. The European Stroke Prevention Study. *Lancet* 1987;2:1351–1354.
365. Taylor DW, Barnett HJM, Haynes RB, et al. Low-dose and high-dose acetylsalicylic acid for patients undergoing carotid endarterctomy: a randomised controlled trial. ASA and Carotid Endarterectomy (ACE) Trial Collaborators. *Lancet* 1999;353:2179–2184.
366. Guiraud-Chaumeil B, Rascol A, David J, Boneu B, Clanet M, Bierme R. Prevention desrecidives des accidents vasculaires cerebraux ischemiques par les anti-aggregants palguettaires. *Rev Neurol* 1982;138:367–385.
367. Holloway RG, Benesch C, Rush SR. Stroke prevention. Narrowing the evidence-practice gap *Neurology* 2000;54:1899–1906.
368. Albers GW, Hart RG, Lutsep HL, Newell DW, Sacco RL. AHA Scientific Statement. Supplement to the guidelines for the management of transient ischemic attacks: A statement from the Ad Hoc Committee on Guidelines for the Management of Transient Ischemic Attacks, Stroke Council, American Heart Association. *Stroke* 1999;30:2502–2511.
369. Ganz DA, Kuntz KM, Jacobson GA, Avorn J. Cost-effectiveness of 3-hydroxy-3-methylglutaryl coenzyme a reductase inhibitor therapy in older patients with myocardial infarction. *Ann Intern Med* 2000;132:780–787.
370. Prosser LA, Stinnett AA, Goldman PA, et al. Cost-effectiveness of cholesterol-lowering therapies according to selected patient characteristics. *Ann Intern Med* 2000;132:769–778.
371. Garber AM. Using cost-effectiveness analysis to target cholesterol reduction. *Ann Intern Med* 2000;132:833–835.
372. Benesch CG, Chimowitz MI, for the WASID Investigators. Best treatment of intracranial arterial stenosis? 50 years of uncertainty. *Neurology* 2000;55:465–466.
373. Thijs VN, Albers GW. Symptomatic intracranial atherosclerosis. Outcome of patients who fail antithrombotic therapy. *Neurology* 2000;55: 490–497
374. The WARSS APASS PICSS HAS and GENESIS Study Groups. The feasibility of a collaborative double-blind study using an anticoagulant. *Cerebrovasc Dis* 1997;7:100–112.
375. Tsai HM, Rice L, Sarode R, Chow TW, Moake JL. Antibody inhibitors to von willebrand factor metallproteinase and increased binding of von willebrand factor to platelets in ticlopidine-associated thrombotic thrombocytopenic purpura. *Ann Intern Med* 2000;132:794–799.
376. Hankey GJ. Clopidogrel and thrombotic thrombocytopenic purpura. *Lancet* 2000;356:269–270.

Chapter 11

SURGICAL THERAPY FOR PREVENTION OF ISCHEMIC STROKE

Several operations are used to improve the blood supply to the brain or to remove a source for embolization[220] (Table 11–1). The most widely studied operation is carotid endarterectomy, and also is the most commonly prescribed surgical procedure used in stroke prophylaxis. Other operations aimed at improving the cervical circulation in either the carotid or the vertebrobasilar circulation have been developed, but clinical studies testing the safety and the efficacy of these procedures are limited. During the last decade, endovascular techniques have been used to treat stenotic lesions in intracranial or extracranial arteries. This field is evolving rapidly, and the endovascular procedures likely will be prescribed for treatment of a large number of patients at risk for stroke. In the future, angioplasty and stenting might complement or replace traditional procedures, such as carotid endarterectomy.

CAROTID ENDARTERECTOMY

Rationale

Carotid endarterectomy was the first vascular operation performed with the aim of preventing ischemic stroke among high-risk patients. Since its inception in the 1950s, the operation has been the subject of controversy and, despite recent advances in knowledge about the safety and efficacy of carotid endarterectomy, it remains a source of dispute. The popularity of the operation has swung widely, and rates of carotid endarterectomy in North America and other parts of the world have differed greatly since the early 1980s.[1,2] The number of operations increased in frequency from 15,000 to approximately 107,000 between 1971 and 1986.[3] Subsequent to a series of commentaries by

Table 11–1. **Local Interventions to Prevent Stroke: Treatment of Arterial or Heart Disease**

Carotid endarterectomy—internal carotid artery
Superficial temporal artery—middle cerebral artery anastomosis
Posterior circulation arterial bypass
Encephaloduroarteriomyosynangiosis
Encephaloduromyosynangiosis
Duroarteriosynagiosis
Plication of internal carotid artery—stump syndrome
Resection of a kink—internal carotid artery
Carotid endarterectomy—external carotid artery
Endarterectomy—middle cerebral artery
Endarterectomy—origin of the vertebral artery
Resection of a dissection—internal carotid artery
Graded dilation of internal carotid artery—fibromuscular dysplasia
Arterial bypass operations—subclavian, innominate, or vertebral arteries
Resection of segment of the ascending or the arch of the aorta
Valve replacement
Cardioversion or pacemaker
Resection of atrial myxoma
Closure of patent foramen ovale
Angioplasty and stenting
Internal carotid artery
Middle cerebral artery
Vertebral artery
Basilar artery

neurologists expressing concern about the procedure, the operations declined in number to 83,000 in 1986. Its rate remained stable at approximately 60,000 until the early 1990s. Since then, the number of operations has increased dramatically, chiefly because of the success of carotid endarterectomy in clinical trials that tested the procedure among both symptomatic and asymptomatic patients with moderate-to-severe stenoses of the internal carotid artery. For example, the number of operations performed at academic medical centers doubled from 1990 to 1995.[4] The most dramatic jump has been in the use of carotid endarterectomy to prevent stroke among asymptomatic persons. Since the report of the Asymptomatic Carotid Atherosclerosis Study, the number of operations in Florida increased by approximately 68%.[5] Increases in the number of operations were found in all age groups but were largely among asymptomatic persons. The rates of endarterectomy are approximately 60% higher among men than among women.[2] This finding probably in part reflects the younger age of men who develop atherosclerotic disease at the internal carotid artery. Operations are less frequently performed among African Americans than among whites.[6,7] In addition to a low rate of extracranial atherosclerosis among African Americans, this group of patients also may have an aversion to surgery.[7] Now, approximately 140,000 operations are performed annually in the United States.[8] In Britain, the rates of carotid endarterectomy vary widely among populations.[9] A British report also demonstrated an increased number of operations since the publication of the results of the clinical trials.[10] The dramatic increase in surgery leads to thoughts about whether carotid endarterectomy is being over-or under-used. Ferris et al[11] concluded that carotid endarterectomy may be under-used in the United Kingdom. The situation is not as clear in the United States and Canada, where the rates for the operation are much higher.

Procedure

Because advanced atherosclerotic disease has a predilection for the origin of the internal carotid artery at the bifurcation and because the atherosclerotic plaque can be the source of thromboemboli that go to the brain, surgical removal of the plaque could lower the risk of stroke. In addition to removing the ulcerated or severely stenotic plaque, which would induce thrombosis of the internal carotid artery or be a source of emboli, the operation also removes the source of atherosclerotic debris (cholesterol emboli). The operation also could change hemodynamics by improving cerebral blood flow. Carotid endarterectomy improves cerebrovascular reactivity.[12] The operation also could improve blood flow distal to the stenosis and obviate flow-related symptoms or areas of borderline perfusion that would potentiate the effects of embolization. The improved flow might "wash out" small emboli before they had the time to cause brain ischemia.

The operation itself is relatively straightforward.[13] A vertical skin incision is made over the carotid artery and parallel and anterior to the sternocleidomastoid muscle. The common external and internal carotid arteries are exposed and isolated. Then, arterial clamps temporarily occlude them. A longitudinal arteriotomy opens the wall of the carotid bifurcation and the first portion of the internal carotid artery. The limits of the plaque are identified, and the surgeon dissects the lesion from the involved segment of the arterial wall. The ends of the resection are tacked to prevent a secondary intramural dissection. The arteriotomy is then closed, the clamps are removed, and the flow is restored. An alternative endarterectomy procedure involves an eversion technique to open the artery at the bifurcation.[14]

Several perioperative procedures have been employed to improve the safety and effectiveness of the operation (Table 11–2). Many of these procedures have generated controversy, and, in general, the decisions about their use or non-use should remain at the discretion of the surgeon. None of these procedures has been established as uniformly effective or as a replacement for meticulous surgical technique. Among the issues is the performance of the operation using either general or regional anesthesia. Most patients have surgery while under general anesthesia; however, local anesthesia can also be used.[15,16] The potential advantages of carotid endarterectomy using local anesthesia include lower rates of stroke, myocardial infarction, pulmonary embolism, and vascular death.[17] Regional anesthesia often has been used when a patient has severe heart disease. Papavasiliou et al[16] reported that nonneurological complications, particularly cardiopulmonary events, are less frequent with the regional anesthesia than with general anesthesia. The patient's neurological status can be monitored clinically during the operation. In contrast, general anesthesia helps protect against ischemia.[18] The metabolic depressant effects of the anesthetic agents may serve a neuroprotective function during the time of ischemia. The downside of general anesthesia is that some patients may have a high risk of complications from the anesthesia. In addition, clinical signs of an acute neurological event can be masked by the anesthesia. As a result, patients having general anesthesia often are monitored during surgery using electroencephalography or evoked potentials. Antiplatelet aggregating agents and anticoagulants are given in the perioperative period in an effort to limit thromboembolism. The assumption is that the trauma can serve as an impetus for platelet aggregation or thrombosis. Unfortunately, heparin can lead to perioperative bleeding, and the reversal of the effects of heparin with protamine can induce arterial thrombosis.[19]

Patches have been used to increase the size of the arteriotomy to prevent postoperative recurrent stenosis.[20] An early report suggested that patch grafting with venous tissue should not be used as a component of carotid endarterectomy because of the high risk of complications.[21] More recently, AbuRahma et al[22] concluded that patch closure was associated with a lower risk of stroke than primary closure of the

Table 11–2. **Perioperative Procedures: Carotid Endarterectomy**

Anesthesia
General anesthesia
Local—regional anesthesia
Monitoring
Electroencephalography
Evoked potentials
Transcranial Doppler ultrasonography
Measuring of carotid artery pressure distal to occlusion
Prevention of thromboembolism
Aspirin
Heparin
Surgical techniques
Placement of a temporary shunt
Patch grafting

surgical site. Patches are more commonly needed among women, whose arteries are smaller.[23,24] Patch closure of the small artery appears to be as safe and effective as primary closure of a larger internal carotid artery.[25,26] Placement of a shunt has been used to provide adequate blood flow to the ipsilateral hemisphere during the operation. Electroencephalographic (EEG) monitoring with selective shunting has been used to avoid ischemia.[27,28] This approach permits selective use of shunting in situations when the electroencephalogram detects changes. In addition, distal arterial pressure monitoring, transcranial Doppler ultrasonography, and cerebral blood flow studies are used to assess the patient's blood flow during the operation. Changes in these ancillary tests also could prompt placement of a shunt. Shunts have been controversial because of the need for punctures of the artery above and below the operative site; these arterial injuries would serve as sites for thromboembolism. A recent report concluded that most patients having carotid endarterectomy do not need placement of shunt if adequate collateral blood flow can be demonstrated through the anterior communicating artery or the ipsilateral posterior communicating artery.[29] Stendel et al[30] concluded that the use of intra-operative Doppler ultrasonography could be used to improve the outcomes of carotid endarterectomy by detecting vascular changes, including vasospasm. In the North American Symptomatic Carotid Endarterectomy Trial, none of these operative procedures, including the use of EEG monitoring, heparin administration, local or general anesthesia, shunt use, or simple or patch closure, affected the overall surgical morbidity.[31] Thus, these ancillary measures seem not to greatly alter safety or efficacy of the operation, and their use remains at the discretion of the surgeon.

Traditionally, the decision for carotid endarterectomy also involved a recommendation for an arteriogram as part of the pre-operative evaluation to determine whether the atherosclerotic lesion was sufficiently severe for surgery. Arteriography usually has been done to define the location and the extent of the atherosclerotic plaque and the presence of collateral channels of blood flow.[32] In addition, arteriography can demonstrate a severe stenosis of the siphon of the internal carotid artery that might alter management plans. A tandem intracranial lesion can be detected in approximately 10% of patients scheduled for carotid endarterectomy.[33] Another argument for arteriography is that it is the best method to assess the presence and extent of intracranial atherosclerosis. Although these results might change decisions for treatment, they also affect prognosis. Surprisingly, Kappelle et al[34] found that the presence of intracranial disease increased the value of carotid endarterectomy. However, arteriography is an invasive procedure and is accompanied by a risk of stroke. In the Asymptomatic Carotid Atherosclerosis Study, the risk of stroke following arteriography was greater than that following the operation.[35] Avoiding arteriography would limit the risk of procedural complications and also reduce costs. For a condition such as an asymptomatic stenosis, the overall management needs to have a very low risk for complications. Thus, the requirement for a preliminary test that is more dangerous than the actual treatment becomes problematic. As a result, non-invasive studies are being used to substitute for arteriography. Carotid endarterectomy can be done safely if the operation is performed only on the basis of the carotid duplex.[36,37] The specificity and sensitivity of these tests are very high and, in centers that have established the reliability of these tests, they can substitute for arteriography.[38–42] Arteriography could be restricted to cases of a subtotal occlusion or findings of string sign.[37] In addition, the procedure could be limited to cases in which the proximal and distal limits of the plaque cannot be determined by the non-invasive studies.[37] As a result of the advances in the sensitivity and specificity of the non-invasive tests, the number of pre-operative arteriograms has declined since 1985.[2,4] Although the combination of duplex and magnetic resonance angiography may not be less expensive than conventional arteriography, their high yield and non-invasive nature mean that increasingly patients will have carotid artery operations without prerequisite arteriography.

Carotid endarterectomy is expensive. It involves surgeon's fees and operating room costs. In addition, the charges for hospitalization and ancillary diagnostic tests are considerable. Thus, ways are needed to limit expenses without reducing the safety and the efficacy of the operation. A strategy that involves an outpatient pre-operative evaluation, admission to the hospital on the day of surgery, a brief period of post-operative observation in the hospital, and convalescence at home when the patient is stable makes economic and medical sense. A study that used no angiography, regional anesthesia, and less care in an intensive care unit than is traditionally used was effective in reducing lengths of stay and costs.[43] Importantly, the mortality rate in this series was 0, and only 0.9% of patients treated with this protocol had strokes. Harbaugh et al[44] concluded that performing the operation under local anesthesia, no post-operative monitoring in an intensive care unit, and early discharge of stable patients can lower the economic costs of the operation. They recommended discharge within 24–48 hours after surgery.[45] Changes in care are occurring.[46] Recent data show that the lengths of stay and the number of cardiac complications that might have mandated intensive unit care have declined.[5]

Safety

Because carotid endarterectomy is being done to prevent an event that might not ever occur even without surgery, the operation must be extraordinarily safe for any benefit to accrue (Table 11–3). The importance of safety is increased because the operative complications occur at the onset of treatment, whereas the events that carotid endarterectomy prevents gradually accumulate over subsequent years. Even patients with severe arterial narrowing will not be helped by carotid endarterectomy unless they have a high risk without surgery and have a low risk of complications from surgery.[47] Safety can be assured by careful patient selection, attention to heart disease, control of blood pressure, reliable monitoring, and meticulous surgical technique.[48] In addition, antiplatelet aggregating agents can lower the risk of post-procedural ischemic events.[221] If the operation can not be done with a very low rate of perioperative morbidity and mortality, then it should not be performed, regardless of the potential indication. Both the surgeon and the institution need to show evidence that the intervention can be done without a high rate of complications. In some situations, a patient who needs the operation badly might need to be referred to another institution where carotid endarterectomy can be performed safely.

Table 11–3. **Common Complications of Carotid Endarterectomy**

Ischemic stroke
Embolization
Hypoperfusion
Recurrent stenosis or occlusion
Post-endarterectomy hyperperfusion syndrome
Headache
Seizures
Intracerebral hemorrhage
Cranial nerve palsies
Myocardial infarction
Cardiac arrhythmias

A study performed in the mid-1970s found a prohibitively high rate of major complications following carotid endarterectomy; the combined morbidity and mortality approached 20%.[222] This appalling result prompted reconsideration about the safety of the operation in a community setting. The results of the Springfield report were buttressed by a 1984 survey of operations performed in Cincinnati, Ohio, which found the combined perioperative morbidity and mortality to be 9.5%.[49] These data also were stimuli for the recent trials. Since then, numerous reports have described the rates of major complications following carotid endarterectomy. In general, the more recent data are not as gloomy as those published previously, but the current results also imply that the room for improvement remains considerable. For example, one recent study at a single hospital found the 30 day rate of stroke or death to be 11.4%.[223] A systemic review of published studies showed that the 30-day post-operative mortality of carotid endarterectomy is approximately 1.6% and that the risk of stroke or death is approximately 5.6%.[50] An interesting aspect of this report was that the frequency of perioperative stroke was calculated to be 7.7% when a neurologist assessed the patient but only 2.3% when a surgeon did the evaluation. The investigators in the North American Symptomatic Carotid Endarterectomy Trial reported that the 30-day mortality was 1.1% and that 1.8% of patients had disabling strokes after surgery among 1415 patients who had surgery as part of the treatment in the trial.[31] These results were from a cadre of skilled surgeons operating at centers with expertise in treatment of stroke. Still, similar data are reported from other groups. A multi-center review found that the risk of ipsilateral stroke, myocardial infarction, or death was 8.5%.[51] A regional study based on 291 operations reported a combined stroke or mortality rate of 5.2% (9/174) among patients who had carotid endarterectomy for treatment of a symptomatic stenosis and 5.1% (6/117) among asymptomatic patients.[52] Early outcome assessments after carotid endarterectomy at one institution found the post-operative mortality to be 1.8% and the stroke rate to be 0.5%.[53]

Several regional or national surveys have been following the safety of carotid endarterectomy when done by a large number of surgeons at multiple institutions. A review of the U.S. Medicare database reported that the perioperative mortality in a general patient care setting was approximately 1.36 times that reported in clinical trials.[54] A statewide survey of carotid endarterectomy among 1945 operations performed on persons >65 found a mortality of 1.9% and a 1.8% rate of moderate-to-severe strokes.[55] The risk of complications was highest among hospitals that did a small number of operations. In a broad-bases data review, Lanska and Kryscio[56] reported that the in-hospital mortality was 1.2% following carotid endarterectomy. The rate increased with advancing age; persons <65 had a mortality of 0.9%, and those ages 75 or older was 1.7%. Among persons having carotid endarterectomy and another operation, usually coronary artery bypass graft surgery, the mortality of 6.1%; among those having carotid endarterectomy as the primary surgical procedure, mortality was 0.9%. O'Neill et al[224] found that low patient volume and older aged surgeons predicted higher rates of poorer outcomes after carotid endarterectomy. A statewide review from Florida found that perioperative mortality was 1.4% at hospitals involved in clinical trials, 1.7% in high-volume institutions, and 2.5% in low-volume hospitals.[57] Another survey from the same state found that the mortality has declined from 1.2% to 0.8% since 1990.[5] A survey done in North Carolina based on 11,973 operations found that a post-operative mortality of 1.2% and a stroke rate of 1.7%.[58] A study from Maine found that post-operative stroke rate was 2.5% and mortality was 0.3%.[59] Complication rates were higher among symptomatic patients. Similar mortality figures were reported in California, New York, and Ontario.[1] A British study found that the number of complications, including stroke or death, has declined in recent years; the combined risk of death or stroke following carotid endarterectomy in Britain had declined to 2%.[10] Thus, these data show a decline in mortality and morbidity following carotid endarterectomy since 1990. Some of the decline probably reflects improvements in surgical techniques and skills, better perioperative care and anesthesia, and focused selection of patients who have the operation. The increased number of asymptomatic patients having surgery also may explain the decline in morbidity and mortality.

A majority of complications are due to technical errors.[60] Thus, the skill of the surgeon is critical for the success of carotid endarterectomy.[61] A physician referring a patient for the operation must know the surgeon's skills as confirmed by his or her rates of perioperative morbidity and mortality. Depending on the nature of the surgeon's practice, the frequency of serious complications could vary. For example, a surgeon who primarily operates on patients who are neurologically unstable likely will have a higher rate of perioperative complications than will a surgeon who specializes in treatment of asymptomatic patients. The number of operations performed by the surgeon and in the hospital also is an important surrogate for the likelihood of major complications.[62,63]

The long-term survival after carotid endarterectomy is influenced by a history of myocardial infarction, the presence of congestive heart failure or diabetes mellitus, or advanced age.[64] (See Table 11–4.) Rothwell et al[65] detected several predictors of stroke or death after carotid endarterectomy. Operative risks are increased among women (relative risk [RR] 1.44) and persons older than 75 (RR 1.36), with systolic hypertension (RR 1.82), with peripheral vascular disease (RR 2.19), with a contralateral internal carotid artery occlusion (RR 1.91), or with intracranial stenosis of the internal carotid artery (RR 1.56). Inversely, they could not find a relationship between the rate of surgical complications and the presence of diabetes mellitus, prior myocardial infarction, angina, smoking, or plaque morphology. McCrory et al[66] found that complications of carotid endarterectomy were greatest among patients older than 75, those with symptomatic stenoses, and those with preoperative diastolic blood pressure >110. The presence of a thrombus in the internal carotid artery or a stenosis near the siphon also increased the chance of complications. In addition, they found that the presence of two or more factors increased the risk of complications by a factor of 1.7. Goldstein et al[51] found that the probability of complications was highest among persons older than 75 and those with intraluminal thrombus or carotid siphon stenosis. They could not find a difference in the rates of major complications as influenced by the severity of arterial narrowing or the presence of contralateral stenosis. The presenting symptoms, race, sex, or the history of angina, myocardial infarction, congestive heart failure, or chronic lung disease also did not influence the risk of complications. Ferguson et al[31] noted that complications were most common among patients having surgery for hemispheric ischemic symptoms, those with a positive computed tomography (CT) scan, and those with either a contralateral occlusion or an ulcerated plaque (see Table 11–4). Buchan et al[67] found that intraluminal clots in the internal carotid artery were associated with stroke and severe narrowing (Fig. 11–1). The presence of a contralateral occlusion of the internal carotid artery was associated with an increased risk of a perioperative stroke.[68] A 1998 report found that the risk of perioperative stroke or death was 5% among patients with contralateral occlusion and 3% among those without the lesion.[69] Samson et al[28] concluded that operation could be done safely even in the presence of a contralateral internal carotid artery occlusion. Thus, this arteriographic finding should not be considered as a contraindication. Medically treated patients also have a high risk for ischemic stroke. The presence of an occlusion of the contralateral internal carotid artery might increase the risk of perioperative stroke following carotid endarterectomy.

Although the risk of post-operative stroke is higher among persons older than

Table 11–4. **Risk Factors for Complications Following Carotid Endarterectomy**

- Contraindications
  - Recent myocardial infarction
  - Unstable angina
  - Recent major hemispheric infarction
- Increased risk
  - Neurologically unstable—recurrent symptoms
  - Extensive vascular disease
    - Contralateral occlusion
    - Tandem lesion
    - Intraluminal thrombus
  - Advanced age
  - Medical diseases
    - History of coronary artery disease
    - Chronic lung disease
    - Hypertension
    - Diabetes mellitus
    - Obesity

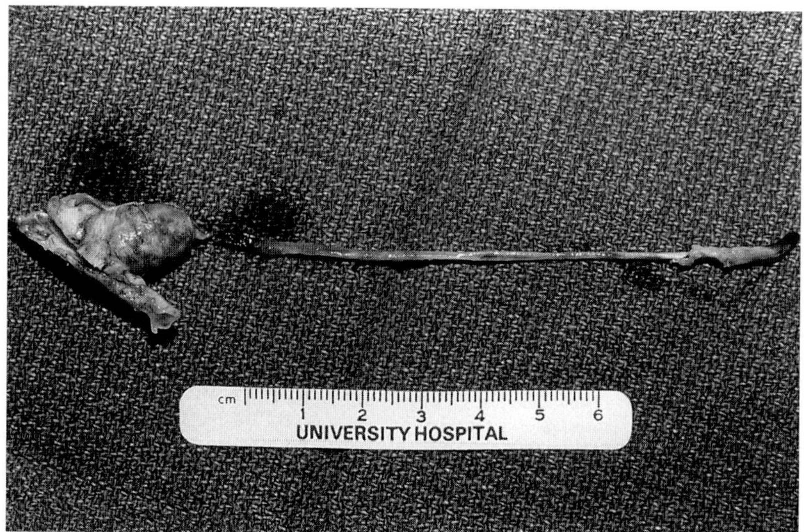

Figure 11–1. A long intraluminal clot removed from the internal carotid artery at the time of carotid endarterectomy.

80, carotid endarterectomy can be performed safely in this agc group.[70,71] O'Hara et al[15] performed 182 operations in 167 persons older than 83, and only 5 adverse events (3 strokes and 2 transient ischemic attacks (TIAs) occurred within 30 days of the surgery. Approximately 85% of the patients were free from stroke up to 5 years after the procedure. Hoballah et al [72] concluded that carotid endarterectomy can be done safely among persons who were older than 80. Conversely, carotid endarterectomy also can be done successful among persons <50 years old.[73] Unfortunately, this group has a higher rate of recurrent stenosis and late re-operations than persons older than 60 who have surgery. Patients with a severe stenosis of the internal carotid artery and an ipsilateral intracranial saccular aneurysm can be treated successfully.[74,75] The risk of subarachnoid hemorrhage seems not to be increased greatly with the operation.

A history of a recent stroke is associated with an increased likelihood of complications following carotid endarterectomy. In the past, surgery was delayed several weeks after a stroke. The concern was that early revascularization could lead to intracranial hemorrhage or worsening of brain edema after infarction. In contrast, a minor stroke may not differ greatly from a hemispheric TIA, particularly one that has an abnormal CT. Delaying surgery might leave a patient at high risk for a disabling event. Several groups have looked at the timing of carotid endarterectomy after stroke. Surgery can be performed within a few days of stroke if the CT scan is negative and the neurological signs are minimal.[76] Blohme et al[225] found that the risk of neurological complications was high if a stroke was found on brain imaging. They reported complications in 9.8% of patients who had a stroke seen on CT and 2.8% among patients whose scans were normal. Hoffman et al[77] included that the morbidity and mortality following surgery is not higher among persons treated within 6 weeks of stroke than among those operated at longer intervals. Early carotid endarterectomy can be recommended if the patient is stable clinically after stroke and if the CT is negative.[76] To date, a minor stroke with minimal CT changes does not contraindicate early carotid endarterectomy. The operation could be delayed for patients with serious neurological impairments and a stroke seen on CT.[76]

The leading complications of carotid endarterectomy are ischemic stroke, intracranial hemorrhage, seizures, cranial nerve palsies, and myocardial infarction (see Table 11–3) Stroke and cardiac events are the leading causes of death. Strokes following carotid endarterectomy can be secondary to ischemia developing during the clamp time, post-operative thromboembolism, or intracranial bleeding; or they may be secondary to other causes not directly related the surgery.[78] Ischemic stroke is the most common neurological complication of carotid endarterectomy. Strokes can be the result of embolization or secondary to poor perfusion to the hemisphere. Embolization to the brain can occur at the time of the initial arterial dissection or at the time that flow is restored at the end of the operation.[79] Intraluminal clots or atherosclerotic debris can be released during manipulation of the artery, and the restoration of flow permits migration to the brain. Post-operative thrombosis at the operative site can cause an acute occlusion of the internal carotid artery. A relatively common scenario is the discovery of a new focal neurological deficit while the patient is in the recovery room. Immediate assessment for an internal carotid occlusion and surgical re-exploration may be needed to restore flow. The most common reason appears to be immediate thrombosis at the arteriotomy site secondary to adhesion and aggregation of platelets on the denuded arterial surface.

Recurrent arterial stenosis can develop several years after carotid endarterectomy.[80] Recurrent stenosis is more common among women and persons with small arteries.[81] The recurrent narrowing usually is not due to reformation of the atherosclerotic plaque. Rather, the changes are due to an inflammatory reaction, myointimal proliferation, and fibrosis. The frequencies of early recurrent stenosis are broad and range from 1.3% to 37% of patients with recurrent symptoms and 0%–8.2% of asymptomatic patients.[82] A recent series of 187 patients followed for an average of 30.4 months found that approximately one-third of the new cerebrovascular events were ipsilateral to the operated artery, and the most common reason was a recurrent stenosis.[83] Symptomatic recurrent stenosis may prompt a second operation.[80] Angioplasty also may be a treatment for post-operative recurrent arterial stenosis.[84]

Cerebral hyperperfusion can follow carotid endarterectomy for treatment of very severe stenosis of the internal carotid artery. The marked hyperperfusion is secondary to impaired autoregulation distal to the original stenosis.[85] Cerebral blood flow increases in both the ipsilateral and the contralateral cerebral hemispheres.[85] The rises in flow can be dramatic and overwhelm normal physiologic responses. The sudden increase in flow also changes dynamics in collateral vessels. Chambers et al[86] found post-operative changes in flow in periorbital branches and the anterior communicating artery. Changes in flow velocities in the ipsilateral middle cerebral artery were detected by transcranial Doppler ultrasonography in 33 of 40 patients who had carotid surgery. Changes in the middle cerebral artery can be detected by magnetic resonance imaging.[87] The resultant increase in flow can produce a situation that mimics hypertensive encephalopathy. Brain edema and microvascular changes are found. In addition, hemorrhage after carotid endarterectomy also is secondary to disturbed baroreceptor function, a volatile blood pressure, and a hypertensive encephalopathy.[88] The symptoms usually occur 2–5 days after surgery. Symptoms include headache, progressively worsening neurological impairments, seizures, and intracranial hemorrhage. In one series of 1472 patients, intracranial hemorrhage was detected in 0.75% of cases. The median time for hemorrhage was 3 days after surgery. The focal neurological signs usually reflect dysfunction of the hemisphere ipsilateral to the endarterectomy. These changes probably resolve during the first several days after surgery. This complication should be anticipated when carotid endarterectomy is performed on a patient with a very severe stenosis. Careful management of arterial blood pressure is the best way to avoid hyperperfusion after surgery. The blood pressure changes also may be less if a regional anesthesia is used during the surgery.[89]

Cranial nerve palsies are a potential complication of carotid endarterectomy. (see Table 11–3.) In one recent series, 51 of 190 operations were complicated by dysfunction of at least one cranial nerve.[90] In another study of 200 patients having surgery, 25 patients had cranial nerve injuries.[91] All were transient, and recovery occurred during the next 5–8 months. The most commonly affected nerves were the hypoglossal, recurrent laryngeal, superior laryngeal, marginal mandibular, and great auricular. Ferguson et al[31] reported post-operative cranial nerve palsies in 8.6% of patients enrolled in a large multi-center clinical trial. The most commonly affected were the hypoglossal, facial, and vagus nerves. The palsies usually are secondary to traction or stretching. Less commonly, a hematoma can compress the nerve and, rarely, a nerve may be sectioned inadvertently. Cranial nerve injuries were most common among patients who had a long plaque in the carotid artery, patching of the artery, or a post-operative neck hematoma. Multiple cranial nerve palsies are most often found as a complication of neck hematomas.[90] Vagal nerve palsies are associated with the presence of long carotid plaques that need extensive dissection. Vocal cord paralysis leading to dysphonia and dysphagia can result from the vagal nerve trauma. The hypoglossal nerve palsy is particularly bothersome. Paralysis of one-half of the tongue is very disabling. Most cranial nerve palsies recover gradually during subsequent months.

The most common non-neurological complications of carotid endarterectomy are cardiac events (see Table 11–3). Although patients with coronary artery disease can have surgery, those with unstable angina pectoris or a recent myocardial infarction should have the carotid operation delayed. Approximately 8% of 1415 patients enrolled in a large trial had medical complications; 14 patients had myocardial infarctions, 101 had other cardiac complications, and 11 had respiratory problems.[92] Most medical complications resolved, but 5 patients died of cardiac events—either sudden death or myocardial infarction. Attention to heart disease is a critical part of the perioperative management of carotid endarterectomy. The staging of operations to treat patients with severe carotid artery and coronary artery disease has been uncertain. Patients having carotid endarterectomy before coronary artery bypass surgery have an increased risk of complications.[66] Conversely, ischemic stroke is a relatively common complication of coronary artery bypass surgery. A potential strategy is to do the two operations simultaneously in a combined operation. In this regard, the data are discouraging. A report from Cleveland, Ohio, noted that the complication rate was 4.2% among patients who had carotid endarterectomy first and 7.8% among patients who had cardiac procedures before or with the carotid operation.[93] A large non-randomized study found that the risk of stroke was 1.4% among patients having coronary artery bypass surgery without carotid endarterectomy and that 2 strokes occurred among 52 patients who had combined carotid and cardiac operations.[94] Coyle et al[95] reported that the 30-day mortality for patients having carotid endarterectomy followed by coronary artery bypass surgery was 6.6%. When the operations were done simultaneously, the 30-day mortality was 26.2%. They recommended delaying cardiac surgery after the carotid operation unless the patient had a very high risk for myocardial infarction. Hertzer et al[53] found that the risk of stroke was 4.3% and mortality was 5.3% when carotid endarterectomy was combined with cardiac revascularization. Plestis et al[96] reported on the results of a combined carotid endarterectomy and coronary bypass grafting operation performed on 213 patients. The in-hospital mortality was 5.6%; 11 patients had post-operative strokes, and 5 had myocardial infarctions. The risks of complications were highest among men, persons older than 62 years, and those with hypertension. Hines et al[97] concluded that prophylactic carotid endarterectomy would be helpful in preventing strokes among patients with severe stenoses who had coronary artery bypass grafting.

Potential Indications

Analyses of several clinical trials of carotid endarterectomy conclusively demonstrated the utility of the operation in preventing stroke, myocardial infarction, or death among patients with a recent TIA or

Table 11–5. **Potential Indications: Carotid Endarterectomy**

Symptomatic patients
- Stenosis >50%—increases with more severe narrowing
- Presence of ulceration increases indication
- Reasonable surgical risk
- Skilled surgeon available
- Overall risk of surgery <3%

Asymptomatic patients
- Stenosis >60%—increases with more severe narrowing
- Reasonable surgical risk
- Skilled surgeon available
- Overall risk of surgery <1.5%

stroke.[98–100] (See Table 11–5.) Although perioperative complications mean that major adverse experiences, including stroke, are more common within 30 days with surgery than with medical treatment, the long-term benefits of operation in reducing stroke are dramatic.[98] One can say with confidence that a patient who has carotid endarterectomy without any complications is greatly helped by surgery. Although carotid endarterectomy is helpful among patients with recent ischemic symptoms ipsilateral to a high-grade stenosis, its value is even greater when the patient has both recent and remote neurological symptoms. These patients had a TIA or ischemic stroke some time in the past and then are seen with a new event. This latter group of patients appears to have a particularly high risk for stroke.[101] Although the efficacy of carotid endarterectomy is most strongly influenced by the severity of arterial narrowing, an ulcerated stenotic plaque also is associated with a high risk for stroke, and carotid endarterectomy is particularly helpful.[102]

After several years of uncertainty about the utility of carotid endarterectomy, the results clinical trials in North America and Europe that prospectively tested the safety and efficacy of the operation now form the basis for the current guidelines about the role of operation in prevention of ischemic stroke (Table 11–6). Overall, the degree of

Table 11–6. **Results of Clinical Trials of Carotid Endarterectomy: Prevention of Ipsilateral Stroke in Treatment of Symptomatic Patients**

Trial	Degree of Stenosis	Surgical Treatment Events/Patients	(%)	Medical Treatment Events/Patients	(%)
NASCET					
	70%–99%				
	50%–69%	57/430	13.2	80/430	18.6
	<50%	89/678	13.1	110/690	15.9
ECST					
	70%–99%	5/455	11.1	27/323	8.4
	50%–69%	58/570	10.1	39/372	10.5
	30%–49%	38/389	9.8	18/259	6.9
	<30%	6/219	2.7	2/155	1.3
VA					
	>50%	4/92	4.3	7/101	6.9

NASCET = α North American Symptomatic Carotid Endarterectomy Trial
ECST = European Carotid Surgery Trial
VA = Veterans Administration Endarterectomy Trial

benefit from surgery was greater in the North American studies than in the European trials. Some of the differences can be attributed to methods used in grading the severity of arterial narrowing. In general, a lesion graded as having a 70% narrowing in Europe was calibrated as being approximately 55% in North America. In 1991, European investigators found that carotid endarterectomy was effective in lessening the risk of stroke among patients with a 70%–90% narrowing of the internal carotid artery.[103] They also found that surgery offered no advantage over medical treatment for patients with mild (<30% stenosis) disease. Simultaneously, the North American Symptomatic Carotid Endarterectomy Trial found that surgery markedly reduced the risk of stroke among persons with severe (>70%) narrowing.[104] (See Fig. 11–2.) Overall, the 2-year risk of ipsilateral stroke was reduced from 26% to 9%. The risk of disabling ipsilateral stroke was reduced from 13.1% to 2.5%. The degree of benefit was greatest among patients with very severe narrowing (>90%). Regardless of the qualifying event, patients seemed to do better with surgery. Patients with either hemispheric TIA or amaurosis fugax were helped.[105] The efficacy was greater among patients with TIA because the risk of stroke rises greatly. A study performed in Veterans Affairs Hospitals in the United States found that carotid endarterectomy was associated with an absolute risk reduction of 17.7% among men with a >70% stenosis and an absolute risk reduction of 11.7% among men with a >50% stenosis.[106] The European investigators reported that surgery was not helpful for patients with moderate narrowing.[107] The European Carotid Surgery Trial subsequently found that found the operation to be effective when the degree of narrowing is approximately the same as the 50% stenosis described in the North American study.[108] The results of the European study complement those in the second major report by the North American Symptomatic Carotid Endarterectomy Trial.[109] This study demonstrated that surgery reduced the risk of ipsilateral stroke over 5 years from 22.2% to 15.7% among patients with a stenosis of 50%–69%. Still, the efficacy was not seen across all groups of patients. Men and patients with recent stroke or hemispheric symptoms seemed to be helped by surgery, whereas no effect was seen in women. The net benefit from surgery was found despite a post-operative stroke or death rate that was 2.1% in this large international trial. A population study compared its long-term results to the North American study.[70] The authors reported that 97% of patients who had surgery because of recent neurological symptoms were free of ipsilateral stroke symptoms at 2 years and at 5 years; 93% of patients had not had an ipsilateral stroke. These data show that the effectiveness of carotid endarterectomy can persist outside the setting of a clinical trial.

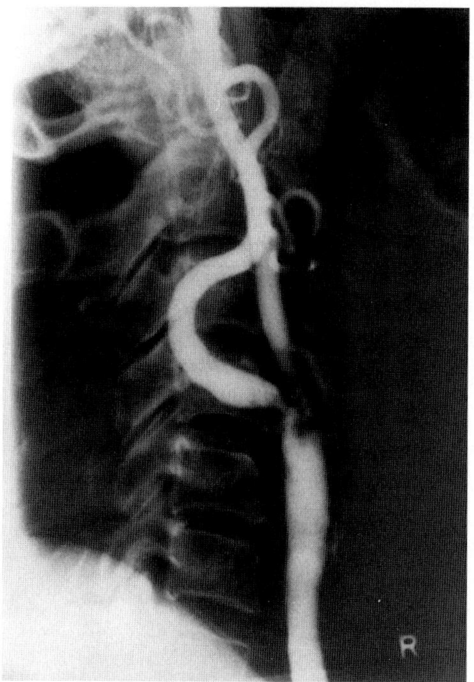

Figure 11–2. Severe stenosis of the origin of the internal carotid artery.

The CASANOVA Study compared the usefulness of medical or surgical treatment among 410 patients with asymptomatic 50%–90% stenosis.[110] (See Table 11–7.) Unfortunately, a large number of patients in the medical group subsequently had an operation and, as a result, the benefit of

Table 11–7. **Results of Clinical Trials of Carotid Endarterectomy: Prevention of Ipsilateral Stroke in Treatment of Asymptomatic Patients**

Trial	Degree of Stenosis	Surgical Treatment Events/Patients	(%)	Medical Treatment Events/Patients	(%)
CASANOVA	50%–90%	7/216	3.2	3/118	2.5
VA	>50%	10/211	4.7	22/233	9.4
ACAS*	>60%				
Actual		33/825	4.0	52/834	6.2
Projected		42	5.1	92	11.0

CASANOVA = Carotid Artery Stenosis with Asymptomatic Narrowing: Operation Versus Aspire
VA = Veterans Administration
ACAS = Asymptomatic Carotid Atherosclerosis Study
*Ipsilateral stroke, perioperative stroke, or death.

surgery in stroke prevention could not be established. A Veterans Affairs cooperative study found a modest effect in prevention of stroke or TIA with surgical treatment of an asymptomatic severe stenosis.[111] A trial performed at the Mayo Clinic involved a comparison of aspirin or carotid endarterectomy among patients with asymptomatic narrowing.[112] The surgically treated patients did not receive aspirin. The trial was halted prematurely because of the high rate of cardiac events in the surgical group—a phenomenon likely due to the absence of antiplatelet aggregating treatment. Libman et al[113] found a 4.7% perioperative risk of complications following carotid endarterectomy for treatment of asymptomatic stenoses. They found no net benefit in reduction of stroke by 5 years when compared to medical therapy. The Asymptomatic Carotid Atherosclerosis Study has provided the most definitive data to date about the usefulness of carotid endarterectomy in preventing ipsilateral stroke among patients with an asymptomatic carotid stenosis.[35] This large trial found that surgery reduced the 5-year risk of stroke from approximately 10% to approximately 5%. The benefit was confined to male patients. One of the reasons for the success of the operation in this trial was the very low rate of surgical morbidity. It is hoped that an ongoing European trial will help clarify the role of carotid endarterectomy in management of patients with severe, asymptomatic stenosis of the internal carotid artery.[114]

An asymptomatic bruit can be detected in approximately 20% of patients with peripheral vascular disease and 10% of patients with severe coronary artery disease.[115] The prevalence of asymptomatic stenoses is approximately the same. Hart and Easton[115] noted that neither an asymptomatic bruit nor stenosis was associated with a perioperative stroke. The presence of an asymptomatic bruit in a patient scheduled for elective, non-cardiac surgery does not carry a high associated risk for perioperative stroke. These patients do not need an evaluation or carotid endarterectomy before the elective operation.[116]

McCormick et al[117] reported that carotid endarterectomy could reopen an *occluded internal carotid artery*. In their series of 42 patients, 24 arteries were reopened and, on follow up, only 1 of the 17 had reoccluded. Morgenstern et al[118] found that carotid endarterectomy can be done relatively safely for treatment of patients with near occlusion of the internal carotid artery. They noted 3 perioperative strokes among 48 patients having the surgery. In comparison, 11.1% of 58 medically treated patients had a stroke within 1 year. The operation has been used to treat progressive narrowing of the internal carotid artery following angioplasty and stent placement.[119]

Surgery also can be performed to prevent recurrent amaurosis fugax or ischemic optic neuropathy. In addition, patients with severe disease of the internal carotid artery who are developing progressive visual loss secondary to poor perfusion might be helped by carotid endarterectomy. The operation can improve both retrobulbar and ophthalmic artery flow. Costa et al[120] found improved flow velocities in the central retinal, ophthalmic, and short posterior ciliary arteries in patients who had the operation. Thus, preserving ocular function is a potential indications for carotid endarterectomy.

Lunn et al[121] reviewed the potential impact of carotid endarterectomy on cognitive functioning. The rationale for the operation is that revascularization will improve blood flow and lessen the evolution of a chronic ischemic process that is leading to a vascular dementia. The operation likely will not sway the course of vascular dementia. To date, surgery has not been established as effective for improving cognition among patients with severe extracranial vascular disease.[122]

Carotid endarterectomy also can be done to treat radiation-associated atherosclerosis. In one series, 20 patients with scarring and radiation-induced fibrosis underwent the operation; no deaths or strokes were noted.[123] Carotid endarterectomy has little or no value in treatment of patients with vertebrobasilar ischemia.[124] No studies have demonstrated that carotid endarterectomy will prevent stroke in persons with vertebrobasilar TIA. This finding is not surprising because the source for emboli in the posterior circulation is not likely to be treated with a carotid operation. The likelihood of improving flow in the vertebrobasilar circulation via the posterior communicating artery ipsilateral to an operated carotid artery also is low.

Summary

The role of carotid endarterectomy in management of patients with severe but asymptomatic disease of the internal carotid artery is controversial.[125–130] (See Fig. 11–2.) Clinical studies have demonstrated that the risk of stroke ipsilateral to an asymptomatic carotid stenosis is much lower than the likelihood of stroke with a recently symptomatic lesion.[131] Thus, the overall benefit from a surgical procedure will be less. Yin and Carpenter[132] outlined criteria for carotid endarterectomy to be cost-effective for management of patients with asymptomatic bruits. Its prevalence should be 4.5%, screening tests should be specific in 91% of cases, the risk of stroke in medically treated patients should be at least 3.3%, and the operation should lower the risk of stroke by 37% with a relatively low operative morbidity. Another study found carotid endarterectomy to be cost-effective for treatment of asymptomatic patients with stenosis >60% if the operation was not offered to the very elderly or those who have a high operative risk.[133] In addition, the chances of operative complications need to be very low for the presence of a net benefit from the operation. A recent study showed the perioperative surgical mortality and morbidity among asymptomatic patients was 1.5%.[134] The risk of stroke or death following arteriography (1.2%) was approximately the same as the operation.

Benavente et al[226] concluded that the benefit from surgery was small and that the surgery should not be recommended for most patients. They advised medical management instead. Perry et al[227] and Hill[228] believed that the data about the usefulness of the operation are insufficiently strong to recommend either screening for carotid stenosis or surgical treatment of a severe lesion. Conversely, based on data from recent clinical trials, Brott and Toole[229] emphasized that carotid endarterectomy was associated with a 5.9% absolute reduction in the risk of stroke within 5 years. They deduced that surgery could be recommended to prevent stroke among asymptomatic patients with severe stenosis of the internal carotid artery. Castaldo[230] stated that endarterectomy was appropriate for carefully selected patients with an asymptomatic stenosis if the surgical morbidity was kept very low. Lee et al[231] decided that surgery offered a modest but real benefit in prevention of stroke but at a substantial economic cost. They recommended development of a way to identify patients with asymptomatic stenosis who were at the highest risk for stroke. Surgery would be restricted to those patients. Another analysis found that surgery could be recommended only if the morbidity and mortality from arteriography and surgery were kept to a minimum.[232] Recent guidelines published in the United States recommend carotid endarterectomy for patients in good condition who have a severe asymptomatic narrowing if a skilled surgeon is available.[100]

Carotid endarterectomy is an important option for the management of advanced atherosclerotic disease of the extracranial internal carotid artery. The operation lowers the risk of ipsilateral ischemic stroke, including disabling stroke, among persons with or without recent neurological symptoms. Because the risk of stroke is high among patients with TIA or minor stroke, the net benefit from carotid endarterectomy is especially high in this group. As a result, there is a consensus about the utility of the operation.

In general, the decision to recommend carotid endarterectomy is based on (*1*) the patient's neurological status, (*2*) the severity of the local arterial pathology, (*3*) the presence of other medical conditions, and (*4*) the availability of a skilled surgeon (see Table 11–5). For carotid endarterectomy to be effective in treatment, it must be done with an extremely low rate of operative complications. Regardless of the presence or absence of ischemic symptoms, the recommendation for carotid endarterectomy should be made on a case-by-case basis using the appraisal of the potential risks and benefits of the operation.

EXTRACRANIAL-INTRACRANIAL ARTERIAL ANASTOMOSIS

Rationale

Because carotid endarterectomy was found not to be effective in reopening an occluded internal carotid artery, other surgical procedures were developed in an effort to improve blood flow to the ipsilateral cerebral hemisphere. The usual scenario was discovery of an internal carotid artery occlusion during the evaluation of a TIA or a minor stroke. In addition to performing the operation on patients with occlusions of the internal carotid artery, bypass procedures also were used to treat patients with occlusions of the middle cerebral artery or stenosis of the distal internal carotid artery or the proximal portion of the middle cerebral artery. As well as the superficial temporal artery–middle cerebral artery anastomosis, other bypass operations are done to provide collateral flow around an occluded artery. Patients with severe disease in the posterior circulation also have been treated with bypass procedures.[135]

Procedure

The most commonly performed operation was the creation of an anastomosis between a branch of the superificial temporal artery and a branch of the middle cerebral artery.[233,234,235] The operation involves the dissection of a branch of the middle cerebral artery from the scalp. The surgeon then transposes the artery through a craniectomy defect and an incision of the dura. The artery is attached to a distal branch of the middle cerebral artery on the lateral surface of the hemisphere using microsurgical techniques. Long saphenous vein bypass grafts to the anterior or the posterior circulation have been performed in patients with a reasonable degree of long-term patency.[136] Laser-assisted, high-flow extracranial–intracranial bypass procedures also are available.[137] Venous and arterial bypass operations for occlusions of the common carotid artery involve a transposition of vessels around the carotid lesion in combination with new collaterals directed to the surface of the hemisphere.[138] The primary purpose for the bypass operations is to improve blood flow to the brain. Unlike carotid endarterectomy, these operations do not eliminate a source for embolization. Ancillary diagnostic studies, including those that measure cerebral blood flow, have demonstrated improvements in the circulation following surgery. The hemodynamic status among patients with occlusive cerebrovascular disease is improved by bypass operations.[139]

Safety

Because of the small caliber of the arteries and relatively low flow in the anastomosis, the bypasses are at high risk for thrombosis. The long-term patency of the extracranial–intracranial bypass operations appears to be relatively poor because of the high propensity for occlusion. Some patients may not derive a long-term benefit from the operation in maintaining blood flow.[140] Because the operation involves a craniotomy and a surgical procedure on the blood vessels on the surface of the brain, the potential for neurological complications is high. For this reason, bypass operations usually are not done on a cerebral hemisphere recently affected by a new infarction. A sudden increase of blood flow in the brain following surgery can lead to an intracranial hemorrhage. Seizures or infections are possible complications. Ischemic stroke is the most frequent adverse experience, especially in patients with a stenosis of the internal carotid artery or the middle cerebral artery.[236] The sudden change and reversal in blood flow may promote stasis. As a result, thrombosis of the proximal portion of the artery may lead to subcortical infarction even though the cortical vessels are patent due to the bypass. Schmiedek et al[141] reported that the mortality and morbidity of bypass operations was as high as 14%. The rates of complications of bypass procedures for patients with posterior circulation atherosclerosis have been high.[142] The very high risk of patients with posterior circulation disease might explain the high rate of poor outcomes. Most of the patients who have been referred for surgery are unstable neurologically and are at a very high risk for stroke whether or not they have surgical treatment.

Potential Indications

A large international study tested the value of extracranial–intracranial bypass procedures to treat patients who were at high risk for stroke.[143] (see Table 11–8.) The trial enrolled 714 patients who were treated medically and 663 patients who had the operation. The 30-day post-operative mortality was 0.6%, and 2.5% of surgically treated patients had a stroke within 1 month. Despite a 96% rate of patency of the bypass procedures, the operation did not reduce the long-term risks of stroke. As a result, the operation was largely abandoned. The trial was severely attacked, and one of the leading criticisms was that the "right" patients were not enrolled in the study.[237] As a result, efforts have focused on patients with occlusions of the internal carotid artery who might be candidates for

Table 11–8. **Mortality and Stroke Rates: International Trial of Extracranial–Intracranial Arterial Anastomosis**

	SURGICAL TREATMENT (N = 663)		MEDICAL TREATMENT (N = 714)	
	n	**%**	**n**	**%**
Death	113	17%	143	20%
Stroke				
ICA occlusion/No symptoms	57/245	23.2%	72/276	26.1%
ICA occlusion/Symptoms	64/140	45.7%	51/147	34.7%
ICA stenosis	29/77	37.7%	26/72	36.1%
MCA stenosis	22/50	44%	14/59	23.7%

ICA = internal carotid artery; MCA = middle cerebral artery.

surgery. Impaired perfusion or abnormal cerebral hemodynamics might identify patients who could respond to a bypass operation.[141,144,145,238] A recent study looked at the prognosis of patients with internal carotid artery occlusions and prior neurological symptoms.[146] They noted that patients who had relatively preserved cerebral blood flow had a relatively low risk for stroke. In contrast, patients with impaired blood flow had a high risk for recurrent ischemic stroke, approximately 10% per year. These results suggest that some patients with occlusions of the internal carotid artery might benefit from an extracranial–intracranial bypass operation. These data could prompt the consideration of another trial to test bypass operations in the subgroup of patients with impaired cerebral blood flow.

Bypass operations have been performed to lessen the severity of ischemic oculopathy distal to an occlusion of the internal carotid artery.[147] Bypass operations have been performed to maintain blood flow to the hemisphere following symptomatic traumatic dissection of the internal carotid artery or the vertebral artery.[148–150]

A variety of bypass procedures have been attempted to improve blood flow among patients with moyamoya disease and moyamoya syndrome.[151–153] (See Table 11–1.) Although no controlled trials have tested the usefulness of these revascularization operations, the anecdotal data suggest that surgery can lessen the risk of ischemic stroke. Among the operations are *encephaloduroarteriomyosynagiosis, encephalomyosynagiosis,* and *duroateriosynagniosis.*[152,154,155] All of these operations involve a craniotomy and the placement of tissue on the surface of the ipsilateral hemisphere through a dural incision. The assumption is that factors are released by the operation that stimulate angiogenesis and new collateral formation through the pial vessels.

Summary

The status of the various extracranial–intracranial arterial bypass procedures is not clear. The results of the large international trial found that the operation was not superior to medical therapy in preventing stroke. Although external critics subjected the trial to considerable fire, its results are valid. Still, the concept of creating a new collateral channel to improve blood flow to the brain has appeal. The operation might be advantageous in preventing stroke among a subgroup of patients with occlusions of the internal carotid artery or the middle cerebral artery. The use of cerebral blood flow and metabolism studies could improve selection of patients with occlusions who could be treated surgically. With the advances in endovascular treatment, the bypass operations likely will not be used for treatment of most patients with stenosis of the internal carotid, middle cerebral, or basilar arteries. Revascularization procedures still will be employed to treat patients with severe occlusive intracranial vascular diseases, such as those with moyamoya disease or syndrome.

OTHER SURGICAL PROCEDURES

Vascular operations are performed to treat patients with atherosclerotic cerebrovascular disease in the subclavian, common carotid, external carotid, or vertebral arteries (see Table 11–1). They might be done in conjunction with other revascularization procedures aimed at the internal carotid artery. Because these procedures are done in a small number of patients and for rather specific indications, information is limited about their safety and efficacy.

Embolization is a potential complication of a *stump syndrome.*[156,157] In this situation, the internal carotid artery is occluded distally to the carotid bifurcation (Fig. 11–3). The residual proximal pouch of the internal carotid artery serves as a blind alley in which thrombi can develop. Pieces of the clot can embolize and could reach the brain via collateral branches. Surgical plication of the stump could be used to prevent stroke in this relatively uncommon situation. The operation can be done with a reasonable degree of safety. The value of the operation has not been established but its indications probably are few.

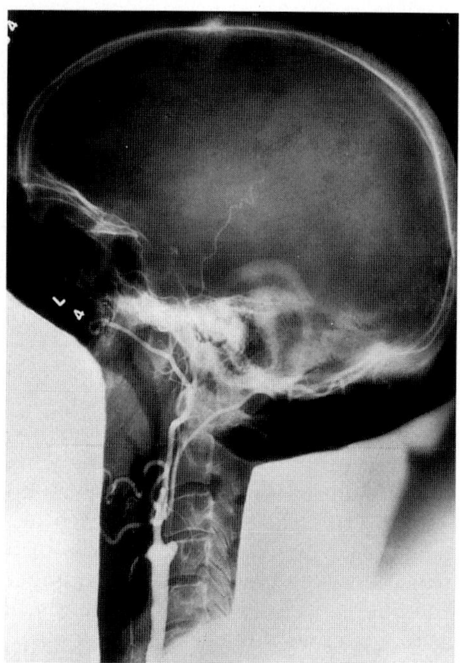

Figure 11–3. Lateral view of left carotid arteriogram demonstrates an occlusion of the internal carotid artery with a stump. The external carotid artery and its branches can be seen distal to the bifurcation.

Severe atherosclerotic disease can lead to the development of kinks or loops of the internal carotid artery. The significance of these findings is unclear and, generally, patients are treated medically. Still, a marked kink of the internal carotid artery might reduce cerebral blood flow. Surgical resection of a segment of the artery that includes the kink can be done to restore normal flow.[158] The necessity for and success of this procedure are unclear. Most affected people probably do not need this operation.

Endarterectomy of the origin of the *external carotid artery* also can be performed alone or in conjunction with surgical treatment of the internal carotid artery.[159] The potential indication would be recurrent neurological symptoms in a patient with an occluded internal carotid artery and who has prominent collateral flow from the external carotid artery. A stenotic lesion could serve as the source of emboli in the same manner as a plaque of the internal carotid artery.

Endarterectomy of the middle cerebral artery also has been performed. Clinical experience with this microsurgical procedure is limited. In the future, stenotic lesions of the middle cerebral artery likely will be treated with endovascular techniques rather than an operation. Endarterectomy of the origin of the vertebral artery also is a possibility.

Surgical resection of the involved segment or ligation of the artery can be performed for treatment of patients with *dissecting aneurysms of the internal carotid artery.* Among 22 patients treated surgically, Schievink et al[150] reported that 2 had postoperative strokes. The benefit from surgical treatment is not known. Because the long-term prognosis of patients with arterial dissections usually is benign, most patients likely will not need surgical treatment.

Graduated dilation of the internal carotid artery has been used to treat patients with *fibromuscular dysplasia.*[160] Surgical resection of a section of the internal carotid or vertebral artery also has been used to treat persons affected by this arteriopathy. Still, the prognosis of patients with fibromuscular dysplasia appears to be more benign than that of atherosclerosis. As a result, the need for surgical treatment remains unclear.

Atherosclerotic disease of the subclavian or innominate artery also can lead to stenosis or occlusion of these vessels. In general, the prognosis is good for patients with subclavian or innominate atherosclerosis causing *subclavian steal syndrome.*[161] The efficacy of surgical repair is not established. Revascularization procedures can be performed on the cervical segment of the vertebral artery.[162] A carotid–subclavian artery bypass also can be performed to treat brachiocephalic occlusive disease. The transposition of the vessels has a better long-term patency than either synthetic or vein grafts.[163] Cervical arteries have been used to bypass occlusions of the common carotid artery, which in turn could serve as the source for an extracranial–intracranial bypass operation.[164] The indications for these operations have not been established.

Advanced *atherosclerotic disease of the aorta* can be the source for embolism. Patients with large, mobile plaques of the ascending aorta or the arch of the aorta can serve as the nidus for thromboembolism or embolism of atherosclerotic debris. Surgical treatment of the aorta may lessen the risk of embolization. Bojar et al[165] performed replacement of the aortic section to remove a highly atherosclerotic lesion. Localized debridement and surgical correction also could be done. In contrast, King et al[166] found that replacement of an atherosclerotic ascending aorta is a high-risk procedure. They reported that 4 of 17 treated patients died following the procedure; 3 patients had strokes, and 9 patients had other types of operative morbidity. The high morbidity of aortic operations means that their use will be limited for the prevention of stroke.

CARDIAC OPERATIONS

Some cardiac operations are performed with the primary goal of preventing embolism (see Table 11–1). Among these are replacement of a severely deformed or stenotic valve. Surgical resection is the usual treatment of a left atrial myxoma that is recognized as a very high-risk source for embolism. In this situation, emboli consist of pieces of the tumor rather than thrombus. Patients with atrial fibrillation can be treated with anti-arrhythmic medications, cardioversion, interruption of the bundle of His, a pacemaker, or an external atrial defibrillator.[167]

Patients with large intra-cardiac shunts via a patent foramen ovale might have a high risk for embolism.[168] Cujec et al[169] and Homma et al[170] concluded that surgical closure of a patent foramen ovale might be superior to either anticoagulants or antiplatelet aggregating agents for preventing recurrent ischemic stroke. Giroud et al[171] successfully treated 8 patients with a large patent foramen ovale with surgical closure of the hole. The operations were performed safely, and the patients did not need anticoagulation post-operatively. Guffi et al[172] reported similar results among 11 patients. Other surgical procedures include transcatheter closure of the fistula.[173] Conversely, Nendaz et al[174] could not find any advantage of a surgical procedure over anticoagulant therapy. In addition, they found that patients who did not receive any specific treatment did as well as patients who received antiplatelet aggregating agents, anticoagulants, or a surgical procedure to close the patent foramen ovale.

ANGIOPLASTY AND STENTING

Rationale

Angioplasty and stenting are commonly used to treat severely stenotic atherosclerotic disease of coronary arteries and other vessels in the body. These procedures now are being used to treat patients at high risk for ischemic stroke. Still, the roles of angioplasty and stenting have not been determined in the management of patients with intracranial or extracranial arterial disease.

Procedure

Angioplasty involves the placement of a microcatheter into the lumen of a stenotic segment of the artery. Once the catheter is in the correct location, a small balloon is inflated to dilate the stenotic section. The goal is to enlarge the residual lumen close to a degree that is normal. To maintain the larger, normal vascular lumen, angioplasty now is complemented by placement of a stent. A stent usually consists of a fine mesh that lies on the endothelial surface of the segment. Its purpose is to give support to the arterial wall so that recurrent stenosis or acute occlusion can be avoided. Angioplasty leads to a compression of connective tissue, stretching of the internal elastic lamina, and compression or stretching on intramural smooth muscle.[175] The angioplasty also can lead to a fracture of the plaque, which could be the source of thrombotic or atherosclerotic emboli. To trap the debris and prevent embolization to the brain, a second, distal balloon can be inflated distal to the stenotic site. At the conclusion of the angioplasty, both the

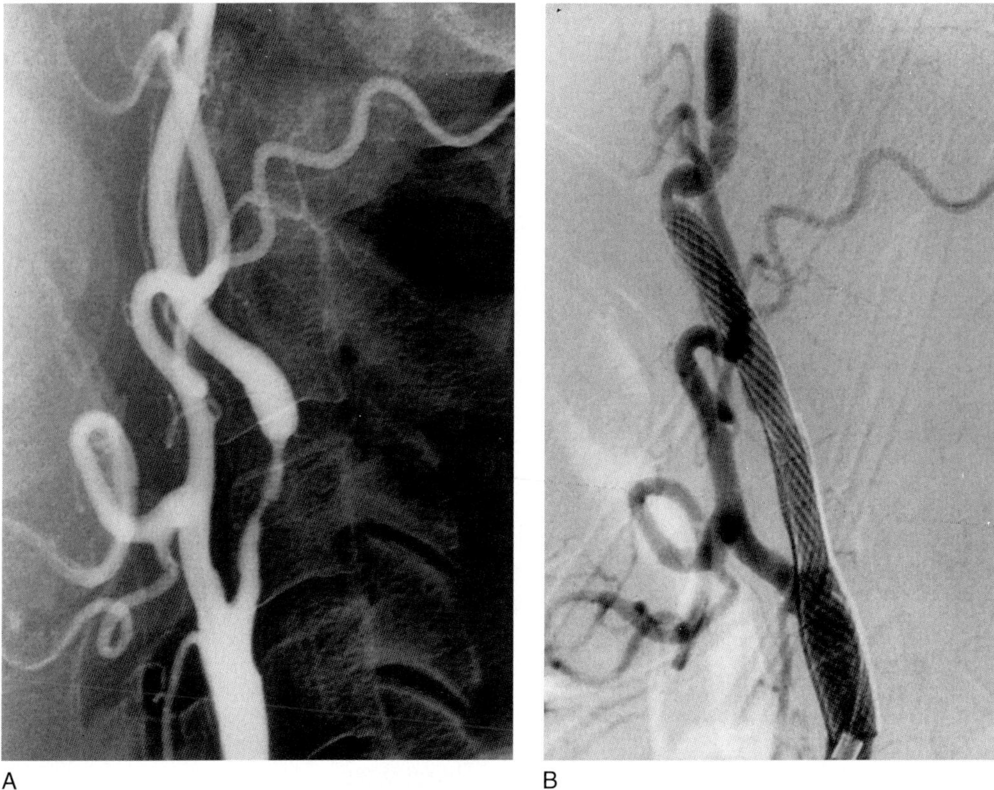

Figure 11–4. (A) A lateral view of a left carotid arteriogram. There is severe stenosis of the left internal carotid artery. (B) A second left carotid arteriogram using subtraction techniques from the same patient. Angioplasty and stenting have resulted in restoration of the normal lumen of the internal carotid artery.

catheter and balloons can be removed while the stent remains (Fig. 11–4).

Markus et al[176] noted that angioplasty of the internal carotid artery is associated with improvement of hemodynamics of blood flow to the ipsilateral hemisphere. The recovery of impaired hemodynamics is similar to that achieved with carotid endarterectomy. Transcranial Doppler ultrasonography has demonstrated a marked increase in flow velocities after angioplasty.[177] Still, McCleary et al[178] concluded that angioplasty and stenting did not have an advantage over carotid endarterectomy in improving cerebral hemodynamics.

Angioplasty has several potential advantages, including the lack of need for general anesthesia or a neck incision.[179] The latter is a bonus because it lessens the likelihood of cervical hematomas and cranial nerve palsies. The procedure also means that the general complications of surgery, in particular cardiac events, are sidestepped. Patients also may prefer the angioplasty and stenting instead of carotid endarterectomy because the former is a non-surgical procedure.[179]

Safety

Beebe and Kritpracha[180] expressed concerns about the responses of ulcerated plaques to angioplasty and stenting. In addition, eccentrically shaped plaques, heavily calcified lesions, and areas of neointimal hyperplasia may not be treated well with angioplasty and stenting. Potential complications of angioplasty include dissection of the artery that causes occlusion of the artery. The tear in the arterial wall can induce formation of an intramural hematoma that compresses the lumen. Vasospasm also can follow angioplasty. A subarachnoid hemorrhage secondary to dissection can be a complication of angioplasty of an intracranial artery. Angioplasty of an intracranial artery also could lead to occlusion of a small penetrating branch vessel. The injury to the plaque or the endothelial surface can stimulate thrombosis. Embolization of atherosclerotic debris also can occur. Sudden arterial occlusion or injury may necessitate emergent surgery. Intra-arterial papaverine has been used to prevent occlusion following angioplasty treatment of basilar artery stenosis.[181] Slow inflation of an under-size balloon appears to improve safety of intracranial angioplasty; the 30-day rate of complications were rated as minor in 6.2% and major in 0.7% among 231 patients who had 271 procedures.[182]

The safety of angioplasty and stenting of the carotid artery has not been established.[183,239] Some authors[239] reported that endovascular treatment is more dangerous than carotid endarterectomy. In a series of 85 patients who had angioplasty for stenoses >70%, the most common adverse experiences were hypotension, bradycardia, asystole, or syncope.[184] Strokes occurred in 4 patients. The risk of stroke appears to be greater among older persons and those who have long segments of narrowing and multiple areas of stenosis.[185] Qureshi et al[240] noted thromboembolic events in 73 of 834 patients (8.8%) among patients who had carotid artery angioplasty and stenting. Jordan et al[186] did a retrospective comparison of angioplasty and stenting versus carotid endarterectomy for treatment of patients with carotid lesions. The carotid operations were performed under regional anesthesia, and only 1 of 109 patients had a stroke and none died. Conversely, 3 of 268 patients having angioplasty died, and 23 patients had stroke. The investigators concluded that the intravascular intervention was inferior to carotid endarterectomy. The same group also found that angioplasty and stenting were more expensive than surgery.[187] A small randomized trial compared carotid endarterectomy and angioplasty and stenting.[188] The study was stopped prematurely when strokes occurred in 5 of 7 patients treated with the endovascular procedure while no complications were reported among the 10 patients having surgery. Conversely, Becquemin et al[189] concluded that carotid artery angioplasty could be performed safely. Querishi et al[241,242] concluded that improved periprocedural treatment, such as using direct thrombin inhibitors or platelet glycoprotein IIb/IIIa receptor blockers, might improve the safety of endovascular procedures.

Recurrent arterial stenosis can follow angioplasty. The placement of the stent is aimed at forestalling this long-term complication. One study reported recurrent stenosis in 6 of 85 patients undergoing angioplasty for treatment severe atherosclerosis.[184] Recurrent stenosis after angioplasty and stenting can be treated with carotid endarterectomy.[119] Robbin et al[190] used carotid artery ultrasound to monitor the integrity of the arteries treated with angioplasty and found a very low rate of recurrent stenosis.

Angioplasty with marked dilation of the vascular stenosis may lead to severe hyperperfusion after the procedure.[177] The symptoms of hyperperfusion after angioplasty and stenting include headache, confusion, vomiting, and seizures.

Potential Indications

The role of angioplasty and stenting of intracranial or extracranial arteries is rapidly evolving (Table 11–9). The procedures are used in treatment of patients with severe stenosis of the internal carotid artery in the neck or in the siphon. Yadav et al[191] treated 22 patients with recurrent stenosis following carotid endarterectomy, and they achieved a reduction in the narrowing in almost all patients. Only one patient had a minor stroke, but recurrent stenosis was found subsequently in approximately 50% of cases. In a second report, Yadav et al[192] reported the results of 126 procedures performed in 107 patients with severe disease, prior carotid operations, or severe medical co-morbid diseases. Patients generally did well, and the arteries were dilated successfully. Seven patients had a

Table 11–9. **Potential Indications for Endovascular Treatment (Angioplasty and Stenting) in Cerebrovascular Disease**

Stenosis of the internal carotid artery
- Not a good candidate for carotid endarterectomy
- Recurrent stenosis after carotid endarterectomy
- Distal extracranial artery or intracranial artery lesion
- Radiation-induced arterial narrowing

Stenosis of the distal vertebral artery
Stenosis of the basilar artery
Stenosis of the proximal segment of the middle cerebral artery

minor stroke, 2 had major strokes, and 1 patient died. The researchers noted a low rate of recurrent stenosis. Another study of 108 patients undergoing 114 procedures found success from angioplasty and stenting in 108 instances.[193] Only 2 patients had major strokes after the procedure. Lanzino et al[194] did endovascular procedures in 21 patients with recurrent stenosis following carotid endarterectomy. No major complications were noted, and the patients had successful dilation of the arterial narrowing. Another series of 259 patients with atherosclerotic disease of the carotid artery had angioplasty and stent placement. Most patients did well, and only 3 patients had embolic events and 2 patients had dissections as complications.[195] Al-Mubarak et al[196] performed carotid stenting in 44 patients with a high risk for neurological complications. The complication rate of stroke or death was 4.5%. No delayed neurological events or need for additional treatment was noted during long-term follow up. An international survey of 2048 cases treated with angioplasty and stenting found technical success in 98.6% of the procedures.[197] Within 30 days, minor or major strokes were reported in 3.08% and 1.32% of treated patients, respectively. The 30-day mortality was 1.37% and, by 6 months, restenosis was found in 4.8% of patients.

Angioplasty also has been used to treat stenotic lesions of the cervical portions of the vertebral arteries.[162] Angioplasty of a stenotic segment of a tandem lesion of the common carotid artery, distal internal carotid artery, or brachiocephalic artery can be done in conjunction with carotid endarterectomy.[198,199] Coronary and carotid artery angioplasty can be done in conjunction.[200]

Angioplasty has been used to treat severe atherosclerotic lesions of the middle cerebral artery or the basilar artery.[201–203] Mori et al[204] treated 27 intracranial stenoses with angioplasty. Complications occurred in 3 patients, and recurrent stenosis was discovered at 3 months in approximately 30% of cases. They concluded that the best lesions to treat with an endovascular intervention are readily accessible and less than 5 mm. long. Concentric lesions with a smooth contour and little or no calcification also could be treated. The presence of a near total occlusion or clot lessened the likelihood of success with angioplasty. Another study reported the results of angioplasty for treatment of 12 patients with severe atherosclerotic disease of the distal vertebral or the basilar arteries.[205] Four patients had complications, 2 had dissections of the artery, and 2 others had thromboembolic events. Callahan et al[206] treated 15 patients with intracranial atherosclerosis who did not respond to treatment with anticoagulants. Balloon angioplasty was successful in the 15 cases, but 2 patients had complications. One patient had a stroke, and another patient had rupture of the vessel. Nakatuska et al[207] concluded that submaximal angioplasty in the basilar artery may be associated with a lower risk of arterial rupture. The angioplasty would permit increase in flow even if some narrowing were still present. Angioplasty has been used in combination with thrombolytic treatment for management of acute occlusion of intracranial vertebrobasilar arteries.[208]

Kellogg et al[202] recommended angioplasty for treatment of fibromuscular dysplasia of the carotid artery. Although dissection is a potential complication of angioplasty, the procedure also has been used to treat arterial dissections leading to a severe stenosis.[209] Hurst et al[210] showed that a stent can be used to treat extracranial aneurysms of the internal carotid artery while maintaining the patency of the parent vessel. Angioplasty has not been successful in reopening arteries narrowed to cerebral vasculitis.[201] Inversely, patients with a severe stenosis secondary to an arterial dissection can be treated successfully with stenting.[211]

Angioplasty and stenting may the preferred therapy for lesions that cannot be readily treated with surgical procedures.[179,212,213] Endovascular treatment may also be indicated for treatment of recurrent stenosis following carotid endarterectomy or non-atherosclerotic lesions leading to stenosis. Stenosis following radiation therapy also may be best treated with an endovascular approach.[179,214] Patients at high surgical risk, including those with severe heart or lung disease, also may benefit from an endovascular treatment.[179]

Summary

The role of angioplasty and stenting is not established.[215] Clinical trials are needed to define the role of angioplasty and stenting in treatment of both intracranial and extracranial vascular disease.[216] The procedure holds great promise for treatment of patients who have not been able to be treated with other local interventions. Angioplasty and stenting may be the best choice for treatment of patients with stenosis of the distal internal carotid artery, proximal middle cerebral artery, the distal vertebral artery, or the basilar artery. Angioplasty and stenting also may become an important option for treatment of patients with diseases of the cervical portions of the carotid or vertebral arteries. To date, endovascular techniques to treat patients with severe intracranial or extracranial disease should be considered to be experimental.

SUMMARY AND ALGORITHM FOR SURGICAL MANAGEMENT

Summary

Carotid endarterectomy should be recommended if the operative morbidity and mortality are minimal. The medical community must ensure that patients forego the procedure if they should not have carotid endarterectomy and those who would benefit from surgery actually do have the operation.[8] A practice guideline recommended that the upper limits be <7% for persons whose most recent symptom was stroke, <5% for patients with TIA, and <3% for asymptomatic patients.[217,218] Another guideline has concluded that surgery is recommended for patients with severe symptomatic stenosis if the patient is stable medically, if the distal ipsilateral carotid artery does not have a more severe narrowing, and if the surgeon's rate of complications is less than 6%.[219] The same group recommended that surgery not be done if the patient has an asymptomatic narrowing <60%.[219]

Algorithm

A patient with a symptomatic or asymptomatic severe stenosis of the internal carotid artery should be considered for surgical treatment (Fig. 10–6). In general, the degree of narrowing should exceed 50%, but the indication for surgery grows with increases in the severity of the stenosis. The presence of ulceration also strengthens the recommendation for carotid endarterectomy. Surgery should be considered only if the patient is judged to have a reasonable operative risk and if a skilled surgeon is available. Carotid artery surgery is not recommended to treat patients with symptoms in the posterior circulation. The indications for extracranial–intracranial vascular anastomoses are limited. Interventional techniques may take a leading role in treatment of stenotic disease of the intracranial or extracranial arteries in either the carotid or the vertebrobasilar circulation. Although angioplasty and stenting show great promise, both safety and efficacy have not been established. The surgical interventions should be supplemented with antiplatelet aggregating agents.

SUMMARY

Carotid endarterectomy in the hands of skilled surgeons at good centers is highly effective in symptomatic patients with a corresponding carotid stenoses of 70%–99%. A modest benefit accrues to some symptomatic patients with stenoses of 50%–69% and none at all to symptomatic patients with stenoses of less than 50%. The benefits of carotid endarterectomy in asymptomatic patients with stenoses of 60% or more are limited.

These results were obtained in high-quality, closely supervised clinical trials guided by strict measures of stenoses. In the larger world, the complication rates from the procedure are higher, the indications looser, and the interpretations of stenoses wider. Extrapolations from ultrasonography, magnetic resonance angiography, and casual measurement of angiographic stenoses result in systematic overeading.

Extracranial–intracranial anastomoses enjoyed a cornucopia of positive reports from clinical series. However, a single controlled, multi-center trial rendered a resounding "no" to the procedure. Now, new techniques have evolved, better methods of assessing brain perfusion have emerged, and once again the rationale for a controlled trial in selected patients exists.

A number of reconstructive procedures around the aortic arch and its vessels have been performed and advocated. Middle cerebral artery endarterectomy, surgery on arterial dissections, and correction of arterial kinks have been performed with inconclusive results.

Surgery on diseased cardiac valves and embolizing atrial myxoma have found their place in stroke prevention. Procedures on patients with patent foramen ovale have yet to prove their worth.

Angioplasty and stenting promise a less invasive alternative to carotid endarterectomy. However, the important comparative questions can be answered only by direct comparison in a randomized clinical trial.

Although surgical therapy remains one of the pillars in stroke prevention, its role needs to be re-examined continuously, not only in the face of increasingly effective medical therapies but also in regard to growing data and sophistication in identifying the individuals most likely to benefit from these interventions.

Any surgical interventions must be considered as an adjunct to measures to control risk factors for atherosclerosis and antithrombotic medications.

REFERENCES

1. Tu JV, Hannan EL, Anderson GM, et al. The fall and rise of carotid endarterectomy in the United States and Canada. *N Engl J Med* 1998;339: 1441–1447.
2. Gillum RF. Epidemiology of carotid endarterectomy and cerebral arteriography in the United States. *Stroke* 1995;26:1724–1728.
3. Pokras R, Dyken ML. Dramatic changes in the performance of endarterectomy for diseases of the extracranial arteries of the head. *Stroke* 1988; 19:1289–1290.
4. Holloway RGJ, Witter DMJ, Mushlin AI, Lawton KB, McDermott MP, Samsa GP. Carotid endarterectomy trends in the patterns and outcomes of care at academic medical centers, 1990 through 1995. *Arch Neurol* 1998;55: 25–32.
5. Huber TS, Wheeler KG, Cuddeback JK, Dame DA, Flynn TC, Seeger JM. Effect of the Asymptomatic Carotid Atherosclerosis Study on carotid endarterectomy in Florida. *Stroke* 1998; 29:1099–1105.
6. Oddone EZ, Horner RD, Sloane R, et al. Race, presenting signs and symptoms, use of carotid artery imaging, and appropriateness of carotid endarterectomy. *Stroke* 1999;30:1350–1356.
7. Oddone EZ, Horner RD, Diers T, et al. Understanding racial variation in the use of carotid endarterectomy: the role of aversion to surgery. *J Nat Med Assoc* 1998;90:25–33.
8. Chassin MR. Appropriate use of carotid endarterectomy. *N Engl J Med* 1998;339: 1468–1471.
9. Oliver SE, Thomson RG. Are variations in the use of carotid endarterectomy explained by population need? A study of health service utilisation in two English health regions. *Eur J Vasc Endovasc Surg* 1999;17:501–506.
10. Brittenden J, Murie JA, Jenkins AM, Ruckley CV, Bradbury AW. Carotid endarterectomy

before and after publication of randomized controlled trials. *Br J Surg* 1999;86:206–210.
11. Ferris G, Roderick P, Smithies A, et al. An epidemiological needs assessment of carotid endarterectomy in an English health region. Is the need being met? *BMJ* 1998;317:447–451.
12. D'Angelo V, Catapano G, Bozzini V, et al. Cerebrovascular reactivity before and after carotid endarterectomy. *Surg Neurol* 1999;51:321–326.
13. Loftus CM. Carotid endarterectomy: how the operation is done. *Clin Neurosurg* 1997;44: 243–265.
14. Shah DM, Darling RC, Chang BB, et al. Carotid endarterectomy by eversion technique: its safety and durability. *Ann Surg* 1998;228:471–478.
15. O'Hara PJ, Hertzer NR, Mascha EJ, et al. Carotid endarterectomy in octogenarians: early results and late outcome. *J Vasc Surg* 1998;27: 860–869.
16. Papavasiliou AK, Magnadottir HB, Gonda T, Franz D, Harbaugh RE. Clinical outcomes after carotid endarterectomy: comparison of the use of regional and general anesthetics. *J Neurosurg* 2000;92:291–296.
17. Tangkanakul C, Counsell CE, Warlow CP. Local versus general anaesthesia in carotid endarterectomy: a systematic review of the evidence. *Eur J Vasc Endovasc Surg* 1997;13:491–499.
18. Deriu GP, Milite D, Mellone G, Cognolato D, Frigatti P, Grego F. Clamping ischemia, threshold ischemia and delayed insertion of the shunt during carotid endarterectomy with patch. *J Cardiovasc Surg* 1999;40:249–255.
19. Levison JA, Faust GR, Halpern VJ, et al. Relationship of protamine dosing with postoperative complications of carotid endarterectomy. *Ann Vasc Surg* 1999;13:67–72.
20. Shi Q, Wu MH, Sauvage LR. Clinical and experimental demonstration of complete healing of porous Dacron patch grafts used for closure of the arteriotomy after carotid endarterectomy. *Ann Vasc Surg* 1999;13:313–317.
21. Yamamoto Y, Piepgras DG, Marsh WR, Meyer FB. Complications resulting from saphenous vein patch graft after carotid endarterectomy. *Neurosurgery* 1996;39:670–675.
22. AbuRahma AF, Robinson PA, Saiedy S, Richmond BK, Khan J. prospective randomized trial of bilateral carotid endarterectomies: primary closure versus patching. *Stroke* 1999;30: 1185–1189.
23. Anderson A, Padayachee TS, Sandison AJ, Modaresi KB, Taylor PR. The results of routine primary closure in carotid endarterectomy. *Cardiovasc Surg* 1999;7:50–55.
24. AbuRahma AF, Robinson PA, Stickler DL. Analysis of regression of postoperative carotid stenosis from prospective randomized trial of carotid endarterectomy comparing primary closure versus patching. *Ann Surgery* 1999;229: 767–772.
25. Bhattacharya V, Ghali R, El-Massry S, et al. A clinical comparison of Dacron patch closure of small-caliber carotids compared with primary closure of large-caliber carotids after endarterectomy. *Am Surg* 1999;65:378–382.
26. Ballotta E, Da Giau G, Saladini M, Abbruzzese E, Renon L, Toniato A. Carotid endarterectomy with patch closure versus carotid eversion endarterectomy and reimplantation: a prospective randomized study. *Surgery* 1999;125: 271–279.
27. Salvian AJ, Taylor DC, Hsiang YN, et al. Selective shunting with EEG monitoring is safer than routine shunting for carotid endarterectomy. *Cardiovasc Surg* 1997;5:481–485.
28. Samson RH, Showalter DP, Yunis JP. Routine carotid endarterectomy without a shunt, even in the presence of a contralateral occlusion. *Cardiovasc Surg* 1998;6:475–484.
29. Wain RA, Veith FJ, Berkowitz BA, et al. Angiographic criteria reliably predict when carotid endarterectomy can be safely performed without a shunt. *J Am Coll Surg* 1999;189: 93–100.
30. Stendel R, Hupp T, al Hassan AA, Brock M. The use of direct intra-operative Doppler ultrasonography in carotid thromboendarteriectomy. A prospective study. *Acta Neurochir* 1998;140: 925–931.
31. Ferguson GG, Eliasziw M, Barr HW, et al. The North American Symptomatic Carotid Endarterectomy Trial. Surgical results in 1415 patients. *Stroke* 1999;30:1751–1758.
32. Bain DJ, Fergie N, Quin RO, Greene M. Role of arteriography in the selection of patients for carotid endarterectomy. *Br J Surg* 1998;85: 768–770.
33. Rouleau PA, Huston J, Gilbertson J, et al. Carotid artery tandem lesions: frequency of angiographic detection and consequences for endarterectomy. *Am J Neuroradiol* 1999;20: 621–625.
34. Kappelle LJ, Eliasziw M, Fox AJ, Sharpe BL, Barnett HJM. Importance of intracranial atherosclerotic disease in patients with symptomatic stenosis of the internal carotid artery. The North American Symptomatic Carotid Endarterectomy Trial. *Stroke* 1999;30:282–286.
35. Executive Committee for the Asymptomatic Carotid Atherosclerosis Study. Endarterectomy for asymptomatic carotid artery stenosis. *JAMA* 1995;273:1421–1428.
36. Shifrin EG, Bornstein NM, Kantarovsky A, et al. Carotid endarterectomy without angiography. *Br J Surg* 1996;83:1107–1109.
37. Loftus IM, McCarthy MJ, Pau H, et al. Carotid endarterectomy without angiography does not compromise operative outcome. *Eur J Vasc Endovasc Surg* 1998;16:489–493.
38. Kuntz KM, Skillman JJ, Whittemore AD, Kent KC. Carotid endarterectomy in asymptomatic patients—is contrast angiography necessary? A morbidity analysis. *J Vasc Surg* 1995;22:706–714.
39. Lustgarten JH, Solomon RA, Quest DO, Khanjdi AG, Mohr JP. Carotid endarterectomy after noninvasive evaluation by duplex ultrasonography and magnetic resonance angiography. *Neurosurgery* 1994;34:612–618.
40. Polak JF, Kalina P, Donaldson MC, et al. Carotid endarterectomy: preoperative evaluation of candidates with combined Doppler sonography and

MR angiography. Work in progress. *Radiology* 1993;186:333–338.
41. Guzman RP. Appropriate imaging before carotid endarterectomy. *Can J Surg* 1998;41:218–223.
42. Hankey GJ, Warlow CP. Symptomatic carotid ischaemic events: safest and most cost effective way of selecting patients for angiography, before carotid endarterectomy. *BMJ* 1990;300:1485–1491.
43. Back MR, Harward TR, Huber TS, Carlton LM, Flynn TC, Seeger JM. Improving the cost-effectiveness of carotid endarterectomy. *J Vasc Surg* 1997;26:456–462.
44. Harbaugh KS, Pikus H.J., Shumaker GH, Perron AD, Harbaugh RE. Increasing the value of carotid endarterctomy. *J Neurovasc Dis* 1996;1:39–46.
45. Harbaugh KS, Harbaugh RE. Early discharge after carotid endarterectomy. *Neurosurgery* 1995;37:219–224.
46. Mukherjee D. Carotid endarterectomy: changing practice patterns. *J Cardiovasc Surg* 1998;39:703–707.
47. Rothwell PM, Warlow CP. Prediction of benefit from carotid endarterectomy in individual patients: a risk-modelling study. European Carotid Surgery Trialists' Collaborative Group. *Lancet* 1999;353:2105–2110.
48. McKinsey JF, Gewertz BL. Improving perioperative management of carotid endarterectomy. *Can J Surg* 1998;41:224–227.
49. Brott T, Thalinger K. The practice of carotid endarterectomy in a large metropolitan area. *Stroke* 1984;15:950–955.
50. Rothwell PM, Slattery J, Warlow CP. A systematic review of the risks of stroke and death due to endarterectomy for symptomatic carotid stenosis. *Stroke* 1996;27:260–265.
51. Goldstein LB, McCrory DC, Landsman PB, et al. Multicenter review of preoperative risk factors for carotid endarterectomy in patients with ipsilateral symptoms. *Stroke* 1994;25:1116–1121.
52. Wong JH, Findlay JM, Suarez-Almazor ME. Regional performance of carotid endarterectomy. Appropriateness, outcomes, and risk factors for complications. *Stroke* 1997;28:891–898.
53. Hertzer NR, O'Hara PJ, Mascha EJ, et al. Early outcome assessment for 2228 consecutive carotid endarterectomy procedures: the Cleveland Clinic experience from 1989 to 1995. *J Vasc Surg* 1997;26:1–10.
54. Stukenborg GJ. Comparison of carotid endarterectomy outcomes from randomized controlled trials and Medicare administrative databases. *Arch Neurol* 1997;54:826–832.
55. Karp HR, Flanders WD, Shipp CC, Taylor B, Martin D. Carotid endarterectomy among Medicare beneficiaries: a statewide evaluation of appropriateness and outcome. *Stroke* 1998;29:46–52.
56. Lanska DJ, Kryscio RJ. In-hospital mortality following carotid endarterectomy. *Neurology* 1998;51:440–447.
57. Wennberg DE, Lucas FL, Birkmeyer JD, Bredenberg CE, Fisher ES. Variation in carotid endarterectomy mortality in the Medicare population: trial hospitals, volume, and patient characteristics. *JAMA* 1998;279:1278–1281.
58. Maxwell JG, Rutledge R, Covington DL, Churchill MP, Clancy TV. A statewide, hospital-based analysis of frequency and outcomes in carotid endarterectomy. *Am J Surg* 1997;174:655–660.
59. Perler BA, Dardik A, Burleyson GP, Gordon TA, Williams GM. Influence of age and hospital volume on the results of carotid endarterectomy: a statewide analysis of 9918 cases. *J Vasc Surg* 1998;27:25–31.
60. Hamdan AD, Pomposelli FBJ, Gibbons GW, Campbell DR, LoGerfo FW. Perioperative strokes after 1001 consecutive carotid endarterectomy procedures without an electroencephalogram: incidence, mechanism, and recovery. *Arch Surg* 1999;134:412–415.
61. Gorelick PB. Carotid endarterectomy. Where do we draw the line? *Stroke* 1999;30:1745–1750.
62. Hannan EL, Popp AJ, Tranmer B, Fuestel P, Waldman J, Shah D. Relationship between provider volume and mortality for carotid endarterectomies in New York state. *Stroke* 1998;29:2292–2297.
63. Kucey DS, Bowyer B, Iron K, Austin P, Anderson G, Tu JV. Determinants of outcome after carotid endarterectomy. *J Vasc Surg* 1998;28:1051–1058.
64. Estes JM, Guadagnoli E, Wolf R, LoGerfo FW, Whittemore AD. The impact of cardiac comorbidity after carotid endarterectomy. *J Vasc Surg* 1998;28:577–584.
65. Rothwell PM, Slattery J, Warlow CP. Clinical and angiographic predictors of stroke and death from carotid endarterectomy: systematic review. *BMJ* 1997;315:1571–1577.
66. McCrory DC, Goldstein LB, Samsa GP, et al. Predicting complications of carotid endarterectomy. *Stroke* 1993;24:1285–1291.
67. Buchan A, Gates P, Pelz D, Barnett HJM. Intraluminal thrombus in the cerebral circulation. Implications for surgical management. *Stroke* 1988;19:681–687.
68. Gasecki AP, Eliasziw M, Ferguson GG, Hachinski V, Barnett HJM. Long-term prognosis and effect of endarterectomy in patients with symptomatic severe carotid stenosis and contralateral carotid stenosis or occlusion: results from NASCET. North American Symptomatic Carotid Endarterectomy Trial (NASCET) Group. *J Neurosurg* 1995;83:778–782.
69. Aungst M, Gahtan V, Berkowitz H, Roberts AB, Kerstein MD. Carotid endarterectomy outcome is not affected in patients with a contralateral carotid artery occlusion. *Am J Surg* 1998;176:30–33.
70. Hallett JWJ, Pietropaoli JAJ, Ilstrup DM, Gayari MM, Williams JA, Meyer FB. Comparison of North American Symptomatic Carotid Endarterectomy Trial and population-based outcomes for carotid endarterectomy. *J Vasc Surg* 1998;27:845–850.
71. Ballotta E, Da Giau G, Saladini M, Abbruzzese E. Carotid endarterectomy in symptomatic and asymptomatic patients aged 75 years or more:

perioperative mortality and stroke risk rates. *Ann Vasc Surg* 1999;13:158–163.
72. Hoballah JJ, Nazzal MM, Jacobovicz C, et al. Entering the ninth decade is not a contraindication for carotid endarterectomy. *Angiology* 1998; 49:275–278.
73. Levy PJ, Olin JW, Piedmonte MR, Young JR, Hertzer NR. Carotid endarterectomy in adults 50 years of age and younger: a retrospective comparative study. *J Vasc Surg* 1997;25:326–331.
74. Kann BR, Matsumoto T, Kerstein MD. Safety of carotid endarterectomy associated with small intracranial aneurysms. *Southern Medical Journal* 1997;90:1213–1216.
75. Pappada G, Fiori L, Marina R, Citerio G, Vaiani S, Gaini SM. Incidence of asymptomatic berry aneurysms among patients undergoing carotid endarterectomy. *J Neurosurg Sci* 1997;41: 257–262.
76. Giordano JM. The timing of carotid endarterectomy after acute stroke. *Semin Vasc Surg* 1998; 11:19–23.
77. Hoffmann M, Robbs JV, Abdool CA. Carotid endarterectomy after recent stroke—how soon? An interim analysis. *South African Journal of Surgery* 1998;36:63–67.
78. Riles TS, Imparato AM, Jacobowitz GR, et al. The cause of perioperative stroke after carotid endarterectomy. *J Vasc Surg* 1994;19:206–214.
79. Gaunt ME. Transcranial Doppler: preventing stroke during carotid endarterectomy. *Annals of the Royal College of Surgeons of England* 1998; 80:377–387.
80. Mansour MA. Recurrent carotid stenosis: prevention, surveillance, and management. *Semin Vasc Surg* 1998;11:30–35.
81. Johnson CA, Tollefson DF, Olsen SB, Andersen CA, McKee-Johnson J. The natural history of early recurrent carotid artery stenosis. *Am J Surg* 1999;177:433–436.
82. Lattimer CR, Burnand KG. Recurrent carotid stenosis after carotid endarterectomy. *Br J Surg* 1997;84:1206–1219.
83. Ganesan V, Cote R, Mackey A. Significance of carotid restenosis following endarterectomy. *Cerebrovasc Dis* 1998;8:338–344.
84. Hobson RW, Goldstein JE, Jamil Z, et al. Carotid restenosis: operative and endovascular management. *J Vasc Surg* 1999;29:228–235.
85. Schroeder T, Sillesen H, Sorensen O, Engell HC. Cerebral hyperperfusion following carotid endarterectomy. *J Neurosurg* 1987;66:824–829.
86. Chambers BR, Smidt V, Koh P. Hyperperfusion in post-endarterectomy. *Cerebrovasc Dis* 1994;4: 32–37.
87. Shinno K, Ueda S, Uno M, Nishitani K, Nagahiro S, Harada M. Hyperperfusion syndrome following carotid endarterectomy: evaluation using diffusion-weighted magnetic resonance imaging—case report. *Neurologia Medico-Chirurgica* 1998; 38:557–561.
88. Ejaz AA, Meschia JF. Thalamic hemorrhage following carotid endarterectomy-induced labile blood pressure: controlling the liability with clonidine—a case report. *Angiology* 1999;50: 327–330.
89. Hartsell PA, Calligaro KD, Syrek JR, Dougherty MJ, Raviola CA. Postoperative blood pressure changes associated with cervical block versus general anesthesia following carotid endarterectomy. *Ann Vasc Surg* 1999;13:104–108.
90. Zannetti S, Parente B, De Rango P, et al. Role of surgical techniques and operative findings in cranial and cervical nerve injuries during carotid endarterectomy. *Eur J Vasc Endovasc Surg* 1998;15:528–531.
91. Ballotta E, Da Giau G, Renon L, et al. Cranial and cervical nerve injuries after carotid endarterectomy: a prospective study. *Surgery* 1999;125:85–91.
92. Paciaroni M, Eliasziw M, Kappelle LJ, et al. Medical complications associated with carotid endarterectomy. *Stroke* 1999;30:1759–1763.
93. Hertzer NR, Loop FD, Beven EG, O'Hara PJ, Krajewski LP. Surgical staging for simultaneous coronary and carotid disease: a study including prospective randomization. *J Vasc Surg* 1989; 9:455–463.
94. Fillinger MF, Rosenberg JM, Semel L, et al. Combined carotid endarterectomy and coronary artery bypass in a community hospital. *Cardiovasc Surg* 1993;1:7–12.
95. Coyle KA, Gray BC, Smith RB, et al. Morbidity and mortality associated with carotid endarterectomy: effect of adjunctive coronary revascularization. *Ann Vasc Surg* 1995;9:21–27.
96. Plestis KA, Ke S, Jiang ZD, Howell JF. Combined carotid endarterectomy and coronary artery bypass: immediate and long-term results. *Ann Vasc Surg* 1999;13:84–92.
97. Hines GL, Scott WC, Schubach SL, Kofsky E, Wehbe U, Cabasino E. Prophylactic carotid endarterectomy in patients with high-grade carotid stenosis undergoing coronary bypass: does it decrease the incidence of perioperative stroke? *Ann Vasc Surg* 1998;12:23–27.
98. Goldstein LB, Hasselblad V, Matchar DB, McCrory DC. Comparison and meta-analysis of randomized trials of endarterectomy for symptomatic carotid artery stenosis. *Neurology* 1995; 45:1965–1970.
99. Easton JD, Wilterdink JL. Carotid endarterectomy: trials and tribulations. *Ann Neurol* 1994; 35:5–17.
100. Biller J, Feinberg WM, Castaldo JE, et al. Guidelines for carotid endarterectomy: a statement for healthcare professionals from a special writing group of the Stroke Council, American Heart Association. *Circulation* 1998;97:501–509.
101. Paddock-Eliasziw LM, Eliasziw M, Barr HW, Barnett HJM. Long-term prognosis and the effect of carotid endarterectomy in patients with recurrent ipsilateral ischemic events. North American Symptomatic Carotid Endarterectomy Trial Group. *Neurology* 1996;47:1158–1162.
102. Eliasziw M, Streifler JY, Fox AJ, et al. Significance of plaque ulceration in symptomatic patients with high-grade carotid stenosis. North American Symptomatic Carotid Endarterectomy Trial. *Stroke* 1994;25:304–308.
103. European Carotid Surgery Trialists' Collaborative Group. MRC European Carotid Surgery Trial:

interim results for symptomatic patients with severe (70–99%) or with mild (0–29%) carotid stenosis. *Lancet* 1991;337:1235–1243.
104. North American Symptomatic Carotid Endarterectomy Trial Collaborators. Beneficial effect of carotid endarterectomy in symptomatic patients with high-grade carotid stenosis. *N Engl J Med* 1991;325:445–453.
105. Streifler JY, Eliasziw M, Benavente OR, et al. The risk of stroke in patients with first-ever retinal vs hemispheric transient ischemic attacks and high-grade carotid stenosis. North American Symptomatic Carotid Endarterectomy Trial. *Arch Neurol* 1995;52:246–249.
106. Mayberg MR, Wilson SE, Yatsu F, et al. Carotid endarterectomy and prevention of cerebral ischemia in symptomatic carotid stenosis. Veterans Affairs Cooperative Studies Program 309 Trialist Group. *JAMA* 1991;266:3289–3294.
107. European Carotid Surgery Trialists' Collaborative Group. Endarterectomy for moderate symptomatic carotid stenosis: interim results from the MRC European Carotid Surgery Trial. *Lancet* 1996;347:1591–1593.
108. European Carotid Surgery Trialists' Collaborative Group. Randomised trial of endarterectomy for recently symptomatic carotid stenosis: final results of the MRC European Carotid Surgery Trial (ECST). *Lancet* 1998;351:1379–1387.
109. Barnett HJM, Taylor DW, Eliasziw M, et al. Benefit of carotid endarterectomy in patients with symptomatic moderate or severe stenosis. North American Symptomatic Carotid Endarterectomy Trial Collaborators. *N Engl J Med* 1998;339: 1415–1425.
110. The CASANOVA Study Group. Carotid surgery versus medical therapy in asymptomatic carotid stenosis. *Stroke* 1991;22:1229–1235.
111. Hobson RW, Weiss DG, Fields WS, et al. Efficacy of carotid endarterectomy for asymptomatic carotid stenosis. The Veterans Affairs Cooperative Study Group. *N Engl J Med* 1993; 328:221–227.
112. Mayo Asymptomatic Carotid Endarterectomy Study Group. Results of a randomized controlled trial of carotid endarterectomy for asymptomatic carotid stenosis. *Mayo Clin Proc* 1992;67:513–518.
113. Libman RB, Sacco RL, Shi T, Correll JW, Mohr JP. Outcome after carotid endarterectomy for asymptomatic carotid stenosis. *Surg Neurol* 1994; 41:443–449.
114. Robless P, Emson M, Thomas D, Mansfield A, Halliday A. Are we detecting and operating on high risk patients in the asymptomatic carotid surgery trial? The Asymptomatic Carotid Surgery Trial Collaborators. *Eur J Vasc Endovasc Surg* 1998;16:59–64.
115. Hart RG, Easton JD. Management of cervical bruits and carotid stenosis in preoperative patients. *Stroke* 1983;14:290–297.
116. Ropper AH, Wechsler LR, Wilson LS. Carotid bruit and the risk of stroke in elective surgery. *N Engl J Med* 1982;307:1388–1390.
117. McCormick PW, Spetzler RF, Bailes JE, Zabramski JM, Frey JL. Thromboendarterectomy of the symptomatic occluded internal carotid artery. *J Neurosurg* 1992;76:752–758.
118. Morgenstern LB, Fox AJ, Sharpe BL, Eliasziw M, Barnett HJM, Grotta JC. The risks and benefits of carotid endarterectomy in patients with near occlusion of the carotid artery. North American Symptomatic Carotid Endarterectomy Trial (NASCET) Group. *Neurology* 1997;48:911–915.
119. Vale FL, Fisher WS, Jordan WDJ, Palmer CA, Vitek J. Carotid endarterectomy performed after progressive carotid stenosis following angioplasty and stent placement. Case report. *J Neurosurg* 1997;87:940–943.
120. Costa VP, Kuzniec S, Molnar LJ, Cerri GG, Puech-Leao P, Carvalho CA. The effects of carotid endarterectomy on the retrobulbar circulation of patients with severe occlusive carotid artery disease. An investigation by color Doppler imaging. *Ophthalmology* 1999;106:306–310.
121. Lunn S, Crawley F, Harrison MJ, Brown MM, Newman SP. Impact of carotid endarterectomy upon cognitive functioning. A systematic review of the literature. *Cerebrovasc Dis* 1999;9:74–81.
122. Irvine CD, Gardner FV, Davies AH, Lamont PM. Cognitive testing in patients undergoing carotid endarterectomy. *Eur J Vasc Endovasc Surg* 1998; 15:195–204.
123. Kashyap VS, Moore WS, Quinones-Baldrich WJ. Carotid artery repair for radiation-associated atherosclerosis is a safe and durable procedure. *J Vasc Surg* 1999;29:90–96.
124. McNamara JO, Heyman A, Silver D, Mandel ME. The value of carotid endarterectomy in treating transient cerebral ischemia of the posterior circulation. *Neurology* 1977;27:682–684.
125. Warlow C. Carotid endarterectomy for asymptomatic carotid stenosis. Better data, but the case is still not convincing. *BMJ* 1998;317:1468.
126. Chaturvedi S. Is carotid endarterectomy appropriate for asymptomatic stenosis. *Arch Neurol* 1999;56:879–881.
127. Barnett HJM, Haines SJ. Carotid endarterectomy for asymptomatic carotid stenosis. *N Engl J Med* 1993;328:276–278.
128. Barnett HJM, Eliasziw M, Meldrum HE, Taylor DW. Do the facts and figures warrant a 10-fold increase in the performance of carotid endarterectomy on asymptomatic patients? *Neurology* 1996;46:603–608.
129. Barnett HJM, Meldrum HE, Eliasziw M. The dilemma of surgical treatment for patients with asymptomatic carotid disease. *Ann Intern Med* 1995;123:723–725.
130. Chaturvedi S, Halliday A. Is another clinical trail warranted regarding endarterctomy for asymptomatic carotid stenosis? *Cerebrovasc Dis* 1998;8: 210–213.
131. The European Carotid Surgery Trialists Collaborative Group. Risk of stroke in the distribution of an asymptomatic carotid artery. *Lancet* 1995;345:209–212.
132. Yin D, Carpenter JP. Cost-effectiveness of screening for asymptomatic carotid stenosis. *J Vasc Surg* 1998;27:245–255.
133. Cronenwett JL, Birkmeyer JD, Nackman GB, et al. Cost-effectiveness of carotid endarterectomy

in asymptomatic patients. *J Vasc Surg* 1997;25: 298–309.
134. Young B, Moore WS, Robertson JT, et al. An analysis of perioperative surgical mortality and morbidity in the asymptomatic carotid atherosclerosis study. ACAS Investigators. Asymptomatic Carotid Artheriosclerosis Study. *Stroke* 1996; 27:2216–2224.
135. Ausman JI, Diaz FG, Vacca DF, Sadasivan B. Superficial temporal and occipital artery bypass pedicles to superior, anterior inferior, and posterior inferior cerebellar arteries for vertebrobasilar insufficiency. *J Neurosurg* 1990;72:554–558.
136. Regli L, Piepgras DG, Hansen KK. Late patency of long saphenous vein bypass grafts to the anterior and posterior cerebral circulation. *J Neurosurg* 1995;83:806–811.
137. Klijn CJ, Kappelle LJ, van der Grond J, van Gijn J, Tulleken CA. A new type of extracranial/intracranial bypass for recurrent haemodynamic transient ischaemic attacks. *Cerebrovasc Dis* 1998; 8:184–187.
138. Sekhar LN, Bucur SD, Bank WO, Wright DC. Venous and arterial bypass grafts for difficult tumors, anuerysms, and occlusive vascular lesions: evolution of surgical treatment and improved graft results. *Neurosurgery* 1999;44: 1207–1224.
139. Iwama T, Hashimoto N, Takagi Y, Tsukahara T, Hayashida K. Predictability of extracranial/intracranial bypass function: a retrospective study of patients with occlusive cerebrovascular disease. *Neurosurgery* 1997;40:53–59.
140. Schick U, Zimmermann M, Stolke D. Long-term evaluation of EC-IC bypass patency. *Acta Neurochir* 1996;138:938–942.
141. Schmiedek P, Piepgras A, Leinsinger G, Kirsch CM, Einhupl K. Improvement of cerebrovascular reserve capacity by EC-IC arterial bypass surgery in patients with ICA occlusion and hemodynamic cerebral ischemia. *J Neurosurg* 1994; 81:236–244.
142. Hopkins LN, Budny JL. Complications of intracranial bypass for vertebrobasilar insufficiency. *J Neurosurg* 1989;70:207–211.
143. The EC/IC Bypass Study Group. Failure of extracranial-intracranial arterial bypass to reduce the risk of ischemic stroke. Results of an international randomized trial. *N Engl J Med* 1985;313:1191–1200.
144. Yamashita T, Kashiwagi S, Nakano S, et al. The effect of EC-IC bypass surgery on resting cerebral blood flow and cerebrovascular reserve capacity studied with stable XE-CT and acetazolamide test. *Neuroradiology* 1991;33:217–222.
145. Vorstrup S, Haase J, Waldemar G, Andersen A, Schmidt J, Paulson OB. EC-IC bypass in patients with chronic hemodynamic insufficiency. *Acta Neurol Scand* 1996;166(Suppl):79–81.
146. Grubb RL, Jr., Derdeyn CP, Fritsch SM, et al. Importance of hemodynamic factors in the prognosis of symptomatic carotid occlusion. *JAMA* 1998;280:1055–1060.
147. Kawaguchi S, Sakaki T, Kamada K, Iwanaga H, Nishikawa N. Effects of superficial temporal to middle cerebral artery bypass for ischaemic retinopathy due to internal carotid artery occlusion/stenosis. *Acta Neurochir* 1994;129:166–170.
148. Vishteh AG, Marciano FF, David CA, Schievink WI, Zabramski JM, Spetzler RF. Long-term graft patency rates and clinical outcomes after revascularization for symptomatic traumatic internal carotid artery dissection. *Neurosurgery* 1998; 43:761–768.
149. Morgan MK, Sekhon LH. Extracranial–intracranial saphenous vein bypass for carotid or vertebral artery dissections: a report of six cases. *J Neurosurg* 1994;80:237–246.
150. Schievink WI, Piepgras DG, McCaffrey TV, Mokri B. Surgical treatment of extracranial internal carotid artery dissecting aneurysms. *Neurosurgery* 1994;35:809–815.
151. Iwama T, Hashimoto N, Miyake H, Yonekawa Y. Direct revascularization to the anterior cerebral artery territory in patients with moyamoya disease: report of five cases. *Neurosurgery* 1998; 42:1157–1161.
152. Ueki K, Meyer FB, Mellinger JF. Moyamoya disease: the disorder and surgical treatment. *Mayo Clin Proc* 1994;69:749–757.
153. Golby AJ, Marks MP, Thompson RC, Steinberg GK. Direct and combined revascularization in pediatric moyamoya disease. *Neurosurgery* 1999; 45:50–60.
154. Kinugasa K, Mandai S, Tokunaga K, et al. Ribbon enchephalo-duro-arterio-myo-synangiosis for moyamoya disease. *Surg Neurol* 1994; 41:455–461.
155. Kinugasa K, Mandai S, Kamata I, Sugiu K, Ohmoto T. Surgical treatment of moyamoya disease: operative technique for encephalo-duro-arterio-myo-synangiosis, its follow-up, clinical results, and angiograms. *Neurosurgery* 1993;32: 527–531.
156. Ryan PG, Day AL. Stump embolization from an occluded internal carotid artery. Case report. *J Neurosurg* 1987;67:609–611.
157. Hankey GJ, Warlow CP. Prognosis of symptomatic carotid artery occlusion. *Cerebrovasc Dis* 1991;1:245–256.
158. Radonic V, Baric D, Giunio L, Buca A, Sapunar D, Marovic A. Surgical treatment of kinked internal carotid artery. *J Cardiovasc Surg* 1998; 39:557–563.
159. Archie JP, Jr. The outcome of external carotid endarterectomy during routine carotid endarterectomy. *J Vasc Surg* 1998;28:585–590.
160. Chiche L, Bahnini A, Koskas F, Kieffer E. Occlusive fibromuscular disease of arteries supplying the brain: results of surgical treatment. *Ann Vasc Surg* 1997;11:496–504.
161. Fields WS, Lemak NA. Joint Study of Extracranial Arterial Occlusion. VII. Subclavian steal—a review of 168 cases. *JAMA* 1972; 222:1139–1143.
162. Molnar RG, Naslund TC. Vertebral artery surgery. *Surg Clin N Am* 1998;78:901–913.
163. Law MM, Colburn MD, Moore WS, Quinones-Baldrich WJ, Machleder HI, Gelabert HA. Carotid-subclavian bypass for brachiocephalic occlusive disease. Choice of conduit and long-term follow-up. *Stroke* 1995;26:1565–1571.

164. Kobayashi T, Houkin K, Ito F, Kohama Y. Transverse cervical artery bypass pedicle for treatment of common carotid artey occlusion: new adjunct for revascularization of the internal carotid artery domain. *Neurosurgery* 1999;45: 299–302.
165. Bojar RM, Payne DD, Murphy RE, et al. Surgical treatment of systemic atheroembolism from the thoracic aorta. *Ann Thorac Surg* 1996;61: 1389–1393.
166. King RC, Kanithanon RC, Shockey KS, Spotnitz WD, Tribble CG, Kron IL. Replacing the atherosclerotic ascending aorta is a high-risk procedure. *Ann Thorac Surg* 1998;66:396–401.
167. Giardina EG. Atrial fibrillation and stroke: elucidating a newly discovered risk factor. *Am J Cardiol* 1997;80:11D–18D.
168. Serena J, Segura T, Perez-Ayuso MJ, Bassaganyas J, Molins A, Davalos. The need to quantify right-to-left shunt in acute ischemic stroke: a case-control study. *Stroke* 1998;29: 1322–1328.
169. Cujec B, Mainra R, Johnson DH. Prevention of recurrent cerebral ischemic events in patients with patent foramen ovale and cryptogenic strokes or transient ischemic attacks. *Can J Cardiol* 1999;15:57–64.
170. Homma S, Di Tullio MR, Sacco RL, Sciacca RR, Smith C, Mohr JP. Surgical closure of patent foramen ovale in cryptogenic stroke patients. *Stroke* 1997;28:2376–2381.
171. Giroud M, Tatou E, Steinmetz E, et al. The interest of surgical closure of patent foramen ovale after stroke: a preliminary open study of 8 cases. *Neurol Res* 1998;20:297–301.
172. Guffi M, Bogousslavsky J, Jeanrenaud X, Devuyst G, Sadeghi H. Surgical prophylaxis of recurrent stroke in patients with patent foramen ovale: a pilot study. *J Thorac Cardiovasc Surg* 1996;112:260–263.
173. Bogousslavsky J, Devuyst G, Nendaz M, Yamamoto H, Sarasin F. Prevention of stroke recurrence with presumed paradoxical embolism. *J Neurol* 1997;244:71–75.
174. Nendaz MR, Sarasin FP, Junod AF, Bogousslavsky J. Preventing stroke recurrence in patients with patent foramen ovale: antithrombotic therapy, foramen closure, or therapeutic abstention? A decision analytic perspective. *Am Heart J* 1998;135:532–541.
175. Zubkov AY, Lewis AI, Scalzo D, Bernanke DH, Harkey HL. Morphological changes after percutaneous transluminal angioplasty. *Surg Neurol* 1999;51:399–403.
176. Markus HS, Clifton A, Buckenham T, Taylor R, Brown MM. Improvement in cerebral hemodynamics after carotid angioplasty. *Stroke* 1996; 27:612–616.
177. Schoser BG, Heesen C, Eckert B, Thie A. Cerebral hyperperfusion injury after percutaneous transluminal angioplasty of extracranial arteries. *J Neurol* 1997;244:101–104.
178. McCleary AJ, Nelson M, Dearden NM, Calvey TA, Gough MJ. Cerebral haemodynamics and embolization during carotid angioplasty in high-risk patients. *Br J Surg* 1998;85:771–774.
179. Chaturvedi S. Medical, surgical, and interventional treatment for carotid artery disease. *Clin Neuropharmacol* 1998;21:205–214.
180. Beebe HG, Kritpracha B. Carotid stenting versus carotid endarterectomy: update on the controversy. *Semin Vasc Surg* 1998;11:46–51.
181. Jimenez C, Duong H, Olarte M, Pile-Spellman J. Recurrent abrupt occlusion after transluminal angioplasty for basilar artery stenosis: case report. *Neurosurgery* 1999;44:210–215.
182. Connors III JJ, Wojak JC. Percutaneous transluminal angioplasty for intracranial atherosclerotic lesions: evolution of technique and short-term results. *J Neurosurg* 1999;91:415–423.
183. Beebe HG, Archie JP, Baker WH, et al. Concern about safety of carotid angioplasty. *Stroke* 1996; 27:197–198.
184. Gil-Peralta A, Mayol A, Marcos JR, et al. Percutaneous transluminal angioplasty of the symptomatic atherosclerotic carotid arteries. Results, complications, and follow-up. *Stroke* 1996;27:2271–2273.
185. Mathur A, Roubin GS, Iyer SS, et al. Predictors of stroke complicating carotid artery stenting. *Circulation* 1998;97:1239–1245.
186. Jordan WDJ, Voellinger DC, Fisher WS, Redden D, McDowell HA. A comparison of carotid angioplasty with stenting versus endarterectomy with regional anesthesia. *J Vasc Surg* 1998;28: 397–402.
187. Jordan WDJ, Roye GD, Fisher WS, Redden D, McDowell HA. A cost comparison of balloon angioplasty and stenting versus endarterectomy for the treatment of carotid artery stenosis. *J Vasc Surg* 1998;27:16–22.
188. Naylor AR, Bolia A, Abbott RJ, et al. Randomized study of carotid angioplasty and stenting versus carotid endarterectomy: a stopped trial. *J Vasc Surg* 1998;28:326–334.
189. Becquemin JP, Qvarfordt P, Castier Y, Melliere D. Carotid angioplasty: is it safe? *J Endovasc Surg* 1996;3:35–41.
190. Robbin ML, Lockhart ME, Weber TM, et al. Carotid artery stents: early and intermediate follow-up with Doppler US. *Radiology* 1997;205: 749–756.
191. Yadav JS, Roubin GS, King P, Iyer S, Vitek J. Angioplasty and stenting for restenosis after carotid endarterectomy. Initial experience. *Stroke* 1996;27:2075–2079.
192. Yadav JS, Roubin GS, Iyer S, et al. Elective stenting of the extracranial carotid arteries. *Circulation* 1997;95:376–381.
193. Wholey MH, Jarmolowski CR, Eles G, Levy D, Buecthel J. Endovascular stents for carotid artery occlusive disease. *J Endovasc Surg* 1997;4: 326–338.
194. Lanzino G, Mericle RA, Lopes DK, Wakhloo AK, Guterman LR, Hopkins LN. Percutaneous transluminal angioplasty and stent placement for recurrent carotid artery stenosis. *J Neurosurg* 1999;90:688–694.
195. Theron JG, Payelle GG, Coskun O, Huet HF, Guimaraens L. Carotid artery stenosis: treatment with protected balloon angioplasty and stent placement. *Radiology* 1996;201:627–636.

196. Al-Mubarak N, Roubin GS, Gomez CR, et al. Carotid artery stenting in patients with high neurologic risks. *Am J Cardiol* 1999;83:1411–1413.
197. Wholey MH, Wholey M, Bergeron P, et al. Current global status of carotid artery stent placement. *Cathet Cardiovasc Diagn* 1998;44:1–6.
198. Levien LJ, Benn CA, Veller MG, Fritz VU. Retrograde balloon angioplasty of brachiocephalic or common carotid artery stenoses at the time of carotid endarterectomy. *Eur J Vasc Endovasc Surg* 1998;15:521–527.
199. Widenka DC, Spuler A, Steiger H. Treatment of carotid tandem stenosis by combined carotid endarterectomy and balloon angioplasty: technical case report. *Neurosurgery* 1999;45:179–182.
200. Mathur A, Roubin GS, Yadav JS, Iyer SS, Vitek J. Combined coronary and bilateral carotid stenting: a case report. *Cathet Cardiovasc Diagn* 1997;40:202–206.
201. McKenzie JD, Wallace RC, Dean BL, Flom RA, Khayata MH. Preliminary results of intracranial angioplasty for vascular stenosis caused by atherosclerosis and vasculitis. *Am J Neuroradiol* 1996;17:263–268.
202. Kellogg JX, Nesbit GM, Clark WM, Barnwell SL. The role of angioplasty in the treatment of cerebrovascular disease. *Neurosurgery* 1998;43:549–555.
203. Suh DC, Sung KB, Cho YS, et al. Transluminal angioplasty for middle cerebral artery stenosis in patients with acute ischemic stroke. *Am J Neuroradiol* 1999;20:553–558.
204. Mori T, Mori K, Fukuoka M, Arisawa M, Honda S. Percutaneous transluminal cerebral angioplasty: serial angiographic follow-up after successful dilatation. *Neuroradiology* 1997;39:111–116.
205. Terada T, Higashida RT, Halbach VV, et al. Transluminal angioplasty for arteriosclerotic disease of the distal vertebral and basilar arteries. *J Neurol Neurosurg Psychiatry* 1996;60:377–381.
206. Callahan AS, Berger BL. Balloon angioplasty of intracranial arteries for stroke prevention. *J Neuroimaging* 1997;7:232–235.
207. Nakatsuka H, Ueda T, Ohta S, Sakaki S. Successful percutaneous transluminal angioplasty for basilar artery stenosis: technical case report. *Neurosurgery* 1996;39:161–164.
208. Nakayama T, Tanaka K, Kaneko M, Yokoyama T, Uemura K. Thrombolysis and angioplasty for acute occlusion of intracranial vertebrobasilar arteries. Report of three cases. *J Neurosurg* 1998;88:919–922.
209. Butterworth RJ, Thomas DJ, Wolfe JHN, Mansfield AO, Al-Kutoubi A. Endovascular treatment of carotid dissecting aneurysms. *Cerebrovasc Dis* 1999;9:242–247.
210. Hurst RW, Haskal ZJ, Zager E, Bagley LJ, Flamm ES. Endovascular stent treatment of cervical internal carotid artery aneurysms with parent vessel preservation. *Surg Neurol* 1998;50:313–317.
211. Coric D, Wilson JA, Regan JD, Bell DA. Primary stenting of the extracranial internal carotid artery in a patient with multiple cervical dissections: technical case report. *Neurosurgery* 1998;43:956–959.
212. Gomez CR. The role of carotid angioplasty and stenting. *Semin Neurol* 1998;18:501–511.
213. Hacein-Bey L, Koennecke HC, Pile-Spellman J, et al. Pilot study for cerebral balloon angioplasty: design considerations and case-control methods. *Cerebrovasc Dis* 1998;8:354–357.
214. Ahuja A, Blatt GL, Guterman LR, Hopkins LN. Angioplasty for symptomatic radiation-induced extracranial carotid artery stenosis: case report. *Neurosurgery* 1995;36:399–403.
215. Joint Officers of the Congress of Neurological Surgeons and the American Association of Neurological Surgeons. Carotid angioplasty and stent: an alternative to carotid endarterectomy. *Neurosurgery* 1997;40:344–345.
216. Bettmann MA, Katzen BT, Whisnant J, et al. Carotid stenting and angioplasty: a statement for healthcare professionals from the Councils on Cardiovascular Radiology, Stroke, Cardiovascular Surgery, Epidemiology and Prevention, and Clinical Cardiology, American Heart Association. *J Vasc Interv Radiol* 1998;9:3–5.
217. Moore WS, Mohr JP, Najafi H, Robertson JT, Stoney RJ, Toole JF. Carotid endarterectomy: practice guidelines. Report of the Ad Hoc Committee to the Joint Council of the Society for Vascular Surgery and the North American Chapter of the International Society for Cardiovascular Surgery. *J Vasc Surg* 1992; 15:469–479.
218. Moore WS, Barnett HJM, Beebe HG, et al. Guidelines for carotid endarterectomy. A multidisciplinary consensus statement from the ad hoc committee, American Heart Association. *Stroke* 1995;26:188–201.
219. Findlay JM, Tucker WS, Ferguson GG, Holness RO, Wallace MC, Wong JH. Guidelines for the use of carotid endarterectomy: current recommendations from the Canadian Neurosurgical Society. *CMAJ* 1997;157:653–659.
220. Albers GW, Hart RG, Lutset HL, Newell DW, Sacco RL. Supplement to the guidelines for the management of transient ischemic attacks. A statement from the Ad Hoc Committee on Guidelines for the Management of Transient Ischemic Attacks, Stroke Council, American Heart Association. *Stroke* 1999;30:2502–2511.
221. Taylor DW, Barnett HJM, Haynes RB, et al. Low-dose and high-dose acetylsalicylic acid for patients undergoing carotid endarterectomy: a ransomised controlled trial. *Lancet* 1999;353:2179–2184.
222. Easton JD, Sherman DG. Stroke and mortality rate in carotid endarterectomy: 228 consecutive operations. *Stroke* 1977;8:565–568.
223. Chaturvedi S, Aggarwal A, Murugappan A. Results of carotid endarterectomy with prospective neurologist follow-up. *Neurology* 2000;55:769–772.
224. O'Neill L, Lanska DJ, Hartz A. Surgeon characteristics associated with mortality and morbidity following carotid endarterectomy. *Neurology* 2000;55:773–781.

225. Blohme L, Sandstrom V, Hellstrom G, Swedenborg J, Takolander R. Complications in carotid endarterectomy are predicted by qualifying symptoms and preoperative CT findings. *Eur J Vasc Endovasc Surg* 1999;17:213–218.
226. Benavente O, Moher D, Pham B. Carotid endarterectomy for asymptomatic carotid stenosis: a meta-analysis. *BMJ* 1998;317:1477–1480.
227. Perry JR, Szalai JP, Norris JW. Consensus against both endarterectomy and routine screening for asymptomatic carotid artery stenosis. Canadian Stroke Consortium. *Arch Neurol* 1997;54:25–28.
228. Hill AB. Should patients be screened for asymptomatic carotid artery stensis? *Can J Surg* 1998; 41:208–213.
229. Brott T, Toole JF. Medical compared with surgical treatment of asymptomatic carotid artery stenosis. *Ann Intern Med* 1995;123:720–722.
230. Castaldo J. Is carotid endarterectomy appropriate for asymptomatic stenosis? Yes. *Arch Neurol* 1999;56:877–879.
231. Lee TT, Solomon NA, Heidenreich PA, Oehlert J, Garber AM. Cost-effectiveness of screening for carotid stenosis in asymptomatic persons. *Ann Intern Med* 1997;126:337–346.
232. Lanska DJ, Kryscio RJ. Endarterectomy for asymptomatic internal carotid artery stenosis. *Neurology* 1997;48:1481–1490.
233. Donaghy RMP. Patch and bypass in microangional surgery. In: *Micro-Vascular Surgery.* Donaghy RMP, Yasargil MG, eds. St. Louis. CV Mosby, 1967:75–86.
234. Yasargil MG. Anastomosis between the supervicial temporal artery and a branch of the middle cerebral artery. In: *Microsurgery Applied to Neurosurgery.* Yasargil MB, ed. Stuttgart: George Thiems Verlag, 1969:105–115.
235. Ratcheson RA, Grubb RL, Jr. Superficial temporalmiddle cerebral cortical artery anastomosis. In: *Stroke and the Extracranial Vessels.* Smith RR, ed. New York. Raven Press, 1984:255–263.
236. Sundt TMJ, Whisnant JP, Fode NC, Piepgras DG, Houser OW. Results, complications, and follow-up of 415 bypass operations for occlusive disease of the carotid system. *Mayo Clin Proc* 1985;60:230–240.
237. Day AL, Rhoton AL, Jr., Little JR. The extracranial-intracranial bypass study. *Surg Neurol* 1986;26:222–226.
238. Yonas H. Predictability of extracranial/intracranial bypass function. A retrospective study of patients with occlusive cerebrovascular disease. *Neurosurgery* 1997;41:1447–1448.
239. Golledge J, Mitchell A, Greenhalgh RM, Davies AH. Systematic comparison of the early outcome of angioplasty and endarterectomy for symptomatic carodis artery disease. *Neurology* 2000;31: 1439–1443.
240. Qureshi AI, Luft AR, Sharma M, Guterman LR, Hopkins LN. Prevention and treatment of thromboembolic and ischemic complications associated with endovascular procedures: Part II - clinical aspects and recommendations. *Neurosurgery* 2000;46:1360–1376.
241. Qureshi AI, Luft AR, Sharma M, Guterman LR, Hopkins LN. Prevention and treatment of thromboembolic and ischemic complications associated with endovascular procedures: Part I - pathophysiological and pharmacological features. *Neurosurgery* 2000;46:1344–1359.
242. Qureshi AI, Suri FK, Khan J, Fessler RD, Guterman LR, Hopkins LN. Abciximab as an adjunct to high-risk carotid or vertebrobasilar angioplasty: preliminary experience. *Neurosurgery* 2000;46:1316–1325.

Chapter 12

MANAGEMENT OF ACUTE ISCHEMIC STROKE

Acute ischemic stroke is a neurological emergency. The first hours after onset are critical for initiation of treatment that can limit the neurological consequences of ischemic stroke. Time limits to define acute ischemic stroke are evolving but, for any effective therapy to ameliorate stroke, it probably must occur within a few hours. Although the first 24 hours might be considered an upper boundary in defining acute ischemic stroke, in reality, the first 3–6 hours are the most crucial. Thus, the focus of this chapter is on components of acute management that can be initiated during this short period. The key elements of emergent management are outlined in Table 12–1. Equal participants in the plans for the modern approach to stroke are the patients and their families, the emergency medical services (EMS) in the community, the hospital, and physicians. Because time

Table 12–1. **Components of the Emergent Management of Patients with Acute Ischemic Stroke**

"Time is brain"
Prompt recognition
Speedy transport
Urgent evaluation
Rapid treatment

is such a critical variable, key decisions about acute treatment are made in an emergency department before a patient is admitted to the hospital. Occasionally, acute stroke therapies might be administered elsewhere in a hospital, such as in an interventional neuroradiology suite, but, even in this case, decisions about treatment are made in the emergency department. Thus, acute treatment of stroke should not be considered as a course of management that is initiated once the patient is hospitalized.

An exception is the urgent management of strokes that occur among patients already in the hospital for treatment of another condition. This scenario accounts for approximately 10% of strokes. Although acute care happens in the area of the hospital in which they are being treated, the principles of acute management are similar to those used in the emergency department.

BRAIN ATTACK

The strategy for managing patients with acute ischemic stroke is modeled on that applied to treating patients with acute myocardial ischemia. The similarities between the two acute vascular illnesses are several. Both are life-threatening diseases that are secondary to thromboembolic arterial occlusions. Both are accompanied by serious complications that require emergent treatment in their own right. The current definitive treatment for both acute myocardial and cerebral ischemia is thrombolytic therapy and, in both instances, the therapy must be started within a few hours for a reasonable chance for success. The emphasis of the current method of treating ischemic stroke is summarized in the term *brain attack.*[1–5] The term *brain attack* obviously imitates the term *heart attack,* and it gives the sense of urgency that is needed to treat stroke successfully.

Although there is parallelism between acute myocardial ischemia and acute cerebral ischemia, important differences also exist (Table 12–2). Many differences involve recognition of the illness and the potentially ominous nature of the symptoms. These differences can be overcome by the concerted effort of the public and health

Table 12–2. **Similarities and Differences: Acute Ischemic Stroke and Acute Myocardial Infarction**

Similarities
Both have sudden onset
Both involve an arterial occlusion secondary to thromboembolism
Both are accompanied by life-threatening complications (ie arrhythmias, seizures, heart failure, brain edema)
Myocardial infarction is a complication of stroke and vice versa
Both can be treated successfully with thrombolytic therapy
Treatment for both is most effective if started within 3 hours
With both, patients may deny that they are having the event
Differences
Pain is an important symptom of myocardial infarction, whereas pain may be absent with stroke
The message can aim at seeking medical attention if severe chest pain occurs, but the symptoms of stroke are less obvious and more varied
Consciousness usually is normal with myocardial infarction, but decreased consciousness is seen with severe stroke
With myocardial infarction, cognition is normal; with stroke, disorders of higher brain function are prominent

care providers. The dictum for stroke care in the new millennium is "time is brain."[6]

An important focus of modern stroke management is attention to issues that lead to delays in diagnosis or treatment. The leading reasons these delays are (*1*) problems in recognition, (*2*) delays in transportation to an appropriate emergency department, (*3*) lags in evaluation, and (*4*) slowness in initiating treatment.[7–10] All of these problems must be tackled simultaneously if the treatment of acute ischemic stroke is to be successful.

This strategy is radically different from the past approach that was predicated on a sense of hopelessness and helplessness.[11] For too many years, stroke was considered to be an unfortunate accident of nature for which nothing could be done to modify outcomes. Physicians approached stroke with a sense of nihilism, and patients and families with a sense that they must be resigned to their fate. Unfortunately, this sense of nihilism still has not been abandoned by some professional organizations that provide leadership in stroke care.[12] In some countries, stroke services are poorly organized and a sizeable percentage of patients are sent to hospitals that do not have available facilities such as computed tomography (CT).[13] Insurance programs, governmental regulations, and health care plans have been slow to support emergent stroke care. In a survey of 28 health maintenance organizations (HMOs) in California, the symptoms of stroke were categorized as those that mandated emergency treatment by only 2.[14] A minority of HMOs had a standard policy of advising their members to call 911 or to go to an emergency department if the signs of an acute vascular event (either myocardial infarction or stroke) were noted.[14] Changes in attitudes among both health care providers and insurance companies are fundamental for success. A public educational program that instructs patients about the importance of seeking medical attention for stroke will go for naught if the medical community does not manage the illness as an emergency or if insurance companies place obstacles infront of treatment. Fortunately, professional groups from around the world are developing strategies to expedite urgent treatment for stroke.[6,15–23] Strategies that emphasize a sense of urgency in treatment are critical because a treatment of proven value is available.[24] A regional stroke code/care system that is available 24 hours/day and 7 days/week will increase the number of patients who can be treated within the first hours after stroke.[25] Treating acute stroke as an emergency every hour of the day and every day of the week must become the norm. The American Heart Association is implementing programs to reach the goal of having 20% of persons with stroke being seen <3 hours of onset by 2003.[26,27] This goal is audacious.

CARE PRIOR TO ARRIVAL IN THE EMERGENCY DEPARTMENT

Recognition

A major hurdle to overcome is the problem of patients and observers not recognizing that a stroke is happening. Most patients and families also do not know the best response to the appearance of neurological symptoms. Improving recognition of stroke is critical, because the potentially useful therapies that are available will be of no avail unless the patient seeks medical attention within the necessary time. The key for success is to see a physician in an emergency department as quickly as possible. Although there is a treatment of proven effectiveness, it is not used widely because most patients are not seen at a medical institution until more than 3 hours after stroke.[28,29] For example, Ferro et al[8] found that only 117 of 309 patients with acute ischemic stroke arrived at medical centers within 6 hours of stroke. Recently, Kothari et al[30] reported that less than 30% of patients arrived at an emergency department within 3 hours; the median time of arrival was 5.7 hours. These latter results are particularly disappointing because the data were from a community that has had a very active regional stroke care program. Several factors are critical for determining early access to acute stroke care. Studies show that patients with mild strokes, those with a gradual evolution, or those with nocturnal events do not arrive in time for treatment, whereas those with severe strokes that occur in the afternoon are most likely to be seen quickly.[31–33] Persons with severe strokes or brain hemorrhage and those transported by ambulance are seen early.[33,34] A decline in consciousness, seizures, or major deficits usually leads to early recognition of stroke.[10,33–35] Women and those who first contacted their primary care physician arrive late.[33,34]

Patients must know the symptoms of stroke. Unfortunately, a sizeable proportion of people at the highest risk does not know the protean manifestations of stroke.[36–38] Pancioli et al[36] found that only 57% of 1880 surveyed persons knew at least one of the five major symptoms of stroke and that the most at-risk persons did not know the full spectrum of neurological presentations. The level of knowledge is lowest among persons older than 75.[36–38] Unfortunately, this age group is at the greatest risk. Younger persons, those in generally poor health, and those with a history of a transient ischemic attack (TIA) or stroke generally have the highest level of knowledge.[37] Still, even patients who have been instructed about stroke often do not seek attention quickly.[39] A concerted educational program is needed to teach the public about the symptoms of stroke. In particular, persons at highest risk, especially the elderly, should be informed about the presentations of the acute illness. Ways to convey information include friends, newspapers, magazines, and the mass media.[40]

Some patients may not recognize that they are having a stroke because the illness is producing neglect, cognitive impairments, or decreased consciousness.[35] An observer may recognize the symptoms of stroke even if the patient is unaware of the problem. As a result, educational programs also should be aimed at families, neighbors, co-workers, and friends as well as patients themselves.[476] Education of spouses, adult children, and neighbors is critical because the interval from stroke until treatment is longer for patients who have a stroke at home than for those who have an event at work.[35,41] A majority of older persons are likely to be at home rather than in a public place at the time of stroke. Many strokes occur during the night. Thus, educating other persons in the household becomes an important strategy to avoid delays in recognition.[476] The importance of advice from friends and family members is highlighted by the experience of Kothari et al.[30] Of 151 patients with stroke seen in an emergency department, 40% said that a relative or a friend told them to seek help. Among patients who did not seek medical attention immediately, the leading reasons for delay were the hope that the symptoms would clear spontaneously and the desire to wait for relatives to come home to obtain assistance or advice.[8] Patients should be encouraged to seek medical attention immediately even if family members or friends are absent.

EDUCATIONAL PROGRAM

An educational program should highlight a limited number of symptoms, which are included in Table 12–3. The message should be straightforward and include features that reflect the culture of the community.

Table 12–3. **Public Educational Program for Increasing Stroke Awareness**

- Emphasize symptoms of stroke
  - Sudden onset
  - Weakness, numbness, clumsiness—usually observed on one side of body
  - Slurred speech or difficulty speaking or understanding others
  - Intense vertigo or imbalance
  - Unusually severe headache
- Emphasize response
  - Seek medical attention immediately
- Program components
  - Television and radio advertisements
  - Fliers, posters, newspaper articles, and brochures
  - One-to-one teaching—medical institutions, visiting nurses, home health care, and social services
  - Public meetings—senior citizens groups, churches, clubs, and health fairs

For example, the term *brain attack* may not be appropriate for a Spanish-speaking community because the term implies epilepsy rather than stroke. The program should emphasize the sudden nature of the onset of symptoms. Prominent or severe signs are likely to draw the most attention. Still, more subtle deficits such as aphasia, visual loss, and incoordination are equally important. The message should be that the sudden occurrence of focal neurological symptoms reflecting a loss of function of one part of the brain might be secondary to a stroke and that the pattern of impairment reflects the area of brain injury.

In addition knowing the symptoms of stroke, patients should be taught to seek medical attention immediately. Many patients do not know that a potentially useful treatment for stroke is available.[42] They need to be informed that acute stroke is not a hopeless situation and that they can be helped if they seek medical attention quickly. Even if neurological symptoms are not due to ischemic stroke, findings may be secondary to another serious disease, such as brain hemorrhage, which also needs urgent treatment. Even if the symptoms begin to resolve spontaneously, the patient still should be seen quickly. A transient episode of neurological dysfunction could be secondary to a TIA, but this event also is an emergency. The TIA might be a warning sign for an impending infarction, and prompt initiation of prophylactic therapies is needed to prevent stroke. The likelihood of patients seeking medical attention for trivial reasons seems low. In one series of 100 patients referred for a possible acute stroke, vascular events were eventually diagnosed in 87.[25] Very few stroke mimickers were found.

RESPONSES TO SYMPTOMS OF STROKE

The best response for patients is to call an emergency access number, such as 911 in the United States.[43–45] Calling an emergency system has several advantages. It means that care and assessment can begin at the patient's location. Transportation is accomplished on an urgent basis, and the receiving emergency department is alerted that a patient with a potential stroke is being transported to the institution. An approach that emphasizes calling such an emergency assistance number can be successful. A public education program in Cincinnati, Ohio, that emphasized use of the 911 system increased the patients with stroke being transferred to emergency departments from 40% to 60%.[46] It also reduced the mean time from stroke until arrival from 3.2 hours to 1.5 hours.

The second-best response is for the patient to go directly to the nearest emergency department as quickly as possible. Because of the neurological impairment, the patient should not drive to the hospital; another person should operate the motor vehicle. The time in transit likely will be longer than with an ambulance, but at least the patient will arrive at an emergency department where treatment might be given. Patients should not call a personal physician. The physician might not be readily available, and subsequent delays likely will preclude treatment.[35] Barsan et al[41] found that the median time from stroke until first medical contact was 84 minutes when 911 was called. It increased to 270 minutes if the patient first called a physician's office. Calling the local hospital switchboard for advice also likely will result in delays.

Many patients live alone and, because of the stroke, may not be able to call for help.[33] Devices that can be activated by a patient during an emergency are available at some retirement communities and homes. Patients should be encouraged to activate this system if they cannot reach a telephone to summon help. Elderly people also should participate in programs that invite relatives or neighbors to check on them at regular intervals. Although this arrangement might not permit treatment within 3 hours of stroke, it improves access to care. Some patients may not want to go to the hospital for personal or financial reasons. Still, they should be encouraged to call for help because of the high potential for death or disability without treatment. A potent argument might be that stroke can be treated if therapy is started soon. This treatment holds the promise of preventing disability and loss of independence, an outcome feared greatly by most patients.

Initial Contact, Evaluation, and Transport

For treatment of stroke to be successful, all components of the health care system must respond to a call for help with alacrity.[45] Each potential choke point for the swift care of patients must be identified and overcome. The person (dispatcher) at the emergency telephone center who receives a call must recognize the importance of the call and the features of stroke. Depending on the community, the person answering the telephone might not have a high level of medical sophistication or know the common symptoms of stroke. One study found that dispatchers correctly recognized the signs of stroke in only 52% of cases.[47] These individuals need to be taught about the presentations of stroke and about the interval from onset of symptoms (See Table 12–3).

Receptionists and telephone operators at physicians' offices and the local hospital also should be taught about the presentations of stroke and the correct advice to provide if a patient calls with complaints suggestive a stroke. The receptionist or nurse should either directly call EMS (911 in the United States) or advise the caller to do so. The goal remains to have the patient arrive in an emergency department as quickly as possible. The receptionist or nurse should inform the patient's physician of the call so that he or she can make plans to see the patient on arrival in the emergency department. Personal physicians also may have important information that otherwise might not be readily available; however, the operator should not delay the patient's treatment by searching for the physician before advising the patient to go to an emergency department. The receptionist or nurse should not advise the patient to stay at home until the physician returns the call.

EMERGENCY MEDICAL SERVICES

The dispatcher should send EMS personnel to the site on a priority basis.[3,44,48] Regional EMS must be organized so that stroke is given the same emphasis as myocardial infarction. In the past, stroke was not considered to be a true medical emergency and ambulances were not sent on a priority basis.[43] Rapid ambulance protocols are used to help transport patients with acute stroke.[43,49] Similar protocols should be adopted universally by rescue squads and EMS.

The initial responses of the paramedics at the time of their arrival at the patient's location also are critical.[43–45] They should assess the patient quickly. In addition to providing initial life support and examining vital signs, paramedics also can do a brief neurological examination. The Glasgow Coma Scale is widely used to rate the severity of brain injury in patients with depressed consciousness following craniocerebral trauma.[50] Most paramedics are very adept in using this rating tool. Although this assessment can be used to examine patients with severe insults, most patients with stroke will not be comatose. Thus, the Glasgow Coma Scale scores usually are close to normal. If a low Glasgow Coma Scale score is recorded, then the patient most likely has either a severe brain stem infarction secondary to basilar artery occlusion or a massive intracranial hemorrhage. This information is important prognostically, and it affects plans for acute care.

A limited neurological examination provides important information supporting the diagnosis of ischemic stroke.[51] Paramedics should not be expected to do a detailed neurological assessment. In addition to rating consciousness, they can look for language or motor impairments. Kothari et al[52] found that the presence of unilateral weakness of the face, unilateral arm weakness, or language/speech abnormalities had a high degree of specificity and sensitivity for stroke. These findings are detected easily, and paramedics can do the assessments reliably and quickly. Using just these findings, paramedics are likely to recognize TIA or stroke correctly in approximately 75% of cases.[47] However, a sizeable proportion of EMS personnel does not know the presentations of stroke or are unaware of the importance of the 3-hour treatment window.[53] Educational programs, such as those written by the American Heart Association and a group in Los Angeles, have been developed to speed the training of EMS personnel.[45,51] These programs allow paramedics to identify both ischemic and hemorrhagic stroke with a reasonably high degree of sensitivity and specificity.[47] Both community EMS systems and hospital emergency medical services should implement these programs.

MANAGEMENT BY EMERGENCY MEDICAL SERVICES

Although paramedics currently cannot give any specific therapy to treat stroke, they do provide the first critical steps in care. If necessary, they secure the patient's airway, provide breathing assistance, and stabilize the patient's cardiovascular status. Depending on the level of their training, they might be able to initiate other emergent care for complications. Some interventions might be given under the remote direction of an emergency medicine physician. For example, they can start intravenous access to give medication and can check a patient's blood glucose concentration. If hypoglycemia is present, a bolus of glucose and 50 mg of thiamine could be given. In some circumstances, paramedics can obtain an electrocardiogram or draw samples of blood that can be sent for analysis when the patient arrives at the hospital. In addition, paramedics can call the hospital to inform staff that a patient with a stroke is being transferred.[48] This message alerts the receiving hospital and gives it time to mobilize resources to rapidly treat the patient.

Patients with cognitive or language impairments may not be able to relate key parts of their history. In this situation, observers or relatives usually become major sources of relevant information. While the patient is being transferred to the hospital via an ambulance, observers usually come by private vehicle. Depending on the distances involved and traffic, they could arrive at the hospital several minutes or longer after the patient. As a result, physicians may not be able to obtain crucial aspects of the history, and critical time can be lost while waiting for relatives to arrive. Thus, paramedics should obtain critical components of the history that might influence treatment on arrival to the hospital. They should ask about the time of onset of stroke, which should be ascertained as closely as possible. Information about any recent medical illnesses, bleeding, trauma, surgery, or strokes also should be sought. They also can inquire about the use of medications—in particular, oral anticoagulants.

TRANSPORTATION TO AN EMERGENCY DEPARTMENT

The patient should be transported to the closest medical facility that has the capabilities to manage a patient with an acute ischemic stroke.[43,45,55] The institution should have physicians who have expertise in the diagnosis and treatment of stroke, facilities that image the brain on an urgent basis, and resources to treat stroke and its potential complications.[48,54] A hospital that cannot handle stroke should be bypassed. In particular, if the closest emergency department does not have the capacity to do a CT scan of the brain on an emergent basis 24 hours/day and 7 days/week, then the patient should be transported to another hospital that does have these capabilities.[55] Going to a local hospital that does not have the capacity to handle acute stroke greatly delays treatment. In one study, transfer to a local health center and then subsequent referral to another emergency department delayed care by approximately 8 hours.[9] This logistical bottleneck must be avoided. In some circumstances, governmental regulations or insurance company guidelines require that a patient go to the closest or a specific hospital. These requirements, which often are based on fiscal rather than clinical considerations, must be changed to expedite emergent medical care. Administrative obstacles to treating acute stroke must be overcome well in advance of an emergent situation.

The time spent in transport is particularly great for persons living in rural or sparsely populated areas.[33] Distances can be vast, and the availability of physicians and medical centers with expertise in stroke care can be limited. A potential approach would be to arrange air transport (fixed wing aircraft or helicopter) to a major medical center.[56] However, the logistics of arranging air transportation also are time consuming, and the time saved by air transport may be marginal, especially for distances less than 100 miles (160 km).

TELEMEDICINE

If the patient arrives at a small hospital that has CT but does not have physicians who commonly deal with stroke, strategies such as a telephone consultation or telemedicine might permit care.[57] Although this tactic has not been implemented extensively, modern technology permits a physician to evaluate a patient, including his or her CT scan, from a remote site and then give advice to the local physician. The National Institutes of Health Stroke Scale (NIHSS) can be assessed reliably using telemedicine, although less experienced examiners might take somewhat longer to perform the assessment.[58] A joint decision about emergent treatment, possibly including the administration of thrombolytic agents, could be made. Subsequently, air or land ambulance transfer could be organized while the patient is receiving the acute treatment. Thereafter, the patient could be moved to a larger hospital for subsequent care. Although these methods currently are expensive and largely untested, they hold great potential and their costs are likely to decline. Technical advances will increase the ease of their use. A major issue may be administrative. Hospital or physician fees and legal implications must be addressed. Telemedicine may be the only way to bring acute stroke care expertise to a sizeable segment of society that does not live in large metropolitan areas. It may be particularly critical for sparsely populated areas in countries such as the United States, Canada, and Australia.[59]

INITIAL STEPS IN EMERGENT CARE

Acute Stroke Treatment Centers

In the future, a limited number of institutions in a geographical region could be designated as acute stroke treatment centers. This designation would serve to denote hospitals that have the necessary expertise to provide modern treatment of persons with acute stroke. The program for certifying these medical facilities likely will require an accreditation process similar to that used to designate acute trauma centers in the United States and other countries. Such a process likely will be needed because many hospitals might not be able to offer a full range of services, including the intra-arterial administration of medications, that might be required to treat stroke. Regional EMS and ambulance services need this type of formal documentation to take patients to the appropriate institution and to bypass uncertified institutions. Pending such a program, however each institution should develop a contingency plan for treatment of patients with stroke.[60]

Stroke Teams

Organizations have developed specific time goals for key steps in the evaluation and treatment of patients with stroke.[45,48,47] (see Table 12–4.) These goals are most

Table 12–4. **Time Goals for Evaluation and Treatment of Patients with Acute Ischemic Stroke**

Step	Time from Arrival at Emergency Treatment Center (min)
Seen by a physician	10
Seen by physician from stroke team	15
Completion of computed tomography study	25
Interpretation of computed tomography study	45
Initiation of treatment	60

Adapted from the guidelines of the American Heart Association.[45,332]

Table 12–5. **Responsibilities of Individual Members of Acute Stroke Care Team**

Physicians
Do emergency assessment of overall condition
Initiate resuscitative measures, if necessary
Review history of event
Ascertain recent medical history for potential contraindications for specific treatments for stroke
Order diagnostic studies, including computed tomography
Perform medical and neurological examinations
Score severity of stroke using the National Institutes of Health Stroke Scale
Review the results of the diagnostic tests, including computed tomography
Decide about initiation of stroke-specific treatments, in particular thrombolytic therapy
Nurses
Perform regular assessments of the patient's vital signs
Perform regular assessments of the patient's neurological status
Prepare and administer ordered medications
Radiology and laboratory personnel
Perform diagnostic tests on an urgent basis
Pharmacy
Prepare ordered medications on an urgent basis

likely to be achieved by implementing a coordinated team approach. Comprehensive stroke services should include this emergency treatment group, which usually is designated as an *acute stroke care team*.[5,61] Emergency department triage personnel should notify the members of the acute stroke care team that a patient with a stroke is arriving or has arrived. If notification is given before the patient reaches the hospital, then the group can be assembled and be ready to evaluate the patient on arrival. The goal is for the members of the acute stroke care team to assemble within 10 minutes.[62]

Personnel

A physician should head the acute stroke care team. In most large hospitals, the leader will be either a neurologist or a neurosurgeon.[62] This physician likely will make primary decisions regarding acute medical treatment, including the administration of thrombolytic agents. Additional members of the team are other physicians (particularly emergency medicine specialists and radiologists), nurses, laboratory personnel, radiology technicians, and pharmacists.[48] Each member of the team has different responsibilities, but the common aim is to evaluate and treat the patient quickly. (see Table 12–4 and 12–5.) The goal is to begin treatment within 1 hour of the patient's arrival at the hospital.[3,7,48,63,64]

Emergency Diagnostic Tests

Necessary baseline diagnostic tests must be obtained quickly (Table 12–6). Blood samples must be examined in the laboratory promptly. For example, it can take up to 20 minutes to perform some coagulation tests. The CT scan must be readily available. In many circumstances, accessibility to CT is the primary reason that an evaluation is not done speedily.[7] Steps to overcome delays in obtaining a CT scan should be implemented in concert with the radiology department. The presence of a scanner within the confines of the emergency department speeds evaluation because delays associated with moving the patient to a remote site are avoided. In addition, urgent treatment and clinical assessments can be continued more easily in the emergency department than in a remotely located radiology suite. In particular, medications that might be needed

Table 12–6. **General Emergency Department Orders for a Patient with Acute Ischemic Stroke**

1. Absolute bed rest
2. Vital signs and blood pressure checked every 15 minutes
3. Temperature checked every 4 hours
4. Neurological checks every 15 minutes
5. Cardiac monitoring and pulse oximetry
6. Nothing given by mouth
7. Intravenous access with normal saline—slow infusion approximately 100 mL/hr
8. Diagnostic studies obtained on an urgent basis
   a. Computed tomography of brain without contrast
   b. Chest x-ray
   c. Electrocardiogram
   d. Complete blood count and platelet count
   e. Prothrombin time and activated partial thromboplastin time
   f. Blood glucose
   g. Serum chemistries, including electrolytes
9. Supplemental oxygen given if patient is hypoxic
10. Elevated temperature treated with antipyretic
11. If temperature is elevated, cultures of blood, urine, and sputum obtained

for treatment of acute complication are more readily available in the emergency department. The radiology service should be informed immediately that a patient with a stroke is expected to arrive in the emergency department or has arrived. Such notification is important. If the necessary technicians are not already in the hospital, then they should be summoned to come to the institution on a priority basis. The CT equipment must be made ready, and the patient with a suspected stroke must take immediate priority for the scan. Because a scan is obtained without contrast enhancement, it can be completed within a few minutes. The radiologist should be immediately available to interpret the results. Fortunately, several diagnostic tests can be done simultaneously. For example, laboratory specimens can be assayed while the patient is being examined or is having a CT study.

Clinical Evaluation

The goals of the physician's initial examination are to assess the patient's neurological status and to look for the presence of any other medical illnesses.[65] One of the aims is to determine whether ischemic stroke is the most likely explanation for the patient's symptoms. The differential diagnosis of acute ischemic stroke is not extensive. In addition to the most common alternative diagnoses that are included in Table 3–8, other conditions that rarely might be confused with stroke include dementia, multiple sclerosis, myasthenia gravis, or Bell's palsy.[66] Some of the alternative diagnoses in Table 3–8 are life-threatening in their own right. Others can be easily treated. For example, hypoglycemia in an insulin-dependent diabetic patient might imitate stroke. Acute hemorrhagic stroke also is confused with ischemic stroke. The two illnesses have a similar course, and both cause prominent focal neurological impairments. The nuances for distinguishing hemorrhagic and ischemic stroke are described in Chapter 3. Other aims of the examination are to screen for acute complications of stroke that need urgent treatment and to look for findings that could affect a decision to administer acute stroke-specific therapies, such as recombinant tissue plasminogen activator (rt-PA.). Although history and examination are discussed individually in this text, in reality, they usually are obtained simultaneously. For example, vital signs and consciousness are evaluated before much history is obtained or the patient's neurological examination is performed. They are then checked at regular intervals.

Vital Signs

CONSCIOUSNESS

The patient's level of consciousness is the first item assessed. A depression in consciousness (stupor or coma) means that the patient has a serious brain illness and is at high risk for compromise of the airway, respiratory problems, or cardiovascular complications. The acute level of consciousness also is a very strong predictor of outcome.[67] During the patient's time in the emergency department, consciousness should be rated repeatedly by nursing personnel to detect changes suggestive of neurological worsening. In general, patients do not develop stupor or coma within the first hours after ischemic stroke. The exception would be patients with occlusion of the basilar artery or the rare patient with bilateral hemispheric infarctions. The presence of stupor or coma within a few hours suggests that the patient had an intracranial hemorrhage, a metabolic disturbance such as hypoglycemia, or seizures secondary to the stroke. A decline in consciousness during the period of observation should prompt a search for an acute complication of stroke, including seizures, hydrocephalus, or a hemorrhagic transformation of the infarction. A decline also mandates the initiation of the emergent life-supporting interventions described subsequently.

AIRWAY, BREATHING, AND CIRCULATION

Other vital signs also provide important information about prognosis and the possible cause of stroke (Table 12–6). The patient's airway should be evaluated because a partial obstruction might be found in a patient with bulbar dysfunction. Disturbances in breathing also are seen among patients with severe strokes or metabolic disturbances. In particular, respiratory dysfunction occurs with lower brain stem infarctions.[68] Both the cardiac rate and rhythm are assessed clinically and with a cardiac monitoring system. Cardiac arrhythmias are a potential complication of acute stroke. The most common arrhythmias that might need to be treated are described subsequently. In addition, the presence of atrial fibrillation supports the diagnosis of cardioembolic stroke.

TEMPERATURE

Most patients with acute stroke do not have an elevated body temperature. Yet, in one series, 15% of patients developed a fever >38.3°C within the first 24 hours of stroke.[69] Another report found at least one episode of fever in 37.6% of 330 patients with recent stroke.[70] The presence of fever in the first hours after stroke is associated with poor neurological outcome.[69,71,72,111,112] Castillo et al[72] found that the 3-month mortality was 1% among patients who were normothermic after stroke and 15.8% among those who developed fever. A fever also is found among older patients with large infarctions.[70] An abnormal temperature also provides clues about the cause of stroke; for example, a fever raises concerns about the diagnosis of infective endocarditis. A fever also could be secondary to an infectious complication. Approximately two-thirds of acute fevers after stroke are secondary to infectious complications.[70] A "central" fever due to disruption of normal thermoregulatory mechanisms of the brain is uncommon after ischemic stroke. Hypothermia is extremely uncommon. It might be seen in an elderly patient, a person who was alone at the time of stroke and has had environmentally induced lowering of the body temperature, or a critically ill patient whose overall status is precarious.

BLOOD PRESSURE

The blood pressure should be checked regularly during the time the patient is in the emergency department. Arterial hypertension is common.[73] Both the systolic and the diastolic blood pressure values influence decisions about acute management. Trends in blood pressure readings are particularly important. For example, a continued rise in blood pressure levels is particularly bothersome, whereas an isolated elevation may be less concerning. An elevated blood pressure can represent the chronic illness that predisposed the patient to stroke. It also can represent a reaction to the acute neurological illness. Arterial hypertension may result from the stress of seizures, headache, pain, nausea, vomiting, or acute neurological symptoms, such as vertigo. Impaired baroreceptor sensitivity may explain hypertension and variability in blood pressure after stroke.[74] Fear or anxiety also can induce hypertension. Events such as emergent transportation in an ambulance and arrival in an emergency department can induce an emotional reaction and a rise in blood pressure. In addition, hypertension could be a physiological response to the acute ischemic process. This response may be needed to maintain adequate perfusion to the brain distal to an arterial occlusion. Increased intracranial pressure also may induce arterial hypertension in an effort to maintain adequate cerebral perfusion pressure. Fortunately, this effect is not as common during the first hours after ischemic stroke as it is following intracranial hemorrhage. Arterial hypertension during the first 24 hours predicts poor outcomes after stroke.[75] Sudden lowering of the blood pressure could induce neurological worsening. Fortunately, blood pressure usually declines spontaneously in most patients.

History

Several key questions need to be asked during the initial evaluation. A recommended sequence is outlined in Table 12–7. The sequence of questions is important because the answers greatly influence decisions about the administration of thrombolytic therapy or other acute interventions. For example, if the patient's stroke began more than 3 hours before arrival in the emergency department, thrombolytic therapy cannot be recommended.

Table 12–7. **Key Questions for the Initial Assessment of Patient with Acute Ischemic Stroke**

When did the symptoms of the stroke begin?
- Has there be any worsening or improvement?
- Were there any prior (warning) events in the past few days?
- Was recovery from those events complete?

What are the symptoms of the new stroke?

Has there been any recent (previous 6 weeks) history of a medical illness?
- Ischemic stroke?
- Other neurological illness?
- Myocardial infarction?
- Major bleeding event?
- Major operation?
- Major trauma?

Did any trauma occur with the new stroke?

What medications are being taken?
- Anticoagulants?
- Antiplatelet aggregating agents?
- Cardiac medications?
- Insulin?

ONSET OF STROKE

The time of onset needs to be defined as precisely as possible. Onset is considered as the time of the first neurological symptom, not the time of recent worsening. To help determine the time of onset, the patient and observers should be asked about the circumstances at the time of onset. Because stroke usually occurs suddenly, they may remember an event (television program, telephone call, etc.) that would give a fairly accurate time for the first symptom. Events that occur in public places probably are more likely to be timed accurately than are those that happen at home. The "embarrassment" of an event occurring in public and the presence of more observers heightens awareness of the onset. The patient and observers may disagree. In such a circumstance, the most prudent course is to assume that the most remote time of onset is correct. Many strokes occur during sleep and, because they usually are not painful, a patient will not be roused from sleep when the stroke occurs. Judging the time of onset becomes problematic in this situation. The most judicious approach is to assume that the stroke happened shortly after the patient went to sleep rather than a few minutes before awakening. Because elderly patients often have nocturia, asking about the presence of neurological problems at the time of rising to go to the toilet might permit a closer definition of the onset. The issue of awakening from sleep with new neurological problems could occur in the setting of a nap.

SYMPTOMS OF STROKE

The patient and observers should be queried about the symptoms of the stroke that are described in Chapter 3. The evolution of symptoms and the time course also are important. They should be asked about worsening or improvement in the symptoms or if the symptoms have been waxing and waning. A disturbance in consciousness, including seizures or syncope, which might confound the diagnosis of stroke, should be sought. The occurrence of headache or pain also can be reviewed. Although most strokes occur spontaneously, the patient should be asked about an inciting incident—such as coughing, sneezing, defecating, turning the head, or falling—that immediately preceded the vascular event.

RECENT MEDICAL HISTORY

The patient's past medical history greatly influences decisions about management. In particular, a history of recent events or serious concomitant illnesses could affect decisions for acute management. Patients with a history of diabetes mellitus should be asked about the use of insulin or oral hypoglycemic medications. Hypoglycemia can mimic acute ischemic stroke, and a bolus of glucose could cure the patient.[76] Patients with a recent myocardial infarction, ischemic stroke, major operation, major trauma, or major bleeding might not be eligible for treatment with thrombolytic agents or other medications that affect coagulation because of a high risk for bleeding complications.

RECENT USE OF MEDICATIONS

The recent use of medications should be surveyed. Most important questions should probe the recent use of anticoagulants and antiplatelet aggregating agents. Although these medications may not contraindicate treatment with thrombolytic agents or other acute stroke therapies, they prompt screening of the results with coagulation tests. The use of cardiovascular medications, in particular digoxin, diuretics, beta-blockers, calcium channel blocking agents and other antihypertensive agents, also influences decisions about ancillary care.

General Examination

The general examination focuses on the cardiovascular system. In particular, cardiac murmurs, cardiac arrhythmias, and cervical bruits should be noted. These findings could represent complications of the stroke or might provide hints about the likely cause of the cerebrovascular event. Auscultation of the chest also might detect evidence of pneumonia or pulmonary congestion. Distal edema of the limbs also points to cardiac failure. Evidence of embolization to other parts of the body (e.g, Roth's spots in the eyes, splinter hemorrhages in the fingers, absent pulses in the limbs, etc.) might explain the cause of stroke. The examination also can detect trauma, bleeding, a recent operative scar, or signs of organ failure that could influence acute management.

Neurological Examination

The goals of the neurological examination are to define the severity and types of impairments that give information about the location and the size of the ischemic stroke (see Chapter 3). The severity provides prognostic information and influences decisions about acute treatment. Patients with mild impairments generally have a good prognosis and might not need treatment with a potentially dangerous medication such as rt-PA. Patients with severe deficits generally have poor prognoses without treatment.[77–79] They also may have the greatest risk for complications of the stroke or its treatment. Several stroke scales, which are described in Chapter 3, are used to quantify neurological impairments.[80] The widely used NIHSS (see Table 3–11) has been validated, and its total score strongly predicts outcomes after stroke.[81–84] The NIHSS can be used to predict subsequent worsening. In general, a base score of 7 or greater predicts neurological deterioration, and most patients with a score of 7 or higher will not be normal at 48 hours after stroke.[85] All physicians actively involved in the urgent management of patients with acute ischemic stroke should become familiar with the NIHSS.

SUBTYPES OF ISCHEMIC STROKE

The emergent diagnosis of a subtype of ischemic stroke is not very accurate. Results of ancillary tests, which strongly influence subtype diagnosis, are not readily available when the patient is in the emergency department.[86] As a result, diagnoses often change after the patient is admitted to the hospital. Even stroke specialists have difficulty making subtype diagnoses and often change their opinions.[87,88] Thus, primary care or emergency medicine physicians should not be expected to diagnose the subtype. Fortunately, subtype diagnoses currently are not critical for decisions about acute care. The scales to differentiate hemorrhagic stroke from ischemic stroke have sensitivity and specificity too low to be useful in emergency situations.[89] These scales should not be used in lieu of brain imaging tests.

NEUROLOGICAL WORSENING

Neurological status should be assessed regularly during the patient's stay in the emergency department. Serial ratings of the NIHSS are an effective way to monitor for changes.[90] Neurological worsening can occur in up to 40% of patients.[85,91–93] Neurological worsening is usually seen among persons with moderate-to-severe strokes, younger persons, and those with posterior circulation strokes.[85,94,95] Neurological deterioration heightens urgency in initiating treatment of the stroke. Outcomes among patients with neurological deterioration are considerably poorer than among those who remain stable.[93,94] One study found that 35% of patients with a deteriorating stroke died, whereas only 8% of patients who did not worsen had fatal outcomes.[91] Neurological worsening during the first hours after stroke may be due to the development of medical or neurological complications, or it may be secondary to propagation of a thrombus, early recurrent embolization, or collateral failure.[71,96] Deterioration due to hemorrhagic transformation of an infarction, hydrocephalus, brain edema, or herniation usually occurs at later time periods. Thus, measures to maintain or improve perfusion or to protect ischemic neurons are key strategies in halting neurological worsening in the first hours after ischemic stroke.

SPONTANEOUS IMPROVEMENT

Conversely, the patient might improve spontaneously during the first hours after admission. Although complete recovery could be compatible with the diagnosis of TIA, the presence of neurological deficits when the patient is being evaluated in the emergency department excludes the diagnosis of TIA for all intents and purposes. However, spontaneous early and partial improvement does occur. Rothrock et al[97] noted that early improvement is seen in approximately one-fourth of patients evaluated during the first hours after stroke. These patients might not completely recover, but improvement could affect decisions about using emergent, stroke-specific therapies. The stroke subtype diagnosis did not affect the rate of early, spontaneous improvement.[97]

In many situations, neurologists likely will not be involved in providing emergent treatment of acute ischemic stroke. Primary care or emergency medicine physicians will make the key decisions, possibly using telephone or telemedicine consultation. Thus, the level of expertise of these physicians must be ascertained. Kothari et al[98] demonstrated that emergency physicians have a high degree of accuracy in diagnosing ischemic stroke and TIA. They correctly identified final diagnoses in 346 of 351 patients who were seen for possible TIA or stroke. This level of accuracy suggests that trained physicians, regardless of their specialty, can make reliable decisions about emergent treatment of stroke.

Diagnostic Studies

The results of the emergent diagnostic tests listed in Table 4–1 influence decisions for management in the emergency department. This battery of tests should be readily available to most emergency departments. Because of the critical nature of early treatment, these tests should be obtained on an urgent basis to meet the timeline outlined in Table 12–4.[17,99] Some tests are aimed at determining whether ischemic stroke is the likely explanation for the patient's neurological symptoms. Others are done to detect potentially serious medical or neurological complications or to assess for factors that could preclude urgent treatment with an agent such as rt-PA.

EMERGENT COMPUTED TOMOGRAPHIC IMAGING

The single most important diagnostic test is CT of the brain. The role of CT in evaluating patients with stroke is described in Chapter 4. Its results are critical to exclude intracranial bleeding. Although a normal CT scan obtained in the first hours after stroke is compatible with the diagnosis, patients with multilobar infarctions likely will have abnormal scans. These changes can be found within the first 3–6 hours (Figs. 12–1, through 12–3). The presence of visible infarction on CT is a predictor of unfavorable outcomes even when adjustments are made for the severity of stroke or the time.[100,478] In addition to providing prognostic information, the findings on the scan affect decisions about emergent treatment of the stroke—in particular, the administration of rt-PA.[101,478] Thus, agreement among physicians in interpreting relevant CT findings must be high. Unfortunately, physicians have only fair to moderate agreement in picking out the early CT changes that influence treatment

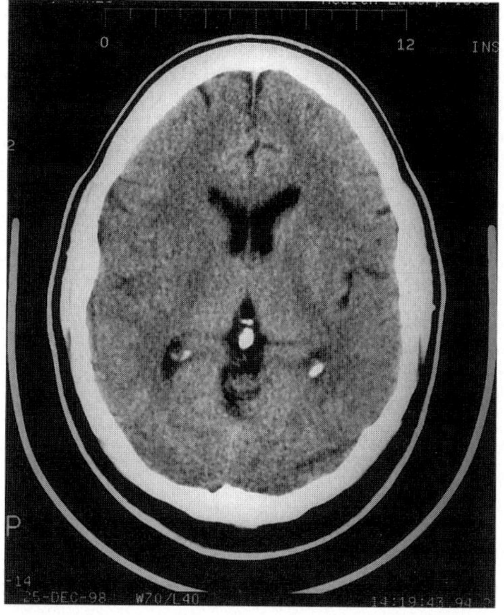

Figure 12–1. Computed tomogram obtained within 3 hours of onset of ischemic stroke of the right hemisphere. Obliteration of the Sylvian fissure, loss of the ribbon of the insular cortex, and hypodensity in the lenticuli striate territory are noted. These findings portend a major infarction and a high risk of bleeding following use of a thrombolytic agent.

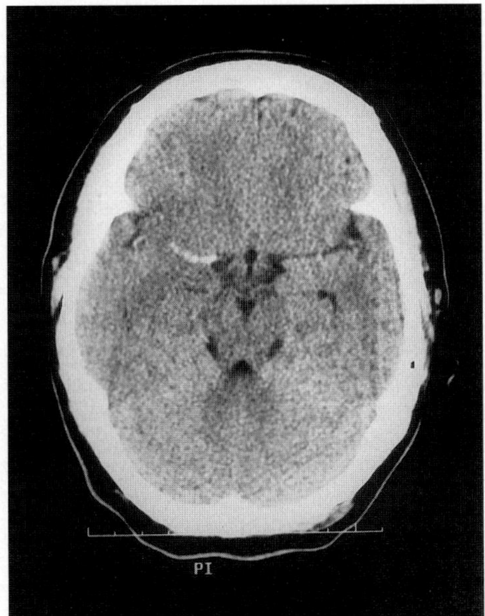

Figure 12–2. A computed tomographic scan of a patient with signs of a major right hemisphere infarction. An embolus (thrombus) in the right middle cerebral artery is present (dense artery sign).

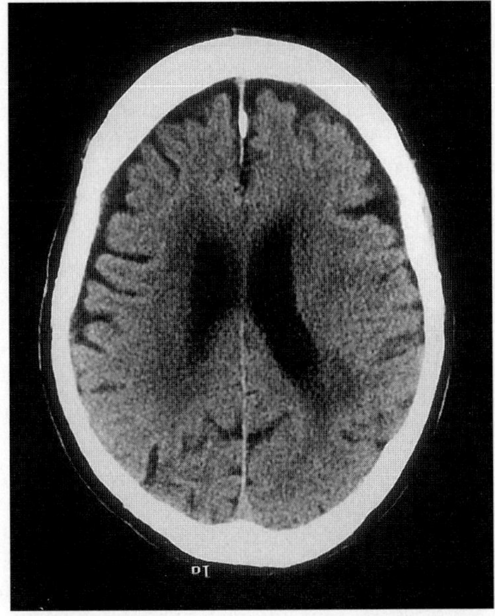

Figure 12–3. The computed tomographic scan shows an acute infarct in the left posterior frontal lobe (slight hypodensity and edema with sulcal effacement.

decisions.[102] In the future, brain imaging tests, such as positron emission tomography, magnetic resonance imaging, or single photon emission computed tomography, might supplant CT. They might shed light on tissue viability and perfusion and further improve the selection of patients to treat.[103]

OTHER DIAGNOSTIC TESTS

Some experts advocate the use of ancillary diagnostic tests, such as arteriography, carotid duplex, or echocardiography, to define the location and nature of the lesion leading to stroke before administering any therapy aimed at treating the acute neurological event.[104,478] Such an approach is necessary if an intervention such as intra-arterial thrombolytic therapy, angioplasty, or surgery is prescribed to treat a local arterial occlusion. These tests might not be needed for a treatment such as intravenous rt-PA or neuroprotective agents. In addition, these tests take time to complete, and delays in treatment may be counterproductive by lessening the chances for an effective response. Evidence is needed that the information from these tests can improve decisions about treatment. At present, the use of these tests as a prelude to acute treatment should not be mandated or recommended.

GENERAL EMERGENT TREATMENT

A model set of the initial orders for a patient being seen in an emergency department is included in Table 12–6. General emergent treatment is affected by the patient's neurological and medical status. For example, the priorities of emergent care of an alert patient with minimal deficits differ from those in an obtunded patient with findings of a multilobar infarction. Similarly, the occurrence of acute complications, such as cardiac arrhythmias or seizures, can take a priority in initial management.

ABCs of Life Support

Airway compromise can complicate major infarctions that affect the cerebral hemisphere, brain stem, or cerebellum.[105] In general, patients with stroke who require intubation have depressed levels of consciousness and scores of 10 or less on the Glasgow Coma Scale. The prognosis of patients who require endotracheal intubation generally is very poor; approximately one-half of them will be dead within 30 days of stroke.[105] Still, these patients need emergent protection of the airway.[20,99,106] Securing the airway avoids obstruction or aspiration pneumonia. In addition, elective intubation can assist in the management of severe brain edema or increased intracranial pressure.[107] Intubation in the emergency department also expedites subsequent acute care once a critically ill patient is admitted to an intensive care unit.

Measuring oxygen saturation concentrations with a pulse oximeter may influence decisions about the use of supplemental oxygen. Hypoxic patients and those with blood oxygen desaturation should be treated.[17,20,99] In contrast, non-hypoxic patients do not need to receive supplemental oxygen as part of emergent treatment.[108] Oxygen usually is given by nasal prongs or via a facemask. Follow-up examination of arterial blood gases may be needed to screen for hypercarbia or acidosis, particularly if the patient has evidence of lung disease.

Screening for pneumonia, sepsis, or a urinary tract infection is indicated if a patient is febrile.[72,109] Because fever may worsen an ischemic brain illness by increasing metabolic demands, antipyretics are indicated to lower body temperature.[17,97,110–112] Lowering an acutely elevated body temperature appears to improve the prognosis of patients with severe strokes.[113] Sustained fevers might mandate therapies, including cooling blankets, to lower the temperature.

Management of Acute Cardiovascular Complications

Cardiac arrhythmias and myocardial ischemia are potential complications that are more common among older persons and those with severe stroke or a history of heart disease.[114] Variabilities in heart rate can complicate infarctions of the cerebral hemisphere or the medulla.[115] Patients with infarction in the insular region have a particularly high rate of cardiovascular complications.[116,117] The relationship between a right or left hemisphere lesion and cardiac complications has not been resolved. Some authors detected a higher rate of cardiac abnormalities with right hemisphere lesions, and others noted more changes among persons with left hemisphere strokes.[116–118] The insular lesions apparently lead to disturbances in sympathetic and parasympathetic nervous system function that subsequently cause cardiac arrhythmias and sudden death.[115,119–121] The circadian rhythm of heart rate variability also is lost temporarily after ischemic stroke.[122] This loss may lead to cardiac arrhythmias.

Electrocardiographic changes secondary to stroke include ST depression prolongation of the QT interval, inverted T waves, and U waves.[117,120,123,124] (See Table 4–8.) Some of the electrocardiographic changes reflect myocardial ischemia and can be secondary to exacerbation of pre-existing ischemic heart disease.[120] Additional changes reflect direct myocardial damage from the release of catecholamines secondary to a rapid rise in intracranial pressure, altered sympathovagal tone, and the stress of the neurological event.[74,125] McDermott et al.[117] found depression of ST segments in 29% of patients within the first 5 days after stroke. They found more cardiac changes among patients with left hemisphere lesions. The presence of neurogenic ST changes among patients with coronary artery disease appears to lead to an increase in severe cardiovascular complications after stroke.[123]

Fortunately, life-threatening cardiac arrhythmias are relatively rare after ischemic stroke.[124,126] Still, monitoring of cardiac rate and rhythm is recommended during the stay in the emergency department.[20,99] Cardiac monitoring most commonly will detect atrial fibrillation, which likely is chronic and was present before the stroke.[126] Still, a sizeable proportion of patients have ventricular arrhythmias that mandate treatment. Sudden death can occur.[120] Medical interventions should be prescribed if serious arrhythmias develop.

Management of Arterial Hypertension

A sizeable proportion of patients have hypertension during the first hours after stroke.[73,127] In one series of 624 patients with acute ischemic stroke, 60% had elevated blood pressures during the first 24 hours.[73] In many cases, the blood pressure can be volatile and the elevations can be marked. Broderick et al[128] assessed early changes in blood pressure in 69 patients seen within minutes of onset of acute ischemic stroke. Twenty-four patients had a systolic blood pressure >160 mm Hg, but 23 of these patients had spontaneous declines in blood pressure levels during the next 90 minutes. The average decline was almost 30 mm Hg. In general, patients have a spontaneous decline in blood pressure of 20%–25% or greater during the first 24 hours.[129]

The urgency in managing arterial hypertension depends on the plans for initiation of therapies to treat the stroke itself. Sustained hypertension (systolic blood pressure >185 mm Hg or diastolic blood pressure >110 mm Hg) precludes the administration of thrombolytic agents.[19] The primary reason is that it increases the risk of hemorrhage after the administration of thrombolytic agents.[130] Presumably, the combination of thrombolysis and high perfusion pressure can worsen hemorrhagic changes. However, rapid control of blood pressure might permit subsequent treatment with rt-PA. Nevertheless, rapid lowering of the blood pressure may decrease perfusion to the brain.[71] The drop in cerebral perfusion pressure may aggravate ischemia because autoregulation is lost and blood flow to the brain is pressure-dependent during stroke.[131] Neurological worsening is a potential complication.

In general, the rule of thumb is to be cautious.[20,73,99,132,478] The goal is to lower blood pressure gradually during the first 24 hours using either oral or intravenous medications.[133] Intravenous medications do act more rapidly and might be indicated if the patient has evidence of concomitant acute myocardial ischemia, acute renal injury, or an arterial dissection. In addition, they may be needed to treat patients who might receive thrombolytic agents (Table 12–8).

Table 12–8. **Management of Arterial Hypertension: Emergent Treatment of Acute Ischemic Stroke**

- Emergent treatment with thrombolytic agents is possible
- Patient cannot be treated if systolic blood pressure >185 mm Hg or diastolic blood pressure >110 mm Hg
- If there is sufficient time to stabilize blood pressure, can attempt to lower to desired values
- Intravenous medications
  - Labetalol
    - Initial dose: 10–20 mg
    - Subsequent doses: 20–80 mg every 10–15 minutes
    - Stop if no response after 150 mg
- Emergent treatment with thrombolytic agents is not possible
- In general, use caution in lowering blood pressure
- Blood pressure usually declines spontaneously
- If myocardial ischemia, renal failure, dissection, or hemorrhagic transformation occur, more aggressive treatment would be needed
- If blood pressure levels that require emergent treatment are not known, treat if calculated mean blood pressure >130 mm Hg or systolic blood pressure >220 mm Hg
- Oral agents preferred
- Intravenous medications if emergent treatment is needed
  - Labetalol
    - Initial dose: 10–20 mg
    - Subsequent doses: 20–80 mg every 10–15 minutes
    - Alternative is to infuse 2–8 mg per minute and adjust dose
    - Stop if no response after 150 mg
  - Nitroprusside intravenous infusion
    - Usual initial dose: 0.5 mcg/kg/min
    - Dose range 0.5–10 µg/kg/min
- Monitor blood pressure carefully during treatment

The choice of medications to lower blood pressure should be made on an individual basis. Sublingual administration of the potent calcium channel blocker nifedipine should be avoided.[20,134] This agent causes deep and prolonged lowering of blood pressure than can be dangerous in an unstable patient with a recent acute ischemic stroke. Angiotensin converting enzyme inhibitors, calcium channel blockers and vasodilators have the potential to increase intracranial pressure among persons with severe strokes, while alpha- and beta-blockers have little effect on intracranial pressure.[135] Captopril should not be given if renal artery stenosis is suspected.[133] Nifedipine and the other dihydropyridine calcium channel blocking medications generally increase heart rate, whereas clonidine and the beta-blockers slow cardiac pulse.[133] These features can effect cardiac output and cerebral perfusion. In general, a short-acting medication should be used if a potent antihypertensive medication is needed. Although the vasodilators nitroglycerine and sodium nitroprusside are not ideal, their short duration of effect makes them the first choice for treatment of malignantly high blood pressure values.

Management of Blood Glucose and Fluids

HYPERGLYCEMIA

An elevated level of blood glucose can aggravate the effects of acute brain ischemia. Presumably, elevated blood glucose concentrations can stimulate formation of lactic acidosis in a hypoxic situation, and acidosis can worsen the brain injury. A high rate of poor outcomes is seen among persons with a history of diabetes mellitus or the presence of hyperglycemia at the time of stroke.[136] The volume of infarction also is higher in hyperglycemic patients. Weir et al[137] found that a blood glucose level >8 mmol/L forecasted a poor prognosis after stroke even when correcting for the patient's age, severity of neurological signs, and the presumed cause. Other studies show that hyperglycemia in the first hours is correlated with neurological worsening and poor outcomes, especially among patients with non-lacunar infarctions.[71,138] Still, the relationships between blood glucose levels and outcomes after stroke are complex. Patients with an increased level of glycosylated hemoglobin (a marker for sustained hyperglycemia) do not have poor outcomes when compared with those with normal levels.[139] In general, the level of blood glucose is correlated with severity of neurological impairment.[140] Elevated blood glucose levels can be a manifestation of a very severe stroke and, thus, hyperglycemia may not be a completely independent risk factor for a poor outcome. The information about hyperglycemia leading to an increased risk of hemorrhagic transformation of the infarction also is unclear. Bruno et al[138] found no relationship. Conversely, Broderick et al[141] concluded that hyperglycemia promotes hemorrhagic changes in the basal ganglia following early reperfusion.

Still, the desired level of blood glucose is not clear. Patients with moderately elevated levels should be treated cautiously. The blood glucose level among patients with marked hyperglycemia should be lowered to at least 300 mg/dL (16.63 mmol/L) or less.[110] Lowering the blood glucose level to normal values can be difficult in a short time, and the usefulness of such rapid lowering is problematic.

HYPOGLYCEMIA

Hypoglycemia can cause focal neurological signs that emulate acute ischemic stroke.[76] An immediate assessment of the blood glucose concentration should permit rapid initiation of glucose-containing fluids to correct hypoglycemia. Because hypoglycemia has a high potential for serious neurological injury, it would be reasonable to intravenously administer a bolus of glucose in conjunction with 50 mg of thiamine to any obtunded patient with signs of a potential stroke. Even if the patient subsequently is found to have hyperglycemia, the additional glucose should not have a major impact on outcome.

FLUID BALANCE

Fluids should be administered carefully during the first hours after stroke.[99,106] Many patients are elderly and have a history of severe heart disease. Thus, there is a fear that administration of a large volume of fluids can precipitate congestive heart failure. This fear is heightened because normal saline is the preferred fluid to be given intravenously. A hypo-osmolar fluid, such as 5% dextrose in water, is avoided because of the potential for aggravating brain edema, and the small amount of glucose probably is not needed for most patients. The potential for inducing congestive heart failure or pulmonary edema probably is quite low because most patients with stroke have some element of dehydration. In fact, expanding the vascular compartment by giving intravenous fluids could be helpful in improving cerebral perfusion.[110] Hypervolemic hemodilution has been used to treat acute brain ischemia. This regimen is discussed subsequently.

Management of Acute Neurological Complications

The most common causes of neurological worsening after stroke include brain edema, hyperthermia, hyperglycemia, or arterial hypertension or hypotension.[71,142] The acute treatment of hypertension, hypotension, hyperthermia, and hyperglycemia was discussed previously in this chapter. Brain edema and secondary increases in intracranial pressure are not common complications within the first few hours. Thus, management of brain edema occurs primarily after the patient is admitted to the hospital (see Chapter 13).

Seizures are a potential acute neurological complication. In one series, seizures at onset of stroke were reported in 50 of 1000 patients.[143] Seizures occur with either thrombotic or embolic infarctions that involve the cerebral cortex.[144,145] They are more common with infarctions that develop hemorrhagic transformation. Early seizures are not benign; they can worsen acute neurological injury and are correlated with poor outcome. In part, these outcomes are associated with the size and the severity of the cortical injury.

Although no study has tested the utility of anticonvulsant treatment in the setting of acute ischemic stroke, anticonvulsants are recommended if early seizures occur.[20] (see Table 12–9.) This recommendation is based on the assumption that seizures can exacerbate brain injury and because of the evidence for the general usefulness of anticonvulsants in treatment of seizures complicating other acute neurological illnesses. Intravenous administration of a short-acting anticonvulsant (diazepam or lorazepam) followed by phenytoin or fosphenytoin usually is recommended to treat patients who are having recurrent seizures. Some anticonvulsants might have neuroprotective effects; however, phenytoin can be associated with serious cardiac

Table 12–9. **Management of Seizures: Emergent Treatment of Acute Ischemic Stroke**

Patient has not had seizures as part of the acute ischemic stroke
Do not start prophylactic anticonvulsants
Patient has had seizures with stroke but currently is not having seizures
If patient can swallow, give oral medication
Phenytoin
Carbamazepine
Valproate
If patient cannot take medications intravenously or by nasogastric tube
Patient is having frequent seizures or status epilepticus
Intravenous therapy
Lorazepam: 0.1 mg/kg (usual dose: 2 mg), or Diazepam: 0.15–0.25 mg/kg (usual dose: 5–10 mg), or Phenytoin: 15–20 mg/kg (usual dose: 1000 mg), or Fosphenytoin: 10–20 mg/kg (usual dose: 1000 mg), or Phenobarbital: 20 mg/kg (usual dose: 120–600 mg)
Start maintenance therapy
Phenytoin
Carbamazepine
Valproate

complications when it is administered intravenously. In particular, patients with pre-existing ischemic heart disease appear to be at high risk of arrhythmias secondary to phenytoin. Thus, the agent should be given slowly—at a rate slower than 50 mg/min. Fosphenytoin is more water soluble and appears to have less cardiac toxicity than phenytoin. Intravenous valproate or phenobarbital could be alternatives. Oral medications, including elixirs administered via a nasogastric tube, could be given to patients who have a history of seizure at the onset of stroke but who are not having seizures at the time of evaluation. Oral medications should be given rapidly to achieve therapeutic concentrations as soon as possible. Prophylactic administration of anticonvulsants is not recommended for treatment of patients who have not had seizures.[20]

Patients with seizures at the time of stroke were not enrolled in the trials that tested thrombolytic therapy because of concern regarding post-ictal paralysis imitating stroke. Still, the history of a seizure with acute stroke should not automatically preclude treatment with rt-PA. If the patient had a seizure at the time of an embolic event and still has neurological impairments during the clinical evaluation, then the patient could be considered for treatment with rt-PA.

EMERGENT TREATMENT OF ACUTE ISCHEMIC STROKE ITSELF

Until recently, management of stroke focused on general supportive therapies to prevent or treat acute or subacute neurological or medical complications.[20,99] Although these components of care are critical in improving outcomes, they are not aimed at directly treating the stroke itself. As late as 1995, no emergent treatment had been shown to be conclusively effective in improving neurological outcomes. Despite the widespread use of emergent anticoagulant treatment, this therapy had not been established as either effective or safe. Guidelines written in 1994 concluded that the value of anticoagulation was uncertain.[20]

Since then, intravenous administration of rt-PA has been proven as effective in improving outcomes, provided it is given within 3 hours of stroke to carefully selected patients.[24] Still, this therapy has serious limitations, and most patients with stroke cannot be treated with rt-PA. Additional therapies are needed to improve outcomes.

In general, interventions aimed at limiting the neurological consequences of ischemic stroke are categorized as those that improve or restore blood flow to the brain and those that provide some neuroprotective benefit (Table 12–10). The therapies that improve cerebral blood flow include thrombolytic agents that speed lysis of the intra-arterial thrombus as well as anticoagulants and antiplatelet aggregating agents that halt propagation of the thrombus or early recurrent embolism. In addition, surgical removal of the clot, administration of vasodilators or vasopressors that alter the hemodynamic state and rheological agents that affect viscosity may improve cerebral perfusion. Several neuroprotective therapies aim to limit the metabolic or cellular consequences of acute brain ischemia by a number of strategies.

Table 12–10. **Interventions for Treatment of Acute Ischemic Stroke**

Restore or improve blood flow—perfusion
- Thrombolytic agents
  - Intra-arterial administration
  - Intravenous administration
- Fibrinogen depleting agent
- Anticoagulants
- Antiplatelet aggregating agents
- Volume expansion and hemodilution
- Carotid endarterectomy
- Embolectomy
- Endovascular procedures

Neuroprotection
- Antagonists to excitatory amino acids, including glutamate
- Calcium channel blocking agents
- Free radical antagonists
- Metabolic depressants
- Membrane stabilizing agents
- Anti-inflammatory agents
- Hyperbaric oxygen

THROMBOLYTIC THERAPY

Pharmacology and Rationale

Natural fibrinolysins are released by the endothelium to halt the propagation of a thrombus and, thus, maintain normal hemostasis. These lysins also lead to a breakup of a thromboembolic arterial occlusion; however, their effects may not produce spontaneous recanalization in sufficient time to permit reperfusion and salvage ischemic but not necrotic brain tissue. Thrombolytic agents thus speed the conversion of inactive plasminogen to plasmin, the potent natural fibrinolytic substance.[146,147] Several different thrombolytic agents have been developed (Table 12–11). Streptokinase and urokinase were the first agents used to treat patients with vascular occlusions. These compounds have a systemic fibrinolytic effect and are associated with bleeding. Because of the high rate of bleeding complications, more fibrin-specific thrombolytic agents were created, including alteplase (rt-PA), reteplase, prourokinase, and anistreplase (anisolyated plasminogen streptokinase activator complex).[146] Staphylokinase is another thrombolytic agent that has high specificity for fibrin, and it appears not to prolong bleeding time to the same degree as rt-PA.[148–150]

Streptokinase is produced by group A beta-hemolytic streptococci. Urokinase is a direct plasminogen activator secreted from human kidney cells. Single-chain urokinase plasminogen activator (prourokinase) is a precursor of urokinase. Prourokinase may have higher fibrin specificity than urokinase, but the two agents appear to have equal thrombolytic effects.[151,152] Reteplase is a single-chain tissue plasminogen activator including the kringle 2-protease domains of tissue plasminogen activator.[153] Alteplase (rt-PA) is a double-chain compound developed by recombinant genetic techniques. It affects the lysine sites of plasminogen to increase binding to fibrin and controls the inhibition of plasmin by alpha-2-antiplasmin.[154,155] Each agent can be given either intravenously or intra-arterially. Most agents are given with an initial bolus dose followed by a continuous intravenous infusion administered over approximately 1 hour. Reteplase has a longer half-life that rt-PA and is administered in two bolus doses approximately 30 minutes apart.[156] Its effects are equal to the rt-PA regimen that includes a relatively larger bolus followed by an infusion given over approximately 1 hour. Twenty units of reteplase have the same thrombolytic effect as approximately 100 units of rt-PA.[156] These thrombolytic agents have been used to treat acute arterial occlusions of the coronary arteries or pulmonary embolism. They also have been used to treat patients with ischemic stroke.

A Japanese study evaluated changes in coagulation and fibrinolysis following intra-arterial administration of a thrombolytic agent in 24 patients.[157] They found elevations in fibrin degradation products, D-dimer, and plasmin inhibitor complex as well as declines in alpha-2-plasmin inhibitor. It appears that rt-PA can activate coagulation and the formation of fibrin and that these effects are not influenced by heparin.[158] Both rt-PA and streptokinase increase pro-thrombin fragment 1 + 2 after administration, a finding that suggests that these agents stimulate generation of thrombin and increase its activity after treatment.[159–163] Both rt-PA and reteplase have interactions that may alter the activity of heparin.[153] Huang et al[164] found that fibrinolytic agents affect platelet adhesion probably by affecting von Willebrand factor and binding at the glycoprotein IIb/IIIa receptor.[163–167] The effects on platelets portend a potentially useful role for ancillary treatment with aspirin or a blocker of the glycoprotein IIb/IIIa receptor, such as abciximab, following use of a

Table 12–11. **Thrombolytic Medications**

Streptokinase
Urokinase
Alteplase (recombinant tissue plasminogen activator)
Reteplase
Prourokinase
Anistreplase (anisoylated plasminogen streptokinase activator complex)
Staphylokinase

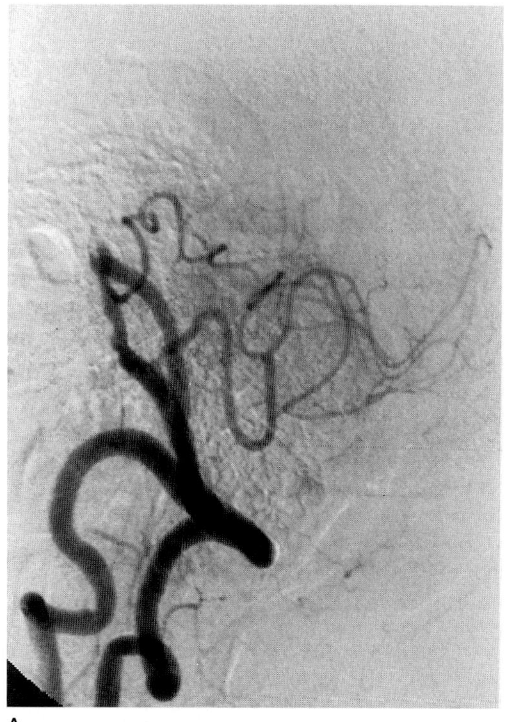

A

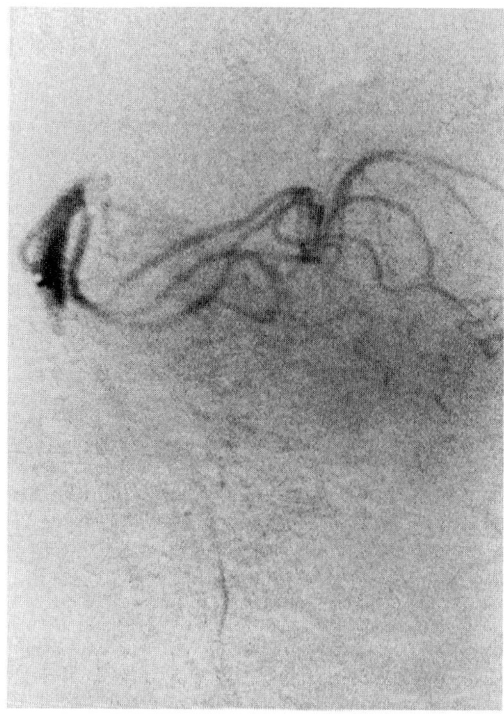

B

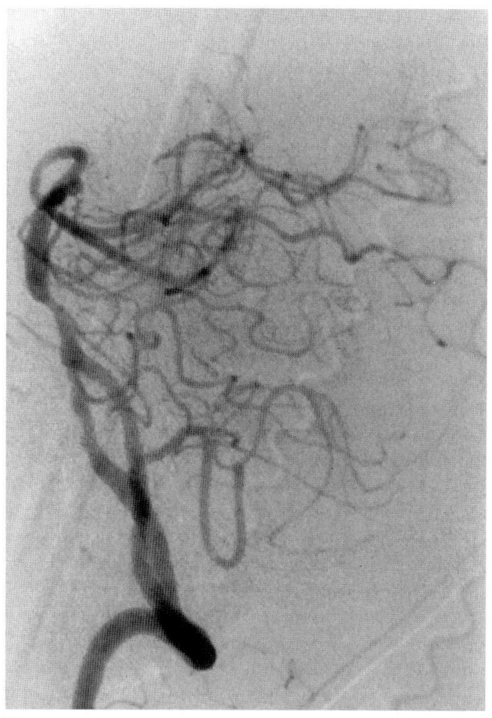

C

Figure 12–4. A series of lateral vertebral arteriograms using subtraction techniques evaluates a basilar artery thrombosis. (A) The proximal basilar artery is demonstrated as occluded just distal to the junction of the vertebral arteries. (B) A fine catheter has been inserted through the basilar thrombus, and another injection of contrast visualizes the distal basilar artery and its branches. (C) A third arteriogram is performed after intra-arterial administration of urokinase. The basilar artery is patent, and flow to distal branches is seen. A residual stenosis of the mid-section of the basilar artery is present. (Courtesy of AJ Fox, MD, London Health Science Center, London, Ontario.)

thrombolytic agent.[168] In contrast, adjunctive treatment with antiplatelet aggregating agents may increase the problem of bleeding. Smooth muscle cell proliferation also can be promoted by rt-PA.[169]

Ancrod is a defibrinogenating enzyme that is a derivative of snake venom. Ancrod cleaves to only A-fibrinopeptides of the fibrin clot.[170] It rapidly lowers blood levels of fibrinogen and, thus, halts propagation of a thrombus.[171] Ancrod increases blood levels of fibrin degradation products and D-dimer.[172] It has been used as an alternative to heparin for treatment of high-risk patients having major operations.[173]

Experimental and clinical studies demonstrate that thrombolytic agents promote recanalization of intracranial arteries and reduce the size of brain infarctions.[174,175] Animal studies show that early administration of rt-PA can reduce the volume of infarction.[176] In addition, experimental studies demonstrate that rt-PA alters the vascular immunoreactivity of inflammatory adhesion molecules in the setting of acute ischemic stroke.[177] This action may produce a neuroprotective effect. Kilic et al[178] found that rt-PA could increase blood flow, decrease infarct volume, decrease brain edema, and increase neurological recovery in an experimental stroke model. They found no evidence of neurotoxicity.

Ancillary tests have shown that intra-arterial thrombolysis can reopen occluded arteries (Fig. 12–4). Using magnetic resonance angiography to monitor responses, Ohue et al[179] demonstrated arterial recanalization in 4 of 6 treated patients. Sequential transcranial Doppler ultrasonography also can be used to monitor flow-related responses to intravenous or intra-arterial thrombolytic treatment.[180,478] Rapid recanalization can be detected. Diffusion- and perfusion-weighted magnetic resonance imaging also has been used to monitor changes in the brain's response to intra-arterial rt-PA.[181] Using diffusion- and perfusion- MRI, Marks et al[182] found that intravenously administered rt-PA improves early reperfusion after ischemic stroke. Using positron emission tomography (PET) studies, Heiss et al[183] found that rt-PA preserves critically ischemic tissue through early reperfusion. Based on single photon emission computed tomography (SPECT), Grotta and Alexandrov[184] and Sasaki et al[185] demonstrated that rt-PA could reduce the size of a hypoperfusion defected following stroke. Another study using SPECT could not find a change in perfusion defect following streptokinase treatment.[186] Baird et al[187] also concluded that SPECT could help select patients who could be treated with thrombolytic agents. They noted that SPECT changes of reperfusion were associated with decreased disability and death and improved neurological outcomes.

Safety

INTRACRANIAL HEMORRHAGE FOLLOWING TREATMENT OF MYOCARDIAL INFARCTION

Brain hemorrhage is a potentially fatal complication of thrombolytic therapy for treating either ischemic stroke or myocardial infarction (Table 12–12). Hillegass et al[188] found the risk of intracranial bleeding to be 0.07% among patients who received streptokinase for treatment of myocardial infarction. Gurwitz et al[189] found that the risk of intracranial hemorrhage was approximately 0.95%. A survey of thrombolytic treatment of acute myocardial infarction reported a rate of complicating intracranial hemorrhage of approximately 0.46%–0.88%.[190] Hemorrhages following thrombolytic therapy are severe, with

Table 12–12. **Complications of Thrombolytic Medications**

Intracranial hemorrhage
Symptomatic hemorrhagic transformation of infarction
Asymptomatic hemorrhagic transformation of infarction
Subarachnoid, intraventricular, or intracerebral hemorrhage
Systemic hemorrhage
Cardiac rupture
Allergic reactions, including anaphylaxis

rapid evolution of hematoma formation. Bleeding can occur in the brain, ventricles, subarachnoid space, or subdural space. Computed tomography often will show multiple fluid levels of blood.[191] Intracranial hemorrhage following thrombolytic treatment for acute myocardial infarction is more common among persons older than 65, women, African Americans, diabetics, hypertensives, those weighing less than 70 kg, those with a history of stroke, and patients receiving anticoagulants as adjunctive treatment.[189,192,193] Gore et al[194] correlated the likelihood of intracranial hemorrhage following thrombolysis with the dose of rt-PA; the risk was 1.3% with a 150 mg dose and 0.4% with a dose of 100 mg. Longstreth et al[195] calculated that thrombolytic therapy would increase the risk of brain hemorrhage following myocardial infarction by a factor of 3.6. These findings conclusively show that intracranial bleeding is a potential complication of treatment with thrombolytic therapy. Although the risk is small following treatment of myocardial infarction, it is a potentially fatal adverse complication. Because of this concern about brain hemorrhage, thrombolytic therapy has not been recommended to treat myocardial ischemia among patients who have a history of stroke.

INTRACRANIAL HEMORRHAGE FOLLOWING TREATMENT OF ISCHEMIC STROKE

Not surprisingly, the risk of major hemorrhage following treatment for acute ischemic stroke is considerable.[196] (See Table 12–13.) Jaillard et al[197] evaluated the risk of hemorrhagic transformation among patients treated with streptokinase or placebo. Asymptomatic hemorrhagic transformation occurred among patients receiving either placebo or the thrombolytic agent, but bleeding associated with neurological worsening was 10 times more common among the patients given streptokinase. The risk of symptomatic hemorrhagic transformation following thrombolytic treatment is more common among elderly persons and those who have atrial fibrillation, diabetes mellitus, a decreased level of consciousness, or severe abnormalities on CT.[196,197] The National Institute of Neurological Disorders and Stroke (NINDS) investigators found that the risk of brain hemorrhage following thrombolytic therapy for treatment of stroke was increased with age, the severity of neurological impairments, or the presence of edema on CT.[198] In particular, patients with a NIHSS score >20 had the highest risk. A 16% rate of hemorrhage was noted in this group. The dose of thrombolytic agent and the presence of an elevated diastolic blood pressure also are markers of an increased risk.[199]

In addition to CT, other tests might be used to predict the risk of bleeding following the administration of a thrombolytic agent. One study using SPECT showed that a marked reduction of baseline cerebral blood flow was associated with an increased risk of hemorrhage following treatment.[200] Trouillas et al[201] correlated the risk of bleeding with the presence of elevated fibrin degradation products in the blood following treatment. Demchuk et al[202] reported that patients with a baseline serum glucose >11.1 mmol/L (200 mg/dL) had an approximately 25% risk of symptomatic intracranial hemorrhage. Some of this high risk may be associated with the severity of neurological impairments among patients with hyperglycemia.

CARDIAC RUPTURE

Cardiac rupture is a potential complication of delayed thrombolytic treatment for patients who have a stroke following an acute myocardial infarction. The risk of fatal cardiac rupture following thrombolytic treatment for acute myocardial ischemia is approximately 1.7%. It is highest in women and persons older than 70.[203] Kasner et al[204] described 3 cases who received rt-PA for acute stroke and subsequently developed hemopericardium and cardiac tamponade. All of the patients had indistinct or mild symptoms that were retrospectively recognized as compatible with a subacute myocardial infarction. The risk of cardiac rupture increases when rt-PA is given more than 12 hours after the cardiac event.[205] However, Katzan et al[206] have safely administered intra-arterial thrombolytic

Table 12–13. **Symptomatic Intracranial Bleeding: Clinical Trials of Thromolytic Agents—Acute Ischemic Stroke**

Agent and Trial	Treatment Events/Patients	%	Control Events/Patients	%
Streptokinase				
MAST-E[237]	33/156	21.2	4/154	2.6
MAST-I*[239]				
Without aspirin	10/157	6	1/156	0.6
With aspirin	15/156	10		
ASK[241]				
< 3 hours	4/41	9.8	0/29	0
3–4 hours	19/133	14.3	5/137	3.6
Alteplase				
ECASS-I[243]	62/313	19.8	20/307	6.5
NINDS[24]	20/312	6.6	2/312	0.6
ECASS-II[250]				
Total	33/407	8.1	3/386	0.8
< 3 hours	6/81	7	1/77	1
3–6 hours	27/326	8.3	2/309	0.6
ATLANTIS[251]	21/307	6.7	4/306	1.3
Prourokinase				
PROACT—II† [229]	11/108	10.	1/54	2

*MAST included four treatment arms: control, aspirin, streptokinase, and both streptokinase and aspirin.

†In the PROACT—II study, enrolled patients received heparin in addition to prourokinase (treatment) or heparin alone (control).

MAST-E = Multicentre Acute Stroke Trial Europe
MAST-I = Multicentre Acute Stroke Trial Italy
ASK = Australian Streptokinase Trial
ECASS = European Cooperative Acute Stroke Study
NINDS = National Institute of Neurological Disorders and Stroke
ATLANTIS = Alteplase Thrombolysis for Acute Noninterventional Therapy in Ischemic Stroke
PROACT = Prolyse in Acute Cerebral Thromboembolism

agents within 2–13 days following open heart surgery.

ALLERGIC REACTIONS

Anaphylaxis is a rare complication of rt-PA.[207,208] Symptoms include respiratory distress and marked edema of the mouth and tongue.[479] Elevated IgE antibodies to rt-PA are the likely explanation of the allergic reaction. Allergic reactions also can complicate treatment with streptokinase.[209]

Results of Clinical Trials in Treatment of Acute Ischemic Stroke

Thrombolytic therapy was tested in clinical trials in the 1960s and early 1970s. The trials were abandoned because of a high rate of complications, particularly involving intracranial hemorrhage that followed treatment. These studies treated patients up to 24 hours after the onset of stroke. Thus, therapy was given long after there was any potential for therapeutic efficacy.

Furthermore, the studies were performed before the development of CT, and it is likely that some patients with de novo brain hemorrhage were given thrombolytic agents, a disastrous scenario. With development of modern brain imaging studies, the creation of new, more selective thrombolytic agents and the success of thrombolytic therapy in treating acute myocardial ischemia in the 1980s, interest was rekindled about the use of these medications for treating stroke. The cardiac studies demonstrated declines in mortality from myocardial infarction. Responses were of greatest benefit when the agent was administered within 2 hours.[210] These results imply a similar scenario for stroke. Both intra-arterial and intravenous administration of thrombolytic agents can be used to treat stroke.

INTRA-ARTERIAL THROMBOLYSIS

Intra-arterial administration has several potential advantages. It involves the administration of a relatively larger dose of agent directly to the site of the arterial thrombus. Because the dose is concentrated, intra-arterial therapy might be more effective than intravenous administration in dissolving large clots in major intracranial arteries.[211] Furthermore, embedding the tip of the catheter in the clot can expedite lysis.[212] Mechanical devices or suction also could be applied directly to the thrombus. Thus, intra-arterial thrombolysis can be combined with physical measures that help to disrupt the clot.[213,214] One review concluded that recanalization could be achieved in 21%–71% of patients who received intra-arterial thrombolysis.[215] The likelihood of recanalization was greatest among patients who had occlusions of small- to medium- caliber arteries, such as the middle cerebral artery or its branches. Because the agent is administered only to patients with intra-arterial occlusions, a concomitant arteriogram may exclude patients from treatment. Because the dose can be smaller, the risk of major bleeding may be less than with intravenous treatment. Intra-arterial thrombolysis has limitations, however. Issues such as technical advances and the experience of the physicians greatly affect the usefulness of intra-arterial therapy.[216]

Sasaki et al[217] found that either rt-PA or *urokinase* could be used to achieve recanalization. Urbach et al[218] administered urokinase to 12 patients with embolic occlusions of the distal internal carotid artery and proximal portions of the anterior cerebral and middle cerebral arteries. They noted that only 4 patients had reasonable outcomes and concluded that the chances of recanalization were poor. In a small, uncontrolled trial testing intra-arterial thrombolysis in 33 patients with very severe strokes secondary to occlusion of the internal carotid artery, recanalization was achieved in 8 patients, and 4 of these had good outcomes.[219] Gonner et al[220] administered thrombolytic agents to 43 patients with a variety of arterial occlusions; 9 had very good outcomes and 17 had residual, nondisabling deficits. Another study examined the usefulness of thrombolytic therapy among 31 patients with occlusions of the internal carotid artery.[221] They found that treatment was not successful. Jahan et al[222] gave urokinase intra-arterially to 26 patients within 6 hours of acute stroke and achieved partial or complete recanalization in 11. Seven patients with some evidence of recanalization had good outcomes. They noted that success was unlikely if a patient had an occlusion at the bifurcation of the internal carotid artery. Schumacher et al[223] gave local intra-arterial fibrinolysis to 5 patients with severe thromboembolic stroke who had no occlusion found by arteriography. The investigators presumed that angiographically occult occlusions of perforating branches were the cause of the ischemic symptoms. The patients did well. Suarez et al[224] administered heparin and intra-arterial urokinase to 54 patients with acute ischemic stroke. Improvements were noted in 43% of patients, and 17% of the patients had hemorrhagic changes on CT done after treatment. Although the authors considered intra-arterial therapy to be promising, they also noted that intra-arterial treatment is expensive and that it delays the initiation of thrombolysis. Gruber et al[480] reported success in giving intra-arterial rt-PA (0.11 mg/kg) to a child with a cardioembolic stroke.

Based on a small study of 34 patients with middle cerebral artery occlusions treated with urokinase, Lanzieri et al[225] concluded that emergent intra-arterial thrombolysis was cost effective. Schumacher et al[226] concluded that advanced age is not a contraindication for intra-arterial thrombolytic therapy.

INTRA-ARTERIAL ADMINISTRATION OF PROUROKINASE

Prourokinase has been used to treat patients with acute myocardial infarction and to reopen occluded coronary arteries.[227] Research has progressed to the treatment of stroke. A phase II, randomized trial of recombinant *prourokinase* showed that the agent in combination with heparin could achieve a high rate of recanalization.[228] However, the use of high doses of adjuvant heparin was associated with a heightened risk of intracranial bleeding. A subsequent trial that tested 9 mg prourokinase plus heparin or heparin alone in patients with occlusions in the middle cerebral artery found that the prourokinase improved outcomes even when the therapy was started up to 6 hours after stroke.[229] (see Table 12–14

Table 12–14. **Mortality: Clinical Trials of Thrombolytic Agents—Acute Ischemic Stroke**

Agent and Trial	Treatment Events/Patients	%	Control Events/Patients	%
Streptokinase				
MAST-E[237]				
10 days	53/156	34.0	28/154	18.2
3 months	70/156	44.9	53/154	34.4
MAST–I*[239]				
Without aspirin				
10 days	30/157	19	20/156	13
6 months	44/157	28	45/156	29
With aspirin				
10 days	53/156	34		
6 months	68/156	44		
ASK[241]				
< 3 hours	11/41	26.8	7/29	24.1
3–4 hours	52/133	39.1	27/137	19.7
Alteplase				
ECASS—I[243]	69/313	22.4	48/307	15.4
NINDS (90 days)	54/312	17.3	64/312	20.5
ECASS—II[250]	43/409	10.5	42/391	10.7
ATLANTIS[251]				
30 Days	23/307	7.6	13/306	4.2
90 Days	33/307	10.9	21/306	6.9
Prourokinase				
PROACT—II† [229]	30/121	25	16/59	27

*MAST included four treatment arms: control, aspirin, streptokinase, and both streptokinase and aspirin.

†In the PROACT—II study, enrolled patients received heparin in addition to prourokinase (treatment) or heparin alone (control).

Table 12–15. **Favorable Outcome Rates: Clinical Trials of Thrombolytic Agents—Acute Ischemic Stroke**

Agent and Trial	Treatment Events/Patients	%	Control Events/Patients	%
Streptokinase				
MAST—E[237]	32/156	20.5	28/154	19.2
MAST—I*[239]				
Without aspirin	60/157	38	50/154	32
With aspirin	57/156	37		
ASK[241]				
< 3 hours	27/41	65.9	14/29	48.3
3–4 hours	63/133	47.4	68/137	49.6
Alteplase				
NINDS[24]	121/312	39	81/312	26
ECASS—II†[250]	165/409	40.3	143/391	36.6
ATLANTIS[251]	128/307	41.7	124/306	40.5
Prourokinase				
PROACT—II‡[229]	31/121	26	10/59	17

*MAST—I included four treatment arms—control, aspirin, streptokinase, and both streptokinase and aspirin.

†ECASS—I data are not included because numbers of patients with favorable outcomes were not listed.

‡In the PROACT—II study, enrolled patients received heparin in addition to prourokinase (treatment) or heparin alone (control)

and Table 12–15.) The rates of favorable outcomes were 40% among the 121 patients who received prourokinase and 25% among the 59 control patients. Symptomatic intracranial hemorrhage developed in 10% of patients treated with prourokinase and in 2% of controls.

INTRA-ARTERIAL THROMBOLYSIS IN TREATMENT OF VERTEBROBASILAR ARTERIAL OCCLUSIONS

Several groups evaluated the potential value of intra-arterial thrombolytic therapy in treating occlusions in the vertebrobasilar circulation.[230–231] Huemer et al[231] achieved recanalization in 10 of 16 patients with acute basilar artery thrombosis; 5 of these patients survived. Brandt et al[233] reported that recanalization of the basilar artery with the use of thrombolytic agents could lessen mortality. In a series of 51 cases, deaths occurred in 12 of 26 patients who had recanalization and 23 of 25 who did not have reopening of the artery. Intra-arterial urokinase was administered to 9 patients within 2–13 hours after acute basilar arterial occlusion.[234] Recanalization was achieved in 7 patients, and 5 of them recovered. Levy et al[235] examined the survival rates among patients who received intra-arterial thrombolytic therapy for treatment of acute vertebrobasilar occlusions and concluded that mortality was increased by a factor of 2.34 or 1.95 if recanalization was not achieved.

INTRAVENOUS THROMBOLYSIS

Based on the results of preliminary studies, a meta-analysis in 1992 concluded that thrombolytic therapy could reduce death and disability without causing an increased risk of hemorrhagic infarction.[236] At approximately the same time, several large trials were launched to test the usefulness of early intravenous administration of thrombolytic agents. Both streptokinase and rt-PA were tested.

STREPTOKINASE

The Multicenter Acute Stroke Trial—Europe was a randomized, placebo-controlled trial evaluating the use of intravenous streptokinase given within 6 hours of acute ischemic stroke.[237] (See Tables 12–14 and 12–15.) The trial was halted prematurely because of an unacceptably high rate of mortality within 10 days of stroke among the patients treated with streptokinase. Most deaths were secondary to intracranial bleeding. The risk of symptomatic hemorrhage was 21.2% among 156 patients treated with streptokinase and 2.6% among 154 patients given placebo. Hommel et al[238] concluded that streptokinase increased the risk of symptomatic hemorrhage by a factor of 5.82.

The Multicentre Acute Stroke Trial—Italy was a complex comparison of streptokinase, aspirin, or the combination against placebo for treatment of acute ischemic stroke.[239] This trial was stopped early because of a high early mortality among persons treated with the combination of aspirin and streptokinase. Based on this study's results, Motto et al[240] found that the presence of bleeding after treatment with streptokinase was associated with a markedly increased risk of unfavorable outcomes.

An Australian trial of streptokinase also was halted because of a high rate of fatal intracranial hemorrhage when patients were treated with streptokinase in the interval of 3–4 hours after onset of stroke.[241] Among those treated after 3 hours, deaths occurred in 52 of 133 patients administered streptokinase and 27 of 137 patients receiving placebo (relative risk: 1.98). However, this trend was not seen if the agent was given at earlier intervals. Among patients treated within 3 hours, deaths occurred in 11 of 41 patients given streptokinase and 7 of 29 given placebo. Using SPECT studies, Infeld et al[242] found that streptokinase increased non-nutritional reperfusion and that the medication might lead to reperfusion injury and poor outcomes.

RECOMBINANT TISSUE PLASMINOGEN ACTIVATOR

Hacke et al[243] treated 620 patients within 6 hours of acute ischemic stroke with either rt-PA (1.1 mg/kg or 100 mg) or placebo (see Tables 12–14 and 12–15). This study included strict CT criteria for entry. Subsequently, approximately one-sixth of the patients were judged to be ineligible largely because of imaging findings of a large, multilobar infarction. Symptomatic intracranial hemorrhages were more common among persons treated with rt-PA, and risk was highest among patients who had baseline CT findings that should have prevented enrollment. After the publication of other trials, a post-hoc analysis looked at the outcomes of 38 patients treated with placebo and 49 treated with rt-PA within 3 hours of onset of stroke.[244] (See Fig. 12–5.) A trend of an increased rate of favorable outcomes was noted with treatment.

In the United States, a series of studies of rt-PA culminated in a large clinical trial that tested the efficacy of the agent in treating acute ischemic stroke. Pilot projects demonstrated that very early treatment was feasible and that a dose greater than 0.9 mg/kg was complicated by a high rate of intracranial bleeding.[245–247] Based on these experiences, Levine and Brott[248] concluded that thrombolytic therapy was

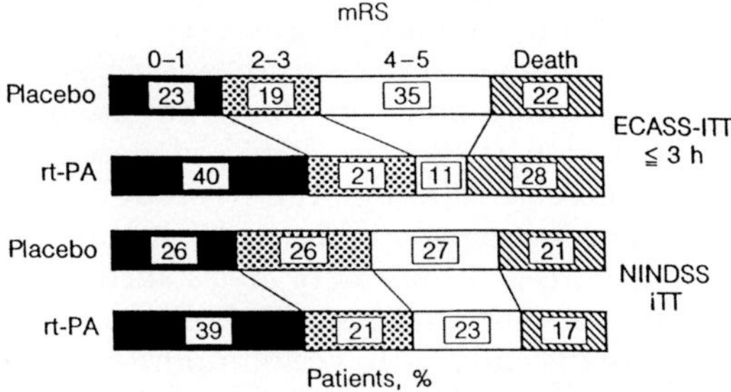

Figure 12–5. Comparisons of outcomes at 3 months using the modified Rankin Scale (mRS) among patients treated within 3 hours of acute ischemic stroke in the European Cooperative Acute Stroke Study (ECASS) intention-to-treat (ITT) population or the National Institute of Neurological Disorders and Stroke Study (NINDSS). (Reprinted from the ECASS 3-Hour Cohort. Secondary analysis of ECASS data by time stratification. *Cerebrovasc Dis* 1998;8:198–203, with permission.)

unlikely to be effective if arterial occlusion persisted more than 4–6 hours.

The NINDS performed two back-to-back randomized, double-blind, placebo-controlled trials.[24] Patients were treated within 3 hours of stroke. One-half of the patients were treated within 90 minutes. Patients with a broad spectrum of neurological impairments were recruited. Despite the very short time window, very few patients had TIA instead of stroke, a finding that implied that only 2% of placebo-treated patients had normal NIHSS scores at 24 hours. By 24 hours, a trend showed a higher rate of improvement among patients treated with rt-PA. At 3 months, several rating instruments showed that the rates of favorable outcomes (normal or very minimal disability) were approximately 15% higher among patients treated with rt-PA. The NINDS investigators concluded that the severity of neurological impairments and the patient's age influenced responses to thrombolytic therapy.[249] Patients younger than 65 and those with a mild-to-moderate stroke had the best outcomes.

Attempts to lengthen the time window for the use of rt-PA have not been successful. The second European and Australian trial used the dose of rt-PA that was administered in the NINDS trials, but patients were treated up to 6 hours after stroke.[250] As part of the trial, investigators participated in intensive training to evaluate the baseline CT findings. As a result, the number of patients with moderate-to-severe strokes was less than in previous studies. Favorable outcomes were noted in 40.3% of patients treated with rt-PA and 36.6% of patients given placebo. Although the trend of more favorable outcomes along with treatment was seen, the results were not statistically significant. The small number of seriously ill patients might have hampered the demonstration of benefit in this trial. Clark et al[481] found no improvement in outcomes among a series of patients treated with rt-PA up to 6 hours after stroke. Because of the very small number of patients treated under 3 hours, no benefit was seen. Another trial in the United States also did not find a benefit from treatment during the 3- to 5-hour time period.[251] At 90 days, 32% of the placebo-treated patients and 34% of the patients receiving rt-PA had made excellent recoveries. Within 10 days of treatment, the rate of symptomatic intracranial hemorrhage was 1.1% among patients given placebo and 7.0% among patients receiving rt-PA. In an uncontrolled study, Trouillas et al[252] showed that intravenous rt-PA could be given successfully up to 7 hours after onset of stroke. In another report, Trouillas et al[201] found that persons with a low (poor) score on a stroke scale, a proximal occlusion of the internal carotid artery, or a positive CT scan had the poorest responses to rt-PA. In particular, CT findings indicating loss of the gray-white matter junction were a strong predictor of a poor response to thrombolytic treatment.

CLINICAL EXPERIENCE WITH INTRAVENOUS THROMBOLYTIC THERAPY

Subsequent to the publication of the NINDS results, intravenous rt-PA has been moved to clinical settings.[253,254] (See Table 12–16.) Grond et al[255] demonstrated that early intravenous administration of rt-PA was associated with favorable outcomes in 10 of 12 patients treated for acute vertebrobasilar circulation stroke. The agent has been used successfully to treat patients with anterior choroidal infarction.[254] Chiu et al[256] reported that rt-PA was given to 6% of patients with acute ischemic stroke in a large metropolitan area in the United States. They noted that 37% of treated patients fully recovered and that the rate of hemorrhage was 10%. Smith et al[257] reported that emergency medicine physicians could effectively treat patients with rt-PA even without consultation with a neurologist. They reported that early identification, rapid CT, and the existence of stroke protocols were the key aspects for success. Strict adherence to protocols is important for the agent to be administered safely.[258,253] A national survey reported the results of treatment of 189 patients; overall, the risk of intracranial hemorrhage was 6%.[259] The investigators reported that following the protocol developed by the NINDS trials was critical.[259] The risk of

Table 12–16. **Clinical Experience with Alteplase in a General Patient-Care Setting**

Study	Patients (N)	Symptomatic Hemorrhage N	Symptomatic Hemorrhage %	Mortality N	Mortality %	Favorable Outcomes N	Favorable Outcomes %
Chiu et al[256]	30	2	6	7	23	11	37
Grond et al[255]	100	5	5	12	12	53	53
Tanne et al[259]	189	11	6	18	9.5	77	46
Egan et al[260]	33	3	9.1	6	18.2	12	36.4
Wirkowski et al[261]	14	1	7	3	21	5	35
Wang et al[473]	57	3	5	6	9	27	47
Albers et al[474]	389	13	3.3	51	13	132	35
Katzan et al[475]	70	11	15.7	11	15.7	20	28.6

bleeding was 4% when the protocol was followed carefully, but it rose to 11% if deviations from the protocol were found. A regional experience of six hospitals in Oregon was similar to that of the NINDS trials; the risk of hemorrhage was restricted to those patients whose NIHSS score was greater than 20.[260] Another institution found that the primary reasons for not giving rt-PA to patients with stroke were delays in arrival, mild impairments, the presence of anticoagulants, or severe concomitant medical illnesses.[261] In general, the risks and benefits from treatment with rt-PA in clinical settings are similar to those reported in the clinical trials.[28] In 1999, Lewandowski et al[262] reported on the safety and possible efficacy of intravenous rt-PA followed by intra-arterial therapy. They noted an improved rate of recanalization with the combination of interventions. Additional research is needed on the usefulness of the combination of intravenous and intra-arterial treatment.

Ancrod

In 1983, a small controlled trial found an improvement in favorable outcomes among patients treated with *ancrod*.[263] A subsequent small trial found that ancrod was safe and that it might improve outcome.[264] A clinical trial suggested that the defibrinogenating agent could improve outcomes after stroke.[265] Patients who had blood fibrinogen levels <100 mg/dL had the best therapeutic responses. A subsequent clinical trial found that ancrod could improve outcomes after stroke.[266,482] However, the agent had to be given within 3 hours of onset of stroke—the same interval for the effective use of rt-PA. A larger trial found that ancrod given as a 72-hour intravenous infusion started within 3 hours of stroke increased the likelihood of favorable outcomes.[483] However, ancord also increased the rate of symptomatic intracranial bleeding.

Summary

In 1997, Wardlaw et al[267] concluded that thrombolytic agents had not been established as effective in treating patients with acute ischemic stroke. This conclusion was based on a meta-analysis that combined results of trials testing rt-PA with those evaluating streptokinase. This approach is not valid because the two compounds differ in their potential for bleeding complications and possible benefits. In addition, combining data from patients treated up to 6 hours after stroke with those who were treated much sooner is problematic.

STREPTOKINASE

The evidence is very clear that streptokinase, in the dose and regimen used in the trials in Europe and Australia, is not safe.[237,239,241] Before this agent can be recommended for treatment of acute stroke, clinical trials will need to establish both its safety and efficacy. The failure of streptokinase might be secondary to the dose, the relatively long interval until treatment, or other variables such as ancillary care or the severity of stroke. The dose of streptokinase used in the trials was the same as that administered to patients with myocardial infarction. It may have been too high. This is an issue because the dose of rt-PA for treatment of stroke is lower than that given to treat myocardial infarction. The two European trials treated patients up to 6 hours after stroke, whereas the Australian trial gave streptokinase within 4 hours.[237,239,241] The latter study found that the risk of bleeding jumped considerably when streptokinase was given more than 3 hours after the stroke. Possibly, streptokinase would be safe and effective if it were given at a lower dose and within 3 hours, but this hypothesis needs testing. The Italian study found that a combination of streptokinase and aspirin was particularly dangerous.[239] Thus, the use of any ancillary agent that affects coagulation could have major impact on safety.

RECOMBINANT TISSUE PLASMINOGEN ACTIVATOR

Some authors have concluded that current evidence does not support the use of rt-PA for treating acute ischemic stroke.[268,269] This opinion is due largely to the differences in results between the NINDS and the other trials. Although all of the trials tested rt-PA, other differences are substantial. Most notably, the time from stroke onset to treatment makes comparisons difficult. The success of the NINDS trial may have been secondary to luck, but it also reflects the short interval to treatment in this trial. The other trials treated most or all of their patients more than 3 hours after stroke. The collective experience of the rt-PA trials shows that time truly is critical when using this agent to treat stroke. Thus, although an inability to expand the time window for treatment beyond 3 hours is disappointing, the data from the NINDS trials are compelling and they are not refuted by the results of other trials. Intravenous rt-PA can be recommended for treatment of carefully selected patients when it can be given within 3 hours of the onset of stroke. Overall, the benefits from treatment with rt-PA clearly outweigh potential risks.[28]

Caplan[270] concluded that decisions for thrombolytic therapy should be individualized and based on the presumed cause of stroke, extent of brain injury, and site of vascular occlusion. Others have pointed out that no other therapy is known to be effective in treating stroke and the results of the NINDS trials were positive regardless of the stroke subtype.[271,272] Some opinion leaders concluded that intra-arterial administration of thrombolytic therapy is superior to intravenous treatment for patients with occlusions in the internal carotid artery, proximal portion of the middle cerebral artery, or the basilar artery.[273] This opinion may be correct, but no trials have tested the relative safety and efficacy of the two approaches in a head-to-head comparison. The burden now is placed on the advocates of intra-arterial treatment to provide evidence that this route of administration is superior.

INTRA-ARTERIAL THROMBOLYSIS

The results of intra-arterial thrombolysis are promising nevertheless; the technique might extend the time window for treatment up to 6 hours or possibly longer. However, intra-arterial thrombolysis should be considered as experimental until definitive data permit regulatory approval. Even if intra-arterial therapy prolongs the time window, it might not expand the number of patients treated. A patient will need to be managed in a large, sophisticated center that has the facilities and medical expertise to administer this treatment. This therapy cannot be given in an emergency department or in most community hospitals. Withholding rt-PA to an eligible patient seen within 3 hours of stroke so that intra-arterial treatment can be given at a later time is problematic. Possibly, this scenario can be recommended when intra-arterial therapy is approved and if this approach is found to be safer and more effective than intravenous administration of rt-PA.

STRATEGIES FOR SELECTING PATIENTS TO TREAT WITH RT-PA

Yuh et al[274] and Ueda et al[275,276] proposed that some patients will not respond to thrombolytic therapy even when it is given within a few hours. Based on the results of SPECT, they suggested that other patients might benefit from treatment even when it is given more than 3 hours after stroke. Albers[277] proposed that a mismatch between diffusion- and perfusion-weighted images on early magnetic resonance imaging (MRI) might help in the identification of patients who can be treated with thrombolytic therapy even if the medication is given more than 3 hours after stroke. This proposition is supported by the finding that diffusion-weighted MRI is much more sensitive than CT in detecting the early changes of brain ischemia.[278] Using MRI, PET, or SPECT to improve the selection of patients treated with intravenous or intra-arterial thrombolysis needs testing before it can be applied to a clinical setting.[279,484] In particular, the time consumed in performing the test and the resultant delay in treating the patient must be justified by the improved ability to select patients who have a too-high risk for complications or too-low chance for success. Additional research on this strategy is needed.

POTENTIAL CONSEQUENCES OF TREATING OR NOT TREATING

Thrombolytic therapy cannot be given with impunity to patients with acute ischemic stroke. It is associated with a real risk of serious bleeding complications. In addition, rt-PA is expensive. Conversely, the economic and human costs of not treating patients are even higher. Based on the results of the NINDS trials, a recent cost-effectiveness study found that reductions in rehabilitation and nursing home costs far exceed expenses in administering rt-PA.[280]

INTRAVENOUS THROMBOLYSIS IS EFFECTIVE BUT NOT VERY USEFUL

Despite the approval of rt-PA for treating ischemic stroke, most patients in Canada and the United States are not being treated. Thus, intravenous rt-PA is an effective therapy that is not very useful because very few patients are receiving the medication. The low use of rt-PA may be secondary to lack of patient awareness, inertia or deficiencies in the health care system, and physician concerns about its potential for complications.[281] Yet, the primary barrier to treatment is the narrow time window.[29,261] Only a concerted public and professional education program will overcome these hurdles. A regional, coordinated stroke care program, as outlined in this chapter, also is needed. Still, even with these efforts, a majority of patients cannot be treated with rt-PA. This conclusion is highlighted by one recent series of 214 patients seen for acute stroke in an emergency department; only 6 of the study's patients were considered eligible for treatment with rt-PA.[282] Ninety-five patients arrived after the time window, 31 had resolution of their symptoms, 20 were judged to have minor strokes that did not need to be treated, and 22 had intracranial hemorrhages.

ALTERNATIVES TO INTRAVENOUS THROMBOLYSIS

To date, intravenous rt-PA is the only medication that reduces the neurological consequences of acute ischemic stroke.[477] It is the only agent that has been approved for treatment of ischemic stroke by regulatory bodies in Europe, the United States, and Canada.[283,477] Although the therapy is not risk-free or a panacea, it does work. It should be given to carefully selected patients by physicians who have expertise in diagnosing and treating stroke and in settings where the patient can receive appropriate supportive care.[54,270,284] The protocol for treatment should be followed to maintain safety.[253] Still, concerns about secondary brain hemorrhage mean that the decision must be made with considerable care.[285]

Guidelines and Algorithm

Several groups have endorsed the use of rt-PA and have published guidelines for its use in treating acute ischemic stroke.[16,19,64,286–288] The guidelines generally parallel the management plan used in the NINDS trials.[24] With the exception of the addition of the CT criteria used by the first European trial of rt-PA, the guidelines used the same features for eligibility and non-eligibility as were used in the NINDS trials.[16,19,287] In particular, all of the statements recommend that the initiation of treatment be restricted to within 3 hours of stroke onset. The recommended dose of rt-PA is 0.9 mg/kg (maximum 90 mg), with 10% given as a bolus and the remainder infused over 1 hour. The recommendations for care after administration of rt-PA are discussed subsequently in this chapter.

An algorithm can be used to ease screening of patients who might be eligible for treatment with rt-PA (Table 12–17). It takes the form of a series of questions, and the sequence of questions is important because it generally parallels stages in screening a patient in the emergency department. For example, the first question involves the determination of the time of onset of stroke. If the onset is within 3 hours, then the remainder of the questions can be addressed. Conversely, if the stroke is older than 3 hours, then the rest of the screening process becomes irrelevant.

WHEN DID THE STROKE OCCUR?

The stroke must have begun within the past 3 hours. If the physician is uncertain about the time of onset or if the time elapsed is longer than 3 hours, then rt-PA should not be given. This short time window excludes treatment of almost all patients whose strokes developed during sleep. An exception might be the occasional patient who awakens from a short nap with signs of a stroke. The rule of assuming that the stroke occurred 1 minute after onset of sleep probably is too restrictive, but it remains the most cautious strategy. The patient and observers often disagree about the time of onset. In these circumstances, the physician should try to clarify the time of the first symptom. If this issue cannot be resolved, then the physician should assume that the longest time is correct. This decision may lead to a patient not being treated with rt-PA.

Table 12–17. **Screening Algorithm: Questions to Address Prior to Treatment with Recombinant Tissue Plasminogen Activator**

When did the stroke occur?
Any recent medical illnesses?
Which medications is the patient taking?
Vital signs, blood pressure, and medical status?
Any other likely explanation for symptoms?
Neurological status?
Results of diagnostic tests?
Results of computed tomogram?
Do the patient and family understand the potential risks and benefits?

DOES THE PATIENT HAVE A HISTORY OF ANY RECENT MEDICAL ILLNESSES?

The patient and family should be queried about any recent (generally <4–6 weeks) illnesses that might increase the risk of hemorrhagic complications from rt-PA. Among these are myocardial infarction, stroke, or trauma—particularly head injury, bleeding, or surgery. Although a recent history of a prior stroke precludes treatment with rt-PA, a TIA does not. Thus, a history of any recent neurological symptoms that could be either a TIA or a stroke should be examined closely. If the patient's symptoms truly cleared in their entirety (a TIA), then rt-PA can be given even if the event happened in the previous 24 hours. In addition to a history of remote trauma, the patient and family should be asked about a fall or any acute trauma at the time of the stroke. A complicating fracture or other major injury may lead to serious bleeding and probably prevents treatment with rt-PA. The issue of recent surgery is a problem. The spectrum of surgical procedures is broad, and chances of serious bleeding vary. In general, caution should be exercised if a post-operative bleeding complication is likely to lead to either mortality or major morbidity. Still, discussing the issue with the surgeon might permit treatment of a patient who otherwise might not have been treated.

WHICH MEDICATIONS IS THE PATIENT TAKING?

Although all medications should be recorded, only a few have an effect on treatment. The most important medication is warfarin. Prolongation of the International Normalized Ratio (INR) level >1.7 secondary to the use of oral anticoagulants eliminates the possibility of treating with rt-PA. If a patient is using warfarin, then laboratory measurement of the INR becomes critical. A patient with a modestly elevated (non-therapeutic) INR of 1.7 or less can be treated. Reversing the effects of warfarin by the administration of vitamin K or clotting factors should not be done to give rt-PA. The use of antiplatelet aggregating agents is not a contraindication for treatment. Diabetic patients should be asked specifically about their use of oral agents or insulin. In particular, any change in the dose of medication or diet could be a warning that a patient's symptoms might be secondary to hypoglycemia. A prompt assessment of the blood glucose concentration and treatment of a low level may obviate the need for rt-PA.

WHAT ARE THE PATIENT'S VITAL SIGNS, BLOOD PRESSURE, AND MEDICAL STATUS?

Acute cardiovascular or pulmonary complications often take precedence. Depending on the severity of the complications and necessary interventions, the patient's condition may not be sufficiently stable in time to give rt-PA.

Sustained hypertension is the most common medical problem that contraindicates treatment with rt-PA. Because the NINDS trials demonstrated safety with rt-PA only when the systolic blood pressure was <185 mm Hg and the diastolic blood pressure was <110 mm Hg, these are the limits contained in the guidelines. If time is sufficient, then the patient can be monitored to see whether the values spontaneously decline to acceptable levels. In addition, short-acting antihypertensive drugs (see Table 12–8) can be used. However, if the blood pressure does not stabilize with these treatments, then rt-PA should not be administered.

Evidence of active bleeding means that the patient cannot be treated with rt-PA. However, screening for minor bleeding, such as microscopic hematuria or occult blood in the stool, is not necessary.

IS THERE ANY OTHER LIKELY EXPLANATION FOR THE PATIENT'S SYMPTOMS?

The differential diagnosis in Table 3–8 should be considered. Both clinical findings and the results of ancillary tests affect the diagnosis of ischemic stroke. If diagnosis of ischemic stroke is in doubt, then rt-PA should not be given.

WHAT IS THE PATIENT'S NEUROLOGICAL STATUS?

Both the history and physical examination evaluate the patient's neurological status. If the course is one of dramatic improvement, then the patient might not need rt-PA. Dramatic improvement could be described as nearly total resolution of the signs. Minimal recovery would include improvement from hemiplegia to moderate weakness or from global aphasia to moderate language impairments. If symptoms are unchanged, fluctuating, improving minimally, or worsening, then rt-PA could be indicated.

In general, the prognosis of a patient with mild deficits (NIHSS <4 points) is good and treatment probably is not needed. An exception would be the rare patient with an isolated severe deficit, such as profound aphasia, that can cause serious disability. Withholding treatment of a mildly affected patient is accompanied by a possibility that the patient will deteriorate at a later time. If this scenario occurs, then the patient likely will not be able to be treated with rt-PA because the 3-hour time period will have expired.

The decision about treating a seriously affected patient is difficult. These patients have very poor prognoses, and the risk of hemorrhage is especially high. Current guidelines advise caution about the prescription of rt-PA to patients with an NIHSS score >20–22 points. Careful examination of the CT becomes especially critical in this situation because of the abnormalities that portend a very high risk of hemorrhage. The risks and benefits of treatment need to be thoroughly discussed with the family because, in this situation, the patient likely will be too seriously ill to give consent.

Thus, the ideal patients for treatment with rt-PA will have an NIHSS score from approximately 6–10 points to approximately 15–20 points. Complete recovery should be the goal of treatment of less seriously ill patients. A goal of partial recovery—maybe achieving mild-to-moderate deficits instead of severe disability—may represent a satisfactory response in more seriously ill patients even if they do not recover completely.

WHAT ARE THE RESULTS OF THE DIAGNOSTIC STUDIES?

The question about results of diagnostic studies is addressed relatively late in the sequence because of the time required to do the tests, which means that the results not available immediately. The results of the urgently performed tests listed in Table 4–1 could affect decisions about the use of rt-PA (Fig. 12–6). The most obvious are abnormalities in the INR, activated partial thromboplastin time, and platelet count, which can forecast an increased risk of bleeding complications. The electrocardiogram may uncover evidence of an undiagnosed, possibly recent, myocardial infarction. In this circumstance, emergent consultation from a cardiologist might clarify the situation. The likelihood is small that results of serum levels of creatine kinase or troponin will be available in sufficient time to administer rt-PA. Thus, the decision about a cardiac reason to prohibit treatment must be made based on clinical and electrocardiographic findings. If there is any doubt that a myocardial infarction may be recent, then rt-PA should not be given.

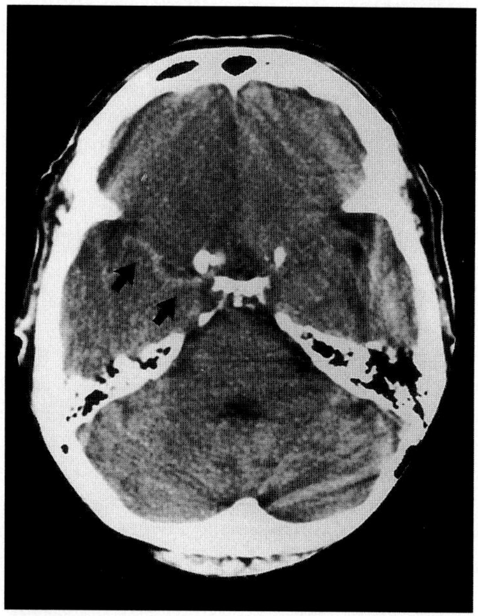

Figure 12–6. Hyperdense middle cerebral artery sign. Unenhanced computed tomographic scan showing thrombus within the right middle cerebral artery (arrows). (Courtesy Dr. D. Lee.)

WHAT ARE THE RESULTS OF THE COMPUTED TOMOGRAM?

The importance of CT is emphasized in Chapter 4 and previously in this chapter. No patient with a suspected acute ischemic stroke should be treated with rt-PA until a CT has been examined. Preferably, it will be interpreted by a radiologist but, if time is short, a skilled neurologist or an emergency medicine physician can read the scan.

A finding of intracranial bleeding on CT is an absolute contraindication to treatment with rt-PA.

Many patients have CT evidence of old strokes. Some of these may have been clinically silent. An older infarction is not a reason to forego rt-PA; however, CT also can estimate the "age" of a new stroke. If the stroke appears relatively dark with well-defined borders and with some evidence of mass effect, then the reported interval from onset of stroke should be reassessed. These CT findings would be uncommon for a stroke <3 hours old. The patient and family should be asked again about the actual time of onset. If the stroke looks older than 3 hours and uncertainty persists, then rt-PA should not be administered.

Several CT findings affect decisions about the use of rt-PA (see Table 4–3). These changes are most commonly found among patients with moderate-to-severe strokes. As a rule of thumb, these abnormalities become very important if the NIHSS score is 15 or greater. The current guidelines reflect the recommendations of von Kummer et al[289–291] that were incorporated in the European trial. These CT findings should be included in making a decision to recommend treatment with rt-PA.

DO THE PATIENT AND FAMILY UNDERSTAND THE POTENTIAL RISKS AND BENEFITS?

Thrombolytic therapy cannot be given with impunity. The data show that its administration is associated with a risk of bleeding complications, including potentially life-threatening intracranial hemorrhage. In contrast, stroke is a dangerous illness that often leads to death or disability. To date, intravenous administration of rt-PA is the only therapy established as effective in improving outcomes of stroke. The net benefit from treatment is present despite a relatively high risk of complications. Some institutions use a detailed information summary and consent that is signed by the patient and family before treatment. Although this formal process may not be necessary because rt-PA is an approved therapy for acute stroke, the patient and family should be given clear information about the risks and benefits of treatment. This is the obligation of the treating physician. Because patients with very severe stroke cannot give consent because of the nature of their illness, informing the next of kin becomes critical. Making decisions about treatment of stroke is very stressful for family members. The family and patient need time to decide about treatment, but they also need to be told that time is a crucial aspect of treatment. The goal remains to start treatment as soon as possible.

The family and patient should be told about the potential bleeding risk from treatment with rt-PA. They need to be aware that the risk of intracranial bleeding is greater with thrombolytic therapy for stroke than for management of myocardial ischemia. Although the overall risk of intracranial hemorrhage is approximately 6%, the risk appears as high as 16% among persons with very severe strokes. The risk of hemorrhage must be balanced against the chances of death or disability without treatment. The natural history of persons with such severe strokes is dismal. Because the natural history of stroke is exceedingly poor among patients with very severe infarctions, families generally are willing to give consent because they recognize that rt-PA is the "only chance" for the patient. They generally appear to be willing to risk the chance of hemorrhage, which could be fatal, to avoid a disabling stroke that might leave their loved one in a nursing home.

ANTICOAGULANTS

Anticoagulants, in particular heparin, are commonly prescribed for the treatment of acute ischemic stroke. Despite their widespread use, anticoagulants remain controversial because of a lack of proven efficacy and the potential for intracranial bleeding.[292] A 1989 survey of American neurologists showed that many physicians did not know whether heparin was helpful in improving outcomes after stroke.[293] Approximately 6% of neurologists thought heparin had been established as effective, whereas 16% thought the agent to be ineffective. The other physicians were unsure about its status. Its use also ranged widely; some physicians prescribed it to all of their acutely ill patients, and others gave it to none of their patients.

Rationale

Propagation of the thrombus and secondary collateral failure are potential mechanisms of neurological worsening after acute ischemic stroke.[71,294] These phenomena following an acute arterial occlusion might be prevented with the emergent administration of anticoagulants. In addition, emergent anticoagulant therapy might forestall early recurrent embolism, particularly among patients with cardiac sources of embolism. For an anticoagulant to be useful in an acute situation, it must have immediate effects on the coagulation cascade. In addition, anticoagulants often are prescribed as an adjunct to thrombolysis for managing patients with acute myocardial ischemia, and these agents might be helpful in treating patients with ischemic stroke.[295]

A medication such as warfarin that has delayed antithrombotic actions will not be useful in an urgent care setting. The indirect thrombin inhibitors (heparin, low molecular weight [LMW] heparins, dermatan sulfate, heparan sulfate, or antithrombin III) generally have immediate anticoagulant effects.[296] Other anticoagulant agents include the direct thrombin inhibitors hirudin, hirulog, and argatroban.[296] Several anticoagulants have been prescribed, but heparin is the most commonly used.[297,298] Low molecular weight heparins and danaparoid also have been used during the last few years. The pharmacology of heparin and the LMW anticoagulants is discussed in Chapter 10. The LMW heparins might have other therapeutic actions in acute stroke that might be independent of their effects on coagulation. Using an experimental model, Li et al[299] showed that LMW heparins can lessen brain edema if they are given within 3 hours of onset stroke. This observation deserves additional study.

Results of Clinical Trials—Acute Ischemic Stroke

An analysis of clinical trials performed before 1993 noted that heparin was effective in preventing deep vein thrombosis after stroke but that it did not improve outcomes, reduce the risk of pulmonary embolism, or lower mortality.[300] This same analysis showed that heparin was associated with an increased risk of bleeding. Alexandrov et al[301] concluded that persons with cardioembolic stroke or proximal occlusion of the middle cerebral artery were at the highest risk for bleeding following treatment with heparin. Another report found that intracerebral hemorrhage following the use of heparin was most common among patients with cardioembolic stroke, those with moderate-to-large infarctions, and when the heparin was given within 24 hours of stroke or if the level of anticoagulation was excessive.[302] In contrast, Toni et al[303] did not correlate symptomatic hemorrhagic transformation of infarction with the administration of heparin.

HEPARIN

In a small trial, the Cerebral Embolism Study Group[304,305] concluded that heparin was effective in reducing early recurrent stroke an improving outcomes (Tables 12–18 and 12–19). They noted that bleeding occurred when patients with large strokes received immediate heparin therapy and also concluded that the use of a bolus dose to initiate treatment might increase the risk of hemorrhagic complications However, this study enrolled only 45 patients, and its conclusions should be viewed with considerable caution. In an uncontrolled study, Chamorro et al[306] administered heparin to 231 patients with recent stroke and atrial fibrillation. Despite treatment, 5 patients had recurrent stroke. Eight patients had hemorrhagic complications and, in 6 cases, these were fatal. Yasaka et al[307] found that full doses of heparin were associated with bleeding in 5 of 26 patients with acute cardioembolic stroke. Clinical outcomes were not described. Camerlingo et al[308] gave heparin to 45 patients within 5 hours of onset of stroke. Two patients had intracerebral hemorrhages, and 23 patients improved. No control group was available for comparison. In an uncontrolled study, another group administered heparin to 52 patients with progressing stroke.[309] In 38 patients, the progression stopped. Improvement was marked in 20, but in 11 others there was worsening despite heparin. Another uncontrolled trial of heparin treatment of 36 patients with progressing ischemic stroke could not find a benefit from treatment.[310] Patients with events in either the carotid or the vertebrobasilar circulations seemed not to respond to the anticoagulant.

A relatively small, placebo-controlled trial tested heparin among 225 patients with acute, partial, stable stroke.[311] No differences in outcomes, rates of neurological worsening, or rates of improvement were noted. However, this study excluded patients with cardioembolism and those with other potential indications for urgent administration of an anticoagulant. The

Table 12–18. **Favorable Outcomes: Clinical Trials of Anticoagulants—Acute Ischemic Stroke**

	Treatment			Control		
	Patients	Favorable Outcomes Events		Patients	Favorable Outcomes Events	
Agent and Trial	**N**	**N**	**%**	**N**	**N**	**%**
Heparin						
IST*[312]						
Lower dose	4861	1776	36.9	9718	3582	37.1
Higher dose	4856	1802	37.4			
Low molecular weight heparin						
FISS[314]						
Low dose	101	47	47	105	37	36
High dose	100	54	54			
Low molecular weight danaparoid						
TOAST[316]	641	482	75.2	634	467	73.7

*Some patients in the heparin treatment and control groups also received aspirin.
IST = International Stroke Trial
FISS = Fraxaparine in Ischemic Stroke Study
TOAST = Trial of Org 10172 in Acute Stroke Treatment

Table 12–19. **Bleeding Events: Clinical Trials of Anticoagulants—Acute Ischemic Stroke**

	Treatment			Control		
Agent and Trial	**Patients**	**Events**	**%**	**Patients**	**Events**	**%**
Heparin						
Duke et al[311]	112	0	0	113	0	0
CESG[304]	24	0	0	21	2	9
IST*[312]						
Lower dose	4861	35	0.7	9718	41	0.4
Higher dose	4856	85	1.8			
Low molecular weight heparin						
FISS[314]						
Low dose	101	0	0	105	1	1
High dose	100	0	0			
FISS—bis[332]	516	25	4.8	250	7	2.8
Low molecular weight heparinoid						
TOAST[314]	638	10	1.5	628	3	0.4

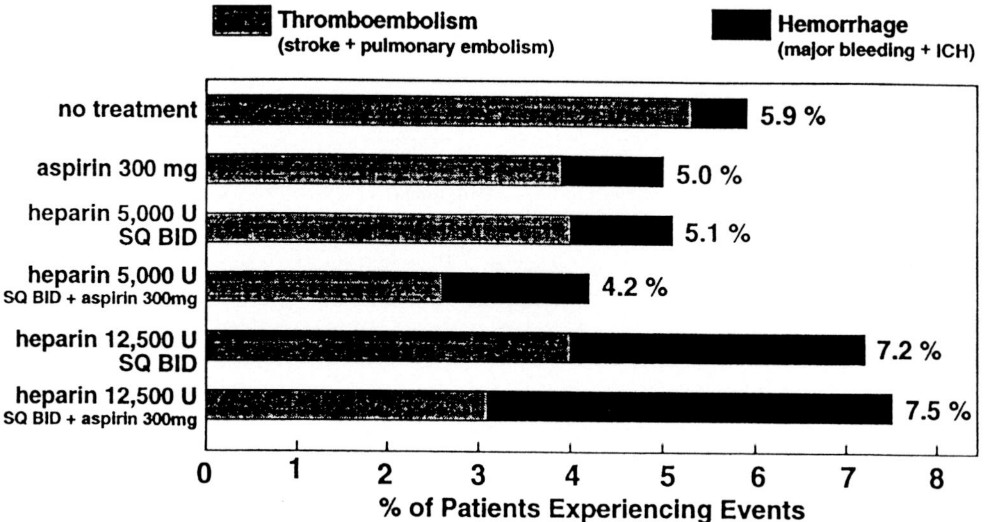

Figure 12–7. Aggregate rates (%) of thromboembolic or major bleeding events among patients enrolled in the International Stroke Trial. (Reprinted from Albers G et al, antithombotic and thorubotytic therapy for ischemic stroke *Chest* 1998,114 [Suppl]:683, with permission of publisher.)

International Stroke Trial tested subcutaneously administered heparin in a large number of patients with ischemic stroke.[312] The medication was given up to 48 hours after stroke in two different doses administered with or without concomitant aspirin (Fig. 12–7). Although the trial enrolled almost 20,000 patients, it does have serious limitations. A sizeable proportion of patients were not evaluated with CT before treatment and, thus, some patients with de novo intracerebral hemorrhage could have been enrolled. The International Stroke Trial was an unblinded trial; as a result, the physicians knew the nature of treatment. Thus, their responses to new neurological symptoms could have been biased by this information. The levels of anticoagulation were not monitored by regular tests, such as the activated partial thromboplastin time. As a result, some patients likely were under-treated with a resultant lack of efficacy, and others were over-treated with a potential for an increase in the risk of bleeding. Not surprisingly, this trial found that heparin did not improve outcomes.

LOW MOLECULAR WEIGHT HEPARINS

A pilot study of nadroparin, an LMW heparin, demonstrated that the agent was safe when given to treat patients with acute ischemic stroke.[313] A subsequent study by the same investigators showed that subcutaneous nadroparin, when given twice a day for a period of 10-days, was effective in improving outcomes at 6 months after stroke.[314] (See Tables 12–18 and 12–19.) However, a benefit from treatment was not seen at either 10 days or 3 months after stroke. The results of another trial of nadroparin have not been published, but presentations at meetings suggested that the medication was not effective. Berge et al[485] found that a LMW heparin was not superior to aspirin in preventing early recurrent events among patients with atrial fibrillation and recent stroke. Other LMW heparins have not been tested for the treatment of stroke. Because of the marked variations between the agents' effects on coagulation, data about the safety and efficacy of nadroparin should not be transferred to other compounds.[315]

DANAPAROID

A U.S. trial evaluated the efficacy of danaparoid when it was given within 24 hours of onset of acute ischemic stroke.[316] (See Tables 12–18 and 12–19.) Patients with a broad spectrum of neurological impairments were recruited, and the agent was given as an intravenous bolus followed by a continuous intravenous infusion for 7 days. Infusions were adjusted in response to levels of inhibition of activated factor X. The investigators found the danaparoid increased the risk of symptomatic intracranial bleeding among patients with severe strokes (NIHSS score >15) and non-neurological bleeding among persons weighing less than 125 lb. Despite a trend of improvement of early outcomes (7 days) with treatment, no sustained benefit in improving outcomes was noted. As a result, danaparoid was not found to be effective. The subgroup of patients with stroke secondary to large artery atherosclerosis appeared to have benefit from treatment. Patients with stroke secondary to occlusions or severe stenosis of the internal carotid artery appeared to have a high rate of poor outcomes, and danaparoid might be beneficial in this group. A post-hoc analysis from this trial suggested that an anticoagulant might be effective if given to patients who have severe internal carotid artery disease detected acutely by carotid duplex ultrasonography.[317] Additional research is needed to determine whether this group of patients truly might benefit from emergent anticoagulation. To date, anticoagulation has not been established as an effective therapy for this indication.

ADJUNCTIVE ANTICOAGULANT TREATMENT

The adjunctive use of anticoagulation following treatment with rt-PA is stimulated by the widespread use of heparin after thrombolytic therapy for management of acute myocardial ischemia. Current guidelines advise that anticoagulants not be started within 24 hours of treatment with rt-PA.[16,19] A small study treated 43 patients within 7 hours of onset of stroke with intravenous rt-PA followed by heparin.[252] A majority of patients made a complete recovery, and 6.9% had hemorrhages. A German study evaluated the combination of rt-PA and heparin among 43 patients with acute stroke; patients were treated using the criteria developed by the NINDS investigators.[318] Despite the concomitant use of the thrombolytic agent and heparin, only 1 patient had a symptomatic hemorrhagic transformation. The PROACT study tested the combination of intravenous heparin and intra-arterial prourokinase in a series of patients with occlusion of the middle cerebral artery.[228] Although the rate of recanalization was greatest among patients who received high doses of heparin and prourokinase, the patients treated with this combination also had the highest rate of intracranial bleeding. Additional research is needed on the role of anticoagulation as an adjunct to thrombolytic therapy. However, in the future, anticoagulation might be replaced by the use of an intravenous antiplatelet aggregating agent, such as abciximab.

OTHER ANTITHROMBOTIC AGENTS

Yasaka et al[307] administered *antithrombin III* to 20 patients with acute cardioembolic stroke; 2 hemorrhages occurred, and no recurrent embolic events were noted. *Hirudin* has been given as an adjunctive therapy with thrombolysis for treatment of patients with acute myocardial ischemia, but the risk of brain hemorrhage with hirudin was as high or higher than for large doses of heparin.[319,320] The agent may be safer when given alone.[321] Because of the high risk of hemorrhage among patients with cardiac ischemia, the medication has not been tested among patients with stroke. *Argatroban* is an immediately acting agent that inhibits thrombin. It might be an alternative to heparin in treating patients with acute ischemic stroke.[322,323] It has been used in treatment of patients with heparin-associated thrombocytopenia.[324] Clinical trials have not tested argatroban in treatment of patients with acute ischemic stroke.

Conclusions

In 1994, a panel of the Stroke Council of the American Heart Association concluded that the data about the usefulness of emergent anticoagulant treatment were insufficient to provide any recommendation about the use of heparin in treating acute ischemic stroke.[20] The panel stated that there was no evidence that heparin had either a positive or a negative effect on outcomes regardless of the presumed cause of stroke or involved vascular territory. The clinical trials reported since then provide additional information. The urgent use of anticoagulants has not been demonstrated as efficacious in preventing early recurrent stroke or in improving neurological outcomes. The trials show that early anticoagulation is potentially dangerous and does increase the likelihood of intracranial bleeding, especially among persons with severe strokes. Thus, recent clinical trials do not provide data to support emergent anticoagulation in the initial management of patients with acute ischemic stroke.[325–329,477]

Despite the largely negative results of the recent trials, anticoagulants still are prescribed widely, and some leaders in the field continue to advise early use of heparin.[330] For example, Caplan[331] recommended emergent heparin treatment for some patients with acute ischemic stroke secondary to cardioembolism. Some authors have advocated that additional clinical trials of heparin be performed.[332] Maybe future trials of anticoagulants will find a role for these agents in improving neurological outcomes or in preventing early recurrent neurological symptoms. For example, the observation that anticoagulants might be effective in improving outcomes with stroke secondary to large artery atherosclerosis might be confirmed by future clinical trials.

Notwithstanding the lack of data showing the usefulness of urgent anticoagulant therapy, many physicians likely will continue to prescribe these medications—possibly out of habit. Some recommendations should be followed if heparin or another acutely acting anticoagulant is to be prescribed (Table 12–20) No data exist to show that unfractionated heparin is either more safe or more dangerous than the LMW heparins or danaparoid. A bolus dose of heparin should be given if the goal is to achieve a therapeutic level of anticoagulation rapidly, the presumable reason for urgent treatment of stroke. Although some advise against the use of bolus dose for safety reasons, information is limited about any special danger from this strategy. A bolus dose of heparin to start treatment should not be considered to be foolhardy; however, intermittent and recurrent intravenous bolus doses of heparin are more dangerous than a continuous infusion. Thus, maintenance of anticoagulation with intravenous therapy should be done via an infusion. Subcutaneous administration of heparin or the LMW heparins results in a gradual antithrombotic effect and probably will be less effective than intravenous

Table 12–20. **Conclusions and Recommendations About the Use of Heparin in Treatment of Patients with Recent Ischemic Stroke**

Effective in preventing deep vein thrombosis after stroke
Not established as effective in preventing early recurrent embolic stroke
Not established as effective in halting neurological worsening
Not established as a safe and effective adjunct to thrombolysis
No data about superiority of any intravenous anticoagulant
Features of stroke that contraindicate treatment with thrombolytic agents probably preclude treatment with anticoagulants
Doses should be calculated on a weight-based nomogram
A bolus dose can be used to initiate treatment
Maintenance should be done via a continuous intravenous infusion.
Subcutaneous administration given to prevent deep vein thrombosis
Should not be given until a computed tomograph excludes brain hemorrhage
Check levels of anticoagulation regularly
Adjust doses in response to level of anticoagulation

therapy. Subcutaneous heparin treatment is not established as being more safe than intravenous therapy; the International Stroke Trial demonstrated that subcutaneous heparin increases the risk of brain hemorrhage.[312]

No patient should receive an anticoagulant for treatment of an acute ischemic stroke unit CT has eliminated primary intracranial hemorrhage as the cause of the neurological symptoms.[333] An anticoagulant should not be prescribed if a CT scan cannot be obtained. The severity of neurological impairments or the size of stroke on CT should influence the decision to start emergent anticoagulant treatment. The features that contraindicate the use of thrombolytic therapy probably also suggest that anticoagulants should not be administered. Recent trials show that emergent anticoagulation is dangerous when given to persons with severe infarctions. As a rule of thumb, anticoagulants should not be given within the first hours after stroke to persons whose baseline NIHSS score is >15.

Excessive levels of anticoagulation cause serious bleeding complications, including symptomatic hemorrhagic transformation of the infarction. Although the treatment regimen described in Chapter 10 (See Table 10–5) should lessen the likelihood of major complications, it does not guarantee safety. A weight-based dosing scheme still requires close monitoring of the level of anticoagulation.[334] Patient responses to anticoagulant therapy vary considerably among individuals, and individual patient's responses also change. As a result, monitoring the patient's level of anticoagulation is a critical component of care. Doses of heparin or LMW compounds need to be adjusted to maintain safety and potential efficacy.

ANTIPLATELET AGGREGATING AGENTS

Antiplatelet aggregating agents are the most commonly prescribed medical therapy to prevent ischemic stroke in high-risk patients. Still, the role of acutely administered antiplatelet aggregating agents in treating acute ischemic stroke is unclear.[335]

Rationale

Platelets are a key component of acute arterial occlusion leading to ischemic stroke.[336] Thus, an agent that immediately halts platelet aggregation could prevent propagation of a thrombosis or prevent recurrent embolism. Platelet activation is ongoing after stroke, and an inhibitory agent might be useful.[337] Dipyridamole, clopidogrel, and ticlopidine are unlikely to be useful in an acute care setting, because their effects on platelet function are delayed. In contrast, aspirin affects platelet activity within a few minutes of administration. Aspirin also affects leukocytes and the vascular endothelium, further the formation of thrombi.[338] Patients are advised to take aspirin while en route to an emergency department because the medication promotes resolution of the coronary artery occlusion and lessens the effects of acute myocardial ischemia. This scenario has not been replicated in acute stroke care.

Antagonists to the glycoprotein IIb/IIIa (GP IIb/IIIa) receptor affect integrins, which influence fibrinogen binding to the platelet.[335,339–341] In experimental models, these antagonists halt the accumulation of platelets and fibrin in microvascular thrombosis in stroke.[342–344] As such, these agents have a potent and immediate affect on thrombosis and can halt propagation of a clot. In addition, these agents could reduce the size of brain infarction, possibly because of their effects on the microcirculation.[343] A bolus dose of the GP IIb/IIIa antagonist abciximab can immediately block more than 80% of platelet receptors and immediately reduce platelet aggregation to less than 20% of normal.[345] A subsequent infusion can maintain this inhibition. Anti-adhesion molecules also can be used as an adjunct to rt-PA to help prevent thrombosis.[346]

Results of Clinical Trials—Acute Ischemic Stroke

ASPIRIN

The International Stroke Trial tested aspirin (300 mg/day) when given alone or in combination with heparin to patients

Table 12–21. **Favorable Outcome Fates: Clinical Trials of Aspirin—Acute Ischemic Stroke**

	Treatment					Control				
	Patients	Bleeding		Favorable Outcomes		Patients	Bleeding		Favorable	
Trials	(N)	N	%	N	%	N	N	%	N	%
MAST—I	153	3	2	59	39	156	1	0.6	50	32
IST*	9720	87	0.9	3639	37.8	9715	74	0.8	3521	36.5
CAST	10335	115	1.1	7139	72	10320	93	0.9	7023	71.3

*Some patients in aspirin-treatment and control groups also received heparin.
MAST = Multicentre Acute Stroke Trial-Italy
IST = International Stroke Trial
CAST = Chinese Acute Stroke Trial

seen within 48 hours of stroke.[312] (See Table 12–21 and Fig.12–7.) Aspirin was associated with a slight increase in the risk of hemorrhagic complications and a modest efficacy in preventing recurrent stroke and in improving outcome. Despite the large size of the trial, results showing aspirin's usefulness were not definitive. Only when the data from the International Stroke Trial were combined with those of the equally large Chinese Acute Stroke Trial was a significant benefit from aspirin therapy found.[347] The results of these studies show that aspirin generally can be given safely within 48 hours of onset of stroke; however, the impact of aspirin is marginal in limiting brain injury after stroke.

Combining aspirin with thrombolytic therapy appears to increase the risk of hemorrhage.[239] Based on data from the Multicentre Acute Stroke Trial—Italy, Ciccone et al[348] noted 22 fatal hemorrhagic strokes among 156 patients who received aspirin and streptokinase and 11 fatal intracranial hemorrhages among 157 patients who were given streptokinase alone. These data suggest that the use of aspirin as an adjunct to thrombolytic therapy may not be safe or effective. The combination of aspirin and an anticoagulant also might be used, but data about the safety and efficacy of this tactic are not available.

Ridogrel, a potent antiplatelet aggregating agent that inhibits thromboxane synthase and a prostaglandin receptor antagonist, has been tested as an adjunct to thrombolysis among patients with acute myocardial infarction.[349] The agent was shown to be more effective than aspirin. Studies of ridogrel to treat acute stroke are not available.

Blockade of the glycoprotein IIb/IIIa receptor is used to treat patients with unstable angina or as an adjunct to coronary artery angioplasty.[350,351] Immediately acting antagonists also are effective in lessening arterial thrombosis and in improving outcomes after acute myocardial ischemia.[352–355,351,486] These agents help to maintain arterial patency while reducing the necessary dose of thrombolytic drug.[356] Thus, this combination might maintain efficacy and increase safety. These agents might have a role in the treatment of acute ischemic cerebrovascular disease. Because thrombolytic agents can affect platelet activity, blockage of the glycoprotein IIb/IIIa receptor may be particularly helpful in preventing reocclusion.[168] Wallace et al[357] found that intravenous administration of *abciximab* could be used to prevent or treat thrombosis of the basilar artery. These agents have been used as adjuncts for treatment of patients having cerebrovascular angioplasty and stenting.[487,488] A pilot study has evaluated the safety of abciximab in treating of patients with acute ischemic stroke. Serious bleeding complications were infrequent, and additional studies are planned.[489] Still, it will be some time before the usefulness of intravenously administered abciximab is known.

Conclusion

These large clinical trials described demonstrate a marginal improvement in patient outcomes. Modest benefits accrue from the emergent administration of aspirin for the treatment of acute ischemic stroke.[327,358] The degree of improvement is so small, however, that aspirin should not be considered as a treatment for acute stroke.[327] The chief attributes of aspirin are that it is relatively safe and that is inexpensive. Although antiplatelet aggregating agents are the mainstays of medical treatment to prevent stroke, their utility in acute care is much less certain. Still, the lack of benefit from early anticoagulation makes the use of antiplatelet aggregating agents attractive. They might be useful as an adjunct to thrombolytic therapy or as a monotherapy, but additional research on early treatment with antiplatelet aggregating agents is needed to better define their role.

OTHER MEDICAL INTERVENTIONS TO IMPROVE CEREBRAL PERFUSION

Other interventions to improve blood flow attempt to increase arterial diameter, augment perfusion pressure, or decrease the blood's viscosity.

Drug-Induced Hypertension

Among patients with stroke, cerebral autoregulation is lost, and flow becomes pressure-dependent. Thus, increasing blood flow through the use of vasopressors could improve flow through collateral channels. Drug-induced hypertension has been used successfully to reverse the ischemic consequences of vasospasm following subarachnoid hemorrhage.[359] Vasopressors and vasodilators have been used to improve blood flow to the brain.[360] Agents, such as phenylephrine, could be administered to increase blood pressure.[361] However, rapidly and profoundly lowering blood pressure during stroke could worsen ischemia by decreasing blood flow. This is a major reason antihypertensive agents are prescribed with considerable caution after stroke.

Results of treatment with drug-induced hypertension among patients with ischemic stroke have been inconclusive. Rordorf et al[361] found that increasing blood pressure did not increase mortality or morbidity and that it might improve outcomes, particularly among patients with multiple arterial stenoses. The combination of hypervolemic hemodilution and iatrogenic hypertension can lead to hypertensive encephalopathy.[362] Thus, the value of induced hypertension is uncertain in treatment of stroke.

Vasodilators

Vasodilators increase blood flow, but their value in treatment of stroke probably is marginal. The vessels in the ischemic area already are dilated maximally, and the vasodilator likely decreases flow to critical areas by diverting blood to other vascular beds. Recently, a review of vinpocetine, a vinka alkaloid that is a vasodilator, found that the agent did not reduce mortality or disability after stroke.[363]

Hemodilution and Hypervolemia

Because blood is a non-Newtonian fluid, ratios of cellular elements and plasma protein concentrations to serum are critical in flow because of their effects on viscosity. Increases in the concentration of red blood cells, white blood cells, or fibrinogen can lessen flow.[364] (See Fig. 12–8). Hypervolemic hemodilution has been used to reduce viscosity.[365] Infusions of crystalloids or LMW dextran alone or in combination with venesection have been used to reduce viscosity. A study of hydroxyethyl starch found that the agent increased cardiac output without affecting heart rate or blood

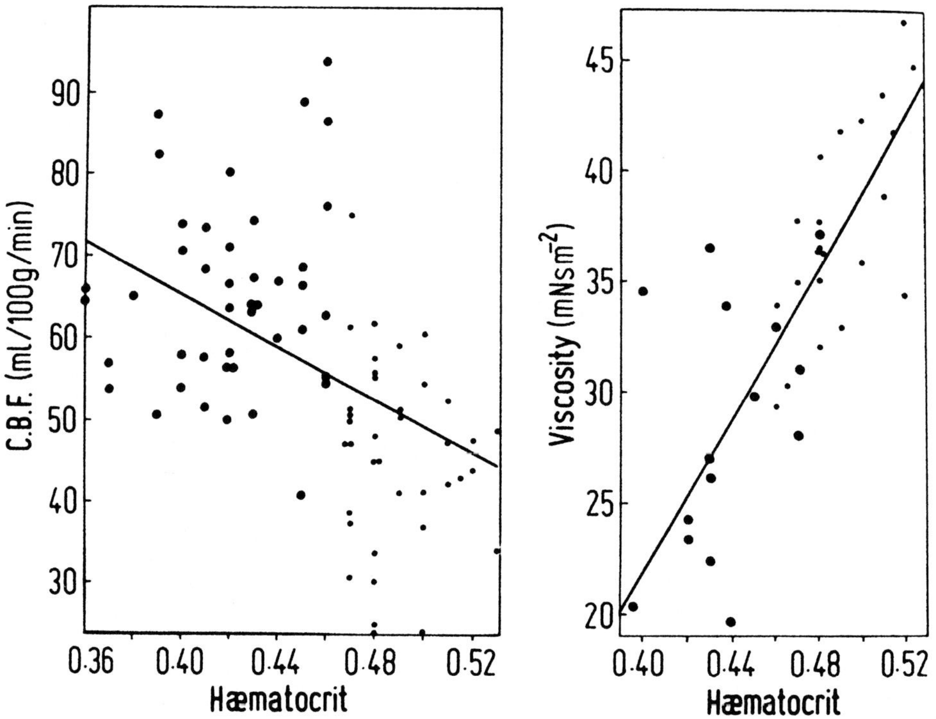

Figure 12–8. Relationship of cerebral flood flow and blood viscosity to hematocrit. (Reprinted from Thomas DJ, et al. Effect of haematocrit on cerebral blood-flow in man. *Lancet* 1977,2:941, with permission.)

pressure, and no decline in cardiac output that could have reduced cerebral perfusion pressure was found.[366] Pentoxifylline improves red blood cell deformability and increases shear stress, but it does not change red blood cell aggregation or viscosity.[367,368] Blood substitutes could improve flow because they reduce viscosity and at the same time maintain the oxygen-carrying capacity of normal blood.[369]

Results of Clinical Trials—Acute Ischemic Stroke

Volume expansion has been used successfully as a preoperative treatment for patients undergoing carotid endarterectomy; the therapy appears to lower the risk of ischemia at the time of arterial clamping.[370] Hemodilution has been tested in several clinical trials (Table 12–22). Matthews et al[371] found no benefit from treatment with LMW dextran. The combination of dexamethasone and LMW dextran was tested in another trial, but no benefit accrued from treatment.[372] Another trial found that hemodilution was associated with an increased mortality secondary to brain edema, although outcomes at 3 months might be better with treatment.[373] Koller et al[374] prescribed LMW dextran, intravenous crystalloid infusions, and venesection, to rapidly and vigorously lowering the hematocrit to a value of 30%–35%. They noted clinical improvements with treatment, but the study's results were not definitive. Based on another small series, Strand[375] believed that the combination of venesection and administration of LMW dextran was safe and could improve outcomes.

Large clinical trials in Italy and Scandinavia found no benefit from hemodilution treatment for acute stroke.[376,377] The Scandinavian study raised the possibility that hemodilution might be associated with increased mortality. These studies' results

Table 12–22. **Results of Clinical Trials of Hemodilution in Patients with Recent Ischemic Stroke**

	Treatment					Control				
	Number	Favorable Outcomes		Mortality		Number	Favorable Outcomes		Mortality	
Study	N	N	%	N	%	N	N	%	N	%
Mathews[371]	52	16	30.8	13	25	48	21	43.8	13	27.1
Strand[375]	52	34	65	13	25	50	22	44	14	28
SSSG[377]	183	—		29	15.8	190	—		24	12.6
Italian[376]	633	289	45.7	175	27.6	634	303	47.7	174	27.4

SSSG = Scandinavian Stroke Study Group

lead to the conclusion that hemodilution is not indicated for treatment of most patients with stroke. In addition to a lack of established efficacy, hemodilution also can be complicated by serious side effects. Osmotic changes could stimulate the development of brain edema, which could be a problem, particularly for patients with multilobar infarctions. Severe allergic reactions or a coagulopathy can accompany use of LMW dextran. In addition, persons with acute ischemic stroke have a high rate of heart disease. The administration of large volumes of fluids could induce acute myocardial ischemia, congestive heart failure, or pulmonary edema. The use of interventions to improve the fluidity of blood is complicated, and they should be used with caution.[364]

Saxena et al[369] tested *diaspirin, a* cross-linked hemoglobin oxygen carrier and potential blood substitute, for treatment of acute ischemic stroke. Mortality and other serious adverse experiences were more common and favorable outcomes were less frequent among patients who received diaspirin. A trial of intravenous *pentoxifylline* followed by oral medications showed that the medication was safe but that it did not improve outcomes.[378] Extracorporeal membrane filtration has been used to treat patients with stroke.[379] The goal is to rapidly improve rheological characteristics of the blood by reducing fibrinogen and macroglobulins without affecting the hematocrit. Clinical experience is limited. One study did not find a difference at 3 months between patients treated with extracorporeal rheophoresis and controls.[380] Retrograde transvenous administration of fluids and possibly medications has been used to improve perfusion in experimental models.[381] The strategy is to send blood to the ischemic area via the veins rather than the arteries. This procedure is invasive and involves the placement of catheters in the major intracranial venous sinuses. Oxygenated blood is removed from the patient and then recirculated via the catheters. Cooling the blood might provide a hypothermic-neuroprotective effect. Clinical experience is limited.

Conclusion

At present, hemodilution should not be used to treat patients with acute ischemic stroke.[382] Current guidelines do not recommend the use of hemodilution for treatment of acute ischemic stroke.[20] Different strategies, including the use of venesection and the administration of LMW dextran, hydroxyethyl starch, or albumin, are not effective. Neither drug-induced vasoconstriction/hypertension nor vasodilation has been determined as useful. Pending additional research, these therapies should be considered to be of unproven value.

SURGICAL AND OTHER INTERVENTIONS TO IMPROVE CEREBRAL PERFUSION

Rationale

Surgical treatment to remove an intraluminal clot or create new collateral channels might restore flow in sufficient time to halt the effects of stroke.[383] However, referral to a center that has this expertise and mobilization of the needed resources on arrival greatly limits the utility of surgical procedures. Overall, clinical experience in the use of surgical procedures to treat stroke is limited.

Carotid Endarterectomy

Meyer et al[384] operated on 34 patients with acute occlusions of the internal carotid artery and achieved a patency rate of 94%. Nine patients completely recovered, and 4 had minimal disability. The remaining patients had severe disability or died. Walters et al[385] performed emergent carotid endarterectomy to manage 64 patients with acute ischemic stroke. They noted that patients with a broad spectrum of neurological impairments seemed to benefit. Ten of the 13 patients who had surgery for treatment of severe strokes either improved or remained stable. Eckstein et al[386] reported on the success of emergent carotid endarterectomy in 71 patients who presented with acute ischemic stroke, stroke-in-evolution, or crescendo TIA. No major complications from surgery were reported. Favorable outcomes were noted in 9 of 16 patients having surgery for acute stroke and in 26 of 34 patients who had operation for stroke-in-evolution. In another study, the same group evaluated emergent carotid endarterectomy in combination with intra-arterial administration of a thrombolytic agent to lyse a distal embolus.[387] Four of 14 patients recovered, and 6 had minor sequelae.

Embolectomy

Embolectomy can be performed to remove a clot from the middle cerebral artery.[388,389] The operation usually is done when the thrombus is in the first segment of the artery or at the bifurcation of the middle cerebral artery. In a small study, Kakinuma et al[389] concluded that embolectomy was superior to medical therapies in improving flow among patients whose pre-operative angiograms show very poor perfusion. They also acknowledged that infarction in the lenticulostriate area might not be avoided by embolectomy.

Endovascular Treatment

Endovascular treatment (angioplasty and stenting) alone or in combination with intra-arterial thrombolytic therapy, is a potential treatment for acute ischemic stroke.[390] The most common location for angioplasty and stenting appears to be the proximal portion of the middle cerebral artery. Anecdotal experience suggests that angioplasty and stenting can be safe and effective.[391] Nakano et al[392] performed direct angioplasty in 10 patients who could not receive other treatment. They were able to crush the embolus manually and establish recanalization in all 10 patients. The combination of angioplasty and thrombolytic therapy could be better than intravenous rt-PA given alone.[42] No controlled trial has tested the usefulness of angioplasty, but this strategy holds promise.

Conclusion

The indications for emergent surgery are unclear. Issues such as the mortality and morbidity related to the operation in comparison to the potential benefits accrued from surgical treatment need careful study.[393] To date, current guidelines do not recommend surgical revascularization procedures to treat stroke.[20] With the expansion of neurointerventional techniques, including intra-arterial administration of thrombolytic agents, these therapies might supplant conventional surgical procedures.

NEUROPROTECTIVE THERAPIES

Neuroprotective agents may protect neurons from ischemia or reperfusion injury. The aim is to improve the brain parenchyma's intrinsic ability to withstand the effects of ischemia.[394] These agents could be combined with thrombolytic therapy or other therapies to maintain or restore circulation.[395] Several agents could potentially limit some metabolic or biochemical consequences. Still, several variables influence the success of neuroprotective therapy. Neuroprotective medications differ widely in terms of pharmacokinetics, mechanisms of action, toxicity, and pharmacologic properties.[396] The safety and tolerability of these compounds and their ease in administration are not uniform.

Among the potential agents are those that reportedly counteract the effects of free radical scavengers, excitatory amino acids, transmembrane fluxes of electrolytes and water, pro-inflammatory interleukins, tumor necrosis factor alpha, or apoptotic factors.[360,397–404] Experimental studies have demonstrated the efficacy of a large number of protective agents. For example, lubeluzole appears to block extracellular glutamate concentrations in animal models of stroke.[405] Some medications reduce the volume of brain infarction and brain edema in experimental models by competitively or non-competitively inhibiting the *n*-methyl-*d*-aspartate (NMDA) receptor and glutamate toxicity.[327,399,403,406,407] The NMDA receptor is critical in looking at the effects of excitatory amino acids and transmembrane fluxes of calcium, sodium, and water. Depletion of cellular potassium may play a role in cell necrosis.[407] The effects of nitric oxide also may be a target of neuroprotective therapy.[408] A controlled metabolic suppression strategy that mimics hibernation might improve tolerance of the brain to ischemia.[409]

Most of these therapies have a primary goal of protecting neurons from the effects of ischemia; however, protection of white matter, oligodendroglia, astrocytes, and axons probably is equally critical.[407,410] The actions of actin, a filament-severing protein, also may be influential in stroke. One of its antagonists, gelsolin, has been tested successfully in murine models of stroke.[411]

Changes in the aggregation of white blood cells may play a role in the evolution of brain ischemia.[412] Inhibitors of inflammatory reactions induced by leucocyte aggregation may protect the brain. Anti-inflammatory agents can limit the release of cytokines, interleukins, and tissue necrosis factor alpha.[413] Gene transfer therapy could be used to modify cellular responses, including apoptosis.[414] Citicoline is an intermediate in phospholipid synthesis, which can be used to help repair membrane damage as the result of ischemic stroke.[415]

The combination of neuroprotective and thrombolytic agents is attractive.[395] The two therapies have independent mechanisms of action that could be complementary. A neuroprotective medication could be given by EMS personnel in the field because it likely will not worsen intracranial bleeding. The neuroprotective agent might extend the window of opportunity for the use of thrombolytic therapy or other measures to restore flow. In addition, neuroprotective therapy could be continued after admission to the hospital. Success in improving blood flow could expedite the delivery of neuroprotective agents to the focus of ischemia. Experimental models have demonstrated success with the use of a combination of a neuroprotective agent and rt-PA.[416] In addition, combinations of neuroprotective agents also might have complementary effects.[327,407]

Results of Clinical Trials—Acute Ischemic Stroke

Although the results of experimental studies have been positive, clinical trials have been disappointing.[417–419,477,490] Several medications have been tested. Many of these trials have been sponsored by pharmaceutical companies and, in some instances, the results of some the trials have not been published despite completion of the research. Apparently, some trials were stopped for lack of efficacy and others were halted prematurely because of high rates of major adverse experiences with active therapy.[402,407] Among the side effects were declines in consciousness, seizures, confusion, delirium, psychosis, and cardiac toxicity.

ANTAGONISTS TO EXCITATORY AMINO ACIDS, INCLUDING GLUTAMATE

Most of the trials testing the antagonists to glutamate or blockers of the NMDA receptor were negative or were stopped prematurely because of side effects.[407,420] *Dizocilpine* (MK801), the first NMDA antagonist to be tested in experimental models, was associated with too many side effects to be used in people.[421] Albers et al[422] tested the safety of oral *dextromethorphan* among patients. No toxicity was noted, but this agent was not tested for efficacy. A study of the safety of the NMDA antagonist *dextrorphan* found a high rate of adverse experiences with the active agent.[423] Almost all patients had signs of neurotoxicity. Other agents that have not been helpful are *selfotel* and *aptiganel*. Trials of selfotel in treating head injury were stopped prematurely in part because of a reported increased mortality with treatment among patients with stroke.[424,425] Davis et al[425] found that selfotel was not effective. A trend towards an increased mortality with treatment among patients with severe stroke raised the possibility of neurotoxicity from the agent. A dose-escalation study of aptiganel found that large doses led to hypertension and central nervous system side effects, including sedation, confusion, agitation, and hallucinations.[426] A study of *ramacemide*, a neuroprotective agent, was found to decrease neurological deficits secondary to coronary artery bypass grafting surgery.[427] The NMDA receptor blocker was evaluated in a pilot dose-escalation study.[428] It appears to be well tolerated, and it might be useful in stroke. A glycine site antagonist at the NMDA receptor GV 50526 appears to be free of hemodynamic and neurological side effects, but it may cause hepatotoxicity.[429] In an experimental study, Stieg et al[421] reported that *memantine* limits NMDA toxicity without behavioral disturbances.

Lubeluzole was tested in a series of clinical trials. Potential side effects of lubeluzole were mainly cardiological—both arrhythmias and changes in cardiac conduction occurred. However, another study found no changes in heart rate or QT interval on the electrocardiogram.[430] A pilot trial of the medication showed that lubeluzole at a daily dose of 10 mg was safe and it appeared to reduce mortality.[431] Grotta et al[432] found improvements in clinical outcomes but no reduction in mortality among patients treated with lubeluzole given within 6 hours of ischemic stroke. A subsequent trial, which has not been reported in the literature but whose results have been described at meetings, apparently found no benefit from treatment.

Magnesium is a neuroprotective agent that causes vasoconstriction and increases regional cerebral blood flow.[433] It also blocks the NMDA receptor, antagonizes the transmembrane ingress of calcium, and stimulates the production of adenosine triphosphate.[433] Magnesium is widely used as a therapy to treat eclampsia and pre-eclampsia. It is an effective anticonvulsant and might stabilize ischemic tissue. Preliminary clinical studies demonstrated that magnesium infusions given to patients with acute stroke do not affect heart rate, blood pressure, or glucose concentrations.[434] Another preliminary study suggested that magnesium might improve outcomes after stroke.[435] Other clinical studies are ongoing.

CALCIUM CHANNEL BLOCKING AGENTS

The potential usefulness of both receptor and voltage calcium channel antagonists have been evaluated.[399] L-type selective and non-selective derivatives of the calcium antagonists have been examined in clinical studies.[436] These agents improve cerebral blood flow and inhibit the effects of excessive intraneuronal concentrations of calcium.[436]

Nimodipine

Nimodipine is the most extensively tested calcium channel blocking agent. It was examined in a series of studies. Kaste et al[437] found that nimodipine did not improve outcomes and that an increased risk of early deaths was secondary to drug-induced hypotension. Another European study was negative.[438] A U.S. study found that nimodipine did not improve outcomes, except in patients who were treated within 18 hours of onset of stroke and who had a negative CT.[439] Wahlgren et al[440] found that the use of nimodipine increased the chances of a poor outcome. The investigators concluded that nimodipine caused hemodynamic effects and hypotension, which may intensify the ischemic process. Infeld et al[441] found that nimodipine did increase reperfusion to the brain but that no net clinical benefit was apparent.

Nicardipine

A pilot study suggested that nicardipine, an intravenously administered calcium channel blocker, might improve outcomes if it was given within 12 hours of onset of stroke.[442] The intravenous dose of nicardipine was titrated to blood pressure levels for approximately 72 hours and then followed by an oral agent for 30 days. No subsequent studies were done, presumably because of the negative results.

Flunarizine

Flunarizine was tested in a double-blind, placebo-controlled trial in Scandinavia and the Netherlands.[443] The medication was given intravenously for 1 week followed by 3 weeks of oral administration. No improvement of neurological status or functional outcomes was found.

FREE RADICAL ANTAGONISTS

Free radical scavengers also have been examined.[399] *Tirilazad,* a 21-aminosteroid that has prominent antioxidant properties without a major glucocorticoid effect, was successful in experimental models of stroke.[444] However, clinical trials of tirilazad gave inconclusive results.[445] One study was halted prematurely after an interim analysis showed that the likelihood of a therapeutic effect from tirilazad was remote.[446]

Other Medications

Administration of medications that depress metabolic function could lessen the effects of acute ischemia. *General anesthetics* and *barbiturates* can be given, but these medications also depress consciousness and cardiovascular activity. *Hypothermia* combined with medications can be successful in limiting the consequences of focal brain ischemia.[447]

Clomethiazole is a neuroprotective agent that increases concentrations of gamma-aminobutyric acid. Unfortunately, clinical studies did not demonstrate an improvement in long-term outcomes with treatment.[448,449] A large trial tested clomethiazole given within 12 hours of stroke; favorable outcomes were noted in 56.1% of patients treated with the agent and 54.8% of patients given placebo.[448]

A pilot study did not report major side effects from large doses of *naloxone.*[450] Nausea, hypotension, hypertension, bradycardia, and myoclonus were uncommon; however, no evidence of a therapeutic effect was found in this study.[451]

A small, placebo-controlled trial compared three possible doses of *citicoline* in treating patients with ischemic stroke.[452] No major side effects were noted. Inexplicably, the doses of 500 mg and 2000 mg of citicoline were associated with improved outcomes, although an intermediate dose of 1000 mg was not effective. A potential advantage of citicoline is that it can be given up to 24 hours after stroke. Unfortunately, a subsequent study of citicoline given in a dose of 500 mg/day did not demonstrate any net benefit from treatment.[453]

Several trials of *GM1-gangliosides* found that this agent, which is a component of neuronal membranes, was not effective in improving outcomes.[360,454–456]

A Japanese study tested *ebselen* among patients with middle cerebral artery stroke.[457] Ebselen's mechanism of action is not clear, although it presumably has a neuroprotective effect. Further research might be indicated to determine whether this medication has a role in treating acute ischemic stroke.

Piracetam affects the phospholipid bilayer of membranes and, thus, could be neuroprotective. It also has effects on platelet function and thrombosis.[458] This medication is used for a variety of indications, including the treatment of dementia. De Deyn et al[459] tested piracetam in a series of patients with acute ischemic stroke. Mortality at 3 months was 23.9% (111/464) among patients treated with the medication and 19.2% (89/463) among those who received placebo. Other studies show that piracetam is safe and might be effective in improving outcomes after stroke.[460–462] Still, the data are not conclusive, and additional research is needed about the possible use of piracetam in acute stroke care.[445]

Administration of an anti-intercellular adhesion molecule 1-antibody (Anti ICAM-1) reduced ischemia in animal models.[463] The anti-ICAM-1 antibody, *enlimomab*, was found to be safe in a pilot study.[464] However, a subsequent randomized trial did not find efficacy of the enlimomab to be effective, and mortality, largely due to infection, resulted in worse outcomes among the treated patients.[445]

HYPERBARIC OXYGEN

Hyperbaric oxygen (HBO) therapy is used to treat patients with Caisson disease or air embolism, but its value in treating persons with strokes of other causes is uncertain.[465] Hyperbaric oxygen could be effective even if it is delayed several hours after air embolism. It can be used to treat increased intracranial pressure after stroke.[466] Side effects have not been reported from HBO therapy.[467,468] The feasibility of using HBO also is unclear.[360,468]

Conclusion

To date, none of the neuroprotective agents is established as useful in lessening the clinical consequences of acute ischemic stroke.[469] Despite their potential benefit in experimental models of stroke, results of clinical trials are largely negative. Some agents have been associated with extraordinarily high rates of neurological complications, and others have not shown evidence of efficacy.

Still, this area of bench and clinical research remains dynamic. As knowledge about the pathophysiology of brain ischemia expands, additional pharmacologic agents likely will be developed to perturb the cellular and metabolic consequence of ischemic stroke. These agents should continue to be tested alone or in combination with interventions that improve or restore blood flow. The persons designing future trials testing neuroprotective agents should be cognizant of the fact that a small (<10%) improvement in outcomes is important if death and disability are to be avoided.

SUBSEQUENT ACUTE CARE

The initial treatment of stroke and management of acute medical and neurological complications influence decisions for subsequent care in both the emergency department and after admission to the hospital. Decisions about admission to the hospital are discussed in Chapter 13. However, all patients who receive emergent treatment of acute ischemic stroke itself should be admitted to a hospital. Some patients might be admitted to units in the hospital, such as the interventional neuroradiology unit, for additional treatment of the stroke. Patients also may be treated in the emergency department of a small hospital and then evacuated to another larger hospital for care in an acute stroke care unit.

Treatment after the administration of thrombolytic agents is especially important. Detailed guidelines for nursing care are available.[470–472] Nurses should use sequential assessments of the NIHSS to detect neurological worsening or improvement.[470] Close observation, including frequent measurements of blood pressure, should be continued during the first hours after treatment. The patient should be admitted to a skilled care unit that includes cardiac monitoring. Arterial hypertension should prompt urgent treatment to lower blood pressure because of the potential risk of hemorrhagic complications (see Table 12–8). Blood pressure should be treated aggressively if arterial hypertension develops while the patient is being transported from one hospital to another. Because of the high risk for bleeding complications, a patient should not have arterial lines, central venous lines, bladder catheters, or nasogastric tubes placed within a few hours of treatment with rt-PA. Patients receiving rt-PA should not receive aspirin, other antiplatelet aggregating agents, heparin, warfarin, or other anticoagulants within 24 hours.[16,19,287]

SUMMARY

Treatment of acute ischemic stroke marks one of the great achievements of the "decade of the brain." Nevertheless, a stroke must be recognized before it can be treated. Great gaps remain in the recognition of the symptoms of stroke, patients' understanding of the urgency of these symptoms, and appropriate management by physicians. Urgent evaluation and prompt imaging have become essential steps in diagnosis leading to therapy. Stroke teams have proven their worth. General measures—such as life support and management of cardiac complications, blood pressure, blood glucose, and fluids—make a big difference in the majority of individuals. A few profit from the proven effectiveness of intravenous thrombolytic therapy. Aspirin has a modest role in acute therapy and a definite role in secondary prevention, as do other antiplatelet agents and warfarin. Attempts to increase cerebral blood flow and outcome by hemodilution, emergent anticoagulation, or surgery have not been successful. Neuroprotectants continue to be evaluated in clinical trials, but the gap between effectiveness in the laboratory and at the bedside has not yet been breached.

Combined therapy with thrombolytics and neuroprotectants is being advocated and tested. The therapeutic age of acute stroke treatment has arrived.

REFERENCES

1. Petit, C. Victims of stroke much more likely to live through it. *San Francisco Chronicle,* 1991.
2. Camarata PJ, Heros PC, Latchaw RE. "Brain attack." The rationale for treating stroke as a medical emergency. *Neurosurgery* 1994;34: 144–158.
3. Adams HP, Jr. Treating ischemic stroke as an emergency. *Arch Neurol* 1998;55:457–461.
4. Heros RC, Camarata PJ, Latchaw RE. Brain attack. Introduction. *Neurosurg Clin N Am* 1997;8:135–144.
5. Alberts MJ. Diagnosis and treatment of ischemic stroke. *Am J Med* 1999;106:211–221.
6. Hill MD, Hachinski V. Stroke treatment: time is brain. *Lancet* 1998;352(Suppl 3):SIII10–SIII14.
7. Barsan WG, Brott TG, Olinger CP, Adams HP, Jr., Haley EC, Jr., Levy DE. Identification and entry of the patient with acute cerebral infarction. *Ann Emerg Med* 1988;17:1192–1195.
8. Ferro JM, Melo TP, Oliveira V, Crespo M, Canhao P, Pinto AN. An analysis of the admission delay of acute strokes. *Cerebrovasc Dis* 1994;4:72–75.
9. Fogelholm R, Murros K, Rissanen A, Ilmavirta M. Factors delaying hospital admission after acute stroke. *Stroke* 1996;27:398–400.
10. Smith MA, Doliszny KM, Shahar E, McGovern PG, Arnett DK, Luepker RV. Delayed hospital arrival for acute stroke: the Minnesota Stroke Survey. *Ann Intern Med* 1998;129:190–196.
11. Biller J, Love BB. Nihilism and stroke therapy. *Stroke* 1991;22:1105–1107.
12. Lees KR. If I had a stroke . . . . *Lancet* 1998;352 (Suppl 3):SIII28–SIII30.
13. Lindley RI, Amayo EO, Marshall J, Sandercock PA, Dennis M, Warlow CP. Hospital services for patients with acute stroke in the United Kingdom: the Stroke Association Survey of consultant opinion. *Ageing* 1995;24:525–532.
14. Neely KW, Norton RL. Survey of health maintenance organization instructions to members concerning emergency department and 911 use. *Ann Emerg Med* 1999;34:19–24.
15. A Working Group on Emergency Brain Resuscitation. Emergency brain resuscitation. *Ann Intern Med* 1995;122:622–627.
16. Quality Standards Subcommittee of the American Academy of Neurology. Practice advisory: thrombolytic therapy for acute ischemic stroke—summary statement. Report of the Quality Standards Subcommittee of the American Academy of Neurology. *Neurology* 1996;47:835–839.
17. The European Ad Hoc Consensus Group. Optimizing intensive care in stroke. A European perspective. *Cerebrovasc Dis* 1997;7:113–128.
18. Adams HP, Jr. The importance of the Helsingborg declaration on stroke management in Europe. *J Intern Med* 1996;240:169–171.
19. Adams HP, Jr., Brott TG, Furlan AJ, et al. Guidelines for thrombolytic therapy for acute stroke: a supplement to the guidelines for the management of patients with acute ischemic stroke. A statement for healthcare professionals from a Special Writing Group of the Stroke Council, American Heart Association. *Circulation* 1996;94:1167–1174.
20. Adams HP, Jr., Brott TG, Crowell RM, et al. Guidelines for the management of patients with acute ischemic stroke. A statement for healthcare professionals from a special writing group of the

Stroke Council, American Heart Association. *Circulation* 1994;90:1588–1601.
21. Organizing Committees (Program advisory, and Local). Asia Pacific consensus forum on stroke management. *Stroke* 1998;29:1730–1736.
22. Lacy CR, Bueno M, Kostis JB. Delayed hospital arrival for acute stroke. *Ann Intern Med* 1999;130:328.
23. Anderson NE, Bonita R, Broad JB. Early management and outcome of acute stroke in Auckland. *Aust N Z J Med* 1997;27:561–567.
24. National Institute of Neurological Disorders and Stroke rt-PA Stroke Study Group. Tissue plasminogen activator for acute ischemic stroke. *N Engl J Med* 1995;333:1581–1587.
25. Zweifler RM, Drinkard R, Cunningham S, Brody ML, Rothrock JF. Implementation of a stroke code system in Mobile, Alabama. Diagnostic and therapeutic yield. *Stroke* 1997; 28:981–983.
26. Fuster V, Smaha L. AHA's new strategic impact goal designed to curb epidemic of cardiovascular disease and stroke. *Circulation* 1999;99:2360.
27. Fuster V. Epidemic of cardiovascular disease and stroke: the three main challenges. Presented at the 71st Scientific Sessions of the American Heart Association. Dallas, Texas. *Circulation* 1999;99:1132–1137.
28. Hacke W. Advances in stroke management: Update 1998. *Neurology* 1999;53(Supp 4):S1–S2.
29. Hacke W, Brott T, Caplan L, et al. Thrombolysis in acute ischemic stroke: Controlled trials and clinical experience. *Neurology* 1999;53 (Supp 4): S3–S14.
30. Kothari R, Jauch E, Broderick J, et al. Acute stroke: delays to presentation and emergency department evaluation. *Ann Emerg Med* 1999; 33:3–8.
31. Streifler JY, Davidovitch S, Sendovski U. Factors associated with the time of presentation of acute stroke patients in an Israeli community hospital. *Neuroepidemiology* 1998;17:161–166.
32. Charatan F. Strokes at night more likely to delay care. *BMJ* 1999;318:959.
33. Wester P, Radberg J, Lundgren B, Peltonen M. Factors associated with delayed admission to hospital and in-hospital delays in acute stroke and TIA: a prospective, multicenter study. Seek-Medical-Attention-in-Time Study Group. *Stroke* 1999;30:40–48.
34. Menon SC, Pandey DK, Morgenstern LB. Critical factors determining access to acute stroke care. *Neurology* 1998;51:427–432.
35. Salisbury HR, Banks BJ, Footitt DR, Winner SJ, Reynolds DJ. Delay in presentation of patients with acute stroke to hospital in Oxford. *QJM* 1998;91:635–640.
36. Pancioli AM, Broderick J, Kothari R, et al. Public perception of stroke warning signs and knowledge of potential risk factors. *JAMA* 1998;279: 1288–1292.
37. Samsa GP, Cohen SJ, Goldstein LB, et al. Knowledge of risk among patients at increased risk for stroke. *Stroke* 1997;28:916–921.
38. Goldstein LB, Gradison M. Stroke-related knowledge among patients with access to medical care in the stroke belt. *J Stroke Cerebrovasc Dis* 1999;8:349–352.
39. Castaldo JE, Nelson JJ, Reed JF, Longenecker JE, Toole JF. The delay in reporting symptoms of carotid artery stenosis in an at-risk population. The Asymptomatic Carotid Atherosclerosis Study experience: a statement of concern regarding watchful waiting. *Arch Neurol* 1997;54: 1267–1271.
40. Cheung RT, Li LS, Mak W, et al. Knowledge of stroke in Hong Kong Chinese. *Cerebrovasc Dis* 1999;9:119–123.
41. Barsan WG, Brott TG, Broderick JP, Haley EC, Levy DE, Marler JR. Time of hospital presentation in patients with acute stroke. *Arch Intern Med* 1993;153:2558–2561.
42. Famularo G, Polchi S, Panegrossi A. Thrombolysis enters the race: a new era for acute ischaemic stroke?. *Eur J Emerg Med* 1998; 5:249–252.
43. Pepe PE, Zachariah BS, Sayre MR, Floccare D. Ensuring the chain of recovery for stroke in your community. *Acad Emerg Med* 1998;5:352–358.
44. Pepe PE, Zachariah BS, Sayre MR, Floccare D. Ensuring the chain of recovery for stroke in your community. Chain of Recovery Writing Group. *Prehospital Emergency Care* 1998;2:89–95.
45. American Heart Association. *Advanced cardiac life support.* American Heart Association, Dallas, 1997.
46. Barsan WG, Brott TG, Broderick JP, Haley EC, Jr., Levy DE, Marler JR. Urgent therapy for acute stroke. Effects of a stroke trial on untreated patients. *Stroke* 1994;25:2132–2137.
47. Kothari R, Barsan W, Brott T, Broderick J, Ashbrock S. Frequency and accuracy of prehospital diagnosis of acute stroke. *Stroke* 1995;26: 937–941.
48. Broderick JP. Logistics in acute stroke management. *Drugs* 1997;54(Suppl 3):109–116.
49. Harbison J, Massey A, Barnett L, Hodge D, Ford GA. Rapid ambulance protocol for acute stroke. *Lancet* 1999;353:1935.
50. Teasdale GM, Pettigrew LE, Wilson JT, Murray G, Jennett B. Analyzing outcome of treatment of severe head injury: a review and update on advancing the use of the Glasgow Outcome Scale. *J Neurotrauma* 1998;15:587–597.
51. Kidwell CS, Starkman S, Eckstein M, Weems K, Saver JL. Identifying stroke in the field. Prospective validation of the Los Angeles Prehospital Stroke Screen (LAPSS). *Stroke* 2000;31:71–76.
52. Kothari R, Hall K, Brott T, Broderick J. Early stroke recognition: developing an out-of-hospital NIH Stroke Scale. *Acad Emerg Med* 1997;4: 986–990.
53. Crocco TJ, Kothari RU, Sayre MR, Liu T. A nationwide prehospital stroke survey. *Prehospital Emergency Care* 1999;3:201–206.
54. Hachinski V. Thrombolysis in stroke. Between the promise and the peril. *JAMA* 1996;276: 995–996.
55. Goldstein LB, Hey LA, Laney R. North Carolina stroke prevention and treatment facilities survey: Statewide availability of programs and services. *Stroke* 2000;31:66–70.

56. Conroy MB, Rodriguez SU, Kimmel SE, Kasner SE. Helicopter transfer offers a potential benefit to patients with acute stroke. *Stroke* 1999; 30:2580–2584.
57. Levine SR, Gorman M. Telestroke. The application of telemedicine for stroke. *Stroke* 1999;30: 464–469.
58. Shafqat S, Kvedar JC, Guanci MM, Chang Y, Schwamm LH. Role for telemedicine in acute stroke. Feasibility and reliability of remote administration of the NIH stroke scale. *Stroke* 1999;30:2141–2145.
59. Scott PA, Temovsky CJ, Lawrence K, Gudaitis E, Lowell MJ. Analysis of Canadian population with potential geographic access to intravenous thrombolysis for acute ischemic stroke. *Stroke* 1998;29:2304–2310.
60. Goldstein LB, Hey LA, Laney R. North Carolina stroke prevention and treatment facilities survey: rt-PA therapy for acute stroke. *Stroke* 1998; 29:2069–2072
61. Langhorne P. Developing comprehensive stroke services: an evidence-based approach. *Postgrad Med* 1995;71:733–737.
62. Alberts MJ, Chaturvedi S, Graham G, et al. Acute stroke teams: results of a national survey. National Acute Stroke Team Group. *Stroke* 1998;29:2318–2320.
63. Lyden PD, Rapp K, Babcock T, Rothrock J. Ultra-rapid identification, triage, and enrollment of stroke patients into clinical trials. *J Stroke Cerebrovasc Dis* 1994;4:106–113.
64. Pessin MS, Adams HP, Jr., Adams RJ, et al. American Heart Association Prevention Conference. IV. Prevention and rehabilitation of stroke. Acute interventions. *Stroke* 1997;28: 1518–1521.
65. Lewandowski CA, Libman R. Acute presentation of stroke. *J Stroke Cerebrovasc Dis* 1999; 8:117–126.
66. Members of the Lille Stroke Program. Misdiagnoses in 1,250 consecutive patients admitted to an acute stroke unit. *Cerebrovasc Dis* 1997;7:284–288.
67. Gladman JR, Harwood DM, Barer DH. Predicting the outcome of acute stroke: prospective evaluation of five multivariate models and comparison with simple methods. *J Neurol Neurosurg Psychiatry* 1992;55:347–351.
68. Vingerhoets F, Bogousslavsky J. Respiratory dysfunction in stroke. *Clin Chest Med* 1994; 15:729–737.
69. Azzimondi G, Bassein L, Nonino F, et al. Fever in acute stroke worsens prognosis. *Stroke* 1995;26: 2040–2043.
70. Georgilis K, Plomaritoglou A, Dafni U, Bassiakos Y, Vemmos K. Aetiology of fever in patients with acute stroke. *J Intern Med* 1999;246:203–209.
71. Davalos A, Castillo J. Potential mechanisms of worsening. *Cerebrovasc Dis* 1997;7(Suppl 5):19–24.
72. Castillo J, Davalos A, Marrugat J, Noya M. Timing for fever-related brain damage in acute ischemic stroke. *Stroke* 1998;29:2455–2460.
73. Brott T, Lu M, Kothari R, et al. Hypertension and its treatment in the NINDS rt-PA Stroke Trial. *Stroke* 1998;29:1504–1509.
74. Robinson TG, James M, Youde J, Panerai R, Potter J. Cardiac baroreceptor sensitivity is impaired after acute stroke. *Stroke* 1997;28: 1671–1676.
75. Robinson T, Waddington A, Ward-Close S, Taub N, Potter J. The predictive role of 24-hour compared to causal blood pressure levels on outcome following acute stroke. *Cerebrovasc Dis* 1997;7:264–272.
76. Wallis WE, Donaldson I, Scott RS, Wilson J. Hypoglycemia masquerading as cerebrovascular disease (hypoglycemic hemiplegia). *Ann Neurol* 1985;18:510–512.
77. Chambers BR, Norris JW, Shurvell BL, Hachinski VC. Prognosis of acute stroke. *Neurology* 1987;37:221–225.
78. Fiorelli M, Alperovitch A, Argentino C, et al. Prediction of long-term outcome in the early hours following acute ischemic stroke. Italian Acute Stroke Study Group. *Arch Neurol* 1995;52:250–255.
79. Fieschi C, Argentino C, Lenzi GL, Sacchetti ML, Toni D, Bozzao L. Clinical and instrumental evaluation of patients with ischemic stroke within the first six hours. *J Neurol Sci* 1989;91: 311–321.
80. Jorgensen HS, Nakayama H, Raaschou HO, Olsen TS. Acute stroke: prognosis and a prediction of the effect of medical treatment on outcome and health care utilization. The Copenhagen Stroke Study. *Neurology* 1997;49: 1335–1342.
81. Muir KW, Weir CJ, Murray GD, Povey C, Lees KR. Comparison of neurological scales and scoring systems for acute stroke prognosis. *Stroke* 1996;27:1817–1820.
82. Adams HP, Jr., Davis PH, Leira EC, et al. Baseline NIH Stroke Scale score strongly predicts outcome after stroke. *Neurology* 1999; 53:126–131.
83. Brott T, Marler JR, Olinger CP, et al. Measurements of acute cerebral infarction: lesion size by computed tomography. *Stroke* 1989;20:871–875.
84. Brott T, Adams HP, Jr., Olinger CP, et al. Measurements of acute cerebral infarction: a clinical examination scale. *Stroke* 1989;20: 864–870.
85. DeGraba TJ, Hallenbeck JM, Pettigrew KD, Dutka AJ, Kelly BJ. Progression in acute stroke: value of the initial NIH stroke scale score on patient stratification in future trials. *Stroke* 1999;30:1208–1212.
86. Adams HP, Jr., Bendixen BH, Kappelle LJ, et al. Classification of subtype of acute ischemic stroke. Definitions for use in a multicenter clinical trial. TOAST. Trial of Org 10172 in Acute Stroke Treatment. *Stroke* 1993;24:35–41.
87. Madden KP, Karanjia PN, Adams HP, Jr., Clarke WR. Accuracy of initial stroke subtype diagnosis in the TOAST study. Trial of ORG 10172 in Acute Stroke Treatment. *Neurology* 1995;45: 1975–1979.
88. Johnson CJ, Kittner SJ, McCarter RJ, et al. Interrater reliability of an etiologic classification of ischemic stroke. *Stroke* 1995;26:46–51.

89. Weir CJ, Murray GD, Adams FG, Muir KW, Grosset DG, Lees KR. Poor accuracy of stroke scoring systems for differential clinical diagnosis of intracranial haemorrhage and infarction. *Lancet* 1994;344:999–1002.
90. Wityk RJ, Pessin MS, Kaplan RF, Caplan LR. Serial assessment of acute stroke using the NIH Stroke Scale. *Stroke* 1994;25:362–365.
91. Davalos A, Cendra E, Teruel J, Martinez M, Genis D. Deteriorating ischemic stroke: risk factors and prognosis. *Neurology* 1990;40: 1865–1869.
92. Donnan GA, Norrving B, Bamford J, Bogousslavsky J. Subcortical infarction: classification and terminology. *Cerebrovasc Dis* 1993;3:248–251.
93. Roden-Jullig A. Progressing stroke. Epidemiology. *Cerebrovasc Dis* 1997;7(Suppl 5): 2–5.
94. Yamamoto H, Bogousslavsky J, Van Melle G. Different predictors of neurological worsening in different causes of stroke. *Arch Neurol* 1998;55:481–486.
95. Toni D. Predictors of stroke deterioration. *Cerebrovasc Dis* 1997;7(Suppl 5):10–13.
96. Alberts MJ, Brass LM. Assessment of early deterioration. *J Stroke Cerebrovasc Dis* 1999;8: 171–175.
97. Rothrock JF, Clark WM, Lyden PD. Spontaneous early improvement following ischemic stroke. *Stroke* 1995;26:1358–1360.
98. Kothari RU, Brott T, Broderick JP, Hamilton CA. Emergency physicians. Accuracy in the diagnosis of stroke. *Stroke* 1995;26:2238–2241.
99. Adams HP, Jr. Management of patients with acute ischaemic stroke. *Drugs* 1997;54(Suppl 3): 60–69.
100. Wardlaw JM, Lewis SC, Dennis MS, Counsell C, McDowall M. Is visible infarction on computed tomography associated with an adverse prognosis in acute ischemic stroke? *Stroke* 1998;29: 1315–1319.
101. Marks MP. CT in ischemic stroke. *Neuroimag Clin N Am* 1998;8:515–523.
102. Grotta JC, Chiu D, Lu M, et al. Agreement and variability in the interpretation of early CT changes in stroke patients qualifying for intravenous rt-PA therapy. *Stroke* 1999;30:1528–1533.
103. Fieschi C, Sette G, Toni D. Assessment of brain tissue viability under clinical circumstances. *Acta Neurochir* 1999;73(Suppl): 73–80.
104. Caplan LR. New therapies for stroke. *Arch Neurol* 1997;54:1222–1224.
105. Bushnell CD, Phillips-Bute BG, Laskowitz DT, Lynch JR, Chilukuri V, Borel CO. Survival and outcome after endotracheal intubation for acute stroke. *Neurology* 1999;52:1374–1381.
106. Hacke W, Krieger D, Hirschberg M. General principles in the treatment of acute ischemic stroke. *Cerebrovasc Dis* 1991;1(Suppl 1):93–99.
107. Grotta J, Pasteur W, Khwaja G, Hamel T, Fisher M, Ramirez A. Elective intubation for neurologic deterioration after stroke. *Neurology* 1995;45:640–644.
108. Ronning OM, Guldvog B. Should stroke victims routinely receive supplemental oxygen? A quasi-randomized controlled trial. *Stroke* 1999;30: 2033–2037.
109. Przelomski MM, Roth RM, Gleckman RA, Marcus EM. Fever in the wake of a stroke. *Neurology* 1986;36:427–429.
110. Lyden PD, Marler JR. Acute medical therapy. *J Stroke Cerebrovasc Dis* 1999;8:139–145.
111. Hajat C, Hajat S, Sharma P. Effects of poststroke pyrexia on stroke outcome. A meta-analysis of studies in patients. *Stroke* 2000;31:410–414.
112. Wang Y, Lim LLY, Levi C, Heller RF, Fisher J, Maths B. Influence of admission body temperature on stroke mortality. *Stroke* 2000;31:404–409.
113. Jorgensen HS, Reith J, Nakayama H, Kammersgaard LP, Raaschou HO, Olsen TS. What determines good recovery in patients with the most severe strokes? The Copenhagen Stroke Study. *Stroke* 1999;30:2008–2012.
114. Myers MG, Norris JW, Hachinski VC, Weingert ME, Sole MJ. Cardiac sequelae of acute stroke. *Stroke* 1982;13:838–842.
115. Korpelainen JT, Sotaniemi KA, Makikallio A, Huikuri HV, Myllyla VV. Dynamic behavior of heart rate in ischemic stroke. *Stroke* 1999;30: 1008–1013.
116. Oppenheimer SM. Neurogenic cardiac effects of cerebrovascular disease. *Curr Opin Neurol* 1994;7:20–24.
117. McDermott MM, Lefevre F, Arron M, Martin GJ, Biller J. ST segment depression detected by continuous electrocardiography in patients with acute ischemic stroke or transient ischemic attack. *Stroke* 1994;25:1820–1824.
118. Lane RD, Wallace JD, Petrosky PP, Schwartz GE, Gradman AH. Supraventricular tachycardia in patients with right hemisphere strokes. *Stroke* 1992;23:362–366.
119. Tokgozoglu SL, Batur MK, Topcuoglu MA, Saribas O, Kes S, Oto A. Effects of stroke localization on cardiac autonomic balance and sudden death. *Stroke* 1999;30:1307–1311.
120. Oppenheimer SM, Hachinski VC. The cardiac consequences of stroke. *Neurol Clin* 1992;10: 167–176.
121. Korpelainen JT, Sotaniemi KA, Huikuri HV, Myllya VV. Abnormal heart rate variability as a manifestation of autonomic dysfunction in hemispheric brain infarction. *Stroke* 1996;27: 2059–2063.
122. Korpelainen JT, Sotaniemi KA, Huikuri HV, Myllyla VV. Circadian rhythm of heart rate variability is reversibly abolished in ischemic stroke. *Stroke* 1997;28:2150–2154.
123. Chua HC, Sen S, Cosgriff RF, Gerstenblith G, Beauchamp NJ, Jr., Oppenheimer SM. Neurogenic ST depression in stroke. *Clin Neurol Neurosurg* 1999;101:44–48.
124. Kocan MJ. Cardiovascular effects of acute stroke. *Progress in Cardiovascular Nursing* 1999; 14:61–67.
125. Kolin A, Norris JW. Myocardial damage from acute cerebral lesions. *Stroke* 1984;15:990–993.
126. Britton M, de Faire U, Helmers C, Miah K, Ryding C, Wester PO. Arrhythmias in patients with acute cerebrovascular disease. *Acta Med Scand* 1979;205:425–428.

127. Morfis L, Schwartz RS, Poulos R, Howes LG. Blood pressure changes in acute cerebral infarction and hemorrhage. *Stroke* 1997;28:1401–1405.
128. Broderick J, Brott T, Barsan W, et al. Blood pressure during the first minutes of focal cerebral ischemia. *Ann Emerg Med* 1993;22: 1438–1443.
129. Phillips SJ. Pathophysiology and management of hypertension in acute ischemic stroke. *Hypertension* 1994;23:131–136.
130. Bowes MP, Zivin JA, Thomas GR, Thibodeaux H, Fagan SC. Acute hypertension, but not thrombolysis, increases the incidence and severity of hemorrhagic transformation following experimental stroke in rabbits. *Exp Neurol* 1996;141:40–46.
131. Powers WJ. Acute hypertension after stroke: the scientific basis for treatment decisions. *Neurology* 1993;43:461–467.
132. Kaplan NM. Management of hypertensive emergencies. *Lancet* 1994;344:1335–1338.
133. Grossman E, Ironi AN, Messerli FH. Comparative tolerability profile of hypertensive crisis treatments. *Drug Saf* 1998;19:99–122.
134. Grossman E, Messerli FH, Grodzicki T, Kowey P. Should a moratorium be placed on sublingual nifedipine capsules given for hypertensive emergencies and pseudoemergencies? *JAMA* 1996; 276:1328–1331.
135. Tietjen CS, Hurn PD, Ulatowski JA, Kirsch JR. Treatment modalities for hypertensive patients with intracranial pathology: options and risks. *Crit Care Med* 1996;24:311–322.
136. Toni D, De Michele M, Fiorelli M, et al. Influence of hyperglycaemia on infarct size and clinical outcome of acute ischemic stroke patients with intracranial arterial occlusion. *J Neurol Sci* 1994;123:129–133.
137. Weir CJ, Murray GD, Dyker AG, Lees KR. Is hyperglycaemia an independent predictor of poor outcome after acute stroke? Results of a long-term follow up study. *BMJ* 1997;314: 1303–1306.
138. Bruno A, Biller J, Adams HP, Jr., et al. Acute blood glucose level and outcome from ischemic stroke. Trial of ORG 10172 in Acute Stroke Treatment (TOAST) Investigators. *Neurology* 1999;52:280–284.
139. Murros K, Fogelholm R, Kettunen S, Vuorela AL, Valve J. Blood glucose, glycosylated haemoglobin, and outcome of ischemic brain infarction. *J Neurol Sci* 1992;111:59–64.
140. Adams HP, Jr., Olinger CP, Marler JR, et al. Comparison of admission serum glucose concentration with neurologic outcome in acute cerebral infarction. A study in patients given naloxone. *Stroke* 1988;19:455–458.
141. Broderick JP, Hagen T, Brott T, Tomsick T. Hyperglycemia and hemorrhagic transformation of cerebral infarcts. *Stroke* 1995;26:484–487.
142. Reith J, Jorgensen HS, Pedersen PM, et al. Body temperature in acute stroke: relation to stroke severity, infarct size, mortality, and outcome. *Lancet* 1996;347:422–425.
143. Davalos A, de Cendra E, Molins A, Ferrandiz M, Lopez-Pousa S, Genis D. Epileptic seizures at the onset of stroke. *Cerebrovasc Dis* 1992;2:327–331.
144. Kilpatrick CJ, Davis SM, Tress BM, Rossiter SC, Hopper JL, Vandendriesen ML. Epileptic seizures in acute stroke. *Arch Neurol* 1990;47:157–160.
145. Kilpatrick CJ, Davis SM, Hopper JL, Rossiter SC. Early seizures after acute stroke. Risk of late seizures. *Arch Neurol* 1992;49:509–511.
146. Bell WR, Jr. Evaluation of thrombolytic agents. *Drugs* 1997;54(Suppl 3):11–16.
147. Lijnen HR, Collen D. Fibrinolytic agents: mechanisms of activity and pharmacology. *Thromb Haemost* 1995;74:387–390.
148. Vanderschueren S, Collen D. Comparative effects of staphylokinase and alteplase in rabbit bleeding time models. *Thromb Haemost* 1996;75: 816–819.
149. Lijnen HR, Stassen JM, Collen D. Differential inhibition with antifibrinolytic agents of staphylokinase and streptokinase induced clot lysis. *Thromb Haemost* 1995;73:845–849.
150. Verstraete M, Lijnen HR, Collen D. Thrombolytic agents in development. *Drugs* 1995;50:29–42.
151. Fox D, Ouriel K, Green RM, Stoughton J, Riggs P, Cimino C. Thrombolysis with prourokinase versus urokinase: an in vitro comparison. *J Vasc Surg* 1996;23:657–666.
152. Credo RB, Burke SE. Fibrinolytic mechanism, biochemistry, and preclinical pharmacology of recombinant prourokinase. *J Vasc Interv Radiol* 1995;6:S8–S18.
153. Rijken DC, Jie AF. Interaction of reteplase with heparin. A comparison between reteplase and alteplase. *Blood Coagulation & Fibrinolysis* 1996;7: 561–566.
154. Collen D, Lijnen HR. Molecular basis of fibrinolysis, as relevant for thrombolytic therapy. *Thromb Haemost* 1995;74:167–171.
155. Koster RW, Cohen AF, Kluft C, et al. The pharmacokinetics of recombinant double-chain t-PA (duteplase): effects of bolus injection, infusions, and administration by weight in patients with myocardial infarction. *Clin Pharmacol Ther* 1991;50:267–277.
156. Martin U, Kaufmann B, Neugebauer G. Current clinical use of reteplase for thrombolysis. A pharmacokinetic–pharmacodynamic perspective. *Clin Pharmacokin* 1999;36:265–276.
157. Ueda T, Hatakeyama T, Sakaki S, Ohta S, Kumon Y, Uraoka T. Changes in coagulation and fibrinolytic system after local intra-arterial thrombolysis for acute ischemic stroke. *Neurologia Medico-Chirurgica* 1995;35:136–143.
158. Fassbender K, Dempfle CE, Mielke O, et al. Changes in coagulation and fibrinolysis markers in acute ischemic stroke treated with recombinant tissue plasminogen activator. *Stroke* 1999; 30:2101–2104.
159. Reganon E, Ferrando F, Vila V, et al. Increase in thrombin generation after coronary thrombolysis with rt-PA or streptokinase with simultaneous heparin versus heparin alone. *Haemostasis* 1998;28:99–105.
160. Eisenberg PR, Sobel BE, Jaffe AS. Activation of prothrombin accompanying thrombolysis with recombinant tissue-type plasminogen activator. *J Am Coll Cardiol* 1992;19:1065–1069.

161. Figueroa BE, Keep RF, Betz AL, Hoff JT. Plasminogen activators potentiate thrombin-induced brain injury. *Stroke* 1998;29:1202–1207.
162. Metz BK, White HD, Granger CB, et al. Randomized comparison of direct thrombin inhibition versus heparin in conjunction with fibrinolytic therapy for acute myocardial infarction: results from the GUSTO-IIb Trial. Global Use of Strategies to Open Occluded Coronary Arteries in Acute Coronary Syndromes (GUSTO-IIb) Investigators. *J Am Coll Cardiol* 1998;31:1493–1498.
163. Paolini R, Casonato A, Boeri G, et al. Effect of recombinant-tissue plasminogen activator, low molecular weight urokinase and unfractionated heparin on platelet aggregation. *J Med* 1993; 24:113–130.
164. Huang TC, Graham DA, Nelson LD, Alevriadou BR. Fibrinolytic agents inhibit platelet adhesion onto collagen type I-coated surfaces at high blood flow conditions. *Blood Coagulation & Fibrinolysis* 1998;9:213–226.
165. Chen H, Wu YI, Hsieh YL, et al. Perturbation of platelet adhesion to endothelial cells by plasminogen activation in vitro. *Thromb Haemost* 1997;78:934–938.
166. Karlberg KE, Chen J, Hagerman I, et al. Streptokinase, but not tissue plasminogen activator, attenuates platelet aggregation in patients with acute myocardial infarction. *J Intern Med* 1993;234:513–519.
167. Kawano K, Aoki I, Aoki N, et al. Human platelet activation by thrombolytic agents: effects of tissue-type plasminogen activator and urokinase on platelet surface P-selectin expression. *Am Heart J* 1998;135:268–271.
168. Gurbel PA, Serebruany VL, Shustov AR, et al. Effects of reteplase and alteplase on platelet aggregation and major receptor expression during the first 24 hours of acute myocardial infarction treatment. GUSTO-III Investigators. Global Use of Strategies to Open Occluded Coronary Arteries. *J Am Coll Cardiol* 1998;31: 1466–1473.
169. Xiaoli M, Wenying H, Mingpeng S. Effects and mechanism of tissue-type plasminogen activator and plasminogen activator inhibitor on vascular smooth muscle cell proliferation. *Internat J Cardiol* 1998;66(Suppl 1):S57–S64.
170. Bell WR, Jr. Defibrinogenating enzymes. *Drugs* 1997;54(Suppl 3):18–30.
171. Atkinson RP. Ancrod in the treatment of acute ischemic stroke. A review of clinical data. *Cerebrovasc Dis* 1998;8(Suppl 1):23–28.
172. Pollak VE, Glas-Greenwalt P, Olinger CP, Wadhwa NK, Myre SA. Ancrod causes rapid thrombolysis in patients with acute stroke. *Am J Med Sci* 1990;299:319–325.
173. Kanagasabay RR, Unsworth-White MJ, Robinson G, et al. Cardiopulmonary bypass with danaparoid sodium and ancrod in heparin-induced thrombocytopenia. *Ann Thorac Surg* 1998;66:567–569.
174. Haley EC, Jr. Thrombolytic therapy for acute ischemic stroke. *Clin Neuropharmacol* 1993;16: 179–194.
175. Shuaib A, Yang Y, Siddiqui MM, Kalra J. Intraarterial urokinase produces significant attenuation of infarction volume in an embolic focal ischemia model. *Exp Neurol* 1998;154: 330–335.
176. Zhang RL, Chopp M, Zhang ZG, Divine G. Early (1 h) administration of tissue plasminogen activator reduces infarct volume without increasing hemorrhagic transformation after focal cerebral embolization in rats. *J Neurol Sci* 1998;160:1–8.
177. Zhang RL, Zhang ZG, Chopp M, Zivin JA. Thrombolysis with tissue plasminogen activator alters adhesion molecule expression in the ischemic rat brain. *Stroke* 1999;30:624–629.
178. Kilic E, Hermann DM, Hossmann KA. Recombinant tissue plasminogen activator reduces infarct size after reversible thread occlusion of middle cerebral artery in mice. *Neuroreport* 1999;10:107–111.
179. Ohue S, Kohno K, Kusunoki K, et al. Magnetic resonance angiography in patients with acute stroke treated by local thrombolysis. *Neuroradiology* 1998;40:536–540.
180. Maurer M, Mullges W, Becker G. Diagnosis of MCA-occlusion and monitoring of systemic thrombolytic therapy with contrast enhanced transcranial duplex-sonography. *J Neuroimaging* 1999;9:99–101.
181. Lansberg MG, Tong DC, Norbash AM, Yenari MA, Moseley ME. Intra-arterial rt-PA treatment of stroke assessed by diffusion- and perfusion-weighted MRI. *Stroke* 1999;30:678–680.
182. Marks MP, Tong DC, Beaulieu C, Albers GW, de Crespigny A, Moseley ME. Evaluation of early reperfusion and IV tPA therapy using diffusion- and perfusion-weighted MRI. *Neurology* 1999; 52:1792–1798.
183. Heiss WD, Grond M, Thiel A, et al. Tissue at risk of infarction rescued by early reperfusion: a positron emission tomography study in systemic recombinant tissue plasminogen activator thrombolysis of acute stroke. *J Cereb Blood Flow Metab* 1998;18:1298–1307.
184. Grotta JC, Alexandrov AV. tPA-associated reperfusion after acute stroke demonstrated by SPECT. *Stroke* 1998;29:429–432.
185. Sasaki O, Takeuchi S, Koizumi T, Koike T, Tanaka R. Complete recanalization via fibrinolytic therapy can reduce the number of ischemic territories that progress to infarction. *Am J Neuroradiol* 1996;17:1661–1668.
186. Yasaka M, O'Keefe GJ, Chambers BR, et al. Streptokinase in acute stroke: effect on reperfusion and recanalization. Australian Streptokinase Trial Study Group. *Neurology* 1998;50:626–632.
187. Baird AE, Donnan GA, Austin MC, Fitt GJ, Davis SM, McKay WJ. Reperfusion after thrombolytic therapy in ischemic stroke measured by single-photon emission computed tomography. *Stroke* 1994;25:79–85.
188. Hillegass WB, Jollis JG, Granger CB, Ohman EM, Califf RM, Mark DB. Intracranial hemorrhage risk and new thrombolytic therapies in acute myocardial infarction. *Am J Cardiol* 1994; 73:444–449.

189. Gurwitz JH, Gore JM, Goldberg RJ, et al. Risk for intracranial hemorrhage after tissue plasminogen activator treatment for acute myocardial infarction. Participants in the National Registry of Myocardial Infarction 2. *Ann Intern Med* 1998;129:597–604.
190. Gore JM, Granger CB, Simoons ML, et al. Stroke after thrombolysis. Mortality and functional outcomes in the GUSTO-I trial. Global Use of Strategies to Open Occluded Coronary Arteries. *Circulation* 1995;92:2811–2818.
191. Wijdicks EF, Jack CR, Jr. Intracerebral hemorrhage after fibrinolytic therapy for acute myocardial infarction. *Stroke* 1993;24:554–557.
192. Alpert JS. Intracranial hemorrhage after thrombolytic therapy: a therapeutic conflict. *J Am Coll Cardiol* 1992;19:295–296.
193. Sloan MA, Gore JM. Ischemic stroke and intracranial hemorrhage following thrombolytic therapy for acute myocardial infarction: a risk–benefit analysis. *Am J Cardiol* 1992;69: A21–A38.
194. Gore JM, Sloan M, Price TR, et al. Intracerebral hemorrhage, cerebral infarction, and subdural hematoma after acute myocardial infarction and thrombolytic therapy in the Thrombolysis in Myocardial Infarction Study. Thrombolysis in Myocardial Infarction, phase II, pilot and clinical trial. *Circulation* 1991;83:448–459.
195. Longstreth WT, Jr., Litwin PE, Weaver WD. Myocardial infarction, thrombolytic therapy, and stroke. A community-based study. The MITI Project Group. *Stroke* 1993;24:587–590.
196. Larrue V, von Kummer R, del Zoppo G, Bluhmki E. Hemorrhagic transformation in acute ischemic stroke. Potential contributing factors in the European Cooperative Acute Stroke Study. *Stroke* 1997;28:957–960.
197. Jaillard A, Cornu C, Durieux A, et al. Hemorrhagic transformation in acute ischemic stroke. *Stroke* 1999;30:1326–1332.
198. The NINDS t-PA Stroke Study Group. Intracerebral hemorrhage after intravenous t-PA therapy for ischemic stroke. *Stroke* 1997;28: 2109–2118.
199. Levy DE, Brott TG, Haley EC, Jr., et al. Factors related to intracranial hematoma formation in patients receiving tissue-type plasminogen activator for acute ischemic stroke. *Stroke* 1994;25: 291–297.
200. Ueda T, Hatakeyama T, Kumon Y, Sakaki S, Uraoka T. Evaluation of risk of hemorrhagic transformation in local intra-arterial thrombolysis in acute ischemic stroke by initial SPECT. *Stroke* 1994;25:298–303.
201. Trouillas P, Nighoghossian N, Derex L, et al. Thrombolysis with intravenous rtPA in a series of 100 cases of acute carotid territory stroke: determination of etiological, topographic, and radiological outcome factors. *Stroke* 1998;29: 2529–2540.
202. Demchuk AM, Morgenstern LB, Krieger DW, et al. Serum glucose level and diabetes predict tissue plasminogen activator-related intracerebral hemorrhage in acute ischemic stroke. *Stroke* 1999;30:34–39.
203. Becker RC, Hochman JS, Cannon CP, et al. Fatal cardiac rupture among patients treated with thrombolytic agents and adjunctive thrombin antagonists: observations from the Thrombolysis and Thrombin Inhibition in Myocardial Infarction 9 Study. *J Am Coll Cardiol* 1999;33: 479–487.
204. Kasner SE, Villar-Cordova CE, Tong D, Grotta JC. Hemopericardium and cardiac tamponade after thrombolysis for acute ischemic stroke. *Neurology* 1998;50:1857–1859.
205. Becker RC, Charlesworth A, Wilcox RG, et al. Cardiac rupture associated with thrombolytic therapy: impact of time to treatment in the Late Assessment of Thrombolytic Efficacy (LATE) study. *J Am Coll Cardiol* 1995;25:1063–1068.
206. Katzan IL, Masaryk TJ, Furlan AJ, et al. Intra-arterial thrombolysis for perioperative stroke after open heart surgery. *Neurology* 1999;52: 1081–1084.
207. Rudolf J, Grond M, Prince WS, Schmulling S, Heiss WD. Evidence of anaphylaxy after alteplase infusion. *Stroke* 1999;30:1142–1143.
208. Pancioli A, Brott T, Donaldson V, Miller R. Asymmetric angioneurotic edema associated with thrombolysis for acute stroke. *Ann Emerg Med* 1997;30:227–229.
209. Stephens MB, Pepper PV. Streptokinase therapy. Recognizing and treating allergic reactions. *Postgrad Med* 1998;103:89–90.
210. Boersma E, Maas AC, Deckers JW, Simoons ML. Early thrombolytic treatment in acute myocardial infarction: reappraisal of the golden hour. *Lancet* 1996;348:771–775.
211. Zivin JA. Thrombolytic stroke therapy. *Neurology* 1999;53:14–19.
212. Casto L, Caverni L, Camerlingo M, et al. Intra-arterial thrombolysis in acute ischaemic stroke: experience with a superselective catheter embedded in the clot. *J Neurol Neurosurg Psychiatry* 1996;60:667–670.
213. Smith TP. Radiologic intervention in the acute stroke patient. *J Vasc Interv Radiol* 1996;7: 627–640.
214. Nesbit GM, Clark WM, O'Neill OR, Barnwell SL. Intracranial intraarterial thrombolysis facilitated by microcatheter navigation through an occluded cervical internal carotid artery. *J Neurosurg* 1996;84:387–392.
215. del Zoppo GJ. Thrombolytic therapy in the treatment of stroke. *Drugs* 1997;54(Suppl 3):90–98.
216. Ferguson RD, Ferguson JG. Cerebral intraarterial fibrinolysis at the crossroads: is a phase III trial advisable at this time? *Am J Neuroradiol* 1994;15:1201–1216.
217. Sasaki O, Takeuchi S, Koike T, Koizumi T, Tanaka R. Fibrinolytic therapy for acute embolic stroke: intravenous, intracarotid, and intra-arterial local approaches. *Neurosurgery* 1995;36: 246–252.
218. Urbach H, Ries F, Ostertun B, Solymosi L. Local intra-arterial fibrinolysis in thromboembolic "T" occlusions of the internal carotid artery. *Neuroradiology* 1997;39:105–110.
219. Endo S, Kuwayama N, Hirashima Y, Akai T, Nishijima M, Takaku A. Results of urgent

thrombolysis in patients with major stroke and atherothrombotic occlusion of the cervical internal carotid artery. *Am J Neuroradiol* 1998;19: 1169–1175.
220. Gonner F, Remonda L, Mattle H, et al. Local intra-arterial thrombolysis in acute ischemic stroke. *Stroke* 1998;29:1894–1900.
221. Jansen O, von Kummer R, Forsting M, Hacke W, Sartor K. Thrombolytic therapy in acute occlusion of the intracranial internal carotid artery bifurcation. *Am J Neuroradiol* 1995;16:1977–1986.
222. Jahan R, Duckwiler GR, Kidwell CS, et al. Intraarterial thrombolysis for treatment of acute stroke: experience in 26 patients with long-term follow-up. *Am J Neuroradiol* 1999;20:1291–1299.
223. Schumacher M, Yin L, Klisch J, Hetzel A. Local intra-arterial fibrinolysis without arterial occlusion? *Neuroradiology* 1999;41:530–536.
224. Suarez JI, Sunshine JL, Tarr R, et al. Predictors of clinical improvement, angiographic recanalization, and intracranialhemorrhage after intraarterial thrombolysis for acute ischemic stroke. *Stroke* 1999;30:2094–2100.
225. Lanzieri CF, Tarr RW, Landis D, et al. Cost-effectiveness of emergency intraarterial intracerebral thrombolysis: a pilot study. *Am J Neuroradiol* 1995;16:1987–1993.
226. Schumacher M, Kraft S, Siekmann R. Is local intra-arterial fibrinolysis contraindicated in elderly patients with cerebral artery occlusion? *Neuroradiology* 1998;40:822–826.
227. Sasahara AA, Barker WM, Weaver WD, et al. Clinical studies with the new glycosylated recombinant prourokinase. *J Vasc Interv Radiol* 1995;6:S84–S93.
228. del Zoppo GJ, Higashida RT, Furlan AJ, Pessin MS, Rowley HA, Gent M. PROACT: a phase II randomized trial of recombinant pro-urokinase by direct arterial delivery in acute middle cerebral artery stroke. PROACT Investigators. Prolyse in Acute Cerebral Thromboembolism. *Stroke* 1998;29:4–11.
229. Furlan A, Higashida R, Wechsler L, et al. Intraarterial prourokinase for acute ischemic stroke. The PROACT II Study: A randomized controlled trial. *JAMA* 1999;282:2003–2011.
230. Becker KJ, Purcell LL, Hacke W, Hanley DF. Vertebrobasilar thrombosis: diagnosis, management, and the use of intra-arterial thrombolytics. *Crit Care Med* 1996;24:1729–1742.
231. Huemer M, Niederwieser V, Ladurner G. Thrombolytic treatment for acute occlusion of the basilar artery. *J Neurol Neurosurg Psychiatry* 1995;58:227–228.
232. Becker KJ, Monsein LH, Ulatowski J, Mirski M, Williams M, Hanley DF. Intraarterial thrombolysis in vertebrobasilar occlusion. *Am J Neuroradiol* 1996;17:255–262.
233. Brandt T, von Kummer R, Muller-Kuppers M, Hacke W. Thrombolytic therapy of acute basilar artery occlusion. Variables affecting recanalization and outcome. *Stroke* 1996;27:875–881.
234. Wijdicks EF, Nichols DA, Thielen KR, et al. Intra-arterial thrombolysis in acute basilar artery thromboembolism: the initial Mayo Clinic experience. *Mayo Clin Proc* 1997;72:1005–1013.
235. Levy EI, Firlik AD, Wisniewski S, et al. Factors affecting survival rates for acute vertebrobasilar artery occlusions treated with intra-arterial thrombolytic therapy: a meta-analytical approach. *Neurosurgery* 1999;45:539–548.
236. Wardlaw JM, Warlow CP. Thrombolysis in acute ischemic stroke: does it work? *Stroke* 1992;23: 1826–1839.
237. Multicenter Acute Stroke Trial—Europe Study Group. Thrombolytic therapy with streptokinase in acute ischemic stroke. *N Engl J Med* 1996;335:145–150.
238. Hommel M, Boissel JP, Cornu C, et al. Termination of trial of streptokinase in severe acute ischaemic stroke. MAST Study Group. *Lancet* 1995;345:57.
239. Multicentre Acute Stroke Trial—Italy (MAST-I) Group. Randomised controlled trial of streptokinase, aspirin, and combination of both in treatment of acute ischaemic stroke. *Lancet* 1995;346: 1509–1514.
240. Motto C, Ciccone A, Aritzu E, et al. Hemorrhage after an acute ischemic stroke. *Stroke* 1999;30: 761–769.
241. Donnan GA, Davis SM, Chambers BR, et al. Streptokinase for acute ischemic stroke with relationship to time of administration: Australian Streptokinase (ASK) Trial Study Group. *JAMA* 1996;276:961–966.
242. Infeld B, Davis SM, Donnan GA, et al. Streptokinase increases luxury perfusion after stroke. *Stroke* 1996;27:1524–1529.
243. Hacke W, Kaste M, Fieschi C, et al. Intravenous thrombolysis with recombinant tissue plasminogen activator for acute hemispheric stroke. The European Cooperative Acute Stroke Study (ECASS). *JAMA* 1995;274:1017–1025.
244. Steiner T, Bluhmki E, Kaste M, et al. The ECASS 3-hour cohort. *Cerebrovasc Dis* 1998;8:198–203.
245. Brott TG, Haley EC, Jr., Levy DE, et al. Urgent therapy for stroke. Part I. Pilot study of tissue plasminogen activator administered within 90 minutes. *Stroke* 1992;23:632–640.
246. Haley EC, Jr., Levy DE, Brott TG, et al. Urgent therapy for stroke. Part II. Pilot study of tissue plasminogen activator administered 91–180 minutes from onset. *Stroke* 1992;23:641–645.
247. Haley EC, Jr., Brott TG, Sheppard GL, et al. Pilot randomized trial of tissue plasminogen activator in acute ischemic stroke. The TPA Bridging Study Group. *Stroke* 1993;24:1000–1004.
248. Levine SR, Brott TG. Thrombolytic therapy in cerebrovascular disorders. *Progress in Cardiovascular Diseases* 1992;34:235–262.
249. The NINDS t-PA Stroke Study Group. Generalized efficacy of t-PA for acute stroke. Subgroup analysis of the NINDS t-PA Stroke Trial. *Stroke* 1997;28:2119–2125.
250. Hacke W, Kaste M, Fieschi C, et al. Randomised double-blind placebo-controlled trial of thrombolytic therapy with intravenous alteplase in acute ischaemic stroke (ECASS II). Second European-Australasian Acute Stroke Study Investigators. *Lancet* 1998;352:1245–1251.
251. Clark WM, Wissman S, Albers GW, et al. Recombinant tissue-type plasminogen activator

(alteplase) for ischemic stroke 3 to 5 hours after symptom onset. The ATLANTIS Study: A randomized controlled trial. *JAMA* 1999;282: 2019–2026.
252. Trouillas P, Nighoghossian N, Getenet JC, et al. Open trial of intravenous tissue plasminogen activator in acute carotid territory stroke. Correlations of outcome with clinical and radiological data. *Stroke* 1996;27:882–890.
253. Buchan AM, Barber PA, Newcommon N, et al. Effectiveness of t-PA in acute ischemic stroke. Outcome relates to appropriateness. *Neurology* 2000;54:679–684.
254. Trouillas P, Derex L, Nighoghossian N, et al. rtPA intravenous thrombolysis in anterior choroidal artery territory stroke. *Neurology* 2000; 54:666–673.
255. Grond M, Stenzel C, Schmulling S, et al. Early intravenous thrombolysis for acute ischemic stroke in a community-based approach. *Stroke* 1998;29:1544–1549.
256. Chiu D, Krieger D, Villar-Cordova C, et al. Intravenous tissue plasminogen activator for acute ischemic stroke: feasibility, safety, and efficacy in the first year of clinical practice. *Stroke* 1998;29:18–22.
257. Smith RW, Scott PA, Grant RJ, Chudnofsky CR, Frederiksen SM. Emergency physician treatment of acute stroke with recombinant tissue plasminogen activator: a retrospective analysis. *Acad Emerg Med* 1999;6:618–625.
258. Osborn TM, LaMonte MP, Gaasch WR. Intravenous thrombolytic therapy for stroke: a review of recent studies and controversies. *Ann Emerg Med* 1999;34:244–255.
259. Tanne D, Bates VE, Verro P, et al. Initial clinical experience with IV tissue plasminogen activator for acute ischemic stroke: a multicenter survey. The t-PA Stroke Survey Group. *Neurology* 1999;53:424–427.
260. Egan R, Lutsep HL, Clark WM, et al. Open label tissue plasminogen activator for stroke: The Oregon experience. *J Stroke Cerebrovasc Dis* 1999; 8:287–290.
261. Wirkowski E, Gottesman MH, Mazer C, Brody GM, Manzella SM. Tissue plasminogen activator for acute stroke in everyday clinical practice. *J Stroke Cerebrovasc Dis* 1999;8:291–294.
262. Lewandowski CA, Frankel M, Tomsick TA, et al. Combined intravenous and intra-arterial r-TPA versus intra-arterial therapy of acute ischemic stroke: emergency management of stroke (EMS) trial. *Stroke* 1999;30:2598–2605.
263. Hossmann V, Heiss WD, Bewermeyer H, Wiedemann G. Controlled trial of ancrod in ischemic stroke. *Arch Neurol* 1983;40:803–808.
264. Olinger CP, Brott TG, Barsan WG, et al. Use of ancrod in acute or progressing ischemic cerebral infarction. *Ann Emerg Med* 1988;17:1208–1209.
265. The Ancrod Stroke Study Investigators. Ancrod for the treatment of acute ischemic brain infarction. *Stroke* 1994;25:1755–1759.
266. Sherman DG, for the STAT Writers Group. Defibrinogenation with Viprinex (ancrod) for the treatment of acute ischemic stroke. *Stroke* 1999;30:234.
267. Wardlaw JM, Warlow CP, Counsell C. Systematic review of evidence on thrombolytic therapy for acute ischaemic stroke. *Lancet* 1997;350:607–614.
268. Bath P. Alteplase not yet proven for acute ischaemic stroke. *Lancet* 1998;352:1238–1239.
269. Hankey GJ. Thrombolytic therapy in acute ischaemic stroke: the jury needs more evidence. *Med J Aust* 1997;166:419–422.
270. Caplan LR. Stroke thrombolysis—growing pains. *Mayo Clin Proc* 1997;72:1090–1092.
271. Grotta J. Should thrombolytic therapy be the first-line treatment for acute ischemic stroke? t-PA—the best current option for most patients. *N Engl J Med* 1997;337:1310–1313.
272. Lyden PD, Grotta JC, Levine SR, Marler JR, Frankel MR, Brott TG. Intravenous thrombolysis for acute stroke. *Neurology* 1997;49:14–20.
273. Caplan LR, Mohr JP, Kistler JP, Koroshetz W. Should thrombolytic therapy be the first-line treatment for acute ischemic stroke? Thrombolysis—not a panacea for ischemic stroke. *N Engl J Med* 1997;337:1309–1310.
274. Yuh WT, Maeda M, Wang AM, et al. Fibrinolytic treatment of acute stroke: are we treating reversible cerebral ischemia? *Am J Neuroradiol* 1995;16:1994–2000.
275. Ueda T, Sakaki S, Yuh WT, Nochide I, Ohta S. Outcome in acute stroke with successful intra-arterial thrombolysis and predictive value of initial single-photon emission-computed tomography. *J Cereb Blood Flow Metab* 1999;19:99–108.
276. Ueda T, Sakaki S, Kumon Y, Ohta S. Multivariable analysis of predictive factors related to outcome at 6 months after intra-arterial thrombolysis for acute ischemic stroke. *Stroke* 1999;30:2360–2365.
277. Albers G. Expanding the window for thrombolytic therapy in acute stroke. The potential role of acute MRI for patient selection. *Stroke* 1999;30:2230–2237.
278. Barber PA, Darby DG, Desmond PM, et al. Identification of major ischemic change. Diffusion-weighted imaging versus computed tomography. *Stroke* 1999;30:2059–2065.
279. Baron JC. Mapping the ischaemic penumbra with PET: Implications for acute stroke treatment. *Cerebrovasc Dis* 1999;9:193–201.
280. Fagan SC, Kertland HR, Tietjen GE. Safety of combination aspirin and anticoagulation in acute ischemic stroke. *Ann Pharmacother* 1994; 28:441–443.
281. Alberts MJ. tPA in acute ischemic stroke: United States experience and issues for the future. *Neurology* 1998;51:S53–S55.
282. O'Connor RE, McGraw P, Edelsohn L. Thrombolytic therapy for acute ischemic stroke: why the majority of patients remain ineligible for treatment. *Ann Emerg Med* 1999;33:9–14.
283. Alberts MJ. Hyperacute stroke therapy with tissue plasminogen activator. *Am J Cardiol* 1997; 80:29D–34D.
284. Koller RL, Anderson DC. Intravenous thrombolytic therapy for acute ischemic stroke. Weighing the risks and benefits of tissue plasminogen activator. *Postgrad Med* 1922;103: 221–224.

285. Furlan AJ, Kanoti G. When is thrombolysis justified in patients with acute ischemic stroke? A bioethical perspective. *Stroke* 1997;28:214–218.
286. Norris JW, Buchan A, Cote R, et al. Canadian guidelines for intravenous thrombolytic treatment in acute stroke. A consensus statement of the Canadian Stroke Consortium. *Can J Neurol Sci* 1998;25:257–259.
287. Norris JW, Buchan A, Cote R, et al. Canadian guidelines for intravenous thrombolytic treatment in acute stroke. A consensus statement of the Canadian Stroke Consortium. *Can J Neurol Sci* 1998;25:257–259.
288. Albers GW, Easton JD, Sacco RL, Teal P. Antithrombotic and thrombolytic therapy for ischemic stroke. *Chest* 1998;114:S683–S698.
289. von Kummer R, Allen KL, Holle R, et al. Acute stroke: usefulness of early CT findings before thrombolytic therapy. *Radiology* 1997;205: 327–333.
290. von Kummer R, Nolte PN, Schnittger H, Thron A, Ringelstein EB. Detectability of cerebral hemisphere ischaemic infarcts by CT within 6 h of stroke. *Neuroradiology* 1996;38:31–33.
291. von Kummer R, Patel S. Neuroimaging in acute stroke. *J Stroke Cerebrovasc Dis* 1999;8:127–138.
292. Phillips SJ. An alternative view of heparin anticoagulation in acute focal brain ischemia. *Stroke* 1989;20:295–298.
293. Marsh EE, Adams HP, Jr., Biller J, et al. Use of antithrombotic drugs in the treatment of acute ischemic stroke: a survey of neurologists in practice in the United States. *Neurology* 1989;39: 1631–1634.
294. Hirsh J, Fuster V. Guide to anticoagulant therapy. Part 1: Heparin. *Circulation* 1994;89:1449–1468.
295. Cantor WJ, Ohman EM. Results of recent large myocardial infarction trials, adjunctive therapies, and acute myocardial infarction: improving outcomes. *Cardiology in Review* 1999;7:232–244.
296. Schubert PJ, Loscalzo J. Antithrombotic therapy. *Compr Ther* 1995;21:344–350.
297. Meschia JF, Biller J. Manipulation of coagulation factors in acute stroke. *Drugs* 1997;54 (Suppl 3): 71–81.
298. Chamorro A, Vila N, Saiz A, Alday M, Tolosa E. Early anticoagulation after large cerebral embolic infarction: a safety study. *Neurology* 1995;45: 861–865.
299. Li PA, He QP, Siddiqui MM, Shuaib A. Posttreatment with low molecular weight heparin reduces brain edema and infarct volume in rats subjected to thrombotic middle cerebral artery occlusion. *Brain Research* 1998;801:220–223.
300. Sandercock PA, van den Belt AG, Lindley RI, Slattery J. Antithrombotic therapy in acute ischaemic stroke: an overview of the completed randomised trials. *J Neurol Neurosurg Psychiatry* 1993;56:17–25.
301. Alexandrov AV, Black SE, Ehrlich LE, Caldwell CB, Norris JW. Predictors of hemorrhagic transformation occurring spontaneously and on anticoagulants in patients with acute ischemic stroke. *Stroke* 1997;28:1198–1202.
302. Babikian VL, Kase CS, Pessin MS, Norrving B, Gorelick PB. Intracerebral hemorrhage in stroke patients anticoagulated with heparin. *Stroke* 1989;20:1500–1503.
303. Toni D, Fiorelli M, Bastianello S, et al. Hemorrhagic transformation of brain infarct: predictability in the first 5 hours from stroke onset and influence on clinical outcome. *Neurology* 1996;46:341–345.
304. Cerebral Embolism Study Group. Immediate anticoagulation of embolic stroke: brain hemorrhage and management options. *Stroke* 1984;15: 779–789.
305. Cerebral Embolism Study Group. Cardioembolic stroke, early anticoagulation, and brain hemorrhage. *Arch Intern Med* 1987;147: 636–640.
306. Chamorro A, Vila N, Ascaso C, Blanc R. Heparin in acute stroke with atrial fibrillation. Clinical relevance of very early treatment. *Arch Neurol* 1999;56:1098–1102.
307. Yasaka M, Yamaguchi T, Moriyasu H, Otta J, Sawada T, Omae T. Antithrombosis III and low-dose heparin in acute cardioembolic stroke. *Cerebrovasc Dis* 1995;5:35–42.
308. Camerlingo M, Casto L, Censori B, et al. Immdiate anticoagulation with heparin for first-ever ischemic strokes in the carotid artery territories observed within 5 hours of onset. *Arch Neurol* 1994;51:462–467.
309. Dahl T, Sandset PM, Abildgaard U. Heparin treatment in 52 patients with progressive ischemic stroke. *Cerebrovasc Dis* 1994;4:101–105.
310. Haley EC, Jr., Kassell NF, Torner JC. Failure of heparin to prevent progression in progressing ischemic infarction. *Stroke* 1988;19:10–14.
311. Duke RJ, Bloch RF, Turpie AG, Trebilcock R, Bayer N. Intravenous heparin for the prevention of stroke progression in acute partial stable stroke. *Ann Intern Med* 1986;105:825–828.
312. International Stroke Trial Collaborative Group. The International Stroke Trial (IST): a randomised trial of aspirin, subcutaneous heparin, both, or neither among 19435 patients with acute ischaemic stroke. *Lancet* 1997;349:1569–1581.
313. Kay R, Wong KS, Woo J. Pilot study of low-molecular-weight heparin in the treatment of acute ischemic stroke. *Stroke* 1994;25:684–685.
314. Kay R, Wong KS, Yu YL, et al. Low-molecular-weight heparin for the treatment of acute ischemic stroke. *N Engl J Med* 1995;333: 1588–1593.
315. Collignon F, Frydman A, Caplain H, et al. Comparison of the pharmacokinetic profiles of three low molecular mass heparins—dalteparin, enoxaparin and nadroparin—administered subcutaneously in healthy volunteers (doses for prevention of thromboembolism). *Thromb Haemost* 1995;73:630–640.
316. The Publications Committee for the Trial of ORG 10172 in Acute Stroke Treatment (TOAST) Investigators. Low molecular weight heparinoid, ORG 10172 (danaparoid), and outcome after acute ischemic stroke: a randomized controlled trial. *JAMA* 1998;279:1265–1272.
317. Adams HP, Jr., Bendixen BH, Leira EC, et al. Antithrombotic treatment of ischemic stroke among patients with occlusion or severe stenosis

of the internal carotid artery. *Neurology* 1999;53:122–125.

318. Grond M, Rudolf J, Neveling M, Stenzel C, Heiss WD. Risk of immediate heparin after rt-PA therapy in acute ischemic stroke. *Cerebrovasc Dis* 1997;7:318–323.
319. The Global Use of Strategies to Open Occluded Coronary Arteries (GUSTO) IIa Investigators. Randomized trial of intravenous heparin versus recombinant hirudin for acute coronary syndromes. *Circulation* 1994;90:1631–1637.
320. Anteman EM. Hirudin in acute myocardial infarction safety. Report from the thrombolysis and thrombin inhibition in myocardial infarction (TIMI) 9A Trial. *Circulation* 1994;90: 1624–1630.
321. Topol EJ, Fuster V, Harrington RA, et al. Recombinant hirudin for unstable angina pectoris. A multicenter, randomized angiographic trial. *Circulation* 1994;89:1557–1566.
322. Lunven C, Gauffeny C, Lecoffre C, O'Brien DP, Roome NO, Berry CN. Inhibition by argatroban, a specific thrombin inhibitor, of platelet activation by fibrin clot-associated thrombin. *Thromb Haemost* 1996;75:154–160.
323. Imiya M, Matsuo T. Inhibition of collagen-induced platelet aggregation by argatroban in patients with acute cerebral infarction. *Thromb Res* 1997;88:245–250.
324. Lewis BE, Walenga JM, Wallis DE. Anticoagulation with Novastan (argatroban) in patients with heparin-induced thrombocytopenia and heparin-induced thrombocytopenia and thrombosis syndrome. *Semin Thromb Hemost* 1997;23:197–202.
325. Samama MM, Desnoyers PC, Conard J, Bousser MG. Acute ischemic stroke and heparin treatments. *Thromb Haemost* 1997;78:173–179.
326. Hankey GJ. Heparin in acute ischaemic stroke. The T wave is negative and it's time to stop. *Med J Aust* 1998;169:534–536.
327. Read SJ, Hirano T, Davis SM, Donnan GA. Limiting neurological damage after stroke: a review of pharmacological treatment options. *Drugs Aging* 1999;14:11–39.
328. Sandercock P. Is there still a role for intravenous heparin in acute stroke? No. *Arch Neurol* 1999; 56:1160–1161.
329. Swanson RA. Intravenous heparin for acute stroke: what can we learn from the megatrials? *Neurology* 1999;52:1746–1750.
330. Grau AJ, Hacke W. Is there still a role for intravenous heparin in acute stroke? Yes. *Arch Neurol* 1999;56:1159–1160.
331. Caplan LR. When should heparin be given to patients with atrial fibrillation-related embolic brain infarcts? *Arch Neurol* 1999;56:1059–1060.
332. Chamorro A. Heparin in acute ischemic stroke: the case for a new clinical trial. *Cerebrovasc Dis* 1999;9(Suppl 3):16–23.
333. Ruff RL, Dougherty JH, Jr. Evaluation of acute cerebral ischemia for anticoagulant therapy: computed tomography or lumbar puncture. *Neurology* 1981;31:736–740.
334. Lackie CL, Luzier AB, Donovan JA, Feras HI, Forrest A. Weight-based heparin dosing: clinical response and resource utilization. *Clin Therap* 1998;20:699–710.
335. Bednar MM, Gross CE. Antiplatelet therapy in acute cerebral ischemia. *Stroke* 1999;30:887–893.
336. del Zoppo GJ. The role of platelets in ischemic stroke. *Neurology* 1998;51:S9–S14.
337. Grau AJ, Ruf A, Vogt A, et al. Increased fraction of circulating activated platelets in acute and previous cerebrovascular ischemia. *Thromb Haemost* 1998;80:298–301.
338. Nagamatsu Y, Tsujioka Y, Hashimoto M, Giddings JC, Yamamoto J. The differential effects of aspirin on platelets, leucocytes and vascular endothelium in an in vivo model of thrombus formation. *Clin Lab Haematol* 1999;21:33–40.
339. Theroux P. Oral inhibitors of platelet membrane receptor glycoprotein IIb/IIIa in clinical cardiology: issues and opportunities. *Am Heart J* 1998;135:S107–S112.
340. Ferguson JJ, Waly HM, Wilson JM. Fundamentals of coagulation and glycoprotein IIb/IIIa receptor inhibition. *Eur Heart J* 1998;19 (Suppl D):D3–D9.
341. Coller BS, Anderson K, Weisman HF. New antiplatelet agents: platelet GPIIb/IIIa antagonists. *Thromb Haemost* 1995;74:302–308.
342. Choudhri TF, Hoh BL, Zerwes HG, et al. Reduced microvascular thrombosis and improved outcome in acute murine stroke by inhibiting GP IIb/IIIa receptor-mediated platelet aggregation. *J Clin Invest* 1998;102: 1301–1310.
343. Kaku S, Umemura K, Mizuno A, Kawasaki T, Nakashima M. Evaluation of the disintegrin, triflavin, in a rat middle cerebral artery thrombosis model. *Eur J Pharmacol* 1997;321:301–305.
344. Cines DB. Glycoprotein IIb/IIIa antagonists: Potential induction and detection of drug-dependent antiplatelet antibodies. *Am Heart J* 1998;135:S152–S159.
345. Tcheng JE, Ellis SG, George BS, et al. Pharmacodynamics of chimeric glycoprotein IIb/IIIa integrin antiplatelet antibody Fab 7E3 in high-risk coronary angioplasty. *Circulation* 1994;90:1757–1764.
346. Chopp M, Zhang RL, Zhang ZG, Jiang Q. The clot thickens—thrombolysis and combination therapies. *Acta Neurochirurgica* 1999;73(Suppl): 67–71.
347. CAST (Chinese Acute Stroke Trial) Collaborative Group. CAST: randomised placebo-controlled trial of early aspirin use in 20,000 patients with acute ischaemic stroke. *Lancet* 1997;349: 1641–1649.
348. Ciccone A, Motto C, Aritzu E, Piana A, Candelise L. Risk of aspirin use plus thrombolysis after acute ischaemic stroke: a further MAST-I analysis. MAST-I Collaborative Group. Multicentre Acute Stroke Trial—Italy. *Lancet* 1998;352:880.
349. The Ridogrel Versus Aspirin Patency Trial (RAPT). Randomized trial of ridogrel, a combined thromboxane A2 synthase inhibitor and thromboxane A2/prostaglandin endoperoxide receptor antagonist, versus aspirin as adjunct to thrombolysis in patients with acute myocardial infarction. *Circulation* 1994;89:588–595.

350. Topol EJ. Prevention of cardiovascular ischemic complications with new platelet glycoprotein IIb/IIIa inhibitors. *Am Heart J* 1995;130: 666–672.
351. Antman EM, Giugliano RP, Gibson CM, et al. Abciximab facilitates the rate and extent of thrombolysis: results of the thrombolysis in myocardial infarction (TIMI) 14 trial. The TIMI 14 Investigators. *Circulation* 1999;21:2720–2732.
352. Simoons ML, de Boer MJ, van den Brand MJ, et al. Randomized trial of a GPIIb/IIIa platelet receptor blocker in refractory unstable angina. European Cooperative Study Group. *Circulation* 1994;89:596–603.
353. Topol EJ, Califf RM, Weisman HF, et al. Randomised trial of coronary intervention with antibody against platelet IIb/IIIa integrin for reduction of clinical restenosis: results at six months. The EPIC Investigators. *Lancet* 1994; 343:881–886.
354. Goto S, Eto K, Ikeda Y, Handa S. Abciximab not RGD peptide inhibits von Willebrand factor-dependent platelet activation under shear. *Lancet* 1999;353:809.
355. Mahaffey KW, Harrington RA, Simoons ML, et al. Stroke in patients with acute coronary syndromes: incidence and outcomes in the platelet glycoprotein IIb/IIIa in unstable angina. Receptor suppression using integrilin therapy (PURSUIT) trial. The PURSUIT Investigators. *Circulation* 1999;99:2371–2377.
356. Califf RM. Glycoprotein IIb/IIIa blockade and thrombolytics: early lessons from the SPEED and GUSTO IV trials. *Am Heart J* 1999;138: S12–S15.
357. Wallace RC, Furlan AJ, Moliterno DJ, et al. Basilar artery rethrombosis: successful treatment with platelet glycoprotein IIB/IIIA receptor inhibitor. *Am J Neuroradiol* 1997;18: 1257–1260.
358. Lindley RI. Drug therapy for acute ischaemic stroke: risks versus benefits. *Drug Saf* 1998; 19:373–382.
359. Mayberg MR, Batjer HH, Dacey R, et al. Guidelines for the management of aneurysmal subarachnoid hemorrhage. A statement for healthcare professionals from a special writing group of the Stroke Council, American Heart Association. *Stroke* 1994;25:2315–2328.
360. Sandercock P, Willems H. Medical treatment of acute ischaemic stroke. *Lancet* 1992;339: 537–539.
361. Rordorf G, Cramer SC, Efird JT, Schwamm LH, Buonanno F, Koroshetz WJ. Pharmacological elevation of blood pressure in acute stroke. Clinical effects and safety. *Stroke* 1997;28: 2133–2138.
362. Amin-Hanjani S, Schwartz RB, Sathi S, Stieg PE. Hypertensive encephalopathy as a complication of hyperdynamic therapy for vasospasm: report of two cases. *Neurosurgery* 1999;44:1113–1116.
363. Bereczki D, Fekete I. A systematic review of vinpocetine therapy in acute ischaemic stroke. *Eur J Clin Pharmacol* 1999;55:349–352.
364. Forconi S, Turchetti V, Cappelli R, Guerrini M, Bicchi M. Haemorheological disturbances and possibility of their correction in cerebrovascular diseases. [Review]. *Journal des Maladies Vasculaires* 1999;24:110–116.
365. Walzl M, Schied G, Walzl B. Effects of ameliorated haemorheology on clinical symptoms in cerebrovascular disease. *Atherosclerosis* 1998;139: 385–389.
366. Stoll M, Treib J, Seltmann A, Anton H, Klaus S. Hemodynamics of stroke patients under therapy with low molecular weight hydroxyethyl starch. *Neurol Res* 1998;20:231–234.
367. Schneider R. Results of hemorheologically active treatment with pentoxifylline in patients with cerebrovascular disease. *Angiology* 1989;40: 987–993.
368. Frampton JE, Brogden RN. Pentoxifylline (oxpentifylline). A review of its therapeutic efficacy in the management of peripheral vascular and cerebrovascular disorders. *Drugs Aging* 1995;7:480–503.
369. Saxena R, Wijnhoud AD, Carton H, et al. Controlled safety study of hemoglobin-based oxygen carrier, DCLHb, in acute ischemic stroke. *Stroke* 1999;30:993–996.
370. Gross CE, Bednar MM, Lew SM, Florman JE, Kohut JJ. Preoperative volume expansion improves tolerance to carotid artery cross-clamping during endarterectomy. *Neurosurgery* 1998;43:222–226.
371. Matthews WB, Oxbury JM, Grainger KM, Greenhall RC. A blind controlled trial of dextran 40 in the treatment of ischaemic stroke. *Brain* 1976;99:193–206.
372. Kaste M, Fogelholm R, Waltimo O. Combined dexamethasone and low-molecular-weight dextran in acute brain infarction: double-blind study. *BMJ* 1976;2:1409–1410.
373. The Hemodilution in Stroke Study Group. Hypervolemic hemodilution treatment of acute stroke. Results of a randomized multicenter trial using pentastarch. *Stroke* 1989;20:317–323.
374. Koller M, Haenny P, Hess K, Weniger D, Zangger P. Adjusted hypervolemic hemodilution in acute ischemic stroke. *Stroke* 1990;21:1429–1434.
375. Strand T. Evaluation of long-term outcome and safety after hemodilution therapy in acute ischemic stroke. *Stroke* 1992;23:657–662.
376. Italian Acute Stroke Study Group. Haemodilution in acute stroke. Results of the Italian haemodilution trial. *Lancet* 1988;1: 318–321.
377. Scandinavian Stroke Study Group. Multicenter trial of hemodilution in acute ischemic stroke. Results of subgroup analyses. *Stroke* 1988;19: 464–471.
378. Hsu CY, Norris JW, Hogan EL, et al. Pentoxifylline in acute nonhemorrhagic stroke. A randomized, placebo-controlled double-blind trial. *Stroke* 1988;19:716–722.
379. Berrouschot J, Barthel H, Scheel C, Koster J, Schneider D. Extracorporeal membrane differential filtration—a new and safe method to optimize hemorheology in acute ischemic stroke. *Acta Neurol Scand* 1998;97:126–130.
380. Berrouschot J, Barthel H, Koster J, et al. Extracorporeal rheopheresis in the treatment of

acute ischemic stroke: A randomized pilot study. *Stroke* 1999;30:787–792.
381. Frazee JG, Luo X, Luan G, et al. Retrograde transvenous neuroperfusion: a back door treatment for stroke. *Stroke* 1998;29:1912–1916.
382. Asplund K. Hemodilution in acute stroke. *Cerebrovasc Dis* 1991;1(Suppl 1):129–138.
383. Najafi H, Javid H, Dye WS, Hunter JA, Wideman FE, Julian OC. Emergency carotid thromboendarterectomy. Surgical indications and results. *Arch Surg* 1971;103:610–614.
384. Meyer FB, Sundt TMJ, Piepgras DG, Sandok BA, Forbes G. Emergency carotid endarterectomy for patients with acute carotid occlusion and profound neurological deficits. *Ann Surg* 1986;203:82–89.
385. Walters BB, Ojemann RG, Heros RC. Emergency carotid endarterectomy. *J Neurosurg* 1987;66:817–823.
386. Eckstein HH, Schumacher H, Klemm K, et al. Emergency carotid endarterectomy. *Cerebrovasc Dis* 1999;9:270–281.
387. Eckstein HH, Schumacher H, Dorfler A, et al. Carotid endarterectomy and intracranial thrombolysis: simultaneous and staged procedures in ischemic stroke. *J Vasc Surg* 1999;29: 459–471.
388. Linskey ME, Sekhar LN, Hecht ST. Emergency embolectomy for embolic occlusion of the middle cerebral artery after internal carotid artery balloon test occlusion. Case report. *J Neurosurg* 1992;77:134–138.
389. Kakinuma K, Ezuka I, Takai N, Yamamoto K, Sasaki O. The simple indicator for revascularization of acute middle cerebral artery occlusion using angiogram and ultra-early embolectomy. *Surg Neurol* 1999;51:332–341.
390. Nakayama T, Tanaka K, Kaneko M, Yokoyama T, Uemura K. Thrombolysis and angioplasty for acute occlusion of intracranial vertebrobasilar arteries. Report of three cases. *J Neurosurg* 1998;88:919–922.
391. Suh DC, Sung KB, Cho YS, et al. Transluminal angioplasty for middle cerebral artery stenosis in patients with acute ischemic stroke. *Am J Neuroradiol* 1999;20:553–558.
392. Nakano S, Yokogami K, Ohta H, Yano T, Ohnishi T. Direct percutaneous transluminal angioplasty for acute middle cerebral artery occlusion. *Am J Neuroradiol* 1998;19: 767–772.
393. Mead GE, O'Neill PA, McCollum CN. Is there a role for carotid surgery in acute stroke?. *Eur J Vasc Endovasc Surg* 1997;13:112–121.
394. Albers GW. Rationale for early intervention in acute stroke. *Am J Cardiol* 1997;80:D4–D10.
395. Steiner T, Hacke W. Combination therapy with neuroprotectants and thrombolytics in acute ischaemic stroke. *Eur Neurol* 1998;40:1–8.
396. Dyker AG, Lees KR. Duration of neuroprotective treatment for ischemic stroke. *Stroke* 1998;29:535–542.
397. Chan PH. Role of oxidants in ischemic brain damage. *Stroke* 1996;27:1124–1129.
398. Clark WM. Cytokines and reperfusion injury. *Neurology* 1997;S10–S14.
399. Fisher M. Clinical pharmacology of cerebral ischemia. Old controversies and new approaches. *Cerebrovasc Dis* 1991;1(Suppl 1):112–119.
400. Nagahiro S, Uno M, Sato K, Goto S, Morioka M, Ushio Y. Pathophysiology and treatment of cerebral ischemia. *J Med Invest* 1998;45:57–70.
401. Morgenstern LB, Pettigrew LC. Brain protection—human data and potential new therapies. *New Horizons* 1997;5:397–405.
402. Zivin JA. Neuroprotective therapies in stroke. *Drugs* 1997;54(Suppl 3):83–88.
403. Dirnagl U, Iadecola C, Moskowitz MA. Pathobiology of ischaemic stroke: an integrated view. *Trends in Neurosciences* 1999;22:391–397.
404. Muir KW, Grosset DG. Neuroprotection for acute stroke: making clinical trials work. *Stroke* 1999;30:180–182.
405. Scheller DK, De Ryck M, Kolb J, et al. Lubeluzole blocks increases in extracellular glutamate and taurine in the peri-infarct zone in rats. *Eur J Pharmacol* 1997;338:243–251.
406. Dogan A, Rao AM, Baskaya MK, et al. Effects of ifenprodil, a polyamine site NMDA receptor antagonist, on reperfusion injury after transient focal cerebral ischemia. *J Neurosurg* 1997; 87:921–926.
407. Lee JM, Zipfel GJ, Choi DW. The changing landscape of ischaemic brain injury mechanisms. *Nature* 1999;399:A7–A14.
408. O'Mahony D, Kendall MJ. Nitric oxide in acute ischaemic stroke: a target for neuroprotection [editorial]. *J Neurol Neurosurg Psychiatry* 1999; 67:1–3.
409. Frerichs KU. Neuroprotective strategies in nature—novel clues for the treatment of stroke and trauma. *Acta Neurochirurgica* 1999;73(Suppl): 57–61.
410. Dewar D, Yam P, McCulloch J. Drug development for stroke: importance of protecting cerebral white matter. *Eur J Pharmacol* 1999;375:41–50.
411. Endres M, Fink K, Zhu J, et al. Neuroprotective effects of gelsolin during murine stroke. *J Clin Invest* 1999;103:347–354.
412. Galante A, Silvestrini M, Stanzione P, et al. Leucocyte aggregation in acute cerebrovascular disease. *Acta Neurol Scand* 1992;86:446–449.
413. Barone FC, Feuerstein GZ. Inflammatory mediators and stroke: new opportunities for novel therapeutics. *J Cereb Blood Flow Metab* 1999; 19:819–834.
414. Heistad DD, Faraci FM. Gene therapy for cerebral vascular disease. *Stroke* 1996;27:1688–1693.
415. Aronowski J, Strong R, Grotta JC. Citicoline for treatment of experimental focal ischemia: histologic and behavioral outcome. *Neurol Res* 1996; 18:570–574.
416. Lekieffre D, Benavides J, Scatton B, Nowicki JP. Neuroprotection afforded by a combination of eliprodil and a thrombolytic agent, rt-PA, in a rat thromboembolic stroke model. *Brain Research* 1997;776:88–95.
417. del Zoppo GJ. Clinical trials in acute stroke: why have they not been successful? *Neurology* 1998; 51:S59–S61.
418. del Zoppo GJ, Wagner S, Tagaya M. Trends and future developments in the pharmacological

treatment of acute ischaemic stroke. *Drugs* 1997;54:9–38.
419. Onal MZ, Fisher M. Acute ischemic stroke therapy. A clinical overview. *Eur Neurol* 1997;38: 141–154.
420. Muir KW, Lees KR. Clinical experience with excitatory amino acid antagonist drugs. *Stroke* 1995;26:503–513.
421. Stieg PE, Sathi S, Warach S, Le DA, Lipton SA. Neuroprotection by the NMDA receptor-associated open-channel blocker memantine in a photothrombotic model of cerebral focal ischemia in neonatal rat. *Eur J Pharmacol* 1999;375:115–120.
422. Albers GW, Saenz RE, Moses JAJ, Choi DW. Safety and tolerance of oral dextromethorphan in patients at risk for brain ischemia. *Stroke* 1991;22:1075–1077.
423. Albers GW, Atkinson RP, Kelley RE, Rosenbaum DM. Safety, tolerability, and pharmacokinetics of the N-methyl-D-aspartate antagonist dextrorphan in patients with acute stroke. Dextrorphan Study Group. *Stroke* 1995;26:254–258.
424. Morris GF, Bullock R, Marshall SB, et al. Failure of the competitive N-methyl-d-aspartate antagonist selfotel (CGS 19755) in the treatment of severe head injury: results of two phase III clinical trials. *J Neurosurg* 1999;91:737–743.
425. Davis SM, Lees KR, Albers GW, et al. Selfotel in acute ischemic stroke. Possible neurotixic effects of an NMDA antagonist. *Stroke* 2000;31: 347–354.
426. Dyker AG, Edwards KR, Fayad PB, Hormes JT, Lees KR. Safety and Tolerability study of aptiganel hydrochloride in patients with an acute ischemic stroke. *Stroke* 1999;30:2038–2042.
427. Arrowsmith JE, Harrison MJ, Newman SP, Stygall J, Timberlake N, Pugsley WB. Neuroprotection of the brain during cardiopulmonary bypass: a randomized trial of remacemide during coronary artery bypass in 171 patients. *Stroke* 1998;29:2357–2362.
428. Dyker AG, Lees KR. Remacemide hydrochloride: a double-blind, placebo-controlled, safety and tolerability study in patients with acute ischemic stroke. *Stroke* 1999;30:1796–1801.
429. Dyker AG, Lees KR. Safety and tolerability of GV150526 (a glycine site antagonist at the N-methyl-D-aspartate receptor) in patients with acute stroke. *Stroke* 1999;30:986–992.
430. Hacke W, Lees KR, Timmerhuis T, et al. Cardiovascular safety of lubeluzole (Prosynap®) in patients with ischemic stroke. *Cerebrovasc Dis* 1998;8:247–254.
431. Diener HC, Hacke W, Hennerici M, Radberg J, Hantson L, De Keyser J. Lubeluzole in acute ischemic stroke. A double-blind, placebo-controlled phase II trial. Lubeluzole International Study Group. *Stroke* 1996;27:76–81.
432. Grotta J. Lubeluzole treatment of acute ischemic stroke. The US and Canadian Lubeluzole Ischemic Stroke Study Group. *Stroke* 1997; 28:2338–2346.
433. Muir KW. New experimental and clinical data on the efficacy of pharmacological magnesium infusions in cerebral infarcts. *Magnesium Research* 1998;11:43–56.
434. Muir KW, Lees KR. Dose optimization of intravenous magnesium sulfate after acute stroke. *Stroke* 1998;29:918–923.
435. Muir KW, Lees KR. A randomized, double-blind, placebo-controlled pilot trial of intravenous magnesium sulfate in acute stroke. *Stroke* 1995;26:1183–1188.
436. Kobayashi T, Mori Y. Ca2+ channel antagonists and neuroprotection from cerebral ischemia. *Eur J Pharmacol* 1998;363:1–15.
437. Kaste M, Fogelholm R, Erila T, et al. A randomized, double-blind, placebo-controlled trial of nimodipine in acute ischemic hemispheric stroke. *Stroke* 1994;25:1348–1353.
438. Bogousslavsky J, Regli F, Zumstein V, Kobberling W. Double-blind study of nimodipine in non-severe stroke. *Eur Neurol* 1990;30: 23–26.
439. American Nimodipine Study Group. Clinical trial of nimodipine in acute ischemic stroke. *Stroke* 1992;23:3–8.
440. Wahlgren NG, MacMahon DG, DeKeyser J, Indredavik B, Ryman T. Intravenous Nimodipine West European Stroke Trial (INWEST) of nimodipine in the treatment of acute ischaemic stroke. *Cerebrovasc Dis* 1994;4: 204–210.
441. Infeld B, Davis SM, Donnan GA, et al. Nimodipine and perfusion changes after stroke. *Stroke* 1999;30:1417–1423.
442. Rosenbaum D, Zabramski J, Frey J, et al. Early treatment of ischemic stroke with a calcium antagonist. *Stroke* 1991;22:437–441.
443. Franke CL, Palm R, Dalby M, et al. Flunarizine in stroke treatment (FIST): a double-blind, placebo-controlled trial in Scandinavia and the Netherlands. *Acta Neurol Scand* 1996;93:56–60.
444. Suzuki H, Kanamaru K, Kuroki M, Sun H, Waga S, Miyazawa T. Effects of tirilazad mesylate on vasospasm and phospholipid hydroperoxides in a primate model of subarachnoid hemorrhage. *Stroke* 1999;30:450–455.
445. Lees KR. Does neuroprotection improve stroke outcome? *Lancet* 1998;351:1447–1448.
446. The RANTTAS Investigators. A randomized trial of tirilazad mesylate in patients with acute stroke (RANTTAS). *Stroke* 1996;27:1453–1458.
447. Schmid-Elsaesser R, Hungerhuber E, Zausinger S, Baethmann A, Reulen HJ. Combination drug therapy and mild hypothermia. A promising treatment strategy for reversible, focal cerebral ischemia. *Stroke* 1999;30:1891–1899.
448. Wahlgren NG, Ranasinha KW, Rosolacci T, et al. Clomethiazole acute stroke study. *Stroke* 1999;30:21–28.
449. Wester P, Strand T, Wahlgren NG, Ashwood T, Osswald G. An open study of clomethiazole in patients with acute cerebral infarction [letter]. *Cerebrovasc Dis* 1998;8:188–190.
450. Barsan WG, Olinger CP, Adams HP, Jr., et al. Use of high dose naloxone in acute stroke: possible side-effects. *Crit Care Med* 1989;17: 762–767.
451. Olinger CP, Adams HP, Jr., Brott TG, et al. High-dose intravenous naloxone for the treatment of acute ischemic stroke. *Stroke* 1990;21:721–725.

452. Clark WM, Warach SJ, Pettigrew LC, Gammans RE, Sabounjian LA. A randomized dose-response trial of citicoline in acute ischemic stroke patients. Citicoline Stroke Study Group. *Neurology* 1997;49:671–678.
453. Clark WM, Williams BJ, Selzer KA, et al. A randomized efficacy trial of citicoline in patients with acute ischemic stroke. *Stroke* 1999;30: 2592–2597.
454. Mohr JP, Biller J, Hilal SK, et al. Magnetic resonance versus computed tomographic imaging in acute stroke. *Stroke* 1995;26:807–812.
455. The SASS Trial. Ganglioside GM1 in acute ischemic stroke. *Stroke* 1994;25:1141–1148.
456. Lenzi GL, Grigoletto F, Gent M, et al. Early treatment of stroke with monosialoganglioside GM-1. Efficacy and safety results of the Early Stroke Trial. *Stroke* 1994;25:1552–1558.
457. Ogawa A, Yoshimoto T, Kikuchi H, et al. Ebselen in acute middle cerebral artery occlusion: a placebo-controlled, double-blind clinical trial. *Cerebrovasc Dis* 1999;9:112–118.
458. Muller WE, Eckert GP, Eckert A. Piracetam: novelty in a unique mode of action. *Pharmacopsychiatry* 1999;32(Suppl)1:2–9.
459. De Deyn PP, Reuck JD, Deberdt W, Vlietinck R, Orgogozo JM. Treatment of acute ischemic stroke with piracetam. Members of the Piracetam in Acute Stroke Study (PASS) Group. *Stroke* 1997;28:2347–2352.
460. De Reuck J, Van Vleymen B. The clinical safety of high-dose piracetam—its use in the treatment of acute stroke. *Pharmacopsychiatry* 1999; 32(Suppl1):33–37.
461. Huber W. The role of piracetam in the treatment of acute and chronic aphasia. *Pharmacopsychiatry* 1999;32(Suppl1):38–43.
462. Orgogozo JM. Piracetam in the treatment of acute stroke. *Pharmacopsychiatry* 1999;32(Suppl1): 25–32.
463. Zhang RL, Chopp M, Jiang N, et al. Anti-intercellular adhesion molecule-1 antibody reduces ischemic cell damage after transient but not permanent middle cerebral artery occlusion in the Wistar rat. *Stroke* 1995;26:1438–1442.
464. Schneider D, Berrouschot J, Brandt T, et al. Safety, pharmacokinetics and biological activity of enlimomab (anti-ICAM-1 antibody): an open-label, dose escalation study in patients hospitalized for acute stroke. *Eur Neurol* 1998; 40:78–83.
465. Bitterman H, Melamed Y. Delayed hyperbaric treatment of cerebral air embolism. *Isr J Med Sci* 1993;29:22–26.
466. Rockswold GL, Ford SE, Anderson DC, Bergman TA, Sherman RE. Results of a prospective randomized trial for treatment of severely brain-injured patients with hyperbaric oxygen. *J Neurosurg* 1992;76:929–934.
467. Nighoghossian N, Trouillas P, Adeleine P, Salord F. Hyperbaric oxygen in the treatment of acute ischemic stroke. A double-blind pilot study. *Stroke* 1995;26:1369–1372.
468. Nighoghossian N, Trouillas P. Hyperbaric oxygen in the treatment of acute ischemic stroke: an unsettled issue. *J Neurol Sci* 1997;150:27–31.
469. Fisher M, Bogousslavsky J. Further evolution toward effective therapy for acute ischemic stroke. *JAMA* 1998;279:1298–1303.
470. Spilker J, Kongable G, Barch C, et al. Using the NIH Stroke Scale to assess stroke patients. The NINDS rt-PA Stroke Study Group. *J Neurosci Nursing* 1997;29:384–392.
471. Braimah J, Kongable G, Rapp K, et al. Nursing care of acute stroke patients after receiving rt-PA therapy. The NINDS rt-PA Stroke Study Group. *J of Neurosci Nursing* 1997;29:373–383.
472. Barch C, Spilker J, Bratina P, et al. Nursing management of acute complications following rt-PA in acute ischemic stroke. The NINDS rt-PA Stroke Study Group. *J Neurosci Nursing* 1997; 29:367–372.
473. Wang DZ, Rose JA, Honings DS, Garwacki DJ, Milbrandt JC, for the OSF Stroke Team. Treating acute stroke patients with intravenous tPA. *Stroke* 2000;31:77–81.
474. Albers GW, Bates VE, Clark WM, Bell R, Verro P, Hamilton SA. Intravenous tissue-type plasminogen activator for treatment of acute stroke: the Standard Treatment with Alteplase to Reverse Stroke (STARS) study. *JAMA* 2000; 283:1145–1150.
475. Katzan IL, Furlan AJ, Lloyd LE, et al. Use of tissue-type plasminogen activator for acute ischemic stroke: the Cleveland area experience. *JAMA* 2000;283:1151–1158.
476. Wein TH, Staub L, Felberg R, et al. Activation of emergency medical servics for acute stroke in a nonurban population. The T.L.L. Temple Foundation Stroke Project. *Stroke* 2000;31: 1925–1928.
477. Brott T, Bogousslavsky J. Treatment of acute ischemic stroke. *N Engl J Med* 2000;343: 710–722.
478. Christou I, Alexandrov AV, Burgin WS, et al. Timing of recanalization after tissue plasminogen activator therapy determined by transcranial doppler correlates with clinical recovery from ischemic stroke. *Stroke* 2000;31: 1812–1816.
479. Rudolf J, Grond M, Schmulling S, Neveling M, Heiss WD. Orolingual angioneurotic edema following therapy of acute ischemic stroke with alteplase. *Neurology* 2000;55:599–600.
480. Gruber A, Nasel C, Lang W, Kitzmuller E, Bavinzski G, Czech T. Intra-arterial thrombolysis for the treatment of perioperative childhood cardioembolic stroke. *Neurology* 2000;54: 1684–1686.
481. Clark WM, Albers GW, Madden KP, Hamilton S, for the Thrombolytic Therapy in Acute Ischemic Stroke Study Investigators. The rtPA (Alteplase) 0- to 6-hour acute stroke trial, part A (A0276g). Results of a double-blind, placebocontrolled, multicenter study. *Stroke* 2000;31:811–816.
482. Mayberg MR, Furlan A. Ancrod-Is snake venom an antidote for stroke? *JAMA* 2000;283: 2440–2441.
483. Sherman DG, Atkinson RP, Chippendale T, et al. Intravenous ancrod for treatment of acute ischemic stroke. The STAT Study: A randomized controlled trial. *JAMA* 2000;283:2395–2403.

484. Schellinger PD, Jansen O, Fiebach JB, et al. Monitoring intravenous recombinant tissue plaminogen activator thrombolysis for acute ischemic stroke with diffusion and perfusion MRI. *Stroke* 2000;31:1318–1328.
485. Berge E, Abdelnoor M, Nakstad PH, Sandset PM, on behalf of the HAEST Study Group. Low molecular-weight heparin versus aspirin in patients with acute inchaemic stroke and atrial fibrillation: a double-blind randomised study. *Lancet* 2000;355:1205–1210.
486. Topol EJ, Mark DB, Lincoff AM, et al. Outcomes at 1 year and economic implications of platelet glycoprotein IIb/IIIa blockade in patients undergoing coronary stenting: results from a multicentre randomised trial. *Lancet* 2000;355:2019–2024.
487. Qureshi AI, Luft AR, Sharma M, Guterman LR, Hopkins LN. Prevention and treatment of thromboembolic and ischemic complications associated with endovascular procedures: Part I-pathophysiological and pharmacological features. *Neurosurgery* 2000;46:1344–1359.
488. Qureshi AI, Suri FK, Khan J, Fessler RD, Guterman LR, Hopkins LN. Abciximab as an adjunct to high-risk carotid or vertebrobasilar angioplasty: preliminary experience. *Neurosurgery* 2000;46:1316–1325.
489. The Abciximab in Ischemic Stroke Investigators. Abciximab in acute ischemic stroke. A randomized, double-blind, placebo-controlled, dose-escalation study. *Stroke* 2000;31:601–609.
490. Clark WM, Raps EC, Tong DC, Kelly RE, for the Cervene Stroke Study Investigators. Cervene (Nalmefene) in acute ischemic stroke. Final results of a phase III efficacy study. *Stroke* 2000; 31:1234–1239.

Chapter 13

MANAGEMENT OF HOSPITALIZED PATIENTS WITH ACUTE ISCHEMIC STROKE

ADMISSION OF PATIENTS TO THE HOSPITAL

Decisions about admission to the hospital should be made on a case-by-case basis. Several variables affect the recommendation for hospitalization in an acute care setting. The most important factors are the severity of neurological impairments and the interval from stroke. In addition, the presence of serious co-morbid diseases, the need for therapies that are best administered in an in-patient setting, and the patient's wishes influence decisions about admission.

A patient with a mild stroke that occurred more than 24 hours before being seen by a physician probably does not need hospitalization. In this situation, the risks of neurological worsening or serious complications are relatively small. The patient likely will not need extensive rehabilitation, and the primary priority in treatment will be the initiation of therapies to prevent recurrent stroke. In addition, a patient with a mild stroke that is several days old likely will decline admission to the hospital—and for good reason: the illness is no longer acute. Admission to the hospital also is not justified if a physician's primary activity is evaluating to determine the cause of stroke. All of the necessary tests can be obtained quickly on an out-patient basis. Hospitalization should be reserved for a situation such as performance of a carotid endarterectomy. The initiation of treatment with oral anticoagulants also probably does not require hospitalization; patients can begin therapy as an out-patient using the regimen described in Chapter 10.

Conversely, a patient with a recent, severe ischemic stroke is critically ill. Chances of life-threatening complications are great. General management should include measures to treat severe co-morbid diseases, such as diabetes mellitus or heart failure, that complicate management.[1,2] If a patient was treated with recombinant tissue plasminogen activator (rt-PA), then close observation is needed. A seriously affected patient probably will not be independent in the near future, and a return to home is unlikely unless rehabilitation is extensive. Such an acutely ill patient needs to be in the hospital, preferably in an acute stroke unit.

Admission to the hospital should involve a smooth transition from the emergency department. In many instances, the physician who treated the patient in the emergency department will continue to supervise care in the hospital. Otherwise, close communication among treating physicians is required so that continuity of care can be maintained after admission. Because most therapies for treatment of the stroke itself likely will have been started in the emergency department, a priority of management after hospitalization is to provide follow-up care.

The main components of management after admission to the hospital differ from those in the emergency department. The patient needs close observation for, and prevention or treatment of, the neurological or medical complications of the stroke. Determination of the likely cause of stroke is followed by starting therapies to prevent recurrent stroke. Rehabilitation is begun to maximize recovery, so that the patient will be able to return to independence. These issues should be addressed simultaneously and in an integrated fashion, although the emphasis in management varies among patients.

STROKE UNITS

During the past several years, the concept of a facility that specializes in the acute treatment of stroke—an acute stroke care unit—has gained popularity. The principles underpinning an acute stroke care unit parallel those that are the foundation of an acute coronary care unit. Just as similarities between stroke and cardiac care exist in the emergent setting—"brain attack" and "heart attack"—the issues of acute stroke care in the hospital are akin to those in acute cardiac care. Patients are seriously ill and have a high risk for serious complications that usually arise in the first days after the event. A stroke unit basically consists of an organized and knowledgeable team of experts who can provide state-of-the-art care to patients with stroke.[3–6] Specialized nurses and rehabilitation professionals complement the activities of physicians who have expertise in the management of stroke. These units improve care by preventing complications and expediting rehabilitative efforts. Personnel in the unit are likely to be able to identify the complications quickly and, thus, be able to intervene rapidly. These steps have the potential to reduce the total economic costs of care and simultaneously improve outcomes.[3] Patients who have been treated with rt-PA or who need close neurological or cardiovascular monitoring could be admitted to a stroke unit.[7] The first 24 hours after stroke are the most critical.

Components of a Stroke Unit

Depending on the institution, the functions and components of management in a stroke unit can vary widely (Table 13–1). Some acute stroke care units are housed in rehabilitation hospitals and focus on measures to speed and maximize recovery after the patient's acute condition is stable. Other stroke units stress acute treatment and can even include services that replicate those found in an intensive care unit. Probably the best description of a modern stroke care unit is an integrated service that provides acute care and then moves smoothly to rehabilitation and long-term treatment. A stroke unit usually includes a geographically defined facility staffed by a cadre of skilled professionals who have the attitude that stroke can be treated and that patients' outcomes can be improved. The attitude that persons with stroke can be helped is the foundation for an effective stroke care unit. It affects all aspects of management.

Table 13–1. **Components of an Acute Stroke Care Unit**

- Geographically defined unit
  - Usually four to eight beds
  - Monitoring capability
    - Cardiac rate and rhythm
    - Blood pressure
    - Pulse oximetry
    - Respiratory rate
    - Intracranial pressure
  - Central nursing station
  - Access to rehabilitation services and diagnostic laboratories
- Personnel
  - Physician—medical director
  - Nurses
  - Rehabilitation specialists
    - Physical therapy
    - Occupational therapy
    - Speech pathology
  - Social worker
  - Neuropsychologist
  - Chaplain
  - Dietician
  - Pharmacist

GEOGRAPHICAL CONSIDERATIONS

Some institutions use a mobile stroke team, consisting primarily of rehabilitation specialists, to provide consultation and treatment for patients housed on general medical units. This approach generally lacks either specialized medical or nursing care. The strategy is not optimal because patients are scattered throughout the hospital, and implementation of special stroke care protocols is hampered by a lack of continuity in staff or care.

Specialized nursing services are especially critical during the first days after stroke, when observation by experienced nurses is instrumental in promptly identifying changes in the patient's neurological condition. Thus, the best arrangement for an acute stroke care unit is a geographically defined facility with beds designated for the treatment of patients with cerebrovascular disease.[4] The number of beds in a unit depends on the number of patients seen annually, but a minimum of four beds likely is needed for the unit to run efficiently.

An acute stroke care unit should have the capability to monitor cardiac rate and rhythm, blood pressure, level of oxygenation, and respiratory rate.[4] The arterial blood pressure can be assessed by non-invasive means or through the use of intra-arterial pressure monitoring. The latter is particularly important if aggressive measures to lower blood pressure, such as intravenous administration of antihypertensive agents, are needed. Patients who need airway protection and ventilatory support likely will need to be admitted to a more intensive care setting.[7] Intracranial pressure monitoring is a possible component of management in a stroke unit, but this capability likely is not needed because most patients with severe intracranial hypertension also need intensive care, including ventilatory assistance. Depending on the level of nursing staff coverage, an acute stroke care unit could handle these critically ill patients. However, a minority of patients with ischemic stroke will need this aggressive treatment. As a result, staff may not possess the expertise to handle ventilators and other intensive care unit treatments. Thus, patients who need very aggressive care or ventilatory assistance may be best treated in an intensive care unit.

A strategy would be to admit a patient into the skilled acute stroke care unit for at least the first 24–48 hours. Thereafter, the patient could be transferred to a less skilled care unit—for example, a neurology in-patient ward—for continued care when his or her status is stable. The ideal situation is for the stroke unit and the neurology ward to be incorporated into the same administrative structure and to be physically adjacent.

The location of the stroke unit should permit easy access to rehabilitation services and diagnostic laboratories. The physical plant should be designed to allow for easy observation of the patients by nursing personnel. A central monitoring facility can permit easy assessment of data from the patients. The patients' rooms and the halls should be adapted to the needs of persons with motor, sensory, or cognitive impairments. Rooms should be lit brightly and have pictures and a television or radio to provide environmental stimuli that help maintain orientation and assist in cognitive and language rehabilitation. The design of the room is important. For example, the bed should be placed so that a patient with a homonymous hemianopia does not have only a blank wall to look at with the normal area of vision. Beds developed to lower the risk of pressure sores should be available for bed-bound patients. Toilet and bathing facilities must be modified to accommodate patients using wheelchairs. The unit also should have devices that ease transfer and mobilization of patients.

PERSONNEL

Physicians, nurses, and other health care professionals (the stroke team) who have special interest and experience in treating persons with cerebrovascular disease staff a modern acute stroke care unit.[8] (See Table 13–1.) Each member of the team has individual responsibilities. To ease communications and expedite management, meetings of the entire group should be held regularly.[8] The patient's progress, schedules for evaluation and treatment, and discharge plans can be reviewed, and integrated management can be adjusted in response to changes in the patient's condition.

A stroke unit is directed by a *physician,* most commonly a neurologist or a neurosurgeon, who sets the policies for the facility. The physician also leads the stroke team. Depending on the institution, physicians of multiple specialties could have admitting privileges, but they should understand that all patients will be treated using standardized stroke protocols or care maps. These physicians remain responsible for all orders for evaluation and treatment.

Nurses are key members of the stroke team. The patient–nurse ratio should not be higher than 4–1.[4] Nurses have frequent interactions with patients throughout the day, perform regular clinical assessments, check monitors, and administer medications. Their role in direct patient care includes assistance in eating, self-care, toileting, and bathing. In addition, nurses work in concert with rehabilitation professionals to start mobilization and to conduct range-of-motion exercises. Nurses are instrumental in teaching the patient and family about stroke, prognosis, acute treatment, rehabilitation, and plans to return to home. Nursing evaluation also is a critical component of discharge planning. A nurse often serves as a case manager and, in this role, facilitates and coordinates the diverse components of management.[9]

Rehabilitation is discussed in more detail in Chapter 14. Still, an effort to maximize functional recovery through early rehabilitation begins as soon as the patient's condition is stable. Baseline rehabilitation assessments generally should be done in the first 24–48 hours after stroke, and a plan for rehabilitation should be formulated. Depending on the institution, this evaluation and plan can be developed by a physician who specializes in rehabilitation, or it can be created by a series of rehabilitation therapists under the direction of the attending physician. In general, *physical therapists* focus on the patient's ability to walk and major movements of the limbs. They also provide assistance in the use of devices, such as a walker, cane, or brace. *Occupational therapists* address fine hand movements and the use of devices that help in activities of daily living. *Speech pathologists* treat impairments in swallowing, articulation, or language. A *neuropsychologist* can assess and treat cognitive impairments. A *recreation therapist* also can assist the patient in addressing activities of daily living. The advice of rehabilitation specialists influences management during the first days after stroke and affects plans for care after discharge. The need for long-term rehabilitation affects decisions about whether the patient will be transferred to an in-patient rehabilitation unit or to an out-patient clinic.

Assistance from social services is particularly helpful in discharge planning. A *social worker* can advise the physician, patient, and family about government or insurance programs or fiscal constraints. In particular, these issues can affect decisions about placement. The social worker also serves the important role of informing the patient and family about resources that might be available to them after discharge. Home health care, transportation, visiting nurse services, and rehabilitation can be addressed. Applications for disability or government aid can be filed.

A *chaplain* can provide solace for patients and families who request religious support. A *dietician* also may help with the patient's hydration and nutrition. Components and consistency of the diet can be modified in response to the patient's needs. Tube feedings are selected for patients needing this form of administration of food and liquids. Diets are modified to treat illnesses such as diabetes mellitus or hypercholesterolemia. A *pharmacist* may give advice on selection and administration of medications.

Activities of a Stroke Unit

Management is multi-factorial (Table 13–2). Medical interventions aimed at treatment of the stroke itself are continued. In the future, new therapies to improve circulation or to provide neuroprotection could be started after admission. The patient's condition can be stabilized so that urgent surgical or endovascular procedures can be performed.

Patients are observed closely, and their neurological and medical status is monitored. In particular, patients are evaluated for development of hypoxia, hyperglycemia, hypotension, fever, or cardiac arrhythmias.[10,11] Any of these complications can add to morbidity or mortality from stroke. Stroke units seem to benefit

Table 13–2. **Components of Acute Care of Patients Hospitalized with Ischemic Stroke**

Continuation of interventions used to treat the stroke
Close observation of the patient's medical and neurological status
Prevention and treatment of medical or neurological complications
Initiation of rehabilitation
Evaluation for the cause of stroke
Initiation of therapies to prevent recurrent stroke
Discharge planning

patients by reducing the number of complications of stroke and by rapidly initiating rehabilitation to maximize recovery from the cerebrovascular event.[12] Stroke units generally have more aggressive mobilization than general wards.[13] The time until mobilization and gait training begin and the time until a stable blood pressure is established are shorter when care is provided in a stroke unit.[14] In addition, the use of parenteral fluids, aspirin, antipyretics, and antibiotics is higher in a stroke unit.[13] Each of these interventions may have modest individual benefits but, in aggregate, they appear to hasten recovery.

Patients in a stroke unit are evaluated for the cause of stroke (see Chapter 4). The results of these studies influence decisions about the use of medical or surgical therapies to prevent recurrent stroke (see Chapters 10 and 11) when these interventions are initiated is influenced by the severity of the stroke. In addition, multidisciplinary and coordinated efforts directed at mobilization and emotional support also have important effects on recovery after stroke.[8,15,16] Finally, the stroke unit can help speed planning for discharge from the hospital.[17]

Care Maps

Bowen and Yaste[18] found that a stroke protocol or care map could reduce the patient's length of stay and improve measures of quality of care, such as the increased use of therapies to prevent deep vein thrombosis. An important aim of stroke protocols is to avoid complications, rather than to focus on acute crisis treatment.[19] Although an integrated multidisciplinary team is at the heart of the care map, the protocol should not restrict the decisions of the patient or the treating physician.[19] The protocol should include orders for general care and observation, diet, activity, evaluation, and therapies aimed at treating the stroke or co-morbid diseases.[4] (See Table 13–3.) Management to limit or treat medical or neurological complications, consultations with rehabilitation services, and strategies for discharge are parts of the care map. Preprinted sets of orders that can be signed by the physician expedite the implementation of the care map. Although this set of orders provides a framework for treating most patients, the physician has the option to add or delete orders to tailor a care map to the individual patient's needs. A care map usually has orders and plans for each of the first 4–7 days of hospitalization. Orders reflect a customary course of stabilization followed by improvement during the first week. Critically ill patients who need intensive care usually cannot be treated using a standard stroke care protocol.

In addition to improving outcomes after stroke, another benefit from care maps could be a reduction in costs. Use of a care map avoids unnecessary interventions or tests. At the same time, the timetable included in the care map can expedite the performance of tests and procedures.

Outcomes of Patients Hospitalized in Stroke Units

Several clinical studies performed primarily in Europe have examined the usefulness of specialized care in a stroke unit.[12–15,20–28] These studies generally have reported a benefit in reductions in mortality, disability, and the need for long-term care after stroke. Strand et al[20] found that treatment in a non-intensive stroke unit reduced disability and long-term hospitalization. Benefits from stroke unit care were present regardless of the patient's age, the severity of stroke, or the patient's medical history.[21] In 1991, Indredavik et al[22] reported that the 6-week mortality among patients in a stroke unit was 7.3% compared with 17.3% mortality among patients on general wards. By 6 weeks, 54% of the patients treated in the stroke unit were home in contrast with 32.7% of the patients treated in a general ward. Langhorne et al[23] found that care in a stroke unit lowered the risk of death within 4 months by approximately 28% and that this reduction in mortality persisted for at least 1 year. A collaborative review found that stroke unit care reduced

Table 13–3. **Components of Acute Care Map for Patients with an Acute Ischemic Stroke**

- Activity
  - Usually on bed rest for the first 24 hours
  - Mobilize the patient when neurologically stable
  - Increase activity as the patient tolerates
  - Prolonged bed rest—measures to avoid pressure sores
  - Range-of-motion exercises
- Vital signs
  - Perform the following assessments at regular intervals
    - Neurological assessments
    - Blood pressure
    - Pulse and respiratory rate
    - Temperature
  - Usually every 4 hours initially
  - Patients given recombinant tissue plasminogen activator initially need more frequent assessments
  - Frequency subsequently adjusted as the patient improves
- Diet
  - Should not be given food and water until swallowing is assessed
  - Adjust consistency of food and liquids to the ability to swallow
  - Modify diet to reflect needs of patient (eg, cholesterol, sodium, glucose)
- General medical care
  - Treat concomitant diseases (eg, hypertension, diabetes, heart disease)
  - Prophylaxis against deep vein thrombosis in bed-bound patients
    - Subcutaneous heparin or low molecular weight heparin/danaparoid
    - Alternating pressure devices and support stockings
  - Avoid placement of indwelling bladder catheter or remove as the patient's condition permits
  - Symptomatic treatment (ie, analgesics, stool softeners, antipyretics)
- Consultation with rehabilitation services
  - Discharge planner—social services
  - Physical therapy
  - Occupational therapy
  - Speech pathology
- Evaluation for the cause of stroke
  - Arterial imaging (ie, carotid duplex, magnetic resonance angiography, arteriography)
  - Cardiac imaging (ie, transesophageal echocardiography)
  - Special coagulation tests (ie, antiphospholipid antibodies, Factor V-Leiden)
  - Tests for autoimmune diseases (ie, antinuclear antibody)
- Initiation of treatment to prevent recurrent stroke
  - Aspirin
  - Ticlopidine
  - Clopidogrel
  - Dipyridamole
  - Warfarin

Note: Components of the care map must be adjusted to the needs of the individual patient.

mortality by approximately 17%, death or disability by approximately 31%, and death or institutionalization by approximately 25%.[24] These are impressive results that are not restricted to a particular subgroup of patients with stroke. Ronning and Guldvog[25] compared outcomes among 364 patients admitted to a stroke unit and 438 patients treated in general wards. The 10-day mortality was 8.2% among patients in the stroke unit and 15.1% among those on the ward. One-year and 18-month survival rates also were greater among patients initially treated in a stroke unit. Another study found that long-term survival and functional recovery were increased by treatment in a stroke unit.[26] The quality of life also was improved among patients who were treated in a stroke unit.[15] Recently, Indredavik et al[27] described a reduction in mortality and an increased likelihood of independence for as long as 10 years after stroke. These sustained benefits are impressive.

A recent Danish study found that care in a stroke unit was associated with a relative risk of death of 0.87, a likelihood of long-term care of 0.94, and the chances of going home of 1.06; in this study, all of these differences were significant.[28] A community-based study found that care in a specialized stroke care unit reduced the risk of early mortality (<1 month) by approximately 50%.[29] Patients in a stroke unit had a 0.61 relative risk of going to a nursing home, and a 1.90 times higher likelihood of going home than did the patients treated in a general patient care setting. In a second report, Jorgensen et al[30] found that mortality at both 1 year and 5 years was lower among patients treated in a stroke unit compared with those hospitalized in a general ward. Care in a stroke unit was associated with a 40% relative reduction in risk of death regardless of age, sex, stroke severity, or the presence of co-morbid diseases.

Van Straten et al[31] reported that coordinated stroke services reduced the length of stay in the hospital and improved the efficiency of discharge planning. Potential logistical issues that would result in delays in discharge can be avoided by implementation of a coordinated team approach. A collaborative review showed that stroke unit care reduced the length of hospitalization by approximately 8% and that the units did not increase the use of acute care resources.[24] Another study showed that well-organized stroke care was associated with economic savings even when therapies were prescribed to elderly patients.[32] Some of these savings can be attributed to the reduction in the number of patients admitted to long-term care facilities. Thus, even if more money might be spent during early care, lower spending later offsets these costs. In addition, stroke unit treatment appears to improve the quality of life of survivors.[15]

Conclusion

Stroke care units make a difference in improving outcomes after stroke.[33] The time has come to implement development of stroke units on a broad basis. Because of the expenses involved and the limited number of skilled professionals available to staff these units, the best strategy is to develop units that can serve a geographical region. Emergency departments in small hospitals can initiate treatment locally and then transfer the patient to another hospital that has a stroke unit so that care can continue.

NEUROLOGICAL COMPLICATIONS OF ISCHEMIC STROKE

In general, neurological worsening occurs within 48 hours of stroke. It develops in up to 40% of patients.[34–39] (Table 13–4) Clinical hallmarks are new neurological impairments reflecting additional brain injury in the region of the original stroke, or a decline in consciousness. The causes of deterioration in neurological condition include early recurrent stroke, symptomatic hemorrhagic transformation of the infarction, brain edema, or metabolic disturbances.[36,40,41] Hemodynamic changes leading to a failure of collateral flow also can cause worsening. Neurological worsening can develop regardless

Table 13–4. **Causes of Neurological Worsening After Acute Ischemic Stroke**

Early recurrent stroke
Symptomatic hemorrhagic transformation of infarction
Brain edema
Metabolic disorders (ie, hypoglycemia or hyponatremia)
Fever
Hemodynamic disorders
Failure of collaterals
Hypotension
Progression of thrombus
Biochemical mechanisms (release of neurotoxic agents)
Infections

of the patient's age or the presumed cause of stroke. Neurological deterioration appears to be more frequent among patients with strokes in the posterior circulation than among patients with strokes in the carotid arterial territory.[42] Patients with cortical infarctions are more likely to deteriorate than are patients with isolated subcortical lesions.[40] Still, the status of up to one-fourth of patients with lacunes can worsen.[35] The outcomes of patients with neurological worsening are poorer than those of patients who do not have deterioration.[36]

Patients with hypertension or hypotension, fever, diabetes mellitus, hyperglycemia, coronary artery disease, or a major abnormality on computed tomography (CT) are at the greatest risk for neurological decline after stroke.[43,44] Chabriat et al[45] evaluated CT factors that predicted neurological deterioration after stroke. The presence of a hyperdense middle cerebral artery increased the likelihood of worsening by a factor of 1.8 (1.1–3.1). The finding of a hypodensity involving more than one-third of the hemisphere increased the odds of neurological deterioration by a factor of 2.5 (1.6–4.0). Development of new neurological signs should prompt a search for the likely cause. Follow-up CT scans usually show an increase in stroke volume among persons who deteriorate.[46] Depending on the presumed etiology, specific interventions are prescribed.

Brain Edema and Increased Intracranial Pressure

Brain edema is the most common cause of a major decline in neurological status once the patient is admitted to the hospital.[5] (See Table 13–5.) Malignant brain edema and neurological deterioration usually appear 2–5 days after a malignant middle cerebral artery territory infarction.[47] (See Fig. 13–1.) Brain edema and secondary increased intracranial pressure account for approximately 78% of deaths that occur within 1 week of stroke.[34] Overall, more than one-fourth of deaths after stroke can be attributed to brain edema and secondary intracranial pressure.[34] Most patients who develop severe and symptomatic brain edema following a major infarction will die as a consequence of herniation.[48] Wijdicks and Diringer[48] found that mortality secondary to brain edema was significantly lower among persons younger than 45 than among older persons; 3 of 11 young patients died compared to 20 of 22 older patients. In another series of 55 patients with malignant hemispheric infarction, 43 died of herniation.[47] All of the survivors had moderate-to-severe disability.

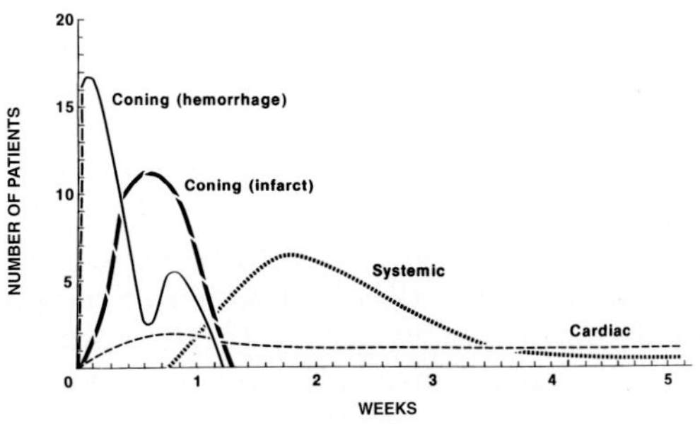

Figure 13–1. Timing of the causes of death following stroke. Herniation (coning) usually leads to death within 1 week of either ischemic or hemorrhagic stroke. Systemic causes of death (most commonly infections or pulmonary embolism) usually peak at 2 weeks.

Table 13–5. **Neurological and Medical Complications Among Patients Hospitalized with Ischemic Stroke**

Brain edema	Cardiac arrhythmias
Increased intracranial pressure	Congestive heart failure
Herniation	Deep vein thrombosis
Cerebellar infarction and hydrocephalus	Pulmonary embolism
Hemorrhagic transformation of the infarction	Respiratory failure
Recurrent ischemic stroke	Pneumonia
Seizures	Urinary incontinence
Dementia	Urinary tract infections
Other neurological disorders	Fecal incontinence
Movement disorders	Constipation
Hemichorea and hemiballism	Gastrointestinal bleeding
Parkinsonism	Disorders of hydration and nutrition
Dystonia	Hyponatremia
Dyskinesia	Dysphagia
Tremors	Pressure sores
Pain	Falls
Allodynia/thalamic pain syndrome	Shoulder pain
Trigeminal neuralgia	Subluxation of the shoulder
Shoulder-hand syndrome	Adhesive capsulitis of the shoulder
Reflex sympathetic dystrophy	Contractures
Gustatory disturbances	Osteoporosis
Hiccups	Depression
Autonomic disorders	Hypomania
Sleep disorders	Anxiety disorders
Cardiovascular complications	Disorders of anger
Ischemic heart disease	Pathological emotionality

PATHOGENESIS

The pathogenesis of brain edema is complex, and a detailed review is beyond the scope of this book. It likely is the result of vasogenic and cytotoxic components. Fluid accumulates in cells and in extracellular spaces, and edema evolves during the first few days after stroke. These changes can be detected by multiparameter magnetic resonance imaging (MRI).[49] In general, edema peaks approximately 5 days after stroke and then gradually abates. It is maximal in the area of the brain affected by the stroke. Because the skull is a closed compartment, a marked increase in brain volume secondary to edema leads to increases in intracranial pressure. Physiological responses to intracranial hypertension include constriction of the intracranial vessels to reduce the intravascular volume and increased absorption of cerebrospinal fluid (CSF) to decrease the volume of the ventricles and subarachnoid space. Fever, hypercarbia, and hypoxia can induce expansion of the volume of the vascular bed. In addition, administration of vasodilating medications also leads to an increase in the blood volume in the cranial vault. Any of these factors can exacerbate intracranial hypertension. In addition, the mass effect of a large infarction in the posterior fossa can compress the fourth ventricle or the aqueduct of Sylvius and block the outflow of CSF. The resultant hydrocephalus also worsens intracranial hypertension. Marked rises in intracranial pressure are dangerous because of their effects on cerebral perfusion. Extreme intracranial hypertension reduces blood flow to such a level that additional ischemia could result. An increase in mean arterial pressure is a physiological response to intracranial hypertension. For this reason, prescription of antihypertensive medications to lower blood pressure can be counterproductive by worsening the brain ischemia. It is possible for intracranial pressure readings to exceed the mean blood pressure and, as a result, perfusion to the brain ceases and brain death results. Still, Frank[50] found that globally elevated intracranial pressure is not a common cause of the initial neurological worsening from large hemispheric infarctions with edema.

The cranial vault is subdivided into three compartments. The falx cerebri separates the left and right cerebral hemispheres. The posterior fossa is delineated from the middle cranial fossa by the tentorium. Because edema generally is restricted to one area of the brain, the localized increase in volume and pressure is greatest in the affected compartment. Differences in volumes and pressures between the three compartments lead to shifts in brain structures—herniation. This herniation leads to secondary neurological injury as the result of distortion and traction. Neurological injuries generally are worst in the rostral brain stem. Extensive brain stem damage leads to coma and a loss of function of vital centers, including those that regulate breathing and cardiovascular function.

PATIENTS AT RISK

Malignant brain edema is not a major problem in patients with lacunar or branch cortical infarctions. Patients with isolated brain stem infarctions also do not develop symptomatic brain edema. Large infarctions secondary to occlusion of the internal carotid artery or proximal portion of the middle cerebral artery are associated with the highest chance of dying.[51] (See Table 13–6.) Risk of serious brain edema can be predicted by the neurological findings at the time of admission to the hospital. Patients with decreased consciousness or with a combination of major motor,

Table 13–6. **Patients at Greatest Risk for Malignant Brain Edema Following Ischemic Stroke**

Clinical findings
Multilobar infarction—cerebral hemisphere
High score on National Institutes of Health Stroke Scale
Decreased consciousness
Combination of major motor, sensory, visual, and cognitive signs
Cardioembolism or artery-to-artery embolism
Seizures
Hyperglycemia
Hypoxia
Hypercarbia
Fever
Brain imaging (computed tomography or magnetic resonance imaging)
Hypodensity involving > one-third of a hemisphere
Early sulcal effacement
Early loss of corticomedullary contrast
Dense artery sign
Vascular imaging (arteriogram, carotid duplex, or transcranial Doppler ultrasonography)
Occlusion of internal carotid artery
Occlusion of proximal portion of middle cerebral artery

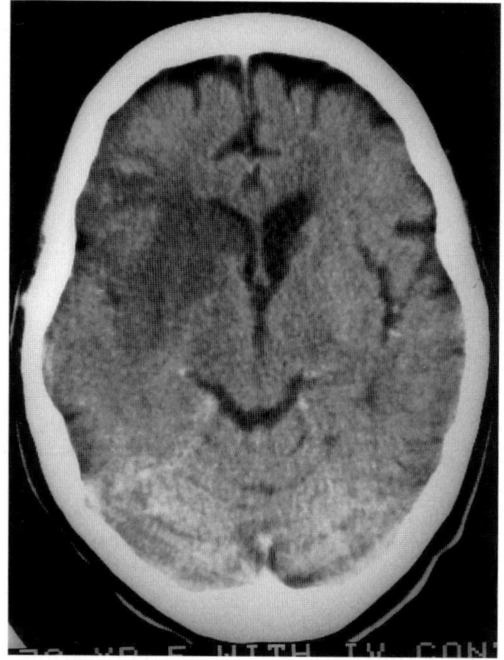

Figure 13–2. Computed tomograph of the brain obtained from a patient with a recent right hemisphere stroke. A large lenticulostriate infarction with compression of the ipsilateral lateral ventricle is seen.

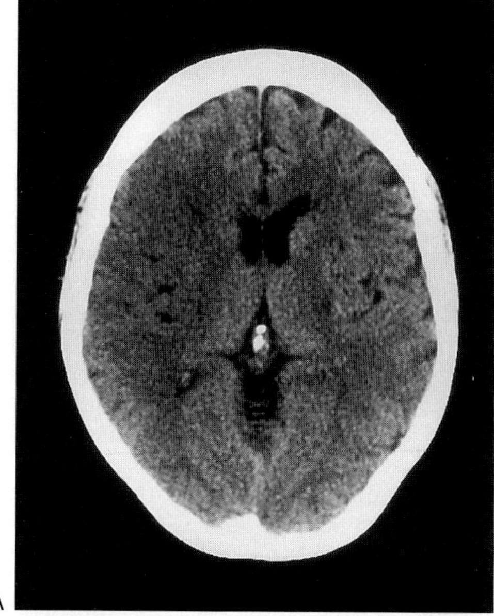

A

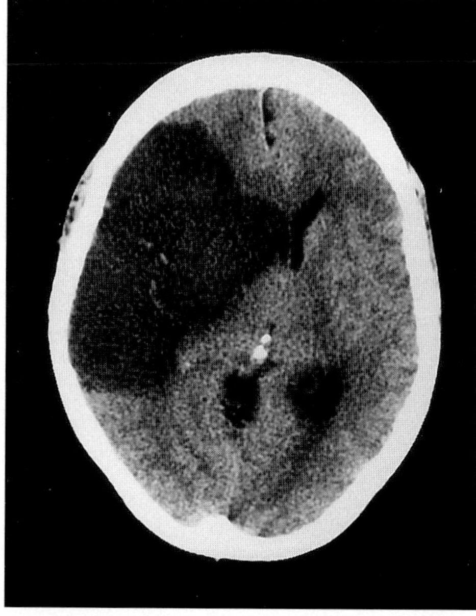

B

Figure 13–3. Cerebral edema with midline shift. This 79-year-old woman with hypertension and type II diabetes presented with vomiting, left hemiparesis, and left-sided neglect. She became increasingly drowsy and developed a right III nerve palsy. She died 3 days later. The computed tomography scan at admission (*A*) shows hypodensity in the right frontal, parietal, and temporal lobes. Two days later (*B*), the infarct is more hypodense, and there is 2 cm. midline shift to the left, compression of the right frontal horn, and effacement of the suprasellar cistern. The enlarged left temporal horn on the later scan suggests the development of an obstructive hydrocephalus. (Courtesy of Dr. B Silver.)

sensory, cognitive, and visual impairments are at greatest risk. The presence of a high score (>15–20 points) on the National Institutes of Health (NIH) Stroke Scale will forecast a high risk.[52] This correlation is made because a high NIH Stroke Scale score is seen among patients with multilobar infarctions of the cerebral hemisphere, and these patients are at the greatest risk for malignant brain edema.

Diagnostic Studies

Early brain imaging studies also forecast which patients are at highest risk. Computed tomography evidence of a multilobar infarction predicts a high risk of serious edema.[52] (See Figs. 13–2 through 13–5.) In general, findings that predict a high risk for intracranial hemorrhage following treatment with rt-PA probably are the same that forecast a high risk for malignant brain edema. In fact, deterioration from brain swelling is most common among patients with occlusion of the middle cerebral artery and early sulcal efface-

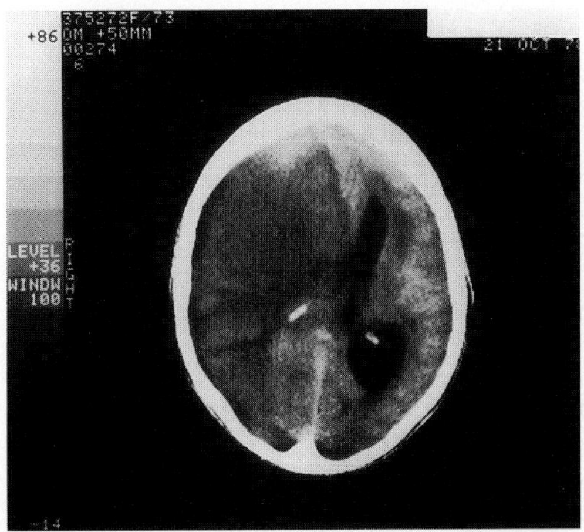

Figure 13–4. Computed tomography scan obtained in a patient with a massive cerebral infarction secondary to occlusion of the internal carotid artery. The area of the posterior cerebral artery is spared. Midline structures are shifted to the left, and the left lateral ventricle is dilated.

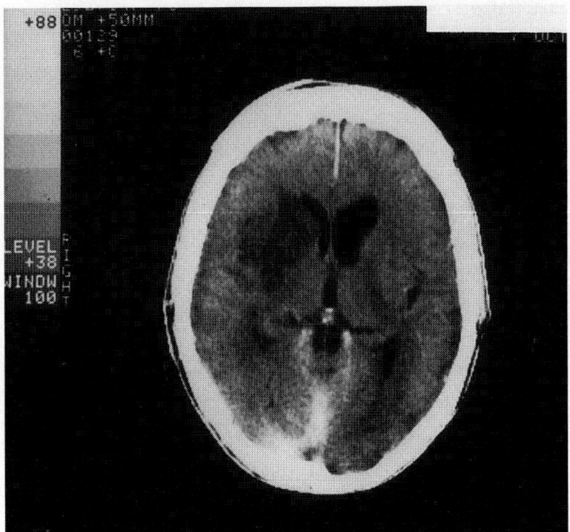

Figure 13–5. A computed tomogram of a patient with a recent infarction of the right hemisphere demonstrates hypodensity in the basal ganglia and mild compression of the ipsilateral lateral ventricle.

ment on CT.[48] Abnormalities on single photon emission computed tomography (SPECT) or cerebral blood flow can predict fatal edema among patients with infarctions in the territory of the middle cerebral artery.[53,54] The arteriographic finding of an occlusion at the bifurcation of the internal carotid artery (the carotid T) predicts a high rate of serious brain edema.[55] In fact, arteriographic changes may be a more important finding than early CT abnormalities.[55] The strong predictive value of arteriographic findings corresponds with findings of multilobar ischemia in the territories of the anterior cerebral and middle cerebral arteries.

Other Factors Predicting Brain Edema

Patients with severe metabolic disorders also may have an increased risk of brain edema. Hyperglycemia, hypoxia, and hypercarbia are the factors most likely implicated (see Table 13–6). Early administration of thrombolytics might increase the risk of brain edema by augmenting reperfusion to an area of tissue that is already irreversibly damaged.[56] This risk is presumably due to a sudden recanalization of the artery, which permits increased flow into the area of previous ischemia. A sudden increase in intravascular pressure promotes the shift of water into extracellular spaces and injured neurons. The risk of serious brain edema as a complication of thrombolytic therapy may be exaggerated. The frequency of serious edema has not increased with thrombolytic therapy among patients in clinical trials. In fact, the high rate of symptomatic bleeding with rt-PA in one trial was counterbalanced by a high frequency of serious brain edema among persons in the control group.[57] Hypervolemic hemodilution can be a contributing factor in the development of brain edema and secondary brain edema; it also can be a partial explanation for the high mortality among patients treated with volume expansion.[58,59]

CLINICAL AND IMAGING FEATURES

Drowsiness and a decline in consciousness are the usual first symptoms of increased intracranial pressure following stroke.[60] (See Table 13–7.) These symptoms usually appear slowly and subtly during the first few days after stroke. The vital signs may become abnormal. In particular, bradycardia and hypertension might be noted. Although papilledema is the traditional

Table 13–7. **Clinical Features of Increased Intracranial Pressure**

General symptoms
- Decrease in level of consciousness
- Waxing and waning of consciousness
- Progression to coma
- Papilledema generally appearing late

Vital signs
- Increase in blood pressure
- Decrease in heart rate

Herniation
- Pupil asymmetry (ipsilateral mydriasis)—III nerve palsy
- Periodic breathing
- New hemiparesis and Babinski sign ipsilateral to stroke

sign of increased intracranial pressure, funduscopic changes can be delayed for hours after the onset of clinically relevant intracranial hypertension. Thus, the absence of papilledema does not exclude the presence of malignant brain edema and increased intracranial pressure. Other signs include asymmetrical pupils, periodic breathing, and a new ipsilateral hemiparesis and Babinski sign.[60] The appearance of hemiparesis ipsilateral to the involved hemisphere is secondary to compression of the contralateral cerebral peduncle against the tentorium (Kernohan notch). These neurological signs appear late and reflect herniation of the brain.

Transcranial Doppler sonography can be used to detect a shift of midline structures among patients with large hemispheric infarctions. Garriets et al[61] found that a 4 mm. shift of the third ventricle or greater predicted herniation and death. They advocated use of sonography to select these patients for decompressive hemicraniectomy.

Imaging of the brain provides important information about the course of brain edema. Early changes involve obliteration of the ipsilateral sulci and compression of the ipsilateral lateral ventricle. Subsequently, midline structures shift to the contralateral hemisphere. The degree of midline shift correlates with changes in the level of consciousness. Acute ventricular dilation of the contralateral ventricle is secondary to obliteration of the foramen of Munro. In general, a shift of the septum pellucidum corresponds to the appearance of coma.[62] Subsequently, distortion of diencephalic and mesencephalic structures is seen. Results of brain imaging studies also predict which patients are likely to die secondary to malignant brain edema.[63] Patients with a volume greater than 400 cu mm., a shift of the septum pellucidum greater than 9 mm., or a pineal displacement greater than 4 mm. are likely to die within 14 days of stroke.[62] Brain imaging can show structural changes with advanced edema and herniation. Magnetic resonance imaging of the brain among patients with acute uncal herniation usually demonstrates compression of the diencephalon with downward displacement of the midbrain and secondary changes in the lateral midbrain.[64] These changes probably correspond to the pathologic finding of Duret hemorrhages in the rostral brain stem.

PREVENTION AND TREATMENT

Prophylaxis includes elevation of the head of the bed to improve venous drainage; avoiding hypoxia, hypercarbia, or hyperthermia; treating fever; and not prescribing potentially hypo-osmolar fluids, such as 5% dextrose in water.[1,34,65] (See Table 13–8.) These measures can be instituted soon after the patient is admitted. Their efficacy has not been tested in clinical trials, yet these conservative interventions generally are recommended for treatment of patients at high risk for malignant brain edema.[66] Schwarz et al[67] reported that a 50 mg bolus of *indomethacin* could reduce intracranial pressure and improve cerebral perfusion pressure for a short time. This therapy likely will receive additional study.

Corticosteroids are widely prescribed to lessen brain edema secondary to brain tumors. Although steroids are effective in this situation, data about their usefulness in stroke treatment are not available. Studies of conventional or large doses of steroids for treatment of stroke have not demonstrated any evidence of efficacy.[68–71] However, the immunosuppressive effects

Table 13–8. **Prevention or Treatment of Brain Edema and Increased Intracranial Pressure Following Stroke**

General prophylaxis
Avoid hypoxia and hypercarbia
Treat hyperthermia
Avoid administration of hypo-osmolar fluids
Improve venous drainage by elevating head of bed
Corticosteroids should not be prescribed
Osmotherapy
Glycerol
Mannitol
Ventilatory assistance and hyperventilation
Intraventricular drainage of cerebrospinal fluid
Hypothermia
Barbiturates
Surgical resection
Surgical decompression

of steroids increase the risk of infectious complications of stroke. Current guidelines recommend that corticosteroids should not be prescribed for treating brain edema among patients with ischemic stroke.[66] Pending new data from clinical trials, these agents should not be prescribed.

Data are limited about the value of hyperosmolar therapy in controlling brain edema after stroke. Hyper-osmotic treatment involves the administration of glycerol, mannitol, or other hypertonic fluids.[65,72,73] Stoll et al[74] recently showed that *osmotherapy* can normalize perfusion to the ischemic focus. Most clinical studies have focused on the utility of *glycerol*.[75–77] Although glycerol can be taken orally, its sweetness makes it intolerable to most patients. Intravenous administration of glycerol has not gained popularity in North America probably because of its potential to induce hemolysis.

Mannitol has been used to treat patients with brain edema after head injuries, and it is administered to patients with stroke. The usual initial dose of mannitol is 0.25–1 gm/kg given intravenously over 20 minutes.[78] The medication usually results in a rapid decline in intracranial pressure, and the effects usually last 4–6 hours. Clinical improvement and improvement in microcirculatory flow can accompany the medication.[79] Patients receiving mannitol will have improvement in their neurological status even without change in the shifts of midline structures.[80] Repeated doses of mannitol can be administered, but the maximal daily dose usually is 2 gm/kg. Repeated infusions of mannitol increase plasma osmolality and decrease water content in the cerebral cortex.[81] This can lead to a relative hyperosmolarity in the brain. A rebound increase in brain water can occur. Repeated doses of mannitol also can affect renal function. Mannitol is recommended for the emergent treatment of patients with neurological worsening secondary to brain edema following stroke.[66] Infusions of 3% saline can reduce intracranial pressure among patients with head injury.[73] Nevertheless, infusions of saline have not worked among patients with stroke, and these fluids can cause pulmonary edema or diabetes insipidus.

Most patients with malignant hemispheric infarctions will need ventilatory assistance.[47] Patients who are deteriorating secondary to brain edema should be intubated to secure the airway and to avoid both hypoxia and hypercarbia. Elective intubation should be done before the patient shows signs of a herniation syndrome.[82] *Hyperventilation* causes hypocarbia and a secondary vasoconstriction of intracranial vessels. Effects on intracranial pressure are almost immediate. Thus, hyperventilation can be performed as an emergent intervention for patients with signs of herniation or severe increases in intracranial pressure.[66] Nevertheless, hyperventilation is of limited benefit and should be considered as an adjunct to other measures to control intracranial pressure.

Despite these measures, a sizeable proportion of patients will develop signs of neurological worsening. Berrouschot et al[83] reported the outcomes of 53 patients with malignant infarctions in the territory of the middle cerebral artery who were treated with anticoagulants, osmotherapy, and mild hyperventilation. Eventually all of the patients became comatose and required mechanical ventilatory support;

37 died in the intensive care unit at an average of 90 hours after stroke. Within 3 months, 42 patients had died.

Intracranial pressure monitoring has been used to assess the course of brain edema following stroke. Monitors can be placed in the subarachnoid space, ventricle, or the substance of the brain. Detections of increases in intracranial pressure can prompt treatment with osmotherapy before neurological worsening occurs. If an intraventricular line is used to monitor pressure, then it could be combined with a system that permits drainage of CSF to lower pressure. This tactic is especially helpful among patients with hydrocephalus secondary to a mass-producing cerebellar infarction. Levels of intracranial pressure have prognostic implications. One recent trial found no survivors among patients who had an intracranial pressure >35 mm Hg.[84] However, the value of intracranial pressure monitoring has been questioned. Schwab et al[84] found that clinical signs of neurological worsening or herniation preceded development of elevations of intracranial pressure detected by monitoring. They concluded that intracranial pressure monitoring was not helpful in the long-term care of high-risk patients and that it did not influence outcomes. This finding should suggest caution about over-reliance on intracranial pressure monitoring to guide treatment of patients with malignant brain edema.

Lowering the body's temperature slows metabolic demands and lessens the development of brain edema. In one large series, elevated body temperature was associated with a very poor prognosis among persons with severe infarctions.[83] Brain temperature is typically higher than body temperature, so monitoring the brain temperature might be helpful in treating patients with severe stroke and severe edema.[85] Moderate *hypothermia* also has been prescribed to treat massive increases in intracranial pressure.[86] Success has been limited. Schwab et al[87] used cooling blankets and intravenous infusions of low-temperature fluids to treat 25 patients with severe middle cerebral infarction. The goal was to lower the body temperature to 33° C. Fourteen patients survived. Pneumonia was an important complication of treatment, and some patients had herniation after the body temperature was returned toward normal. The value of iatrogenic-induced hypothermia remains undetermined.

Barbiturates also have been used to lower intracranial pressure among patients with malignant brain edema.[88,89] They lower metabolic activity but must be given in sufficiently high doses to induce coma and a burst-suppression pattern on electroencephalography. This treatment regimen is complex and difficult. It requires intensive ancillary care, including cardiorespiratory support. It has not been shown to be effective in improving neurological outcomes and, because of the associated high risk for complications, is not recommended.

Surgical resection of a large area of necrotic brain tissue (most commonly the temporal or frontal lobe) can be done to save a patient's life.[65,90–92,39,37,39,35] External decompression of the skull allows the necrotic tissue to herniate through the defect rather than causing intracranial herniation. Experimental models have shown that *decompressive craniectomy* can reduce mortality and improve outcomes by early reduction in the size of the infarction.[93] (See Table 13–9.) Rieke et al[94] performed hemicraniotomy in 32 patients with space-occupying cerebral infarctions and compared their outcomes with 21 medically treated patients. They reported good outcomes in 6 patients having surgery and in none of the medically treated patients. The mortality was 16/21 (76.2%) for patients treated medically and 11/32 (34.4%) for those having surgical decompression. Carter et al[95] reported the 1 year outcomes of 14 patients who had decompressive hemicraniectomy for treatment of a massive infarction of the right hemisphere. Eleven patients survived a procedure that was used as a life-saving operation, and 8 of these patients were able to return home; the 3 other patients had severe disability. All of the patients were younger than 50. Schwab et al[96] performed early hemicraniectomy in 63 patients with acute infarctions involving the entire vascular territory of the middle cerebral artery. They found that the results of surgery were

Table 13–9. **Results of Clinical Series: Surgical Treatment of Malignant Brain Edema Following Acute Hemisphere Infarction**

Author	Patients Treated N	Survivors N	Independent or Good Outcomes
Kondziolka and Fazl[91]	5	5	5
Delashaw et al[356]	9	8	3
Steiger[92]	8	6	4
Kaila and Yonas[90]	4	4	4
Rieke et al[94]	32	21	15
Carter et al[95]	14	11	8
Sakai et al[97]	24	16	0
Schwab et al[96]	63	46	46
Mori et al[98]	13	11	3

surprisingly good when it was performed before signs of herniation had appeared. In a Japanese study, 24 patients with massive strokes were treated with external decompression; 16 patients survived, but all had severe residual disability.[97] Wijdicks and Diringer[48] recommended decompressive hemicraniotomy for the treatment of young patients with deterioration secondary to malignant brain edema. Mori et al[98] used *uncoparahippocampectomy* for direct surgical treatment of downward transtentorial herniation in 13 patients. At the time of surgery, the oculomotor nerve, the posterior cerebral artery, and the midbrain were directly decompressed using an approach via the middle temporal gyrus. They found that the operation could be a life-saving procedure.

The decision to recommend surgical decompression should be made cautiously. Patients who likely will be treated usually have extensive brain injury secondary to the original stroke. The risk of severe neurological residuals is considerable, and the patient has a high risk for profound disability if he or she survives the acute stroke. In general, surgery should be restricted to patients ages 50 years or younger. One can question the appropriateness of resecting a major portion of the dominant hemisphere if a major stroke has occurred. Global aphasia or other severe cognitive impairments could lead to a poor quality of life. The patient will not be able to give consent in this situation; thus, the family must be fully informed about the potential outcomes of this aggressive treatment. They need to realize that survival might be achieved but at the possible cost of a very poor quality of life thereafter. They may not agree to an operation.

Large Cerebellar Infarction and Hydrocephalus

Large cerebellar infarctions present a special management problem. The mass effect of a cerebellar lesion can lead to compression of the brain stem, leading to a progressive decline in consciousness and new focal neurological impairments or obliteration of the fourth ventricle, leading to hydrocephalus.[99,100] Neurological deterioration secondary to the mass effects usually begins within the first 3 days of the infarction. The signs can progress to coma.[101] Changes in the patient's examination correlate with the development of a mass effect.[102,103] (See Table 13–10.) In addition to developing signs of brain stem dysfunction by direct compression from the cerebellar lesion, *acute obstructive hydrocephalus* also leads to a decline in consciousness.[100,104,105] Patients with large cerebellar infarction should be monitored closely during the first 48–72 hours after admission. Follow-up brain

Table 13–10. **Clinical Findings of Mass Effect from Large Cerebellar Infarctions**

Early signs of cerebellar infarction and secondary mass effect
Ipsilateral limb ataxia
Nystagmus
Dysarthria
Stiff neck
Signs of secondary brain stem dysfunction
Trigeminal or facial nerve involvement
Gaze impairments, including bilateral "pseudo" abducens palsy
Bilateral Babinski signs
Small pupils
Late signs of brain stem dysfunction
Pinpoint pupils
Ataxic to agonal respiratory pattern

imaging studies (either CT or MRI) should be done to screen for the development of secondary hydrocephalus or signs of mass effect in the posterior fossa. In particular, the subarachnoid space at the base of the pons can become obliterated. Any decline in consciousness or brain stem dysfunction should prompt consideration of early surgical treatment to remove the cerebellar mass.

Conservative treatment includes measures to lessen edema and placement of a *ventricular drain* to relieve the hydrocephalus. Medical measures to treat cerebellar edema, including fluid restriction and osmotherapy, can be prescribed.[99] Ventricular drainage can help lower intracranial pressure among patients who have secondary hydrocephalus.[105,106] In one series of 52 patients with space-occupying cerebellar infarctions, 16 patients were treated medically and 10 needed ventriculostomy.[101] Thirty patients needed surgical procedures to remove the cerebellar mass. With medical and surgical treatment, 29 of the patients made a good recovery, 15 were disabled, and 8 died. In another series of 11 patients with large cerebellar infarctions with secondary brain stem compression, surgical management and ventriculostomy were life-saving measures.[107] In general, patients with cerebellar infarctions >3 cm. in diameter may need surgical resection.[106]

Hemorrhagic Transformation of Infarction

Hemorrhagic transformation can occur as a spontaneous complication of infarction. Hemorrhagic transformation results from vascular rupture or transvascular wall spread of fluid and red blood cells that follow reperfusion to the ischemic locus.[108] (See Figs. 13–6 and 13–7.) The likelihood of hemorrhagic transformation is strongly related to the size of the infarction and the presumed cause. Hemorrhagic lesions typically occur in large infarctions that involve the cortex of the cerebral or cerebellar hemispheres.[109–113] These are the same patients at high risk for serious brain edema. This complication appears to be more common among patients with

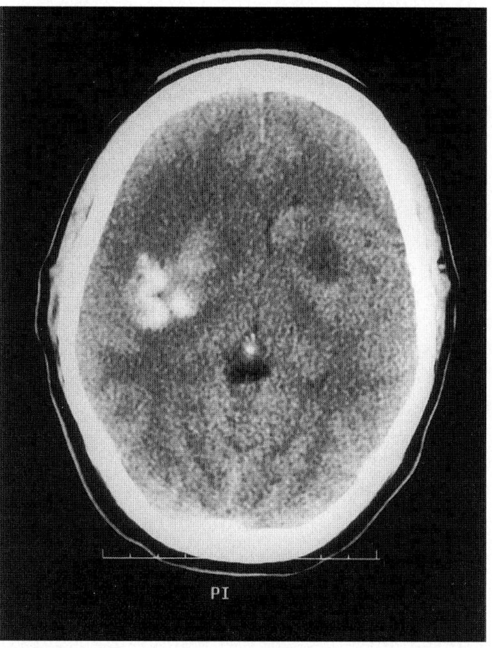

Figure 13–6. Computed tomographic scan with embolic events in both hemispheres secondary to cardioembolism. An area of hypodensity in basal ganglia is noted in the left hemisphere. An area of hemorrhage into the infarction of the right hemisphere also is present.

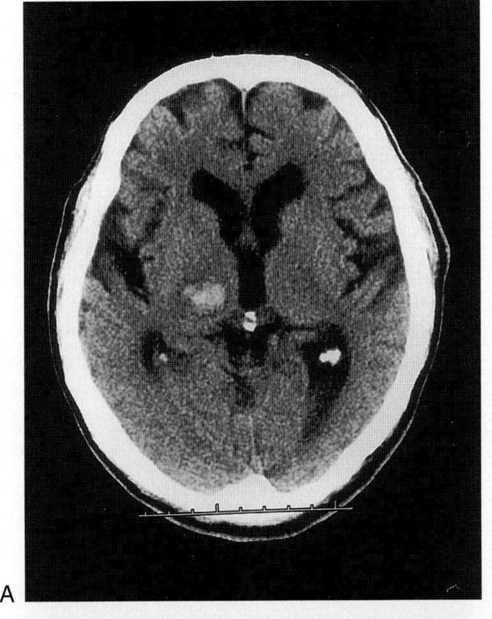

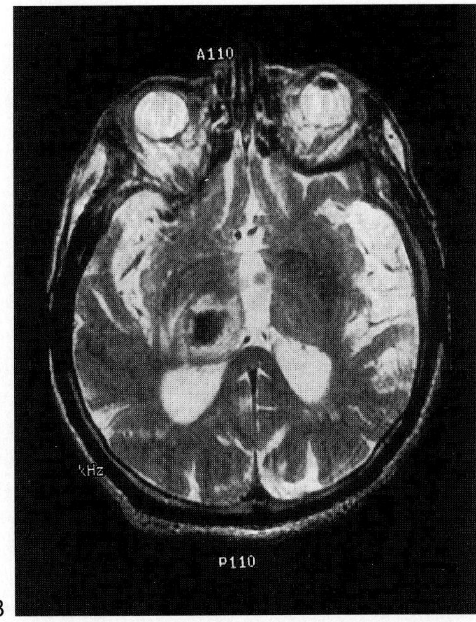

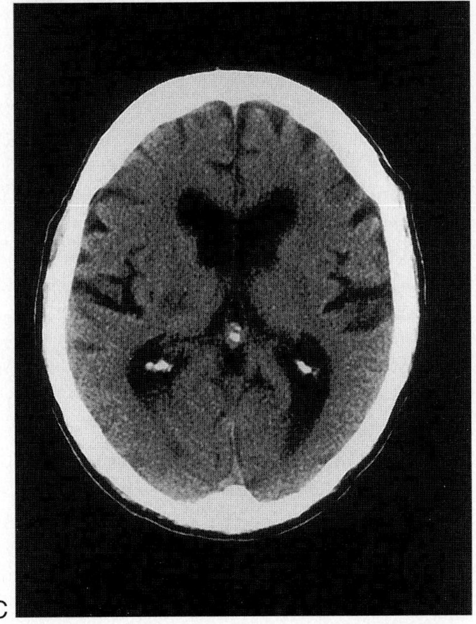

Figure 13–7. Evolution of a right thalamic haemorrhagic infarct. The computed tomography scan (*A*) shows a 1.5 cm. diameter hemorrhage in the lateral right thalamus with mild edema and mass effect. On a T_2-weighted magnetic resonance imaging (*B*) performed 3 days later, the hematoma appears dark because of the intracellular doxy-hemoglogin, but the surrounding edema appears bright. At 2 weeks, the hematoma has been resorbed, and there is a residual hypodense infarct on the computed tomography scan (*C*). (Courtesy of Dr. E. Wong.)

cardioembolic or artery-to-artery emboli from an atherosclerotic plaque than among persons with lacunar strokes.[109,114–116] Elderly patients and those with spontaneous increases in arterial blood pressure, diabetes mellitus, or infective endocarditis appear to have a particularly high risk.[108,117] Patients with severe deficits and major changes on CT or SPECT also have a high risk for bleeding complications.[118,119]

In general, spontaneous hemorrhagic transformation occurs within 1 week of stroke.[110,113] Bleeding appears to increase in blood pressure and recirculation after the artery is recanalized.[120] Hemorrhagic transformation of part of the infarction can be detected by brain imaging in a sizeable proportion of patients and, in most cases, these changes are not associated with neurological worsening. Minor abnormalities, including petechiae and small confluent areas of bleeding, also are detected.[113] In general, the presence and severity of hemorrhagic transformation also can be detected reliably by CT or MRI.[121] In one study of 160 patients with moderate-to-large infarctions secondary to embolism, the frequency of hemorrhagic changes detected by brain imaging was 40.6%.[117] Symptomatic hemorrhagic transformation can occur in up to 10% of patients.[34] The clinical features of hemorrhagic transformation of an infarction are headache, a decline of consciousness, and progression of focal neurological impairments. The leading alternative diagnoses to symptomatic hemorrhagic transformation are recurrent stroke, progression of the original thromboembolic event, or development of brain edema. The latter is the most likely.

Using medications that affect coagulation strongly influence the rate of this complication. Risk of symptomatic bleeding is highest among patients receiving antithrombotic or thrombolytic agents.[119,122,123] In addition, the presence of a volatile or markedly elevated blood pressure after thrombolytic therapy also predicts a high risk for symptomatic intracranial hemorrhage. The risk appears to be the greatest with thrombolytic agents, intermediate with anticoagulants, and lowest with the use of antiplatelet aggregating agents.[114] Hemorrhagic transformation leading to formation of a hematoma and neurological worsening is the most feared adverse experience in treating with either anticoagulants or thrombolytic agents.[124] Three clinical trials of streptokinase were stopped prematurely primarily because of this complication.[125–127] This potential for symptomatic hemorrhagic change is the primary reason for vigorously controlling blood pressure following the administration of rt-PA (see Chapter 12). Symptomatic hemorrhage also is a complication of urgent anticoagulant treatment, especially in patients with large infarctions.[128]

A large symptomatic hemorrhage after stroke causes a markedly increased likelihood of death.[129] There is no specific treatment of symptomatic hemorrhagic transformation. Administering coagulation factors, platelets, or other antidotes might reverse the effects of an anticoagulant or thrombolytic agent. Surgical evacuation of a large symptomatic hematoma can be performed. In general, the prognosis of a patient with a serious symptomatic intracranial hemorrhage is poor, in part because of the bleeding and in part because of the presence of a massive underlying infarction. The best ways to prevent bleeding include careful selection of patients who are treated with thrombolytic or antithrombotic agents and scrupulous management of arterial hypertension.

Early Recurrent Ischemic Stroke

Early recurrent ischemic stroke is a potential cause of neurological worsening in the first days after stroke.[130] In the past, the risk of early recurrent stroke was considered to be exceptionally high, especially among persons with cardioembolic stroke. An early recurrent embolic event was a primary indication for urgent anticoagulation. Recent clinical trials have shown that the risk of recurrent stroke is approximately 2%–3% in the first 2 weeks after stroke.[34,131–133] The risk appears to be the same regardless of stroke subtype, and patients with cardioembolic stroke do not have a significantly higher risk of recurrent embolism. Although the risk of recurrent stroke is much lower than previously perceived, a second stroke is associated with an increased likelihood of death or disability.[134] Thus, measures to prevent recurrent stroke are important. These medications should be started as soon as the patient's neurological condition permits.

Seizures

Overall, seizures complicate approximately 4%–6% of ischemic strokes.[34,135] A majority of seizures occur within 48 hours of stroke.[135–137] Seizures are not benign. They can worsen neurological outcome because of the increased metabolic demands at the time of ischemia.[138] Status epilepticus can occur.[137] In addition, patients who are having frequent seizures likely will need to be admitted to an intensive care unit for respiratory care. Wijdicks and Scott[139] reported that one-fourth of patients who needed mechanical ventilation after hemispheric stroke needed this treatment because of recurrent seizures. Sung and Chu[140] evaluated 118 patients who had seizures and stroke. The first seizure usually occurred within 2 weeks of stroke. Simple, partial seizures are more common than partial, complex, or generalized tonic-clonic seizures. Approximately 30%–40% of patients who have seizures with the onset of stroke subsequently will have recurrent seizures.[34,138,141] Early seizures predict the likelihood of recurrences and the diagnosis of epilepsy.[141]

Seizures are most common among patients with cortical or borderzone infarctions.[135,142] Patients with brain stem or subcortical infarctions have a low risk. The risk also does not correlate with the size of infarction or the presumed cause.[138] Burn et al[143] recently concluded that seizures were most common among patients with major infarctions of the cerebral hemispheres. In addition to hemodynamic factors at the time of stroke, metabolic disturbances during the first few days after the event also may induce seizures.[144] Electrolyte disorders, hypoglycemia, hypoxia, or sepsis are potential contributing factors.

Patients with a delayed onset of seizures are most likely to have recurrent events.[140] Seizures beginning more than 1 year after stroke are most likely to occur among patients with large cortical lesions that have an apparent area of preserved cerebral tissue within the infarcted area.[145]

Seizures are a possible cause of an alteration in consciousness or an encephalopathy following stroke. Overt involuntary tonic-clonic motor activity might not be found. The patient may have non-convulsive seizures. Periodic lateralizing epileptiform discharges (PLED) often will be detected by electroencephalography.[142] Findings of non-convulsive status epilepticus also might be detected by electroencephalography.

Patients who have had seizures following stroke should receive anticonvulsants as prophylaxis against recurrent attacks. No preferred medication has been identified, so the choice should be made on a case-by-case basis.[146]

Dementia

Confusional states can be detected after stroke in approximately one-fourth of patients older than 40.[147] Confusion can be secondary to pre-existing cognitive decline; the stroke; or complications of the stroke, such as an infection or metabolic derangement. A non-convulsive status or a post-ictal state also can present as confusion following stroke.

Cognitive and intellectual decline is relatively common after stroke and often is independent of depression.[148] *Dementia* is also relatively common after stroke. It can appear after the first diagnosed infarction.[149] Overall, stroke is a potent risk factor for dementia. The risk is nine times higher among persons with a history of stroke than it is among persons without ischemic symptoms.[150] In one series of 251 patients older than 60 with ischemic stroke, 66 had dementia.[151] The likelihood of dementia increases among elderly patients and among those with hyperglycemia.[152–154] Race and educational level also appear to be associated with the chances of dementia; minorities and those with low educational achievement seem to have a high risk.[151] Risk of dementia is also increased among persons with a history of prior stroke, diabetes mellitus, left hemisphere lesions, and major dominant hemispheric syndromes.[153] Memory disorders are more common among patients with severe stroke and are associated with poor recovery from stroke.[155,156] In many cases, findings of dementia are most pronounced among patients with aphasia.[149] The development of dementia forecasts a poor prognosis for recovery. It influences decisions about rehabilitation and therapies to prevent recurrent stroke.

Vascular dementia can be secondary to atherothrombotic or cardioembolic stroke, Binswanger's disease, hemodynamic events, amyloid angiopathy, hematologic disorders, or non-atherosclerotic vasculopathies.[157–164] The most widely accepted vascular cause of cognitive decline is multi-infarction dementia, which is most commonly associated with lacunar infarctions in the cerebral hemispheres.[152] Patients with lacunar infarctions have risk of dementia increased 4–12 times over persons with other types of stroke.[165] In most cases of multi-infarction dementia, multiple small or large subcortical infarctions are found.[153,166] Multiple strokes might not be the most important etiology of cognitive decline, but they likely contribute to dementia by causing a loss of neurons, disrupting protein synthesis, and altering synapses.[167]

The diagnosis of vascular dementia can be difficult, and misdiagnoses are common. Erkinjuntti and Hachinski[157] estimated that the accuracy of the diagnosis of vascular dementia is approximately 21%–45%. The primary alternative diagnosis is Alzheimer disease.[168] Patients with Alzheimer disease usually are elderly, and many have risk factors for stroke or have had ischemic events. Many patients likely have a combination of degenerative and vascular dementia. The Hachinski scale (see Table 1–5) is used to expedite the diagnosis of multi-infarction dementia.[169] Although the Hachinski scale is not infallible, it has a sensitivity of 89% and specificity of 90% in differentiating multi-infarction dementia from Alzheimer disease.[170,171] The most useful components of the Hachinski scale in predicting vascular dementia are 1) a stepwise deterioration of deficits, 2) a fluctuating course, 3) a history of hypertension, 4) a history of stroke, and 5) the presence of focal neurological impairments.[170] The scale is sensitive in differentiating multi-infarction dementia from a mixed vascular–Alzheimer dementia, but its specificity is fairly low.[170] In general, brain imaging studies that demonstrate multiple areas of subcortical infarctions support the diagnosis of vascular dementia.[163] A failure to demonstrate abnormalities other than cortical atrophy by either CT or MRI should make a physician doubt this diagnosis. The best management includes treating risk factors for atherosclerosis and using medications to prevent recurrent thromboembolism.

Hydrocephalus is an uncommon chronic complication of ischemic stroke; it is much more frequently diagnosed among patients who have had intracranial bleeding—in particular, subarachnoid hemorrhage. Still, cerebrovascular disease appears to contribute to the development of the syndrome of *normal-pressure hydrocephalus*.[172] Normal-pressure hydrocephalus should be considered if a patient develops signs of cognitive impairments, gait apraxia, and incontinence several months after a stroke.

Other Neurological Complications

MOVEMENT DISORDERS

Less common neurological complications of stroke include movement disorders, such as *hemiballism* or *hemichorea*.[173–175] These disorders are most commonly found among patients with infarctions involving the subthalamic nucleus. Ballistic movements can be violent and very tiring. A prolonged period of hemiballism can lead to exhaustion and death. Treatment usually involves the administration of haloperidol or a phenothiazine to suppress the movement. Other movement disorders are even less frequent. Unilateral *Parkinsonism* can follow large infarctions in the territory of the lenticulostriate arteries.[176] A *focal dystonia* can follow hemiplegia secondary to infarctions in the basal ganglia.[177] Kostic et al[178] found symptomatic dystonias in 16 patients. Dystonia was generalized in 3 patients, segmental in 4, one-sided in 4, and focal in 6. Infarctions in the caudate and lenticular nuclei were the cause of dystonia in 7 of these patients. Focal dystonias appear to be more common among children than adults.[179] *Shoulder girdle dyskinesia* has been associated with infarctions in the thalamus.[180] *Focal tremors* have followed an infarction in the striatum.[181] Head tremor can complicate infarctions in the paramedian region of the pontomesencephalic portion of the brain stem.[182] Grant et al[183] reported four patients with stuttering following infarction. The locations of the stroke differed among the patients.

PAIN

Abnormal pain from innocuous stimulation (*allodynia*) most commonly follows infarction in the ventral posterior lateral nucleus of the thalamus or the dorsolateral medulla.[184–186] Chest wall discomfort with burning, flashes, and cold sensation can follow infarction in the thalamus, corona radiata, or brain stem.[187] Abnormal pain, sometimes called *thalamic pain syndrome,* is most common with lesions in the right thalamus.[188] The area of pain usually corresponds to the region of decreased sensation to pain or temperature. Pontine or medullary infarctions can lead to painful *trigeminal neuralgia* or a "*central pain*" syndrome.[189,190] Treatment of allodynia or neuralgic pain after stroke usually involves the prescription of tricyclic antidepressants, carbamazepine, phenytoin, valproate, or other medications that can suppress irritable membranes.

Shoulder-hand syndrome also can occur after stroke.[191] Typical findings are pain, tenderness, and edema in the arm, wrist, and hand. In addition, the color and temperature of the skin can change. Braus et al[191] found that shoulder-hand syndrome developed in 36 of 132 patients (27%) with hemiplegia following stroke. Wanklyn et al[192] found that coldness of the hemiplegic arm could be associated with vasomotor changes and *reflex sympathetic dystrophy.*

AUTONOMIC DYSFUNCTION

Autonomic nervous system dysfunction can be found following stroke, and cardiac arrhythmias can result.[193] Loss of skin temperature can be the consequence of failure of the autonomic nervous system, which occurs in conjunction with pyramidal dysfunction.[194] *Hypohidrosis* and *decreased sweating response* can be seen in association with autonomic failure among patients with brain stem infarction.[195] Autonomic nervous system disturbances can be prominent during sleep.[196]

Gustatory disturbances can complicate ipsilateral infarctions of the pons or the midbrain.[197] Rousseaux et al[198] found that disorders of smell, taste, and food intake occur in some patients with thalamic infarctions.

HICCUPS

Hiccups occur most frequently with infarctions in the dorsolateral medulla. They can be intractable and extremely distressing to the patient and family. Hiccups also can lead to aspiration pneumonia, respiratory problems, and nutritional problems.[199] They even can be fatal. Treatment options include chlorpromazine, haloperidol, baclofen, and anticonvulsants. Medications used to treat hiccups can cause sedation, which interferes with other activities.[199]

SLEEP DISORDERS

Sleep disorders frequently develop following stroke. Disturbances in the stages of sleep are also common. *Obstructive sleep apnea* and hypopnea are more likely to occur among patients with habitual snoring.[200–202] *Hypersomnia* can complicate infarctions in the paramedian thalamic nuclei.[203] Affected patients can sleep up to 20 hours per day. The defect in arousal appears to involve non–rapid eye movement sleep. Bassetti and Aldrich[204] correlated sleep apnea after stroke with advanced age, obesity, diabetes, and severe neurological impairment. They also reported that sleep apnea can affect both acute treatment and rehabilitation after stroke.

MEDICAL COMPLICATIONS OF ISCHEMIC STROKE

Prevention and treatment of medical complications are critical components of care to prevent death and disability after stroke. Medical complications account for approximately 30% of deaths after stroke, and these deaths usually occur more than 5–7 days after the cerebrovascular event.[205–207] The leading non-neurological causes of death are pneumonia, pulmonary embolism, myocardial infarction, and sepsis. The latter usually arises from a urinary tract infection or an infected pressure sore.[205] Because these complications are leading causes of morbidity or mortality after stroke, their management must be considered as a critical component of

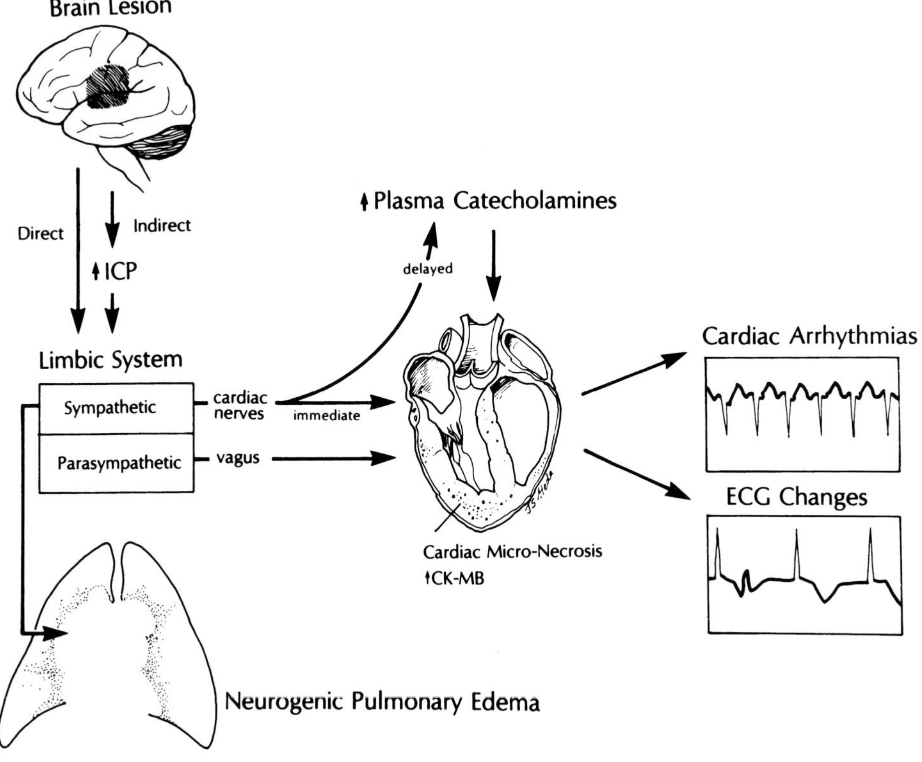

Figure 13–8. Suggested mechanisms of cardiac effects of acute cerebral lesions. (Reprinted from Norris JW. The effects of cerebrovascular lesions upon the heart. *Neurol Clin* 1983;1:87, with permission.)

management.[1] Neither the patient nor society is served well if aggressive therapies to treat stroke, including the administration of thrombolytic therapy, are negated because the patient develops a medical complication that could have been prevented or easily treated. Fortunately, therapies of proven value are available to prevent or treat medical complications of stroke.

Cardiovascular Complications

Ischemic heart disease is present in a sizeable proportion of patients. Coronary artery disease can co-develop or be the underlying cause for cardioembolic stroke. Many patients with stroke have other evidence of atherosclerosis in multiple vascular territories, including coronary artery disease. The cardiovascular complications that occur within the first 24 hours of stroke are described in Chapters 6 and 12. Among the cardiac changes are electrocardiographic findings, abnormal cardiac enzymes, and ventricular arrhythmias that point to *myocardial ischemia*.[34,193,207–219] (See Figs. 13–8 and 13–9.) Cardiac events account for a sizeable proportion of deaths after stroke and include events that are recorded as *sudden deaths*.[212] Noda et al[220] and Tokgozoglu et al[221] found that cardiac arousal is impaired and that these changes can worsen sleep apnea syndrome following brain infarction seen in some elderly patients. Clinical monitoring of the patient's cardiac status should be a part of management. Unless specific contraindications exist, cardiac medications should be restarted as soon as possible. Cardiological consultation may be necessary if adjustments in medications are needed. Attention to a patient's heart disease should be part of a rehabilitation program because cardiac disorders can affect specific interventions, especially physical therapy.

Congestive heart failure is a potential complication.[207,222,223] A sizeable proportion of

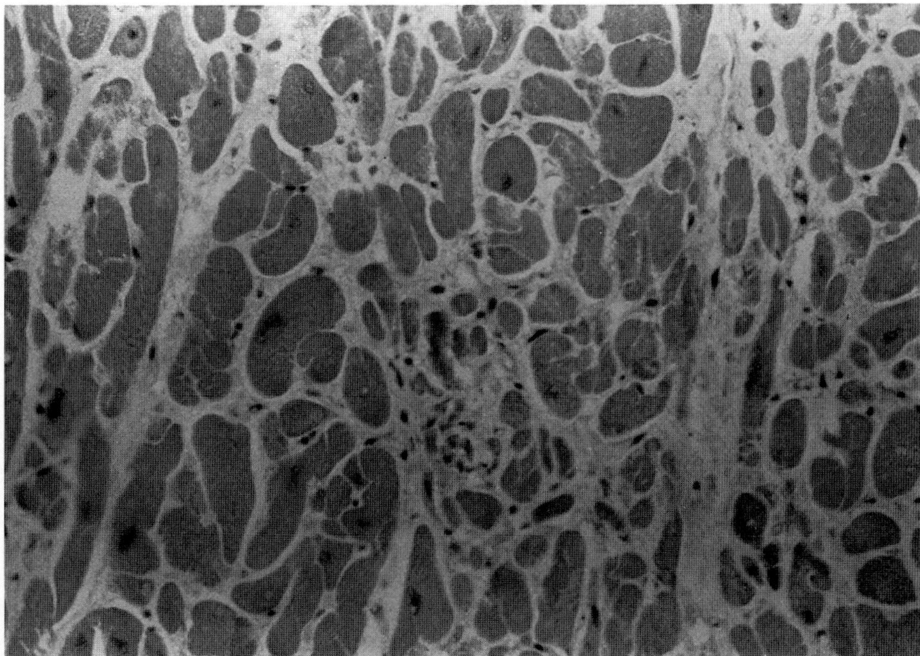

Figure 13–9. Hematoxylin and eosin-stained section of myocardium from a patient who died of a brain stem infarction. Focal areas of myocardial neurosis.

patients with stroke will have underlying heart diseases, such as a dilated cardiomyopathy, which can predispose to congestive heart failure. In addition, neurogenic factors may affect cardiac function including myocardial contractility and rhythm. Management to avoid both dehydration and excessive volumes of fluids are critical among patients with heart disease. The consequences of congestive heart failure after stroke are ominous. Pulmonary edema can lead to hypoxia or hypercarbia that worsens neurological function and brain edema (Table 13–11). Wijdicks and Scott[139] found that *pulmonary edema* or severe congestive heart failure was the cause of respiratory failure in 10 of 24 patients who needed mechanical ventilation after stroke (Fig. 13–10).

Table 13–11. **Causes of Hypoxia or Respiratory Failure After Acute Ischemic Stroke**

Airway compromise
Atelectasis
Pneumonia
Pulmonary embolism
Pulmonary edema—congestive heart failure

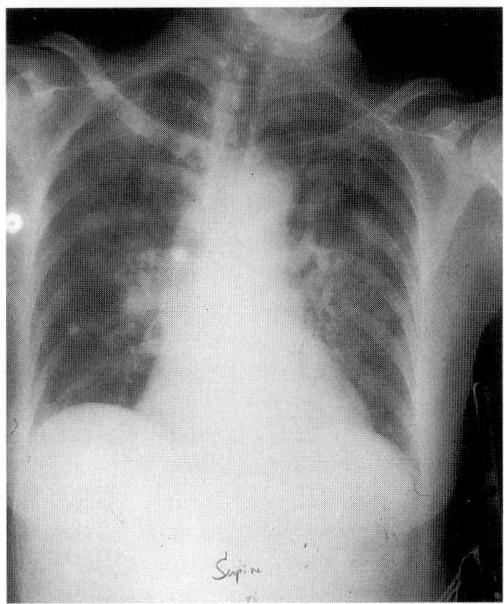

Figure 13–10. This chest x-ray shows severe neurogenic pulmonary edema in a patient with an acute stroke.

Deep Vein Thrombosis and Pulmonary Embolism

PATIENTS AT RISK

Deep vein thrombosis is relatively common among persons with ischemic stroke, and it is costly in terms of additional health care expenses and patient morbidity.[224,225] Deep vein thrombosis is most common among bed-bound patients with severe stroke and a paralyzed lower limb.[34,226] Oppenheimer and Hachinski[212] reported that approximately 53% of bed-bound patients with stroke develop deep vein thrombosis. In many cases, proximal deep vein thrombosis may be occult. In one series of 105 patients with recent stroke undergoing plethysmography following admission to a rehabilitation hospital, thrombi were found in 34 cases.[226] Only 2 patients had symptoms that would have prompted a clinical evaluation. In addtion to prolonged immobility, pertubation of coagulation and fibrinolytic pathways occur with acute stroke.[227,228] These hematologic changes may combine with neurological impairments to lead to a high risk for venous thrombosis.

Deep vein thrombosis causes swelling and pain in the affected limb. These symptoms can hamper rehabilitation and limit activity. In addition, deep vein thrombosis is the underlying factor that promotes pulmonary embolism, a potentially fatal complication of stroke. It accounts for approximately 5% of deaths.[212] Thus, a goal of prevention or treatment of deep vein thrombosis is to prevent life-endangering *pulmonary embolism,* which can occur within a few days after stroke to up to several months later. In one series of 30 patients with pulmonary embolism, the median interval from stroke until diagnosis was 20 days.[229] One-half of these patients presented with sudden death, whereas the remaining patients had chest pain and dyspnea (see Table 13–11). In this series, 11 of the patients had deep vein thrombosis found in the paralyzed lower limb. The primary alternative diagnoses to pulmonary embolism are congestive heart failure/pulmonary edema or pneumonia. A combination of a chest x-ray and nuclide perfusion scan of the lungs usually is done. A mismatch between the two tests suggests an area of hypoperfusion and points to pulmonary embolism. A pulmonary arteriogram can be done to confirm the presence of a thrombus.

PREVENTION AND TREATMENT

Mobilization of patients within the first 24 hours after stroke is an effective way to prevent deep vein thrombosis.[230] (See Table 13–12.) Patients with mild impairments should be allowed out of bed almost immediately. Most patients with moderate deficits also can be mobilized within 24 hours. Initial steps in mobilization involve transfer to a chair, standing, and walking short distances. Measures to avoid falls are crucial. The degree of assistance (use of devices or help of nursing personnel) will depend on the patient's impairments and the presence of co-morbid diseases. Blood pressure should be checked during the first stages of mobilization. A sudden drop in blood pressure could aggravate neurological symptoms. Patients who have severe neurological signs or are unstable neurologically may need prolonged bed rest, and these patients will need additional measures to prevent deep vein thrombosis. Anti-embolism stockings, pneumatic

Table 13–12. **Prevention or Treatment of Deep Vein Thrombosis and Pulmonary Embolism**

Acute prevention
Mobilization
Heparin
Low molecular weight heparins
Danaparoid
Aspirin
Pneumatic calf compression devices
Long-term prevention
Oral anticoagulants
Treatment of pulmonary embolism
Heparin
Thrombolytic agents
Filter in inferior vena cava
Plication of inferior vena cava

Table 13–13. **Prevention of Deep Vein Thrombosis Following Acute Ischemic Stroke**

Author	Heparin Events/Patients N	Low Molecular Weight Heparin/Danaparoid Events/Patients N	Control
McCarthy and Turner[236]	32/144	—	117/161
Turpie et al[238]	—	2/50	7/25
Sandset et al[237]	—	17/52	15/51
Turpie et al[240]	13/43	4/44	—

compression devices, and subcutaneous administration of heparin are effective and widely used ways to prevent deep vein thrombosis.[231]

Antithrombotic agents are *the mainstays in preventing and treating venous* thromboembolic disease.[146,232–238] (See Table 13–13.) A meta-analysis concluded that unfractionated heparin and low molecular weight (LMW) compounds are effective and that either can be recommended.[239] Subcutaneous administration of LMW heparins and danaparoid appears to be safer and more effective than conventional heparin in preventing deep vein thrombosis in a number of situations, including stroke.[240–246] Levine et al[247] compared the safety and efficacy of heparin and LMW heparin in the prevention of proximal deep vein thrombosis in high-risk patients. No differences in the frequency of thromboembolic events or hemorrhages were noted despite the fact that patients received LMW heparin at home, whereas the patients given heparin had to remain in the hospital for treatment. The ability to be treated at home is a major potential advantage for the long-term use of LMW heparin. This feature might not be critical during acute care, but it could be important for discharge planning. Additional advantages of the LMW heparins include better and more predictable responses to subcutaneous injections, a longer half-life, and a lessened need for laboratory monitoring.[248] Gould et al[249] found that LMW heparins were more effective than unfractionated heparin in preventing mortality from venous thromboembolism. Koopman and Buller[250] concluded that LMW heparins might be the best treatment to prevent deep vein thrombosis and pulmonary embolism in immobilized, high-risk patients. Presumably this recommendation would extend to treatment of patients with recent stroke. Gould et al[251] found that costs of treatment with either conventional heparin or LMW heparins were equal. The higher costs of the LMW compounds were offset by the lower expenses generated by complications that are more frequent with traditional unfractionated heparin. Aspirin also has been used to prevent deep vein thrombosis.[357]

External pneumatic calf compression devices can reduce the frequency of deep vein thrombosis among bed-bound patients who cannot be treated with anticoagulants.[252] Compression devices usually are combined with *antiembolic stockings* to help keep compression on the veins in the lower limbs. Kamran et al[253] found deep vein thrombosis among 22 of 83 non-ambulatory patients who received heparin. Six patients had pulmonary emboli. Another 148 nonambulatory patients received the combination of heparin and pneumatic sequential compression devices. One patient had a deep vein thrombosis, and no pulmonary emboli were diagnosed. Oral anticoagulants can be prescribed as a long-term prophylaxis against deep vein thrombosis. This therapy is given to patients with a high degree of likelihood for prolonged immobility.

Intravenous administration of heparin in a continuous infusion is the usual treatment for patients who have a deep vein thrombosis. The infusion usually is continued for 5–10 days and then is followed by a course of oral anticoagulants for several months.[232] Patients who cannot be treated with anticoagulants likely will need either a filter placed in the inferior vena cava or to have the vessel plicated. A prolonged course of anticoagulation is prescribed to most patients with pulmonary embolism.[232] Thrombolytic agents also have been administered. These agents might need to be prescribed to prevent death even at the risk of intracranial bleeding complications.

Respiratory Failure and Pneumonia

Respiratory failure is a potential cause for death after ischemic stroke. It may be secondary to direct injury to the respiratory centers in the brain stem or to a decline in consciousness.[254] Respiratory failure also can be secondary to aspiration, pneumonia, congestive heart failure, or pulmonary embolism (see Table 13–11). Regardless of the underlying cause, the prognosis of patients who need mechanical ventilation after stroke is extraordinarily poor. El-Ad et al[255] report that in-hospital mortality is more than 90% among this group of patients. Bushnell et al[256] found that the 30-day survival rate was approximately 50% among patients who needed intubation. Grotta et al[82] reported on the outcomes of 20 patients who needed elective intubation 3 hours to 7 days after an ischemic stroke; 14 died and only 1 had a favorable outcome.

Pneumonia is a leading cause of death following ischemic stroke; it is estimated to be the cause of death in approximately 35% of fatal cases.[206,212] In one series of 607 patients, pneumonia was a complication of stroke in approximately 12% of patients.[257] Risk is particularly high among elderly patients with infarctions in the basal ganglia.[258] Pneumonia can be an early complication secondary to either aspiration or atelectasis. Its importance as a cause of death or disability increases during the first weeks after stroke. Most cases of fatal pneumonia occur after 1 week following stroke. Pneumonia presumably secondary to silent aspiration during sleep can lead to death among elderly patients with stroke.[258]

Table 13–14. **Leading Causes of New Onset Fever Following Acute Ischemic Stroke**

Pneumonia
Urinary tract infection
Thrombophlebitis
Sepsis
Drug-induced fever
Central fever
Seizures

Prevention is crucial. Protection of the airway helps prevent early aspiration among acutely ill patients who have bulbar dysfunction or vomiting. Subsequently, the careful management of swallowing, nutrition, and hydration becomes a form of prophylaxis. Encouragement to take deep breaths or respiratory therapy can help prevent atelectasis. Early mobilization helps lower the risk of pneumonia.[146,230] Physical therapy also helps lessen the likelihood of pneumonia.

The appearance of hypoxia, a productive cough, fever, pleuritic chest pain, or respiratory distress should prompt evaluation for pneumonia (Table 13–14). The alternative diagnoses are pulmonary edema or pulmonary embolism. A chest X-ray usually is diagnostic, and it and sputum cultures should be obtained. Supplemental oxygen can be prescribed to patients who have hypoxia secondary to pneumonia or other pulmonary complications afterstroke.[230] Antibiotics are critical to manage pneumonia after stroke.[230]

Incontinence, Indwelling Bladder Catheters, and Urinary Tract Infections

Disturbances in bladder control are very frequent following stroke. Most patients recover bladder control relatively quickly. Still, *urinary incontinence* usually is a problem among bed-bound patients with severe strokes.[259] Incontinence can be the result of either a hypertonic bladder or a hypotonic bladder with overflow. In addition, motor, cognitive, or communicative impairments may mean that the patient is unable to reach a toilet or is unaware of the need to void.[260] In general, placement of a chronic indwelling bladder catheter should be avoided; however, nursing or medical needs may mandate the use of a catheter. For example, strict measurements of urinary output may be needed to treat a patient with severe heart failure or increased intracranial pressure. A catheter also can help prevent skin breakdown among bed-bound patients. Unfortunately, it serves as a provocation for the development of urinary tract infections.

Although urinary tract infections occur among patients with stroke who do not have catheters, especially among women, early removal of an indwelling bladder catheter is the most effective tactic to lessen the likelihood of serious infectious complication. Intermittent catheterization scheduled at regular intervals among patients with a neurogenic bladder may be an alternative way to avoid infections and urinary retention. A condom catheter can be used to treat incontinent male patients, but condom catheters do not appear to be safer than indwelling bladder catheters. In addition, condom catheters can cause uncomfortable penile skin irritation. As a result, patients regularly remove the catheters, and the issue of incontinence to subsequent voiding is not avoided. If a patient needs an indwelling catheter, then ancillary care must be careful and aimed at avoiding infectious complications.

In one recent report, *urinary tract infections* developed in 16% of patients with recent ischemic stroke.[5,207,223,257,261,358] A urinary tract infection is uncomfortable because of bladder irritation. It also leads to fever that might cause neurological worsening (see Table 13–14). Urinary tract infections or pneumonia can lead to sepsis that accounts for death in approximately 5% of patients.[212] The presence of a fever should prompt screening of the urine to check for the presence of infection. Antibiotics can be given in response to the results of the urine culture. Prophylactic administration of antibiotics should be avoided. Acidification of the urine can be achieved by adding 500 mg of vitamin C to the diet or fluids.

Gastrointestinal Complications

FECAL INCONTINENCE

Fecal incontinence and bowel care also are important issues in management.[222] They generally are not as acute as urinary incontinence. Still, a bed-bound patient might not be able to maintain anal sphincter control. The presence of fecal incontinence is distressing to the patient, family, and the nurses. It also is irritating to the skin and is a major potential source for infection. Medical therapies, such as antibiotics given orally, may cause *diarrhea.* Because many of the feedings given via nasogastric tube are relatively hyperosmolar, diarrhea also can complicate this form of nutrition. Measures to slow bowel motility or treat *diarrhea* usually are avoided because of the high risk for constipation. Still, prescription of antidiarrhea medications may be needed if the condition is severe. Rarely, a rectal tube may be needed.

CONSTIPATION

Constipation also is a potential complication of stroke because patients often are immobile or dehydrated. Medications, such as opiates, also may slow bowel function. Severe constipation can lead to patient distress, pain, or fecal impaction. Thus, measures to prevent constipation are part of the ancillary treatment of patients with stroke. Stool softeners or laxatives are ordered depending on the needs of the individual patient. Increasing fluids, food, and mobilization also are effective tactics to prevent or treat constipation after stroke.

GASTROINTESTINAL BLEEDING

In a series of 607 patients with acute stroke, *upper gastrointestinal hemorrhage* was a complication in 18 patients.[262] In 9 cases, bleeding was severe. In general, the risk of gastrointestinal bleeding is greatest among elderly patients and those with severe strokes.[262] Several sources of bleeding have been identified. *Stress ulcers* can lead to gastrointestinal bleeding after stroke.[222] Both acute and chronic *peptic ulcers* can occur.[263] Recurrent vomiting secondary to a brain stem infarction may lead to a tear in the esophagus or the stomach. Gastrointestinal bleeding also can be due to stress-induced *erosive gastritis* or ulcers and may be secondary to medications.[207,262–264] Aspirin and non-steroidal anti-inflammatory agents can lead to irritation of the stomach or the small intestine. Antiplatelet aggregating agents or anticoagulants also can lead to worsening of bleeding from an otherwise relatively occult upper gastrointestinal source. Severe blood loss can cause anemia or hypotension that in turn has the potential to worsen the neurological effects of the stroke. In general, gastrointestinal bleeding usually can be treated, and it rarely will lead to death.[264] Measures for treatment include antacids, histamine blocking agents, and sucralfate. Histamine blocking agents should be prescribed with caution to patients with decreased consciousness because these agents can have central nervous system depressant effects. Occasionally, severe blood loss could prompt the need for a transfusion or surgical intervention to treat the source of the gastrointestinal hemorrhage.

Electrolyte Disturbances, Nutrition, and Hydration

Even in the absence of stroke, elderly patients have anemia and low concentrations of serum albumin. The presence of a neurological event aggravates these conditions.[265] The acute and subacute effects of stroke have a major effect on nutrition. Patients with decreased consciousness or bulbar dysfunction cannot swallow. Many patients are intentionally not given food or water during the first 24 hours after stroke because of the uncertain stability of their neurological condition. In addition, delays in starting nutrition may result in the interim period before the swallowing study can be performed. Under-nutrition is common after stroke.[266,267] Declines in nutrition appear to be related to inactivity and dependence on feeding.[265] The loss in fat and proteins leads to a further decreased energy level and a loss of body mass. Axelsson et al[267] reported that nutritional status was abnormal in 16% of patients on admission for stroke. This percentage increased to 22% by the time of discharge. Elderly patients, women, and persons with atrial fibrillation were the most likely to have malnutrition. Patients with malnutrition are less likely to return home, have a higher risk for poor outcomes, and have an increased risk of infection.[267,268]

DEHYDRATION

Many patients are dehydrated when they are first examined. Disturbances in consciousness, swallowing, or mobility often preclude the patient from drinking during the first hours after stroke. Insensible water loss from fever or a warm environment can potentiate the dehydration. The use of medications, such as diuretics to treat hypertension, also can lead to dehydration. In addition, patients with severe stroke often have fluid restriction prescribed in an attempt to lessen brain edema. Dehydration can alter blood viscosity and affect the propensity for deep vein thrombosis or renal failure. Thus, measures to ensure adequate nutrition and hydration should be a fundamental component of managing patients with stroke.[2] They should be initiated as soon as possible. Intravenous administration of fluids, most commonly normal saline, is important to avoid dehydration following stroke.[230] Patients generally receive a minimum of 1.8–2.4 L of normal saline daily. The volume of fluid can be reduced as the patient receives liquids from drinking or tube feedings. If congestive heart failure is likely to occur secondary to the use of normal saline, then it can be substituted with 5% dextrose in 0.45 saline. Potassium supplementation also be added to address electrolyte disturbances.

HYPONATREMIA

Hyponatremia can be secondary to the *syndrome of inappropriate release of antidiuretic hormone* (*SIADH*) or *cerebral salt wasting*. The former is secondary to a relative loss of sodium against water, whereas the latter is associated with loss of both salt and water. Approximately 10% of stroke patients will have SIADH.[212] Cerebral salt wasting is an important complication of subarachnoid hemorrhage.[269] It is due to renal loss of sodium and extracellular fluid volume.[270] Findings of cerebral salt wasting differ from those seen with SIADH. Patients have weight loss, reduced pulmonary wedge pressures, decreased central venous pressure, increased hematocrit, and increased blood urea nitrogen/creatinine ratio. The treatment for cerebral salt wasting is the opposite for SIADH. Rather than restricting fluid administration, which is the usual treatment for SIADH, patients should receive intravenous fluids, including normal saline.

SWALLOWING AND DYSPHAGIA

The neuroanatomy of swallowing is complex; it involves both supranuclear and brain stem regulation of the muscles of the tongue, mouth, throat, and esophagus.[271,272] Both pharyngeal dysfunction and constrictor paresis appear to be critical in causing oral disturbances in swallowing after stroke.[273] In addition to bulbar dysfunction, lingual incoordination can lead to swallowing difficulties. Lingual incoordination is most common among patients with strokes in the subcortical, periventricular white matter of the cerebral hemispheres.[274] Many patients will not be able to swallow effectively during the first days after stroke. Oppenheimer and Hachinski[212] estimated that approximately 50% of patients have some component of dysphagia after stroke. Aphagia (the inability to initiate swallowing) can occur with medullary infarctions.[275] Fortunately, this problem is very rare. Sudden death secondary to airway obstruction can occur in dysphagic patients.[276] In addition, patients with dysphagia have a relatively high risk for aspiration and pneumonia.[277] Difficulty in eating and drinking also leads to malnutrition and dehydration.

The risk of *dysphagia* is not uniform among patients with stroke. The presence of clinically important dysphagia is very low among persons with minor hemispheric strokes. However, patients with infarctions of the brain stem causing cranial nerve palsies and secondary pharyngeal paralysis and those with large hemisphere infarctions with secondary bulbar dysfunction have a very high risk for dysphagia. It is most commonly found among patients with focal facial weakness, a weak cough, or dysarthria.[278] Horner et al[279] found aspiration and dysphagia in 15 of 23 patients with pontine or medullary strokes. Dysphagia occurs in approximately 30% of patients with unilateral hemispheric strokes, and it is most commonly associated with signs of facial weakness or aphasia.[278,280] Aspiration and difficulty swallowing occur in approximately 87% of patients with bilateral hemispheric strokes.[281]

Early assessment of swallowing is critical.[260,277,282] Examination by a speech pathologist within the first 24 hours is useful in identifying swallowing disturbance and documenting levels of hydration and nutrition.[283] Clinical and videofluoroscopy can be used to assess oral transit time, delay or absence in the swallowing reflex, and penetrance.[284,285] Examination of the cough reflex provides an estimate of the risk of aspiration or pneumonia.[286] An intact reflex means that the airway likely is protected. An abnormal response may identify the patient as having a high risk of aspiration secondary to an unprotected airway.[287] This risk is increased by a factor of 8.36 if the patient aspirates more than 10% of a bolus during videofluoroscopy.[288] The 3-oz. water-swallowing test also can be used to identify aspiration. Among patients with severe dysphagia, it has a sensitivity of 94% and specificity of 26%.[289] The bedside swallow can be used to rate dysphagia to food of thicker consistencies. The risk of pneumonia is increased by a factor of 5.57 among those who have silent aspiration compared with those who cough with swallowing.[288]

Pulse oximetry can be used to detect aspiration in most dysphagic patients.[290] A fall in oxygen saturation also is common following swallowing among patients with dysphagia.[291] This finding is a potential marker of severe but otherwise silent aspiration. Pulse oximetry should be used with caution in elderly patients, those who smoke, and those with chronic obstructive lung disease.[290]

In general, the return of swallowing is associated with recovery or improvement of the pharyngeal reflexes.[292] Oral motor exercises are used to expedite a recovery in swallowing. Swallowing techniques, positioning of the head, and diet modification are used as the patient begins to eat.[293] Changing the texture of the foods (using puréed or semisolid food or thickening liquids) is a potentially effective tactic. Decreasing the amount of food consumed with each swallow or administering food by syringe are other ways to re-start eating.[260]

A *nasogastric tube* should be placed if a patient cannot eat. The goal is to start feeding as soon as the patient is stable.[294] Nasogastric tubes are relatively non-invasive and are associated with relatively few complications.[295] Still, lower esophageal sphincter or peristaltic dysfunction may leave the patient at risk for aspiration of tube feedings.[296] Lucas et al[297] reported that vomiting with aspiration secondary to esophageal sphincter disturbances is common after acute stroke. *Percutaneous endoscopic gastrostomy* (*PEG*) is an important alternative for persons with severe stroke.[298] Those who need a PEG generally have a high mortality.[299] If a patient likely will need a prolonged course of tube feeding, then a PEG should be placed as soon as possible. In general, a PEG should be inserted if the patient's dysphagia is likely to persist for longer than 14 days.[295] The likelihood of aspiration pneumonia is less with a PEG than with a nasogastric tube. Placement of a PEG does require trained personnel and has a risk of complications, including peritonitis, skin breakdown, or pneumonia.[294,295] It is, however, better tolerated than a nasogastric tube by many patients and the risk of operative complications with placement of a PEG is relatively low.[299,300] In addition, many long-term care facilities prefer a PEG to a nasogastric tube. Thus, placement may be a needed to allow for transfer to a nursing facility. The PEG can be removed when the patient is able to eat.[294]

Dermatologic and Orthopedic Complications

DECUBITUS ULCERS (PRESSURE SORES)

Skin breakdown occurs in approximately 18% of patients with stroke.[257] Changes in skin integrity can appear rapidly. Bedridden patients can develop pressure sores within the first days after stroke.[5,222,261] Elderly patients with severe neurological deficits and severe concomitant disease are at higher risk. Pressure sores are most common among patients who have diarrhea, fecal incontinence, light body weight, low serum albumin concentrations, urinary catheters, or dementia.[301]

Steps to maintain the integrity of the skin are outlined in practice guidelines.[260] The skin, especially at the sites of bony prominences, should be evaluated daily to look for areas of potential breakdown. It should be cleaned regularly and gently and should be protected from moisture (eg, urine, perspiration). A bedridden patient should be positioned properly and turned regularly. Barrier sprays, lubricants, special mattresses, dressings, and padding may help. Special beds, including those that rotate or change pressure against dependent areas of the body, can be prescribed. Still, the most effective measure to prevent pressure sores is to mobilize the patient.

FALLS

Falls are relatively common as patients with moderate-to-severe deficits begin mobilization.[261] Falls are the most common cause of injury after stroke, and a fractured hip is the potential result.[260] Tutuarima et al[302] estimated that the incidence of falls after stroke is approximately 8.9 per 1000 patient-days. Nyberg et al[303] reported that 62 of 162 patients with stroke had 153 falls after being admitted to a rehabilitation unit. Falls occur during ambulation, transfer, sitting in a wheelchair, or sitting in a chair.[303] In a series of 607 patients with stroke, falls were recorded in 22% of cases.[257] They are more common among men and persons who have cognitive impairments, visual or sensory loss, or incontinence.[302,304–306] Impulsive behavior seems to lead to falls among patients with strokes in the right hemisphere.[307] Patients with impaired postural stability, bilateral motor impairments, bilateral cortical or white matter lesions, neglect, and poor activities of daily living also have a high risk for falls.[305] The use of diuretic, anticonvulsant, or antidepressant medications is correlated with an increased fall risk.[305] A fall can induce bleeding among patients who are receiving anticoagulants. Fortunately, the frequency of serious bleeding seems to be relatively low.[308]

Risk factors and potential hazards in the hospital environment should be assessed before a patient is allowed to stand or ambulate.[260] Among the issues are lighting, the surface of the floors, and location and access to the toilet and bathing facilities. High-risk patients should be supervised and assisted in ambulation or transfer. As the patient's balance and mobility improve with rehabilitation, the supervision and assistance by nursing staff can be reduced. Other strategies include nurse-call systems and bed monitors. Taking the patient to the toilet at regular intervals might deter an unexpected walk by the patient. Encouraging family members to seek the assistance of the nursing staff in mobilizing the patient, rather than having them do the activity without supervision, also can help. Physical restraints should be avoided whenever possible.[306]

SHOULDER PAIN AND ADHESIVE CAPSULITIS OF THE SHOULDER

Shoulder pain is relatively common after stroke.[309] The shoulder is relatively vulnerable to changes in muscle strength and tone following stroke. Dislocation or *subluxation of the shoulder* also is a potential complication.[264,310] The presence of subluxation may not be directly related to the presence of shoulder pain.[311] Movement of the patient in bed, such as pulling on the shoulder, can aggravate the development of shoulder subluxation. This relatively common measure to reposition a patient must be avoided. Having the patient lie on a pad or a blanket that can be lifted or pulled to reposition the patient reduces the temptation to pull the patient by the shoulder. Electrical stimulation to maintain tone of the muscles of the shoulder may help in preventing subluxation.[312] Chronic immobility leads to changes in the joint (*adhesive capsulitis*), causing chronic pain and a loss of the range of motion of the shoulder. Passive external rotation of the shoulder should be part of an evaluation of patients with hemiplegia.[313] Passive range-of-motion exercises are started soon after stroke to avoid changes in the shoulder joint. Attention to shoulder mobility and pain is critical in physical therapy aimed at the upper limbs. The goal is to avoid loss of limb function secondary to orthopedic complications. In addition to physical therapy, anti-inflammatory agents, local injections of corticosteroids, or surgical treatments may be prescribed to patients with painful shoulders after stroke.

CONTRACTURES

Contractures of the muscles on the paretic side begin to develop relatively early after stroke.[222] They can limit movement of the involved joint and are painful. As a result, their presence impairs the patient's ability to recover and tolerate rehabilitation. The correction of contractures involves splinting and casting the involved joints with the goal of positioning them to the most anatomically correct position.

OSTEOPOROSIS

Osteoporosis is a delayed complication of stroke that leads to pathologic fractures, including fractured hips. Hemiplegic patients have a high risk for osteoporosis that develops in the bones of paralyzed limbs.[314,315] Progressive loss of bone mineral density and bone re-absorption are seen in the paralyzed limb during the first year after stroke.[316,317] Osteoporosis combined with the propensity for falls means that patients with stroke have a very high risk for fractures. In addition to the effects of disuse, the development of osteoporosis may be accelerated by the administration of vitamin K antagonist oral anticoagulants.[318,319] Supplementing the diet with vitamin D and calcium can lessen the risk of pathologic fractures.[320] Sato et al[321,322] also found that ipriflavone or exogenous Calcitrol can help maintain bone mass.

Following stroke, the unaffected arm can develop *carpal tunnel syndrome* because of overuse.[323]

Depression and Other Psychiatric Disorders

DEPRESSION

Major depression is relatively common among survivors of stroke.[212,324–328] Depression is both an acute and a long-term consequence of stroke. It occurs in approximately one-fourth of patients during the acute stage.[329] Approximately 20%–40% of patients will have symptoms as long as 3 years after the event.[329–331] Kauhanen et al[331] recently estimated that approximately 10% of patients have major depression.

Depression can be a reaction to the tremendous change in an individual's life or a direct neurological complication of the stroke itself. It can be associated with otherwise-silent cerebral infarction in older persons.[332] The severity of depression and the duration of hospitalization required for treatment were prolonged among patients with extensive imaging evidence of silent infarctions of the brain.[332] Depression also is more common among women, highly educated patients, young persons, and those with large infarctions of the left hemisphere.[325,328,329,333–335] Depression also is more likely in patients who live alone or who have few social contacts.[329] Major depression can lead to both decreased physical and cognitive functioning.[324] Depression also can lead to declines in memory, attention, and problem-solving skills.[331] Patients with psychiatric symptoms, including depression, have a longer length of stay in the hospital, and their rehabilitation is more difficult.[336,337] Depression also is associated with increased mortality or dependence after stroke.[326,338] Treatment with either tricyclic antidepressants or selective serotonin reuptake inhibitors can improve outcome.[337,339,340]

HYPOMANIA AND ANXIETY

Hypomania can complicate infarctions in the non-dominant cerebral hemisphere or the thalamus.[333,341,342] Other acute affective disorders include apathy and catastrophic reactions.[333] A generalized anxiety disorder can occur during the first days after stroke in up to one-fourth of patients.[327,343] In many cases, a chronic anxious state can be a sustained complication of stroke. It can be associated with depression among patients with strokes of the left cerebral hemisphere, but anxiety usually occurs in isolation among patients with right hemisphere lesions.[343] At times, the emotional distress of the stroke may be confused with either depression or anxiety.[344] Counseling and anti-anxiety medications may be needed. In general, minor tranquilizers are avoided because they can depress alertness or cognition. These medications also may influence recovery after stroke (see Chapter 14).

DISORDERS OF ANGER AND EMOTIONALITY

Disorders of anger control are potential complications of stroke.[345] Disinhibition and exaggerated responses to stimuli can occur with frontal lobe or paramedian thalamic infarctions.[346] Pathologic emotionality is an important complication of stroke that can influence recovery.[333] The pseudobulbar syndrome often includes marked swings in behavior that mimic depression or elation. Pathologic crying is most severe with bilateral lesions in the posterior portions of the cerebral hemispheres.[347] In addition, pathologic laughing and crying can complicate hemispheric or subcortical infarctions, including those in the territory of the anterior choroidal artery.[333,348,349] Brown et al[350] reported that fluoxetine is effective in treating emotionalism after stroke. Mukand et al[348] reported that sertraline helped relieve severe bouts of crying and laughter. Derex et al[349] concluded that the serotonin reuptake inhibitor paroxetine can reverse a severe emotional state. Andersen et al[351] recommended citalopram, another serotonergic neurotransmitter, to treat pathologic crying.

COMPONENTS OF TREATMENT IN THE HOSPITAL

Management of patients in an acute care setting is multifaceted, and several activities happen simultaneously. Coordination and close communication are critical for effective care. Scheduling diagnostic tests and consultations must be interdigitated with ongoing medical and nursing care. The priorities in care vary among patients. Evaluation for the presumed cause and initiation of therapies to prevent recurrent stroke are likely to be the primary issues in early treatment of patients with minor strokes. Initiation of rehabilitation may be paramount for treatment of a patient with moderate neurological impairments but who is stable medically. In contrast, nursing and medical treatment to control or prevent complications often is a chief problem in managing a bed-bound patient with a multilobar infarction.

Prevention and Treatment of Complications of Stroke

The complications of stroke have been described in this chapter. Neurological complications likely will peak during the first days after admission. Medical complications appear during the 7–10 days following the event. Measures such as antipyretic medications, antibiotics, treatment of diabetes, and mobilization are critical components of care.[230] Nurses working on general medical wards may miss declines in consciousness.[352] In addition, issues should as decreased proprioception, incontinence, or neglect must be addressed during hospitalization.[352]

Evaluation for the Cause of Stroke

As described in Chapter 4, determining the most likely cause of stroke is done on a case-by-case basis. Many potential diagnostic tests are listed in Table 4–2. Most patients do not need a large number of these tests. In some cases, the cause is obvious clinically, and no ancillary diagnostic test is needed. The primary reason for doing these tests is to have the necessary information to make a decision about long-term treatment to prevent recurrent stroke. If a patient's condition precludes specific medical or surgical therapies to prevent recurrent stroke, then evaluation might become irrelevant. For example, if a patient cannot be treated with either anticoagulants or carotid endarterectomy because of profound impairments or other diseases, then the urgency for early echocardiography or carotid imaging studies becomes low. These tests could be ordered at a subsequent time if the patient improves and these therapies become viable options for treatment.

Initiation of Treatment to Prevent Recurrent Stroke

Several medications (see Table 10–4) are of proven value in preventing recurrent stroke. Virtually all patients should receive medical therapy to prevent recurrent ischemic events initiated before discharge. Failure to prescribe medication to prevent recurrent stroke should be considered as a deviation from standard care unless the physician documents a strong contraindication for treatment. The presumed cause of stroke affects the choice of medical treatment. In general, patients with cardioembolism and most pro-thrombotic states are prescribed oral anticoagulants. Patients with stroke secondary to atherosclerosis and other arterial diseases usually are treated with antiplatelet aggregating agents. Some patients may need a combination of medications.

The timing of initiation of treatment while the patient is hospitalized is not clear. In general, therapies are started as soon as possible after the patient's condition has become stable. Current guidelines for the use of intravenous thrombolytic therapy advise that prophylactic agents not be given until 24 hours after administration of rt-PA.[353,354] In most patients, aspirin can be started with a reasonable degree of safety within 48 hours of stroke.[131,132] A reasonable regimen would be a single dose of 300–325 mg of aspirin followed by daily doses of 75–81 mg. Presumably, other antiplatelet aggregating agents also can be started during this period. The lag in inhibition of platelet aggregation with clopidogrel or ticlopidine has prompted some physicians to supplement these medications with aspirin for the first week. Long-term anticoagulation is an important part of plans to prevent recurrent stroke among patients with atrial fibrillation.[355] Oral anticoagulants probably can be started within 48 hours after stroke for most patients. Exceptions would be patients judged to have a high risk for hemorrhagic transformation of the infarction. Presence of bleeding on CT usually prompts delaying the initiation of anticoagulant treatment for approximately 5–7 days. Some physicians prescribe heparin as an adjunctive therapy while starting treatment with oral anticoagulants. The usefulness of this tactic, which is described in Chapter 10, has not been determined. Most patients probably do not need an interim course of heparin. Treatment with antiplatelet aggregating agents might be delayed if the patient is receiving anticoagulants for treatment of venous thromboembolic disease.

Surgical treatments to prevent recurrent stroke generally are not performed during the period of acute hospitalization. Traditionally, carotid endarterectomy was delayed until at least 6 weeks after stroke. In recent years, this prohibition against early surgery has been challenged because of the range of neurological sequelae caused by ischemic events. In addition, the distinction between a transient ischemic attack and a minor ischemic stroke has become increasingly murky. A patient with minimal neurological impairments after stroke and an imaging test that shows little or no brain injury probably can have surgery during acute hospitalization. Antiplatelet aggregating agents should be prescribed after surgery. If surgery is delayed, plans for re-admission should be spelled out at the time of discharge.

Interventions to treat risk factors for atherosclerosis and ischemic stroke should be started before discharge. These therapies must be tailored to the individual patient's needs. Long-term treatments to forestall myocardial infarction also are components of care after stroke.

Initiation of Rehabilitation

Virtually all patients should be assessed to determine whether they need rehabilitation following stroke. Exceptions include patients at the two extremes of neurological illness. Patients with very mild impairments might not need any specific rehabilitation intervention. Conversely, comatose patients and those with profound cognitive changes cannot undergo rehabilitation because of their inability to participate in the process. Consultations are obtained most commonly from physical therapy, speech pathology, and occupational therapy services. A goal is to have baseline assessments from these services as soon as the patient is stable. Timely assessments are critical for discharge planning. For example, transfer to an inpatient rehabilitation setting cannot be accomplished until plans for rehabilitation have been finalized. Rehabilitation services also should start active therapy aimed at ameliorating disability from the stroke. In some cases, rehabilitation consultants provide a plan that the patient can follow after discharge to home.

Patient and Family Education

During acute hospitalization, the patient and family should receive intensive education about stroke, its consequences, and its treatment.[8,260] The goals of this education are to provide information about the nature of stroke, the neurological signs, and the overall prognosis. In addition, the patient and family should be informed about treatments to prevent recurrent stroke, control complications of stroke, and maximize recovery from the event. Issues such as discharge planning, transfer to rehabilitation settings, and problems faced when returning home also need to be addressed.

Discharge Planning

For most patients, planning for discharge from an acute care setting can begin shortly after admission.[260] Except for critically ill patients who are neurologically unstable, a time for discharge and the likely next residence can be predicted with a reasonably high degree of accuracy. Starting discharge planning soon after admission allows for the participation of the patient, the family, and all members of the stroke team. Hasty planning and precipitous discharges are avoided.

In general, patients with mild strokes can be discharged to return to their homes as soon as three conditions are met: (*1*) their neurological condition is stable; (*2*) treatment for prevention of recurrent stroke has been started; and (*3*) the patient will be safe at home alone or with a caregiver, and outpatient rehabilitation, if necessary, is arranged. Patients with moderate-to-severe strokes usually are in the hospital for 3–7 days during which their neurological condition stabilizes, any medical or surgical complications are treated, rehabilitation is started, and therapies to prevent recurrent stroke are started. Most of these patients will not be discharged to their homes. Instead, they likely will need a course of intensive rehabilitation—usually in an inpatient setting. The active collaboration of the patient and the family is instrumental for discharge planning in this situation. The decision to transfer to an inpatient rehabilitation unit should be made with considerable care; once admitted, patients are monitored at regular intervals for signs of improvement. If improvement is minimal, then the patient may be discharged to a long-term care facility and he or she might not be eligible for readmission to an intensive rehabilitation program; the opportunity for aggressive rehabilitation may have been squandered. The best choice for some severely affected patients may be a transfer to a long-term care facility and then subsequent admission to a rehabilitation hospital if their condition improves. Options in post-hospital care for severely injured patients who survive a multilobar infarction are limited. These patients usually cannot be discharged to home because of their requirement for continued medical and surgical care. An exception to this rule might be the occasional patient who receives terminal hospice care at home. Many severely affected patients cannot be transferred to an inpatient rehabilitation setting because of the serious nature of their residual impairments. These patients likely will go to a skilled nursing facility for continued nursing care and rehabilitation.

SUMMARY

Admission to hospital is no longer an automatic decision for patients with stroke. Recency, severity and concomitant disease contribute to this decision. Care organized around a stroke unit improves all important outcomes, from mortality to morbidity and a higher percentage of eventual discharges to home as opposed to nursing homes or chronic facilities. Stroke care maps facilitate the patient's smooth transition through the different stages of the admission and early discharge planning, paying off in efficiencies and satisfaction.

In about one-third of patients with acute stroke, the condition worsens after admission. The causes can be neurological, systemic, and, occasionally, iatrogenic. Cerebral edema peaks in the first 72 hours after stroke; and hemorrhagic transformation of infarction, early recurrence, and seizures can complicate the course.

Cardiovascular complications are common in a population with a high prevalence of latent or overt coronary artery disease. Pulmonary and urinary tract infections threaten the bed-bound, and immobility is the breeding ground for deep vein thrombosis and pulmonary embolism. Depression is insidious and common, and dementia afflicts about one-quarter of stroke survivors. Hospitalization allows prevention and treatment of stroke complications, investigation of the cause of the stroke, initiation of treatment to prevent recurrent stroke, and the beginning of rehabilitation.

REFERENCES

1. Hacke W, Krieger D, Hirschberg M. General principles in the treatment of acute ischemic stroke. *Cerebrovasc Dis* 1991;1(Suppl 1):93–99.
2. The European Ad Hoc Consensus Group. Optimizing intensive care in stroke. A European perspective. *Cerebrovasc Dis* 1997;7:113–128.

3. Dennis M, Langhorne P. So stroke units save lives: where do we go from here? *BMJ* 1994; 1273–1277.
4. Dayno JM, Mansbach HH. Acute stroke units. *J Stroke Cerebrovasc Dis* 1999;8:160–170.
5. Norris JW, Hachinski VC. Intensive care management of stroke patients. *Stroke* 1976;7:573–577.
6. Bertram M, Schwarz S, Hacke W. Acute and critical care in neurology. *Eur Neurol* 1997;38: 155–166.
7. Mitsias P. Ischemic stroke management in the critical care unit: the first 24 hours. *J Stroke Cerebrovasc Dis* 1999;8:151–159.
8. Reddy MP, Reddy V. After a stroke: strategies to restore function and prevent complications. *Geriatrics* 1971;52:59–62.
9. Baker CM, Miller I, Sitterding M, Hajewski CJ. Acute stroke patients comparing outcomes with and without case management. *Nursing Case Management* 1998;3:196–203.
10. Sulter G, De Keyser J. From stroke unit care to stroke care unit. *J Neurol Sci* 1999;162:1–5.
11. Hund E, Grau A, Hacke W. Neurocritical care for acute ischemic stroke. *Neurosurg Clin N Am* 1997;8:271–282.
12. Stroke Unit Trialists Collaboration. How do stroke units improve patient outcomes? A collaborative systematic review of the randomized trials. *Stroke* 1997;28:2139–2144.
13. Ronning OM, Guldvog B. Stroke unit versus general medical wards. II: neurological deficits and activities of daily living: a quasi-randomized controlled trial. *Stroke* 1998;29:586–590.
14. Indredavik B, Bakke F, Slordahl SA, Rokseth R, Haheim LL. Treatment in a combined acute and rehabilitation stroke unit. *Stroke* 1999;30: 917–923.
15. Indredavik B, Bakke F, Slordahl SA, Rokseth R, Haheim LL. Stroke unit treatment improves long-term quality of life: a randomized controlled trial. *Stroke* 1998;29:895–899.
16. Lincoln NB, Willis D, Philips SA, Juby LC, Berman P. Comparison of rehabilitation practice on hospital wards for stroke patients. *Stroke* 1996;27:18–23.
17. Patel M, Potter J, Perez I, Kalra L. The process of rehabilitation and discharge planning in stroke: a controlled comparison between stroke units. *Stroke* 1998;29:2484–2487.
18. Bowen J, Yaste C. Effect of a stroke protocol on hospital costs of stroke patients. *Neurology* 1994;44:1961–1964.
19. Awad IA, Fayad P, Abdulrauf SI. Protocols and critical pathways for stroke care. *Clin Neurosurg* 1999;45:86–100.
20. Strand T, Asplund K, Eriksson S, Hagg E, Lithner F, Wester PO. A non-intensive stroke unit reduces functional disability and the need for long-term hospitalization. *Stroke* 1985;16: 29–34.
21. Strand T, Asplund K, Eriksson S, Hagg E, Lithner F, Wester PO. Stroke unit care—who benefits? Comparisons with general medical care in relation to prognostic indicators on admission. *Stroke* 1986;17:377–381.
22. Indredavik B, Bakke F, Solberg R, Rokseth R, Haaheim LL, Holme I. Benefit of a stroke unit: a randomized controlled trial. *Stroke* 1991;22: 1026–1031.
23. Langhorne P, Williams BO, Gilchrist W, Howie K. Do stroke units save lives? *Lancet* 1993;342: 395–398.
24. Stroke Unit Trialists' Collaboration. Collaborative systematic review of the randomised trials of organised inpatient (stroke unit) care after stroke. *BMJ* 1997;314:1151–1159.
25. Ronning OM, Guldvog B. Stroke units versus general medical wards. I: twelve- and eighteen-month survival: a randomized, controlled trial. *Stroke* 1998;29:58–62.
26. Indredavik B, Slordahl SA, Bakke F, Rokseth R, Haheim LL. Stroke unit treatment. Long-term effects. *Stroke* 1997;28:1861–1866.
27. Indredavik B, Bakke F, Slordahl SA, Rokseth R, Haheim LL. Stroke unit treatment. 10-year follow-up. *Stroke* 1999;30:1524–1527.
28. Stegmayr B, Asplund K, Hulter-Asberg K, et al. Stroke units in their natural habitat. *Stroke* 1999;30:709–714.
29. Jorgensen HS, Nakayama H, Raaschou HO, Larsen K, Hubbe P, Olsen TS. The effect of a stroke unit: reductions in mortality, discharge rate to nursing home, length of hospital stay, and cost. A community-based study. *Stroke* 1995;26:1178–1182.
30. Jorgensen HS, Kammersgaard LP, Nakayama H, et al. Treatment and rehabilitation on a stroke unit improves 5-year survival. A community-based study. *Stroke* 1999;30:930–933.
31. van Straten A, van der Meulen JH, van den Bos GA, Limburg M. Length of hospital stay and discharge delays in stroke patients. *Stroke* 1997;28:137–140.
32. Kaste M, Palomaki H, Sarna S. Where and how should elderly stroke patients be treated? A randomized trial. *Stroke* 1995;26:249–253.
33. van Gijn J, Dennis MS. Issues and answers in stroke care. *Lancet* 1998;352(Suppl 3): SIII23–SIII27.
34. van der Worp HB, Kappelle LJ. Complications of acute ischaemic stroke. *Cerebrovasc Dis* 1998;8:124–132.
35. Nakamura K, Saku Y, Ibayashi S, Fijishima M. Progressive motor deficits in lacunar infarction. *Stroke* 1999;52:29–33.
36. Roden-Jullig A. Progressing stroke. Epidemiology. *Cerebrovasc Dis* 1997;7(Suppl 5):2–5.
37. Davalos A, Cendra E, Teruel J, Martinez M, Genis D. Deteriorating ischemic stroke: risk factors and prognosis. *Neurology* 1990;40: 1865–1869.
38. Donnan GA, Norrving B, Bamford J, Bogousslavsky J. Subcortical infarction: classification and terminology. *Cerebrovasc Dis* 1993;3:248–251.
39. Davalos A, Castillo J. Potential mechanisms of worsening. *Cerebrovasc Dis* 1997;7(Suppl 5): 19–24.
40. Castillo J. Deteriorating stroke: diagnostic criteria, predictors, mechanisms and treatment. *Cerebrovasc Dis* 1999;9(Suppl 3): 1–8.

41. Castillo J, Davalos A, Noya M. Progression of ischaemic stroke and excitotoxic aminoacids. *Lancet* 1997;349:79–83.
42. Yamamoto H, Bogousslavsky J, Van Melle G. Different predictors of neurological worsening in different causes of stroke. *Arch Neurol* 1998;55:481–486.
43. Wang Y, Lim LLY, Levi C, Heller RF, Fisher J, Maths B. Influence of admission body temperature on stroke mortality. *Stroke* 2000;31: 404–409.
44. Hajat C, Hajat S, Sharma P. Effects of poststroke pyrexia on stroke outcome. A meta-analysis of studies in patients. *Stroke* 2000;31:410–414.
45. Chabriat H, Pappata S, Poupon C, et al. Neurological deterioration in acute ischemic stroke: Potential predictors and associated factors in the European Cooperative Acute Stroke Study (ECASS) I. *Stroke* 1999;30:2631–2636.
46. Pantano P, Caramia F, Bozzao L, Dieler C, von Kummer R. Delayed increase in infarct volume after cerebral ischemia. *Stroke* 1999;30:502–507.
47. Hacke W, Schwab S, Horn M, Spranger M, De Georgia M, von Kummer R. 'Malignant' middle cerebral artery territory infarction: clinical course and prognostic signs. *Arch Neurol* 1996; 53:309–315.
48. Wijdicks EF, Diringer MN. Middle cerebral artery territory infarction and early brain swelling: progression and effect of age on outcome. *Mayo Clin Proc* 1998;73:829–836.
49. Matsumoto K, Lo EH, Pierce AR, Wei H, Garrido L, Kowall NW. Role of vasogenic edema and tissue cavitation in ischemic evolution on diffusion-weighted imaging: comparison with multiparameter MR and immunohistochemistry. *Am J Neuroradiol* 1995;16:1107–1115.
50. Frank JI. Large hemispheric infarction, deterioration, and intracranial pressure. *Neurology* 1995;45:1286–1290.
51. Heinsius T, Bogousslavsky J, Van Melle G. Large infarcts in the middle cerebral artery territory. Etiology and outcome patterns. *Neurology* 1998;50:341–350.
52. Krieger DW, Demchuk AW, Kasner SE, Jauss M, Hantson L. Early clinical and radiological predictors of fatal brain swelling in ischemic stroke. *Stroke* 1999;30:287–292.
53. Firlik AD, Yonas H, Kaufmann AM, et al. Relationship between cerebral blood flow and the development of swelling and life-threatening herniation in acute ischemic stroke. *J Neurosurg* 1998;89:243–249.
54. Berrouschot J, Barthel H, von Kummer R, Knapp WH, Hesse S, Schneider. 99m technetium-ethyl-cysteinate-dimer single-photon emission CT can predict fatal ischemic brain edema. *Stroke* 1998;29:2556–2562.
55. Kucinski T, Koch C, Grzyska U, Freitag HJ, Kromer H, Zeumer H. The predictive value of early CT and angiography for fatal hemispheric swelling in acute stroke. *Am J Neuroradiol* 1998; 19:839–846.
56. Rudolf J, Grond M, Stenzel C, Neveling M, Heiss WD. Incidence of space-occupying brain edema following systemic thrombolysis of acute supratentorial ischemia. *Cerebrovasc Dis* 1998; 8:166–171.
57. Hacke W, Kaste M, Fieschi C, et al. Randomised double-blind placebo-controlled trial of thrombolytic therapy with intravenous alteplase in acute ischaemic stroke (ECASS II). Second European-Australasian Acute Stroke Study Investigators. *Lancet* 1998;352:1245–1251.
58. Scandinavian Stroke Study Group. Multicenter trial of hemodilution in acute ischemic stroke. Results of subgroup analyses. *Stroke* 1988;19: 464–471.
59. The Hemodilution in Stroke Study Group. Hypervolemic hemodilution treatment of acute stroke. Results of a randomized multicenter trial using pentastarch. *Stroke* 1989;20:317–323.
60. Ropper AH, Shafran B. Brain edema after stroke. Clinical syndrome and intracranial pressure. *Arch Neurol* 1984;41:26–29.
61. Gerriets T, Stolz E, Modrau B, Fiss I, Seidel G, Kaps M. Sonographic monitoring of midline shift in hemispheric infarctions. *Neurology* 1999; 52:45–49.
62. Pullicino PM, Alexandrov AV, Shelton JA, Alexandrova NA, Smurawska LT, Norris JW. Mass effect and death from severe acute stroke. *Neurology* 1997;49:1090–1095.
63. Haring H-P, Dilitz E, Pallua A, et al. Attenuated corticomedullary contrast: an early cerebral computed tomography sign indicating malignant middle cerebral artery infarction. *Stroke* 1999;30:1076–1082.
64. Wijdicks EF, Miller GM. MR imaging of progressive downward herniation of the diencephalon. *Neurology* 1997;48:1456–1459.
65. Mayer SA, Coplin WM, Raps EC. Cerebral edema, intracranial pressure, and herniation syndromes. *J Stroke Cerebrovasc Dis* 1999;8:183–191.
66. Adams HP, Jr., Brott TG, Crowell RM, et al. Guidelines for the management of patients with acute ischemic stroke. A statement for healthcare professionals from a special writing group of the Stroke Council, American Heart Association. *Circulation* 1994;90:1588–1601.
67. Schwarz S, Bertram M, Aschoff A, Schwab S, Hacke W. Indomethacin for brain edema following stroke. *Cerebrovasc Dis* 1999;9:248–250.
68. Bauer RB, Tellez H. Dexamethasone as treatment in cerebrovascular disease. 2. A controlled study in acute cerebral infarction. *Stroke* 1973;4:547–555.
69. Norris JW. Steroid therapy in acute cerebral infarction. *Arch Neurol* 1976;33:69–71.
70. Norris JW, Hachinski VC. High dose steroid treatment in cerebral infarction. *BMJ* 1986;292: 21–23.
71. Mulley G, Wilcox RG, Mitchell JR. Dexamethasone in acute stroke. *BMJ* 1978;2:994–996.
72. Qureshi AI, Wilson DA, Traystman RJ. Treatment of elevated intracranial pressure in experimental intracerebral hemorrhage: comparison between mannitol and hypertonic saline. *Neurosurgery* 1999;44:1055–1064.
73. Qureshi AI, Suarez JI, Bhardwaj A, et al. Use of hypertonic (3%) saline/acetate infusion in the treatment of cerebral edema: Effect on

intracranial pressure and lateral displacement of the brain. *Crit Care Med* 1998;26:440–446.
74. Stoll M, Hagen T, Bartylla K, Weber M, Jost V, Treib J. Changes of cerebral perfusion after osmotherapy in acute cerebral edema assessed with perfusion weighted MRI. *Neurol Res* 1998;20:474–478.
75. Mathew NT, Rivera VM, Meyer JS, Charney JZ, Hartmann A. Double-blind evaluation of glycerol therapy in acute cerebral infarction. *Lancet* 1972;2:1327–1329.
76. Larsson O, Marinovich N, Barber K. Double-blind trial of glycerol therapy in early stroke. *Lancet* 1976;1:832–834.
77. Bayer AJ, Pathy MS, Newcombe R. Double-blind randomised trial of intravenous glycerol in acute stroke. *Lancet* 1987;1:405–408.
78. Marshall LF, Smith RW, Rauscher LA, Shapiro HM. Mannitol dose requirements in brain-injured patients. *J Neurosurg* 1978;48:169–172.
79. Onar M, Arik Z. The evaluation of mannitol therapy in acute ischemic stroke patients by serial somatosensory evoked potentials. *Electromyography & Clinical Neurophysiology* 1997;37: 213–218.
80. Manno EM, Adams RE, Derdeyn CP, Powers WJ, Diringer MN. The effects of mannitol on cerebral edema after large hemispheric cerebral infarct. *Neurology* 1999;52:583–587.
81. Paczynski RP, He YY, Diringer MN, Hsu CY. Multiple-dose mannitol reduces brain water content in a rat model of cortical infarction. *Stroke* 1997;28:1437–1443.
82. Grotta J, Pasteur W, Khwaja G, Hamel T, Fisher M, Ramirez A. Elective intubation for neurologic deterioration after stroke. *Neurology* 1995;45: 640–644.
83. Berrouschot J, Sterker M, Bettin S, Koster J, Schneider D. Mortality of space-occupying ("malignant") middle cerebral artery infarction under conservative intensive care. *Intensive Care Medicine* 1998;24:620–623.
84. Schwab S, Aschoff A, Spranger M, Albert F, Hacke W. The value of intracranial pressure monitoring in acute hemispheric stroke. *Neurology* 1996;47:393–398.
85. Schwab S, Spranger M, Aschoff A, Steiner T, Hacke W. Brain temperature monitoring and modulation in patients with severe MCA infarction. *Neurology* 1997;48:762–767.
86. Schwab S, Schwarz S, Aschoff A, Keller E, Hacke W. Moderate hypothermia and brain temperature in patients with severe middle cerebral artery infarction. *Acta Neurochirurgica* 1998;71 (Suppl):131–134.
87. Schwab S, Schwarz S, Spranger M, Keller E, Bertram M, Hacke W. Moderate hypothermia in the treatment of patients with severe middle cerebral artery infarction. *Stroke* 1998;29:2461–2466.
88. Woodcock J, Ropper AH, Kennedy SK. High dose barbiturates in non-traumatic brain swelling: ICP reduction and effect on outcome. *Stroke* 1982;13:785–787.
89. Schwab S, Spranger M, Schwarz S, Hacke W. Barbiturate coma in severe hemispheric stroke: useful or obsolete? *Neurology* 1997;48:1608–1613.
90. Kalia KK, Yonas H. An aggressive approach to massive middle cerebral artery infarction. *Arch Neurol* 1993;50:1293–1297.
91. Kondziolka D, Fazl M. Functional recovery after decompressive craniectomy for cerebral infarction. *Neurosurgery* 1988;23:143–147.
92. Steiger H-J. Outcome of acute supratentorial cerebral infarction in patients under 60. *Acta Neurochir* 1991;111:73–79.
93. Doerfler A, Forsting M, Reith W, et al. Decompressive craniectomy in a rat model of "malignant" cerebral hemispheric stroke: experimental support for an aggressive therapeutic approach. *J Neurosurg* 1996;85:853–859.
94. Rieke K, Schwab S, Krieger D, et al. Decompressive surgery in space-occupying hemispheric infarction: results of an open, prospective trial. *Crit Care Med* 1995;23:1576–1587.
95. Carter BS, Ogilvy CS, Candia GJ, Rosas HD, Buonanno F. One-year outcome after decompressive surgery for massive nondominant hemispheric infarction. *Neurosurgery* 1997;40: 1168–1175.
96. Schwab S, Steiner T, Aschoff A, et al. Early hemicraniectomy in patients with complete middle cerebral artery infarction. *Stroke* 1998;29: 1888–1893.
97. Sakai K, Iwahashi K, Terada K, Gohda Y, Sakurai M, Matsumoto Y. Outcome after external decompression for massive cerebral infarction. *Neurologia Medico-Chirurgica* 1998;38:131–135.
98. Mori K, Ishimaru S, Maeda M. Unco-parahippocampectomy for direct surgical treatment of downward transtentorial herniation. *Acta Neurochir* 1998;140:1239–1244.
99. Mathew P, Teasdale G, Bannan A, Oluoch-Olunya D. Neurosurgical management of cerebellar haematoma and infarct. *J Neurol Neurosurg Psychiatry* 1995;59:287–292.
100. Macdonell RA, Kalnins RM, Donnan GA. Cerebellar infarction: natural history, prognosis, and pathology. *Stroke* 1987;18:849–855.
101. Hornig CR, Rust DS, Busse O, Jauss M, Laun A. Space-occupying cerebellar infarction. Clinical course and prognosis. *Stroke* 1994;25:372–374.
102. Rieke K, Krieger D, Aschoff A, Meyding-Lamade V, Hacke W. Therapeutic strategies in space-occupying cerebellar infarction based on clinical, neuroradiological, and neurophysical logical data. *Cerebrovasc Dis* 1993;3:45–55.
103. Kanis KB, Ropper AH, Adelman LS. Homolateral hemiparesis as an early sign of cerebellar mass effect. *Neurology* 1994;44: 2194–2197.
104. Horwitz NH, Ludolph C. Acute obstructive hydrocephalus caused by cerebellar infarction. Treatment alternatives. *Surg Neurol* 1983;20: 13–19.
105. Greenberg J, Skubick D, Shenkin H. Acute hydrocephalus in cerebellar infarct and hemorrhage. *Neurology* 1979;29:409–413.
106. Brandt T, Grau AJ, Hacke W. Severe stroke. *Baillieres Clin Neurol* 1996;5:515–541.
107. Chen HJ, Lee TC, Wei CP. Treatment of cerebellar infarction by decompressive suboccipital craniectomy. *Stroke* 1992;23:957–961.

108. Moulin T, Crepin-Leblond T, Chopard JL, Bogousslavsky J. Hemorrhagic infarcts. *Eur Neurol* 1994;34:64–77.
109. Chaves CJ, Pessin MS, Caplan LR, et al. Cerebellar hemorrhagic infarction. *Neurology* 1996;46:346–349.
110. Hornig CR, Dorndorf W, Agnoli AL. Hemorrhagic cerebral infarction—a prospective study. *Stroke* 1986;17:179–185.
111. Alexandrov AV, Black SE, Ehrlich LE, Caldwell CB, Norris JW. Predictors of hemorrhagic transformation occurring spontaneously and on anticoagulants in patients with acute ischemic stroke. *Stroke* 1997;28:1198–1202.
112. Lodder J, Krijne-Kubat B, Broekman J. Cerebral hemorrhagic infarction at autopsy: cardiac embolic cause and the relationship to the cause of death. *Stroke* 1986;17:626–629.
113. Toni D, Fiorelli M, Bastianello S, et al. Hemorrhagic transformation of brain infarct: predictability in the first 5 hours from stroke onset and influence on clinical outcome. *Neurology* 1996;46:341–345.
114. Ott BR, Zamani A, Kleefield J, Funkenstein HH. The clinical spectrum of hemorrhagic infarction. *Stroke* 1986;17:630–637.
115. Hart RG, Putnam C. Hemorrhagic transformation of cardioembolic stroke. *Stroke* 1989;20:1117.
116. Beghi E, Bogliun G, Cavaletti G, et al. Hemorrhagic infarction: risk factors, clinical and tomographic features, and outcome. A case-control study. *Acta Neurol Scand* 1989;80:226–231.
117. Okada Y, Yamaguchi T, Minematsu K, et al. Hemorrhagic transformation in cerebral embolism. *Stroke* 1989;20:598–603.
118. Ueda T, Hatakeyama T, Kumon Y, Sakaki S, Uraoka T. Evaluation of risk of hemorrhagic transformation in local intra-arterial thrombolysis in acute ischemic stroke by initial SPECT. *Stroke* 1994;25:298–303.
119. Larrue V, von Kummer R, del Zoppo G, Bluhmki E. Hemorrhagic transformation in acute ischemic stroke. Potential contributing factors in the European Cooperative Acute Stroke Study. *Stroke* 1997;28:957–960.
120. Lyden PD, Zivin JA. Hemorrhagic transformation after cerebral ischemia: mechanisms and incidence. *Cerebrovasc Brain Metab Rev* 1993;5: 1–16.
121. Motto C, Aritzu E, Boccardi E, De Grandi C, Piana A, Candelise L. Reliability of hemorrhagic transformation diagnosis in acute ischemic stroke. *Stroke* 1997;28:302–306.
122. Bogousslavsky J, Regli F. Anticoagulant-induced intracerebral bleeding in brain ischemia. *Acta Neurol Scand* 1985;71:464–471.
123. Teal PA, Pessin MS. Hemorrhagic transformation. The spectrum of ischemia-related brain hemorrhage. *Neurosurg Clin N Am* 1992;3: 601–610.
124. Jaillard A, Cornu C, Durieux A, et al. Hemorrhagic transformation in acute ischemic stroke. *Stroke* 1999;30:1326–1332.
125. Multicentre Acute Stroke Trial—Italy (MAST-I) Group. Randomised controlled trial of streptokinase, aspirin, and combination of both in treatment of acute ischaemic stroke. *Lancet* 1995;346:1509–1514.
126. The Multicenter Acute Stroke Trial—Europe Study Group. Thrombolytic therapy with streptokinase in acute ischemic stroke. *N Engl J Med* 1996;335:145–150.
127. Donnan GA, Davis SM, Chambers BR, et al. Streptokinase for acute ischemic stroke with relationship to time of administration: Australian Streptokinase (ASK) Trial Study Group. *JAMA* 1996;276:961–966.
128. Organizing Committees (Program AaL. Asia Pacific consensus forum on stroke management). *Stroke* 1998;29:1730–1736.
129. Fiorelli M, Bastianello S, von Kummer R, et al. Hemorrhagic transformation within 36 hours of a cerebral infarct. Relationships with early clinical deterioration and 3-month outcome in the European Cooperative Acute Stroke Study I (ECASS I) cohort. *Stroke* 1999;30:2280–2284.
130. Samsa GP, Bian J, Lipscomb J, Matchar DB. Epidemiology of recurrent cerebral infarction: a medicare claims-based comparison of first and recurrent strokes on 2-year survival and cost. *Stroke* 1999;30:338–349.
131. CAST (Chinese Acute Stroke Trial) Collaborative Group. CAST: randomised placebo-controlled trial of early aspirin use in 20,000 patients with acute ischaemic stroke. *Lancet* 1997;349: 1641–1649.
132. International Stroke Trial Collaborative Group. The International Stroke Trial (IST): a randomised trial of aspirin, subcutaneous heparin, both, or neither among 19435 patients with acute ischaemic stroke. *Lancet* 1997;349: 1569–1581.
133. The Publications Committee for the Trial of ORG 10172 in Acute Stroke Treatment (TOAST) Investigators. Low molecular weight heparinoid, ORG 10172 (danaparoid), and outcome after acute ischemic stroke: a randomized controlled trial. *JAMA* 1998;279:1265–1272.
134. Jorgensen HS, Nakayama H, Reith J, Raaschou HO, Olsen TS. Stroke recurrence: predictors, severity, and prognosis. The Copenhagen Stroke Study. *Neurology* 1997;48:891–895.
135. Kilpatrick CJ, Davis SM, Tress BM, Rossiter SC, Hopper JL, Vandendriesen ML. Epileptic seizures in acute stroke. *Arch Neurol* 1990;47: 157–160.
136. Davalos A, de Cendra E, Molins A, Ferrandiz M, Lopez-Pousa S, Genis D. Epileptic seizures at the onset of stroke. *Cerebrovasc Dis* 1992;2:327–331.
137. Rumbach L, Sablot D, Berger E, Tatu L, Vuillier F, Moulin T. Status epilepticus in stroke. Report on a hospital-based stroke cohort. *Neurology* 2000;54:350–354.
138. Kilpatrick CJ, Davis SM, Hopper JL, Rossiter SC. Early seizures after acute stroke. Risk of late seizures. *Arch Neurol* 1992;49:509–511.
139. Wijdicks EF, Scott JP. Causes and outcome of mechanical ventilation in patients with hemispheric ischemic stroke. *Mayo Clin Proc* 1997; 72:210–213.
140. Sung CY, Chu NS. Epileptic seizures in thrombotic stroke. *J Neurol* 1990;237:166–170.

141. So EL, Annegers JF, Hauser WA, O'Brien PC, Whisnant JP. Population-based study of seizure disorders after cerebral infarction. *Neurology* 1996;46:350–355.
142. Pohlmann-Eden B, Cochius JI, Hoch DB, Hennerici M. Stroke and epilepsy: critical review of the literature. *Cerebrovasc Dis* 1997;7:2–9.
143. Burn J, Dennis M, Bamford J, Sandercock P, Wade D, Warlow C. Epileptic seizures after a first stroke: the Oxfordshire Community Stroke Project. *BMJ* 1997;315:1582–1587.
144. Daniele O, Mattaliano A, Tassinari CA, Natale E. Epileptic seizures and cerebrovascular disease. *Acta Neurol Scand* 1989;80:17–22.
145. Awada A, Omojola MF, Obeid T. Late epileptic seizures after cerebral infarction. *Acta Neurol Scand* 1999;99:265–268.
146. Adams HP, Jr. Management of patients with acute ischaemic stroke. *Drugs* 1997;54(Suppl 3): 60–69.
147. Henon H, Lebert F, Durieu I, et al. Confusional state in stroke: relation to preexisting dementia, patient characteristics, and outcome. *Stroke* 1999;30:773–779.
148. Kase CS, Wolf PA, Kelly-Hayes M, Kannel WB, Beiser A, D'Agostino RB. Intellectual decline after stroke: the Framingham Study. *Stroke* 1998;29:805–812.
149. Censori B, Manara O, Agostinis C, et al. Dementia after first stroke. *Stroke* 1996;27: 1205–1210.
150. Kokmen E, Whisnant JP, O'Fallon WM, Chu CP, Beard CM. Dementia after ischemic stroke: a population-based study in Rochester, Minnesota (1960–1984). *Neurology* 1996;46:154–159.
151. Tatemichi TK, Desmond DW, Mayeux R, et al. Dementia after stroke: baseline frequency, risks, and clinical features in a hospitalized cohort. *Neurology* 1992;42:1185–1193.
152. Ross GW, Petrovitch H, White LR, et al. Characterization of risk factors for vascular dementia. *Neurology* 1999;53:337–343.
153. Tatemichi TK, Desmond DW, Paik M, et al. Clinical determinants of dementia related to stroke. *Ann Neurol* 1993;33:568–575.
154. Foster NL, Hickenbottom SL. When do strokes cause dementia. Effects of subcortical cerebral infarction on cortical glucose metabolism and cognitive function. *Arch Neurol* 1999;56: 778–779.
155. Wade DT, Parker V, Langton HR. Memory disturbance after stroke: frequency and associated losses. *Int Rehabil Med* 1986;8:60–64.
156. Bowler JV, Eliasziw M, Steenhuis R, et al. Comparative evolution of Alzheimer disease, vascular dementia, and mixed dementia. *Arch Neurol* 1997;54:697–703.
157. Erkinjuntti T, Hachinski V. Rethinking vascular dementia. *Cerebrovasc Dis* 1993;3:3–23.
158. Caplan L, Schoene WC. Clinical features of subcortical arteriosclerotic encephalopathy (Binswanger disease). *Neurology* 1978;28: 1206–1215.
159. Chui HC, Victoroff JI, Margolin D, Jagust W, Shankle R, Katzman R. Criteria for the diagnosis of ischemic vascular dementia proposed by the State of California Alzheimer's Disease Diagnostic and Treatment Centers. *Neurology* 1992;42:473–480.
160. Gorelick PB. Status of risk factors for dementia associated with stroke. *Stroke* 1997;28:459–463.
161. Hachinski V. Binswanger's disease: neither Binswanger's nor a disease. *J Neurol Sci* 1991; 103:1.
162. Kinkel WR, Jacobs L, Polachini I, Bates V, Heffner RR, Jr. Subcortical arteriosclerotic encephalopathy (Binswanger's disease). Computed tomographic, nuclear magnetic resonance, and clinical correlations. *Arch Neurol* 1985;42:951–959.
163. Choi SH, Na DL, Chung CS, Lee KH, Na DG, Adair JC. Diffusion-weighted MRI in vascular dementia. *Neurology* 2000;54:83–89.
164. Pasquier F, Leys D. Why are stroke patients prone to develop dementia? *J Neurol* 1997;244: 135–142.
165. Loeb C, Gandolfo C, Croce R, Conti M. Dementia associated with lacunar infarction. *Stroke* 1992;23:1225–1229.
166. Hachinski VC, Lassen NA, Marshall J. Multi-infarct dementia. A cause of mental deterioration in the elderly. *Lancet* 1974;2:207–210.
167. Hachinski VC. Multi-infarct dementia: a reappraisal. *Alzheimer Dis Assoc Disord* 1991;5:64–68.
168. Roman GC, Tatemichi TK, Erkinjuntti T, et al. Vascular dementia: diagnostic criteria for research studies. Report of the NINDS-AIREN International Workshop. *Neurology* 1993;43: 250–260.
169. Hachinski VC, Iliff LD, Zilhka E, et al. Cerebral blood flow in dementia. *Arch Neurol* 1975;32: 632–637.
170. Moroney JT, Bagiella E, Desmond DW, et al. Meta-analysis of the Hachinski Ischemic Score in pathologically verified dementias. *Neurology* 1997;49:1096–1105.
171. Moroney JT, Bagiella E, Hachinski VC, et al. Misclassification of dementia subtype using the Hachinski Ischemic Score: results of a meta-analysis of patients with pathologically verified dementias. *Ann N Y Acad Sci* 1997;826:490–492.
172. Boon AJ, Tans JT, Delwel EJ, et al. Dutch Normal-Pressure Hydrocephalus Study: the role of cerebrovascular disease. *J Neurosurg* 1999; 90:221–226.
173. Johnson WG, Fahn S. Treatment of vascular hemiballism and hemichorea. *Neurology* 1977;27:634–636.
174. Kase CS, Maulsby GO, deJuan E, Mohr JP. Hemichorea-hemiballism and lacunar infarction in the basal ganglia. *Neurology* 1981;31:452–455.
175. Goldblatt D, Markesbery W, Reeves AG. Recurrent hemichorea following striatal lesions. *Arch Neurol* 1974;31:51–54.
176. Fenelon G, Houeto JL. Unilateral parkinsonism following a large infarct in the territory of the lenticulostriate arteries. *Movement Disorders* 1997;12:1086–1090.
177. Apaydin H, Ozekmekci S, Yeni N. Posthemiplegic focal limb dystonia: a report of two cases. *Clin Neurol Neurosurg* 1998;100:46–50.
178. Kostic VS, Stojanovic-Svetel M, Kacar A. Symptomatic dystonias associated with structural

brain lesions: report of 16 cases. *Can J Neurol Sci* 1996;23:53–56.
179. Krauss JK, Jankovic J. Hemidystonia secondary to carotid artery gunshot injury. *Childs Nervous System* 1997;13:285–288.
180. Wali GM. Shoulder girdle dyskinesia associated with a thalamic infarct. *Movement Disorders* 1999;14:375–377.
181. Brannan T, Yahr MD. Focal tremor following striatal infarct—a case report. *Movement Disorders* 1999;14:368–370.
182. Kim JS. Head tremor and stroke. *Cerebrovasc Dis* 1997;7:175–179.
183. Grant AC, Biousse V, Cook AA, Newman NJ. Stroke-associated stuttering. *Arch Neurol* 1999; 56:624–627.
184. Peyron R, Garcia-Larrea L, Gregoire MC, et al. Allodynia after lateral-medullary (Wallenberg) infarct. A PET study. *Brain* 1998;121:345–356.
185. Silverman IE. Central poststroke pain associated with lateral medullary infarction [letter; comment]. *Neurology* 1998;50:836–837.
186. Bowshear D, Leijon G, Thuomas KA. Central poststroke pain. *Neurology* 1998;51:1352–1358.
187. Gorson KC, Pessin MS, DeWitt LD, Caplan LR. Stroke with sensory symptoms mimicking myocardial ischemia. *Neurology* 1996;46: 548–551.
188. Canavero S, Bonicalzi V. Pain after thalamic stroke: right diencephalic predominance and clinical features in 180 patients [letter; comment]. *Neurology* 1998;51:927–928.
189. Kim JS, Kang JH, Lee MC. Trigeminal neuralgia after pontine infarction. *Neurology* 1998;51: 1511–1512.
190. MacGowan DJ, Janal MN, Clark WC, et al. Central poststroke pain and Wallenberg's lateral medullary infarction: frequency, character, and determinants in 63 patients. *Neurology* 1997; 49:120–125.
191. Braus DF, Krauss JK, Strobel J. The shoulder-hand syndrome after stroke: a prospective clinical trial. *Ann Neurol* 1994;36:728–733.
192. Wanklyn P, Forster A, Young J, Mulley G. Prevalence and associated features of the cold hemiplegic arm. *Stroke* 1995;26:1867–1870.
193. Korpelainen JT, Sotaniemi KA, Huikuri HV, Myllya VV. Abnormal heart rate variability as a manifestation of autonomic dysfunction in hemispheric brain infarction. *Stroke* 1996;27: 2059–2063.
194. Korpelainen JT, Sotaniemi KA, Myllyla VV. Asymmetrical skin temperature in ischemic stroke. *Stroke* 1995;26:1543–1547.
195. Korpelainen JT, Sotaniemi KA, Myllyla VV. Ipsilateral hypohidrosis in brain stem infarction. *Stroke* 1993;24:100–104.
196. Giubilei F, Strano S, Lino S, et al. Autonomic nervous activity during sleep in middle cerebral artery infarction. *Cerebrovasc Dis* 1998;8: 118–123.
197. Onoda K, Ikeda M. Gustatory disturbance due to cerebrovascular disorder. *Laryngoscope* 1999; 109:123–128.
198. Rousseaux M, Muller P, Gahide I, Mottin Y, Romon M. Disorders of smell, taste, and food intake in a patient with a dorsomedial thalamic infarct. *Stroke* 1996;27:2328–2330.
199. Kumar A, Dromerick AW. Intractable hiccups during stroke rehabilitation. *Arch Phys Med Rehabil* 1998;79:697–699.
200. Dyken ME, Somers VK, Yamada T, Ren ZY, Zimmerman MB. Investigating the relationship between stroke and obstructive sleep apnea. *Stroke* 1996;27:401–407.
201. Bassetti C, Aldrich MS, Chervin RD, Quint D. Sleep apnea in patients with transient ischemic attack and stroke: a prospective study of 59 patients. *Neurology* 1996;47:1167–1173.
202. Good DC, Henkle JQ, Gelber D, Welsh J, Verhulst S. Sleep-disordered breathing and poor functional outcome after stroke. *Stroke* 1996;27:252–259.
203. Bassetti C, Mathis J, Gugger M, Lovblad KO, Hess CW. Hypersomnia following paramedian thalamic stroke: a report of 12 patients. *Ann Neurol* 1996;39:471–480.
204. Bassetti C, Aldrich MS. Sleep apnea in acute cerebrovascular diseases: final report on 128 patients. *Sleep* 1999;22:217–223.
205. Brott T. Prevention and management of medical complications of the hospitalized elderly stroke patient. *Clin Geriatr Med* 1991;7:475–482.
206. Bamford J, Dennis M, Sandercock P, Burn J, Warlow C. The frequency, causes, and timing of death within 30 days of a first stroke. The Oxfordshire Community Stroke Project. *J Neurol Neurosurg Psychiatry* 1990;53:824–829.
207. Johnston KC, Li JY, Lyden PD, et al. Medical and neurological complications of ischemic stroke: experience from the RANTTAS trial. RANTTAS Investigators. *Stroke* 1998;29: 447–453.
208. Jaster JH, Smith TW. Arrhythmia mechanism of unexpected sudden death following lateral medullary infarction. *Tennessee Medicine* 1998; 91:284.
209. Lane RD, Wallace JD, Petrosky PP, Schwartz GE, Gradman AH. Supraventricular tachycardia in patients with right hemisphere strokes. *Stroke* 1992;23:362–366.
210. McDermott MM, Lefevre F, Arron M, Martin GJ, Biller J. ST segment depression detected by continuous electrocardiography in patients with acute ischemic stroke or transient ischemic attack. *Stroke* 1994;25:1820–1824.
211. Chua HC, Sen S, Cosgriff RF, Gerstenblith G, Beauchamp NJ, Jr., Oppenheimer SM. Neurogenic ST depression in stroke. *Clin Neurol Neurosurg* 1999;101:44–48.
212. Oppenheimer S, Hachinski V. Complications of acute stroke. *Lancet* 1992;339:721–724.
213. Oppenheimer SM. Neurogenic cardiac effects of cerebrovascular disease. *Curr Opin Neurol* 1994; 7:20–24.
214. Oppenheimer SM, Hachinski VC. The cardiac consequences of stroke. *Neurol Clin* 1992;10: 167–176.
215. Svigelj V, Grad A, Tekavcic I, Kiauta T. Cardiac arrhythmia associated with reversible damage to insula in a patients with subarachnoid hemorrhage. *Stroke* 1994;25:1053–1055.

216. Kolin A, Norris JW. Myocardial damage from acute cerebral lesions. *Stroke* 1984;15: 990–993.
217. Korpelainen JT, Sotaniemi KA, Huikuri HV, Myllyla VV. Circadian rhythm of heart rate variability is reversibly abolished in ischemic stroke. *Stroke* 1997;28:2150–2154.
218. Korpelainen JT, Sotaniemi KA, Makikallio A, Huikuri HV, Myllyla VV. Dynamic behavior of heart rate in ischemic stroke. *Stroke* 1999;30: 1008–1013.
219. Yoon BW, Morillo CA, Cechetto DF, Hachinski V. Cerebral hemispheric lateralization in cardiac autonomic control. *Arch Neurol* 1997;54: 741–744.
220. Noda A, Okada T, Katsumata K, Yasuma F, Nakashima N, Yokota M. Suppressed cardiac and electroencephalographic arousal on apnea/hypopnea termination in elderly patients with cerebral infarction. *J Clin Neurophysiol* 1997;14:68–72.
221. Tokgozoglu SL, Batur MK, Topcuoglu MA, Saribas O, Kes S, Oto A. Effects of stroke localization on cardiac autonomic balance and sudden death. *Stroke* 1999;30:1307–1311.
222. Zorowitz RD, Tietjen GE. Medical complications after stroke. *J Stroke Cerebrovasc Dis* 1999;8: 192–196.
223. Tirschwell DL, Kukull WA, Longstreth WT, Jr. Medical complications of ischemic stroke and length of hospital stay: experience in Seattle, Washington. *J Stroke Cerebrovasc Dis* 1999;8: 336–343.
224. Bergqvist D, Jendteg S, Johansen L, Persson U, Odegaard K. Cost of long-term complications of deep venous thrombosis of the lower extremities: an analysis of a defined patient population in Sweden. *Ann Intern Med* 1997;126: 454–457.
225. Hamilton MG, Hull RD, Pineo GF. Venous thromboembolism in neurosurgery and neurology patients: a review. *Neurosurgery* 1994;34: 280–296.
226. Sioson ER, Crowe WE, Dawson NV. Occult proximal deep vein thrombosis: its prevalence among patients admitted to a rehabilitation hospital. *Arch Phys Med Rehabil* 1988;69:183–185.
227. Altes A, Abellan MT, Mateo J, Avila A, Marti-Vilalta JL, Fontcuberta J. Hemostatic disturbances in acute ischemic stroke: a study of 86 patients. *Acta Haematologica* 1995;94:10–15.
228. Kilpatrick TJ, Matkovic Z, Davis SM, McGrath CM, Dauer RJ. Hematologic abnormalities occur in both cortical and lacunar infarction. *Stroke* 1993;24:1945–1950.
229. Wijdicks EF, Scott JP. Pulmonary embolism associated with acute stroke. *Mayo Clin Proc* 1997;72:297–300.
230. Langhorne P. Measures to improve recovery in the acute phase of stroke. *Cerebrovasc Dis* 1999;9 (Suppl 5):2–5.
231. Stephens PH, Healy MT, Smith M, Jewkes DA. Prophylaxis against thromboembolism in neurosurgical patients: a survey of current practice in the United Kingdom. *Br J Neurosurg* 1995;9: 159–163.
232. Hyers TM, Agnelli G, Hull RD, et al. Antithrombotic therapy for venous thromboembolic disease. *Chest* 1998;114:S561–S578.
233. Desmukh M, Bisignani M, Landau P, Orchard TJ. Deep vein thrombosis in rehabilitating stroke patients. Incidence, risk factors and prophylaxis. *Am J Phys Med Rehabil* 1991;70: 313–316.
234. McCarthy ST, Turner JJ, Robertson D, Hawkey CJ, Macey DJ. Low-dose haparin as a prophylaxis against deep-vein thrombosis after acute stroke. *Lancet* 1977;2:800–801.
235. Dumas R, Woitinas F, Kutnowski M, et al. A multicentre, double-blind, randomized study to compare the safety and efficacy of once-daily ORG 10172 and twice-daily low dose heparin in preventing deep-vein thrombosis in patients with acute ischaemic stroke. *Ageing* 1994;23: 512–516.
236. McCarthy ST, Turner J. Low-dose subcutaneous heparin in the prevention of deep-vein thrombosis and pulmonary emboli following acute stroke. *Ageing* 1986;15:84–88.
237. Sandset PM, Dahl T, Stiris M, Rostad B, Scheel B, Abildgaard U. A double-blind and randomized placebo-controlled trial of low molecular weight heparin once daily to prevent deep-vein thrombosis in acute ischemic stroke. *Semin Thromb Hemost* 1990;16(Suppl):25–33.
238. Turpie AG, Levine MN, Hirsh J, et al. Double-blind randomised trial of Org 10172 low-molecular-weight heparinoid in prevention of deep-vein thrombosis in thrombotic stroke. *Lancet* 1987;1:523–526.
239. Clagett GP, Anderson FA, Jr., Geerts W, et al. Prevention of venous thromboembolism. *Chest* 1998;114:S531–S560.
240. Turpie AG, Gent M, Cote R, et al. A low-molecular-weight heparinoid compared with unfractionated heparin in the prevention of deep vein thrombosis in patients with acute ischemic stroke. A randomized, double-blind study. *Ann Intern Med* 1992;117:353–357.
241. Lensing AW, Prins MH, Davidson BL, Hirsh J. Treatment of deep venous thrombosis with low-molecular-weight heparins. A meta-analysis. *Arch Intern Med* 1995;155:601–607.
242. Prandoni P, Lensing AW, Buller HR, et al. Comparison of subcutaneous low-molecular-weight heparin with intravenous standard heparin in proximal deep-vein thrombosis. *Lancet* 1992;339:441–445.
243. Bergqvist D. Low molecular weight heparins. *J Intern Med* 1996;240:63–72.
244. Green D, Hirsh J, Heit J, Prins M, Davidson B, Lensing AW. Low molecular weight heparin: a critical analysis of clinical trials. *Pharmacol Rev* 1994;46:89–109.
245. Hull RD, Raskob GE, Pineo GF, et al. Subcutaneous low-molecular-weight heparin compared with continuous intravenous heparin in the treatment of proximal-vein thrombosis. *N Engl J Med* 1992;326:975–982.
246. Samama MM, Cohen AT, Darmon JY, et al. A comparison of enoxaparin with placebo for the prevention of venous thromboembolism in

acutely ill medical patients. *N Engl J Med 341* 1999;793:800.

247. Levine M, Gent M, Hirsh J, et al. A comparison of low-molecular-weight heparin administered primarily at home with unfractionated heparin administered in the hospital for proximal deep-vein thrombosis. *N Engl J Med* 1996;334: 677–681.
248. Martineau P, Tawil N. Low-molecular-weight heparins in the treatment of deep-vein thrombosis. *Ann Pharmacother* 1960;32:588–598.
249. Gould MK, Dembitzer AD, Doyle RL, Hastie TJ, Garber AM. Low-molecular-weight heparins compared with unfractionated heparin for treatment of acute deep venous thrombosis. A meta-analysis of randomized, controlled trials. *Ann Intern Med* 1999;130:800–809.
250. Koopman MM, Buller HR. Low-molecular-weight heparins in the treatment of venous thromboembolism. *Ann Intern Med* 1998;128: 1037–1039.
251. Gould MK, Dembitzer AD, Sanders GD, Garber AM. Low-molecular-weight heparins compared with unfractionated heparin for treatment of acute deep venous thrombosis. A cost-effectiveness analysis. *Ann Intern Med* 1999;130:789–799.
252. Black PM, Crowell RM, Abbott WM. External pneumatic calf compression reduces deep venous thrombosis in patients with ruptured intracranial aneurysms. *Neurosurgery* 1986;18:25–28.
253. Kamran SI, Downey D, Ruff RL. Pneumatic sequential compression reduces the risk of deep vein thrombosis in stroke patients. *Neurology* 1998;50:1683–1688.
254. Vingerhoets F, Bogousslavsky J. Respiratory dysfunction in stroke. *Clin Chest Med* 1994;15: 729–737.
255. el-Ad B, Bornstein NM, Fuchs P, Korczyn AD. Mechanical ventilation in stroke patients—is it worthwhile? *Neurology* 1996;47:657–659.
256. Bushnell CD, Phillips-Bute BG, Laskowitz DT, Lynch JR, Chilukuri V, Borel CO. Survival and outcome after endotracheal intubation for acute stroke. *Neurology* 1999;52:1374–1381.
257. Davenport RJ, Dennis MS, Wellwood I, Warlow CP. Complications after acute stroke. *Stroke* 1996;27:415–420.
258. Nakagawa T, Sekizawa K, Arai H, Kikuchi R, Manabe K, Sasaki H. High incidence of pneumonia in elderly patients with basal ganglia infarction. *Arch Intern Med* 1997;157:321–324.
259. Ween JE, Alexander MP, D'Esposito M, Roberts M. Incontinence after stroke in a rehabilitation setting: outcome associations and predictive factors. *Neurology* 1996;47:659–663.
260. Gresham GE, Duncan PW, Stason WB, et al. Post-stroke rehabilitation. U.S. Department of Health and Human Services, 1995.
261. Dromerick A, Reding M. Medical and neurological complications during inpatient stroke rehabilitation. *Stroke* 1994;25:358–361.
262. Davenport RJ, Dennis MS, Warlow CP. Gastrointestinal hemorrhage after acute stroke. *Stroke* 1996;27:421–424.
263. Jura E. Gastrointestinal disturbances in stroke. *Acta Neurol Scand* 1987;76:168–171.
264. Wijdicks EF, Fulgham JR, Batts KP. Gastrointestinal bleeding in stroke. *Stroke* 1994; 25:2146–2148.
265. Unosson M, Ek AC, Bjurulf P, von Schenck H, Larsson J. Feeding dependence and nutritional status after acute stroke. *Stroke* 1994;25: 366–371.
266. Choi-Kwon S, Yang YH, Kim EK, Jeon MY, Kim JS. Nutritional status in acute stroke: undernutrition versus overnutrition in different stroke subtypes. *Acta Neurol Scand* 1998;98:187–192.
267. Axelsson K, Asplund K, Norberg A, Alafuzoff I. Nutritional status in patients with acute stroke. *Acta Med Scand* 1988;224:217–224.
268. Gariballa SE, Parker SG, Taub N, Castleden CM. Influence of nutritional status on clinical outcome after acute stroke. *Am J Clin Nutr* 1998;68:275–281.
269. Sivakumar V, Rajshekhar V, Chandy MJ. Management of neurosurgical patients with hyponatremia and natriuresis. *Neurosurgery* 1994;34:269–274.
270. Harrigan MR. Cerebral salt wasting syndrome: a review. *Neurosurgery* 1996;38:152–160.
271. Zald DH, Pardo JV. The functional neuroanatomy of voluntary swallowing. *Ann Neurol* 1999;46: 281–286.
272. Robbins J. The evolution of swallowing neuroanatomy and physiology in humans: a practical perspective. *Ann Neurol* 1999;46:279–280.
273. Elmstahl S, Bulow M, Ekberg O, Petersson M, Tegner H. Treatment of dysphagia improves nutritional conditions in stroke patients. *Dysphagia* 1999;14:61–66.
274. Daniels SK, Brailey K, Foundas AL. Lingual discoordination and dysphagia following acute stroke: analyses of lesion localization. *Dysphagia* 1999;14:85–92.
275. Vigderman AM, Chavin JM, Kososky C, Tahmoush AJ. Aphagia due to pharyngeal constrictor paresis from acute lateral medullary infarction. *J Neurol Sci* 1998;155:208–210.
276. Finestone HM, Fisher J, Greene-Finestone LS, Teasell RW, Craig ID. Sudden death in the dysphagic stroke patient—a case of airway obstruction caused by a food bolus: a brief report. *Am J Phys Med Rehabil* 1998;77:550–552.
277. Smithard DG, O'Neill PA, Parks C, Morris J. Complications and outcome after acute stroke. Does dysphagia matter? *Stroke* 1996;27: 1200–1204.
278. Horner J, Massey EW. Silent aspiration following stroke. *Neurology* 1988;38:317–319.
279. Horner J, Buoyer FG, Alberts MJ, Helms MJ. Dysphagia following brain-stem stroke. Clinical correlates and outcome. *Arch Neurol* 1991; 48:1170–1173.
280. Barer DH. The natural history and functional consequences of dysphagia after hemispheric stroke. *J Neurol Neurosurg Psychiatry* 1989;52: 236–241.
281. Horner J, Brazer SR, Massey EW. Aspiration in bilateral stroke patients: a validation study. *Neurology* 1993;43:430–433.
282. Bath PMW, Bath FJ, Smithard DG. Interventions for dysphagia in acute stroke. The

Cochrane Database of Systemic Reviews. 2000, Volume 3.

283. Lucas C, Rodgers H. Variation in the management of dysphagia after stroke: does SLT make a difference? *Internat J Lang Comm Disord* 1998;33(Suppl):284–289.
284. Mann G, Hankey GJ, Cameron D. Swallowing function after stroke: prognosis and prognostic factors at 6 months. *Stroke* 1999;30:744–748.
285. Domenech E, Kelly J. Swallowing disorders. *Med Clin N Am* 1999;83:97–113.
286. Addington WR, Stephens RE, Gilliland K, Rodriguez M. Assessing the laryngeal cough reflex and the risk of developing pneumonia after stroke. *Arch Phys Med Rehabil* 1999;80:150–154.
287. Addington WR, Stephens RE, Gilliland KA. Assessing the laryngeal cough reflex and the risk of developing pneumonia after stroke: an interhospital comparison. *Stroke* 1999;30:1203–1207.
288. Holas MA, DePippo KL, Reding MJ. Aspiration and relative risk of medical complications following stroke. *Arch Neurol* 1994;51:1051–1053.
289. DePippo KL, Holas MA, Reding MJ. Validation of the 3-oz water swallow test for aspiration following stroke. *Arch Neurol* 1992;49:1259–1261.
290. Collins MJ, Bakheit AM. Does pulse oximetry reliably detect aspiration in dysphagic stroke patients? *Stroke* 1997;28:1773–1775.
291. Zaidi NH, Smith HA, King SC, Park C, O'Neill PA, Connolly MJ. Oxygen desaturation on swallowing as a potential marker of aspiration in acute stroke. *Ageing* 1995;24:267–270.
292. Hamdy S, Aziz Q, Rothwell JC, et al. Recovery of swallowing after dysphagic stroke relates to functional reorganization in the intact motor cortex. *Gastroenterology* 1998;115:1104–1112.
293. DePippo KL, Holas MA, Reding MJ, Mandel FS, Lesser ML. Dysphagia therapy following stroke: a controlled trial. *Neurology* 1994;44:1655–1660.
294. Klor BM, Milianti FJ. Rehabilitation of neurogenic dysphagia with percutaneous endoscopic gastrostomy. *Dysphagia* 1999;14:162–164.
295. O'Mahony D, McIntyre AS. Artificial feeding for elderly patients after stroke. *Ageing* 1995;24:533–535.
296. Aithal GP, Nylander D, Dwarakanath AD, Tanner AR. Subclinical esophageal peristaltic dysfunction during the early phase following a stroke. *Digest Dis Sci* 1999;44:274–278.
297. Lucas CE, Yu P, Vlahos A, Ledgerwood AM. Lower esophageal sphincter dysfunction often precludes safe gastric feeding in stroke patients. *Arch Surg* 1999;134:55–58.
298. Norton B, Homer-Ward M, Donnelly MT, Long RG, Holmes GK. A randomised prospective comparison of percutaneous endoscopic gastrostomy and nasogastric tube feeding after acute dysphagic stroke. *BMJ* 1996;312:13–16.
299. James A, Kapur K, Hawthorne AB. Long-term outcome of percutaneous endoscopic gastrostomy feeding in patients with dysphagic stroke. *Ageing* 1998;27:671–676.
300. Wijdicks EF, McMahon MN. Percutaneous endoscopic gastronomy after acute stroke. Complications and outcome. *Cerebrovasc Dis* 1999; 9:109–111.
301. Allman RM, Laprade CA, Noel LB, et al. Pressure sores among hospitalized patients. *Ann Intern Med* 1986;105:337–342.
302. Tutuarima JA, van der Meulen JH, de Haan RJ, van Straten A, Limburg M. Risk factors for falls of hospitalized stroke patients. *Stroke* 1997;28:297–301.
303. Nyberg L, Gustafson Y. Patient falls in stroke rehabilitation. A challenge to rehabilitation strategies. *Stroke* 1995;26:838–842.
304. Mayo NE, Korner-Bitensky N, Becker R, Georges P. Predicting falls among patients in a rehabilitation hospital. *Am J Phys Med Rehabil* 1989;68:139–146.
305. Nyberg L, Gustafson Y. Fall prediction index for patients in stroke rehabilitation. *Stroke* 1997;28:716–721.
306. Schleenbaker RE, McDowell SM, Moore RW, Costich JF, Prater G. Restraint use in inpatient rehabilitation: incidence, predictors, and implications. *Arch Phys Med Rehabil* 1994;75:427–430.
307. Rapport LJ, Webster JS, Flemming KL, et al. Predictors of falls among right-hemisphere stroke patients in the rehabilitation setting. *Arch Phys Med Rehabil* 1993;74:621–626.
308. Stein J, Viramontes BE, Kerrigan DC. Fall-related injuries in anticoagulated stroke patients during inpatient rehabilitation. *Arch Phys Med Rehabil* 1995;76:840–843.
309. Gamble GE, Jones AK, Tyrrell PJ. Shoulder pain after stroke: case report and review. *Ann Rheum Dis* 1999;58:451.
310. Zorowitz RD, Hughes MB, Idank D, Ikai T, Johnston MV. Shoulder pain and subluxation after stroke: correlation or coincidence? *Am J Occup Ther* 1996;50:194–201.
311. Arsenault AB, Bilodeau M, Dutil E, Riley E. Clinical significance of the V-shaped space in the subluxed shoulder of hemiplegics. *Stroke* 1991;22:867–871.
312. Linn SL, Granat MH, Lees KR. Prevention of shoulder subluxation after stroke with electrical stimulation. *Stroke* 1999;30:963–968.
313. Mngoma NF, Culham EG, Bagg SD. Resistance to passive shoulder external rotation in persons with hemiplegia: evaluation of an assessment system. *Arch Phys Med Rehabil* 1999;80:531–535.
314. Sato Y, Kaji M, Saruwatari N, Oizumi K. Hemiosteoporosis following stroke: importance of pathophysiologic understanding and histologic evidence. *Stroke* 1999;30:1978–1979.
315. Ramnemark A, Nyberg L, Lorentzon R, Olsson T, Gustafson Y. Hemiosteoporosis after severe stroke, independent of changes in body composition and weight. *Stroke* 1999;30:755–760.
316. Ramnemark A, Nyberg L, Lorentzon R, Englund U, Gustafson Y. Progressive hemiosteoporosis on the paretic side and increased bone mineral density in the nonparetic arm the first year after severe stroke. *Osteoporosis International* 1999;9:269–275.
317. Sato Y, Kuno H, Kaji M, Ohshima Y, Asoh T, Oizumi K. Increased bone resorption during the first year after stroke. *Stroke* 1998;29:1373–1377.
318. Sato Y, Tsuru T, Oizumi K, Kaji M. Vitamin K deficiency and osteopenia in disuse-affected

limbs of vitamin D–deficient elderly stroke patients. *Am J Phys Med Rehabil* 1999;78:317–322.
319. Sato Y, Honda Y, Kunoh H, Oizumi K. Long-term oral anticoagulation reduces bone mass in patients with previous hemispheric infarction and nonrheumatic atrial fibrillation. *Stroke* 1997;28:2390–2394.
320. Sato Y, Maruoka H, Oizumi K. Amelioration of hemiplegia-associated osteopenia more than 4 years after stroke by 1 alpha-hydroxyvitamin D3 and calcium supplementation. *Stroke* 1997;28: 736–739.
321. Sato Y, Kuno H, Asoh T, Honda Y, Oizumi K. Effect of immobilization on vitamin D status and bone mass in chronically hospitalized disabled stroke patients. *Ageing* 1999;28:265–269.
322. Sato Y, Kuno H, Kaji M, Saruwatari N, Oizumi K. Effect of ipriflavone on bone in elderly hemiplegic stroke patients with hypovitaminosis D. *Am J Phys Med Rehabil* 1999;78:457–463.
323. Sato Y, Kaji M, Tsuru T, Oizumi K. Carpal tunnel syndrome involving unaffected limbs of stroke patients. *Stroke* 1999;30:414–418.
324. Sharpe M, Hawton K, Seagroatt V, et al. Depressive disorders in long-term survivors of stroke. Associations with demographic and social factors, functional status, and brain lesion volume. *Br J Psychiatry* 1994;164:380–386.
325. House A, Dennis M, Molyneux A, Warlow C, Hawton K. Emotionalism after stroke. *BMJ* 1989;298:991–994.
326. Pohjasvaara T, Leppavuori A, Siira I, Vataja R, Kaste M, Erkinjuntti T. Frequency and clinical determinants of poststroke depression. *Stroke* 1998;29:2311–2317.
327. O'Rourke S, MacHale S, Signorini D, Dennis M. Detecting psychiatric morbidity after stroke: comparison of the GHQ and the HAD Scale. *Stroke* 1998;29:980–985.
328. Paradiso S, Robinson RG. Minor depression after stroke: an initial validation of the DSM-IV construct. *Am J Geriatr Psychiatry* 1999;7:244–251.
329. Astrom M, Adolfsson R, Asplund K. Major depression in stroke patients. *Stroke* 1993;24: 976–982.
330. Palomaki H, Kaste M, Berg A, et al. Prevention of poststroke depression: 1 year randomised placebo controlled double blind trial of mianserin with 6 month follow up after therapy. *J Neurol Neurosurg Psychiatry* 1999;66:490–494.
331. Kauhanen M-L, Korpelainen JT, Hiltunen P, et al. Poststroke depression correlates with cognitive impairment and neurological deficits. *Stroke* 1999;30:1875–1880.
332. Fujikawa T, Yokota N, Muraoka M, Yamawaki S. Response of patients with major depression and silent cerebral infarction to antidepressant drug therapy, with emphasis on central nervous system adverse reactions. *Stroke* 1996;27:2040–2042.
333. Ghika-Schmid F, Bogousslavsky J. Affective disorders following stroke. *Eur Neurol* 1997;38: 75–81.
334. Paolucci S, Antonucci G, Pratesi L, Traballesi M, Grasso MG, Lubich S. Poststroke depression and its role in rehabilitation of inpatients. *Arch Phys Med Rehabil* 1999;80:985–990.
335. Shimoda K, Robinson RG. The relationship between poststroke depression and lesion location in long-term follow-up. *Biological Psychiatry* 1999;45:187–192.
336. Galynker I, Prikhojan A, Phillips E, Focseneanu M, Ieronimo C, Rosenthal R. Negative symptoms in stroke patients and length of hospital stay. *J Nervous Mental Dis* 1997;185: 616–621.
337. van de Weg FB, Kuik DJ, Lankhorst GJ. Post-stroke depression and functional outcome: a cohort study investigating the influence of depression on functional recovery from stroke. *Clin Rehabil* 1999;13:268–272.
338. Everson SA, Roberts RE, Goldberg DE, Kaplan GA. Depressive symptoms and increased risk of stroke mortality over a 29-year period. *Arch Intern Med* 1998;158:1133–1138.
339. Teasell RW, Merskey H, Deshpande S. Antidepressants in rehabilitation. *Phys Med Rehabil Clin N Am* 1999;10:237–253.
340. Reding MJ, Orto LA, Winter SW, Fortuna IM, Di Ponte P, McDowell FH. Antidepressant therapy after stroke. A double-blind trial. *Arch Neurol* 1986;43:763–765.
341. Vuilleumier P, Ghika-Schmid F, Bogousslavsky J, Assal G, Regli F. Persistent recurrence of hypomania and prosopoaffective agnosia in a patient with right thalamic infarct. *Neuropsychiatry, Neuropsychology, & Behavioral Neurology* 1998; 11:40–44.
342. Fujikawa T, Yamawaki S, Touhouda Y. Silent cerebral infarctions in patients with late-onset mania. *Stroke* 1995;26:946–949.
343. Astrom M. Generalized anxiety disorder in stroke patients. A 3-year longitudinal study. *Stroke* 1996;27:270–275.
344. Schramke CJ, Stowe RM, Ratcliff G, Goldstein G, Condray R. Poststroke depression and anxiety: different assessment methods result in variations in incidence and severity estimates. *J Clin Exp Neuropsychology* 1998;20:723–737.
345. Everson SA, Kaplan GA, Goldberg DE, Lakka TA, Sivenius J, Salonen JT. Anger expression and incident stroke. *Stroke* 1999;30:523–528.
346. Eslinger PJ, Warner GC, Grattan LM, Easton JD. "Frontal lobe" utilization behavior associated with paramedian thalamic infarction. *Neurology* 1991;41:450–452.
347. Andersen G, Ingeman-Nielsen M, Vestergaard K, Riis JO. Pathoanatomic correlation between poststroke pathological crying and damage to brain areas involved in serotonergic neurotransmission. *Stroke* 1994;25:1050–1052.
348. Mukand J, Kaplan M, Senno RG, Bishop DS. Pathological crying and laughing: treatment with sertraline. *Arch Phys Med Rehabil* 1996; 77:1309–1311.
349. Derex L, Ostrowsky K, Nighoghossian N, Trouillas P. Severe pathological crying after left anterior choroidal artery infarct. Reversibility with paroxetine treatment. *Stroke* 1997;28: 1464–1466.
350. Brown KW, Sloan RL, Pentland B. Fluoxetine as a treatment for post-stroke emotionalism. *Acta Psychiatrica Scandinavica* 1998;98:455–458.

351. Andersen G, Vestergaard K, Riis JO. Citalopram for post-stroke pathological crying. *Lancet* 1993;342:837–839.
352. Kidd D, Stout RW. The assessment of acute stroke in general medical wards. *Disability & Rehabilitation* 1996;18:205–208.
353. Adams HP, Jr., Brott TG, Furlan AJ, et al. Guidelines for thrombolytic therapy for acute stroke: a supplement to the guidelines for the management of patients with acute ischemic stroke. A statement for healthcare professionals from a Special Writing Group of the Stroke Council, American Heart Association. *Circulation* 1996;94:1167–1174.
354. Norris JW, Buchan A, Cote R, et al. Canadian guidelines for intravenous thrombolytic treatment in acute stroke. A consensus statement of the Canadian Stroke Consortium. *Can J Neurol Sci* 1998;25:257–259.
355. Anderson DC. Primary and secondary stroke prevention in atrial fibrillation. *Semin Neurol* 1998;18:451–459.
356. Delashaw JB, Broaddus WC, Kassell NF, et al. Treatment of right hemispheric cerebral infarction by hemicraniectomy. *Stroke* 1990;21: 874–881.
357. Pulmonary Embolism Prevention (PEP) Trial Collaborative Group. Prevention of pulmonary embolism and deep vein thrombosis with low dose aspirin: Pulmonary Embolism Prevention (PEP) trial. *Lancet* 2000;355:1295–1302.
358. Langhorne P, Stott DJ, Robertson L, et al. Medical complications after stroke. A multicenter study. *Stroke* 2000;31:1223–1229.

Chapter 14

REHABILITATION AND RECOVERY AFTER ISCHEMIC STROKE

GUIDELINES FOR REHABILITATION

Most physicians focus on the acute treatment of patients with stroke and leave the subsequent convalescence and recovery activities to the direction of specialists in rehabilitation. Still, physicians should know about the goals and guidelines for rehabilitation of survivors of stroke. Rehabilitation is a key component in the comprehensive array of stroke services.[1,2] Successful rehabilitation is critical for successful recovery of many patients who have survived stroke. In many ways, rehabilitation is a learning process; it is an activity that requires the patient and family to relearn the activities that they once took for granted. The spectrum of stroke-related services is broad, and choices for treatment are influenced by an individual patient's needs. In addition to preventing death and disability, another goal of modern treatment of acute ischemic stroke is to avoid the necessity of undergoing a prolonged program of rehabilitation that is time-consuming and expensive.

Several terms are important in assessing stroke rehabilitation and long-term care.[3] *Impairment* reflects the types and severity of neurological deficits. *Disability* reflects the behavioral consequences of the impairment and involves a change in the patient's interaction with the environment and daily activities. *Handicap* refers to the social and societal consequences of the disability, leading to changes in the patient's role.[3,4] These nuances are critical because disability and handicap after stroke will vary considerably among patients with similar neurological impairments. Career and occupation before stroke, living environment, family support system, and cultural or societal norms all influence the individual patient's status with regard to disability or handicap.

Several stages are included in the rehabilitation process.[2,3,5,6] (See Table 14–1. Fig. 14–1 and) Rehabilitation usually begins as soon as the patient is stable medically and then progresses in response to the patient's improvements.[7,8] Rehabilitation is more than just a collection of individual activities dealing with the motor, sensory, language, and cognitive sequelae of stroke. An integrated, interdisciplinary approach seems to have a greater effect on outcomes than do special treatment modalities or a great intensity of therapy.[9] Comprehensive services can be used to assess impairment, improve communication, and speed mobility.[7,10] A randomized trial evaluating rehabilitation found that a team approach with coordinated activities improved outcomes, especially among men.[11] To date, a stroke-team strategy that imitates the in-patient model probably has the best chance for increasing the likelihood of meaningful recovery after stroke.

Table 14–1. **Steps in the Process of Rehabilitation**

Baseline and subsequent assessments
Severity of neurological impairments
Responses to treatments
Medical condition
Goal planning
Accommodation and occupation
Personal support
Needed interventions selected
Organization of rehabilitation efforts
Plans for long-term care

Goals for Rehabilitation

The ultimate goal of rehabilitation is have the patient return to his or her status before the stroke. This lofty goal might be achieved among patients who have minimal neurological deficits following their stroke; however, many patients with stroke cannot achieve this level of recovery. As a result, goals set for rehabilitation should be audacious but still achievable. They should reflect the severity of the patient's neurological impairments, the patient's age, the presence of severe co-morbid diseases, and the social situation. For example, elderly patients and those with bilateral signs are the least likely to be independent and to be discharged to a community setting after rehabilitation.[12] Goals should not be unrealistic because the patient and family may be disappointed if the goals are not achieved. This sense of failure can exacerbate many social and emotional problems that follow stroke.

A sizeable proportion of patients are dissatisfied with their experience in rehabilitation; among the complaints are insufficient therapy, lack of information, and poor recovery.[10] To avoid this dissatisfaction, the patient and family must be fully informed throughout the rehabilitation process. Decisions must be made jointly by health care providers, the patient, and the family.[2] These decisions include selection of the types of and setting for rehabilitation, the need for ancillary services, and plans for discharge to the community. Specific plans for rehabilitation management should include types of treatments and their sequence, intensity, frequency, and expected duration.[2] These decisions should not be considered irrevocable and may be modified during the rehabilitation process. Because the sequelae of stroke can affect the patient and family for the rest of their lives, long-term plans for re-integration into society should be included.

Monitoring Responses to Rehabilitation

Patients should be assessed at regular intervals throughout the rehabilitation process. Guidelines have recommended

Clinical evaluation during acute care
Purposes
Determine etiology, pathology, and severity of stroke
Assess co-morbidities
Document clinical course
When
On admission and during acute hospitalization
By whom
Acute care physician
Nursing staff
Rehabilitation consultants

Screening for rehabilitation
Purposes
Identify patients who may benefit from rehabilitation
Determine appropriate setting for rehabilitation
Identify problems needing treatment
When
As soon as patient is medically stable
By whom
Rehabilitation clinicians

Not referred for rehabilitation
- No or minimal disability
- Too severely disabled to participate in rehabilitation. Provide supportive services; consider rescreening at a future date if condition improves

Referred for individual rehabilitation services (rehabilitation nurse, occupational therapist, physical therapist, psychologist, speech-language pathologist)
- Same assessment stages as for interdisciplinary program

Referred to interdisciplinary rehabilitation program in out-patient facility, home, inpatient unit or facility, or nursing facility

Assessment on admission to rehabilitation
Purposes
Validate referral decision
Develop management plan
Provide baseline for monitoring progress
When
Within 3 working days for an intense program;
1 week for a less intense inpatient program;
or three visits for an outpatient or home program
By whom
Rehabilitation clinicians/team

Assessment during rehabilitation
Purposes
Monitor progress
Adjust treatment regimen
Provide basis for discharge decision
When
Weekly for intense program
At least bi-weekly for less intense programs
By whom
Rehabilitation clinicians/team

Assessment after discharge from rehabilitation
Purposes
Evaluate adaptation to home environment
Determine need for continued rehabilitation services
Assess caregiver burden
When
Within 1 month of discharge
Regular intervals during first year
By whom
Rehabilitation clinicians
Principal physician

Figure 14–1. Stages of assessment for post-stroke rehabilitation. (Reprinted from Gresham GE, Duncan PW, Stason WB, et al. *Post stroke rehabilitation* [Clinical Practice Guideline, No. 16]. Rockville, MD: US Department of Health and Human Services, Public Health Service, Agency for Health Care Policy and Research. AHCPR Publication No. 95-0662. May, 1995.)

that a patient's progress be assessed weekly during an intense rehabilitation program in either an in-patient rehabilitation unit or a high-level nursing facility.[2] Progress should be documented at least every 14 days for patients who are being treated in less intense nursing units, as an out-patient, or in a home program.[2] A detailed program using standard rating instruments should be applied to the evaluation of responses to rehabilitation.[13] However, criteria for monitoring responses to rehabilitation vary among inpatient units, skilled nursing facilities, and home health care programs.[14] In general, standardized measures administered at baseline are re-examined at these points in time. Measures are selected to target the impairments and disabilities that have been the focus of treatment.[2] Changes in responses can prompt transfer from one type of rehabilitation setting to another. For example, a patient who is improving rapidly while in a skilled nursing facility might be moved to an inpatient rehabilitation unit to receive more intensive and concentrated services. As the patient improves and rehabilitation interventions become less frequent, the timing of the assessments can become less frequent.

SELECTION OF PATIENTS FOR REHABILITATION

Rehabilitation is an expensive process. An intensive program involves the participation of a large number of professionals. It is time-consuming and requires special and limited resources. Thus, the selection of patients to undergo rehabilitation becomes a critical initial step. A goal of modern stroke treatment is to limit neurological injury so that the patient does not have impairments, disability, or handicap after stroke. Patients who recover from stroke do not need any rehabilitation. Patients with very mild impairments may need very little, if any, rehabilitation. A brief period of instruction from a physician or a rehabilitation specialist may suffice—the patient could receive a series of activities to do independently. Another group of patients are not good candidates for rehabilitation because of their poor neurological status. For example, nursing care and supportive measures likely will be the only long-term treatment for patients who are in a prolonged coma following stroke. Still, a sizeable proportion of patients with mild-to-severe neurological sequelae will need rehabilitation. It is critical to focus on the patients who have the best chances for maximizing recovery (Fig. 14–2).

Several groups have evaluated factors that predict poor or good responses to rehabilitation.[15–25] (See Table 14–2.)

Location of Stroke and Severity of Neurological Impairments

Miyai et al[26] found that patients with hemispheric infarctions in the basal

Table 14–2. **Clinical Factors that Predict a Poor Response to Rehabilitation after Ischemic Stroke**

Strong negative predictors	Probably negative predictors
Coma or prolonged decreased consciousness	Advanced age
Poor cognition	Low intellect
Urinary or bowel incontinence for more than 2 weeks after stroke	Language impairments
Severe motor impairments	Sensory loss greater on left than right side
Little motor recovery within 1 month after stroke	Homonymous hemianopia
Previous strokes	Absence of spouse or close family member
Presence of perceptual-visual-spatial defects	Positive predictors
Poor sitting balance	Strong family support
Neglect	Strong financial support
Severe apraxia	High socioeconomic class
Heart or other co-morbid diseases	High level of education
	Early initiation of rehabilitation
	Comprehensive rehabilitation program

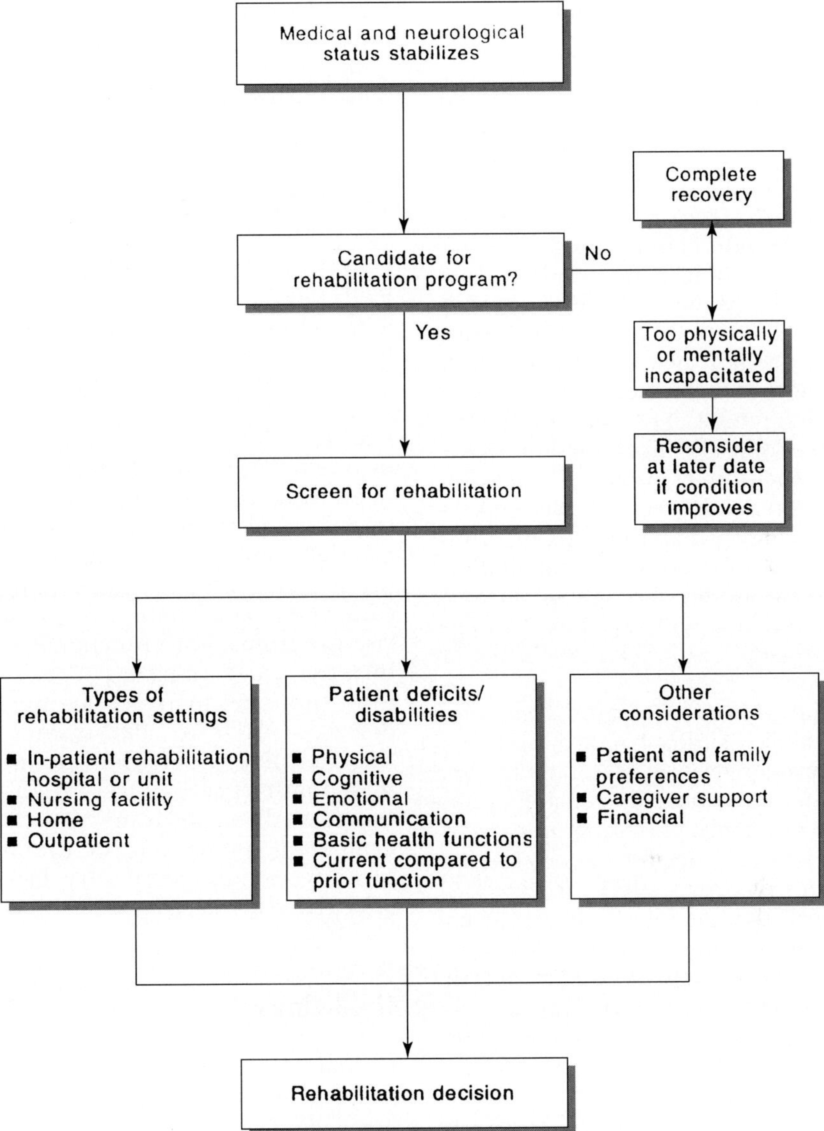

Figure 14–2. Framework for rehabilitation decisions. (Reprinted from Gresham GE, Duncan PW, Stason WB, et al. Post stroke rehabilitation [Clinical Practice Guideline, No. 16]. Rockville, MD: US Department of Health and Human Services, Public Health Service, Agency for Health Care Policy and Research. AHCPR Publication No. 95-0662. May, 1995.)

ganglia and the internal capsule may not respond well to rehabilitation because of the persistent loss of interactions between subcortical structures, which impede relearning and the restoration of neural connections. Although the presence of these findings does not mean that rehabilitation is contraindicated or that rehabilitation efforts will be unsuccessful, they do forecast poorer recovery. Another study found that a cortical infarction and involvement of the right hemisphere predicted poorer responses to rehabilitation.[27] In contrast, patients with brain stem infarctions improve rapidly, and many can regain nearly full functional independence.[28]

Galski et al[29] found that cognitive impairments, including changes in comprehension, judgement, verbal memory, and abstract thinking, affect responses to rehabilitation. Cassvan et al[30] found that patients with a right hemiparesis recovered ambulation more quickly than did patients with left-sided weakness. Wade et al[31] did not find a real difference between recovery from right or left hemiplegia. Paolucci et al[32] found that the presence of cognitive impairments, global aphasia, or hemineglect increased the likelihood of poor outcomes, including impaired mobility after stroke. In another report, these investigators concluded that the patients who responded best to in-patient rehabilitation included those under the age of 65 and those who did not have aphasia or neglect.[33] Depression also affects responses to rehabilitation.[34,35]

Wade and Hewer[36,37] found that age, functional ability, sitting balance, and urinary incontinence were important factors in predicting responses to rehabilitation. Urinary incontinence persisting more than 7–10 days is a very negative predictor for survival or recovery after stroke.[38,39] Bonita and Beaglehole[40] noted that recovery of motor function after stroke correlated with the severity of impairments at the time of the event. Age was not as important a predictor of outcomes. The chances of recovery were 10 times greater among patients with mild strokes than for those with severe strokes. In contrast, Alexander[41] concluded that recovery was strongly related to the combination of a patient's age and severity of neurological signs. He noted that 100% of his patients younger than 55 were able to return home, and 96% of patients who had mild deficits were discharged to home after rehabilitation.

Interval from Stroke

The time from stroke until the onset of rehabilitation probably affects responses. Still, the time window is not as important as other factors in predicting the affects of rehabilitation.[42] Early rehabilitation and minor impairments also increased the likelihood of good functional outcomes.[33]

Co-morbid Diseases

Severe co-morbid diseases, including heart disease, arthritis, diabetes mellitus, and lung disease, influence choices for rehabilitation and predict the utilization of resources.[43–46] (See Table 14–3.) In particular, the development of congestive heart failure, urinary tract infections, or pneumonia can affect the length of stay in an acute care setting and delay transfer to a rehabilitation center.[47] Heart disease can delay initiation of rehabilitation, complicate the clinical course and ancillary care, limit participation in physical exercise programs, limit functional status, and increase early mortality.[45,48,49] In addition, non-cerebrovascular neurological diseases, such as Parkinson's disease, degenerative dementia, or peripheral neuropathy, can affect rehabilitation. Issues such as insurance coverage, governmental regulations, or the availability of beds at subsequent care facilities also affect transfer decisions.[50]

Guidelines

Guidelines provide detailed recommendations for screening eligibility for rehabilitation.[2] (See Tables 14–3 and 14–4. and Fig. 14–3.) The first step in screening involves the patient's neurological and medical condition. Thereafter, the patient's pre-morbid medical history and social and environmental factors should be assessed. Based on these factors, a group of rehabilitation specialists can advise about the type and setting of continued rehabilitation. Baseline assessment, which includes consultation from rehabilitation specialists (physical therapy, speech pathology, and occupational therapy at a minimum), is required before the patient can be moved to a rehabilitation program.

Table 14–3. **Screening for Rehabilitation: Neurological and Medical Factors**

- Neurological impairments assessed by a standard rating instrument—National Institutes of Health Stroke Scale
  - Consciousness
    - Altered consciousness eliminates rehabilitation
- Cognitive and mental status assessed by a standard rating instrument—Mini Mental Status
  - Cognitive impairments
    - Severe deficits likely eliminate rehabilitation
    - Moderate deficits may impede rehabilitation
    - Mild-to-moderate deficits usually a focus of rehabilitation
  - Language impairments
    - Severe deficits may impede rehabilitation
    - Mild-to-severe deficits usually a focus of rehabilitation
  - Neglect
    - Severe deficits may impede rehabilitation
  - Depression
    - Unless treated, may impede rehabilitation
  - Vision
    - Severe deficits impede rehabilitation
  - Articulation
    - Mild-to-severe deficits usually a focus of rehabilitation
  - Swallowing
    - Severe deficits may not respond to rehabilitation
    - Mild-to-moderate deficits usually a focus of rehabilitation
  - Pain
    - Generally impedes rehabilitation and needs treatment
  - Sensory loss
    - Generally impedes rehabilitation
    - Usually is a focus of rehabilitation
  - Motor loss
    - Severe deficits (paralysis) have poor responses
    - Mild-to-moderate deficits (paresis) a focus of rehabilitation
  - Balance and coordination
    - Severe deficits (ataxia) impede rehabilitation
    - Mild-to-moderate deficits a focus of rehabilitation
- Presence of other neurological diseases evaluated
  - Peripheral neuropathy
  - Movement disorders, such as Parkinson disease
  - Dementia, such as Alzheimer disease
- Presence of serious co-morbid diseases evaluated
  - Heart disease
  - Lung disease
  - Diabetes mellitus
  - Poor vision or hearing
  - Psychiatric disease
  - Arthritis
  - Functional health patterns
    - Nutrition and hydration
    - Ability to swallow
    - Urinary or fecal incontinence
    - Skin integrity
    - Activity tolerance
    - Sleep patterns

SELECTION OF SITE FOR REHABILITATION

Patients can be transferred to several different sites for rehabilitation after discharge from an acute care setting (Fig. 14–3 and Table 14–5). The factors that portend responses to rehabilitation also affect the selection of location for these treatment modalities. The patient's and family's wishes also influence options for treatment. For example, a patient may opt to be transferred to a skill nursing facility close to home to have strong family support, rather than go to an in-patient rehabilitation facility in a more remote city.

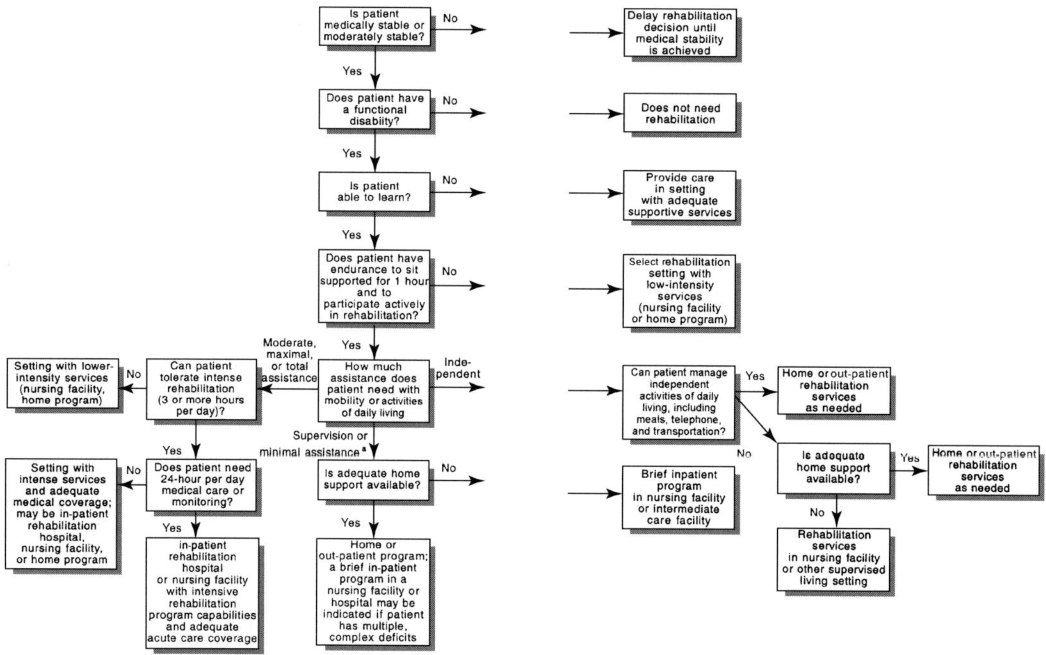

Figure 14–3. Selection of setting for rehabilitation program after hospitalization for acute stroke. (Reprinted from Gresham GE, Duncan PW, Stason WB, et al. *Post stroke rehabilitation* [Clinical Practice Guideline, No. 16]. Rockville, MD: US Department of Health and Human Services, Public Health Service, Agency for Health Care Policy and Research. AHCPR Publication No. 95-0662. May, 1995.)

Table 14–4. **Screening for Rehabilitation: Demographic, Social, and Environmental Factors of the Patient, Family, and Caregivers**

Age
Gender
Race and ethnicity or cultural beliefs
Primary language
Level of education
Financial resources and health insurance
Size of community and availability of resources
Memberships in religious groups, special interest groups, etc.
Members in the household and relationship to patient
Other potential caregivers within reasonable distances
Developmental stage and structure of family
Prior activities, including work
Prior socialization, leisure activities, and hobbies
History of mental illness, alcoholism, or other drug abuse
Ability to cope with illness, disability, and treatment
Expectations regarding outcomes, including rehabilitation
Willingness to seek assistance
Living environment—building, living quarters, facilities
Availability of community resources—health care, rehabilitation, transportation, home care agencies

In-Patient Rehabilitation Unit

In-patient rehabilitation hospitals, or units that function as part of another hospital, offer a full range of specialists in rehabilitation, who form an interdisciplinary team.[2,51] A physician who has expertise in rehabilitation directs the program. In

Table 14–5. **Sites for Rehabilitation**

In-patient rehabilitation unit
Free-standing in-patient rehabilitation unit
In-patient rehabilitation unit as part of another hospital
Skilled nursing facility
Outpatient
Home based
Day hospital programs
Out-patient clinics

general, the rehabilitation team meets regularly to review a patient's progress, adjust the rehabilitation regimen, and organize discharge plans. The usual members of the team are listed in Table 14–6. In-patient treatment is the most expensive and intense form of rehabilitation after stroke. In general, the patient transferred to an in-patient rehabilitation program should need at least two forms of traditional rehabilitation (physical therapy, speech pathology, or occupational therapy). The patient must have a reasonable chance of responding to rehabilitation and have the stamina to be able to participate in it for at least 3 hours per day.[2] Most patients who transfer to in-patient rehabilitation settings also need medical care and monitoring.

Table 14–6. **Rehabilitation Professionals**

Physician
Physiatrist
Neurologist
Other
Nurse care manager
Physical therapist
Occupational therapist
Speech pathologist
Recreation therapist
Vocational counselor
Social worker
Neuropsychologist

COMPLICATIONS DURING IN-PATIENT REHABILITATION

Patients in an in-patient rehabilitation setting are at risk for the same complications of stroke described in Chapter 13. With the pressure to transfer patients from an acute care hospital to a rehabilitation setting within a few days of stroke, many patients admitted to in-patient rehabilitation are at high risk for subacute neurological and medical complications. As a result, the interventions aimed at preventing or treating the complications described in Chapter 13 remain important parts of medical management in the rehabilitation unit. In one series, 147 medical complications developed during the rehabilitation of 245 patients; most complications were among patients with severe stroke.[52] Urinary tract infections, falls, musculoskeletal pain, aspiration pneumonia, and skin problems were the most common complications.[45,52–54] Concomitant heart disease, hypertension, sleep apnea, deep vein thrombosis, malnutrition, and seizures also may need to be addressed during rehabilitation in the hospital.[45,46] In general, the likelihood of a patient developing complications in rehabilitation settings correlates with the severity of the stroke and the length of hospital stay.[53]

ADMISSION TO IN-PATIENT REHABILITATION

Most patients with moderate-to-severe deficits following their first stroke should be admitted to an in-patient rehabilitation center.[43] These patients have the best chances for maximal recovery. Younger patients (in general under the age of 75) benefit the most from in-patient rehabilitation (Table 14–7).[55] A focused stroke-rehabilitation unit improves both the degree and the rapidity of recovery while reducing mortality and the likelihood of a patient being transferred to a skilled nursing facility for long-term care.[56–59] A comparison of in-patient to out-patient rehabilitation found that intensive care within a housed unit reduced the likelihood of death or disability from 38% to 23%.[51]

Table 14–7. **Admission to an In-Patient Rehabilitation Program**

Moderate-to-severe neurological impairments
Normal consciousness and restricted cognitive impairments
Need for at least two of three major rehabilitation therapies (physical, occupational, speech)
Younger age (usually <80, but flexible)
Absence of severe co-morbid medical or neurological diseases
Stamina for at least 3 hours of therapy per day
Relatively good functional status before stroke
Well-motivated patient and family

This same study found that patients with moderate-to-severe strokes seemed to benefit the most from intensive inpatient rehabilitation.

DISCHARGE FROM IN-PATIENT REHABILITATION

Once a patient has gained maximal benefit from in-patient rehabilitation, he or she should be transferred to another setting (see Fig. 14–3). Patients who have achieved independence or who need only minimal assistance or supervision usually can be discharged to home. Patients may need subsequent home or out-patient rehabilitation services tailored to their residual impairments. Those who do not improve after in-patient rehabilitation likely will be transferred to a nursing facility that has a lower intensity of medical and rehabilitation services.

Skilled Nursing Facility

The capabilities of long-term care nursing facilities for rehabilitation vary widely. Many long-term care facilities provide supportive nursing care and very low levels of rehabilitation. Much of the care is primarily custodial. However, in response to the need for patients to have rehabilitation in a less intense environment than an in-patient rehabilitation hospital, many nursing facilities have developed coordinated rehabilitation programs.[2] In general, rehabilitation in a skilled nursing care facility is less expensive than in a hospital setting. Still, these services can be very effective in improving outcomes after stroke.[60]

ADMISSION TO A SKILLED NURSING FACILITY

Skilled nursing care facilities can handle patients who need some component of medical care and some level of rehabilitation. Skilled nursing facility rehabilitation must be distinguished from long-term care, and the patient and family must understand this difference. Although these facilities are less aggressive than inpatient rehabilitation hospitals, the rehabilitation program still has a goal of returning the patient to home. Patients who cannot return home but have neurological impairments that require only one type of rehabilitation therapy can be treated in a skilled nursing unit. For example, a patient who needs only gait training for poor balance can be admitted. In addition, patients whose health will not permit several hours of therapy per day can be treated in a skilled care nursing facility. A patient with heart disease and poor stamina might receive rehabilitative care in a skilled care nursing facility. Patients who have completed in-patient rehabilitation at a hospital might be transferred to a skilled nursing facility when their medical condition no longer requires close medical supervision. In general, a patient's progress is monitored every 1 or 2 weeks.

LONG-TERM NURSING CARE

Elderly patients and those with very severe stroke likely will be admitted to a nursing home.[61] In one population study, approximately 25% of survivors of stroke were located in a nursing home at 90 days after stroke.[61] More than one-half of patients with poor scores on standardized disability scales were transferred.[61] Patients most likely to be admitted to a long-term care facility include those with advanced age, severe lower or upper limb weakness, or language deficits.[62] Unless a patient has profound deficits from the stroke or severe co-morbid diseases that preclude rehabilitation, he or she should not be transferred directly from an acute care setting to a nursing home (see Fig. 14–3). Thus, most patients who are admitted to a long-term care facility have been transferred from another rehabilitation setting. Even those in a long-term care facility should receive access to rehabilitative efforts. Admittedly, efforts are not as intense or coordinated as in other rehabilitation settings. Still, improvements in mobility or language could greatly improve the quality of these patients' lives even if they are not able to return to independence or home.

Out-Patient Rehabilitation

Out-patient rehabilitation can involve therapy prescribed in the patient's home or another community setting or measures administered to a patient who travels to a rehabilitation center.[51] (See Table 14–5.) Out-patient rehabilitation is less expensive than in-patient or skilled nursing facility treatment because it can lessen the costs of nursing and medical care. It can follow a period of in-patient therapy, increasing the gains achieved in this initial period of treatment.[63] (see Fig. 14–3.)

Out-Patient rehabilitation requires that the patient travel to the site for treatment. If transportation is a problem, then an in-home program might be needed. Out-patient facilities provide the same comprehensive battery of services provided in an in-patient setting. It has several advantages, including access to an interdisciplinary program and equipment. The out-patient clinic also provides for social contact and peer support for patients who are living at home.[2] Day hospital programs are variations on out-patient rehabilitation that usually are more intense. In fact, the day hospital program mimics in-patient rehabilitation except that the patient is housed at home, receiving several hours of therapy per day for several days a week.[2] Frequent physician contact and the weekly monitoring system used in in-patient settings is applied to day hospital programs.

The use of out-patient therapy varies widely among patients. Some patients may have sporadic visits to one therapist, whereas others may be seen several times a week. The interval from stroke and prior rehabilitation activities influences choices for out-patient rehabilitation. A common scenario is more frequent visits early in the course of rehabilitation and then a gradual tapering of the number of encounters. At times, out-patient rehabilitation can be combined with services provided at home.[218] For example, a patient may be seen in an out-patient clinic once a week but receive other therapies at home on a more frequent basis.

Most home rehabilitation programs are designed for medically stable patients who require only intermittent contact with rehabilitation services.[2,218–220] Care usually is coordinated by a home health care agency. Depending on the patient's needs, services that can be provided include nursing, physical therapy, speech therapy, occupational therapy, social services, and home assistance. Assistance with meals and self-care can be provided. A major advantage of home care rehabilitation is that learning takes place in the location where the skills will be used.[2] Patients also benefit from the psychological support of being home with family. Nevertheless, home rehabilitation can increase the responsibility and burden on a family member or other caregiver. Some rehabilitation equipment may not be available, and substitutes might need to be found. For example, parallel bars will not be present in a home. Bars might need to be attached to the walls of a patient's home so that the patient can practice walking. In addition, in-home rehabilitation programs deprive the patient of social interactions and peer support from other patients, which might aggravate a sense of isolation. Thus, although home rehabilitation has many attributes, its use as a solitary treatment site should be restricted to patients who do not have the ability to travel to an out-patient program.

Information about the usefulness of long-term out-patient rehabilitation is mixed. One survey found that focused stroke rehabilitation programs did not produce a strong benefit in improving outcomes.[64] Conversely, Marsh[65] found that a day rehabilitation stroke program, in which the patient receives therapy approximately 6 hours a day for several days a week, could improve outcomes. Baskett et al[66] and Young and Forster[67] recently noted that supervised, home-based programs are as effective as out-patient or day hospital rehabilitation.

Costs of home care programs are considerable. The expense of providing coordinated medical, nursing, and rehabilitative services in a home setting are high. In addition, home care does not eliminate the need for subsequent in-patient care. Thus, home care or domiciliary care programs do not seem to help reduce use of hospital resources.[68]

INDIVIDUAL REHABILITATION SERVICES

Physical Therapy

When most physicians consider rehabilitation, their primary focus is on physical therapy. In most situations, physical therapy is a key component in efforts to maximize recovery after stroke (Table 14–8). Recovery of mobility and motor skills is key to regaining independence in performing self-care activities. The goal of physical therapy is to teach the patient to manage impaired mobility and sensorimotor deficits by the use of exercise, functional training, compensatory techniques, and assistive devices.[2] Physical therapy usually is prescribed as part of a coordinated team approach. It can be done in either an in-patient or an out-patient setting. Skilled care nursing facilities and home health programs have physical therapists as part of their group of rehabilitation specialists. A meta-analysis showed that relatively intensive physical therapy significantly reduces mortality or neurological worsening and enhances recovery after stroke.[69]

Table 14–8. **Physical Therapy Activities: Treatment of Patients with Ischemic Stroke**

Sensory impairments
Develop methods to accommodate for diminished sensory input
Teach compensatory strategies for loss of proprioception and position sense
Pain
Position the upper limb using slings or supports
Elevate upper limb to reduce edema of the upper limb
Use ice, heat, or ultrasound to treat musculoskeletal pain
Avoid exercises that can increase shoulder pain
Range of motion
Use passive or active range-of-motion exercises
Motor function
Use modalities that assist in contraction of muscles
Assist in isokinetic, isometric, eccentric, or concentric exercises
Exercise agonist and antagonist muscle groups
Increase complexity of muscle actions as condition improves
Mobility and balance
Practice sitting, standing, transferring, walking
Practice reaching, turning, changing directions, carrying objects
Practice going up and down stairs and ramps

PERSONNEL

Often, several individuals will be part of a physical therapy team. A physical therapist has completed at least 4 years of college and has a master's degree in physical therapy. Physical therapists must pass a licensure examination. Just as among physicians, physical therapists often specialize in particular aspects of physical rehabilitation. Some physical therapists have a special interest in cardiac, orthopedic, or rheumatologic rehabilitation, whereas others develop expertise in neurological care. This distinction is important because approaches to rehabilitation differ.[70] A physical therapist who frequently treats patients with sequelae of brain disease usually will be a member of a stroke rehabilitation team. Their experience is critical for optimal physical therapy. In comparison, a physical therapy assistant usually has 2 years of college education, and a physical therapy aide has had training by a local program. The assistant and aide work under the direction of the physical therapist. A usual physical therapy session will last approximately 45 minutes.[71]

INTERVAL FROM STROKE

The timing of physical therapy is critical. It should be started as soon as the patient is medically stable and, thus, will begin while the patient still is in an acute care setting. The timing of the initiation of physical therapy corresponds with a period of spontaneous recovery after the acute neurological event. Milestones in improvement of mobility are available. A study of 238 patients with stroke showed that sitting balance usually can be achieved on the day of stroke, standing balance can be reached by 3 days, and 10-step walking can be accomplished by 6 days in most cases.[72] Motor recovery is most rapid within 30 days after stroke.[73] Still, Bonita and Beaglehole[40] noted that approximately 70% of stroke survivors had some motor impairment at 1 month. By 6 months, this number had dropped to approximately 60%. A majority of the recovery after stroke occurs within the first 3 months. The rate of improvement is slow thereafter.[34,74] In general, patients with severe motor dysfunction will not achieve independence in activities of daily living, but those with moderate motor impairments will have major increases in recovery.[75] However, motor deficits usually are mild or absent among most patients who survive more than 6 months after stroke.[40] Although recovery of sensorimotor function and mobility is most dramatic during the first weeks after stroke, patients can benefit from physical therapy prescribed months later. Wade et al[76] reported that physical therapy prescribed 1 year following stroke could improve mobility and gait. Thus, patients may benefit from a program of physical therapy that involves long-term follow up and care.

RECOVERY FROM MOTOR AND SENSORY IMPAIRMENTS

The patterns and types of motor and sensory impairments greatly influence decisions about physical therapy. In general, the rapidity of recovery of the motor function in the upper and lower limbs occurs at approximately the same rate in both limbs.[73] However, many patients, especially those with infarctions in the territory of the middle cerebral artery, have more severe deficits in the upper limbs than in the lower ones. As a result, the amount of functional recovery of the upper limbs often is less than in the lower. In particular, recovery of useful fine movement of the hand can be limited. Some patients with severe motor impairment in the arm have little improvement, regardless of the level of physical therapy.[77]

The process of recovery of motor or sensory function after stroke is complex.[78,79] This is an area of ongoing research, and information about the mobilization of neural structures to help in the relearning process will expand considerably in the future. To date, some information is available about the events that lead to the return of useful motor skills following stroke. Motor recovery seems to involve the activation of brain structures remote from the stroke, including the motor cortex, sensory cortex, visual cortex, cerebellum, thalamus, and basal ganglion.[80] Motor recovery may involve the activation of unaffected corticomotor projections from the contralateral hemisphere to stimulate pre-existing uncrossed motor pathways or activate midline muscles.[81] For example, uncrossed cortico-spinal fibers from the right hemisphere might become active in an attempt to improve right-sided function following a left hemisphere stroke. Imaging evidence of the presence of Wallerian degeneration of the pyramidal tract may slow functional recovery, but it does not limit outcome after rehabilitation among patients with hemiparesis.[82] Thus, even if some pathologic–anatomic consequences of stroke are irreversible, the brain appears to be able to develop compensatory mechanisms to maximize physiological responses. These compensatory mechanisms must be realized by the physical therapist to reach the highest degree of functional recovery possible.

RECOVERY OF GAIT AND COORDINATION

Gait disturbances are relatively common after ischemic stroke. They can be secondary to motor or sensory impairments or due to disorders of balance and coordination. The spectrum of disorders of station and gait will reflect the location and extent of brain injury and include ataxic, apraxic, or hemiparetic disturbances. Occasionally, a patient will have a freezing episode while walking; in this situation, the motor function of the paralyzed side suddenly halts.[83] Low rates of increase in force and postural swaying with changes in position identify a patient as being at high risk for falling during the initiation of gait training.[84] Abnormal movements of the upper limb, trunk, pelvis, and lower limb are seen on the ipsilateral side and the unaffected contralateral side during walking.[85,86] Measures that involve synchronous activation of axial trunk muscles on both sides of the body appear to be critical in recovering mobility and motor function.[87] Disorders in balance greatly limit the recovery of mobility. Intact balance reactions are correlated strongly with the ability to walk.[88] Good balance depends on several neural systems, including vestibular, cerebellar, proprioception, and motor control. Astasia-abasia (the inability to sit unassisted and falling backward) can occur in patients with thalamic infarctions.[89]

RECOVERY OF SPECIFIC MOTOR FUNCTIONS

Several components of muscle function affect the ability to move the paretic limbs and restoration of mobility. Slowness in developing torque usually contributes to the weakness of the paretic muscles.[90] As the velocity of movements improves, the abnormal movements decrease. Focusing physical therapy on strength and coordination of the hemiplegic side appears to be an important goal for maximizing recovery.[85] Extensor muscle overactivity is a component of gait disorders after stroke. It must be addressed in rehabilitating patients with hemiparesis.[91] An evaluation of repetitive movements of the side of the body ipsilateral to a hemispheric infarction also is important.[92] Deficiencies in movement were seen with right (non-dominant) hemisphere lesions but not left (dominant) hemisphere strokes. This observation may explain some of the problems in rehabilitation and recovery of balance in patients with right hemisphere events. Decreased proximal motor function can amplify other motor impairments, including defects in sequencing movements. These findings can affect responses to physical therapy.[93] The control and execution of motor skills are affected and involve more than learning these functions.[94]

IMPORTANCE OF SENSORY LOSS IN RECOVERY

Intact sensory function is associated with good motor recovery.[34] In particular, a loss of position and vibratory sense decreases mobility and hampers the efficacy of physical therapy. Very severe sensory loss leads to syndromes such as *the alien hand,* in which patients feel that their hand is foreign and driven by an external agent. This sign occurs in association with strokes involving the frontal and callosal regions.[95] The presence of an alien hand syndrome limits recovery from physical or occupational therapy. Visuospatial function also affects arm motor recovery after stroke.[96] Patients may not be able to participate in physical exercises because of visual loss or more complex visually mediated disturbances, such as optic ataxia. A distortion of perceived space may exacerbate the motor and sensory problems among patients with right hemisphere stroke.[97,98] Including measures focusing on neglect as part of the physical therapy program also may improve motor and functional recovery.[99] Lin[100] reported that using lateralized task, limb activation, and controlled sensory stimulation approaches can help in the treatment of sensorimotor impairments among patients with neglect. The use of mirrors might lessen neglect.[101] Sensorimotor stimulation can increase muscle activity.[102] This intervention is most effective in patients with severe deficits, including patients with hemi-anopia or hemi-inattention.

OTHER FACTORS THAT AFFECT RECOVERY

Orthopedic complications can complicate physical therapy. Contractures or adhesive capsulitis can limit limb function. Severe shoulder pain can impede responses to rehabilitation.[34] Changes in motor tone can lead to spasticity that in turn reduces mobility. Spasticity with unilateral hemispheric stroke is associated with modulation of muscle stretch reflexes.[103] The changes likely will affect the patient's ability to improve walking.

ACTIVITIES OF PHYSICAL THERAPY

Physical therapists focus on improving posture control, walking, standing, balance, and upper limb function.[71,104] (See Table 14–8.) Coordinating physical therapy with other rehabilitative activities increases motor performance.[11,105] A review of physical therapy concluded that there is strong information to support its use as a component of rehabilitation after stroke; patients having rehabilitation had better motor recovery than would be anticipated with spontaneous improvement.[106] Ernst[106] concluded that even a small benefit could mean the difference in living at home or in a long-term care institution. A comparison of rehabilitation programs that focused efforts on improving either upper or lower limb function recently showed that an emphasis on leg training was likely to improve activities of daily living, walking, and dexterity.[107] Therefore, the net benefit of a physical therapy program focusing on improving leg activity is greater than one that aims at improving arm function. Patients with severe arm impairment generally do not improve with physical therapy regardless of the intensity of the intervention.[108] However, intensive treatment of patients with some motor recovery of the upper limb is effective.[108] Adults with stroke have improvements in the less affected upper limb.[109]

MODES OF PHYSICAL THERAPY

Several models of physical therapy are used (Table 14–9). The remedial approach involves traditional physical therapy exercises and neuromuscular facilitation.[2] *Remediation* involves forced sensory stimulation modalities, exercises, and resistance training to enhance motor recovery. Using the *compensatory model*, the goal of therapy is to achieve independence in activities of daily living by trying to improve function rather than stimulating motor recovery.[2] *Constraint-induced movement* and forced use therapies can be applied to improve function among patients with chronic motor impairments.[110,111] Compensatory techniques may be used to improve function after motor recovery has reached a plateau. It also may be the preferred approach when a patient has severe motor impairments. A third model is based on the concept that motor control entails complex interactions among the neurological and musculoskeletal systems and the environment.[2] The concept involves task-specific motor control. Data are not available to suggest that treatment based on one theory of physical

Table 14–9. **Modes and Ancillary Techniques of Physical Therapy**

Remediation
Compensation
Constraint-induced movement
Intermittent pneumatic compression devices
Acupuncture
Sensory stimulation
Biofeedback
Robot training
Electric stimulation

therapy is superior to other strategies.[2] A large number of therapeutic interventions have been used to improve motor recovery and neuromuscular function (see Table 14–5). These activities are labor intensive and expensive, and additional research is needed to study their utility. Aerobic exercises can improve sensorimotor function.[112,113] Low-intensity treadmill exercises can be used to help improve walking among hemiparetic patients who have heart disease.[114] Increasing the level or time of physical therapy sessions has not been associated with a corresponding increase in recovery when compared with results of conventional levels of therapy.[115]

ANCILLARY TECHNIQUES

Because of a loss of autonomic innervation of the fine arteries of the paralyzed limb, trophic changes, including edema, can occur. Edema of the dependent limbs (hand and foot) can be considerable and cause pain. *Intermittent pneumatic compression devices* have been used to reduce edema in a paralyzed hand. Roper et al[116] found that such devices do not assist in eliminating this aspect of chronic paralysis. To date, elevation of the hand and increasing mobility appear to be the best ways to reduce distal limb edema. Pain and dysesthesias in the affected arm and leg can complicate subcortical infarctions and limit the effects of rehabilitation. *Acupuncture* has been used in conjunction with rehabilitation.[117] Although limited data suggest that acupuncture might relieve pain and spasticity, it is not a standard form of treatment following stroke.

Sensory stimulation has been used as an adjunct to improve recovery and posture.[118] *Biofeedback* also has used as an ancillary technique to improve function beyond traditional physical therapy.[119] Goals have focused on improving balance and increasing range of motion, speed of walking, and integrated movements. The results of studies of biofeedback have been inconclusive.[2,120] *Robot training* has been used to enhance motor outcomes after stroke.[121] The use of this newly developed assistive device has not been tested in clinical trials. Cyclic *electric stimulation* of the wrist can improve function of the extensors and limit upper limb disability.[122] Neuromuscular stimulation causes contraction of the paralyzed muscles of the hand and reduces hand edema.[123,124] It can produce short-term increases in muscle strength and motor control and relieve spasticity.[125] However, the effects on functional recovery are unclear.[2] Hummelsheim et al[125] found that electrical stimulation did not help either biomechanical or functional movement.

ADAPTIVE AND ORTHOTIC DEVICES

Adaptive and orthotic devices should be prescribed only if other ways of performing a task are not available or cannot be learned.[2] (See Table 14–10.) Any device

Table 14–10. **Orthotic Devices and Equipment to Improve Activities of Daily Living**

Transportation
Manual or electrically powered wheelchair
Single or quad cane
Pickup or rolling walker
Transfer board to assist in movement to and from bed, chair, shower, automobile
Gait/transfer belt
Hydraulic lifts or electric stair lift
Higher seats on toilet and chairs
Bedside commode, urinal, or bedpan
Toilet seat with rails or bars
Shower chair with rails or bars
Non-skid mats in shower
Other devices
Large handles on eating utensils
Rocker knife
Non-skid mats, plate guards, or scoop dishes
Cups
Long-handled sponge
Adapted razor, toothbrush and brush
Self-adhesive closures for clothes and shoes
Elastic shoestrings
Long-handled shoe horn
One-handed buttoning device
Communication devices
Communication board or book
Pacing boards
Electronic communication devices

should have proven safety and efficacy. The patient, family, and other caregivers must be trained in the proper use of these devices. Prescription of a device should be considered as a supplement to, rather than a substitute for, other measures to recover function. Many of these devices are expensive. Financial issues, including insurance payments, should be reviewed before they are prescribed.

Several assistive and orthotic devices can be used to improve sensorimotor function after stroke (see Table 14–6). A *wheelchair* can be used if a patient has severe motor impairments or poor stamina.[2] It should be adapted to the patient's individual needs. The use of a *cane* when walking can improve spatial variables among patients with hemiparetic gaits.[126] Lower limb orthotic devices are prescribed if the knee or ankle needs to be stabilized for the patient to walk. These devices can be used to facilitate gait training and reduce the energy cost of walking.[2] Because of the potential for spasticity and clonus, spring-loaded ankle braces usually are not prescribed to patients with hemispheric stroke. Other orthotic devices are given to stabilize the wrist or improve fine-motor function of the hand. Other devices can assist in activities of daily living (see Table 14–6). These devices usually are recommended by an occupational therapist.

Treatment of Spasticity

Spasticity can greatly impede the recovery of mobility and motor function after stroke.[45] To limit the effects of spasticity, physical therapists emphasize range-of-motion activities and placement of the limbs in positions that antagonize the usual patterns. In addition, a number of medications can be prescribed to limit the effects of spasticity. Most of these medications cause some element of muscle weakness, and the decision to prescribe these agents must consider this potential side effect.

The most promising treatment involves the local injection of *botulinum toxin*. The medication, which is widely used to treat dystonias, can be used to ease restricted areas of spasticity following stroke.[127] Burbaud et al[128] reported that botulinum toxin was useful in treating lower limb spasticity during the first year after stroke. Patients often have excessive plantar flexion and inversion at the ankle that limits the ability to walk. Injections led to clear symptomatic improvement in spasticity of the foot, improving both movements of the ankle and ambulation.[129,130] Cromwell and Paquette[131] successfully administered injections of botulinum toxin to the biceps and quadriceps femoris muscles in a patient with quadriparesis and involuntary movements following a brain stem infarction. After the injections, the patient's mobility increased considerably. Similar experiences have been reported with treatment of spasticity in the upper limbs. Bhakta et al[132] found that botulinum toxin could be injected safely into the biceps, forearm flexors, and finger flexors to relieve spasticity of the upper limbs. They noted less disability and improved hand function following the injections. The effects of the botulinum toxin injection usually last several weeks to a few months. Repeated injections may be needed, and some patients will develop antibodies to the toxin and the effective of the agent will be lost.

Baclofen is used orally or by intrathecal injection to lessen spasticity. It acts by potentiating the effects of the inhibitory neurotransmitter gamma aminobutyric acid in the spinal cord. Baclofen can cause generalized weakness and drowsiness as well as reduce motor tone. Sudden discontinuance of baclofen also can lead to seizures, hallucinations, and psychosis.[133] Most patients will receive oral doses of baclofen that are gradually escalated until the patient's symptoms are improved or unless side effects appear. Intrathecal

Table 14–11. **Medical Treatment of Spasticity**

Botulinum toxin injections
Baclofen
Dantrolene
Alcohol or phenol nerve blocks
Surgical cutting of nerves

infusions of baclofen have been used to treat severe spasticity in patients with multiple sclerosis, spinal cord injury, or cerebral palsy.[134] Patients will have relief of spasticity, improved range of motion in both the upper and lower limbs, and improved abilities for activities of daily living. The pain and involuntary movements associated with the spasticity also can be relieved. Treatment involves the placement of an intrathecal catheter, and the baclofen is administered continuously via a pump. Intrathecal infusions of baclofen can be used to treat severe spasticity after serious brain diseases, including stroke.[135,136] Still, the number of patients treated with intrathecal infusions of baclofen following stroke is limited.

Dantrolene sodium inhibits the intracellular transport of calcium in muscle cells and, as a result, muscle contractility is lessened.[137] Dantrolene affects the strength of muscles in both the paralyzed and unaffected limbs, and weakness is a common complaint. It also can lead to hepatotoxicity. Limited evidence is available to show that dantrolene is effective in reducing spasticity and improving outcomes after stroke.[138] Still, it is an option if the patient cannot tolerate baclofen or does not respond to local injections of botulinum toxin.

Diazepam has been used to relax hypertonic muscles, but the medication appears not to be as effective as baclofen. In addition, the potential for abuse of diazepam is a strike against long-term administration of the agent for treatment of spasticity. Nerve blocks with *phenol* or *alcohol* can be used to treat severe spasticity. However, the effects of these agents are irreversible, and their use should be restricted to treatment of severely affected, bed-bound patients. Chronic *epidural stimulation* of the *spinal cord* or stimulation of antagonist muscles and nerves, *surgical rhizotomy*, and *myelotomy* are potential options for treatment of profound spasticity.[139] These surgical procedures are very rarely done to treat patients after stroke.

Occupational Therapy

Occupational therapy involves measures that improve functional independence, including improvement of hand and finger function. The usual goals are to improve functional recovery of the upper limbs, to achieve independence in activities of daily living, and to help in the patient's return to the community.[140] An occupational therapist can prescribe devices to assist in meeting these goals.[71]

PERSONNEL

A registered occupational therapist has had 4 years of education and an internship.[2] A certified occupational therapy assistant has had 4 years of education and a 12-week internship. An assistant usually works under the direction of a registered occupational therapist.

OCCUPATIONAL THERAPY MODALITIES

Occupational therapy after stroke was tested in a small, randomized trial.[141] Patients who had occupational therapy had higher recovery on standard disability scales and less handicap and caregiveer strain than did those who did not have treatment. The presence of apraxia can slow the relearning of self-care skills.[142] A number of assistive and orthotic devices can improve functional independence (see Table 14–10). The use of objects in a functional context will improve coordinated movements and goal-directed actions.[143] Out-patient occupational therapy has been shown to increase the activities of daily living, reduce handicap, and lessen strain on caregivers.[144] A key activity of the occupational therapist is to assess the patient's ability to function independently or under supervision. This assessment is critical when deciding whether a patient can be discharged to home alone or with family members.

Speech Pathology

PERSONNEL

Speech and language pathologists treat patients with disorders of language, articulation, or swallowing (Table 14–12). In the United States, these professionals have had

Table 14–12. **Rehabilitation Activities of Speech Pathologist**

Assess swallowing, speech, and language
Assist in improving swallowing
Assist in improving articulation
Use communication assistance devices
Assist in improving language
Aural comprehension
Oral production
Reading
Writing

4 years of college and have earned a master's degree in speech-hearing-language pathology.[2] In addition, the speech pathologist must undergo supervised clinical observation and perform a clinical fellowship before obtaining a certificate of clinical competence. Many speech pathologists concentrate their practices in educational settings and treat children who have disorders of articulation. A smaller number of speech pathologists have extensive experience in dealing with acquired language or articulation problems in adults. Fortunately, the speech pathologist in a stroke team usually has considerable expertise. However, persons with the same level of experience may not be available to facilitate subsequent outpatient speech therapy in small communities. Some studies have demonstrated that trained volunteers can be as effective as a trained speech pathologist in improving language function following stroke.[145] However, a detailed, accurate evaluation of language impairments remains a prerequisite for effective therapy, and this evaluation can best be done by a trained speech pathologist.

SWALLOWING

Issues that are related to treating patients with swallowing deficits are discussed in Chapter 13. The interventions started in an acute care setting likely will be continued during rehabilitation. The goal is for the patient to return to normal eating and drinking and to achieve normal levels of hydration and nutrition.

ARTICULATION

The goals of speech therapy in treating disorders of articulation are to restore the normal intelligibility of speech or to use other strategies or devices when speech remains unintelligible.[2] Sensory stimulation; exercises to strengthen the muscles of the pharynx, mouth, lips, and tongue; positioning; and improving respiratory capacity can be prescribed with the goals of improving respiration, phonation, resonation, articulation, and prosody.[2] Several devices can be used to assist severely dysarthric patients with communication (see Table 14–10).

APHASIA

Severe disorders of language (aphasia) lead to severe disability and handicap after stroke. Most aphasic patients cannot be employed, and the inability to convey one's thoughts greatly lessens quality of life. Fortunately, most patients will have some recovery of language function. Several factors, including the patient's age, sex, handedness, and level of education, affect recovery from aphasia.[146] In addition, the patient's emotional and motivational levels, severity and type of aphasia, and location of the brain lesion also influence the recovery of language function. Aftonomos et al[147] reported that improvement in language function did not differ greatly among functional levels or types of aphasia. Recovery from aphasia can occur rapidly, and it appears to be concomitant with activation of changes in brain activity from the left hemisphere to homologous regions of the right hemisphere.[148] Basso et al[149] found that rehabilitation could improve language skills, but responses to speech therapy were affected by the severity of the language impairments and the time after stroke. Selnes[150] found that the degree of recovery was not associated with the volume of the lesion but did seem to be correlated with destruction in the posterior, superior temporal lobe. These findings of plasticity may be important in organizing rehabilitative efforts to regain language. Changes in prosody and language are independent and mediated by different hemispheres.[151] This dissociation can be used to modulate language recovery.

TREATMENT OF APHASIA

The goals of treating aphasia are several and include restoration of the patient's ability to speak, comprehend aural speech, read, and write.[2] The speech pathologist assists the patient in developing tactics to deal with language problems and to deal with the psychological consequences of aphasia. A speech pathologist also can help family members and caregivers in their communication with the patient.[2] Data about the usefulness of speech and language therapy are mixed, and the role of language rehabilitation is unclear.[152–154] Regular support and encouragement appear to be a key component of efforts to speed recovery of language.[145]

Cognitive Rehabilitation

Efforts to improve cognition also can be prescribed. Treatments emphasize retraining, substitution of intact abilities, and compensatory approaches.[2] The results of psychological testing correlate closely with improvements in self-care found after stroke.[155] In addition, the severity of behavioral impairments is directly related to the status of the patient on admission to either an acute care hospital or a rehabilitation unit.[155] Patients with right hemisphere stroke may have difficulty in understanding pragmatic and social nuances that affect efforts to recover after stroke.[156] Behavioral therapy can be added to traditional physical therapy for treatment after stroke.[157] The usefulness of cognitive rehabilitation has not been established for improving outcomes after ischemic stroke.

Treatment of Depression

Depression may persist for months and years after stroke.[158] It can be the result of a normal reaction to the changes in an individual's life caused by the stroke or a manifestation of a specific brain injury (see Chapter 13). In addition, pre-existing psychiatric disease, concomitant medical conditions, and side effects of medications also can lead to depression. Treatment of depression remains an important component of rehabilitation after stroke. Abnormal behavior, including depression, forecasts poor functional competence and performance after discharge from rehabilitation.[159,160] Mild depression can respond to increased attention and encouragement from the family or staff.[2] More severe depression can be treated with psychotherapy, tricyclic antidepressants, or selective serotonin reuptake inhibitors.

RESTORATIVE THERAPIES

A number of medications are being evaluated to determine their usefulness in speeding recovery after stroke.[161,162,221] Agents that may assist in improving outcome can modulate relearning and recovery.[163] Among the medications that might enhance recovery are neurotrophic growth factors, amphetamines, antidepressants, gamma aminobutyric acid agonists, and citicoline.[161] Crisostomo et al[164] reported that amphetamines promote the recovery of motor function following stroke. Another study showed that concomitant administration of amphetamines paired with physical therapy accelerated recovery after stroke.[165] Dam et al[166] tested the value of fluoxetine and maprotine in improving patients with hemiplegia who were undergoing rehabilitation. They found that fluoxetine, a selective serotonin reuptake inhibitor, improved recovery. The other medication did not offer any benefit. Wiart et al[222] reported that fluoxetine was efficacious in treating post-stroke depression. Another study tested the effect of nimodipine on recovery of memory following ischemic stroke.[167] Patients who were given the medication for 7–14 days after stroke had improved memory function at 3 months.

In contrast, some medications can have a negative influence on motor responses or other outcomes after ischemic stroke (Table 14–13). Among the medications that might adversely affect recovery are clonidine, prazosin, neuroleptics, dopamine antagonists, phenytoin, benzodiazepines, and phenobarbital.[161,168,169] Additional research

Table 14–13. **Medications that Might Impede Recovery After Stroke**

Clonidine
Prazosin
Neuroleptic medications
  Pheothiazines
  Haloperidol
Phenytoin
Benzodiazepines
Phenobarbital

is needed to determine whether restorative medications can be used to improve outcomes after ischemic stroke. Cell transplants have been used in an attempt to improve motor recovery after stroke.[223,224]

RETURN TO SOCIETY

Although the focus of treatment of patients with stroke is on acute care and rehabilitation, one should not lose sight of the long-term consequences of the illness. A sizeable proportion of patients will live for many years after a cerebrovascular event. Some of the consequences of stroke will affect the patient and the family for the rest of their lives. Even patients with mild stroke will have sequelae that affect their lives. Thus, the physician, other health care providers, the patient, and the family need to plan for the patient's return to everyday society. The importance of these activities is highlighted by the studies of long-term outcomes. During a follow-up evaluation 14 years after stroke, Tuomilehto et al[170] found that 19.4% of 1241 patients were still living and that 80% of these persons were at home. In a survey of patients with stroke followed for 20 years, Gresham et al[171] reported that the overall functional status of patients was good and that mortality rates were similar to that found among patients with no history of stroke.

Thus, the approach to care of patients must include plans for long-term treatment. The physician treating the patient with stroke should anticipate and address several issues in medical and nursing care. Management should include plans for the long-term treatment of risk factors for stroke and prescription of medications that can prevent recurrent stroke. In some instances, continued nursing care and home health services, including rehabilitation, might be needed on a long-term basis. A strategy to modify services and reduce their intensity as the patient improves might be included in the treatment plan. Re-integration into the family and community must be addressed. Several of the issues listed in Table 14–4 affect plans for returning to society. In particular, addressing the emotional consequences of stroke and the change in life are important for both a patient's and family's well-being. Some patients will need assistance in applying for worker's compensation, welfare, or disability benefits. In addition, issues such as returning to work, leisure activities, sex, and driving should be included.

Discharge from Rehabilitation

Discharge from either an acute care hospital or an in-patient rehabilitation unit often is accompanied by considerable stress for the patient and family. This change in status is particularly traumatic for a stroke patient. The patient has had a serious, potentially life-threatening brain illness. Fear of another event is very real. The stroke may have caused motor, sensory, or cognitive impairments that affect the lives of all family members. Although, at this point, the acute and subacute treatment of stroke and its consequences are completed, issues of long-term care are only beginning. Adjustments to the realities of the new situation are critical for the patient's smooth transition back to society. Several steps in planning are required, and active collaboration of the patient and family is critical. Keeping the patient and family informed and vested in the transition to new care settings is critical for success.

LONG-TERM NURSING CARE

Several variables affect decisions about discharge and return to society (see Table 14–4). In general, the choices are to return home or to go to a housed, long-term care facility (nursing home). Most patients dread being placed in nursing homes, and they and their families will want to consider a return home as a preferred option. Still, a sizeable percentage of patients with stroke will require chronic institutionalized care.[172] A report by Gresham et al[173] found that 16% of stroke survivors were institutionalized. Another 31% of patients were dependent in self-care, and 20% had impaired mobility after stroke. Thus, changes in life-style or independence are prominent even if a patient is not in a nursing home. Patients who move to nursing homes generally are elderly and have had severe strokes causing motor or cognitive impairments that preclude independence in a usual living situation (see Table 14–14). Because many elderly women live alone, they have a higher risk of going to a nursing home than do similarly aged men.[174] Some patients require care that is beyond the capability of the family or visiting medical service providers to offer in home settings. In particular, many elderly patients have an equally frail spouse who cannot assume a role as primary caregiver. Other family members might not be readily available. In these circumstances, the patient may need to be admitted to a nursing home. Because these patients have such severe neurological impairments, their survival is reduced and the quality of their life is poor. They remain at high risk for complications of a chronic debilitating illness, such as infection, pressure sores, or orthopedic problems. Nursing home care is expensive and patients and families often worry that personal financial resources will be consumed to provide care for a loved one. A patient's financial status and health insurance coverage are important variables in deciding to transfer a patient to an extended-care facility. Governmental programs or welfare might be needed to pay for the costs of long-term institutionalized care.

Table 14–14. **Factors that Often Lead to Admission into Long-Term Nursing Care Units Following Stroke**

Severe neurological impairments
Decreased consciousness
Major cognitive impairments
Dementia
Major sensorimotor impairments
Severe co-morbid medical or neurological diseases
Dementia
Movement disorders
Neuropathy
Heart disease
Orthopedic diseases
Blindness
Limited independence before stroke
Advanced age
Living alone
Close family members not available
Close family members cannot provide care

Family members might feel guilty about not taking a patient home. Some cultures and religions emphasize the importance of family support and caring for relatives, particularly parents. Thus, a move to a nursing home may be very traumatic for the entire family. The sense of failure and economic implications of the stroke may affect all members of the family. This situation also means that family members may have a number of social problems that require attention. Education of the family and, if necessary, counseling may ease the transition to a nursing home.

RETURN TO A PATIENT'S HOME

Several levels of out-patient assistance are available depending on the community. Issues such as home health care services, transportation, home care assistance, and the living environment must be addressed (Table 14–15). If these services are readily available, then a patient might be discharged to home rather than to an extended-care institution. Home health care services will receive referrals from several sources, including hospitals, physicians, nurses, community groups, families, or patients.[175,176,219] The size of a community and its resources are critical. Many small communities may not have public transportation or other support services to permit living at home. However, the social

Table 14–15. **Issues to be Addressed Before Discharge to Home**

Severity of neurological impairments
Mild-to-moderate—home
Severe—care facility
Severity of co-morbid diseases
Required medical therapies
Living situation in patient's home
Family or other caregiver
Physical situation at home
Stairs/floors
Bath and toilet
Lights
Meal preparation
Community and neighbor support
Availability of home health care services
Nursing
Rehabilitation
Household/meals
Transportation
Medical and rehabilitation clinic visits
Recreation
Socialization

support of neighbors, friends, fellow church members, and relatives in a small community might be better than in a more urban area.

LIVING SITUATION IN THE PATIENT'S HOME

The discharge to home can follow several patterns. The patient could return to living alone. He or she may or may not need the assistance of professional home and health care services. Depending on the nature of the patient's disability and desires, services could include assistance in home making, delivery or preparation of meals, transportation to appointments, home-based rehabilitation, or home-based nursing care. Single patients and those with poor social support have poor outcomes after stroke.[160] Patients who live alone often achieve a high degree of activities of daily living but poor levels of socialization after stroke, whereas those living with another person will have the opposite findings.[177] The patient also could be placed in a household with family members or other persons. Patients may need to be placed in a living situation that includes support, or they may need the assistance of relatives or home health services.[176,178] The members of the household and their relationship to the patient should be clear before discharge. If the patient lives in a household, then another person—most commonly a spouse or adult child—assumes the role of primary caregiver. For example, assistance with meals or activities of daily living would be the responsibility of the primary caregiver. Ancillary professional health services could be involved in providing additional support in this environment. For example, a day care program, respite care, or nursing or home health services could be included in a management program after discharge.[179] Adult day care programs or respite care may be implemented to allow the primary caregiver time to work outside of the home or to have some independent social time.

Patient-Related Issues, Including Quality of Life

Most patients rate their health as being worse after a stroke.[180] This finding should not be surprising. Still, some patients and families report that stroke devastated their lives.[181] The affects of stroke are protean. In addition to the loss of independence, a stroke affects the patient's status in the family and in society. All aspects of normal life, from work to social activities, are affected. A patient may not be able to do usual recreational activities because of the impairments. A majority of patients with stroke report a rapid decline in the quality and quantity of leisure pursuits.[182] Sjogren[183] found that most patients have decreased leisure activities. Even if a decline in leisure activities might not be disabling in the traditional sense, it does affect the patient's sense of well-being. Gresham et al[173] found that 62% of stroke survivors had reduced socialization.

FACTORS THAT AFFECT INDEPENDENCE AFTER STROKE

Limitations after stroke can be influenced by several patient-specific variables. The patient's age and gender are important. An elderly patient who already is retired will have different goals from a younger patient who has dependent children. In the latter situation, a parent may want to work to provide financial support for his or her children or want to resume child-rearing activities. Still, these goals may differ among patients and will reflect the basic structure of the family. Other patient-specific factors that can influence return to home include race, ethnicity, cultural beliefs, primary language, and level of education. Although these factors often are not considered, they have a major impact on the ability of the patient to be at home. Physicians and other health care providers must be sensitive to these factors. For example, a patient whose primary language is not English may have severe problems in dealing with English-speaking caregivers unless the need for a translator is anticipated. Some cultures and ethnic groups resist the intrusion of non-family members in a home caregiving setting. In addition, the desire of family members to assist the patient in activities of daily living is very strong in some cultures. Although the family's assistance generally is positive, an over-solicitous approach may impede the patient's ability to practice skills for recovery from stroke.

The nature of neurological residuals after stroke also affects long-term outcomes. Self-care activities and involvement in social activities relate most strongly to arm function and visuospatial abilities.[96] Cognitive or language impairments also can cause disability or handicaps that affect the patient's activity in society. Disorders of comprehension, judgment, memory, or abstract thinking increase the likelihood of the need for home health care services after discharge from a rehabilitation unit.[29] Still, the types and severity of impairments do not directly predict a patient's status months or years after stroke. For example, types of impairments at 6 months do not correlate well with functional disability of psychosocial handicaps.[184]

LONG-TERM PSYCHOLOGICAL CONSEQUENCES OF STROKE

A sizeable proportion of severely affected patients have persistent complaints, such as pain, anxiety, decreased self-esteem, decreased energy, confusion, low mood, or urinary incontinence that cause a poor quality of life.[185–188] (See Chapter 13.) These affects are secondary to brain disease or psychological or emotional consequences of the stroke. In addition, a presence of depression or anxiety after return to home is associated with more disability and a poorer quality of life.[189] The prevalence of depression actually increases in the first year after stroke.[190] Severe depression in the first year after stroke can lead to agoraphobia, social withdrawal, apathy, self-neglect, irritability, or emotionalism.[191–193] Psychosocial handicaps and decreased sexual activity also lessen the quality of life.[192–194]

QUALITY OF LIFE—IMPLICATIONS IN LONG-TERM CARE

In general, the quality of life improves in the months after stroke, but it remains impaired for most patients. A poor quality of life is strongly associated with depression and the severity of neurological defects.[195] The many consequences of stroke must be considered in the plans for a patient's return to society. The cognitive, motor, and sensory impairments must be assessed, and plans must be made to help the patient to overcome them. In addition, the social and psychological sequelae are equally important. In many ways, these issues are even more important than the more obvious neurological impairments. Social re-integration involves changes in physical and financial environments.[196] A physician should seek help from psychiatry, social services, and rehabilitation teams to address these problems. Long-term measures to improve psychological symptoms and psychosocial support are critical.[181,197] Medications or counseling may be needed. Psychosocial interventions and education about stroke and its consequences for both the patient and the family are important ways to smooth the transition to society.[197,198] In particular, close communications among the patient, the family, and professionals remain important.[185] These communications should be ongoing.

Family Issues

Changes in family roles are common, and they have a major impact on recovery.[186] (See Table 14–15.) The functioning of the family affects the patient's course on return to home.[159] The family's ability to handle the issues related to stroke must be assessed, and family-specific plans should be developed before discharge.[199] (See Table 14–4.) Issues such as the other members in the household and the structure of the family should be addressed. The health and age of the primary caregiver can be critical. An elderly spouse who has poor health often cannot assume responsibilities for long-term care. Additional support services will be needed, particularly if other potential family caregivers do not live within a reasonable distance. The presence of small children or another person with a disability in the household also can affect decisions about a return to home. A history of mental illness, alcoholism, or other drug abuse in family members also can affect the ability of the patient to return home. The emotional status of family members and their ability to cope with the illness, its treatment, and residual disabilities are important. These features influence discharge planning because family caregivers often have anxiety or acute or chronic depression that affects their physical health and their sense of well-being.[181,200–202] The patient's family needs both educational and social support. Mobilization of social services, religious groups, neighbors, friends, or neighbors could provide help for the family.

PATIENT AND FAMILY EDUCATION

Education of the patient and the family about stroke and rehabilitation, including clear expectations about responses and complications, is critical for achieving a good outcome.[159] Family members should be encouraged to participate in the patient's effort to recover after stroke. They can assume several roles—caregiver, therapist, coach, and cheerleader. Involvement of community social services also should be encouraged. The presence of high social support appears to increase the speed and degree of recovery after stroke.[203] Glass et al[204] found that those patients with severe stroke but high support recovered better than did patients with mild stroke but little emotional support from relatives. The involvement of a stroke-family caseworker was tested in a randomized, controlled trial.[205] The presence of the social worker was associated with increased satisfaction of the patient and family and improved social outcomes. Caregivers' stress is an important factor in recovery after stroke.[206]

Recovery after stroke is a tedious process that can take years. Many friends and neighbors are available for assistance during the first months after the event; however, involvement in care may diminish during subsequent months. The primary caregiver and family members may develop a sense of isolation as support from volunteers declines. Thus, social services and other professional providers need to continue to be available for long-term care and support of the family.

Home Environment

In general, the patient's living arrangements before stroke correlates to the likelihood of being able to return to home.[207] A survey of 492 patients found that 301 survivors were at home with someone else in the household at 1 year after stroke.[208] Another 82 patients were living alone, and 53 were in long-term care facilities. Still, 147 patients living at home needed community services, including nursing interventions, home health aides, day care centers, and delivery of meals.[208] Because of the need for these services in the home, long-term economic costs of stroke are considerable. Leibson et al[209] calculated that the costs of care during the first year after stroke are approximately 3.4 times the medical costs the person needed in the year before the cerebrovascular event.

LIVING ENVIRONMENT

The patient's living quarters must be assessed (see Table 14–15). Location is critical. For example, an apartment on a second floor can make transportation into and out of the home difficult. A building with an elevator is a more acceptable location for a patient than a building with only a stairway. A two-story house can present problems for a patient who is relatively immobile. In many homes, the bedroom and bathroom may be on a different floor than other living spaces. The size of the house may result in the patient being in a relatively remote part of the building from where other members of the family usually are located. For example, persons who are watching television in the living room might not hear calls for help from a patient who has fallen in a distant bedroom. A narrow hallway may limit the ability of a patient to move easily in a wheelchair or a walker. Home adjustments and assistive devices often are needed to improve transfers and self-care activities.[178] The patient may need a hospital bed or a lift to be moved from a bed to a chair (see Table 14–10). A bedside commode, urinal, or bedpan may need to be purchased. Bathroom modifications may include an elevated seat on the toilet and rails with the toilet and shower. The kitchen and living room may involve changes in chairs, tables, and so forth. Rails could be added to hallways. Lighting and floor surfaces should be evaluated for the risk for falls. Assistive devices for activities of daily living can help the patient to regain independence.

Returning to Work

A sizeable proportion of persons with stroke are elderly. Thus, the issue of returning to work may not be paramount. However, younger patients often want to return to work (Table 14–16). Because patients' conditions often improve in the first weeks after stroke, governmental bodies often will not immediately declare that a patient is disabled as a consequence of stroke. Some patients will have such severe strokes that a return to work is an unattainable goal. The patient and family should not be given the unrealistic expectation that a patient with multiple cognitive, motor, and sensory impairments likely will return to pre-stroke vocational activity.

Table 14–16. **Factors that Influence Return to Work After Stroke**

Age
Occupation and level of income
Level of education
Severity and types of impairments
Ability to return to occupation before stroke
Ability to learn a new occupation
Types and severity of co-morbid medical and neurological diseases
Required medical therapies
Requirement to drive to work and availability of other forms of transportation
Social welfare system and types of disability programs
Personal motivation

The likelihood of a return to work can be predicted by several clinical factors. Black-Schaffer and Osberg[210] found that patients without aphasia and those who needed a short course of rehabilitation were most likely to be able to return to work. Wozniak et al[211] found that a return to work was most likely among patients with higher incomes and less severe stroke. Some patients may not be able to return to their pre-stroke jobs because of the nature of their residual impairments. For example, a person might not be able to manipulate heavy or dangerous equipment.

VOCATIONAL REHABILITATION

Vocational rehabilitation is an important part of activities to ease a patient's return to society.[198] Patients should be referred for this service. The importance of vocational rehabilitation is highlighted in the report by Gresham et al.[173] They found that 71% of patients had a reduction in vocational function after stroke. A reduction in status at work and in salary can follow. Follow-up information about outcomes was available from 65 of 71 young patients with ischemic stroke at least 1 year before evaluation.[194] Approximately two-thirds of the patients reported no major problems. Forty-six patients (73%) had returned to work. Still, occupational adjustments were required for 12 patients, and almost half of the patients had symptoms of depression. In other series of 30 young patients with stroke, 81% were able to return to work.[212] The status of a group of young adults was surveyed at an average of 6 years after ischemic stroke.[213] Only 42% of these patients had been able to return to work; most had residual emotional, social, and physical impairments.

Driving

For almost all adults, the ability to return to *driving* is a marker of independence and reintegration into social activities. Driving may not be a major problem for patients with mild strokes; however, the presence of cognitive, motor, and sensory impairments makes driving difficult. The required reaction times may be beyond the patient's motor skills. Prominent visual field impairments, visual loss, or neglect can mean that the patient cannot see hazards on the road or may miss road signs. The propensity for seizures also can affect a patient's driving status. Most patients are unable to return to driving after stroke.[214] On occasion, assistive devices might be used to help a patient drive; however, a patient should be evaluated by a licensing body before he or she starts operating a motor vehicle. An inability to drive can affect a patient's likelihood of returning to work. The consequences of not being able to drive are felt most keenly among persons who live in areas where public transportation is not readily available.

Sexual Dysfunction

Sexual dysfunction and dissatisfaction are common among both men and women with stroke and their spouses.[215] Issues include changes in general attitudes toward sexuality, impotence, and a lack of desire to participate in sexual activity.[215,216] Decreased libido, sexual arousal, and satisfaction appear to be related to hemisensory loss.[217] Male patients can have impaired erection and ejaculation, whereas female patients have impaired vaginal lubrication.[216,217] In addition, fear that sex might cause hypertension that induces another stroke is an issue.[216] Psychological and social factors are key problems related to sexuality that must be addressed.

SUMMARY

Stroke is remarkable not for the damage that it inflicts but for the recovery that it allows. All stroke survivors recover to some degree. The best results are obtained when the patients are carefully selected for the appropriate type of rehabilitation, goals are set, and responses to rehabilitation are monitored. Rehabilitation can take place in a range of settings, including in-patient rehabilitation hospitals, nursing facilities, and outpatient departments. The type and timing of rehabilitation are crucial. Physical, occupational, and speech therapy all have their optimal time and intensity. Although the evidence favors rehabilitation overall, component interventions are based more on practice than on proof. The advent of sophisticated brain imaging, the development of clinical trial methodology, and pilot data on promising drugs and interventions place us at the threshold of scientific restorative therapy. Return and reintegration into society are beset by many obstacles. Diminished capacity, financial issues, stress, and depression complicate recovery. Stroke affects the whole family; however, the very difficulties that the patient and family face can also be the beginning of a fruitful re-examination of life and relationships as well as a source of fulfillment and hope.

REFERENCES

1. Dennis M. Stroke services. *Lancet* 1992;339: 793–795.
2. Gresham GE, Duncan PW, Stason WB, et al. *Post-stroke rehabilitation.* U.S. Department of Health and Human Services, 1995.
3. Wade DT. Stroke: rehabilitation and long-term care. *Lancet* 1992;339:791–793.
4. Clarke PJ, Black SE, Badley EM, Lawrence JM, Williams JI. Handicap in stroke survivors. *Disability & Rehabilitation* 1999;21:116–123.
5. Pessin MS, Adams HP, Jr., Adams RJ, et al. American Heart Association Prevention Conference. IV. Prevention and rehabilitation of stroke. Acute interventions. *Stroke* 1997;28: 1518–1521.
6. Stewart DG. Stroke rehabilitation. 1. Epidemiologic aspects and acute management. *Arch Phys Med Rehabil* 1999;80:S4–S7.
7. Dombovy ML, Basford JR, Whisnant JP, Bergstralh EJ. Disability and use of rehabilitation services following stroke in Rochester, Minnesota, 1975–1979. *Stroke* 1987;18:830–836.
8. Jorgensen HS, Kammersgaard LP, Houth J, et al. Who benefits from treatment and rehabilitation in a stroke unit? A community-based study. *Stroke* 2000;31:434–439.
9. Cifu DX, Stewart DG. Factors affecting functional outcome after stroke: a critical review of rehabilitation interventions. *Arch Phys Med Rehabil* 1999;80:S35–S39.
10. Tyson SF, Turner G. The process of stroke rehabilitation: what happens and why. *Clin Rehabil* 1999;13:322–332.
11. Wood-Dauphinee S, Shapiro S, Bass E, et al. A randomized trial of team care following stroke. *Stroke* 1984;15:864–872.
12. Granger CV, Hamilton BB, Fiedler RC. Discharge outcome after stroke rehabilitation. *Stroke* 1992;23:978–982.
13. Granger CV, Hamilton BB. Measurement of stroke rehabilitation outcome in the 1980s. *Stroke* 1990;21:II46–II47.
14. Forbes SA, Duncan PW, Zimmerman MK. Review criteria for stroke rehabilitation outcomes. *Arch Phys Med Rehabil* 1997;78: 1112–1116.
15. Dombovy ML, Sandok BA, Basford JR. Rehabilitation for stroke: a review. *Stroke* 1986; 17:363–369.
16. Heinemann AW, Roth EJ, Cichowski K, Betts HB. Multivariate analysis of improvement and outcome following stroke rehabilitation. *Arch Neurol* 1987;44:1167–1172.
17. Jongbloed L. Prediction of function after stroke: a critical review. *Stroke* 1986;17:765–776.
18. Anderson TP. Studies up to 1980 on stroke rehabilitation outcomes. *Stroke* 1990;21:II43–II45.
19. Lofgren B, Nyberg L, Osterlind P, Mattsson M, Gustafson Y. Stroke rehabilitation—discharge predictors. *Cerebrovasc Dis* 1997;7:168–174.
20. Macciocchi SN, Diamond PT, Alves WM, Mertz T. Ischemic stroke: relation of age, lesion location, and initial neurologic deficit to functional outcome. *Arch Phys Med Rehabil* 1998;79: 1255–1257.
21. Dromerick AW, Reding MJ. Functional outcome for patients with hemiparesis, hemihypesthesia, and hemianopsia. Does lesion location matter? *Stroke* 1995;26:2023–2026.
22. Kwakkel G, Wagenaar RC, Kollen BJ, Lankhorst GJ. Predicting disability in stroke—a critical review of the literature. *Ageing* 1996;25:479–489.
23. Liu M, Domen K, Chino N. Comorbidity measures for stroke outcome research: a preliminary study. *Arch Phys Med Rehabil* 1997;78:166–172.
24. Olsen TS. Arm and leg paresis as outcome predictors in stroke rehabilitation. *Stroke* 1990;21: 247–251.
25. Pohjasvaara T, Erkinjuntti T, Vataja R, Kaste M. Correlates of dependent living 3 months after ischemic stroke. *Cerebrovasc Dis* 1998;8:259–266.
26. Miyai I, Blau AD, Reding MJ, Volpe BT. Patients with stroke confined to basal ganglia have diminished response to rehabilitation efforts. *Neurology* 1997;48:95–101.
27. Chae J, Zorowitz R. Functional status of cortical and subcortical nonhemorrhagic stroke survivors and the effect of lesion laterality. *Am J Phys Med Rehabil* 1998;77:415–420.
28. Nelles G, Contois KA, Valente SL, et al. Recovery following lateral medullary infarction. *Neurology* 1998;50:1418–1422.
29. Galski T, Bruno RL, Zorowitz R, Walker J. Predicting length of stay, functional outcome, and aftercare in the rehabilitation of stroke patients. The dominant role of higher-order cognition. *Stroke* 1993;24:1794–1800.
30. Cassvan A, Ross PL, Dyer PR, Zane L. Lateralization in stroke syndromes as a factor in ambulation. *Arch Phys Med Rehabil* 1976;57: 583–587.
31. Wade DT, Hewer RL, Wood VA. Stroke: influence of patient's sex and side of weakness on outcome. *Arch Phys Med Rehabil* 1984;65: 513–516.
32. Paolucci S, Antonucci G, Gialloreti LE, et al. Predicting stroke inpatient rehabilitation outcome: the prominent role of neuropsychological disorders. *Eur Neurol* 1996;36:385–390.
33. Paolucci S, Antonucci G, Pratesi L, Traballesi M, Lubich S, Grasso MG. Functional outcome in stroke inpatient rehabilitation: predicting no, low and high response in patients. *Cerebrovasc Dis* 1998;8:228–234.
34. Broeks JG, Lankhorst GJ, Rumping K, Prevo AJ. The long-term outcome of arm function after stroke: results of a follow-up study. *Disabil Rehabil* 1999;21:357–364.
35. Pohjasvaara T, Leppavuori A, Siira I, Vataja R, Kaste M, Erkinjuntti T. Frequency and clinical determinants of poststroke depression. *Stroke* 1998;29:2311–2317.
36. Wade DT, Hewer RL. Outlook after an acute stroke: urinary incontinence and loss of consciousness compared in 532 patients. *Q J Med* 1985;56:601–608.
37. Wade DT, Hewer RL. Functional abilities after stroke: measurement, natural history and prognosis. *J Neurol Neurosurg Psychiatry* 1987;50: 177–182.

38. Wade DT, Wood VA, Hewer RL. Recovery after stroke—the first 3 months. *J Neurol Neurosurg Psychiatry* 1985;48:7–13.
39. Gross JC. A comparison of the characteristics of incontinent and continent stroke patients in a rehabilitation program. *Rehabilitation Nursing* 1998;23:132–140.
40. Bonita R, Beaglehole R. Recovery of motor function after stroke. *Stroke* 1988;19:1497–1500.
41. Alexander MP. Stroke rehabilitation outcome. A potential use of predictive variables to establish levels of care. *Stroke* 1994;25:128–134.
42. Novack TA, Satterfield WT, Lyons K, Kolski G, Hackmeyer L, Connor M. Stroke onset and rehabilitation: time lag as a factor in treatment outcome. *Arch Phys Med Rehabil* 1984;65: 316–319.
43. Giaquinto S, Buzzelli S, Di Francesco L, et al. On the prognosis of outcome after stroke. *Acta Neurol Scand* 1999;100:202–208.
44. Harvey RL, Roth EJ, Heinemann AW, Lovell LL, McGuire JR, Diaz S. Stroke rehabilitation: clinical predictors of resource utilization. *Arch Phys Med Rehabil* 1998;79:1349–1355.
45. Black-Schaffer RM, Kirsteins AE, Harvey RL. Stroke rehabilitation. 2. Co-morbidities and complications. *Arch Phys Med Rehabil* 1999;80: S8–S16.
46. Liu M, Tsuji T, Tsujiuchi K, Chino N. Comorbidities in stroke patients as assessed with a newly developed comorbidity scale. *Am J Phys Med Rehabil* 1999;78:416–424.
47. Tirschwell DL, Kukull WA, Longstreth WT, Jr. Medical complications of ischemic stroke and length of hospital stay: Experience in Seattle, Washington. *J Stroke Cerebrovasc Dis* 1999;8: 336–343.
48. Roth EJ. Heart disease in patients with stroke. Part II: Impact and implications for rehabilitation. *Arch Phys Med Rehabil* 1994;75:94–101.
49. Roth EJ, Mueller K, Green D. Stroke rehabilitation outcome: impact of coronary artery disease. *Stroke* 1988;19:42–47.
50. Gubitz G, Phillips S, Aguilar E. Discharge disposition of patients on an acute stroke unit. *J Stroke Cerebrovasc Dis* 1999;8:330–335.
51. Ronning OM, Guldvog B. Outcome of subacute stroke rehabilitation: a randomized controlled trial. *Stroke* 1998;29:779–784.
52. Kalra L, Yu G, Wilson K, Roots P. Medical complications during stroke rehabilitation. *Stroke* 1995;26:990–994.
53. Dromerick A, Reding M. Medical and neurological complications during inpatient stroke rehabilitation. *Stroke* 1994;25:358–361.
54. Kong KH, Chua KS, Tow AP. Clinical characteristics and functional outcome of stroke patients 75 years old and older. *Arch Phys Med Rehabil* 1998;79:1535–1539.
55. Kalra L. Does age affect benefits of stroke unit rehabilitation? *Stroke* 1994;25:346–351.
56. Kalra L. The influence of stroke unit rehabilitation on functional recovery from stroke. *Stroke* 1994;25:821–825.
57. Kalra L, Dale P, Crome P. Improving stroke rehabilitation. A controlled study. *Stroke* 1993;24:1462–1467.
58. Kramer AM, Steiner JF, Schlenker RE, et al. Outcomes and costs after hip fracture and stroke. A comparison of rehabilitation settings. *JAMA* 1997;277:396–404.
59. Kalra L, Eade J. Role of stroke rehabilitation units in managing severe disability after stroke. *Stroke* 1995;26:2031–2034.
60. Gladman JR, Lincoln NB, Barer DH. A randomised controlled trial of domiciliary and hospital-based rehabilitation for stroke patients after discharge from hospital. *J Neurol Neurosurg Psychiatry* 1993;56:960–966.
61. Brown RD, Jr., Ransom J, Hass S, et al. Use of nursing home after stroke and dependence on stroke severity: a population-based analysis. *Stroke* 1999;30:924–929.
62. Lai SM, Alter M, Friday G, Lai SL, Sobel E. Disposition after acute stroke: who is not sent home from hospital? *Neuroepidemiology* 1998;17:21–29.
63. Werner RA, Kessler S. Effectiveness of an intensive outpatient rehabilitation program for postacute stroke patients. *Am J Phys Med Rehabil* 1996; 75:114–120.
64. Dobkin BH. Focused stroke rehabilitation programs do not improve outcome. *Arch Neurol* 1989;46:701–703.
65. Marsh M. A day rehabilitation stroke program. *Arch Phys Med Rehabil* 1984;65:320–323.
66. Baskett JJ, Broad JB, Reekie G, Hocking C, Green G. Shared responsibility for ongoing rehabilitation: a new approach to home-based therapy after stroke. *Clin Rehabil* 1999;13: 23–33.
67. Young JB, Forster A. The Bradford Community Stroke Trial: results at six months. *BMJ* 1992; 304:1085–1089.
68. Wade DT, Langton-Hewer R, Skilbeck CE, Bainton D, Burns-Cox C. Controlled trial of a home-care service for acute stroke patients. *Lancet* 1985;323–326.
69. Langhorne P, Wagenaar R, Partridge C. Physiotherapy after stroke: more is better? *Physiotherapy Research International* 1996;1:75–88.
70. Driessen MJ, Dekker J, Lankhorst G, van der Zee J. Occupational therapy for patients with chronic diseases: CVA, rheumatoid arthritis and progressive diseases of the central nervous system. *Disabil Rehabil* 1997;19:198–204.
71. Ballinger C, Ashburn A, Low J, Roderick P. Unpacking the black box of therapy—a pilot study to describe occupational therapy and physiotherapy interventions for people with stroke. *Clin Rehabil* 1999;13:301–309.
72. Smith MT, Baer GD. Achievement of simple mobility milestones after stroke. *Arch Phys Med Rehabil* 1999;80:442–447.
73. Duncan PW, Goldstein LB, Horner RD, et al. Similar motor recovery of upper and lower extremities after stroke. *Stroke* 1994;25: 1181–1188.
74. Skilbeck CE, Wade DT, Hewer RL, Wood VA. Recovery after stroke. *J Neurol Neurosurg Psychiatry* 1983;46:5–8.
75. Chiu L, Shyu WC, Chen TR. A cost-effectiveness analysis of home care and community-based

nursing homes for stroke patients and their families. *J Advanced Nursing* 1997;26:872–878.
76. Wade DT, Collen FM, Robb GF, Warlow CP. Physiotherapy intervention late after stroke and mobility. *BMJ* 1992;304:609–613.
77. Parry RH, Lincoln NB, Vass CD. Effect of severity of arm impairment on response to additional physiotherapy early after stroke. *Clin Rehabil* 1999;13:187–198.
78. Marque P, Felez A, Puel M, et al. Impairment and recovery of left motor function in patients with right hemiplegia. *J Neurol Neurosurg Psychiatry* 1997;62:77–81.
79. Silvestrini M, Cupini LM, Placidi F, Diomedi M, Bernardi G. Bilateral hemispheric activation in the early recovery of motor function after stroke. *Stroke* 1998;29:1305–1310.
80. Seitz RJ, Azari NP, Knorr U, Binkofski F, Herzog H, Freund HJ. The role of diaschisis in stroke recovery. *Stroke* 1999;30:1844–1850.
81. Muellbacher W, Artner C, Mamoli B. The role of the intact hemisphere in recovery of midline muscles after recent monohemispheric stroke. *J Neurol* 1999;246:250–256.
82. Miyai I, Suzuki T, Kii K, Kang J, Kubota K. Wallerian degeneration of the pyramidal tract does not affect stroke rehabilitation outcome. *Neurology* 1998;51:1613–1616.
83. Bussin JL, Abedin H, Tallis RC. Freezing episodes in hemiparetic stroke: results of a pilot survey. *Clin Rehabil* 1999;13:207–210.
84. Cheng PT, Liaw MY, Wong MK, Tang FT, Lee MY, Lin PS. The sit-to-stand movement in stroke patients and its correlation with falling. *Arch Phys Med Rehabil* 1998;79:1043–1046.
85. De Q, I, Simon SR, Leurgans S, Pease WS, McAllister D. Gait pattern in the early recovery period after stroke. *Journal of Bone & Joint Surgery—American Volume* 1996;78:1506–1514.
86. Sunderland A, Bowers MP, Sluman SM, Wilcock DJ, Ardron ME. Impaired dexterity of the ipsilateral hand after stroke and the relationship to cognitive deficit. *Stroke* 1999;30:949–955.
87. Dickstein R, Heffes Y, Laufer Y, Ben-Haim Z. Activation of selected trunk muscles during symmetric functional activities in poststroke hemiparetic and hemiplegic patients. *J Neurol Neurosurg Psychiatry* 1999;66:218–221.
88. Keenan MA, Perry J, Jordan C. Factors affecting balance and ambulation following stroke. *Clin Orthop* 1984;165–171.
89. Masdeu JC, Gorelick PB. Thalamic astasia: inability to stand after unilateral thalamic lesions. *Ann Neurol* 1988;23:596–603.
90. Canning CG, Ada L, O'Dwyer N. Slowness to develop force contributes to weakness after stroke. *Arch Phys Med Rehabil* 1999;80:66–70.
91. Yelnik A, Albert T, Bonan I, Laffont I. A clinical guide to assess the role of lower limb extensor overactivity in hemiplegic gait disorders. *Stroke* 1999;30:580–585.
92. Baskett JJ, Marshall HJ, Broad JB, Owen PH, Green G. The good side after stroke: ipsilateral sensory-motor function needs careful assessment. *Ageing* 1996;25:239–244.
93. Miyai I, Suzuki T, Kang J, Kubota K, Volpe BT. Middle cerebral artery stroke that includes the premotor cortex reduces mobility outcome. *Stroke* 1999;30:1380–1383.
94. Winstein CJ, Merians AS, Sullivan KJ. Motor learning after unilateral brain damage. *Neuropsychologia* 1999;37:975–987.
95. Tow AM, Chua HC. The alien hand sign—case report and review of the literature. *Ann Acad Med Singapore* 1998;27:582–585.
96. Sveen U, Bautz-Holter E, Sodring KM, Wyller TB, Laake K. Association between impairments, self-care ability and social activities 1 year after stroke. *Disabil Rehabil* 1999;21:372–377.
97. Irving-Bell L, Small M, Cowey A. A distortion of perceived space in patients with right-hemisphere lesions and visual hemineglect. *Neuropsychologia* 1999;37:919–925.
98. Harvey M, Milner AD. Residual perceptual distortion in "recovered" hemispatial neglect. *Neuropsychologia* 1999;37:745–750.
99. Paolucci S, Antonucci G, Guariglia C, Magnotti L, Pizzamiglio L, Zoccolotti P. Facilitatory effect of neglect rehabilitation on the recovery of left hemiplegic stroke patients: a cross-over study. *J Neurol* 1996;243:308–314.
100. Lin KC. Right-hemispheric activation approaches to neglect rehabilitation poststroke. *Am J Occup Ther* 1996;50:504–515.
101. Ramachandran VS, Altschuler EL, Stone L, Al-Aboudi M, Schwartz E, Siva N. Can mirrors alleviate visual hemineglect? *Medical Hypotheses* 1999;52:303–305.
102. Feys HM, De Weerdt WJ, Selz BE, et al. Effect of a therapeutic intervention for the hemiplegic upper limb in the acute phase after stroke: a single-blind, randomized, controlled multicenter trial. *Stroke* 1998;29:785–792.
103. Faist M, Ertel M, Berger W, Dietz V. Impaired modulation of quadriceps tendon jerk reflex during spastic gait: differences between spinal and cerebral lesions. *Brain* 1999;122:567–579.
104. Benaim C, Perennou DA, Villy J, Rousseaux M, Pelissier JY. Validation of a standardized assessment of postural control in stroke patients. The postural assessment scale for stroke patients (PASS). *Stroke* 1999;30:1862–1868.
105. Hesse SA, Jahnke MT, Bertelt CM, Schreiner C, Lucke D, Mauritz KH. Gait outcome in ambulatory hemiparetic patients after a 4-week comprehensive rehabilitation program and prognostic factors. *Stroke* 1994;25:1999–2004.
106. Ernst E. A review of *stroke* rehabilitation and physiotherapy. *Stroke* 1990;21:1081–1085.
107. Kwakkel G, Wagenaar RC, Twisk JW, Lankhorst GJ, Koetsier JC. Intensity of leg and arm training after primary middle-cerebral-artery stroke: a randomised trial. *Lancet* 1999;354:191–196.
108. Parry RH, Lincoln NB, Vass CD. Effect of severity of arm impairment on response to additional physiotherapy early after stroke. *Clin Rehabil* 1999;13:187–198.
109. Pohl PS, Winstein CJ. Practice effects on the less-affected upper extremity after stroke. *Arch Phys Med Rehabil* 1999;80:668–675.

110. Miltner WH, Bauder H, Sommer M, Dettmers C, Taub E. Effects of constraint-induced movement therapy on patients with chronic motor deficits after stroke: a replication. *Stroke* 1999; 30:586–592.
111. van der Lee JH, Wagenaar RC, Lanakhorst GJ, Vogelaar TW, Deville WL, Bouter LM. Forced use of upper extremity in chronic stroke patients. *Stroke* 1999;30:2369–2375.
112. Potempa K, Lopez M, Braun LT, Szidon JP, Fogg L, Tincknell T. Physiological outcomes of aerobic exercise training in hemiparetic stroke patients. *Stroke* 1995;26:101–105.
113. Smith GV, Silver KH, Goldberg AP, Macko RF. "Task oriented" exercises improves hamstring strength and spastic reflexes in chronic stroke patients. *Stroke* 1999;30:2112–2118.
114. Macko RF, DeSouza CA, Tretter LD, et al. Treadmill aerobic exercise training reduces the energy expenditure and cardiovascular demands of hemiparetic gait in chronic stroke patients. A preliminary report. *Stroke* 1997;28: 326–330.
115. Lincoln NB, Parry RH, Vass CD. Randomized, controlled trial to evaluate increased intensity of physiotherapy treatment of arm function after stroke. *Stroke* 1999;30:573–579.
116. Roper TA, Redford S, Tallis RC. Intermittent compression for the treatment of the oedematous hand in hemiplegic stroke: a randomized controlled trial. *Ageing* 1999;28:9–13.
117. Wong AM, Su TY, Tang FT, Cheng PT, Liaw MY. Clinical trial of electrical acupuncture on hemiplegic stroke patients. *Am J Phys Med Rehabil* 1999;78:117–122.
118. Magnusson M, Johansson K, Johansson BB. Sensory stimulation promotes normalization of postural control after stroke. *Stroke* 1994;25: 1176–1180.
119. Wolf SL. Use of biofeedback in the treatment of stroke patients. *Stroke* 1990;21:II22–II23.
120. Glanz M, Klawansky S, Stason W, et al. Biofeedback therapy in poststroke rehabilitation: a meta-analysis of the randomized controlled trials. *Arch Phys Med Rehabil* 1995;76: 508–515.
121. Volpe BT, Krebs HI, Hogan N, Edelsteinn L, Diels CM, Aisen ML. Robot training enhanced motor outcome in patients with stroke maintained over 3 years. *Neurology* 1999;53: 1874–1876.
122. Powell J, Pandyan AD, Granat M, Cameron M, Stott DJ. Electrical stimulation of wrist extensors in poststroke hemiplegia. *Stroke* 1999;30: 1384–1389.
123. Faghri PD. The effects of neuromuscular stimulation-induced muscle contraction versus elevation on hand edema in CVA patients. *J Hand Therapy* 1997;10:29–34.
124. Kraft GH, Fitts SS, Hammond MC. Techniques to improve function of the arm and hand in chronic hemiplegia. *Arch Phys Med Rehabil* 1992;73:220–227.
125. Hummelsheim H, Maier-Loth ML, Eickhof C. The functional value of electrical muscle stimulation for the rehabilitation of the hand in stroke patients. *Scand J Rehabil Med* 1997;29:3–10.
126. Kuan TS, Tsou JY, Su FC. Hemiplegic gait of stroke patients: the effect of using a cane. *Arch Phys Med Rehabil* 1999;80:777–784.
127. Simpson DM, Alexander DN, O'Brien CF, et al. Botulinum toxin type A in the treatment of upper extremity spasticity: a randomized, double-blind, placebo-controlled trial. *Neurology* 1996;46:1306–1310.
128. Burbaud P, Wiart L, Dubos JL, et al. A randomised, double blind, placebo controlled trial of botulinum toxin in the treatment of spastic foot in hemiparetic patients. *J Neurol Neurosurg Psychiatry* 1996;61:265–269.
129. Yablon SA, Agana BT, Ivanhoe CB, Boake C. Botulinum toxin in severe upper extremity spasticity among patients with traumatic brain injury: an open-labeled trial. *Neurology* 1996;47:939–944.
130. Hesse S, Krajnik J, Luecke D, Jahnke MT, Gregoric M, Mauritz KH. Ankle muscle activity before and after botulinum toxin therapy for lower limb extensor spasticity in chronic hemiparetic patients. *Stroke* 1996;27:455–460.
131. Cromwell SJ, Paquette VL. The effect of botulinum toxin A on the function if a person with poststroke quadriplegia. *Physical Therapy* 1996; 76:395–402.
132. Bhakta BB, Cozens JA, Bamford JM, Chamberlain MA. Use of botulinum toxin in stroke patients with severe upper limb spasticity. *J Neurol Neurosurg Psychiatry* 1996;61:30–35.
133. Rivas DA, Chancellor MB, Hill K, Freedman MK. Neurological manifestations of baclofen withdrawal. *J Urol* 1993;150:1903–1905.
134. Ochs GA. Intrathecal baclofen. *Baillieres Clin Neurol* 1993;2:73–86.
135. Rawicki B. Treatment of cerebral origin spasticity withcontinuous intrathecal baclofen delivered via an implantable pump: long-term follow-up review of 18 patients. *J Neurosurg* 1999;91: 733–736.
136. Albright AL, Barron WB, Fasick MP, Polinko P, Janosky J. Continuous intrathecal baclofen infusion for spasticity of cerebral origin. *JAMA* 1993;270:2475–2477.
137. Ward A, Chaffman MO, Sorkin EM. Dantrolene. A review of its pharmacodynamic and pharmacokinetic properties and therapeutic use in malignant hyperthermia, the neuroleptic malignant syndrome and an update of its use in muscle spasticity. *Drugs* 1986;32:130–168.
138. Katrak PH, Cole AM, Paulos CJ, McCauley JC. Objective assessment of spasticity, strength, and function with early exhibition of dantrolene sodium after cerebrovascular accident: a randomized double-blind study. *Arch Phys Med Rehabil* 1992;73:4–9.
139. Dimitrijevic MR, Sherwood AM. Spasticity: medical and surgical treatment. *Neurology* 1980;30: 19–27.
140. Chang LH, Hasselkus BR. Occupational therapists' expectations in rehabilitation following stroke: sources of satisfaction and dissatisfaction. *Am J Occup Ther* 1998;52:629–637.
141. Walker MF, Gladman JR, Lincoln NB, Siemonsma P, Whiteley T. Occupational therapy for stroke

patients not admitted to hospital: a randomised controlled trial. *Lancet* 1999;354: 278–280.

142. Bjorneby ER, Reinvang IR. Acquiring and maintaining self-care skills after stroke. The predictive value of apraxia. *Scand J Rehabil Med* 1985;17:75–80.
143. Trombly CA, Wu CY. Effect of rehabilitation tasks on organization of movement after stroke. *Am J Occup Ther* 1999;53:333–344.
144. Walker MF, Gladman JR, Lincoln NB, Siemonsma P, Whiteley T. Occupational therapy for stroke patients not admitted to hospital: a randomised controlled trial. *Lancet* 1999;354: 278–280.
145. David R, Enderby P, Bainton D. Treatment of acquired aphasia: speech therapists and volunteers compared. *J Neurol Neurosurg Psychiatry* 1982;45:957–961.
146. Ferro JM, Mariano G, Madureira S. Recovery from aphasia and neglect. *Cerebrovasc Dis* 1999;9 (Suppl 5):6–22.
147. Aftonomos LB, Appelbaum JS, Steele RD. Improving outcomes for persons with aphasia in advanced community-based treatment programs. *Stroke* 1999;30:1370–1379.
148. Thulborn KR, Carpenter PA, Just MA. Plasticity of language-related brain function during recovery from stroke. *Stroke* 1999;30:749–754.
149. Basso A, Capitani E, Vignolo LA. Influence of rehabilitation on language skills in aphasic patients. A controlled study. *Arch Neurol* 1979;36: 190–196.
150. Selnes OA. Recovery from aphasia: activating the "right" hemisphere. *Ann Neurol* 1999;45: 419–420.
151. Barrett AM, Crucian GP, Raymer AM, Heilman KM. Spared comprehension of emotional prosody in a patient with global aphasia. *Neuropsychiatry, Neuropsychology, & Behavioral Neurology* 1999;12:117–120.
152. Greener J, Grant A. Beliefs about effectiveness of treatment for aphasia after stroke. *Int J Lang Commun Disord* 1998;33(Suppl):162–163.
153. Greener J, Enderby P, Whurr R, Grant A. Treatment for aphasia following stroke: evidence for effectiveness. *Int J Lang Commun Disord* 1998;33(Suppl):158–161.
154. Lincoln NB, McGuirk E, Mulley GP, Lendrem W, Jones AC, Mitchell JR. Effectiveness of speech therapy for aphasic stroke patients. A randomised controlled trial. *Lancet* 1984;1197–1200.
155. Bourestom NC, Howard MT. Behavioral correlates of recovery of self-care in hemiplegic patients. *Arch Phys Med Rehabil* 1968;49: 449–454.
156. Happe F, Brownell H, Winner E. Acquired "theory of mind" impairments following stroke. *Cognition* 1999;70:211–240.
157. Basmajian JV, Gowland CA, Finlayson MA, et al. Stroke treatment: comparison of integrated behavioral-physical therapy vs traditional physical therapy programs. *Arch Phys Med Rehabil* 1987;68:267–272.
158. Astrom M, Adolfsson R, Asplund K. Major depression in stroke patients. A 3-year longitudinal study. *Stroke* 1993;24:976–982.
159. Clark MS, Smith DS. Psychological correlates of outcome following rehabilitation from stroke. *Clin Rehabil* 1999;13:129–140.
160. Kim P, Warren S, Madill H, Hadley M. Quality of life of stroke survivors. *Q Life Res* 1999;8: 293–301.
161. Fisher M, Finkelstein S. Pharmacological approaches to stroke recovery. *Cerebrovasc Dis* 1999;9(Suppl 5):29–32.
162. Goldstein LB, Davis JN. Restorative neurology. Drugs and recovery following stroke. *Stroke* 1990;21:1636–1640.
163. Wahlgren NG, Martinsson L. New concepts for drug therapy after stroke. Can we enhance recovery? *Cerebrovasc Dis* 1998;8(Suppl 5): 33–38.
164. Crisotomo EA, Duncan PW, Propst M, Dawson DV, Davis JN. Evidence that amphetamine with physical therapy promotes recovery of motor function in stroke patients. *Ann Neurol* 1988;23: 94–97.
165. Walker-Batson D, Smith P, Curtis S, Unwin H, Greenlee R. Amphetamine paired with physical therapy accelerates motor recovery after stroke. Further evidence. *Stroke* 1995;26:2254–2259.
166. Dam M, Tonin P, De Boni A, et al. Effects of fluoxetine and maprotiline on functional recovery in poststroke hemiplegic patients undergoing rehabilitation therapy. *Stroke* 1996;27: 1211–1214.
167. Sze KH, Sim TC, Wong E, Cheng S, Woo J. Effect of nimodipine on memory after cerebral infarction. *Acta Neurol Scand* 1998;97:386–392.
168. Goldstein LB. Common drugs may influence motor recovery after stroke. The Sygen in Acute Stroke Study Investigators. *Neurology* 1995;45: 865–871.
169. Goldstein LB. Potential effects of common drugs on stroke recovery. *Arch Neurol* 1998;55: 454–456.
170. Tuomilehto J, Nuottimaki T, Salmi K, et al. Psychosocial and health status in stroke survivors after 14 years. *Stroke* 1995;26:971–975.
171. Gresham GE, Kelly-Hayes M, Wolf PA, et al. Survival and functional status 20 or more years after first stroke: the Framingham Study. *Stroke* 1998;29:793–797.
172. Leibson CL, Ransom JE, Brown RD, O'Fallon WM, Hass SL, Whisnant JP. Stroke-attributable nursing home use: a population-based study. *Neurology* 1998;51:163–168.
173. Gresham GE, Fitzpatrick TE, Wolf PA, et al. Residual disability in survivors of stroke—the Framingham study. *N Engl J Med* 1975;293: 954–956.
174. Smurawska LT, Alexandrov AV, Bladin CF, Norris JW. Cost of acute stroke care in Toronto, Canada. *Stroke* 1994;25:1628–1631.
175. Maheswaran R, Davis S. Experience of an open referral system for stroke rehabilitation in the community. *Clin Rehabil* 1998;12:265–271.
176. Thorngren M, Westling B, Norrving B. Outcome after stroke in patients discharged to independent living. *Stroke* 1990;21:236–240.
177. Schmidt SM, Herman LM, Koenig P, Leuze M, Monahan MK, Stubbers RW. Status of stroke

patients: a community assessment. *Arch Phys Med Rehabil* 1986;67:99–102.
178. Lofgren B, Nyberg L, Mattsson M, Gustafson Y. Three years after in-patient stroke rehabilitation: a follow-up study. *Cerebrovasc Dis* 1999;9: 163–170.
179. Forster A, Young J. Specialist nurse support for patients with stroke in the community: a randomised controlled trial. *BMJ* 1996;312: 1642–1646.
180. Duncan PW, Samsa GP, Weinberger M, et al. Health status of individuals with mild stroke. *Stroke* 1997;28:740–745.
181. Lawrence L, Christie D. Quality of life after stroke: a three-year follow-up. *Ageing* 1979;8: 167–172.
182. Parker CJ, Gladman JR, Drummond AE. The role of leisure in stroke rehabilitation. *Disabil Rehabil* 1997;19:1–5.
183. Sjogren K. Leisure after stroke. *Int Rehabil Med* 1982;4:80–87.
184. De Haan R, Horn J, Limburg M, Van Der Meulen J, Bossuyt P. A comparison of five stroke scales with measures of disability, handicap, and quality of life. *Stroke* 1993;24:1178–1181.
185. Addington-Hall J, Lay M, Altmann D, McCarthy M. Symptom control, communication with health professionals, and hospital care of stroke patients in the last year of life as reported by surviving family, friends, and officials. *Stroke* 1995;26:2242–2248.
186. Williams LS, Weinberger M, Harris LE, Biller J. Measuring quality of life in a way that is meaningful to stroke patients. *Neurology* 1999;53: 1839–1843.
187. Chang AM, Mackenzie AE. State self-esteem following stroke. *Stroke* 1998;29:2325–2328.
188. Astrom M. Generalized anxiety disorder in stroke patients. A 3-year longitudinal study. *Stroke* 1996;27:270–275.
189. Ahlsio B, Britton M, Murray V, Theorell T. Disablement and quality of life after stroke. *Stroke* 1984;15:886–890.
190. Palomaki H, Kaste M, Berg A, et al. Prevention of poststroke depression: 1 year randomised placebo controlled double blind trial of mianserin with 6 month follow up after therapy. *J Neurol Neurosurg Psychiatry* 1999;66:490–494.
191. House A, Dennis M, Mogridge L, Warlow C, Hawton K, Jones L. Mood disorders in the year after first stroke. *Br J Psychiatry* 1991;158:83–92.
192. Angeleri F, Angeleri VA, Foschi N, Giaquinto S, Nolfe G. The influence of depression, social activity, and family stress on functional outcome after stroke. *Stroke* 1993;24:1478–1483.
193. Kauhanen M-L, Korpelainen JT, Hiltunen P, et al. Poststroke depression correlates with cognitive impairment and neurological deficits. *Stroke* 1999;30:1875–1880.
194. Neau JP, Ingrand P, Mouille-Brachet C, et al. Functional recovery and social outcome after cerebral infarction in young adults. *Cerebrovasc Dis* 1998;8:296–302.
195. Jonkman EJ, de Weerd AW, Vrijens NL. Quality of life after a first ischemic stroke. Long-term developments and correlations with changes in neurological deficit, mood and cognitive impairment. *Acta Neurol Scand* 1998; 98:169–175.
196. Trigg R, Wood VA, Hewer RL. Social reintegration after stroke: the first stages in the development of the Subjective Index of Physical and Social Outcome (SIPSO). *Clin Rehabil* 1999;13: 341–353.
197. Evans RL, Bishop DS. Psychosocial outcomes in stroke survivors. Implications for research. *Stroke* 1990;II48–II49.
198. Flick CL. Stroke rehabilitation. 4. Stroke outcome and psychosocial consequences. *Arch Phys Med Rehabil* 1999;80:S21–S26.
199. Bishop DS, Evans RL. Family functioning assessment techniques in stroke. *Stroke* 1990;21: II50–II51.
200. Han B, Haley WE. Family caregiving for patients with stroke. *Stroke* 1999;30:1478–1485.
201. Noonan WC, Evans RL, Hendricks R. Using personal and family variates to predict patients' adjustment after stroke. *Psychol Rep* 1988;63: 247–251.
202. Dennis M, O'Rourke S, Lewis S, Sharpe M, Warlow C. A quantitative study of the emotional outcome of people caring for stroke survivors. *Stroke* 1998;29:1867–1872.
203. Lofgren B, Gustafson Y, Nyberg L. Psychological well-being 3 years after severe stroke. *Stroke* 1999;30:567–572.
204. Glass TA, Matchar DB, Belyea M, Feussner JR. Impact of social support on outcome in first stroke. *Stroke* 1993;24:64–70.
205. Dennis M, O'Rourke S, Slattery J, Staniforth T, Warlow C. Evaluation of a stroke family care worker: results of a randomised controlled trial. *BMJ* 1997;314:1071–1076.
206. McClenahan R, Weinman J. Determinants of carer distress in non-acute stroke. *Int J Lang Commun Disord* 1998;33(Suppl):138–143.
207. Wilson DB, Houle DM, Keith RA. Stroke rehabilitation: a model predicting return home. *West J Med* 1991;154:587–590.
208. Legh-Smith J, Wade DT, Langton-Hewer R. Services for stroke patients one year after stroke. *J Epidemiol Community Health* 1986;40:161–165.
209. Leibson CL, Hu T, Brown RD, Hass SL, O'Fallon WM, Whisnant JP. Utilization of acute care services in the year before and after first stroke: A population-based study. *Neurology* 1996;46:861–869.
210. Black-Schaffer RM, Osberg JS. Return to work after stroke: development of a predictive model. *Arch Phys Med Rehabil* 1990;71:285–290.
211. Wozniak MA, Kittner SJ, Price TR, Hebel JR, Sloan MA, Gardner JF. Stroke location is not associated with return to work after first ischemic stroke. *Stroke* 1999;30:2568–2573.
212. Adunsky A, Hershkowitz M, Rabbi R, Asher-Sivron L, Ohry A. Functional recovery in young stroke patients. *Arch Phys Med Rehabil* 1992;73:859–862.
213. Kappelle LJ, Adams HP, Jr., Heffner ML, Torner JC, Gomez F, Biller J. Prognosis of young adults

with ischemic stroke. A long-term follow-up study assessing recurrent vascular events and functional outcome in the Iowa Registry of Stroke in Young Adults. *Stroke* 1994;25: 1360–1365.

214. Legh-Smith J, Wade DT, Hewer RL. Driving after a stroke. *J R Soc Med* 1986;79:200–203.
215. Korpelainen JT, Nieminen P, Myllya VV. Sexual functioning among stroke patients and their spouses. *Stroke* 1999;30:715–719.
216. Monga TN, Lawson JS, Inglis J. Sexual dysfunction in stroke patients. *Arch Phys Med Rehabil* 1986;67:19–22.
217. Korpelainen JT, Kauhanen M-L, Kemola H, Malinen U, Myllyla VV. Sexual dysfunction in stroke patients. *Acta Neurol Scand* 1998;98: 400–405.
218. Anderson C, Rubenach S, Mhurchu CN, Clark M, Spencer C, Winsor A. Home or hospital for stroke rehabilitation? Results of a randomized controlled trial. I: Health outcomes at 6 months. *Stroke* 2000;31:1024–1031.
219. Mayo NE, Wood-Dauphinee S, Cote R, et al. There's no place like home. An evaluation of early supported discharge for stroke. *Stroke* 2000; 31:1016–1023.
220. Anderson C, Mhurchu CN, Rubenach S, Clark M, Spencer C, Winsor A. Home or hospital for stroke rehabilitation? Results of a randomized controlled trial. II: Cost minimization analysis at 6 months. *Stroke* 2000;31:1032–1037.
221. Gladstone DJ, Black SE. Enhancing recovery after stroke with noradrenergic pharmacotherapy: a new frontier? *Can J Neurol Sci* 200;27: 97–105.
222. Wiart L, Petit H, Joseph PA, Mazaux JM, Barat M. Fluoxetine in early poststroke depression. A double-blind placebo-controlled study. *Stroke* 2000;31:1829–1832.
223. Zivin JA. Cell transplant therapy for stroke. Hope or hype. *Neurology* 200Ø;55:467.
224. Kondziolka D, Wechsler L, Goldstein S, et al. Transplantation of cultured human neuronal cells for patients with stroke. *Neurology* 2000;55: 565–569.

INDEX

ISCHEMIC CEREBROVASCULAR DISEASE

Series Editor:
Sid Gilman, M.D.
William J. Herdman Professor of Neurology
Chair, Department of Neurology
University of Michigan Medical Center

Contemporary Neurology Series Available:

19 THE DIAGNOSIS OF STUPOR AND COMA, EDITION 3
Fred Plum, M.D., and Jerome B. Posner, M.D.

32 CLINICAL NEUROPHYSIOLOGY OF THE VESTIBULAR SYSTEM, EDITION 2
Robert W. Baloh, M.D., and Vincente Honrubia, M.D.

42 MIGRAINE: MANIFESTATIONS, PATHOGENESIS, AND MANAGEMENT
Robert A. Davidoff, M.D.

43 NEUROLOGY OF CRITICAL ILLNESS
Eelco F.M. Wijdicks

44 EVALUATION AND TREATMENT OF MYOPATHIES
Robert C. Griggs, M.D., Jerry R. Mendell, M.D., and Robert G. Miller, M.D.

45 NEUROLOGIC COMPLICATIONS OF CANCER
Jerome B. Posner, M.D.

46 CLINICAL NEUROPHYSIOLOGY
Jasper R. Daube, M.D., *Editor*

47 NEUROLOGIC REHABILITATION
Bruce H. Dobkin, M.D.

48 PAIN MANAGEMENT: THEORY AND PRACTICE
Russell K. Portenoy, M.D., and Ronald M. Kanner, M.D., *Editors*

49 AMYOTROPHIC LATERAL SCLEROSIS
Hiroshi Mitsumoto, M.D., D.Sc., David A. Chad, M.D., F.R.C.P., and
Eric P. Pioro, M.D., D. Phil, F.R.C.P.

50 MULTIPLE SCLEROSIS
Donald W. Paty, M.D., F.R.C.P.C., and George C. Ebers, M.D., F.R.C.P.C., *Editors*

51 NEUROLOGY AND THE LAW: PRIVATE LITIGATION AND PUBLIC POLICY
H. Richard Beresford, M.D., J.D.

52 SUBARACHNOID HEMORRHAGE: CAUSES AND CURES
Bryce Weir, M.D.

53 SLEEP MEDICINE
Michael S. Aldrich, M.D.

54 BRAIN TUMORS
Harry S. Greenburg, M.D., and William F. Chandler, M.D., and Howard M. Sandler, M.D.

55 THE NEUROLOGY OF EYE MOVEMENTS, EDITION 3
R. John Leigh, M.D., and David S. Zee, M.D.

56 MYASTHENIA GRAVIS AND MYASTHENIC DISORDERS
Andrew Engel, M.D., *Editor*

57 NEUROGENETICS
Stefan-M. Pulst, M.D., *Editor*

58 DISEASES OF THE SPINE AND SPINAL CORD
Thomas N. Byrne, M.D., Edward C. Benzel, M.D., and Stephen G. Waxman, M.D., Ph.D.

59 DIAGNOSIS AND MANAGEMENT OF PERIPHERAL NERVE DISORDERS
Jerry R. Mendell, M.D., David R. Cornblah, M.D., and John T. Kissel, M.D.

60 THE NEUROLOGY OF VISION
Jonathan D. Trobe, M.D.

61 HIV NEUROLOGY
Bruce James Brew, M.B.B.S., M.D., F.R.A.C.P.